Pharmacy

CLINICAL PHARMACY

Volume 4, Number 1
January-February 1985

Enalapril

Patient-controlled analgesia

AMERICAN SOCIETY OF HOSPITAL PHARMACISTS

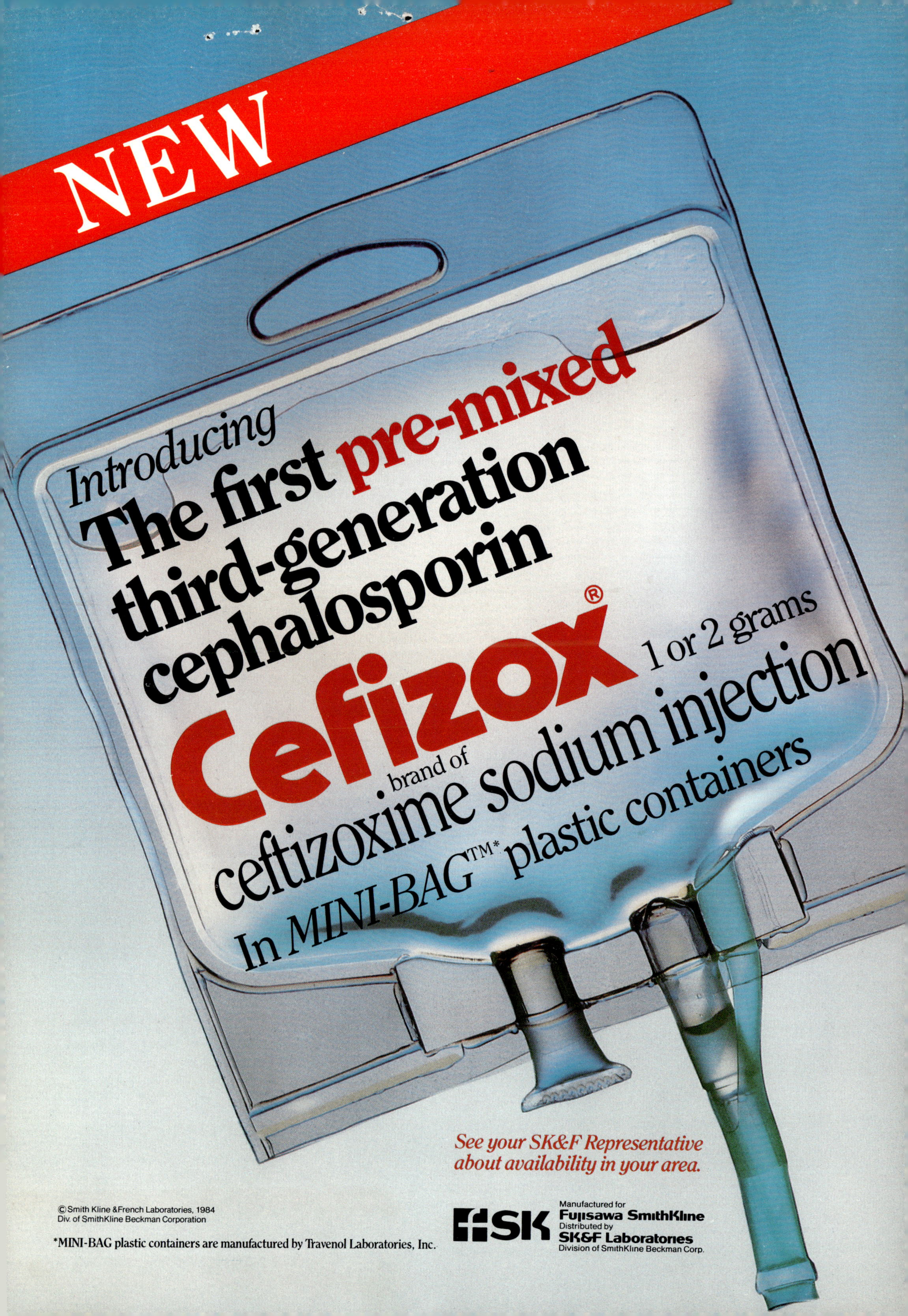
NEW
Introducing
The first pre-mixed
third-generation
cephalosporin
Cefizox®
1 or 2 grams
brand of
ceftizoxime sodium injection
In MINI-BAG™* plastic containers
See your SK&F Representative
about availability in your area.
©Smith Kline &French Laboratories, 1984
Div. of SmithKline Beckman Corporation
*MINI-BAG plastic containers are manufactured by Travenol Laboratories, Inc.
Manufactured for
Fujisawa SmithKline
Distributed by
SK&F Laboratories
Division of SmithKline Beckman Corp.

January–February 1985 Volume 4, Number 1 Coden: CPHADV ISSN: 0278-2677

CLINICAL PHARMACY

Drug Review

27 **Enalapril, a nonsulfhydryl angiotensin-converting enzyme inhibitor**
Peter H. Vlasses, Ghassem E. Larijani, Dale P. Conner, and Roger K. Ferguson

Research

41 **Relationship between plasma morphine concentrations and pharmacologic effects in postoperative patients using patient-controlled analgesia**
David A. Graves, Janice M. Arrigo, Thomas S. Foster, Terry J. Baumann, and Randal L. Batenhorst

48 **Efficacy of patient-controlled analgesia versus conventional analgesia for postoperative pain**
Stephen J. Bollish, Carol L. Collins, Duane M. Kirking, and Robert H. Bartlett

53 **Analgesia with oral narcotics and added ibuprofen in cancer patients**
Wendy A. Weingart, Christine A. Sorkness, and Robert H. Earhart

59 **Prediction of theophylline clearance using condition correction factors**
Mark J. Haumschild and John E. Murphy

Research Notes

65 **Managing hypertension with captopril and hydrochlorothiazide using two versus three daily doses**
Arthur A. Schuna, Gary R. Schmidt, Michael E. Pitterle, Theodore L. Goodfriend, Gregory J. Beirne, and A. Vishnu Moorthy

67 **Salivary penetration of moxalactam**
Daniel T. Casto, Peter Gal, Jack D. McCue, and Alicia A. Zumwalt

70 **Amikacin pharmacokinetics in morbidly obese patients undergoing gastric-bypass surgery**
Robert A. Blouin, Kim L. Rowse Brouwer, Kenneth E. Record, Ward O. Griffen, Jr., Patricia M. Plezia, and William John

72 **Lack of effect of ceftazidime on serum glucose in patients with liver disease**
Thomas R. Beam, Jr., Mary T. Pasko, Jody A. Spooner, and Daniel S. Camara

74 **Predicting serum gentamicin concentrations in patients undergoing hemodialysis**
Michael J. Melby, Joseph F. Heissler, Eugene C. Grochowski, and Richard A. Stockmar

77 **Evaluation of two methods for predicting initial lithium dosages without measuring serum concentrations**
John M. Patrias and Fred H. Moore

Editorials

80 **Progress and problems with pain**
Arthur G. Lipman

81 **How reliable are serum digoxin assays?**
Martha L. Hyneck

82 **Volume 4**

Pharmacokinetics in Drug Therapy

84 **Choosing optimal sampling times for therapeutic drug monitoring**
Gerald E. Schumacher

Grand Rounds

93 **Treatment of trigeminal neuralgia: Use of baclofen in combination with carbamazepine**
Karen A. Baker, Jerry E. Taylor, and Gilbert E. Lilly

Drug Experience

97 **Toxicity and elimination of trazodone after overdose**
Erkan Hassan and Delwyn D. Miller

100 **Clonidine and naloxone in ultrashort opiate detoxification**
Philip W. Holman

102 **Metoclopramide-induced tetanus-like dystonic reaction**
Robert DellaValle, James L. Wielenga, and Owen Taylor

---

3 **News**
Applying pharmacodynamics in patient care, L. Michael Posey . . . Tocainide marketed in U.S. . . . Study shows little change in microbial resistance patterns . . . Pentamidine now available commercially . . . Ceforanide approved for twice-daily dosing . . . NIH panel recommends decreased use of frozen plasma . . . Wyeth's triphasic oral contraceptive marketed

19 **Letters**
Severe hypersensitivity secondary to extended carbamazepine administration, S. J. Rose . . . Origins of aztreonam resistance, B. L. Ashby; David L. Dworzack, Margaret A. Bartelt, Robert T. Bailey, Jr., Robert J. Fitzgibbons, Jr., Jack W. Reich, George D. Picetti III . . . Update on the new triphasic oral contraceptives, Lucinda Glantz Miller

25 **Correction**

105 **Procedure for Submission of Manuscripts to Journals Published by the American Society of Hospital Pharmacists**

111 **CP Continuing Education**

113 **Current Literature**
Book Reviews: *Antacids and Other Drugs in Gastrointestinal Diseases* (*Ritschel*), Rosemary R. Berardi . . . *Antimicrobial Prescribing, Second Edition* (*Meyers*), Marc H. Stranz . . . *A Clinical Companion to Biochemical Studies, Second Edition* (*Schwarz*), Joseph T. DiPiro . . . *Manual of Antibiotics and Infectious Diseases, Fifth Edition* (*Conte, Barriere*), Teresa A. Tartaglione . . . *Side Effects of Drugs, Annual 8, 1984* (*Dukes*), Ronald B. Stewart . . . Books Received

118 **Advertising Index**

Instructions to Authors

CLINICAL PHARMACY gives priority to (1) studies that objectively evaluate drug effects in human trials, (2) evaluative review articles on the clinical uses of new drugs, and (3) evaluations of the current status of drug therapy in selected diseases. Contributions to the following sections are invited:

Drug Reviews: Detailed, analytical reviews on the clinical use of specific drugs, with preference given to new drugs and to evaluative rather than descriptive literature reviews.

Therapy Reviews: Articles that focus primarily on a disease state (rather than on a drug or drug class) and its treatment. These reviews foster an understanding of the pathophysiology of a disease and the related treatment.

Research: Reports of well-conducted original research on drug effects in humans.

Research Notes: Short research reports, such as updates on previously published work, confirmations of previous findings, or original research of modest scope.

Grand Rounds: Patient case reports and literature reviews combined in a way that gives them high educational value.

Drug Experience: Straightforward reports, with selected literature references, of unusual drug experiences.

Therapy Consultation: Brief advice, in a question-and-answer format, on how to handle specific drug-therapy problems. Readers are invited to submit questions, which the editor will forward to appropriate consultants for answering.

Letters: Short comments on previously published work or about potential problems, apparent trends, or controversies in drug therapy or clinical research.

Commentaries: Well-reasoned expressions of opinion on drug-therapy or clinical-research issues.

The editors have the sole authority to decide in which section to publish an accepted manuscript.

Manuscripts are subject to review by qualified outside reviewers, as well as by the editors, and will be accepted for publication only if they are believed to represent an important contribution to the literature. All papers submitted for publication must be accompanied by a completed copy of a manuscript checklist. The checklist appears on page 105 of the January–February 1985 issue. Authors of especially important original work may request "fast-track" review of their papers. Authors may suggest appropriate reviewers for their papers.

Accepted materials become the permanent and sole property of ASHP and may not be published or reprinted elsewhere without written permission from both the author and the editor.

The editors reserve the right to revise all materials submitted, if necessary. The publisher assumes no responsibility for the statements and opinions advanced by contributors to CLINICAL PHARMACY.

CLINICAL PHARMACY accepts manuscripts prepared according to the specifications of the Uniform Requirements for Manuscripts Submitted to Biomedical Journals (*Am J Hosp Pharm.* 1982; 38:1538–43). CLINICAL PHARMACY's manuscript checklist (page 105, January-February 1985 issue) generally conforms to the Uniform Requirements.

Under the terms of the Copyright Revision Act of 1976 (Public Law 94-553) it is necessary to have the rights of the authors transferred to the publisher in order to provide for the widest possible dissemination of professional and scientific literature. Accordingly, all transmittal letters accompanying manuscripts submitted for publication, including contributions for the Letters column, must contain the following language: "In consideration of the American Society of Hospital Pharmacists (ASHP) taking action in reviewing and editing my (our) submission, the author(s) undersigned hereby transfer(s), assign(s), or otherwise convey(s) all ownership rights in the submission and all copyright ownership to ASHP. In the event that such work is not published by ASHP, all said rights shall be released." We regret that we cannot consider manuscripts for publication that are not accompanied with transmittal letters containing the above language signed by all authors.

Authors must certify in their letter of transmittal that none of the material in their manuscript has been published previously nor is under consideration or been accepted for publication elsewhere. If this certification cannot be made, suitable explanation must be offered.

Six copies of all manuscripts should be submitted. Manuscripts should be typewritten with double spacing (including tables) on one side of good quality, 21.6 × 27.9-cm white paper, and with margins of at least 2.5 cm. For guidance on style, authors should consult the manuscript checklist, recent issues of CLINICAL PHARMACY, and the *Council of Biology Editors Style Manual*, fifth edition. *The American Heritage Dictionary of the English Language* and the AMA's *Manual for Authors and Editors* contain helpful advice on correct usage.

Galley proofs are sent to authors for inspection against the original manuscript and for correction. Unnecessary alterations in galley proof must be avoided. Extensive alterations will be charged to the author. An order form for reprints is sent to the corresponding author after galley proofs have been cleared.

CLINICAL PHARMACY (ISSN 0278-2677) is published bimonthly by the American Society of Hospital Pharmacists, 4630 Montgomery Avenue, Bethesda, MD 20814. Joseph A. Oddis, Executive Vice President. Second class postage is paid at Washington, DC, and at additional mailing offices. **Postmaster: Send address changes to: ASHP, 4630 Montgomery Avenue, Bethesda, MD 20814.**

Annual Subscription Rate:	*USA*	*Non-USA*
ASHP Member	$35	$40
ASHP Student Member	$25	$30
Institutions and Nonmembers	$55	$60

The cost of single copies is $9. Airmail delivery outside of the continental United States is available for an additional charge of $36 per year. Requests to replace missing issues free of charge are honored only up to six months after date of issue.

Microfilm and microfiche editions are available for purchase. Contact University Microfilms, 300 N. Zeeb Road, Ann Arbor, MI 48106.

Articles in CLINICAL PHARMACY are abstracted and indexed in *Current Contents, Clinical Sciences, Excerpta Medica, Index Medicus, Inpharma, International Pharmaceutical Abstracts*, and *Reactions*.

March–April 1985 Volume 4, Number 2 Coden: CPHADV ISSN: 0278-2677

CLINICAL PHARMACY

Therapy Reviews

149 **Allogeneic bone marrow transplantation in the treatment of hematologic diseases**
Gary C. Yee and Timothy R. McGuire

161 **Management of maldigestion associated with pancreatic insufficiency**
Richard S. Perry and Jeff Gallagher

170 **Nontraditional analgesics for the management of postherpetic neuralgia**
Michael Thompson and Michelle Bones

Research

177 **Pharmacokinetics of ceftriaxone in subjects with renal insufficiency**
Steven F. Kowalsky, Roger M. Echols, and Marie A. Parker

182 **Altered gentamicin pharmacokinetics during the perioperative period**
Dwight D. Kloth, Bernard R. Tegtmeier, Clifford Kong, Michael P. Akahoshi, Stacie Hayase Leach, J. David Beatty, and John A. Zaia

186 **Predicting plasma procainamide concentrations resulting from a sustained-release preparation**
David M. DiPersio and Moses S. S. Chow

191 **Phenytoin therapy and immune response to influenza vaccine**
Marc Levine, B. Lynn Beattie, Donald M. McLean, and David Corman

195 **Intermittent dobutamine hydrochloride infusions in outpatients with chronic congestive heart failure**
David S. Roffman, Mark M. Applefeld, William R. Grove, Barry S. Talesnick, Frederick J. Sutton, Kathryn A. Newman, and William P. Reed

199 **Bioavailability assessment of a new liquid controlled-release pseudoephedrine product**
David A. Graves, Keith S. Rotenberg, James R. Woodworth, Lewis P. Amsel, and Orville N. Hinsvark

Research Note

204 **Treatment of cancer-associated hypercalcemia with mithramycin and oral etidronate disodium**
Daniel H. Shevrin, Linda R. Bressler, William P. McGuire, Subhash C. Kukreja, Lawrence J. Kukla, and Thomas E. Lad

Grand Rounds

206 **Immune globulin in the treatment of autoimmune thrombocytopenic purpura**
Cindy J. Wordell, Elizabeth A. Stubits, Karen J. Tietze, Janice A. Gaska, and Ellen M. Cosgrove

214 **Propranolol-induced depression and psychosis**
William A. Parker

Drug Experience

219 **Life-threatening anaphylaxis following subcutaneous administration of isosulfan blue 1%**
Stephen M. Longnecker, Michael M. Guzzardo, and Lee P. Van Voris

221 **Carbamazepine-induced thrombocytopenia in a young child**
Joan Marie Bradley, Rosalie Sagraves, and Anthony C. Kimbrough

123 **News**
Dietary modifications recommended for reducing heart disease, Olin H. Welsh, Jr. . . . Drug-induced blood disorders very rare . . . Long-acting third-generation cephalosporin ceftriaxone reaches U.S. market . . . Nomifensine, a second-generation antidepressant, approved by FDA . . . Naltrexone approved by FDA . . . Panel considers treatment of travelers' diarrhea . . . Oral acyclovir approved for treatment of genital herpes . . . Combination product approved for deep-vein thrombosis . . . Long-acting bronchodilator marketed . . . Isotretinoin associated with new adverse effects . . . Cardioselective β blocker acebutolol approved by FDA . . . Injectable agent approved for urinary-tract infections

145 **Letters**
Cimetidine-induced alopecia, Carl J. Tullio, Mark A. Roberts . . . Putting amoxicillin–potassium clavulanate in perspective, Allen J. Vaida . . . I. V. amantidine sulfate for extrapyramidal crisis. N. Gadoth, H. Sroka, G. Goldhammer, J. Alcalay, M. Bechar

224 **CP Continuing Education**

228 **Current Literature**
Book Reviews: *Clinical Pharmacy and Therapeutics, Third Edition (Herfindal, Hirschman)* Michael E. Ward . . . *Guide to Clinical Studies and Developing Protocols (Spilker)* Catherine Angell Sohn . . . *New Drugs Annual: Cardiovascular Drugs (Volume 2) (Scriabine)* Bradley G. Wulf . . . Books Received

240 **Advertising Index**

Instructions to Authors

CLINICAL PHARMACY gives priority to (1) studies that objectively evaluate drug effects in human trials, (2) evaluative review articles on the clinical uses of new drugs, and (3) evaluations of the current status of drug therapy in selected diseases. Contributions to the following sections are invited:

Drug Reviews: Detailed, analytical reviews on the clinical use of specific drugs, with preference given to new drugs and to evaluative rather than descriptive literature reviews.

Therapy Reviews: Articles that focus primarily on a disease state (rather than on a drug or drug class) and its treatment. These reviews foster an understanding of the pathophysiology of a disease and the related treatment.

Research: Reports of well-conducted original research on drug effects in humans.

Research Notes: Short research reports, such as updates on previously published work, confirmations of previous findings, or original research of modest scope.

Grand Rounds: Patient case reports and literature reviews combined in a way that gives them high educational value.

Drug Experience: Straightforward reports, with selected literature references, of unusual drug experiences.

Therapy Consultation: Brief advice, in a question-and-answer format, on how to handle specific drug-therapy problems. Readers are invited to submit questions, which the editor will forward to appropriate consultants for answering.

Letters: Short comments on previously published work or about potential problems, apparent trends, or controversies in drug therapy or clinical research.

Commentaries: Well-reasoned expressions of opinion on drug-therapy or clinical-research issues.

The editors have the sole authority to decide in which section to publish an accepted manuscript.

Manuscripts are subject to review by qualified outside reviewers, as well as by the editors, and will be accepted for publication only if they are believed to represent an important contribution to the literature. All papers submitted for publication must be accompanied by a completed copy of a manuscript checklist. The checklist appears on page 105 of the January–February 1985 issue. Authors of especially important original work may request "fast-track" review of their papers. Authors may suggest appropriate reviewers for their papers.

Accepted materials become the permanent and sole property of ASHP and may not be published or reprinted elsewhere without written permission from both the author and the editor.

The editors reserve the right to revise all materials submitted, if necessary. The publisher assumes no responsibility for the statements and opinions advanced by contributors to CLINICAL PHARMACY.

CLINICAL PHARMACY accepts manuscripts prepared according to the specifications of the Uniform Requirements for Manuscripts Submitted to Biomedical Journals (*Am J Hosp Pharm.* 1982; 38:1538–43). CLINICAL PHARMACY's manuscript checklist (page 105, January-February 1985 issue) generally conforms to the Uniform Requirements.

Under the terms of the Copyright Revision Act of 1976 (Public Law 94-553) it is necessary to have the rights of the authors transferred to the publisher in order to provide for the widest possible dissemination of professional and scientific literature. Accordingly, all transmittal letters accompanying manuscripts submitted for publication, including contributions for the Letters column, must contain the following language: "In consideration of the American Society of Hospital Pharmacists (ASHP) taking action in reviewing and editing my (our) submission, the author(s) undersigned hereby transfer(s), assign(s), or otherwise convey(s) all ownership rights in the submission and all copyright ownership to ASHP. In the event that such work is not published by ASHP, all said rights shall be released." We regret that we cannot consider manuscripts for publication that are not accompanied with transmittal letters containing the above language signed by all authors.

Authors must certify in their letter of transmittal that none of the material in their manuscript has been published previously nor is under consideration or been accepted for publication elsewhere. If this certification cannot be made, suitable explanation must be offered.

Six copies of all manuscripts should be submitted. Manuscripts should be typewritten with double spacing (including tables) on one side of good quality, 21.6 × 27.9-cm white paper, and with margins of at least 2.5 cm. For guidance on style, authors should consult the manuscript checklist, recent issues of CLINICAL PHARMACY, and the *Council of Biology Editors Style Manual*, fifth edition. *The American Heritage Dictionary of the English Language* and the AMA's *Manual for Authors and Editors* contain helpful advice on correct usage.

Galley proofs are sent to authors for inspection against the original manuscript and for correction. Unnecessary alterations in galley proof must be avoided. Extensive alterations will be charged to the author. An order form for reprints is sent to the corresponding author after galley proofs have been cleared.

CLINICAL PHARMACY (ISSN 0278-2677) is published bimonthly by the American Society of Hospital Pharmacists, 4630 Montgomery Avenue, Bethesda, MD 20814. Joseph A. Oddis, Executive Vice President. Second class postage is paid at Washington, DC, and at additional mailing offices. **Postmaster: Send address changes to: ASHP, 4630 Montgomery Avenue, Bethesda, MD 20814.**

Annual Subscription Rate:	*USA*	*Non-USA*
ASHP Member	$35	$40
ASHP Student Member	$25	$30
Institutions and Nonmembers	$55	$60

The cost of single copies is $9. Airmail delivery outside of the continental United States is available for an additional charge of $36 per year. Requests to replace missing issues free of charge are honored only up to six months after date of issue.

Advertising for CLINICAL PHARMACY is accepted in accordance with the Statement of Advertising Policy of the American Society of Hospital Pharmacists (see *Am J Hosp Pharm.* 1981; 38:1045). For additional information, contact the Advertising Representative (William McCausland Associates, Inc., P.O. Box 189, Pitman, NJ 08071. Phone 609-589-5454).

All articles published, including editorials, letters, and book reviews, represent the opinions of the authors and do not reflect the official policy of the American Society of Hospital Pharmacists or the institution with which the author is affiliated, unless this is clearly specified.

Microfilm and microfiche editions are available for purchase. Contact University Microfilms, 300 N. Zeeb Road, Ann Arbor, MI 48106.

Articles in CLINICAL PHARMACY are abstracted and indexed in *Current Contents, Clinical Sciences, Excerpta Medica, Index Medicus, Inpharma, International Pharmaceutical Abstracts*, and *Reactions.*

May–June 1985 Volume 4, Number 3 Coden: CPHADV ISSN: 0278-2677

CLINICAL PHARMACY

Therapy Reviews

279 **Pathophysiology and treatment of deep-vein thrombosis and pulmonary embolism**
Barry L. Carter, Mark E. Jones, and L. Anthony Waickman

297 **Management of bronchiolitis**
Milap C. Nahata, Julie A. Johnson, and Dwight A. Powell

304 **Management of antibiotic-associated pseudomembranous colitis**
Mark H. Gross

Research

311 **Evaluation of the vancomycin-clearance:creatinine-clearance relationship for predicting vancomycin dosage**
Gary R. Matzke, John M. Kovarik, Michael J. Rybak, and Steve C. Boike

316 **Twice-daily moxalactam versus gentamicin and clindamycin in patients with penetrating abdominal trauma**
Larry D. Crots, Farouck N. Obeid, H. Mathilda Horst, and Brack A. Bivins

Research Notes

320 **Acyclovir pharmacokinetics in a patient on continuous ambulatory peritoneal dialysis**
Shiv K. Seth, James A. Visconti, Lee A. Hebert, and Harvey C. Krasny

322 **Appearance of ranitidine in breast milk following multiple dosing**
Gregory L. Kearns, Richard F. McConnell, Jr., John M. Trang, and Ronald B. Kluza

325 **Warfarin absorption in a patient with short-bowel syndrome**
Mark E. Lehman, Kenneth W. Kolb, Glenn R. Barnhart, Lawrence D. Wagman, and William H. Barr

Drug Experience

327 **Gentamicin elimination in a patient undergoing continuous ultrafiltration**
Mark E. Lehman and Kenneth W. Kolb

330 **Pentobarbital coma for treating intractable seizures in a neonate**
Timothy E. Welty and Robert L. Kriel

332 **Potentiation of warfarin anticoagulation by topical testosterone ointment**
Sarah McQuade Lorentz and Robert T. Weibert

334 **Dermatologic reaction to a sustained-release theophylline product**
Stephen Mendel, Charles A. Beck, Jr., and Jean A. Rumsfield

245 **News**
Phospholipids may hold key to allergic and immunologic reactions, Linda M. McManus . . . AIDS tests reach market as cases increase . . . I.V. indomethacin marketed for patent ductus arteriosus . . . Patients, professionals good guessers in double-blind trial

255 **Letters**
Acetylcysteine for severe atelectasis in premature infants, Jacob Amir, Eliahu Wilunsky, Israel Zelikovic, Salomon H. Reisner . . . Pharmacologic effects of the triazolo group, George Taniguchi . . . Venoconstriction by angiotensin II, Joseph T. Rackson

336 **CP Continuing Education**

340 **ASHP CE Instructions and Enrollment Form**

342 **Current Literature**
Book Reviews: *Antimicrobial Therapy (Ristuccia, Cunha)*, Steven L. Barriere . . . *Critical Care: A Comprehensive Approach (Bone)*, Erkan Hassan . . . *The Psychopharmacology of Lithium (Johnson)*, Janet L. Kinney . . . Books Received . . . New Periodical

354 **Advertising Index**

Instructions to Authors

CLINICAL PHARMACY gives priority to (1) studies that objectively evaluate drug effects in human trials, (2) evaluative review articles on the clinical uses of new drugs, and (3) evaluations of the current status of drug therapy in selected diseases. Contributions to the following sections are invited:

Drug Reviews: Detailed, analytical reviews on the clinical use of specific drugs, with preference given to new drugs and to evaluative rather than descriptive literature reviews.

Therapy Reviews: Articles that focus primarily on a disease state (rather than on a drug or drug class) and its treatment. These reviews foster an understanding of the pathophysiology of a disease and the related treatment.

Research: Reports of well-conducted original research on drug effects in humans.

Research Notes: Short research reports, such as updates on previously published work, confirmations of previous findings, or original research of modest scope.

Grand Rounds: Patient case reports and literature reviews combined in a way that gives them high educational value.

Drug Experience: Straightforward reports, with selected literature references, of unusual drug experiences.

Therapy Consultation: Brief advice, in a question-and-answer format, on how to handle specific drug-therapy problems. Readers are invited to submit questions, which the editor will forward to appropriate consultants for answering.

Letters: Short comments on previously published work or about potential problems, apparent trends, or controversies in drug therapy or clinical research.

Commentaries: Well-reasoned expressions of opinion on drug-therapy or clinical-research issues.

The editors have the sole authority to decide in which section to publish an accepted manuscript.

Manuscripts are subject to review by qualified outside reviewers, as well as by the editors, and will be accepted for publication only if they are believed to represent an important contribution to the literature. All papers submitted for publication must be accompanied by a completed copy of a manuscript checklist. The checklist appears on page 105 of the January–February 1985 issue. Authors of especially important original work may request "fast-track" review of their papers. Authors may suggest appropriate reviewers for their papers.

Accepted materials become the permanent and sole property of ASHP and may not be published or reprinted elsewhere without written permission from both the author and the editor.

The editors reserve the right to revise all materials submitted, if necessary. The publisher assumes no responsibility for the statements and opinions advanced by contributors to CLINICAL PHARMACY.

CLINICAL PHARMACY accepts manuscripts prepared according to the specifications of the Uniform Requirements for Manuscripts Submitted to Biomedical Journals (*Am J Hosp Pharm.* 1982; 38:1538–43). CLINICAL PHARMACY's manuscript checklist (page 105, January-February 1985 issue) generally conforms to the Uniform Requirements.

Under the terms of the Copyright Revision Act of 1976 (Public Law 94-553) it is necessary to have the rights of the authors transferred to the publisher in order to provide for the widest possible dissemination of professional and scientific literature. Accordingly, all transmittal letters accompanying manuscripts submitted for publication, including contributions for the Letters column, must contain the following language: "In consideration of the American Society of Hospital Pharmacists (ASHP) taking action in reviewing and editing my (our) submission, the author(s) undersigned hereby transfer(s), assign(s), or otherwise convey(s) all ownership rights in the submission and all copyright ownership to ASHP. In the event that such work is not published by ASHP, all said rights shall be released." We regret that we cannot consider manuscripts for publication that are not accompanied with transmittal letters containing the above language signed by all authors.

Authors must certify in their letter of transmittal that none of the material in their manuscript has been published previously nor is under consideration or been accepted for publication elsewhere. If this certification cannot be made, suitable explanation must be offered.

Six copies of all manuscripts should be submitted. Manuscripts should be typewritten with double spacing (including tables) on one side of good quality, 21.6 × 27.9-cm white paper, and with margins of at least 2.5 cm. For guidance on style, authors should consult the manuscript checklist, recent issues of CLINICAL PHARMACY, and the *Council of Biology Editors Style Manual*, fifth edition. *The American Heritage Dictionary of the English Language* and the AMA's *Manual for Authors and Editors* contain helpful advice on correct usage.

Galley proofs are sent to authors for inspection against the original manuscript and for correction. Unnecessary alterations in galley proof must be avoided. Extensive alterations will be charged to the author. An order form for reprints is sent to the corresponding author after galley proofs have been cleared.

CLINICAL PHARMACY (ISSN 0278-2677) is published bimonthly by the American Society of Hospital Pharmacists, 4630 Montgomery Avenue, Bethesda, MD 20814. Joseph A. Oddis, Executive Vice President. Second class postage is paid at Bethesda, MD, and at additional mailing offices. **Postmaster: Send address changes to: ASHP, 4630 Montgomery Avenue, Bethesda, MD 20814.**

Annual Subscription Rate:	*USA*	*Non-USA*
ASHP Member	$35	$40
ASHP Student Member	$25	$30
Institutions and Nonmembers	$55	$60

The cost of single copies is $9. Airmail delivery outside of the continental United States is available for an additional charge of $36 per year. Requests to replace missing issues free of charge are honored only up to six months after date of issue.

All articles published, including editorials, letters, and book reviews, represent the opinions of the authors and do not reflect the official policy of the American Society of Hospital Pharmacists or the institution with which the author is affiliated, unless this is clearly specified.

Microfilm and microfiche editions are available for purchase. Contact University Microfilms, 300 N. Zeeb Road, Ann Arbor, MI 48106.

Articles in CLINICAL PHARMACY are abstracted and indexed in *Current Contents, Clinical Sciences, Excerpta Medica, Index Medicus, Inpharma, International Pharmaceutical Abstracts*, and *Reactions*.

September–October 1985 Volume 4, Number 5 Coden: CPHADV ISSN: 0278-2677

CLINICAL PHARMACY

Drug Reviews

507 **Pentamidine isethionate in the treatment of *Pneumocystis carinii* pneumonia**
Susan Drake, Victor Lampasona, Harold L. Nicks, and Stephen W. Schwarzmann

516 **Aztreonam, a new monobactam antimicrobial**
David R. P. Guay and Christopher Koskoletos

527 **Product selection criteria for intravascular ionic contrast media**
Dennis P. Swanson, Terry J. Dick, Stuart M. Simms, and James H. Thrall

Therapy Reviews

539 **Treatment of infectious complications of acquired immunodeficiency syndrome**
Melissa M. Furio and Cindy J. Wordell

555 **Therapeutic management of cystic fibrosis**
Robert J. Kuhn and Milap C. Nahata

Grand Rounds

566 **Recognition and management of acute suppurative parotitis**
Richard S. Perry

Drug Experience

572 **Failure of creatinine clearance to predict gentamicin half-life in a renal-transplant patient with diabetes mellitus**
Katherine A. Michael, James L. Mohler, Robert A. Blouin, Bruce A. Lucas, and Robert P. Rapp

475 **News**
Researchers discuss promising drugs for AIDS at Atlanta conference, William A. Check . . . Data on dose-dumping of sustained-release theophylline published . . . Synthetic THC approved by FDA . . . Study shows benefit in treating elderly hypertensive patients . . . Adjuvant chemotherapy useful in osteosarcoma, says NIH Panel . . . Ceftazidime reaches U.S. market . . . Captopril approved for all degrees of hypertension

488 **Letters**
Use of 0.9% sodium chloride injection without heparin for maintaining indwelling intermittent injection sites, Terry Dean, Pam Ridley; Joseph M. Ferraro, Robert F. Guanci, Robert J. Stoneburner; Edward L. Epperson . . . The opioid-nonadrenergic link in Gilles de la Tourette's syndrome, R. Sandyk . . . Beneficial hemodynamic effects of oral levodopa in a patient with cardiomyopathy, Ronald W. Maddox, W. Stanley Arnold, Van Odell Sliger . . . Procainamide-induced hypotension during CPR, Edgar R. Gonzalez, Joseph P. Ornato . . . Potentiation of opiate analgesia with ibuprofen, R. Sandyk

576 **CP Continuing Education**

583 **Current Literature**
Book Reviews: *The Aging Process: Therapeutic Implications* (*Butler, Bearn*), Judi B. Shor . . . *Beta Blockers in the Treatment of Cardiovascular Disease* (*Kostis, De Felice*), Renee P. Tannenbaum . . . *Clinical Guide to Parenteral Micronutrition* (*Baumgartner*), David F. Driscoll . . . *Evaluation and Treatment of Chronic Pain* (*Aronoff*), Stephen J. Bollish . . . *Pediatric Medications: An Emergency and Critical Care Reference* (*Stewart, Stewart*), Kathleen M. Reilly . . . Books Received

590 **Advertising Index**

Instructions to Authors

CLINICAL PHARMACY gives priority to (1) studies that objectively evaluate drug effects in human trials, (2) evaluative review articles on the clinical uses of new drugs, and (3) evaluations of the current status of drug therapy in selected diseases. Contributions to the following sections are invited:

Drug Reviews: Detailed, analytical reviews on the clinical use of specific drugs, with preference given to new drugs and to evaluative rather than descriptive literature reviews.

Therapy Reviews: Articles that focus primarily on a disease state (rather than on a drug or drug class) and its treatment. These reviews foster an understanding of the pathophysiology of a disease and the related treatment.

Research: Reports of well-conducted original research on drug effects in humans.

Research Notes: Short research reports, such as updates on previously published work, confirmations of previous findings, or original research of modest scope.

Grand Rounds: Patient case reports and literature reviews combined in a way that gives them high educational value.

Drug Experience: Straightforward reports, with selected literature references, of unusual drug experiences.

Therapy Consultation: Brief advice, in a question-and-answer format, on how to handle specific drug-therapy problems. Readers are invited to submit questions, which the editor will forward to appropriate consultants for answering.

Letters: Short comments on previously published work or about potential problems, apparent trends, or controversies in drug therapy or clinical research.

Commentaries: Well-reasoned expressions of opinion on drug-therapy or clinical-research issues.

The editors have the sole authority to decide in which section to publish an accepted manuscript.

Manuscripts are subject to review by qualified outside reviewers, as well as by the editors, and will be accepted for publication only if they are believed to represent an important contribution to the literature. All papers submitted for publication must be accompanied by a completed copy of a manuscript checklist. The checklist appears on page 105 of the January–February 1985 issue. Authors of especially important original work may request "fast-track" review of their papers. Authors may suggest appropriate reviewers for their papers.

Accepted materials become the permanent and sole property of ASHP and may not be published or reprinted elsewhere without written permission from both the author and the editor.

The editors reserve the right to revise all materials submitted, if necessary. The publisher assumes no responsibility for the statements and opinions advanced by contributors to CLINICAL PHARMACY.

CLINICAL PHARMACY accepts manuscripts prepared according to the specifications of the Uniform Requirements for Manuscripts Submitted to Biomedical Journals (*Am J Hosp Pharm.* 1982; 38:1538–43). CLINICAL PHARMACY's manuscript checklist (page 105, January-February 1985 issue) generally conforms to the Uniform Requirements.

Under the terms of the Copyright Revision Act of 1976 (Public Law 94-553) it is necessary to have the rights of the authors transferred to the publisher in order to provide for the widest possible dissemination of professional and scientific literature. Accordingly, all transmittal letters accompanying manuscripts submitted for publication, including contributions for the Letters column, must contain the following language: "In consideration of the American Society of Hospital Pharmacists (ASHP) taking action in reviewing and editing my (our) submission, the author(s) undersigned hereby transfer(s), assign(s), or otherwise convey(s) all ownership rights in the submission and all copyright ownership to ASHP. In the event that such work is not published by ASHP, all said rights shall be released." We regret that we cannot consider manuscripts for publication that are not accompanied with transmittal letters containing the above language signed by all authors.

Authors must certify in their letter of transmittal that none of the material in their manuscript has been published previously nor is under consideration or been accepted for publication elsewhere. If this certification cannot be made, suitable explanation must be offered.

Six copies of all manuscripts should be submitted. Manuscripts should be typewritten with double spacing (including tables) on one side of good quality, 21.6 × 27.9-cm white paper, and with margins of at least 2.5 cm. For guidance on style, authors should consult the manuscript checklist, recent issues of CLINICAL PHARMACY, and the *Council of Biology Editors Style Manual,* fifth edition. *The American Heritage Dictionary of the English Language* and the AMA's *Manual for Authors and Editors* contain helpful advice on correct usage.

Galley proofs are sent to authors for inspection against the original manuscript and for correction. Unnecessary alterations in galley proof must be avoided. Extensive alterations will be charged to the author. An order form for reprints is sent to the corresponding author after galley proofs have been cleared.

CLINICAL PHARMACY (ISSN 0278-2677) is published bimonthly by the American Society of Hospital Pharmacists, 4630 Montgomery Avenue, Bethesda, MD 20814. Joseph A. Oddis, Executive Vice President. Second class postage is paid at Bethesda, MD, and at additional mailing offices. **Postmaster: Send address changes to: ASHP, 4630 Montgomery Avenue, Bethesda, MD 20814.**

Annual Subscription Rate:	*USA*	*Non-USA*
ASHP Member	$38	$43
ASHP Student Member	$28	$33
Institutions and Nonmembers	$60	$65

The cost of single copies is $10. Airmail delivery outside of the continental United States is available for an additional charge of $72 per year. Requests to replace missing issues free of charge are honored only up to six months after date of issue.

Microfilm and microfiche editions are available for purchase. Contact University Microfilms, 300 N. Zeeb Road, Ann Arbor, MI 48106.

Articles in CLINICAL PHARMACY are abstracted and indexed in *Current Contents, Clinical Sciences, Excerpta Medica, Index Medicus, Inpharma, International Pharmaceutical Abstracts,* and *Reactions.*

November–December 1985 Volume 4, Number 6 Coden: CPHADV ISSN: 0278-2677

CLINICAL PHARMACY

Drug Review

625 **Nomifensine maleate: A new second-generation antidepressant**
Janet L. Kinney

Therapy Reviews

637 **Preventing *Haemophilus influenzae* type b disease**
Daniel T. Casto and Deborah L. Edwards

649 **Use of antihypertensive agents in patients with glucose intolerance**
James M. McKenney, Robert P. Goodman, and Jackson T. Wright, Jr.

657 **Drug-induced systemic lupus erythematosus**
Mark A. Stratton

Research

664 **Pharmacokinetics of high-dose azlocillin sodium in patients with cystic fibrosis**
Roger A. Woolf, Jeffrey R. Koup, Arnold L. Smith, Bettina C. Hilman, Donald Goldmann, and Judy Williams-Warren

Research Note

669 **Clearance of procainamide and *N*-acetylprocainamide in patients undergoing continuous ambulatory peritoneal dialysis**
Cynthia L. Raehl, A. Vishnu Moorthy, Gregory J. Beirne, and Michael E. Pitterle

Editorial

673 **Nomifensine: An antidepressant with a difference?**
Larry Ereshefsky

Grand Rounds

675 **Drug-induced torsade de pointes**
Cynthia L. Raehl, Ashvin K. Patel, and Marie LeRoy

595 **News**
Conference outlines challenges in the treatment of cocaine abuse, Carla J. Brink . . . New NIH recommendations for adjuvant therapy for breast cancer, Jane L. Miller . . . Leuprolide approved for palliative treatment of advanced prostatic cancer . . . New β blocker for glaucoma approved by FDA . . . Studies of bepridil in use against arrhythmias halted

615 **Letters**
Successful treatment of cerebellar tremor with clonazepam, R. Sandyk . . . Phenytoin injection precautions, Peter D. Reeme . . . Drug clearance in patients undergoing continuous arteriovenous hemofiltration, Michael Rubino . . . Effect of warfarin on activated partial thromboplastin time, Thomas G. Burnakis; Barry L. Carter, Mark E. Jones

691 **Acknowledgment to Reviewers**

692 **CP Continuing Education**

696 **CP Continuing Education Enrollment Form**

703 **Current Literature**
Book Reviews: *AMA Handbook of Poisonous and Injurious Plants* (*Lampe, McCann*), Michael D. Ellis . . . *Blue Book of Pharmacologic Therapeutics* (*Johnson*), Karen J. Klamerus . . . *Interpretation of Clinical Laboratory Tests* (*Siest, Henry, Schiele et al.*), Ralph E. Small . . . Books Received . . . New Periodical

706 **Advertising Index**

707 **Annual Index**

Instructions to Authors

CLINICAL PHARMACY gives priority to (1) studies that objectively evaluate drug effects in human trials, (2) evaluative review articles on the clinical uses of new drugs, and (3) evaluations of the current status of drug therapy in selected diseases. Contributions to the following sections are invited:

Drug Reviews: Detailed, analytical reviews on the clinical use of specific drugs, with preference given to new drugs and to evaluative rather than descriptive literature reviews.

Therapy Reviews: Articles that focus primarily on a disease state (rather than on a drug or drug class) and its treatment. These reviews foster an understanding of the pathophysiology of a disease and the related treatment.

Research: Reports of well-conducted original research on drug effects in humans.

Research Notes: Short research reports, such as updates on previously published work, confirmations of previous findings, or original research of modest scope.

Grand Rounds: Patient case reports and literature reviews combined in a way that gives them high educational value.

Drug Experience: Straightforward reports, with selected literature references, of unusual drug experiences.

Therapy Consultation: Brief advice, in a question-and-answer format, on how to handle specific drug-therapy problems. Readers are invited to submit questions, which the editor will forward to appropriate consultants for answering.

Letters: Short comments on previously published work or about potential problems, apparent trends, or controversies in drug therapy or clinical research.

Commentaries: Well-reasoned expressions of opinion on drug-therapy or clinical-research issues.

The editors have the sole authority to decide in which section to publish an accepted manuscript.

Manuscripts are subject to review by qualified outside reviewers, as well as by the editors, and will be accepted for publication only if they are believed to represent an important contribution to the literature. All papers submitted for publication must be accompanied by a completed copy of a manuscript checklist. The checklist appears on page 105 of the January–February 1985 issue. Authors of especially important original work may request "fast-track" review of their papers. Authors may suggest appropriate reviewers for their papers.

Accepted materials become the permanent and sole property of ASHP and may not be published or reprinted elsewhere without written permission from both the author and the editor.

The editors reserve the right to revise all materials submitted, if necessary. The publisher assumes no responsibility for the statements and opinions advanced by contributors to CLINICAL PHARMACY.

CLINICAL PHARMACY accepts manuscripts prepared according to the specifications of the Uniform Requirements for Manuscripts Submitted to Biomedical Journals (*Am J Hosp Pharm.* 1982; 38:1538–43). CLINICAL PHARMACY's manuscript checklist (page 105, January-February 1985 issue) generally conforms to the Uniform Requirements.

Under the terms of the Copyright Revision Act of 1976 (Public Law 94-553) it is necessary to have the rights of the authors transferred to the publisher in order to provide for the widest possible dissemination of professional and scientific literature. Accordingly, all transmittal letters accompanying manuscripts submitted for publication, including contributions for the Letters column, must contain the following language: "In consideration of the American Society of Hospital Pharmacists (ASHP) taking action in reviewing and editing my (our) submission, the author(s) undersigned hereby transfer(s), assign(s), or otherwise convey(s) all ownership rights in the submission and all copyright ownership to ASHP. In the event that such work is not published by ASHP, all said rights shall be released." We regret that we cannot consider manuscripts for publication that are not accompanied with transmittal letters containing the above language signed by all authors.

Authors must certify in their letter of transmittal that none of the material in their manuscript has been published previously nor is under consideration or been accepted for publication elsewhere. If this certification cannot be made, suitable explanation must be offered.

Six copies of all manuscripts should be submitted. Manuscripts should be typewritten with double spacing (including tables) on one side of good quality, 21.6 × 27.9-cm white paper, and with margins of at least 2.5 cm. For guidance on style, authors should consult the manuscript checklist, recent issues of CLINICAL PHARMACY, and the *Council of Biology Editors Style Manual*, fifth edition. *The American Heritage Dictionary of the English Language* and the AMA's *Manual for Authors and Editors* contain helpful advice on correct usage.

Galley proofs are sent to authors for inspection against the original manuscript and for correction. Unnecessary alterations in galley proof must be avoided. Extensive alterations will be charged to the author. An order form for reprints is sent to the corresponding author after galley proofs have been cleared.

CLINICAL PHARMACY (ISSN 0278-2677) is published bimonthly by the American Society of Hospital Pharmacists, 4630 Montgomery Avenue, Bethesda, MD 20814. Joseph A. Oddis, Executive Vice President. Second class postage is paid at Bethesda, MD, and at additional mailing offices. **Postmaster: Send address changes to: ASHP, 4630 Montgomery Avenue, Bethesda, MD 20814.**

Annual Subscription Rate:	*USA*	*Non-USA*
ASHP Member	$38	$43
ASHP Student Member	$28	$33
Institutions and Nonmembers	$60	$65

The cost of single copies is $10. Airmail delivery outside of the continental United States is available for an additional charge of $72 per year. Requests to replace missing issues free of charge are honored only up to six months after date of issue.

Microfilm and microfiche editions are available for purchase. Contact University Microfilms, 300 N. Zeeb Road, Ann Arbor, MI 48106.

Articles in CLINICAL PHARMACY are abstracted and indexed in *Current Contents, Clinical Sciences, Excerpta Medica, Index Medicus, Inpharma, International Pharmaceutical Abstracts,* and *Reactions.*

News

Applying pharmacodynamics in patient care

Using drug effects rather than serum concentrations in monitoring drug therapy was the subject of an interesting two-part symposium at the APhA Academy of Pharmaceutical Sciences meeting in Philadelphia on October 29–30. The session, which was cosponsored by the American College of Clinical Pharmacy, attracted a large audience that heard how pharmacodynamics is being correlated with pharmacokinetics in clinical research and practice.

The limitations of pharmacokinetics have been known for many years, but recently the application of kinetic principles has come under more and more criticism as practitioners sometimes "treat the serum level, not the patient." Among the other factors speakers mentioned that are leading to increased favor for pharmacodynamics were the following:

- Biological variation produces a large amount of variability in concentration–response relationships.
- Active metabolites confound accurate determination of the adequacy of some drug dosages based on serum concentrations of the parent drug.
- Diseases cause changes in drug receptors in the body and change the way the body responds to therapeutic agents.
- Microorganisms have a large variability in susceptibility to anti-infective agents, even within species.
- Drugs may be present in serum but may distribute to sites of action slowly.

Each of these factors makes conclusions based solely on serum concentration data suspect. However, if the effects of drugs could be measured, the clinician or researcher could be much more confident of appropriate courses of action regarding drug regimens.

Finding Appropriate Measures of Drug Action. The tough part about using pharmacodynamics is that each type of drug has a completely different action. Hence, a unique means of assessment is required for each drug. Speakers at the symposium discussed a variety of methods for looking at the effects of psychoactive agents, calcium-channel blockers, antibiotics, diuretics, β blockers, and H_2-receptor antagonists. The most elaborate models were for the antibiotics.

Jerome J. Schentag of the State University of New York at Buffalo discussed a model his group is testing called the dynamic response concentration (a play on the "minimum inhibitory concentration") for antibiotics. The group relies on a microcomputer-based system such as Abbott's MS2 Research System, which is a computerized spectrophotometer that measures bacterial growth over time as a function of drug concentration.

In a series of computer simulations designed to assess the reasons for variability in bacterial response, Schentag and coworkers found that pharmacokinetic factors accounted for only one half of the variability in dosage requirements. Differences in bacterial susceptibility accounted for the other half of the variability, and when that pharmacodynamic variation was considered with the pharmacokinetic variability, antibiotic dosage requirements varied up to fivefold. The group concluded that a new concept incorporating both factors was needed, and they called this approach dual individualization.

A group of 14 patients with stage III pneumonia was treated with cefmenoxime dosages based on both pharmacokinetic factors and the dynamic response concentration data from the MS2 system. When time above the dynamic response concentration in vivo was plotted against days to eradication of the infection, a consistent relationship was observed regardless of the species of bacteria involved. The group also observed that the disease process had more effect on blood concentrations of the drug than it did on the relationship between the drug and the bacteria.

Another approach to integrating pharmacodynamics and pharmacokinetics in the treatment of infectious diseases was described by Steven L. Barriere of The University of Michigan in Ann Arbor. By combining serum concentration–time data with known bactericidal concentrations from in vitro work, his group has come up with calculations they call area under the bactericidal titer curve (AUBC). The methodology has been tested in three investigations, and factors such as cefotaxime's active metabolite and decreased clearance of cefotaxime in the presence of mezlocillin have been considered in determining drug effects and dose.

Applying the Principles to Other Drugs. Antibiotics are unique in therapeutics, in that a specific diagnosis can often be made complete with in vitro testing of the effects of various therapeutic agents on the "receptor." However, when one attempts to extend the principles, say, to cardiovascular agents, the situation is much more complicated; people usually are not as willing to allow a cardiac biopsy as they might be a throat swab or even a blood sample.

Other speakers at the symposium described the status of work on pharmacodynamic measurements of drug action. John A. Pieper of the University of Tennessee discussed work on verapamil, the pharmacodynamics of which are complicated by the drug's active metabolite, norverapamil. In a study of i.v., single oral, and multiple oral doses to five healthy volunteers, Pieper found good correlations between serum concentrations and PR interval; data collected supported the theory of preferential elimination of the L isomer of verapamil presystemically following oral administration and for a contribution of

Continued on page 11

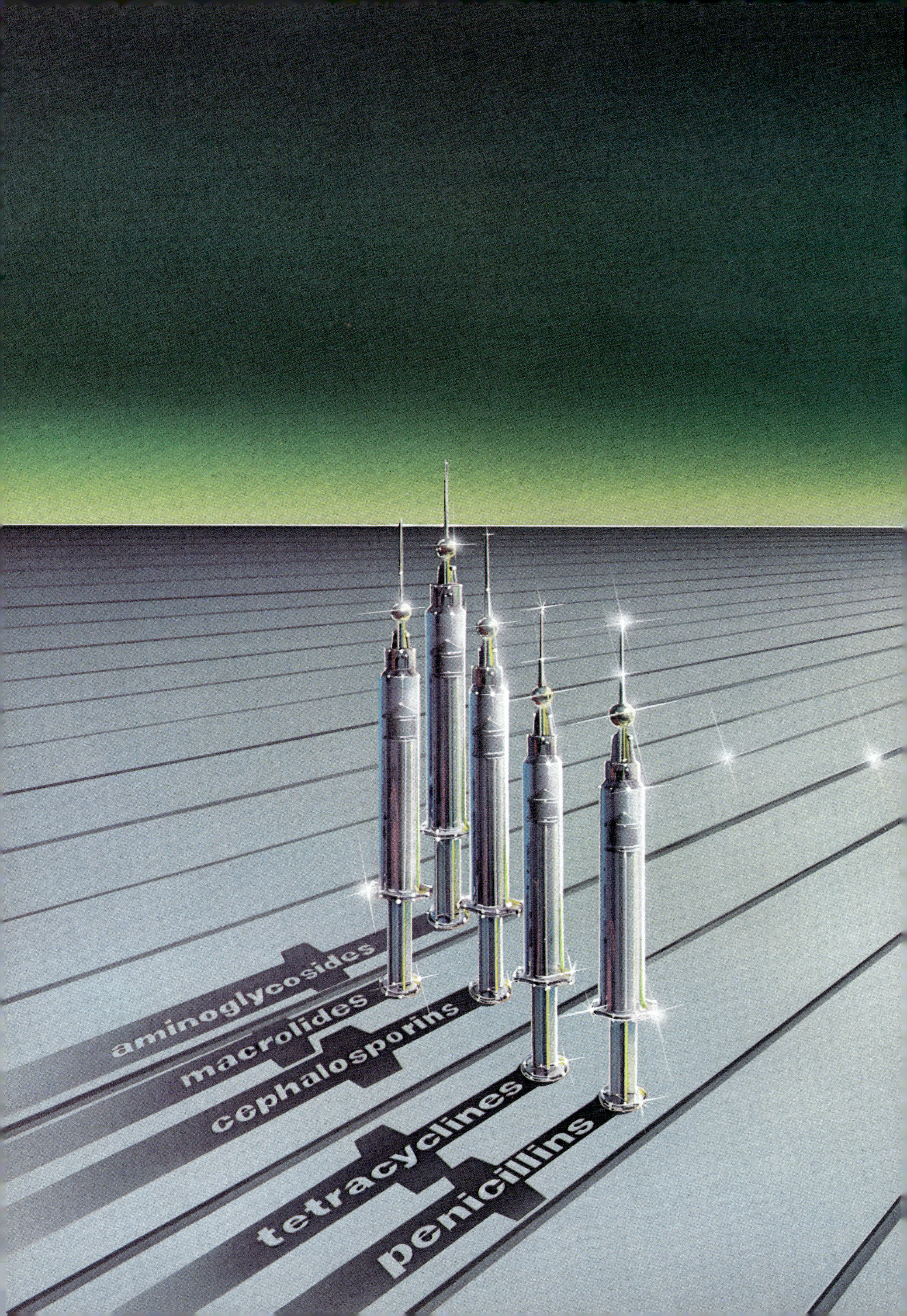
aminoglycosides
macrolides
cephalosporins
tetracyclines
penicillins

Continued from page 3

norverapamil to the AV node effect of this calcium-channel blocker.

In an excellent summary of the role of pharmacodynamics in day-to-day patient care, Leslie V. Benet of the University of California–San Francisco pointed out that correlations between pharmacodynamics and pharmacokinetics may not be useful for a specific patient. However, he noted, such correlations provide an important tool in the understanding of drug–drug and drug–disease interactions in various populations. In discussing diuretics specifically, he noted that the pharmacodynamic response—albeit an easy one to measure for diuretics—would be preferred over a pharmacokinetic analysis. It appears that, at least initially on a research level, many clinical pharmacists will be turning increasingly to pharmacodynamics instead of serum concentration data to analyze drug regimens.

L. MICHAEL POSEY

Tocainide marketed in U.S.

Tocainide hydrochloride (Tonocard, Merck Sharp & Dohme), the first new antiarrhythmic agent approved for marketing in the U.S. in eight years and the first orally active congener of lidocaine, was approved by the Food and Drug Administration on November 9. Tocainide was one of the antiarrhythmic agents reviewed in *Clinical Pharmacy* in the July–August 1983 issue.[1]

The availability of an oral agent chemically similar to lidocaine is expected to offer a smooth transition to ambulatory care for patients whose arrhythmias are controlled by lidocaine injection in the hospital. Tocainide has accumulated more than 3.5 million prescription days of use abroad since 1981, and more than 1100 U.S. physicians have treated patients under a compassionate-use protocol before the drug was approved by FDA.

Tocainide is a type 1 antiarrhythmic compound similar to lidocaine electrophysiologically but different from quinidine, procainamide, and disopyramide. Following oral administration, peak plasma tocainide concentrations occur in 0.5–2.0 hours, and the mean plasma half-life is 15 hours. The usual therapeutic plasma concentration range is 4–10 μg/mL; tocainide undergoes negligible first-pass metabolism, and it has no active metabolites.

The labeled indications for tocainide are for the suppression of symptomatic ventricular arrhythmias, including frequent premature ventricular contractions (unifocal or multifocal), couplets, and ventricular tachycardia. It is contraindicated for patients sensitive to local anesthetics of the amide type and patients with second- or third-degree block who do not have an artificial ventricular pacemaker.

The side effects of tocainide include lightheadedness and dizziness (15.3%), nausea (14.5%), paresthesia and numbness (9.2%), and tremor (8.4%). These reactions have typically been mild, transient, dose related, and reversible upon decreased dosage, taking the drug with food, or drug discontinuation. In long-term controlled trials, therapy was stopped in 21% of patients because of side effects.

The usual adult dose of tocainide is 400 mg every eight hours; up to 1800 mg/day may be given in three divided doses, and doses of more than 2400 mg/day have been used infrequently. Patients who tolerate the t.i.d. regimen may try b.i.d. dosing with careful monitoring. The drug is supplied as 400- and 600-mg tablets in bottles of 100 and unit dose packages of 100. Tocainide costs wholesalers and community pharmacies $33.61 and $42.85 for 100 of the 400- and 600-mg tablets, respectively. Unit dose packages of the two strengths cost $35.50 and $44.74 per 100 tablets, respectively.

1. Wulf BG. Mexiletine and tocainide: two orally active congeners of lidocaine. *Clin Pharm.* 1983; 2:340–6.

Study shows little change in microbial resistance patterns

A recently published study of six million strains of bacteria isolated in U.S. hospitals between 1971 and 1982 shows that there has been remarkably little change in resistance patterns during this period.[1] The study showed that only *Streptococcus faecalis* and *Staphylococcus epidermidis* have developed additional resistance to antibiotics.

The authors obtained data on almost 10 million strains of bacteria from the Bac-Data Medical Information Systems in Clifton, NJ; they analyzed the susceptibilities of 5,828,243 strains that are frequently isolated or that commonly cause deaths. Resistance patterns to 16 commonly used antibiotics were studied. Further data were obtained from two hospitals and analyzed.

The most common organism isolated was *Escherichia coli*, which accounted for 19.2% of strains, followed by *Staphylococcus aureus* at 10.5% and *Strep. faecalis* at 6.3%. Strains of *E. coli*, *Staph. aureus*, *H. influenzae*, and *Pseudomonas aeruginosa* showed virtually identical resistance patterns over the 12 years studied, although there were small variations of a percentage point or two. The two organisms with markedly increased resistance were *Strep. faecalis* and *Staph. epidermidis*.

The authors conclude that, while "local outbreaks of bacterial resistance do arise . . . bacterial resistance on a national scale has remained virtually unchanged during the last decade." They continued, "This may, perhaps, be credited to the continuous efforts in U.S. hospitals to achieve balanced usage of antibiotics."

1. Atkinson BA, Lorian V. Antimicrobial agent susceptibility patterns of bacteria in hospitals from 1971 to 1982. *J Clin Microbiol.* 1984; 20:791–6.

Pentamidine now available commercially

A mainstay of treatment of a common infection in patients with acquired immunodeficiency syndrome (AIDS) is available commercially following an October 24 approval by FDA. Pentamidine (Pentam 300, LyphoMed) was approved after only six months of review by the federal agency for treatment of *Pneumocystis carinii* infections, which are contracted by 60% of AIDS patients.

Pentamidine was previously available only through sources such as the Centers for Disease Control or the New York State Department of Health. FDA has designated pentamidine an orphan drug, meaning that LyphoMed

Continued on page 14

An advance in the
management of type II diabetes

Micronase®

glyburide, **5 mg** tablets

Once-a-day therapy for type II diabetic patients who do not respond to diet alone.

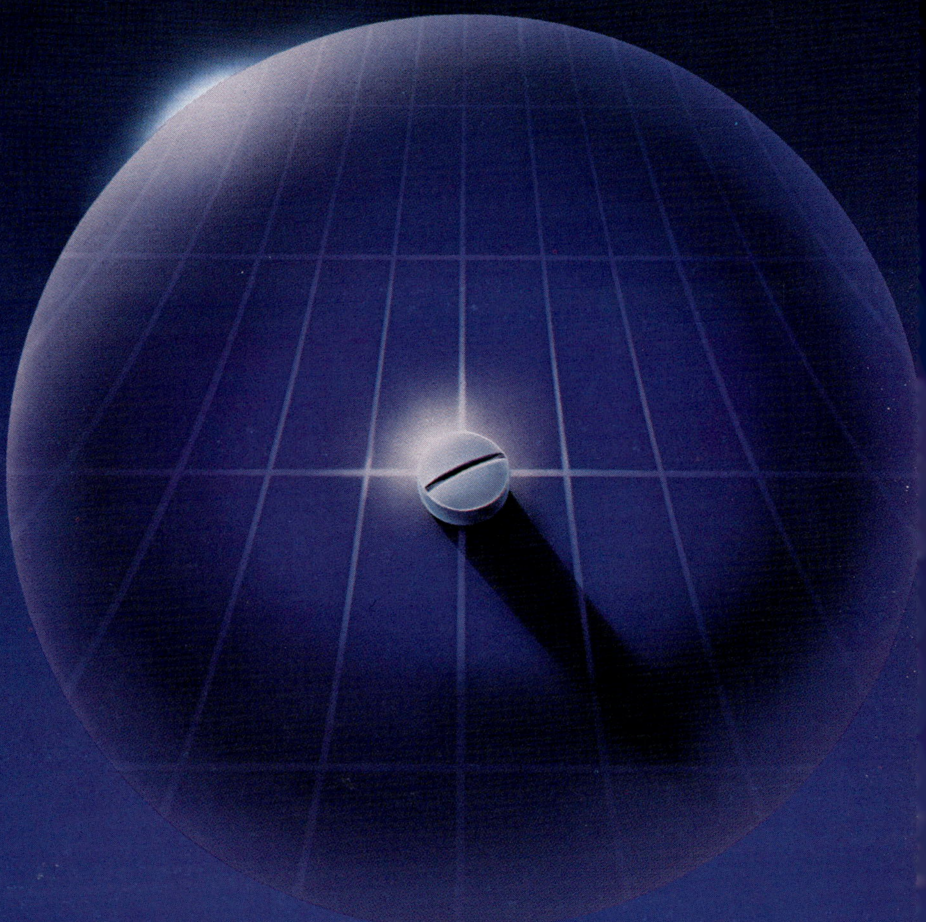

- One dose of *Micronase* each day provides effective 24-hour control of blood glucose. Usual starting dose is 2.5 to 5.0 mg daily.
- Unique dual-excretion pattern...*Micronase* is eliminated 50% in urine and 50% in bile. The plasma clearance of *Micronase* is prolonged only in severe renal impairment.
- *Micronase* helps normalize tissue response to endogenous insulin.[1]
- *Micronase* does *not* cause water retention; may produce slight diuresis.[2]

...has *no* deleterious effect on lipid levels.

...does *not* significantly affect patient weight.

...rarely causes disulfiram-like reactions.

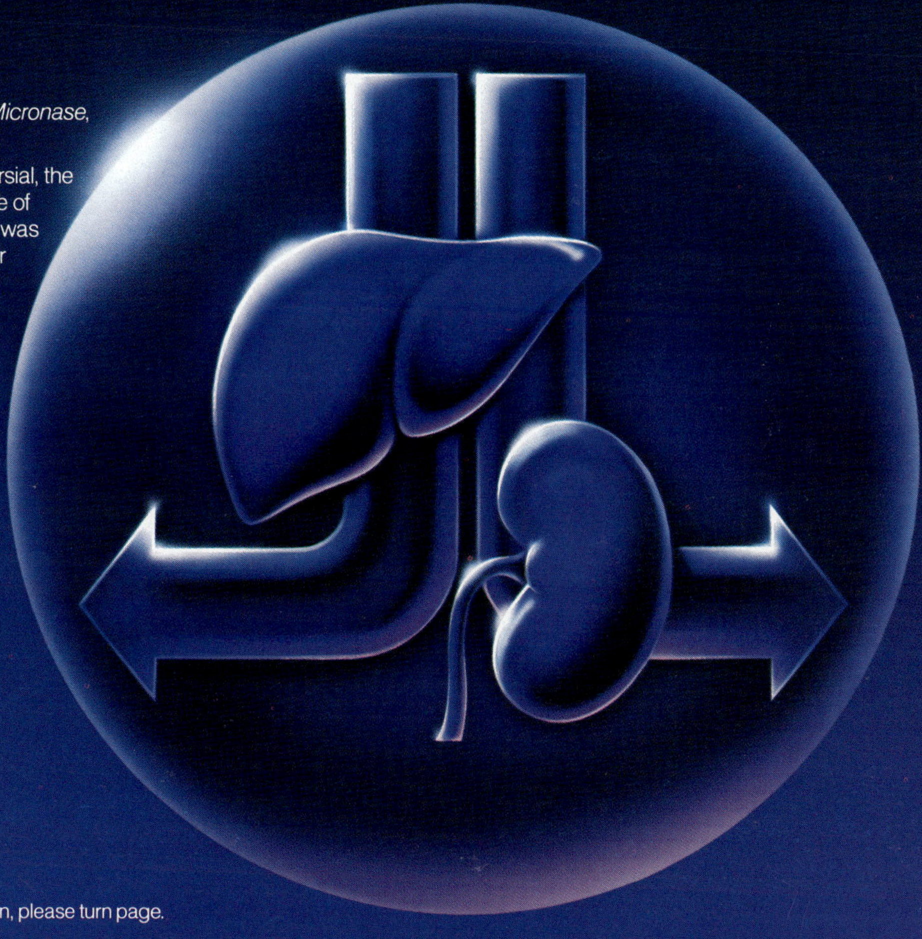

Additional considerations

Overdosage of sulfonylureas, including *Micronase*, can cause hypoglycemia.

Although the interpretations are controversial, the UGDP study reported in 1970 that the use of tolbutamide, an oral hypoglycemic drug, was associated with increased cardiovascular mortality.

References:

1.
Kolterman OG, Prince MJ, Olefsky JM: Insulin resistance in noninsulin-dependent diabetes mellitus: Impact of sulfonylurea agents in vivo and in vitro. *Am J Med* 1983; 74(A):82-101.

2.
Moses AM, Howanitz J, Miller M: Diuretic action of three sulfonylurea drugs. *Ann Intern Med* 1973; 78:541-544.

Upjohn The Upjohn Company
Kalamazoo, MI 49001

For a brief summary of prescribing information, please turn page.

News *Continued from page 11*

can gain certain tax advantages related to the development costs and income.

The injectable drug is supplied in 300-mg vials that cost hospitals $24.95 each. A 24-hour hotline has been established to answer inquiries from health-care practitioners about the product; the number is 312-34-LYPHO.

Ceforanide approved for twice-daily dosing

Ceforanide (Precef, Bristol Laboratories), a recently approved second-generation cephalosporin, is the latest entry into the surgical prophylaxis market. This drug, with a half-life of about three hours, is approved for b.i.d. dosing, meaning that a single dose can provide protection during most surgical procedures.

The antibiotic is active against many of the gram-positive and gram-negative organisms that cefamandole, cefuroxime, and cefonicid are, but it does not have particularly good activity against *Haemophilus influenzae* or *Staphylococcus aureus* in comparison with these other agents. It also does not cover the gram-negative organisms controlled by most third-generation agents.[1]

The approved labeling includes indications for treatment of a variety of infections and for perioperative prophylaxis. The drug's side effects are similar to those of other cephalosporins, and the usual dose is 0.5–1.0 g b.i.d.

Bristol has priced Precef at $9.95 per gram. It is available in 500-mg and 1-g vials and in 500-mg and 1-g StrapKap piggyback containers.

1. Anon. Ceforanide (Precef). *Med Lett Drugs Ther.* 1984; 26:91–2.

NIH panel recommends decreased use of frozen plasma

A consensus development panel, meeting September 24–26 at the National Institutes of Health in Bethesda, MD, recommended that the use of fresh frozen plasma be reduced because of the risks of hypersensitivity and of acquiring disease. The panel said that the risks often outweigh the benefits of use of the product and that alternative techniques can provide safer and more effective therapy.

The panel said there was no justification for use of fresh frozen plasma as a volume expander. It concluded

> [Fresh frozen plasma] is indicated for some documented coagulation protein deficiencies as well as for selected patients who require massive transfusions. It is indicated for patients with multiple coagulation defects as in liver disease, in conjunction with therapeutic plasma exchange for thrombotic thrombocytopenic purpura, for infants with protein-losing enteropathy, and for selected patients with other immune deficiencies. Its use in most other cases should be discouraged.

Among suggested alternatives were autologous dona-

Continued on page 18

1 One-dose protection that lasts longer than the surgery*

12-hour protection eliminates the need for intraoperative dosing

Precef should usually be administered 1 hour before the operation to achieve an effective concentration in the wound tissues

1 One-dose protection against the most common surgical pathogens

Excellent coverage of both gram-negative and gram-positive pathogens*

Well tolerated IM or IV

- Excellent safety record, less than 2% incidence of adverse reactions in 1,534 patients treated with Precef†
- No cases of drug-related pseudomembranous colitis have been reported; however, this condition has been reported with the use of other cephalosporins and other broad-spectrum antibiotics, and its occurrence should be borne in mind

1 One-dose economy

Lower drug acquisition costs than with multi-dose regimens

Lower costs for infusion sets and diluents

1 One-dose simplicity

Simplest possible dosage for most general surgical prophylactic procedures – one gram, one dose – which means fewer IVs

Gives you more control; eliminates potential problems with follow-up doses and helps prevent inappropriate use

Reduces chance of administration errors

*Against possible infections due to susceptible pathogens.
†Refer to Official Package Circular for complete information on side effects.

full prescribing information.

News *Continued from page 14*

tion (patients' own blood) before elective surgery, infusion of shed blood, and the use of specific plasma fractions (e.g., albumin or plasma protein). The panel noted the risks of viral hepatitis and acquired immunodeficiency syndrome in discouraging use of frozen plasma.

Wyeth's triphasic oral contraceptive marketed

The third of the triphasic oral contraceptive products was approved on November 1 by the Food and Drug Administration. Wyeth's Triphasil joins Ortho's Ortho-Novum 7/7/7 and Syntex's Tri-Norinyl, which were approved last April. All three products were discussed in the September–October *CP* article by Smith and Youngkin,[1] and this approach to contraception is the subject of a letter in this issue.[2]

Triphasil combines estrogen and progestogen in the following respective ratios: 30 μg and 50 μg during days 1–6; 40 μg and 75 μg during days 7–11; and 30 μg and 125 μg during days 12–21. This is the only triphasic product that varies the estrogen content; the others vary only the progestogen content over the 21-day cycle. Triphasil is begun on the first day of menstruation rather than on a Sunday, as the other products are.

The drug is priced to pharmacies at $29.64 for three one-month compacts and $58.08 for a six-month supply.

1. Smith MA, Youngkin EQ. Current perspectives on combination oral contraceptives. *Clin Pharm.* 1984; 3:485–96.
2. Miller LG. Update on the new triphasic oral contraceptives. *Clin Pharm.* 1985; 4:24. Letter.

News Briefs

• Marketing of Merck Sharp & Dohme's investigational agent **imipenem-cilastatin** has been delayed in West Germany because of concern over potential neurologic toxicities and deaths similar to those reported in the September–October issue of *CP* (page 536). The drug has a wide spectrum of antibacterial activity, and Merck notes that the drug is often used in gravely ill patients, which makes analyses of circumstances surrounding the toxicities difficult.

• E. R. Squibb has received approval for labeling **captopril** (Capoten) for twice-daily treatment of hypertension; a research study on this dosage of captopril is reported in this issue of *CP* (see page 65).

• **Quinacrine hydrochloride** has been designated an orphan drug by FDA. Principally used in patients with a high risk of recurrent pneumothorax (such as cystic fibrosis patients), quinacrine will be marketed by LyphoMed if FDA approves the product.

• A 23-minute film on **hospital-acquired urinary-tract infections** is available from Norwich–Eaton Pharmaceuticals; "Prevention and Treatment of Nosocomial Infections in the Catheterized Urinary Tract" may be borrowed in 16-mm or Super 8-mm format from Norwich-Eaton Audiovisual Library, 17 Eaton Avenue, Norwich, NY 13815.

Letters

The Letters *column is a forum for rapid exchange of ideas among readers of* CP. *Liberal criteria are applied in the review of submissions to encourage contributions to this column.*

The Letters *column includes the following types of contributions: (1) comments, addenda, and minor updates on previously published work, (2) alerts on potential problems related to drug therapy or clinical research, (3) observations or comments on trends in drug therapy or clinical research, and (4) brief expressions of opinion about controversies in drug therapy or clinical research.*

Letters need not be submitted with the journal's manuscript checklist. The following conditions, however, must be adhered to: (1) the body of the letter must be no longer than two typewritten pages, (2) the use of references, tables, and illustrations should be minimized, (3) the authors' names, affiliations, and mailing addresses must be typed at the end of the letter in the format used by CP, *and (4) the entire letter (including references, tables, and authors' names) must be typed double spaced on plain white paper (not letterhead). Following acceptance of a letter, the authors are required to sign an exclusive publication statement and a copyright-transferral form.*

Severe hypersensitivity secondary to extended carbamazepine administration

Carbamazepine has been used extensively and effectively in the control of both generalized and psychomotor epilepsy with an apparent lack of the behavioral side effects recognized with other anticonvulsants.[1] However, systemic side effects have been described affecting all the body systems; dizziness, nausea, skin reactions, and asthenia are involved in 56% of all reported adverse reactions.[2,3] Skin reactions occur in less than 3% of patients, but only 0.5% of patients with such reactions develop the serious side effects of exfoliative dermatitis or erythroderma.[2] Cases have been reported in both adults[4] and children,[5] and one fatality has been reported.[2] Most effects appear to be caused by drug accumulation, but rarely hypersensitivity reactions occur.[6] We report the case of a child who suffered a previously unreported combination of side effects secondary to carbamazepine.

Case Report. A 12-year-old boy with a history of seizures was seen in the outpatient clinic. Neurologic examination was normal, and an electroencephalogram was reported as compatible with generalized epilepsy. Sodium valproate produced no improvement, so therapy was changed to carbamazepine 200 mg t.i.d. with rapid decrease in seizure occurrence. Three weeks later the child developed an erythematous macular rash, pyrexia, and cough, which was diagnosed as measles. No treatment was given and the rash resolved spontaneously two days later. However, eight days thereafter the child developed suffused conjunctivae and a generalized erythematous macular rash. A drug-sensitivity rash was considered,[2] and the child was treated with chlorpheniramine maleate (Piriton; Allen & Hanburys) 4 mg t.i.d., but the carbamazepine was not stopped. Chlorpheniramine produced no improvement and was discontinued, and the child presented 11 days later with a diffuse, desquamative, erythematous rash affecting his entire body with the exception of his scalp, palms, and soles while still taking carbamazepine. The carbamazepine was stopped and the chlorpheniramine restarted. *Staphylococcus aureus* was cultured from skin and eye swabs, and therapy with Neosporin eye drops (neomycin sulfate, gramicidin, polymyxin B sulfate; Burroughs Wellcome), erythromycin ethyl succinate 500 mg q.i.d. (Abbott Laboratories) orally, and Vioform HC cream (clioquinol and hydrocortisone; Ciba) topically were begun. Over the next two days he developed extensive exfoliative dermatitis, severe arthralgia and joint swelling in his knees and ankles, plus generalized edema. He was then treated with prednisolone 10 mg q.i.d. for 10 days. His blood pressure was normal as was his urinary output, no proteinuria nor diarrhea was noted, serum protein was 53 g/L (normal 68–82 g/L), and serum albumin was 36 g/L (normal 36–52 g/L). The patient's hemoglobin was 13.1 g/dL, and white blood count was 22×10^9/L with a marked neutrophilia (66%) and eosinophilia (7%) but with lymphopenia (6%). Electrolytes and urea were normal, as were the immunoglobulins and viral titers (including measles). Immune complexes were negative, C-reactive protein 53.0 mg/L (normal <5 mg/L) and autoantibodies were negative except for antismooth-muscle protein, which was weakly positive at a dilution of 1 in 10.

The exfoliative dermatitis improved rapidly, and the patient made an uneventful recovery over the next 10 days except for transient conjunctivitis and blurring of vision.[7]

Discussion. Exfoliative dermatitis is a well-recognized albeit rare problem,[2,4,5] but generalized edema and severe, bilateral, symmetrical arthralgia have not previously been reported. Mild facial edema was reported in patients with abnormal lymphocyte function accompanied by generalized lymphadenopathy[6]; this patient, however, appears to have developed an immediate hypersensitivity as evidenced by eosinophilia. No drugs other than carbamazepine and chlorpheniramine had been used, and the introduction of erythromycin did not exacerbate the rash, suggesting that carbamazepine was the most likely causative agent.

It is interesting to speculate whether the initial transient rash represented the preliminary sensitization period to carbamazepine, with the severe reaction resulting from continued use of the drug. There can be little doubt that

Continued on page 23

900 mg q8h

efficacy plus convenience

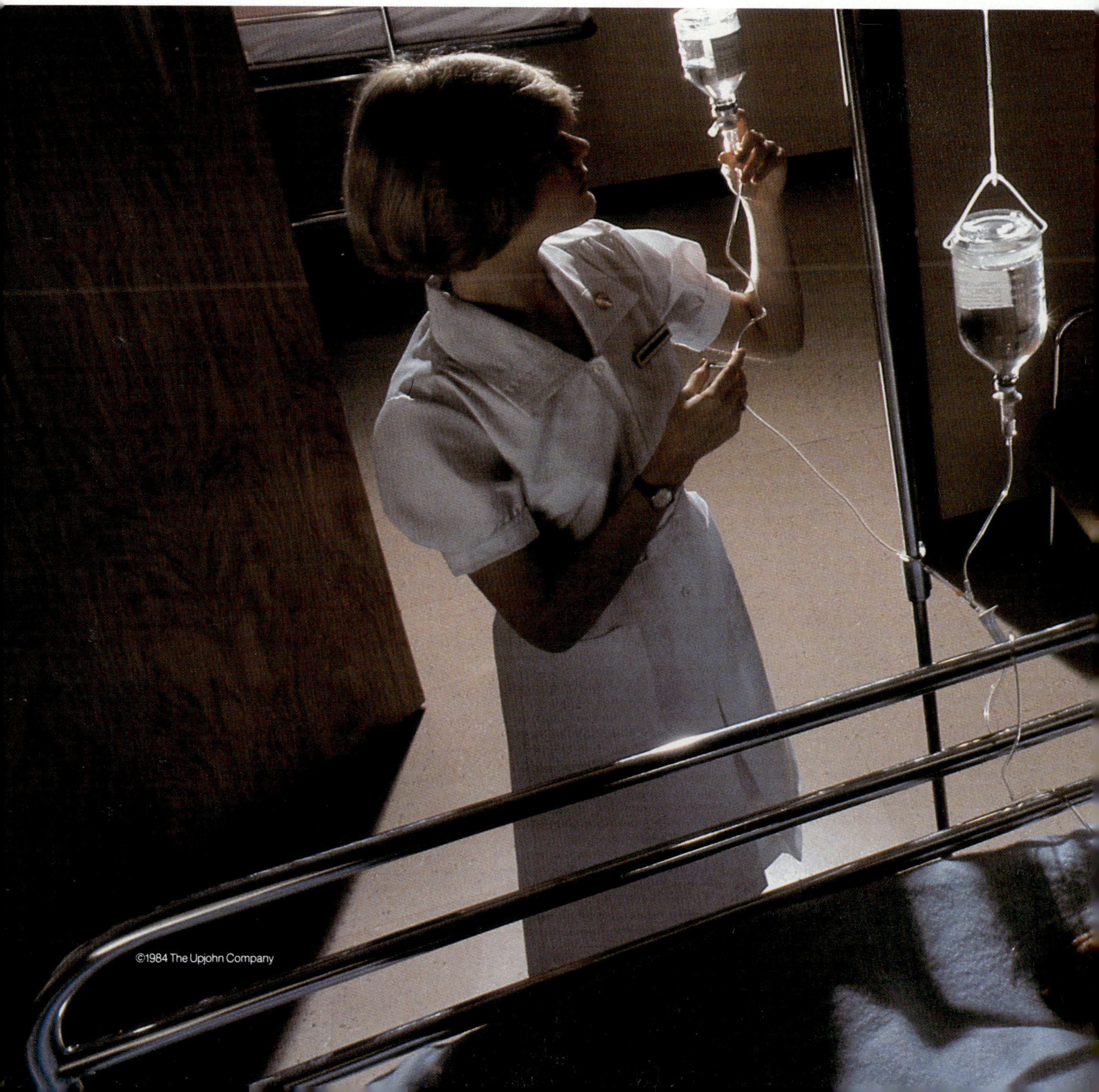

Continued from page 19

this problem would have been minimized had carbamazepine been discontinued after the first rash, but this case illustrates not only the difficulty in differentiating childhood exanthemata from drug-induced skin rashes, but also a therapeutic dilemma. The incidence of mild skin rashes induced by carbamazepine is approximately 3%, but the incidence of severe problems is extremely low; the danger of immediate cessation of an anticonvulsant drug, even if another is substituted, can cause a dangerous increase in seizure frequency.

1. Bacon CJ, Cranager JD, Hierons AM. Behavioral effects of phenobarbital and phenytoin in small children. *Arch Dis Child.* 1981; 56:836–9.
2. Sillanää M. Carbamazepine, pharmacology and clinical uses. 25. Toxic and unwanted effects. *Acta Neural Scand.* 1981; 64(suppl 88):145–63.
3. Steven-Johnson J. Alvarlige bivirkninger ved bruk ar karbamazepin. *T Norske Laegerforen.* 1970; 90:1631–50.
4. Ford GR, Bieder L. Exfoliative dermatitis due to carbamazepine (Tegretol). *NZ Med J.* 1968; 68:386–7.
5. Reed MD, Bertino JS, Blumer JL. Carbamazepine-associated exfoliative dermatitis. *Clin Pharm.* 1982; 1:78–9.
6. Houwerzijl J, DeGast GL, Nater JP et al. Lymphocyte stimulation tests and patch tests in carbamazepine hypersensitivity. *Clin Exp Immunol.* 1977; 29:272–7.
7. Livingston S, Pauli LL, Berman W. Carbamazepine (Tegretol) in epilepsy. *Dis Nerv Syst.* 1974; 35:103–7.

S. J. ROSE, Lecturer in Child Health
University of Aberdeen
Ward 17, Raigmore Hospital
Inverness, Scotland

Origins of aztreonam resistance

Recently Dworzack and colleagues[1] reported a patient who, after exposure to three antibiotics (cefazolin, nafcillin, aztreonam), had a resistant strain of *Enterobacter cloacae.* A sensitive *E. cloacae* had been cultured between the cefazolin therapy and the use of nafcillin–aztreonam. The authors implied that aztreonam may have been responsible for this development of resistance.

I am concerned that this is a nonscientific and anecdotal conclusion. Cultures of cutaneous organisms are not a good way to determine the entire flora present, and the resistant strain of *Enterobacter* may well have been present before the use of aztreonam but not cultured. In addition, since we are all aware that there is no such thing in the real world as a microbial void, only organisms not killed will be left to multiply and hence will assume the role of the dominant flora present in subsequent cultures. After three weeks of "broad" spectrum antibiotic therapy, the isolation of an organism that is relatively resistant to the antibiotics used does not necessarily mean that the organism underwent mutation to *become* resistant. Rather it may well mean the organism was there in the first place. Additionally, the use of cefazolin for perioperative prophylaxis in the patient disallows any conclusion as to the cause, source, or explanation of the secondary culture of a more resistant strain.

1. Dworzack DL, Bartelt MA, Bailey RT Jr et al. Emergence of resistance to aztreonam. *Clin Pharm.* 1984; 3:467, 470. Letter.

B. L. ASHBY, M.D., Associate Medical Director
E.R. Squibb & Sons, Inc.
P.O. Box 4000
Princeton, NJ 08540

We would like to clarify further our observations about aztreonam and the role of inducible β lactamases in causing multiple resistance to the newer β-lactam antibiotics.

A number of new β-lactam antibiotics with expanded spectra of activity have been developed, including the so-called second- and third-generation cephalosporins, the broad-spectrum penicillins, and most recently the monobactams (aztreonam) and the penems. These drugs have in common a relative resistance to hydrolysis by β lactamases, to which they owe in part their expanded spectra of activity.

It has been assumed, until recently, that the sole mechanism for β-lactamase-mediated resistance was the hydrolysis of the β-lactam ring and subsequent inactivation of the antibiotic molecule. However, with the recent release of many of the new enzyme-stable β-lactam agents onto the market, cases have been reported in which multiple β-lactam resistance has developed during or shortly following therapy. In fact, there have already been a greater number of such case reports in association with second- and third-generation cephalosporins than with the older, first-generation cephalosporins.[1–4]

Certain genera (e.g., *Enterobacter*, indole-positive *Proteus, Serratia*, and *Pseudomonas*) characteristically possess inducible β lactamases.[1,2] These organisms, which are frequently initially susceptible to the newer β-lactam antibiotics, may rapidly develop multiple resistance when the gene for the β lactamase is induced. Most β-lactam antibiotics, including the antipseudomonal penicillins, the second- and third-generation cephalosporins, and even the new monobactams, appear to be substrates for these derepressed enzymes and are either hydrolyzed or inactivated by a nonhydrolytic barrier mechanism.[5] Normally, these enzymes are not produced to any great extent, but two mechanisms can lead to induction and subsequent production. One is spontaneous mutation to a stable derepressed state. This mutation occurs at a rate of one in 10^6–10^7 cells.[6] The second mechanism involves the reversible induction of β lactamase by an enzyme inducer[7]; cefoxitin has been clearly demonstrated to be a potent inducer of β lactamases.[5] Other newer β-lactam antibiotics have also been reported to induce production of these enzymes.[8,9]

In order to determine which patients are at risk for developing resistance during therapy to a β-lactam agent, a simple cefoxitin disk-induction test has been designed that will readily detect inducible β lactamases.[2] As we reported, we tested isolate 1 (pretherapy pathogen) for the presence of an inducible β lactamase with the cefoxitin disk-induction test. When isolate 1 was tested by this test, resistance was induced to aztreonam, cefamandole, cefotaxime, and moxalactam, but not to mezlocillin.

Dr. Ashby questions whether isolates 1 and 2, which had the same biochemical profile (API 20E Kit, Analytical Products, Inc., Plainview, NY), were in fact the same isolate of *E. cloacae.* After our original letter was submitted, isolates 1 and 2 were subjected to plasmid analysis by Richard Goering (Department of Medical Microbiology, Creighton University School of Medicine, Omaha, NE) using a modification of the method described by Holmes and Quigley.[10] Lysates of isolates 1 and 2, when analyzed by agarose-gel electrophoresis, possessed identical plasmid profiles. Each isolate contained two distinct plasmids, one with a molecular weight $>10^7$ daltons; the other with a molecular weight <10^7 daltons. These data provide substantial additional evidence that the two isolates represented the same strain, which was present at the onset of aztreonam–nafcillin therapy and subsequently developed resistance to aztreonam as well as to the other β-lactam antibiotics after induction of the β-lactamase enzyme.

We believe it is unlikely that the initial cefazolin therapy contributed to the acquisition of resistance seen in this bacterium. Isolate 1, obtained just before aztreonam–nafcillin therapy (at the conclusion of cefazolin therapy) showed the typical susceptibility pattern of *E. cloacae*. First-generation cephalosporins have rarely been implicated in the development of resistance during therapy, probably because relatively few genera of gram-negative bacilli susceptible to these antibiotics lack β lactamases capable of hydrolyzing them. *Enterobacter* and the other bacteria possessing inducible β lactamases constitutively produce β lactamases active against first-generation cephalosporins and are therefore naturally resistant to these agents.

Although we agree that "cultures of cutaneous organisms are not a good way to determine the entire flora present," the *E. cloacae* isolates in purulent drainage from our patient's surgical wound infection cannot be considered to represent cutaneous flora. The patient clearly demonstrated clinical findings consistent with infection. Cultures of purulent wound drainage are the accepted means of determining the bacterial etiology of such infections and are used for this purpose in clinical practice as well as in investigational antibiotic protocols such as the one followed in this patient's care.

1. Sanders CC, Sanders WE Jr. Emergence of resistance during therapy with the newer β-lactam antibiotics: role of inducible β-lactamases and implications for the future. *Rev Infect Dis.* 1983; 5:639–48.
2. Sanders CC, Sanders WE Jr. Emergence of resistance to cefamandole: possible role of cefoxitin-inducible beta-lactamases. *Antimicrob Agents Chemother.* 1979; 15:792–7.
3. Preheim LC, Penn RG, Sanders CC et al. Emergence of resistance to β-lactam and aminoglycoside antibiotics during moxalactam therapy of *Pseudomonas aeruginosa* infections. *Antimicrob Agents Chemother.* 1982; 22:1037–41.
4. Beckwith DG, Jahre JA. Role of a cefoxitin-inducible β-lactamase in a case of breakthrough bacteremia. *J Clin Microbiol.* 1980; 12:517–20.
5. Sanders CC. Novel resistance selected by the new expanded-spectrum cephalosporins: a concern. *J Infect Dis.* 1983; 147:585–9.
6. Gootz TD, Sanders CC, Goering RV. Resistance to cefamandole: derepression of β-lactamases by cefoxitin and mutation in *Enterobacter cloacae. J Infect Dis.* 1982; 146:34–42.
7. Sanders CC, Sanders WE Jr, Goering RV. In vitro antagonism of beta-lactam antibiotics by cefoxitin. *Antimicrob Agents Chemother.* 1982; 21:968–75.
8. Minami S, Yotsuji A, Inoue M et al. Induction of β-lactamase by various β-lactam antibiotics in *Enterobacter cloacae. Antimicrob Agents Chemother.* 1980; 18:382–5.
9. Sanders CC. Failure to detect resistance in antimicrobial susceptibility tests. *Antimicrob Newsl.* 1984; 1:27–34.
10. Holmes DS, Quigley M. A rapid boiling method for the preparation of bacterial plasmids. *Anal Biochem.* 1981; 114: 193–7.

DAVID L. DWORZACK, M.D., Assistant Professor of Medical Microbiology and Medicine
School of Medicine
Creighton University
Omaha, NE 68131

MARGARET A. BARTELT, PH.D., Director of Microbiology Laboratory
University of Arkansas for Medical Sciences
Little Rock, AR 72205

ROBERT T. BAILEY, JR., PHARM.D., Director of Surgical Research and Development and Assistant Professor of Surgery
Department of Surgery
School of Medicine

ROBERT J. FITZGIBBONS, JR., M.D., F.A.C.S., Assistant Professor of Surgery
Department of Surgery
School of Medicine

JACK W. REICH, M.S., PH.D., Assistant Dean
School of Pharmacy and Allied Health Professions

GEORGE D. PICETTI III, Medical Student
School of Medicine

Creighton University
Omaha, NE 68178

Update on the new triphasic oral contraceptives

In an excellent review of oral contraceptives, Smith and Youngkin[1] mentioned the recently marketed triphasic agents. The triphasic oral contraceptives contain 98.7% less total steroid content than the first oral contraceptive, Enovid (Searle), which became available in the United States in 1960. The amount and severity of side effects have decreased accordingly. Two triphasic products, Tri-Norinyl (Syntex) and Ortho-Novum 7/7/7 (Ortho) differ in their progestin content. Tri-Norinyl has increased progestin content at midcycle to reduce breakthrough bleeding (BTB) at the time it is most frequent.[2] Ortho-Novum 7/7/7 provides increasing progestin gradually in three increments in an effort to more closely mimic the normal ovulation cycle.[3] Both manufacturers chose norethindrone for the progestin as it has been shown to induce fewer metabolic changes than other progestins.[4] A third agent, Wyeth's Triphasil, uses midcycle increases in estrogen dose with progressively larger doses of norgestrel throughout the drug-dosage cycle.

Regardless of which product is used, patients should be counseled on the proper procedure when a dose is missed. When three pills are missed by users of standard (1/50) products, the use of another contraceptive method is recommended. An even smaller margin of error is present with a low-dose product (1/35). For patients on those products, another method of contraception is recommended after missing only two pills.[5]

The triphasic oral contraceptives introduce an even smaller margin of error. Basal concentrations of follicle-stimulating hormone (FSH) and luteinizing hormone (LH) are only partially depressed during the last three days of therapy, producing substantially less inhibition than a standard oral contraceptive dose. Ovulation *is* effectively inhibited, but after missed doses the FSH and LH concentrations recover more quickly.

If a dose has been missed, it is also of the utmost importance to determine at what phase of the patient's cycle. Contrary to popular belief, the time of greatest risk is not at midcycle. Rather, missing a dose immediately before or after the oral contraceptive-free week is the most critical time.[5] During this time, estradiol concentrations increase in a preovulatory state; if this time is extended, the chances for ovulation are increased. During the seven days following a cycle of triphasic therapy, FSH, LH, and estradiol concentrations recover earlier than during standard therapy.[6] Thus the risk is all the more increased in this patient population, and once again, judicious counseling is in order.

This lessened inhibition may be used to advantage in a young woman susceptible to amenorrhea after completion of the 21-day drug cycles (usually those with a history of irregular menstrual cycles). If oral contraception is the only acceptable choice for these patients, then triphasic products should be considered. Because of triphasics' gentle suppression of pituitary-gonadotropin responsiveness, concentrations of endogenous hormones quickly return to normal. Complete pituitary responsiveness can be attained in as few as 10 days.[7] As stated by Upton,[7] "The lesser suppression is sufficient to maintain contraceptive efficacy without the threatened consequence of prolonged post-pill amenorrhea."

As mentioned by Smith and Youngkin,[1] oral contraceptives are not always used for contraception. One such noncontraceptive use is for endometriosis.[5] Unlike standard oral contraceptives, triphasic combinations may not find as much use in this area. As has been noted,[1,7] menstrual bleeding may be increased from that seen with standard oral contraceptives, a reflection of greater endometrial development with the triphasic products. Although the exact etiology of endometriosis is unknown, it is thought that oral contraceptives may be beneficial because of their ability to decrease blood flow, thus decreasing the proposed reflux associated with endometriosis.[5] With the relative increase in flow following triphasic use, this "protection" may be compromised. The patient may be better served by use of another oral contraceptive.

1. Smith MA, Youngkin EQ. Current perspectives on combination oral contraceptives. *Clin Pharm.* 1984; 3:485–96.
2. Syntex (F.P.), Inc. Tri-Norinyl: a new triphasic oral contraceptive. Product Information. Palo Alto, CA; 1984 Apr.
3. Ortho Pharmaceutical Corporation. Ortho-Novum 7/7/7: a triphasic regimen; product information. Raritan, NJ: 1984 Feb.
4. Pasquale SA. Rationale for a triphasic oral contraceptive. *J Reprod Med.* 1984; 29:560–7.
5. Porter CW, Waife RS, Holtrop HR. Oral contraceptives. In: Contraception. New York, NY: Grune and Stratton, Inc.; 1983:21–74.
6. Gaspard UJ, Dubois M, Gillain D et al. Ovarian function is effectively inhibited by a low-dose triphasic oral contraceptive containing ethinyl estradiol and levonorgestrel. *Contraception.* 1984; 29:305–18.
7. Upton GV. The phasic approach to oral contraception: the triphasic concept and its clinical application. *Int J Fertil.* 1983; 28:121–40.

LUCINDA GLANTZ MILLER, PHARM.D., Assistant Director
Turner Drug Information Center
College of Pharmacy
University of Houston
1441 Moursund Street
Houston, TX 77030

Correction

Dietary interaction with phenytoin (March–April 1984, Letters). In the figure on page 110, the axes labels for phenytoin and phenobarbital were reversed for both serum concentrations and daily dosages.

Drug Review

Enalapril, a nonsulfhydryl angiotensin-converting enzyme inhibitor

PETER H. VLASSES, GHASSEM E. LARIJANI, DALE P. CONNER, AND ROGER K. FERGUSON

Abstract: The chemistry, pharmacology, pharmacokinetics, clinical efficacy, adverse effects, and dosage of enalapril maleate, a nonsulfhydryl angiotensin-converting enzyme (ACE) inhibitor, are reviewed.

Enalapril is rapidly converted by ester hydrolysis to enalaprilat, a potent ACE inhibitor; enalapril itself is only a weak ACE inhibitor. Enalapril lowers peripheral vascular resistance without causing an increase in heart rate. In patients with congestive heart failure, enalapril has beneficial hemodynamic effects based on reduction of both cardiac preload and afterload. Approximately 60% of a dose of enalapril is absorbed after oral administration. Excretion of enalaprilat is primarily renal. Accumulation of enalaprilat occurs in patients with creatinine clearances less than 30 mL/min.

Enalapril 10–40 mg per day orally has shown efficacy comparable to that of captopril in treating patients with mild, moderate, and severe hypertension, hypertension caused by renal-artery stenosis, and in congestive heart failure resistant to digitalis and diuretics. When given alone for hypertension, enalapril has efficacy comparable to that of thiazide diuretics and β blockers. Side effects observed with enalapril have generally been minor. Captopril-associated side effects such as skin rash, loss of taste, and proteinuria have been observed in a small number of patients receiving enalapril to date; neutropenia < 300/mm^3 has been noted with captopril but not enalapril. The incidence of these side effects has been noted to be greatly decreased in patients on low doses of captopril.

Enalapril appears to be similar in efficacy to captopril for treating hypertension and congestive heart failure. Whether enalapril is safer than low-dose captopril in patients at high risk for captopril-associated side effects will require further investigation.

Index terms: Dosage; Enalaprilat; Enalapril maleate; Heart failure; Hypertension; Hypotensive agents; Mechanism of action; Metabolism; Pharmacokinetics; Toxicity
Clin Pharm. 1985; 4:27–40

Enalapril (MK-421) is expected to receive Food and Drug Administration approval soon for the treatment of hypertension and congestive heart failure. Enalapril would then become the second agent marketed in a new class of pharmacologic compounds—the angiotensin-converting enzyme (ACE) inhibitors. The first agent, captopril (Capoten, E. R. Squibb & Sons) was marketed in 1980 for use in treatment-resistant hypertension and subsequently received approval in 1981 for use in patients with congestive heart failure responding poorly to digitalis and diuretics.[1] Enalapril will be available as the maleate salt and will be marketed under the trade name Vasotec by Merck Sharp & Dohme.

The purpose of this paper is to review the available information on the clinical pharmacology and therapeutic utility of enalapril in hypertension and congestive heart failure. In addition, the role of ACE inhibitors versus agents in other pharmacologic classes and the similarities and differences between enalapril and captopril will be evaluated to assist practitioners in rational drug selection.

PETER H. VLASSES, PHARM.D., is Associate Director and Associate Professor of Medicine and Pharmacology; GHASSEM E. LARIJANI, PHARM.D., is Fellow in Clinical Pharmacology; DALE P. CONNER, PHARM.D., is Merck Post-Pharm.D. Fellow in Clinical Pharmacology; and ROGER K. FERGUSON, M.D., is Director and Professor of Medicine and Pharmacology, Division of Clinical Pharmacology, Department of Medicine, Jefferson Medical College, Philadelphia, PA.

Address reprint requests to Dr. Vlasses at the Division of Clinical Pharmacology, Department of Medicine, Jefferson Medical College, M-502, 11th and Walnut Streets, Philadelphia, PA 19107.

The assistance of Barbara Leventon in the preparation of this manuscript and of Jerome Feinberg is acknowledged.

This is **article 680-204-8502** in the **ASHP Continuing Education System.** See page 111 for learning objectives and test questions.

Chemistry

The USAN chemical name of enalapril maleate is L-Proline, 1-[*N*-[1-(ethoxycarbonyl)-3-phenylpropyl]-L-alanyl]-, (*S*)-, (*Z*)-2-butenedioate (1:1); its structure is depicted in Figure 1. Enalapril was developed as the result of a careful search for compounds that would inhibit ACE but would be devoid of a sulfhydryl moiety such as that found in captopril (Figure 1). The sulfhydryl moiety has been implicated in some of the side effects of captopril, such as skin rash, loss of taste, proteinuria, and leukopenia.[1] These side effects have also been noted to occur with other sulfhydryl-containing compounds such as D-penicillamine[2] and methimazole.[3]

Although enalapril itself is a weak ACE inhibitor, it is rapidly converted by ester hydrolysis to enalaprilat (MK-422) (Figure 1), a potent ACE inhibitor.[4] Thus, enalapril is considered a prodrug in that its principal biologic activity resides in its metabolite. Administration of enalapril as the maleate salt allows for better oral absorption. The molecular weights of enalapril maleate, the free base, and enalaprilat are approximately 493, 376, and 348, respectively.

The lysine analog of enalapril (lisinopril, MK-521) is currently in clinical trials.[5] Lisinopril is a nonsulfhydryl compound that is well absorbed and does not have to be converted to an active metabolite for biologic activity.

Figure 1. The chemical structures of three angiotensin-converting enzyme inhibitors. Enalapril undergoes esterolysis (-OC_2H_5 → -OH) to become the active form, enalaprilat. Captopril contains a sulfhydryl (-SH) group.

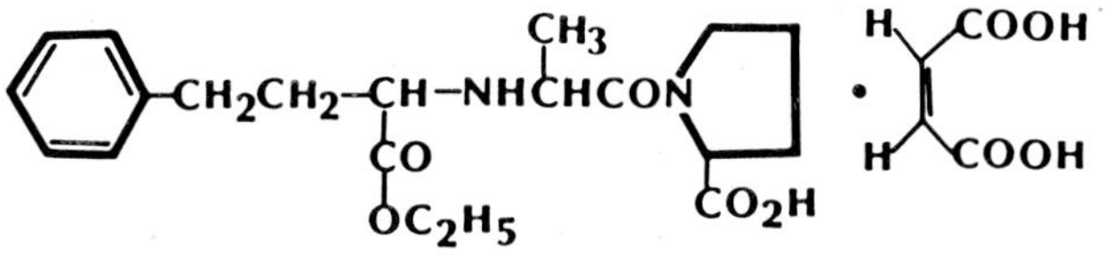

enalapril maleate

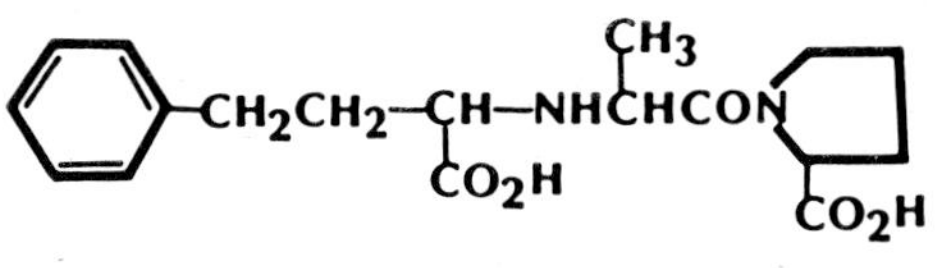

enalaprilat

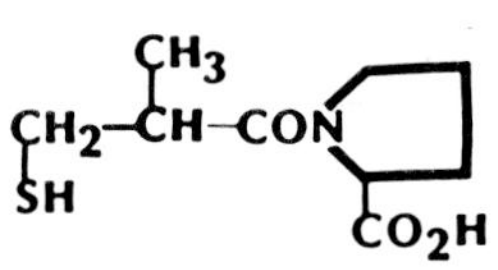

captopril

Pharmacology

There is little doubt that enalaprilat, the active metabolite of enalapril, is a potent ACE inhibitor based on in vitro studies and studies in animals and in man. More controversial, however, is whether ACE inhibition in serum per se is the predominant reason for the therapeutic benefit observed with compounds in this class. Interrelationships between the renin–angiotensin–aldosterone system and other blood pressure control mechanisms involving the sympathetic nervous system, kinins, and prostaglandins may be playing an important role. In addition, pharmacologic actions unrelated to ACE inhibition may be operable. A detailed evaluation of these issues as they relate to captopril has been previously published.[1]

ACE Inhibition. Enalapril and enalaprilat inhibition of hog plasma ACE was studied in vitro. The concentration that inhibited ACE by 50% (I50) was 1.2 nM for enalaprilat, while enalapril had an I50 of 1200 nM in this same model, in which it is poorly de-esterified.[4] In contrast, both enalapril and enalaprilat were potent inhibitors of ACE when administered by the intravenous and oral routes to rats and dogs.[4] In normal volunteers, enalapril in oral doses of 1.25, 2.5, 10, and 20 mg produced dose-related decreases in plasma angiotensin II and aldosterone concentrations and caused increases in plasma renin activity; the latter action was caused by decreased negative feedback by angiotensin II.[6] In this same study, enalapril shifted the angiotensin I dose–systolic blood pressure response curves to the right without altering the angiotensin II response curves. These changes, observed most clearly and comparably after the 10 and 20 mg oral doses, are indicative of ACE inhibition. Enalaprilat was much less active in similar experiments, presumably because of poorer absorption.

The enalaprilat–plasma converting-enzyme complex is stable for months after blood collection and refrigeration.[7] Measurement of serum or plasma ACE activity[8] before and after enalapril administration allows for an objective measure of drug compliance. As with captopril, induction of angiotensin-converting enzyme activity has been reported after enalapril administration in rats,[9,10] dogs,[10] and man.[8,11] The clinical importance of this reported induction is unclear.

Effects in Hypertension. Enalapril lowers blood pressure primarily by decreasing peripheral vascular resistance while, in the absence of congestive heart failure, having little or no effect on cardiac output.[12,13] Heart rate is usually unchanged despite marked falls in arterial pressure,[12,13] though exceptions have been noted.[14] Renal blood flow is maintained or increased,[12,15-17] while glomerular filtration rate generally does not change.[16] Orthostatic hypotension is uncommon.[12,15]

A modest natriuresis has been noted early in

treatment with enalapril.[15,18,19] Plasma volume has been reported to remain the same or increase slightly.[15,20] The baroreceptor reflex is unaffected by enalapril.[20] The antihypertensive effects of enalapril are more pronounced with sodium deprivation[21] and correlate with the height of the pretreatment blood pressure.[13] In one study, regression of left-ventricular hypertrophy was observed without impaired myocardial contractility.[12,22] Enalapril has not been reported to alter plasma lipids. Once a response in blood pressure has been observed, raising the dose from 5 to 40 mg will not usually increase the magnitude of the peak fall in blood pressure but will extend its duration.[23,24]

Effects in Congestive Heart Failure. The beneficial effects of enalapril in congestive heart failure are related to acute and long-term increases in cardiac index and stroke volume and to decreases in pulmonary-capillary wedge, right atrial, and mean arterial pressures and systemic vascular resistance.[25-30] These changes imply decreases in both cardiac preload and afterload. Exercise capacity increases, while heart rate, pulmonary artery pressure, and pulmonary vascular resistance are usually unaffected. Renal and forearm blood flow may increase acutely without a substantial change in hepatic blood flow, suggesting regional blood flow effects.[29] In one study, long-term administration has been associated with systemic venous hypertension in some subjects, requiring increased doses of diuretics[25]; this is contrary to the expected effect, and the mechanism is unclear. Marked drops in blood pressure may occur early in treatment, especially in volume-depleted patients[25]; though occasionally causing symptoms, these drops in blood pressure have usually been well tolerated.

Other Possible Effects. In many studies of enalapril in hypertension and congestive heart failure, the biochemical correlates of ACE inhibition, i.e., decreases in serum ACE activity, serum angiotensin II, and plasma aldosterone concentration, and an increase in plasma renin activity, have been observed.[23,24,31] These changes have not always been found,[21] however, even though enalapril was demonstrating beneficial effects. In some studies, the time course of these humoral effects was not well correlated with that of the beneficial effects. The response to enalapril has been correlated with pretreatment plasma renin activity by some[32,33] but not others,[20,23,24] and enalapril has been reported to be effective in low-renin essential hypertension.[34] It should be noted here, however, that precise, reproducible measurements of angiotension II concentrations and plasma renin activity are difficult and, therefore, subject to interlaboratory variability. In addition, measurement of plasma aldosterone concentrations may not accurately reflect changes in aldosterone secretion.[35] Furthermore, measuring the ability of serum to break down a substrate such as P-(^{3}H)-hippuryl-glycyl-glycine in vitro (i.e., the ACE-inhibiting activity of serum[8]) before and after enalapril may not adequately reflect the inhibitory activity of enalaprilat on angiotension I, the biologic substrate for conversion to angiotensin II. Serum ACE activity may not be reflective of lung or tissue ACE inhibition, where enalapril may be exerting its therapeutic effects.

Nonetheless, the above-noted discrepancies among studies have led investigators to hypothesize additional effects of enalapril beyond those recognized to be associated with inhibition of serum ACE activity.[36] Such effects also seem plausible, since angiotensin II has not been shown to have venoconstrictive effects, yet enalapril has produced substantial effects on preload in patients with congestive heart failure.

Because ACE, also known as kininase II, is involved in the breakdown of bradykinin, a vasodilator, augmented kinin activity has been proposed as a possible mechanism of action of enalapril. Though kinin measurements in plasma or urine are difficult and may not reflect local effects, most studies have not found consistent changes in the kinins that would suggest an important role in the therapeutic effect of enalapril.[31,37] Similarly, alterations in plasma or urinary vasodilatory prostaglandins have been suggested as contributory, but again, studies do not provide adequate biochemical evidence of these effects.[21,38,39] That changes in angiotensin II formation at the local tissue level are not reflected by serum ACE inhibition is a viable theory,[40] but one that is difficult to substantiate in man. Another theory is that decreases in angiotensin II concentrations result in a decrease in sympathetic effects, as angiotensin II is known to augment neurogenic vasoconstriction.[36] In animal studies, high-dose enalapril directly interfered with sympathetic neurotransmission, presumably by inhibiting presynaptic norepinephrine release and postsynaptic alpha$_2$-adrenoceptor action.[41] The importance of these findings to humans is unclear.

Pharmacokinetics

Assay Methods. Enalaprilat concentrations have been measured in serum or urine, either by radioimmunoassay[42] or a fluoroenzymatic method.[43] In the latter method, enalapril concentrations have been estimated by subtraction of the actual measured enalaprilat concentration from the total enalaprilat concentration measured after alkaline or enzymatic hydrolysis of enalapril to enalaprilat in serum or urine. Unlike captopril, enalaprilat is stable in serum under standard sample processing procedures.

Absorption. We compared the serum concentration–time profiles and urinary recovery of enalaprilat in healthy, fasting men after oral doses of 5, 10, 20, and 40 mg of enalapril and after intravenous 5-mg doses of enalapril and enalaprilat, administered on separate occasions.[44] Based on dose-adjusted urinary recovery of total drug (enalapril plus enalaprilat), absorption was estimated at 59–73% with no apparent relationship to dose. These values compare favorably with the 61% absorption reported after a 10-mg dose[45] and the 53–58% absorption we observed in another study after a 40-mg oral dose.[46] After intravenous enalapril maleate, 31–46% of the dose was recovered in the urine as enalaprilat in our study,[44] while a 72–99% recovery was observed after intravenous enalaprilat. Enalaprilat urinary recoveries of 36–44% were noted after oral enalapril. This comparable bioactivation after intravenous and oral dosing suggests that the conversion of enalapril to enalaprilat is primarily a postabsorptive process. First-pass metabolism to enalaprilat was estimated at approximately 18%. Other studies[45,46] have reported comparable urinary enalaprilat recoveries as a percentage of enalapril dose. The 27% fecal recovery of enalaprilat after oral enalapril in one study[45] indicates either esterolysis of unabsorbed enalapril or enterohepatic circulation of enalaprilat, or both. Some day-to-day variability in the absorption of enalapril maleate or its hydrolysis to enalaprilat, or both, has been suggested.[47]

Mean peak serum enalaprilat concentrations in our study[44] after oral doses of 5, 10, 20, and 40 mg of enalapril were 15.3, 37.4, 70.8, and 123.1 ng/mL, respectively. These values occurred between 3.2 and 4.8 hours after dosing and suggest dose proportionality. Peak concentrations of enalapril were near or above these values and occurred within the first hour after dosing. In other studies, Ulm[45] discovered a mean peak enalaprilat concentration of 39 ng/mL after a 10-mg oral dose of enalapril maleate, while Swanson[46] found a value of 154 ng/mL after a 40-mg dose; similar times to reach peak concentrations were observed for enalaprilat.[45,46] In the Swanson study,[46] the area under the serum concentration–time curves for enalaprilat and its urinary recoveries did not differ when 40 mg of enalapril maleate was administered in both the fasting and fed states. Serum concentration–time profiles showed little accumulation of enalaprilat after eight daily doses of enalapril maleate 10 mg in healthy subjects.[47] This finding contrasts with that in patients with renal insufficiency, in whom accumulation of enalaprilat has been observed.[48]

In our initial study in hypertensive patients,[23] mean peak serum concentrations were approximately 28 ng/mL after 5-mg oral doses of enalapril and 50 ng/mL after 10-mg doses; these peak concentrations were somewhat higher than predicted from the cited normal-volunteer experiments.[44–47] Similar findings have been noted in other studies in hypertensive patients.[49] The reasons for this are unclear.

Distribution. We[44,50] and others[45,47] have observed an extended terminal elimination phase for enalaprilat after administration of enalapril. Following intravenous doses of enalaprilat (2.5, 5, and 10 mg) in healthy subjects, all doses produced serum concentration–time curves that converged at the same terminal concentrations.[50] This extended phase is presumably caused by extensive serum binding of enalaprilat to angiotensin converting enzyme. This binding appears to involve a fixed amount of drug, regardless of the dose administered.[50] Enalaprilat exhibits biphasic binding to human plasma.[49] At concentrations less than 8 ng/mL, high-affinity binding predominates, apparently related to attachment of plasma ACE; high-capacity, low-affinity binding to plasma protein occurs at higher concentrations and is approximately 60%. Studies in dogs suggest that neither enalapril nor enalaprilat effectively crosses the blood–brain barrier.[49]

Metabolism. As noted previously, enalapril is primarily converted to enalaprilat by ester hydrolysis (Figure 1). Based on the mass-balance study of Ulm,[45] 94% of an administered 10-mg oral dose was accounted for as enalapril or enalaprilat in urine and feces suggesting little, if any, additional metabolism. The major site of bioactivation appears to be the liver; human plasma was devoid of esterolytic activity while human liver homogenates did have such activity.[51] After intravenous enalapril maleate, serum enalaprilat concentrations were observed within 15 minutes but did not peak until two to six hours after a dose.[44]

Pang and co-workers[52] evaluated enalapril metabolism in a perfused rat-liver preparation. Enalapril had a high extraction ratio (~0.86), while enalaprilat had a low value (~0.05). These authors suggested that a diffusion barrier exists for enalaprilat penetration into the hepatocyte, and therefore, hepatic elimination of enalaprilat was a function of enalapril hepatocyte uptake. Enalaprilat in bile accounted for 18% of the dose.

Elimination. Ulm et al.[45] reported a 61% urinary recovery (18% as enalapril and 43% as enalaprilat) and a 33% fecal recovery (6% as enalapril and 27% as enalaprilat) after administration of a 10-mg oral dose in healthy subjects. The mean renal clearance of enalaprilat was 158 mL/min with a range of 97 to 256 mL/min. This suggests that tubular secretion may contribute to the renal elimination of this diacid metabolite.

The terminal phase half-life of enalaprilat elimination has been estimated to be 35 hours.[45] Another group of investigators have reported mean half-lives of enalapril and enalaprilat to be 1.3 and 5.9 hours, respectively.[53] However, the meaning of these enalaprilat half-life values, which do or do not take into account the tight binding of a small quantity of the metabolite to serum ACE, is of dubious value in predicting the achievement of steady-state conditions. Based on an evaluation of the urine data of repeated single oral doses of enalapril maleate in healthy men, Till and co-workers[47] have reported an effective accumulation half-life for enalaprilat of approximately 11 hours.

Correlation Between Serum Concentration and Effect. In vitro, Swanson et al.[8] noted dose-response curves generated by adding enalaprilat to serum to have an I50 for ACE of 3 n*M* to 6 n*M* with 10 to 15% of the initial activity being nonsuppressible. Subsequently, dose-response curves for serum samples collected following single doses of enalapril in hypertensive patients in the same assay for ACE activity were similar in shape to the in vitro curves and revealed an I50 of approximately 6×10^{-9} *M*.[8] Biollaz and co-workers[54] reported that serum concentrations of enalaprilat in normal volunteers closely correlated with both percentage inhibition of plasma ACE activity and the ratio of plasma angiotensin II to angiotensin I (a measure of ACE blockade).

We demonstrated that a mean enalaprilat concentration of approximately 10 ng/mL is associated with near-maximal achievable suppression of ACE activity.[23] After long-term enalapril administration, we observed a small decrease in inhibitory potency of similar serum concentrations of enalaprilat,[8] a finding compatible with previous reports of ACE induction.[9–11]

Nonetheless, though these associations have been observed, the hemodynamic effects of enalapril in hypertension and congestive heart failure are only poorly associated with serum concentrations of enalaprilat. Though the onset of action and maximal hemodynamic effect correlate well with the appearance of enalaprilat in serum and with peak serum concentrations of enalaprilat, respectively, the magnitude of the long-term hemodynamic response is not predicted by the trough serum concentration.[23,49] This may reflect the activation of other homeostatic blood pressure control mechanisms, the importance of antihypertensive effects unrelated to serum concentration, or other unknown factors.

Influence of Disease States. Enalaprilat accumulates in renal disease. Saris and co-workers[55] found that after a single 10-mg dose of enalapril maleate in 29 patients with varying degrees of renal insufficiency, impairment of renal function resulted in elevated serum concentrations of enalaprilat and a decreased urinary recovery of enalapril and enalaprilat. Kelley and co-workers[56] made similar observations after a single dose of enalapril. We administered 5 mg of enalapril maleate once daily for 12 days in 23 hypertensive patients with varying degrees of renal insufficiency and noted accumulation as a function of the degree of renal impairment. Though blood pressure response was somewhat better in the group with the worst renal function and the highest serum concentrations of enalaprilat, this improved response was not believed to be related to the high serum concentrations as these patients also had the highest aldosterone concentrations before enalapril.[48] Enalaprilat is hemodialyzable.[48,55]

No data are currently available regarding the effects of liver disease or congestive heart failure on the disposition of enalapril maleate. We are currently evaluating enalapril disposition in patients with cirrhosis.

Clinical Use and Efficacy

Hypertension. The details of selected studies of the antihypertensive effects of enalapril maleate are listed in Table 1. In addition, Davies et al.[57] have recently reviewed previously unpublished results of large-scale (Phase III) clinical trials of enalapril. In general, the hypertension studies in Table 1 range from open, uncontrolled trials to well-designed experiments with placebo and positive controls. Though the report of Davies provides large quantities of interesting data, most of the information to date has not been published in peer-reviewed journals and must be evaluated in this context. Nonetheless, based on a review of this published information and our own experience with enalapril, we will discuss the clinical utility of enalapril in hypertension. Selected well-designed studies will be highlighted.

Mild to Moderate Hypertension. In a randomized, double-blind, parallel-group study in 100 patients with mild to moderate hypertension, Sassano et al.[58] compared enalapril 20 mg once daily with placebo. After 15 days of treatment, enalapril induced a significant reduction in mean systolic (161 to 145 mm Hg, $p < 0.001$) and diastolic (103 to 93 mm Hg, $p < 0.001$) blood pressure; the magnitude of the fall in blood pressure was similar after 30 days of treatment. Overall, 57% of patients treated with enalapril achieved a diastolic pressure below 90 mm Hg. Davies et al.[57] report similar findings in another study in which enalapril reduced blood pressure to a greater extent than placebo when administered either once or twice daily in total doses up to 40 mg. Blood pressures of 85 mm Hg or less or a decrease of greater than 10 mm Hg in pressure were observed in 13% of the placebo group, 61% of the twice-daily enalapril group, and 54% of the once-daily group.

In general, the effects of enalapril alone have proven to be comparable to those of hydrochlorothiazide,[57–59] propranolol,[57,60] and metoprolol.[57] When used as monotherapy, any of these agents controls the blood pressure of between 40 and 70% of treated patients. Alone, enalapril has been reported to be somewhat less effective in blacks than in whites and in the old versus the young.[57,61] These findings may be related to the propensity for these groups to have low-renin hypertension.

For a group of patients, the response to the first dose of enalapril alone is usually predictive of the long-term response. However, within the group, a small number of patients with large initial falls in blood pressure will demonstrate an attenuated response with continued treatment.[23] In such cases, greater attention to sodium restriction is suggested. Likewise, a smaller number of patients with modest initial falls in blood pressure will manifest a greater fall with continued administration. A comparison of serum angiotensin-converting enzyme activity before and after enalapril[8] offers an objective measure of patient compliance.[23,24]

The combination of enalapril and hydrochlorothiazide is rational for several reasons. Effective blood pressure control can be increased markedly in comparison to the results achieved with either agent alone. This was especially true in a study we undertook in a group of predominantly black patients who had exhibited some resistance to diuretics alone (Table 1).[62] Secondary increases in aldosterone contribute to the resistance of some patients to diuretics and to the propensity to develop hypokalemia. Combination therapy with enalapril reduces this mechanism for resistance and tends to attenuate diuretic-induced hypokalemia.[62] The order of addition for this combination affects the acute response, i.e., enalapril added to hydrochlorothiazide is more likely to result in sharp, symptomatic falls in blood pressure than vice versa or simultaneous combination of these agents in moderate hypertension.[63] This may reflect the renin dependence of the blood pressure in diuretic-treated patients.

Moderate to Severe Hypertension. The published experience with enalapril in moderate to severe hypertension is more limited. In a randomized, double-blind, parallel-treatment trial in 24 patients with moderate to severe hypertension, Fernandez and co-workers[64] compared enalapril 10–40 mg per day, plus hydrochlorothiazide and methyldopa if needed, with standard titration of triple therapy, i.e., a diuretic, propranolol, and hydralazine (Table 1). Blood pressure control was achieved with enalapril alone in nine patients, in two more with double therapy, and in one patient on triple therapy. In the other group, only one patient received monotherapy, nine patients required double therapy, and two patients received triple therapy. Heart rate was significantly decreased only in the latter group, and side effects were more frequent in this group.

One group has reported encouraging results using intravenous boluses of enalaprilat in seven patients with hypertensive emergencies.[65] However, experience with enalapril in this setting is limited. In-

Table 1.
Clinical Studies of Enalapril in Patients with Hypertension (*table spreads across two pages*)

Study	Study Design	No. Patients/ Treatment Group[a]	Daily Drug Dose[a] (mg)	Length of Therapy (wk)
Mild to Moderate Essential Hypertension				
Ferguson et al.[23]	Open	10	E 5–20	12
deLeeuw et al.[15]	Open	6	E 5–40	12
Dunn et al.[12]	Open	8	E 5–40	12
Wilkins et al.[34]	Randomized, double-blind, placebo controlled, parallel group	Placebo ($n = 7$) E b.i.d. ($n = 8$) E q.d. ($n = 8$)	E 10–40	12
Sassano et al.[58]	Randomized, double-blind, placebo controlled, parallel group	Placebo ($n = 47$) E ($n = 53$)	E 20	4
Enalapril Hypertension group[92]	Randomized, double-blind, propranolol comparison, parallel group	E ($n = 28$) Pr ($n = 26$)	E 10–40 Pr 80–240	12
Vlasses et al.[62]	Single-blind, consecutive treatment	14	E 40 HCTZ 50 E 40 mg + HCTZ 50 mg	2
Moderate to Severe Essential Hypertension				
Fernandez et al.[64]	Randomized, double-blind, parallel treatment group	Group I ($n = 12$)	E 10–40 HCTZ 0–50 MD 0–500	26
		Group II ($n = 12$)	HCTZ 50 Pr 0–240 HZ 0–100	
Hypertension Secondary to Renal Artery Stenosis				
Hodsman et al.[66]	Open	Group I ($n = 10$)	E 10–40	12
		Group II ($n = 10$)	E 10–40 plus other antihypertensive agents	

[a] E = enalapril, Pr = propranolol, HCTZ = hydrochlorothiazide, MD = methyldopa, HZ = hydralazine.
[b] Not reported.
[c] Significantly different ($p < 0.05$) from control(s).

travenous enalaprilat is still an investigational preparation; it will not be marketed at the same time as the oral preparation.

Secondary Forms of Hypertension. Enalapril has been found to be of value in the hypertension associated with renal artery stenosis.[32,66] However, patients with bilateral disease or vascular disease in a solitary kidney may be at risk for renal failure secondary to ACE inhibition (see Adverse Effects). Smith et al.[67] found enalapril useful in captopril-intolerant patients with hypertensive crisis in systemic sclerosis.[67] Isolated reports have suggested usefulness in idiopathic hyperaldosteronism.[68] To our knowledge, enalapril has not been used to date in patients with eclampsia.

Congestive Heart Failure. Table 2 summarizes selected studies of enalapril in congestive heart failure. All of these studies evaluated enalapril as add-on therapy in patients in New York Heart Association Classes II–IV receiving digitalis and diuretics. Overall, enalapril has been effective in both acute and long-term use.

In a randomized, double-blind, parallel-group study, Sharpe and co-workers[69] compared enalapril 5 mg b.i.d. with placebo for three months (Table 2). Enalapril produced objective and symptomatic improvement. Beneficial changes included decreases in systemic vascular resistance and pulmonary capillary wedge pressure, increases in cardiac index and exercise time, and improvement in New York Heart Association Class. In contrast, Dunkman et al.[30] noted somewhat less impressive results in eight patients. The response to enalapril appears to be more dramatic as the degree of heart failure increases, perhaps reflecting the activation of the renin–angiotensin system known to accompany a low cardiac output. The dosage of diuretics should be monitored carefully when enalapril is instituted. Though dosage reductions have been successfully undertaken in some studies, the development of systemic venous hypertension necessitated increases in diuretic dosage in some patients.[25]

Use in Pregnancy and Lactation

There is no experience to date with enalapril in pregnant or breast-feeding women. There was no fetotoxicity in rats treated with up to 200 mg/kg/day

Mean Blood Pressure Response (mm Hg)		% Patients Achieving Diastolic Blood Pressure ≤90 mm Hg	Side Effects	Comments
Systolic	Diastolic			
−14	−8	20	. . .[b]	Five patients received HCTZ 50 mg/day
−28[c]	−15[c]	67	. . .	
−28[c]	−17[c]	100	. . .	Three patients received HCTZ
. . .	+2	15	. . .	All patients had low-renin hypertension; no significant difference between q.d. and b.i.d. blood pressure changes
	−6	62		
	−12[c]	38		
−2	−4	. . .		
−17[c]	−12[c]	57	Increased liver function tests in one patient	
−31[c]	−20[c]	61	29% (mild)	E reduced blood pressure significantly more than Pr ($p < 0.001$)
−20[c]	−12[c]	50	42% (mild)	
. . .	−3	14	. . .	Blood pressure change after E versus after HCTZ alone not significantly different
	−4	7		
	−19[c]	79		
−16[c]	−17[c]	100	0	Nine patients in group I received E alone; 11 patients in group II received more than one drug
−20[c]	−17[c]	100	66%	
−22[c]	−25[c]	100	Two patients needed β blocker therapy for tachycardia; Raynaud's phenomenon developed de novo in one patient and became more severe in another patient with pre-existing disease	Group II had more severe hypertension and worse renal function
−28[c]	−21[c]	100		

Table 2.
Clinical Studies of Enalapril in Patients with Congestive Heart Failure

Study	Study Design	Patient Population	Enalapril Regimen	Mean Drug-Induced Change in Hemodynamic Indicators and Exercise Tolerance[a]						Side Effects	Comments
				HR	MAP	PCWP	CI	SVR	ETT		
Levine et al.[29]	Open	*n* = 7, NYHA[b] III–IV	5–20 mg/day for four weeks	NS[c]	−72%	NS	+19%	NS	NS	. . .[d]	72% of patients had symptomatic improvement
Cody et al.[27]	Open	*n* = 7, NYHA III–IV	10–50 mg/day for four weeks	NS	−10%	NS	+18%	−21%	+182%	. . .	86% improved by one to two NYHA classes
Dunkman et al.[30]	Open	*n* = 8, NYHA II–IV	20–40 mg/day for four weeks	NS	−9%	NS	NS	−17%	+23%	Mild orthostatic hypotension in one patient	25% improved by one NYHA class
Dickstein et al.[93]	Open	*n* = 12, NYHA III–IV	10 mg/day for 12 weeks	NS	NS	−22%	NS	NS	. . .	. . .	All patients had symptomatic improvement; 92% improved by at least one NYHA class
Sharpe et al.[69]	Randomized, double-blind, placebo controlled, parallel group	Enalapril (*n* = 18), placebo (*n* = 18), NYHA II–III	10 mg/day or placebo for 12 weeks	NS	NS	−44%	+27%	−23%	+89%	Skin rash or itch in three patients	All patients had symptomatic improvement; 89% improved by one NYHA class

[a] HR = heart rate, MAP = mean arterial pressure, PCWP = pulmonary-capillary wedge pressure, CI = cardiac index, SVR = systemic vascular resistance, ETT = exercise tolerance time.
[b] New York Heart Association classification; all patients were receiving digitalis and diuretics.
[c] Not significant ($p > 0.05$).
[d] Not reported.

of enalapril, but maternal and fetal toxicity occurred in rabbits treated with 1 mg/kg/day or more.[49] No teratogenicity was observed in rats or rabbits.[49]

Use in Pediatrics

There is no published experience with enalapril in children. We are currently collaborating with another group in such a study, including an assessment of the pharmacokinetics.

Adverse Effects

Enalapril use in over 2000 patients was well tolerated based on data presented as part of its FDA submission.[57] We have treated approximately 75 patients with enalapril in various studies for periods of up to several months and have observed only minor side effects.

As noted previously, hypotension, sometimes symptomatic, may occur three to four hours after initial dosing when enalapril is administered to sodium-deprived or overdiuresed patients.[25,62,63] Placing the patient in Trendelenburg position (legs higher than head) is usually all that is necessary to reverse this, with intravenous 0.9% sodium chloride injection used when the hypotension is excessive or prolonged. Skin rash has been noted in 1.2% of cases with discontinuation required in 0.3%.[57] This incidence of rash was approximately twice that observed in the placebo group but comparable to that of other antihypertensive drugs employed as controls in these trials. Taste disturbances were similar to those noted with the control drugs and did not require drug discontinuation. We described one patient who experienced a burning sensation (hyperesthesia) of the mouth during enalapril treatment that dissipated on dechallenge and reappeared on rechallenge.[70] White blood cell counts were found to be between 1000 and 2500/mm^3 in four patients without a clear relationship to enalapril being established.[57] No cases of neutropenia or agranulocytosis have been encountered with enalapril based on the captopril package insert criterion (less than 300 neutrophils/mm^3).

Mild and reversible increases in serum creatinine were reported in 0.6% of enalapril-treated patients versus 0.26% of patients on control drugs.[57] Azotemia was encountered in eight patients with bilateral renovascular hypertension, six of whom were also receiving diuretics.[57] As noted, this complication may occur with inhibition of angiotensin converting enzyme in approximately 25% of these patients and in those with vascular disease of a solitary kidney.[71,72] The proposed mechanism for the deterioration in renal function in these patients is selective glomerular efferent-arteriolar dilatation resulting in interference with the autoregulatory capacity of the kidney.[72] The incidence of proteinuria with enalapril (0.66%) was comparable to that of control drug therapy (0.53%). No cases of nephrotic syndrome or membranous glomerulonephritis have been reported with enalapril. One case of renal glycosuria and azotemia has been reported.[73]

Other miscellaneous side effects include hyperkalemia and eosinophilia.[74] Rebound hypertension or withdrawal reactions have not been observed. Reactions of unestablished relationship to enalapril observed during clinical trials include myocardial infarction, transient ischemic attacks, and dystonia.[49] Waeber and co-workers[75] described a 46-year-old woman who attempted suicide by ingesting 300 mg of enalapril and 225 mg of oxazepam. Her serum enalaprilat concentration on admission was 1450 ng/mL. She responded to supportive therapy and fluids to correct her hypotension.

Drug Interactions

Enalapril should be used with caution in patients receiving potassium-sparing diuretics or potassium supplementation especially if they have decreased renal function, because these patients have an increased risk of developing hyperkalemia. Enalapril may have pharmacodynamic interactions with other drugs that affect blood pressure, e.g., antihypertensive drugs, nitrates, and anesthetic agents. Other than these additive effects on blood pressure, there are no known contraindications to using enalapril with other antihypertensive drugs.

Dosage

In most trials, enalapril maleate was administered in daily doses of 5 to 40 mg administered either once or twice daily. The usual starting dose in patients with good renal function is 10 mg. Once a response is observed, increasing the dose of enalapril will infrequently lower blood pressure further, though it will extend the duration of the drug's antihypertensive effect.[23,24] Because enalaprilat accumulates in patients with renal disease, a reduced initial dosage of enalapril maleate (5 mg once daily) is recommended in patients with creatinine clearances less than 30 mL/min.[48,49] Hemodialysis patients may be given the usual dose of enalapril maleate on dialysis days.[48,49]

Cost and Availability

Enalapril will be available as 5 mg (white), 10 mg (red), 20 mg (peach), and 40 mg (yellow) barrel-shaped tablets coded as MSD 712 to 715, respectively. No cost figures are currently available.

Instructions to Patients

When counseling patients about to be treated with enalapril, pharmacists should discuss the patient's dietary habits. Excessive sodium restriction (<50 meq/day) could predispose to hypotension when enalapril is initially administered; excess sodium consumption (>200 meq/day) may counteract the antihypertensive effects of enalapril. Excessive potassium consumption, including occult use of potassium-containing salt substitutes, could predispose to hyperkalemia, especially in patients with compromised renal function. Patients may take enalapril before or with meals,[46] presumably without an alteration in its antihypertensive efficacy. Patients should be counseled that excessive fluid loss from prolonged episodes of diarrhea may lead to volume depletion and possibly predispose to enalapril-induced hypotension; holding the dosage may be indicated until the patient's baseline state is regained. Because enalapril is a relatively new medication, patients should be encouraged to report how they are feeling and the occurrence of any adverse effects. Likewise, concomitant medications should be reviewed for the possible occurrence of previously undescribed drug interactions. Enalapril tablets should be differentiated from other medications that the patient may be taking.

FDA-Labeled Indications

Enalapril is expected to be approved by the FDA for the treatment of essential and renovascular hypertension of all degrees of severity and for the management of congestive heart failure. Whether both indications will be approved at the time of initial marketing of enalapril is unknown. Initially, it will only be marketed in the oral form.

Overall Comparison of Enalapril and Captopril

Comparative Efficacy of Enalapril and Captopril. Captopril was initially approved by the FDA only for use in treatment-resistant hypertension because of concerns regarding the incidence of skin rash, taste loss, leukopenia, and proteinuria associated with its use. As data were analyzed, it became apparent that these side effects were dose related and more common in patients with renal failure and autoimmune disease.[1] Results of a recent, large-scale Veterans Administration cooperative trial in patients with mild to moderate hypertension receiving low doses of captopril (e.g., 37.5 mg b.i.d.) revealed that captopril's antihypertensive effects were comparable to those of hydrochlorothiazide.[76] Combination therapy with hydrochlorothiazide resulted in further blood pressure reductions. No leukopenia or frank proteinuria was observed. Skin rash and taste disturbances were observed but in a much lower incidence than previously reported. Primarily on the basis of this data, FDA is considering approving the use of captopril in mild to moderate essential hypertension.

Enalapril and captopril appear very similar in antihypertensive action. In one large-scale study of patients with supine diastolic blood pressures of 100 to 120 mm Hg while receiving hydrochlorothiazide 50 mg/day, enalapril 10–40 mg/day in two divided doses produced similar antihypertensive effects as captopril 75–300 mg/day in three divided doses.[57] We have compared enalapril 20 mg b.i.d. with captopril 200 mg b.i.d. in a double-blind, parallel-group study in 20 patients with mild to moderate hypertension.[77] These agents demonstrated comparable antihypertensive effects, both alone and in combination with hydrochlorothiazide. Of note, we coadministered captopril and enalapril and observed no further reduction in blood pressure than that produced by either agent alone. This would suggest that these agents, at effective doses, are reducing blood pressure by similar mechanisms. Responses to these two agents in congestive heart failure appear similar, though comparative trials are lacking.

Comparative Efficacy of Enalapril and Captopril versus Other Antihypertensive Agents. Recent concerns about the arrhythmogenic potential and lipid-elevating effects of diuretics in some patients,[78] as well as the varied side effects and contraindications of other antihypertensive agents such as the β blockers, make angiotensin-converting enzyme inhibitors attractive alternatives. In this regard, enalapril and captopril lack CNS side effects, do not alter sexual function, are not associated with rebound hypertension, and can be used safely in patients with diabetes, asthma, peripheral vascular disease, congestive heart failure, and psychiatric disorders. These properties make them an attractive alternative for first-line therapy. Many of these properties are shared by the calcium-channel blocking agents, which are also being heavily promoted as antihypertensive agents.[79] An important difference between ACE inhibitors and calcium-channel blockers is the clearer therapeutic advantages of the former in patients with concomitant congestive heart failure. However, the information on these new agents must be counterbalanced to some degree by the extensive clinical experience with thiazide diuretics and β blockers. The 1984 Joint National Committee report on hypertension provides suggestions for rational use of these agents.[80]

As second-line agents to diuretics, ACE inhibitors may help in conserving potassium, a matter of growing concern. They should replace hydralazine in triple therapy, where they are often effective in previously resistant cases.

In the treatment of congestive heart failure resistant to digitalis and diuretics, enalapril or captopril may offer considerable therapeutic benefit. They compare favorably with other vasodilators such as hydralazine and prazosin, as dosage adjustment of the former is difficult in patients in the absence of invasive hemodynamic monitoring and tolerance has been frequently reported with the latter.[81] Future research will consider earliest use of ACE inhibitors in milder forms of congestive heart failure and combined use of vasodilators in resistant cases. It should be noted that no data to date substantiate that mortality is delayed by using ACE inhibitors in congestive heart failure. The quality of life, however, is improved.

Comparative Pharmacokinetics of Enalapril and Captopril. The pharmacokinetics of enalapril and captopril are compared in Table 3. Enalapril has a greater affinity for ACE[82] and is a more potent ACE inhibitor. Captopril can be dosed two to three times per day while enalapril should be administered once or twice daily.

Adverse Effects of Enalapril versus Captopril. The major question today concerns whether important differences exist between enalapril and captopril, especially in low doses, in their relative propensity to cause adverse effects. Table 4, as compiled by Davies and co-workers,[57] summarizes the relative incidence of skin rash, taste disturbances, neutropenia, and proteinuria for these two agents. As can be seen, low-dose captopril in patients with normal renal function appears to be quite similar to enalapril. A higher incidence of side effects with captopril is related to dose and renal dysfunction, especially in patients with underlying autoimmune disease. This experience resulted from the initial investigations of captopril in many patients with resistant hypertension and poor renal function who were subsequently shown to accumulate captopril and its renally cleared metabolites.[1] At this point, experience with enalapril is limited in this type of patient. In addition, studies with enalapril in patients with renal dysfunction were initiated with lower doses in anticipation of accumulation. Thus, whether absence of the sulfhydryl group in enalapril results in a markedly different side-effect profile from that of captopril in high-risk patients is still controversial. Enalapril will need to be studied further in such patients before an accurate assessment can be made. We reported an interesting case of a patient with a previous skin rash during methimazole treatment who developed a severe, unrelenting total body rash during captopril treatment; both of these agents contain a sulfhydryl group.[83] Substituting enalapril for captopril resulted in prompt resolution of the rash with maintenance of blood pressure control. We thought in this patient

Table 3.
Comparative Pharmacokinetics of Captopril, Enalapril, and Enalaprilat

Variable	Captopril	Enalapril	Enalaprilat
Bioavailability	62–68%[89,90]	59–73%[44–46]	...[a]
Effect of food on bioavailability	↓30–40%[46]	None[46]	...
Time to peak serum concentration	0.5–1.5 hr[86–90]	0.5–1.5 hr[45,54]	2–8 hr[44,45,54]
Volume of distribution (steady state)	0.7 L/kg[89]	...	...
Urinary excretion	50% of dose[89]	18% of dose[45]	43% of dose[45]
Total body clearance	0.76 L/kg·hr[89]		9.48 L/hr[45]
Half-life (normal)	0.75–2 hr[86–89]	1.3[53]	5.9–35 hr[45,47,53,b]
(renal dysfunction)	3.5–32 hr[91]		increased[48]

[a] No data.
[b] See text (Pharmacokinetics/Elimination).

Table 4.
Relative Incidence of Adverse Experiences[a]

Adverse Effect	Enalapril NDA Experience (Incidence/Discontinued)	Captopril: Labeling (Incidence)	Captopril: Current Literature[b] (Discontinued): Normal Renal Function, Dose Low-High	Captopril: Current Literature[b] (Discontinued): Impaired Renal Function, Dose Low-High
Rash	1.2%/0.3%	10.0%	1.4–2.1%	2.5–5.1%
Dysgeusia	0.5%/0	7.0%	0.5–1.3%	0.7–2.9%
Neutropenia (<300/mm³)	0	0.3%	0.02%	0.5%, 7.2%[c]
Proteinuria	0.66%[d]	1.2%	0.2–1.0%	1.0–3.5%
(> g/24 hours)	One case[e]	0.3%[e]		

[a] From reference 57 (reprinted with permission).
[b] Discontinued cases—overall incidence not reported.
[c] With collagen disease.
[d] Isolated values only.
[e] >3.0 g/24 hours.

that the sulfhydryl moiety could be incriminated. Similar cases have been reported by others,[84] including two patients with hypertensive crisis related to systemic sclerosis.[67] However, in contrast to these cases, Kuboi[85] described one patient with a rash attributed to enalapril that resolved after substitution of captopril.

Formulary Recommendations

Because of the potential difference in adverse effects in the complicated patient likely to be treated in the hospitalized setting, enalapril should be added to the formulary, preferably in a "clinical-trial" status. A predetermined date (e.g., one year later) should be set for re-evaluation of the adverse effect question. Captopril should be maintained on the formulary. If enalapril is proven to be safer, then captopril could be deleted at a future date. If enalapril and low-dose captopril are deemed equally safe and effective, then total cost per treatment day should be the basis for comparison. The cost, which has been a deterrent to prescribing captopril, may be reduced in the future because of competition in the marketplace.

Conclusion

Angiotensin-converting enzyme inhibitors are an important new class of agents for the treatment of hypertension and congestive heart failure. Enalapril is a nonsulfhydryl ACE inhibitor that appears very similar in efficacy to captopril. These agents will need to be differentiated on the basis of adverse effects, cost, and ease of administration. Whether enalapril is safer than low-dose captopril will be answered after further experience is gained with enalapril in patients with renal dysfunction and autoimmune disease.

References

1. Vlasses PH, Ferguson RK, Chatterjee K. Captopril: clinical pharmacology and benefit-to-risk ratio in hypertension and congestive heart failure. *Pharmacotherapy.* 1982; 2:1–7.
2. Levine WG. Heavy metals and heavy-metal antagonists. In: Goodman and Gilman's the pharmacological basis of therapeutics. 5th ed. Gilman AG, Goodman LS, Gilman A, eds. New York: Macmillan Publishing Co., Inc.; 1975:912–23.
3. Gilman AG, Murad F. Thyroid and antithyroid drugs. In: Goodman and Gilman's the pharmacological basis of therapeutics. 5th ed. Gilman AG, Goodman LS, Gilman A, eds. New York: Macmillan Publishing Co., Inc.; 1975:1398–1422.
4. Sweet CS. Pharmacological properties of the converting enzyme inhibitor, enalapril maleate (MK-421). *Fed Proc.* 1983; 42:167–70.
5. Rotmensch HH, Vlasses PH, Swanson BN et al. Antihypertensive efficacy of once daily MK-521, a new nonsulfhydryl angiotensin converting enzyme inhibitor. *Am J Cardiol.* 1984; 53:116–9.
6. Biollaz J, Burnier M, Turini, GA et al. Three new long-acting converting enzyme inhibitors: relationship between plasma converting enzyme activity and response to angiotensin I. *Clin Pharmacol Ther.* 1981; 29:665–70.
7. Brunner DB, Desponds G, Biollaz J et al. Effect of a new angiotensin converting enzyme inhibitor MK-421 and its lysine analogue on the components of the renin system in healthy subjects. *Br J Clin Pharmacol.* 1981; 11:461–7.
8. Swanson BN, Hichens M, Mojaverian P et al. Angiotensin converting enzyme activity in human serum: relationship to enzyme inhibitor in vivo and in vitro. *Res Commun Chem Pathol Pharmacol.* 1981; 33:525–36.
9. Forslund T, Fyhrquist F, Gronhagen-Riska C et al. Induction of angiotensin-converting enzyme with the ACE inhibitory compound MK-421 in rat lung. *Eur J Pharmacol.* 1982; 80: 121–5.
10. Ulm EH, Vassil TC. Total serum converting enzyme activity in rats and dogs after enalapril maleate (MK-521). *Life Sci.* 1982; 30:1225–30.
11. Johnston CI, Jackson B, Cubela R et al. Mechanism for hypotensive action of angiotensin converting enzyme inhibitors. *Clin Exp Hypertens.* 1984; 6:551–61.
12. Dunn FG, Oigman W, Ventury HO et al. Enalapril improves systemic and renal hemodynamics and allows regression of left ventricular mass in essential hypertension. *Am J Cardiol.* 1984; 53:105–8.
13. Gavras H, Biollaz J, Waeber B et al. Effects of the oral angiotensin converting enzyme inhibitor MK-421 in human hypertension. *Clin Sci.* 1981; 61 (Suppl):281S–83S.
14. Biollaz J, Brunner HR, Gavras I et al. Antihypertensive therapy with MK-421: angiotensin II–renin relationships to evaluate efficacy of converting enzyme blockade. *J Cardiovasc Pharmacol.* 1982; 4:966–72.
15. de Leeuw PW, Hoogma RP, van Soest GA et al. Humoral and renal effect of MK-421 (enalapril) in hypertensive subjects. *J Cardiovasc Pharmacol.* 1983; 5:731–6.
16. Navis GJ, de Jong PE, Donker AJ et al. Effects of enalapril on blood pressure and renal haemodynamics in essential hypertension. *Proc Eur Dial Transplant Assoc.* 1983; 20:577–81.
17. Simon G, Morioka S, Snyder DK et al. Increased renal plasma flow in long-term enalapril treatment of hypertension. *Clin Pharmacol Ther.* 1983; 34:459–65.
18. Millar JA, Derkx FHM, McLean K et al. Pharmacodynamics of converting enzyme inhibition: the cardiovascular, endocrine, and autonomic effects of MK-421 (enalapril) and MK-521. *Br J Clin Pharmacol.* 1982; 14:347P.
19. Hodsman GP, Zabludowski JR, Zoccali C et al. Enalapril (MK-421) and its lysine analogue (MK-521): a comparison of acute and chronic effects on blood pressure, renin–angiotensin system and sodium excretion in normal man. *Br J Clin Pharmacol.* 1984; 17:233–41.
20. Fouad FM, Tarazi RC, Bravo EL et al. Hemodynamic and antihypertensive effects of the new oral angiotensin converting enzyme inhibitor MK-421 (enalapril). *Hypertension.* 1984; 6:167–74.
21. Shoback DM, Williams GH, Swartz SL et al. Time course and effect of sodium intake on vascular and hormonal responses to enalapril (MK-421) in normal subjects. *J. Cardiovasc Pharmacol.* 1983; 5:1010–8.
22. Nakashima Y, Fouad FM, Tarazi RC. Regression of left ventricular hypertrophy from systemic hypertension by enalapril. *Am J Cardiol.* 1984; 53:1044–9.
23. Ferguson RK, Vlasses PH, Swanson BN et al. Effects of enalapril, a new converting enzyme inhibitor, in hypertension. *Clin Pharmacol Ther.* 1982; 32:48–53.
24. Gavras H, Biollaz J, Waeber B et al. Effects of the new oral angiotensin converting enzyme inhibitor MK-421 in human hypertension. *Clin Exp Hypertens.* 1982; 4:303–14.
25. DiCarlo L, Chatterjee K, Parmley WW et al. Enalapril: a new angiotensin-converting enzyme inhibitor in chronic heart failure. Acute and chronic hemodynamic evaluations. *J Am Coll Cardiol.* 1983; 2:865–71.
26. Turini GA, Waeber B, Brunner HR. The renin–angiotensin system in refractory heart failure: clinical, hemodynamic and hormonal effects of captopril and enalapril. *Eur Heart J.* 1983; 4:189–97.

27. Cody RJ, Covit AB, Schaer GL et al. Evaluation of a long-acting converting enzyme inhibitor (enalapril) for the treatment of chronic congestive heart failure. *J Am Coll Cardiol.* 1983; 1:1154–9.
28. Fitzpatrick D, Nicholls MG, Ikram H et al. Haemodynamic, hormonal, and electrolyte effects of enalapril in heart failure. *Br Heart J.* 1983; 50:163–9.
29. Levine TB, Olivari MT, Garberg U et al. Hemodynamic and clinical response to enalapril, a long-acting converting enzyme inhibitor, in patients with congestive heart failure. *Circulation.* 1984; 69:548–53.
30. Dunkman WB, Wilen M, Franciosa JA. Enalapril (MK-421), a new angiotensin converting enzyme inhibitor: acute and chronic effects in heart failure. *Chest.* 1983; 84:539–45.
31. Jackson B, McGrath BP, Johnston CI. Correlation between angiotensin converting enzyme inhibition and the acute hypotensive response to MK-421 in essential hypertension. *Clin Exp Pharmacol Physiol.* 1982; 7:99–104.
32. Hodsman GP, Brown JJ, Cumming AM et al. Enalapril in the treatment of hypertension with renal artery stenosis. *Br Med J.* 1983; 287:1413–7.
33. Weinberger MH, Fineberg NS. Variables predicting blood pressure response to enalapril. *Clin Pharmacol Ther.* 1984; 35:281. Abstract.
34. Wilkins LH, Dustan HP, Walker JF et al. Enalapril in low-renin essential hypertension. *Clin Pharmacol Ther.* 1983; 34: 297–302.
35. Griffing GT, Sindler BH, Aurecchia SA et al. Temporal enhancement of renin-aldosterone blockade by enalapril, an angiotensin converting enzyme inhibitor. *Clin Pharmacol Ther.* 1982; 32:592–8.
36. Unger T, Ganten D, Lang RE. Converting enzyme inhibitors: antihypertensive drugs with unexpected mechanisms. *Trends Pharmacol Sci.* 1983; 4:514–9.
37. Odya CE, Wilgis FP, Walker JF et al. Immunoreactive bradykinin and [des-Arg9]-bradykinin in low-renin essential hypertension—before and after treatment with enalapril (MK-421). *J Lab Clin Med.* 1983; 102:714–21.
38. Vlasses PH, Ferguson RK, Smith JB et al. Urinary excretion of prostaglandin and thromboxane A2 metabolites after angiotensin converting enzyme inhibition in hypertensive patients. *Prostaglandins Leukotrienes Med.* 1983; 11:143–50.
39. Atlas SA, Niarchos AP, Case DB. Inhibitors of the renin-angiotensin system: effects on blood pressure, aldosterone secretion and renal function. *Am J Nephrol.* 1983; 3:118–27.
40. Cohen ML, Kurz KD. Angiotensin converting enzyme inhibition in tissues from spontaneously hypertensive rats after treatment with captopril or MK-421. *J Pharmacol Exp Ther.* 1982; 220:63–9.
41. De Jonge A, Wilffert B, Kalkman HO et al. Captopril impairs the vascular smooth muscle contraction mediated by postsynaptic alpha$_2$-adrenoceptors in the pithed rat. *Eur J Pharmacol.* 1981; 74:385–6.
42. Hichens M, Hand EL, Mulcahy WS. Radioimmunoassay for angiotensin converting enzyme inhibitors. *Ligand Q.* 1981; 4:43–8.
43. Method on file, Merck Sharp & Dohme, Div. Merck & Co., Inc., West Point, PA 19486.
44. Irvin JD, Till AE, Vlasses PH et al. Bioavailability of enalapril maleate. *Clin Pharmacol Ther.* 1984; 35:248. Abstract.
45. Ulm EH, Hichens M, Gomez HJ et al. Enalapril maleate and a lysine analogue (MK-521): disposition in man. *Br J Clin Pharmacol.* 1982; 14:357–62.
46. Swanson BN, Vlasses PH, Ferguson RK et al. Influence of food on the bioavailability of enalapril. *J. Pharm Sci.* 1984; 73: 1655–7.
47. Till AE, Gomez HJ, Hichens M et al. Pharmacokinetics of repeated single doses of enalapril maleate (MK-421) in normal volunteers. *Biopharm Drug Disp.* 1984; 5:273–80.
48. Fruncillo RJ, Rocci ML Jr, Shepley K et al. Enalaprilat accumulates after chronic enalapril dosing in renal failure. *Clin Pharmacol Ther.* Abstract. In press.
49. Data on file, Merck Sharp & Dohme.
50. Till AE, Irvin JD, Hichens M et al. Pharmacodynamics and disposition of intravenous MK-422, the diacid metabolite of enalapril maleate. *Clin Pharmacol Ther.* 1982; 31:275. Abstract.
51. Tocci DJ, de Luna FA, Duncan AEW et al. The physiological disposition and metabolism of enalapril maleate (MK-421) in laboratory animals. *Drug Metab Dispos.* 1982; 10:15–9.
52. Pang KS, Cherry WF, Terrel JA et al. Disposition of enalapril and its diacid metabolite, enalaprilat, in a perfused rat liver preparation: presence of a diffusional barrier for enalaprilat into hepatocytes. *Drug Metab Dispos.* 1984; 12:309–13.
53. Shionoiri H, Gotah E, Akiba N et al. Blood concentration and effect of enalapril on blood pressure, renin angiotensin system and kallikrein kinin system in patients with essential hypertension. *Circulation.* 1983; 68 (Suppl III):348. Abstract.
54. Biollaz J, Schelling JL, Jacot Des Combes B et al. Enalapril maleate and a lysine analogue (MK-521) in normal volunteers; relationship between plasma drug levels and the renin angiotensin system. *Br J Clin Pharmacol.* 1982; 14:363–8.
55. Saris S, Lowenthal D, Klein L et al. Enalapril maleate in renal failure. *Clin Pharmacol Ther.* 1984; 35:272. Abstract.
56. Kelley, J, Doyle G, Donohue J et al. The pharmacokinetic profile of enalaprilat in normal subjects and patients with renal impairment. *Br J Clin Pharmacol.* 1984; 18:274P.
57. Davies RO, Irvin JD, Kramsch DK et al. Enalapril worldwide experience. *Am J Med.* 1984; 77 (Suppl 2A):23–35.
58. Sassano P, Chatellier G, Alhenc-Gelas F et al. Antihypertensive effect of enalapril as first-step treatment of mild and moderate uncomplicated essential hypertension. *Am J Med.* 1984; 77(Suppl 2A):18–22.
59. Bauer JH, Jones LB. Comparative studies: enalapril versus hydrochlorothiazide as first-step therapy for the treatment of primary hypertension. *Am J Kidney Dis.* 1984; 4:55–62.
60. Simon AC, Levenson JA, Bouthier JD et al. Comparison of oral MK-421 and propranolol in mild to moderate essential hypertension and their effects on arterial and venous vessels of the forearm. *Am J Cardiol.* 1984; 53:781–5.
61. Chrysant SG, Brown RD, Ken DC et al. Antihypertensive and metabolic effects of a new converting enzyme inhibitor, enalapril. *Clin Pharmacol Ther.* 1983; 33:742–6.
62. Vlasses PH, Rotmensch HH, Swanson BN et al. Comparative antihypertensive effects of enalapril maleate and hydrochlorothiazide, alone and in combination. *J Clin Pharmacol.* 1983; 23:227–33.
63. Ferguson RK, Vlasses PH, Irvin JD et al. A comparative pilot study of enalapril, a new converting enzyme inhibitor, and hydrochlorothiazide in essential hypertension. *J Clin Pharmacol.* 1982; 22:281–9.
64. Fernandez PG, Kim BK, Galway AB. An appraisal of antihypertensive efficacy and adverse reactions with two drug regimens: enalapril maleate as part of triple therapy compared to conventional triple therapy in moderate to severe hypertension. *Pharmatherapeutica.* 1984; 3:505–14.
65. Evans R, Ferraro J, Martin M et al. Enalaprilat (MK-422) an intravenous angiotensin converting enzyme inhibitor in hypertensive emergencies. *Clin Pharmacol Ther.* 1984; 35:238. Abstract.
66. Hodsman GP, Brown JJ, Davies DL et al. Converting enzyme inhibitor enalapril (MK-421) in treatment of hypertension with renal artery stenosis. *Br Med J.* 1982; 285:1697–9.
67. Smith CD, Smith RD, Korn JH. Hypertensive crisis in systemic sclerosis: treatment with the new oral angiotensin converting enzyme inhibitor MK-421 (enalapril) in captopril intolerant patients. *Arthritis Rheum.* 1984; 27:826–8.
68. Griffing GT, Sindler BH, Aurecchia SA et al. The therapeutic effect of a new angiotensin-coverting enzyme inhibitor, enalapril maleate, in idiopathic hyperaldosteronism. *Clin Res.* 1982; 30:692A. Abstract.
69. Sharpe DN, Murphy J, Coxon R et al. Enalapril in patients with chronic heart failure: a placebo-controlled, randomized, double-blind study. *Circulation.* 1984; 70:271–8.
70. Vlasses PH, Rotmensch HH, Ferguson RK et al. "Scalded mouth" caused by angiotensin converting enzyme inhibitors.

Br Med J. 1982; 284:1672–3.
71. Hricik DE, Browning PJ, Kopelman R et al. Captopril-induced functional renal insufficiency in patients with bilateral renal-artery stenosis or renal-artery stenosis in a solitary kidney. *N Engl J Med.* 1983; 308:373–6.
72. Bender W, Lafrance N, Walker NG. Mechanism of determination in renal function in patients with renovascular hypertension treated with enalapril. *Hypertension.* 1984; 6: I193–I197.
73. Cressman MD, Vidt DG, Acker C. Renal glycosuria and azotemia after enalapril maleate (MK-421). *Lancet.* 1982; 2:440. Letter.
74. Barnes JN, Davies ES, Gent CB. Rash, eosinophilia, and hyperkalemia associated with enalapril. *Lancet.* 1983; 2:41–2. Letter.
75. Waeber B, Nussberger J, Brunner HR. Self-poisoning with enalapril. *Br Med J.* 1984; 288:287–8.
76. Veterans Administration Cooperative Study Group on Antihypertensive Agents. Low-dose captopril in the treatment of mild to moderate hypertension. *Hypertension.* 1983; 5(Suppl III):319–44.
77. Vlasses PH, Rotmensch HH, Rocci ML Jr et al. Double-blind comparison of captopril and enalapril in hypertensive patients. *Clin Pharmacol Ther.* 1984; 35:280. Abstract.
78. Kaplan NM. Mild hypertension: when and how to treat. *Arch Intern Med.* 1983; 143:255–9.
79. Spivack C, Ocken S, Frishman WH. Calcium antagonists: clinical use in the treatment of systemic hypertension. *Drugs.* 1983; 25:154–77.
80. Joint National Committee on Detection, Evaluation, and Treatment of High Blood Pressure. The 1984 report of the Joint National Committee on Detection, Evaluation, and Treatment of High Blood Pressure. *Arch Intern Med.* 1984; 144:1045–57.
81. Packer M. Selection of vasodilator drugs for patients with severe chronic heart failure: a new approach based on a new classification. *Drugs.* 1982; 24:64–74.
82. Patchett AA, Harris E, Tristan EW. A new class of angiotensin converting enzyme inhibitors. *Nature.* 1980; 288:280–3.
83. Rotmensch HH, Vlasses PH, Ferguson RK. Resolution of captopril-induced rash after substitution of enalapril. *Pharmacotherapy.* 1983; 3:131–3.
84. Gavras I, Gavras H. Captopril and enalapril. *Ann Intern Med.* 1983; 98:556. Letter.
85. Kuboi SH, Cody RJ. Enalapril, a rash, captopril. *Ann Intern Med.* 1984; 100:616. Letter.
86. Cody RJ, Shaer GL, Covit AB et al. Captopril kinetics in chronic congestive heart failure. *Clin Pharmacol Ther.* 1982; 32:721–6.
87. Cody RJ, Covit A, Shaer G et al. Captopril pharmacokinetics and the acute hemodynamic and hormonal response in patients with severe chronic congestive heart failure. *Am Heart J.* 1982; 104:1180–3.
88. Jarrott B, Drummer O, Hooper R et al. Pharmacokinetic properties of captopril after acute and chronic administration to hypertensive subjects. *Am J Cardiol.* 1982; 49:1547–9.
89. Duchin KL, Sighvi SM, Willard DA et al. Captopril kinetics. *Clin Pharmacol Ther.* 1982; 31:452–8.
90. Kripalani KJ, McKinstry DN, Singhvi SM et al. Disposition of captopril in normal subjects. *Clin Pharmacol Ther.* 1980; 27:636–41.
91. Duchin KL, Pierides AM, Heald A et al. Elimination kinetics of captopril in patients with renal failure. *Kidney Int.* 1984; 25:942–7.
92. Enalapril in Hypertension Study Group (UK). Enalapril in essential hypertension: a comparative study with propranolol. *Br J Clin Pharmacol.* 1984; 18:51–6.
93. Dickstein K, Soyland E, Gundersen T et al. Acute and chronic hemodynamic effects of enalapril (MK-421) in congestive heart failure. *Int J Cardiol.* 1984; 6:445–56.

"

Indications for Hydergine

Although the treatment of dementia is the best known as well as the most controversial indication, hydergine is widely prescribed in many countries for peripheral vascular disease and for hypertension. In France and Italy, about one third of the prescriptions are for use as a hypotensive. While the efficacy of hydergine in peripheral vascular disease is questionable, it does seem to be a safe and effective antihypertensive agent, particularly in the elderly. Hydergine may also be effective in some patients with tardive dyskinesia. In the United Kingdom the data sheet for hydergine gives its sole indication as "an adjunct in the management of mild to moderate mental impairment in the elderly." The obvious question is, should the drug be prescribed to these patients? It is frustrating that, after 30 years and many trials, the answer is still not clear. For instance, direct comparison of hydergine with antidepressants would be valuable. It is unlikely in the extreme that hydergine, or any other existing drug, will greatly alter the quality of life of a severely demented elderly patient. Even in those less severely affected, cure is out of the question, and this should be made very clear to the patients' relatives before the question of drug treatment is even raised. Therapeutic objectives must therefore be rather modest, and many doctors may feel that they do not warrant the cost of therapy or the, admittedly small, risk of side effects. Others, however, will judge that a course of hydergine, at least 4.5 mg a day, probably for at least three months, is justified. Patients with multi-infarct dementia may be less likely to benefit than those with Alzheimer's. Even if, as many believe, the effect of the drug is on mood rather than on cognition, the benefits to the patients and their families may still be worthwhile. We must add that other drugs, such as naftidrofuryl [nafronyl oxalate] and pentoxifylline, have shown promising results in clinical trials, though the evidence is not as extensive as that for hydergine.

—Anon. Ergot for dementia? *Lancet.* 1984; 2:1313–4. Editorial.

"

Research

Relationship between plasma morphine concentrations and pharmacologic effects in postoperative patients using patient-controlled analgesia

DAVID A. GRAVES, JANICE M. ARRIGO, THOMAS S. FOSTER, TERRY J. BAUMANN, AND RANDAL L. BATENHORST

Abstract: In postoperative patients using patient-controlled analgesia (PCA) to administer i.v. doses of morphine sulfate, respiratory rates and subjective rankings of pain, sedation, and liking for the drug were correlated with plasma morphine concentrations.

In 12 patients selected before surgery, the initial morphine sulfate dose of 0.6 mg/sq m was increased or decreased as needed. Every two hours, cumulative morphine sulfate dose, respiratory rate, and sedation were recorded by the nurse, along with the patient's evaluation of pain and liking for the drug. Plasma was collected in the morning and evening during PCA therapy for morphine analysis. Data were analyzed by analysis of covariance.

Dosing rates and rankings of pain, sedation, and liking decreased as a function of time postoperatively, but respiratory rates did not. Sedation and respiratory rates were independent of morphine concentration. Liking of the drug increased directly with plasma morphine concentration but decreased with time. A high level of pain was directly related to morphine use. For all significant relationships, there was high interpatient variability, with the exception of changes in pain rankings induced by morphine. Patients defined a minimum effective plasma morphine concentration of 20–40 ng/mL. The maximum plasma morphine concentration achieved by self-administration was 82 ng/mL.

These postoperative patients used patient-controlled analgesia to deliver morphine sulfate i.v. for pain relief, not for euphoria, and did not exhibit sedation or respiratory depression. Morphine was consistently effective at plasma concentrations of 40 ng/mL or greater.

Index terms: Analgesics and antipyretics; Blood levels; Dosage; Drug abuse; Drug administration; Morphine; Morphine sulfate; Pain; Tolerance
Clin Pharm. 1985; 4:41–7

While developing and testing a patient-controlled analgesia (PCA) device at the University of Kentucky, we found that PCA provides benefits beyond safe and effective pain relief. With PCA, behavior patterns associated with injectable narcotic requirements can be evaluated for both desirable and untoward effects of narcotic administration. Practitioners have expressed concern about addiction liability associated with the self-administration of opiate analgesics. Although a great deal of infor-

DAVID A. GRAVES, PHARM.D., is Clinical Pharmacist, Clinical Pharmacology Department, Pennwalt Pharmaceutical Division, Rochester, NY. JANICE M. ARRIGO, PHARM.D., is Clinical Research Associate, Division of Clinical Research, Marion Laboratories, Kansas City, MO; at the time of this study, she was Chief Resident in Pharmacy, University of Kentucky Medical Center, Lexington, KY. THOMAS S. FOSTER, PHARM.D., is Professor, College of Pharmacy, University of Kentucky, Lexington, KY. TERRY J. BAUMANN, PHARM.D., is Assistant Professor of Pharmacy, College of Pharmacy and Allied Health Professions, Wayne State University, and Clinical Pharmacist, Henry Ford Hospital, Detroit, MI. RANDAL L. BATENHORST, PHARM.D., is Assistant Professor and Director of Drug Information and Clinical Research, College of Pharmacy, University of Illinois, Chicago, IL.

Address reprint requests to Dr. Foster at the Department of Pharmacy, Room C–114–b, University of Kentucky Medical Center, 800 Rose Street, Lexington, KY 40536.

The assistance of the following persons and institute in various aspects of the research is acknowledged: Richard L. Bennett, M.D., Ward O. Griffen, M.D., George E. Bigelow, Ph.D., John A. Dougherty, Ph.D., Loren L. Miller, Ph.D., Giraud V. Foster, M.D., Ph.D., and the Research Triangle Institute, Research Triangle Park, NC.

Supported in part by grant No. R03-DA03433 from the National Institute of Drug Abuse.

Presented in part at the Tenth Annual Nebraska Residents' Conference and at the Clinical Research Forum of the 19th Annual ASHP Midyear Clinical Meeting, Dallas, TX, December 4, 1984.

mation has been gathered in studies of PCA, none of the studies has assessed prospectively the risk of addiction.

The objective of our study was to determine the impetus for narcotic self-administration. To delineate self-dosing mechanisms, we measured plasma concentrations of morphine and β endorphin and used subjective ranking scales that measured patient pain, sedation, and liking of the drug.

Methods

Twelve patients who were scheduled to undergo surgical procedures were selected for study. Informed consent was obtained from each patient. None of the patients was treated with narcotic drugs of any kind before surgery.

The methods and applications of PCA have been previously described.[1-4] The patients were permitted to begin using PCA in the postoperative recovery room and to continue using PCA when they were transferred to their regular ward beds. Morphine sulfate was administered by a syringe-driven infusion pump electronically connected to a timing device. The timing switchbox was programmed to impose an inactivation interval of six minutes between doses. A chart recorder (Model A, Esterline–Angus Event Recorder, Esterline–Angus, Indianapolis, IN 46224) was connected to the PCA device to permit recording of injection times. Every two hours, the nurse responsible for the patient's care recorded the respiratory rate and the cumulative morphine dose delivered. The cumulative morphine dose was used to determine a weight-corrected morphine dosing rate (mg/kg/hr).

Patients activated the system for delivery of each dose of morphine sulfate by depressing a button on a cord that extended from the device to the bedside. Each dose was delivered over 10–15 seconds into an i.v. line that was already present for fluid therapy. Patients were instructed preoperatively and again in the postoperative recovery room to balance comfort (analgesia) and sleepiness (sedation). Initially, each morphine sulfate dose was 0.6 mg/sq m for all patients. One of the investigators increased the available morphine dose by 50% if inadequate analgesia was reported and decreased the dose by 50% if sedation occurred.

Subjective Assessments. Subjective assessments of pain, sedation, and liking of the drug were made every two hours. A modified Keele scale was used as in previous studies[2,3] to rank the amount of pain experienced by the patient. Patients were asked to respond to the question, "Over the last two hours, how would you describe how you have felt?" with one of the following choices: (1) comfortable, (2) mild discomfort, (3) in pain, (4) in bad pain, or (5) in very bad pain. We used this scale because our patients did not consistently understand the McGill–Melzack Pain Questionnaire or other ranking scales that used large words.[5,6]

Sedation was assessed as the overall degree of sleepiness during a two-hour period. The nurse responsible for the patient's care assigned a sedation ranking using the following scale: (1) wide awake, (2) drowsy, (3) dozing intermittently, (4) mostly sleeping, or (5) only awakens when aroused.

The pain and sedation rankings were used to determine a relative dose indicator (RDI),[7] which was the difference between the sedation and pain rankings (sedation ranking minus pain ranking equals RDI). Positive RDI values represented relative overdosage of morphine, since sedation rankings were greater than pain rankings. Negative RDI values were an indication of relative underdosage of morphine.

A liking scale adapted from addiction research was applied at the same time that pain and sedation were assessed. The Addiction Research Center Inventory[8-11] was originally designed to detect "euphorigenic"[a] properties of abusable drugs in addicts. Direct application of the inventory to our patients was not possible, since many of the responses (e.g., "I have a pleasant feeling in my stomach.") were inappropriate for patients who had recently undergone abdominal surgery. Therefore, patients were asked to complete the statement, "My degree of liking for this drug is . . . " with one of the following responses: (1) not at all, (2) a little, (3) a lot, (4) very much, or (5) as much as possible. This open-ended statement permitted patient interpretation.

Although patients used PCA on the day of surgery, data for that day were not included because of possible residual effects of anesthetic drugs. No data obtained during the night hours (2200 to 0600) were used in any analysis. Analgesia was not assumed if the patient was asleep at the time of data collection. Therefore, no pain ranking or RDI value was available for analysis if the patient was asleep at the time of a nursing evaluation.

Plasma Collection and Analysis. Plasma was collected preoperatively but not on the day of surgery for the purposes of this study. On the morning of the first postoperative day, a single 10-mL blood sample from each patient was withdrawn into a heparinized tube (No. 6527, Becton Dickinson and Co., Rutherford, NJ 07070) at least 10 minutes after a PCA-administered morphine dose. Subsequent samples were drawn at 0700 and 1900 hours every postoperative day that the patient used PCA. After centrifugation, plasma was split into two aliquots and frozen at −70 °C until analysis.

Plasma morphine concentrations were analyzed by the stability-indicating radioimmunoassay developed by Murphy and Hug.[13] The sensitivity of this assay was 1.5 ng/mL. Concentration standards ranging from 1 to 100 ng/mL gave R^2 values greater than 95%. Because all samples were subjected to two separate extractions before exposure to the antigen, cross-reactivity to inactive conjugated (glucuronidated) morphine was minimal.[13]

Plasma β-endorphin concentrations were measured by radioimmunoassay using a kit from ImmunoNuclear Corporation (Catalog No. 46-L2, Stillwater, MN 55082). Minimum sensitivity that we considered acceptable with our plasma sample size was 5 pg/mL. When drawn into tubes (No. 6457, Becton Dickinson and Co.) containing EDTA as an anticoagulant, the normal range for this procedure is 7–15 pg/mL with a coefficient of variation of 6–14% and less than 5% cross-reactivity to β-lipotropin.[b] This assay did not cross-react with α or γ endorphin, dynorphin, Leu- or Met-enkephalin, adrenocorticotropic hormone, α melanocyte-stimulating hormone, prolactin, luteinizing hormone, follicle-stimulating hormone, thyroid-stimulating hormone, vasopressin, or oxytocin,[b] and previous work indicates that the assay is stability indicating for β endorphin.[c]

Statistical Analysis. All data were analyzed using the Statistical Analysis System (SAS).[14] A p value of less than 0.05 was used as the a priori level of significance.

Because of the wide interpatient variability for variables measured in this study, we used the parametric statistical method, analysis of covariance (ANACOVA).[15,16] This test allowed data for all 12 patients to be considered simultaneously while maintaining overall p values; Type I error was thus controlled. We believe this was a reasonable compromise despite normality considerations present with subjective ranking scales. Nonparametric tests would not have allowed ANACOVA-type inferences to be made, and other nonparametric characteristics (Type II errors) would have further weakened overall conclusions.

Results

The characteristics of the 12 patients studied are presented in Table 1. The mean (± standard deviation) age was 35 ± 11 years, and the mean weight was 64.1 ± 14.4 kg. The pain and sedation rankings are presented in a three-dimensional histogram (Figure 1), as in other studies.[1,2,4]

Temporal Findings. The scales for pain, sedation, and liking and the weight-corrected dosing rates were dependent on both time and patient ($p < 0.05$). All three of the subjective ranking scales, as well as dosing rates, diminished as a function of postoperative day with significant interpatient variability. RDI was independent of patient and time, while respiratory rate was shown to be patient-dependent only.

Endorphin and Morphine Concentrations. The majority of β-endorphin concentrations were below assay sensitivity (84% were below 5 pg/mL). Therefore, no correlations were performed.

Morphine concentrations were inversely related to time since surgery and directly related to dosing rate (Figure 2). There was significant interpatient variability. Morphine concentrations varied a great deal, probably as a function of administration times. ANACOVAs were performed on postdistribution morphine concentrations without postinjection time as a factor.

A significant direct patient-dependent relationship existed between plasma morphine concentrations and pain rankings. Sedation, respiratory rate, and RDI were independent of morphine concentration. Liking rankings varied directly with plasma morphine concentration (Table 2).

The difference between pain rankings one hour after and one hour before plasma sampling was calculated for each patient and found to be significantly and inversely related to plasma morphine concentration. Because this relationship was patient-independent, a simple linear regression was applied. Plasma morphine concentration was the independent variable and change in pain rankings

Table 1.
Patient Characteristics[a]

Surgical Procedure	Age (yr)	Weight (kg)
Total abdominal hysterectomy, bilateral oophorectomy	32	70.9
Total abdominal hysterectomy, bilateral oophorectomy	50	57.3
Colostomy	19	38.6
Exploratory laparotomy	28	67.7
Cholecystectomy	58	70.9
Radical hysterectomy	43	85.5
Cholecystectomy	38	86.4
Total abdominal hysterectomy	29	54.1
Nephrectomy	27	75.0
Total abdominal hysterectomy	35	55.9
Cholecystectomy	29	51.4
Exploratory laparotomy	31	55.9

[a] All patients were women except the one who underwent nephrectomy.

Figure 1. Pain versus sedation frequency histogram. Block heights are proportional to observation counts (n = 267).

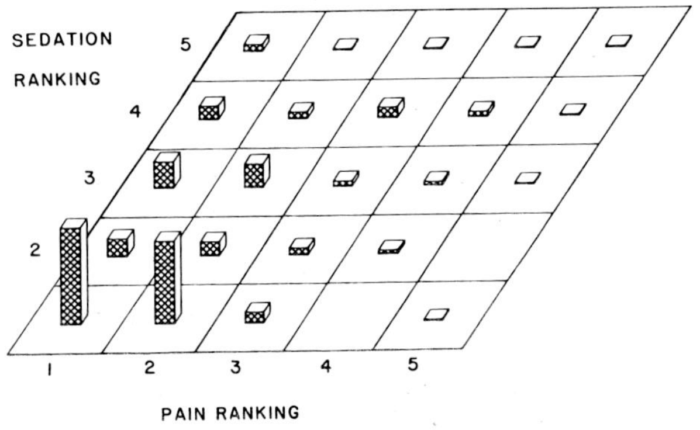

Figure 2. Plasma morphine concentration versus time for 12 individual patients.

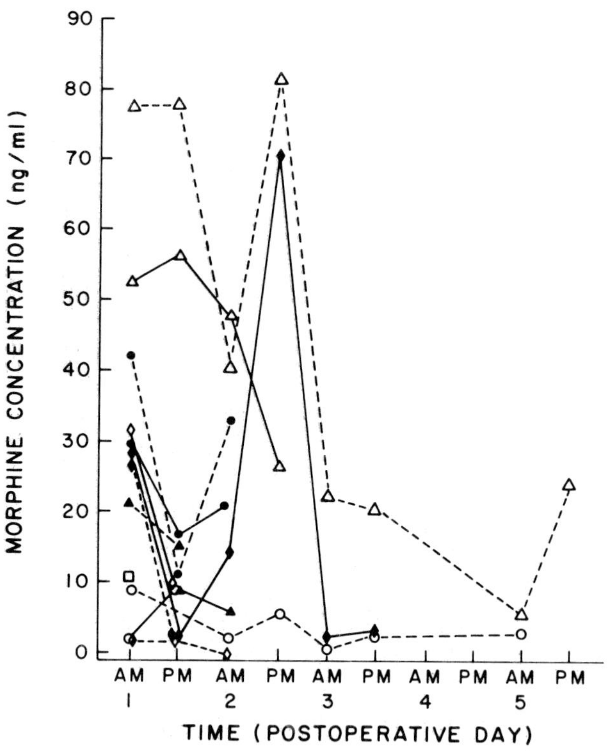

Table 2.
Liking Scale Responses and Changes in Pain Rankings

Variables	Morphine Concentrations (ng/mL, mean ± S.D.)	No. Observations
Liking Scale[a]		
1	. . .	0
2	17.2 ± 17.9	5
3	12.4 ± 14.2	16
4	30.0 ± 29.8	8
5	56.5 ± 36.7	3
Change in Pain Rankings[b]		
No change	18.3 ± 22.0	18
Worsening of pain	14.6 ± 11.1	17
Fall in pain (pain relief)	40.3 ± 30.6	10

[a] Scale ranges from 1 to 5, where 1 = not at all liking the drug and 5 = liking the drug as much as possible.

[b] Calculated as the difference between pain rankings one hour before and one hour after plasma sampling.

was the dependent variable. The slope estimate was significantly different from zero (0.014 pain units per ng/mL of morphine, $R^2 = 0.16$). The intercept term of the regression line was not significantly different from zero. Mean plasma morphine concentrations in patients who experienced a drop in pain rankings (i.e., pain relief) were more than twice those of patients who experienced no change or a worsening of their pain (Table 2). However, the changes seen in respiratory rates, RDIs, sedation rankings, and liking rankings were all independent of plasma morphine concentrations and individual patient.

Discussion

Our results show that postoperative patients, given more than ample opportunity, do not overuse, misuse, or abuse morphine in a self-dosing situation. The group of 12 patients we studied administered morphine to themselves safely and effectively, as evidenced by their consistently low pain and sedation rankings (Figure 1). Initial trepidation associated with introducing PCA into the clinical setting is often because of practitioners' conceptions of dependence liability. Clinicians are often taught the "exposure" theory of addiction, which states that opiate addiction occurs when opiate drug use engenders a powerful tendency toward subsequent, compulsive use.[17] Carried to extremes, this theory implies that narcotic drugs are the cause of opiate dependence and that frequent exposure is likely to cause addiction. Although this theory has some merit in that an individual would be hard-pressed to become addicted to a substance to which he has never been exposed, a second theory appears reasonable. The "adaptive" theory of drug abuse states that addiction occurs when a person attempts to adapt to chronic distress through habitual use of drugs.

The literature supports the fact that patients use morphine more appropriately with PCA than with other therapies.[4,18] We recently reported a patient who used up to 56 mg/hr of morphine via a PCA device; this patient showed neither signs of sedation during dosing nor signs of dependence six months later.[19] The 12 patients in this study reported liking scales that diminished as a function of time. Coupled with the direct relationship between liking of the drug and plasma morphine concentrations, this indicated that if a postoperative patient had a positive feeling about the opiate being administered, that feeling was because of the pain relief associated with its administration. Patients required less morphine as the pain stimulus decreased with time, and liking rankings decreased along with drug use. Other researchers[20] have reported a low incidence of dependence following opiate analgesia. We believe this is fair support for the adaptive orientation theory of opiate addiction.

In our study, sedation and respiratory rates were unrelated to plasma morphine concentrations in either absolute measurements or changes seen during the two-hour interval. We conclude from these findings that there was no drug-induced sedation or respiratory depression in the 12 patients. This supports previous research that described the behavior of PCA dosing as a "closed-loop system,"with patients continuously balancing the need for comfort and the need for a clear sensorium.[4,21,22] The RDI was not helpful in these analyses since there was no drug-induced sedation.

Minimum Effective Concentration of Morphine. Pain rankings correlated directly with plasma morphine concentrations in our study. It appears that high pain rankings caused patients to self-administer morphine, resulting in increased plasma morphine concentrations. In effect, these patients defined a minimum effective plasma concentration (MEC) of morphine. The nature of this minimum concentration, however, should be qualified. We propose that there is no level of comfort that can be maintained at any morphine concentration (short of coma). Rather, we define MEC as the concentration that causes a perceptible decrease in a patient's pain status. Although most other variables were patient dependent, the MEC and subsequent morphine-induced changes in pain status (i.e., pain relief) were the same for all patients.

Dahlstrom et al.[23] reported an MEC of 20 ng/mL for morphine during the postoperative period. While our results do not conflict with this conclusion, Dahlstrom derived the 20-ng/mL concentration using an iterative regression method to predict the concentrations at which redosing occurred in PCA patients; the MEC was defined as the concentration at which patients redosed. Unfortunately, no pain or sedation rankings were collected during this study or similar studies conducted by these researchers.[24-26] We suggest that patients permit morphine concentrations to drop, in some cases, because they have no pain stimulus. This would falsely lower the mean MECs reported by Dahlstrom's group[23-26] and may explain why others have not seen a significant correlation between pharmacologic effect and narcotic concentration.[27,28]

Nayman[29] suggested that a different drug requirement exists for different surgical procedures. Although we believe this is probably true, this question could not be addressed in our study of only 12 patients.

We propose a dynamic, not static, definition of analgesia. The reason that morphine use drops as a function of time postoperatively is not because the MEC falls, but because the patient has less pain and, therefore, needs to be above this MEC less often. Our results imply a patient-independent MEC; the interpatient variability seen with previously reported morphine doses was not because of variation in the MEC between patients, but because of differences in pain perception between patients.[3,4,21,30] For patients who feel the need to alleviate pain, the MEC is above 20–40 ng/mL. The diurnal character of PCA dosing is probably because of an increased number of pain stimuli in the morning hours, not a higher MEC.[3] The reason for the association of certain surgical procedures with higher postoperative analgesic requirements is that some operations are more painful than others, causing patients to stay above the MEC more often by increasing overall doses.[29] This is somewhat different than therapeutic plasma concentrations for other drugs in which a steady biologic state is implied by an MEC. A constant morphine concentration of 40 ng/mL, however, does not guarantee a comfortable state; this concentration would induce an analgesic effect, but if the pain stimulus were great enough, only higher concentrations of morphine would immediately make the patient comfortable.

The patient-independent relationship between pain relief (defined as a drop in pain rankings) and morphine concentrations was dose dependent. Theoretically, any morphine concentration should exert an analgesic effect, but apparently the effect was not perceivable at concentrations below 20 ng/mL; patients whose plasma morphine concentrations were below 20–30 ng/mL generally reported no change or a worsening of pain. Also, our patients did not self-dose to a morphine concentration greater than 82 ng/mL. Since the patients we studied did not exhibit drug-induced sedation or respiratory depression, we conclude that concentrations of at least 90 ng/mL can be safely achieved in patients experiencing postoperative pain. The literature reports that plasma concentrations of morphine are much higher following a single intramuscular dose,[7,27,31] and sedation commonly encountered following intramuscular doses corroborates this.[1,4] It is possible that the upper range might be above 100 ng/mL, but our patients did not achieve such a high plasma concentration even though the opportunity for greater self-dosing existed.

The establishment of an MEC for morphine implies that morphine doses might be determined on the basis of this MEC. The literature describes morphine pharmacokinetics in many different patient populations.[23,32-34] Unfortunately, plasma clearances reported for morphine vary greatly among investigators. While some of these discrepancies may be because of assay affinities for metabolized morphine, there are some differences that have not been explained adequately. Dahlstrom et al.[23] reported a mean clearance of 1.26 L/kg/hr and mean volumes of distribution of 3.7 and 6.3 L/kg for preoperative and postoperative periods, respectively, based on conclusions drawn from an intraoperative dose of morphine given while the patient was still under anesthesia. According to the defined MEC of 20 ng/mL, a dosing rate of approximately 2 mg/hr would be required to maintain an analgesic response (calculated as the product of clearance and the target MEC in a 70-kg patient[35]). While this is not an unreasonable dosing rate, we suspect that the given clearance estimate is somewhat high. Accordingly, dosing rates of 2 mg/hr in the postoperative patient might result in plasma concentrations closer to 40 ng/mL. In normal volunteers weighing 70 kg, a dosing rate of 2.5 mg/hr would result in plasma morphine concentrations of 40 ng/mL.[34] In cancer patients with substantial hepatic disease, a dosing rate of only 1.6 mg/hr would be needed to maintain plasma morphine concentrations of 40 ng/mL in a 70-kg patient.[32] Stanski et al.[33] reported vastly different clearance estimates, which indicated that a dosing rate of less than 1 mg/hr would be required; however, it is suspected that this assay also measured morphine glucuronide, which falsely lowered reported values for clearance.[13]

The estimates just described assume that dosing occurs repeatedly and results in steady-state conditions, but most morphine administration does not occur in this way. Using various volumes of distribution, single doses that would result in a plasma morphine concentration of 40 ng/mL were calculated using the quotient of dose divided by volume of distribution.[35] These doses were 10.4 mg, 9.0 mg, and 5.8 mg for 70-kg postoperative,[23] healthy normal,[34] and oncologic[32] patients, respectively. While these estimates are also reasonable, this is a very simplistic approach that does not take large peripheral compartments into account.[13] Additional work will be required to define morphine pharmacokinetics appropriately during the postoperative period.

Plasma β-Endorphin Concentration. We saw diminished β-endorphin concentrations, many of which were below the sensitivity of our assay. There are three potential explanations for this finding. The first possibility is that morphine influenced the binding of endorphins and changed their distribution. If this were the case, however, normal β-endorphin concentrations should have been observed before surgery. The second possibility is heparin interference with the assay method, and the third possibility is that preoperative and postoperative patients actually do have abnormally low amounts of β endorphin in plasma. There is evidence to support the latter two theories.[a,36,37] We could not delineate a relationship between these β-endorphin concentrations and the variables measured in this study.

While it was disconcerting that analysis of plasma β endorphin was not successful, the absence of these data did not substantially affect our results. We originally planned to use plasma β endorphin as an indicator to define a therapeutic concentration range for morphine, because we believed that the MEC varied among patients. However, while pain rankings, morphine concentrations, and dosing rates were all patient-dependent, the MEC for morphine to induce changes in pain rankings was patient-independent. Pain perception is probably an indication of patients' central endorphin-like activity.[27,37,38] Even if plasma β-endorphin activity had varied among patients, our results would lead us to propose a single MEC for all patients. Total dose requirements were dependent upon each patient's perceived need to alleviate pain and, therefore, to maintain a plasma morphine concentration above 40 ng/mL.

Morphine Dosing Requirements. P.R.N. dosage regimens (such as PCA) are an excellent way to give the patient only as much drug as is required. It is possible that a continuous morphine concentration of 40 ng/mL (maintained by constant intravenous infusion) might prevent pain from becoming unbearable by providing sustained analgesic concentrations and anticipating pain stimuli. This research, however, also supports safely maintaining plasma morphine concentrations as high as 80 ng/mL in selected patients.

The small number of patients in this study and the fact that most patients were women limit the extent of our conclusions. The study results, however, substantiate our inference that the impetus for narcotic self-dosing during the postoperative period is primarily one of analgesia. If a patient reports pain and has no sedation or respiratory depression, studies suggest that withholding a dose of analgesic drug is not sensible and may compromise the patient's prognosis.[4,18,29]

Conclusion

Sedation, euphoria, and respiratory depression were not endpoints for self-dosing during the postoperative period in our study patients. This supports the concept that opiate use in the postoperative period will not lead to addiction. Total dose requirements of morphine were dependent upon the patients' perceived need to alleviate pain and, therefore, to maintain plasma morphine concentrations of at least 40 ng/mL. Adequate doses of narcotic analgesics should be made available to patients so that discomfort caused by undertreatment of pain does not occur.

---

[a] Euphoria is used in the vague but commonly understood sense of a feeling of well-being and implies a "high" feeling associated with recreational drug use.[12]

[b] ImmunoNuclear Corporation. Product information on plasma β endorphin by RIA. Stillwater, MN: 1983.

[c] Arrigo JM, Graves DA, Foster TS. College of Pharmacy, University of Kentucky. Manuscript in preparation. 1984 Nov.

References

1. Bennett RL, Batenhorst RL, Bivins BA et al. Patient-controlled analgesia: a new concept in postoperative pain relief. *Ann Surg.* 1982; 195:700–5.
2. Bennett RL, Batenhorst RL, Graves DA et al. Morphine titration in postoperative laparotomy patients using patient-controlled analgesia. *Curr Ther Res.* 1982; 8232:45–52.
3. Graves DA, Batenhorst RL, Bennett RL et al. Morphine requirements using patient-controlled analgesia: influence of diurnal variation and morbid obesity. *Clin Pharm.* 1983; 2: 49–53.
4. Graves DA, Foster TS, Batenhorst RL et al. Patient-controlled analgesia. *Ann Intern Med.* 1983; 99:360–6.
5. Keele KD. The pain chart. *Lancet.* 1948; 2:6–8.

6. Sriatanakul K, Kelvie W, Lasagna L. The quantification of pain: an analysis of words used to describe pain and analgesia in clinical trials. *Clin Pharmacol Ther.* 1982; 32:143–8.
7. Graves DA, Baumann TJ, Batenhorst RL et al. The relative dose indicator: a novel tool for clinical narcotic research. *Curr Ther Res.* 1984; 36:751–9.
8. Fraser HF, Van Horn GD, Martin WR et al. Methods for evaluating addiction liability. (A) "Attitude" of opiate addicts toward opiate-like drugs. (B) A short-term "direct" addiction test. *J Pharmacol Ther.* 1961; 133:371–87.
9. Haertzen CA, Hill HE, Belleville RE. Development of the addiction research center inventory (ARCI): selection of items that are sensitive to the effects of various drugs. *Psychopharmacologia.* 1963; 4:155–66.
10. Hill HE, Haertzen CA, Wolbach AB. The addiction research center inventory: standardization of scales which evaluate subjective effects of morphine, amphetamine, pentobarbital, alcohol, LSD-25, pyrahexyl, and chlorpromazine. *Psychopharmacologia.* 1963; 4:167–83.
11. Hill HE, Haertzen CA, Wolbach AB. The addiction research center inventory: appendix. *Psychopharmacologia.* 1963; 4: 183–205.
12. Martin WR, Fraser HF. A comparative study of physiological and subjective effects of heroin and morphine administered intravenously to postaddicts. *J Pharmacol Exp Ther.* 1961; 133:388–99.
13. Murphy MR, Hug CC. Pharmacokinetics of intravenous morphine in patients anesthetized with enflurane–nitrous oxide. *Anesthesiology.* 1981; 54:187–92.
14. Freund RJ, Littell RC. Covariance and heterogenicity of slopes. In: SAS for Linear Models. Cary, NC: Statistical Analysis System Institute, Inc.; 1981:187–205.
15. Davie IT, Slawson KB, Burt RA. A double-blind comparison of parenteral morphine, placebo, and oral fenoprofen in management of postoperative pain. *Anesth Analg.* 1982; 61: 1002–5.
16. Lanz E, Theiss D, Riess W et al. Epidural morphine for postoperative analgesia: a double-blind study. *Anesth Analg.* 1982; 61:236–40.
17. Alexander BK, Hadaway PF. Opiate addiction: the case for an adaptive orientation. *Psychol Bull.* 1982; 92:367–81.
18. Bennett RL, Batenhorst RL, Foster TS et al. Postoperative pulmonary function with patient-controlled analgesia. *Anesth Analg.* 1982; 61:171. Abstract.
19. Graves DA, Baumann TJ, Bennett RL et al. Extraordinary analgesic requirement in a patient previously unexposed to narcotics. *Drug Intell Clin Pharm.* 1984; 18:598–600.
20. Porter J, Jick H. Addiction rare in patients treated with narcotics. *N Engl J Med.* 1980; 302:123. Letter.
21. Keeri-Szanto M. Drugs or drums: what relieves postoperative pain? *Pain.* 1979; 6:217–30.
22. Peeters M, Brugmans J. Postoperative pain relief by demand analgesia. *Acta Anaesthesiol Belg.* 1980; 31 (Suppl):233–7.
23. Dahlstrom B, Tamsen A, Paalzow L et al. Patient-controlled analgesic therapy, part IV: pharmacokinetics and analgesic plasma concentrations of morphine. *Clin Pharmacokinet.* 1982; 7:266–79.
24. Tamsen A, Hartvig P, Fagerlund C et al. Patient-controlled analgesic therapy, part I: pharmacokinetics of pethidine in the pre- and postoperative periods. *Clin Pharmacokinet.* 1982; 7:149–63.
25. Tamsen A, Hartvig P, Fagerlund C et al. Patient-controlled analgesic therapy, part II: individual analgesic demand and analgesic plasma concentrations of pethidine in postoperative pain. *Clin Pharmacokinet.* 1982; 7:164–75.
26. Tamsen A, Hartvig P, Fagerlund C et al. Patient-controlled analgesic therapy, part III: pharmacokinetics and analgesic plasma concentrations of ketobemidone. *Clin Pharmacokinet.* 1982; 7:252–65.
27. Laitinen L, Kanto J, Vapaavuori M et al. Morphine concentrations in plasma after intramuscular administration. *Br J Anaesth.* 1975; 47:1265–7.
28. Sawe J, Dahlstrom B, Rane A. Steady-state kinetics and analgesic effect of oral morphine in cancer patients. *Eur J Clin Pharmacol.* 1983; 24:537–42.
29. Nayman J. Measurement and control of postoperative pain. *Ann R Coll Surg Engl.* 1979; 61:419–26.
30. Tamsen A, Sakurada T, Wahlstrom A et al. Postoperative demand for analgesic in relation to individual levels of endorphins and substance P in cerebrospinal fluid. *Pain.* 1982; 13:171–83.
31. Pannuti F, Rossi AP, Iafelice G et al. Control of chronic pain in very advanced cancer patients with morphine hydrochloride administered by oral, rectal, and sublingual routes. *Pharmacol Res Commun.* 1982; 14:369–81.
32. Sawe J, Dahlstrom B, Paalzow L et al. Morphine kinetics in cancer patients. *Clin Pharmacol Ther.* 1981; 30:629–35.
33. Stanski DR, Greenblatt DJ, Lappas DG et al. Kinetics of high-dose intravenous morphine in cardiac surgery patients. *Clin Pharmacol Ther.* 1976; 24:752–6.
34. Stanski DR, Greenblatt DJ, Lowenstein E. Kinetics of intravenous and intramuscular morphine. *Clin Pharmacol Ther.* 1978; 24:52–9.
35. Gibaldi M, Perrier D. Pharmacokinetics. 2nd ed. New York: Marcel Dekker, Inc.; 1982.
36. Terenius L. Clinical aspects. In: Malick JB, Bell RMS, eds. Endorphins: chemistry, physiology, pharmacology, and clinical relevance. New York: Marcel Dekker, Inc.; 1983: 229–49.
37. Oyama T, Jin T, Yamaya R. Profound analgesic effects of beta endorphin in man. *Lancet.* 1980; 1:122–4.
38. Rossier J, French ED, Rivier C et al. Foot-shock-induced stress increases beta endorphin levels in brain but not blood. *Nature.* 1977; 270:618–20.

Efficacy of patient-controlled versus conventional analgesia for postoperative pain

STEPHEN J. BOLLISH, CAROL L. COLLINS, DUANE M. KIRKING, AND ROBERT H. BARTLETT

Abstract: Patient-controlled i.v. administration and intramuscular administration of morphine sulfate were compared in a crossover study to determine their relative effectiveness in relieving postoperative pain.

Twenty adult patients scheduled for abdominal surgery were randomly assigned to one of two groups; one group received i.v. morphine sulfate for 24 hours using a patient-controlled analgesia (PCA) device, after which they were given morphine sulfate i.m. for 24 hours. The treatment order was reversed for the other group. Amount of narcotic administered, respiratory rate, and levels of discomfort, activity, and sedation were assessed by the nursing staff every two hours. At the end of each 24-hour treatment phase, patients ranked their level of pain, amount of pain relief, level of sedation, ability to sleep, and ability to perform pulmonary toilet. Patients were also asked whether they preferred PCA or i.m. analgesic therapy for future surgery.

Patients reported significantly less discomfort while using PCA than during i.m. morphine administration. No significant differences in amount of narcotic used, respiratory rate, nausea and vomiting, or levels of activity or sedation were noted for the two regimens. Patients' rankings of the two treatment modes did not differ significantly, but a majority of patients indicated a preference for future use of PCA.

In these postoperative patients, administration of i.v. morphine sulfate by PCA was as safe as i.m. administration and possibly more effective in relieving pain.

Index terms: Analgesics and antipyretics; Drug administration; Drug administration routes; Morphine sulfate; Pain; Toxicity
Clin Pharm: 1985; 4:48–52

Recent reviews have documented the inadequacy of the current standard methods of administering injectable narcotics.[1–3] Patient-controlled analgesia (PCA) is a relatively new and promising technique for administering injectable narcotic analgesics. In this technique, patients activate an electronic syringe pump connected to their i.v. line when they feel the need for analgesia. The frequency of administration is controlled by an adjustable lockout mechanism that prevents the patient from receiving drug for a predefined period (usually 5–10 minutes) following each dose.

Published studies regarding PCA have shown that the technique offers excellent analgesic efficacy and safety, minimal sedation, decreased narcotic requirement, and little or no respiratory depression.[4–7] In their recent review of 41 studies on PCA, Graves et al[1] found numerous studies examining the efficacy of PCA. However, few investigations compared the effectiveness of PCA with the effectiveness of conventional analgesia; none of the investigations compared the two methods using a crossover design. In most comparative studies, the use of PCA was limited to the postoperative recovery room or the labor and delivery room.[8,9] Such limitations prevent application of the results of those studies to the general patient population.

In a recent prospective trial of PCA, 24 patients scheduled for abdominal surgical procedures were randomly assigned to receive morphine either by the intramuscular route or by PCA for 60 hours beginning in the postoperative recovery room and continuing in the general-care ward.[10] The group using PCA maintained an adequate state of analgesia without sedation with a significantly greater frequency than did the group receiving morphine intramuscularly. Another study of the same patient sample revealed potentially improved pulmonary function during the postoperative period in the group using PCA.[11]

Because of the lack of comparative trials, we used a crossover study design to compare the effective-

STEPHEN J. BOLLISH, PHARM.D., is Pharmacy Services Coordinator, IMED Corporation, San Diego, CA; at the time of this study, he was Clinical Pharmacist—Surgery, University of Michigan Hospitals, and Clinical Assistant Professor of Pharmacy, College of Pharmacy, University of Michigan, Ann Arbor. CAROL L. COLLINS, PHARM.D., is Clinical Pharmacist—Home Care, and Clinical Instructor, College of Pharmacy, University of Michigan; at the time of this study, she was a Clinical Pharmacy Resident, University of Michigan Hospitals, Ann Arbor. DUANE M. KIRKING, PHARM.D., PH.D., is Assistant Professor of Pharmacy Administration, College of Pharmacy, and Assistant Professor of Medical Care Organization, School of Public Health, University of Michigan. ROBERT H. BARTLETT, M.D., is Section Head, General Surgery, and Professor of Surgery, College of Medicine, University of Michigan.

Address reprint requests to Dr. Collins at the Department of Pharmacy Services, University of Michigan Hospitals, Box 006, 1405 East Ann Street, Ann Arbor, MI 48109.

Presented at the Clinical Research Forum, 19th Annual ASHP Midyear Clinical Meeting, Dallas, TX, December 4, 1984.

ness of PCA with the effectiveness of conventional intramuscular administration of narcotic analgesics for the relief of postoperative pain in patients on the general-care ward. Specific factors evaluated were differences in narcotic use, side effects, sedation, relief of pain, and overall patient preference for PCA or conventional therapy.

Methods

The protocol for this study was approved by the human investigations committee of the University of Michigan Hospitals. Twenty adult patients scheduled for elective abdominal surgery under general anesthesia were admitted to the study. Written informed consent was obtained from each patient. Patients were excluded from the study for the following reasons:

- Impaired mental status during a preoperative interview conducted by the primary investigators in consultation with the medical and nursing staffs,
- History of chronic obstructive pulmonary disease,
- Marked metabolic disorders, such as sepsis or severe fluid or electrolyte abnormalities,
- Use of psychoactive drugs within 72 hours before surgery,
- Psychologic disorders,
- History of narcotic drug abuse,
- Allergy to morphine sulfate, or
- An expected postoperative course in the intensive-care unit.

The amount of prestudy narcotic use was recorded as milligrams of morphine sulfate or morphine-sulfate equivalent given to each patient preoperatively, intraoperatively, and in the postoperative recovery room. Meperidine hydrochloride 100 mg or fentanyl citrate 0.2 mg was considered equipotent with 10 mg of morphine sulfate.[12] The study period began immediately upon the patient's return to the ward from the recovery room. Patients were assigned alternately into one of two groups. Patients in group 1 used PCA to administer morphine for 24 hours, after which they were given morphine i.m. for 24 hours. The treatment order was reversed for patients in group 2.

Patients were instructed in the proper use of the PCA device the night before surgery and again at the time the device was connected to their i.v. line. The PCA device[a] consisted of a 50-mL syringe pump filled with morphine sulfate 2 mg/mL. The device was activated by a push button similar to a nurse call button. The device could be set to deliver from 0.25 to 4.0 mg of morphine sulfate per activation with a lockout period of 0–10 minutes. The initial setting for all patients in this study was a dose of morphine sulfate 1 mg per activation with a 10-minute lockout period. The device recorded the number of administration attempts and the number of doses actually given. If a patient attempted two more injections than were allowed per two-hour dosing interval, the lockout period was reduced to five minutes.

During the 24 hours of conventional morphine administration, house physicians were instructed to prescribe morphine sulfate according to their usual custom. Typically, orders were written for morphine sulfate 6–10 mg i.m. every four to six hours as needed. No sedatives, hypnotics, or antiemetic drugs were allowed during the study period.

The nursing staff completed a bedside assessment of each patient every two hours throughout the 48-hour study period. Using a 10-point scale, the nurses assessed patient sedation (1 = wide awake, 10 = deep sleep) and activity (1 = sleeping, 10 = active as if had no surgery). Discomfort was assessed by orally asking patients to rank their pain on a scale of 1 to 10 (1 = very comfortable, 10 = severe pain). The nursing staff did not awaken the patient to determine discomfort level if the patient was obviously sleeping. The nurses also noted the number of narcotic doses given and the respiratory rate. Following each nursing assessment, the "attempts" and "doses given" recorders on the PCA device were set back to zero. The nursing staff also noted any nausea, vomiting, or hypotension.

At the end of each 24-hour treatment period, each patient was asked (orally) to rank on a 10-point scale the level of pain, degree of pain relief, level of sedation, ability to sleep, and ability to carry out routine postoperative pulmonary toilet. At the end of the 48-hour study period, the patients also indicated on a similar 10-point scale their preference of PCA or conventional analgesic therapy for a future surgery.

Demographic characteristics of patients in group 1 and group 2 were compared using a two-tailed Student's t test for paired data. Objective data concerning narcotic use and respiratory rates were evaluated using a two-tailed analysis of variance for crossover design. Mean subjective nursing and patient rankings were evaluated using a two-tailed Wilcoxon rank sum test for two-period crossover design.[13] Results were considered statistically significant at $p < 0.05$.

Results

One patient did not need i.v. therapy by the second postoperative day and was excluded from evaluation. Another patient was then included. No patient required adjustment of the lockout interval based on need for more drug.

Characteristics of the patients in groups 1 and 2 are presented in Table 1. There were no significant intergroup differences in age, weight, body surface area, or prestudy use of morphine sulfate or its equivalent. The mean (±S.D.) age was 49.8 ± 14.2 years for group 1 and 48.9 ± 22.3 years for group 2. The mean weight was 62.7 ± 12.2 kg for group 1 and 67.1 ± 14.9 kg for group 2. The mean body surface area was 1.68 ± 0.14 sq m for group 1 and 1.74 ± 0.14

sq m for group 2.

Data for patient morphine use and respiratory rate and nursing assessments of patient sedation, activity, and discomfort are summarized in Table 2. Patients using PCA reported significantly less discomfort than did patients receiving i.m. morphine. Activity level was significantly different between day 1 and day 2 for all patients. Figure 1 illustrates the results of the nursing assessments of patient activity, discomfort, and sedation during PCA and conventional analgesia. Sixty-five percent of the patients had discomfort rankings of 1–3 while receiving PCA, but only 38% of patients had rankings of 1–3 during conventional analgesia. Discomfort rankings of 4–6 were reported for 28% of patients receiving PCA and 45% of patients receiving conventional analgesia. Discomfort rankings were in the range of 7–10 in 6% of patients using PCA and 17% using conventional analgesia.

The results of the patient questionnaire are shown in Table 3. Mean responses did not differ significantly by treatment type, treatment sequence, or study day. Patients indicated a preference for using PCA during future surgery (Table 4); the mean ranking (±S.D.) for preference of PCA versus conventional analgesic therapy was 3.1 ± 2.49.

Nausea and vomiting were reported by three (15%) patients using PCA and seven (35%) patients receiving conventional analgesia. Euphoria was reported by two (10%) patients using PCA versus four (20%) patients receiving conventional analgesia. No incidents of respiratory depression or hypotension were reported during either treatment. Nausea was reported by the nurse on one occasion with PCA and three occasions with conventional administration.

Table 1.
Characteristics of Study Patients

Age (yr)	Weight (kg)	BSA[a] (sq m)	Prestudy Narcotic Use (mg)[b]	Surgical Procedure
Group 1				
27	45.0	1.45	20.0	Colostomy revision
52	56.8	1.55	4.0	Anal sphinctero-plasty and colostomy
47	74.1	1.77	9.0	Colostomy closure
30	55.5	1.64	12.0	Ileostomy revision and ileal resection
56	80.7	1.95	16.3	Takedown of jejuno-ileo bypass
58	65.4	1.64	42.0	Partial gastrectomy
67	56.4	1.57	0	Enterolysis, exploratory laparotomy
55	82.7	2.09	13.0	Splenectomy, staging laparotomy
38	52.7	1.52	8.0	Choledochoduo-denostomy
68	60.9	1.65	17.5	Cholecystectomy
Group 2				
25	79.5	2.0	22.0	Appendectomy
67	96.4	1.99	2.5	Choledochoje-junostomy
75	59.1	1.58	9.0	Proctocolectomy
30	68.2	1.79	10.0	Highly selective vagotomy
25	47.7	1.49	26.0	Vagotomy and antrectomy
69	54.5	1.55	15.5	Hepatic artery catheter pump placement
64	63.6	1.69	12.0	Cholecystectomy
73	52.0	1.51	24.5	Sigmoid colectomy
25	77.7	1.82	6.0	Cholecystectomy
36	71.8	1.97	11.0	Cholecystectomy

[a] Body surface area.

[b] Prestudy narcotic use is reported as the total morphine sulfate equivalent given preoperatively, intraoperatively, and in the recovery room. Mean (±S.D.) values were 14.2 ± 11.5 mg for group 1 and 13.9 ± 7.9 for group 2.

Discussion

The results of this study indicate that PCA is a promising alternative to conventional intramuscular administration of narcotics for the relief of postoperative pain. Meaningful comparisons of narcotic use, side effects, sedation, pain relief, and patient preferences were possible in this study because each patient received both treatments. A possible limitation of this and all similar comparative studies to date is that neither patients nor nurses were blinded to study treatment, a condition that would be almost impossible to achieve.

Patients' rankings of amount of pain relief, col-

Table 2.
Nurses' Assessments of Patient Morphine Use, Respiratory Rate, Discomfort, Sedation, and Activity[a]

Variable	Treatment: PCA[b]	Treatment: Conventional	Group: 1	Group: 2	Period: Day 1	Period: Day 2
Morphine use (mg/24 hr)	34.1 ± 22.4	37.3 ± 21.4	29.1 ± 17.9	42.3 ± 23.5	38.0 ± 21.5	33.3 ± 22.2
Respiratory rate (per min)	18.5 ± 2.1	18.6 ± 2.0	19.2 ± 2.1	17.9 ± 1.6	18.6 ± 2.0	18.5 ± 2.1
Discomfort[c]	3.2 ± 1.1	4.2 ± 1.6	3.2 ± 1.2	4.2 ± 1.5	3.8 ± 2.5	3.6 ± 1.3
Sedation[c]	2.4 ± 0.9	2.5 ± 0.8	2.6 ± 0.8	2.4 ± 0.9	2.7 ± 1.0	2.3 ± 0.8
Activity[c]	3.6 ± 1.1	3.5 ± 1.0	3.4 ± 1.0	3.8 ± 1.1	3.2 ± 1.0	3.9 ± 1.0

[a] Values reported as mean ± S.D.

[b] Patient-controlled analgesia.

[c] As measured on a 10-point scale where 1 is less and 10 is greater, as explained in detail in the text.

Figure 1. Nursing assessment of patient discomfort (A), sedation (B), and activity (C) during □ PCA and ▧ conventional analgesia.

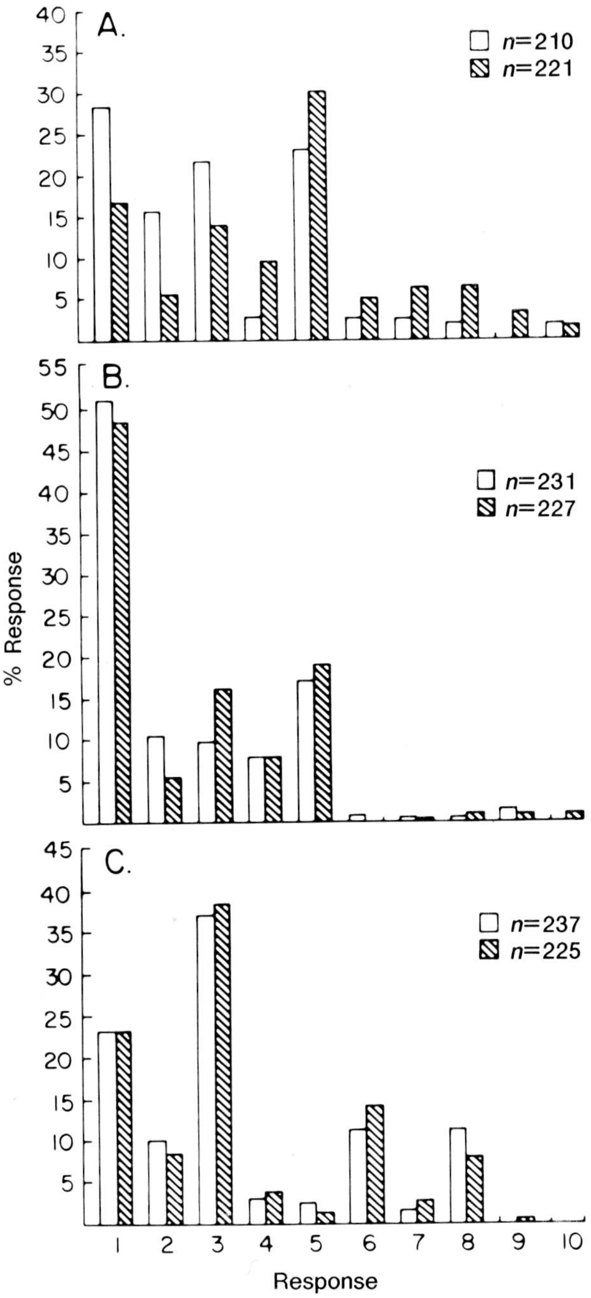

lected at the end of each treatment period, were not consistent with the every-two-hour assessments reported by the patients to the nurses. It is reasonable to hypothesize, however, that data collected in close temporal proximity to the pain experienced provide a more accurate assessment of that pain.

Patients using PCA received 9% less morphine than did patients receiving i.m. therapy, but this difference was not statistically significant. Because there was a large intersubject variation in narcotic use, a significant difference in the mean amount of morphine used during the two treatments would be difficult to detect in a small patient population unless the differences between the treatments were marked. The lack of difference in narcotic use between the two treatments confirmed a previous report.[7]

PCA was found to be a safe alternative to conventional intramuscular administration of narcotic analgesics in this study. No member of either treatment group suffered severe respiratory depression or hypotension. Nausea and vomiting occurred less frequently with PCA. However, care must be used in interpreting the incidence of nausea and vomiting since both conditions are common following abdominal surgery and may be related to residual effects of general anesthesia or mechanical problems with the nasogastric tube.

In contrast to a previous study that analyzed observations made between the hours of 0600 and 2200,[10] no differences in nursing evaluations of sedation and activity were found. Although this study reports results obtained during 24-hour periods, an analysis using only the 0600–2200 observations also revealed no significant differences between the two treatment groups. A significant improvement in activity for all patients on day 2 was noted by the nursing staff. This result is not surprising because patients are generally noted to be more active as they recover from surgery.

The responses to the patient questionnaire (Table 3) failed to show a significant difference between PCA and conventional analgesia; this may be related to the inability of a study with a small sample size to detect differences in treatments with large intersubject variation. Despite our inability to show a difference in the two treatments, most patients indicated that they would prefer to use PCA for future surgery. Patients particularly liked the ability to control their own level of analgesia without having to rely on the nursing staff.

Conclusion

In this study population, i.v. morphine administration by PCA was shown to be as safe as i.m. administration and possibly more effective in relieving pain. No differences in amount of narcotic use, side effects, sedation, or activity level were noted, and the majority of patients preferred PCA for a future surgery. Studies examining the effect of PCA versus conventional therapy on nursing time requirements, postoperative complication rate, and length of hospital stay are needed to determine the cost-effectiveness of PCA.

[a] Med Fusion Inc., 2009 Flightway Drive, Atlanta, GA 30341. This device is not currently commercially available.

Table 3.
Results of Patient Questionnaire[a]

Variable	Treatment		Group		Period	
	PCA[b]	Conventional	1	2	Day 1	Day 2
Level of pain[c]	6.4 ± 2.0	6.2 ± 2.3	5.7 ± 1.5	6.8 ± 2.5	6.7 ± 2.4	5.9 ± 1.9
Pulmonary toilet[d]	4.3 ± 2.4	4.8 ± 2.7	3.8 ± 2.2	5.2 ± 2.3	5.2 ± 2.5	4.0 ± 2.0
Ability to sleep[e]	5.8 ± 1.7	5.7 ± 2.5	5.5 ± 1.4	5.9 ± 2.7	5.5 ± 2.5	6.0 ± 1.6
Relief of pain[f]	4.1 ± 1.6	4.8 ± 1.9	4.3 ± 2.1	4.5 ± 1.4	4.4 ± 1.6	4.4 ± 1.9
Level of sedation[g]	4.9 ± 1.0	5.4 ± 1.9	4.6 ± 1.2	5.7 ± 1.6	5.5 ± 1.7	4.8 ± 1.2

[a] Reported as mean ± S.D.
[b] Patient-controlled analgesia.
[c] Measured on a scale of 1–10 where 1 is "normal or no pain" and 10 is "worst pain I have ever felt."
[d] Measured on a scale of 1–10 where 1 is "able to do pulmonary toilet with no pain" and 10 is "unable to do pulmonary toilet because of pain."
[e] Measured on a scale of 1–10 where 1 is "sleep much more than normal" and 10 is "unable to sleep because of pain."
[f] Measured on a scale of 1–10 where 1 is "very good, no pain" and 10 is "pain intolerable."
[g] Measured on a scale of 1–10 where 1 is "wide awake" and 10 is "sleep all the time."

Table 4.
Patient Preference of Patient-Controlled or Conventional Analgesia for Future Surgery

Ranking	No. Patients (% of Total)
1—Much prefer PCA	6 (30)
2	5 (25)
3	3 (15)
4	2 (10)
5	1 (5)
6	1 (5)
7	0 (0)
8	1 (5)
9	0 (0)
10—Much prefer conventional therapy	1 (5)

References

1. Graves DA, Foster TS, Batenhorst RL et al. Patient-controlled analgesia. *Ann Intern Med.* 1983; 99:360–6.
2. Bennett RL, Griffen WO. Patient controlled analgesia. *Contemp Surg.* 1983; 23:75–89.
3. Austin KL, Stupelton JU, Mather LE. Multiple intramuscular injections: a major source of variability in analgesic response to meperidine. *Pain.* 1980; 8:47–62.
4. Chakravarty K, Tucker W, Rosen M. Comparison of buprenorphine and pethidine given intravenously on demand to relieve postoperative pain. *Br Med J.* 1979; 2:895–7.
5. Tamsen A, Hartvig P, Dahlstrom B et al. Patient controlled analgesic therapy in the early postoperative period. *Acta Anaesthesiol Scand.* 1979; 23:462–70.
6. Bennett RL, Batenhorst RL, Graves DA et al. Morphine titration in postoperative laparotomy patients using patient-controlled analgesia. *Curr Ther Res.* 1982; 32:45–52.
7. Bennett RL, Batenhorst RL, Bivins BA et al. Drug use pattern in patient-controlled analgesia. *Anesthesiology.* 1982; 57:210. Abstract.
8. Keeri-Szanto M, Heaman S. Postoperative demand analgesia. *Surg Gynecol Obstet.* 1952; 134:647–51.
9. Robinson JO, Rosen M, Evans JM et al. Self administered intravenous and intramuscular pethidine: a controlled trial in labour. *Anaesthesia.* 1950; 35:763–70.
10. Bennett RL, Batenhorst RL, Bivins BA et al. Patient-controlled analgesia: a new concept of postoperative pain relief. *Ann Surg.* 1982; 195:700–5.
11. Bennett RL, Batenhorst RL, Foster TS et al. Postoperative pulmonary function with patient-controlled analgesia. *Anesth Analg.* 1982; 61:171. Abstract.
12. Evans RP, DuBé JE. Pain. In: Katcher BS, Young LY, Koda-Kimble MA, eds. Applied therapeutics: the clinical use of drugs. San Francisco: Applied Therapeutics, Inc; 1983:52.
13. Koch GG. The use of non-parametric methods in the statistical analysis of the two-period changeover design. *Biometrics.* 1972; 28:577–84.

Analgesia with oral narcotics and added ibuprofen in cancer patients

WENDY A. WEINGART, CHRISTINE A. SORKNESS, AND ROBERT H. EARHART

Abstract: A scheduled regimen of oral narcotic analgesics was compared with a regimen of oral narcotic analgesics plus ibuprofen for analgesic efficacy in patients with cancer.

Ten patients with metastatic cancer were randomly assigned to receive either ibuprofen 400 mg or a look-alike placebo four times daily in addition to each patient's existing regimen of scheduled oral narcotics. A two-period changeover study design was used. The 24-hour narcotic intake equated to injectable morphine was computed for each patient at baseline and during the nine study days. A visual analogue scale was used to evaluate pain relief, nausea, mood depression, daytime drowsiness and nighttime sleeplessness.

The analgesic efficacy of the narcotic–ibuprofen combination was significantly greater than the analgesic efficacy of the narcotic–placebo combination. Eight patients demonstrated a positive treatment effect with added ibuprofen; the overall improvement in analgesia averaged 39.1% in these patients. There was no significant increase from baseline in the incidence of nausea, mood depression, daytime drowsiness or nighttime sleeplessness.

At the doses used in this study, a treatment regimen of oral narcotic analgesics plus ibuprofen was more effective than oral narcotics alone in relieving pain associated with cancer.

Index terms: Analgesics and antipyretics; Combined therapy; Ibuprofen; Opiates; Pain; Toxicity
Clin Pharm. 1985; 4:53–8

Pain associated with terminal cancer is usually chronic, and the presence of pain has an important adverse influence on the quality of life for patients with cancer. The perception of pain is a function of two characteristics: the actual physical neoplastic insult experienced by the patient, and the psychological and environmental influences, age, and sex of the patient.[1]

In one of the few published studies of the prevalence and severity of cancer pain, Cleeland and Daut[2] found that 17% and 56% of the 123 and 341 patients with nonmetastatic and metastatic cancer, respectively, reported pain caused by their cancer. Patients with metastatic disease generally reported greater severity of pain than patients with nonmetastatic cancer. Some degree of interference with daily activities and enjoyment of life was reported by 34% of patients with metastatic breast or prostate cancer. These findings exemplify the depth of the problems of pain experienced by patients with cancer.

Narcotic analgesics have been the mainstay of pharmacologic therapy for moderate to severe chronic cancer pain. The adverse effects of chronic narcotic use are well known; they include severe constipation and drowsiness that may be serious enough to hinder the ability of patients to perform daily activities. Narcotics used for treatment of cancer pain may be administered on an as-needed or a scheduled basis depending upon the severity and duration of the patient's pain and the philosophy of the prescriber. The as-needed administration of narcotic medications can create an operant conditioning effect, in which patients require increasingly larger total daily doses of narcotic for adequate pain relief, and patients subsequently may develop an increased tolerance to the narcotics.[1,3–5] Thus, a "roller-coaster" effect of pain relief and inadequate pain relief may be established. Patients anticipate the recurrence of pain, and this anticipation creates increased anxiety and can increase the perceived pain itself.

The administration of narcotics on a time-contingent (scheduled) basis does not result in operant conditioning.[3–5] Because patients are not required to re-experience pain before each dose of the narcotic is administered, the reduction in anxiety may decrease the amount of analgesic required to alle-

WENDY A. WEINGART, M.S., is Clinical Data Coordinator, Medical College of Wisconsin, Milwaukee, WI; at the time of this study, she was Clinical Assistant Professor of Pharmacy, University of Wisconsin–Madison. CHRISTINE A. SORKNESS, PHARM.D., is Clinical Associate Professor of Pharmacy, University of Wisconsin–Madison. ROBERT H. EARHART, M.D., is Clinical Research Physician, Cancer Research Unit, The Upjohn Company, Kalamazoo, MI; at the time of this study, he was Assistant Professor of Medicine, Division of Oncology, University of Wisconsin–Madison.

Address reprint requests to Dr. Sorkness at the University of Wisconsin School of Pharmacy, 425 North Charter Street, Madison, WI 53706.

The assistance of Jim M. Koeller, M.S.; Joseph A. Theisen; the Department of Pharmacy, University of Wisconsin Hospital and Clinics; the Department of Biostatistics, Clinical Cancer Center, University of Wisconsin; and The Upjohn Company is acknowledged.

Supported in part by The Upjohn Company.

Presented at the Clinical Research Forum, 19th Annual ASHP Midyear Clinical Meeting, Dallas, TX, December 4, 1984.

viate the pain. The scheduled administration of narcotic analgesics by themselves, however, may not provide adequate analgesia for moderate to severe chronic cancer pain. The total daily dose of narcotic may be limited by the appearance of side effects; alternatively, patients with metastatic pain, especially pain caused by bony metastases, may not receive adequate pain relief from even the largest therapeutic doses of narcotics.[3-7]

Because narcotics frequently provide inadequate analgesia in patients with chronic pain from malignancy, health practitioners have investigated other avenues of analgesic therapy. One alternative to traditional narcotic therapy involves the concurrent use of nonsteroidal anti-inflammatory drugs (NSAIDs). The objective of this study was to determine the relative oral analgesic efficacy of a scheduled regimen of narcotic analgesics versus the same scheduled narcotic regimen plus ibuprofen in chronic cancer pain.

Methods

The study was conducted at the Unviersity of Wisconsin Hospital and Clinics (UWHC) in Madison, WI, in accordance with the ethical standards of the hospital's human subjects committee. The subjects were hospitalized patients and ambulatory patients under the medical supervision of the oncology department. Informed consent was obtained from each patient by the patient's primary physician before the patient was permitted to participate in the study.

Men and women between 16 and 70 years of age with malignant solid tumors and no previous history of allergy or severe adverse reactions to any of the study drugs were eligible to participate in the study. Patients younger than 16 years or older than 70 years were permitted to participate if specific permission was granted by the primary physician. Patients whose pain was not ideally controlled on their current scheduled oral narcotic regimens were eligible for study participation. Patients receiving chemotherapy were not excluded. General medical criteria for patients entering the study included adequate hepatic function, defined as a serum bilirubin concentration ≤ 2.0 mg/dL and serum glutamic oxaloacetic transaminase (SGOT) and lactic acid dehydrogenase (LDH) concentrations less than two times normal values; adequate renal function, defined as a serum blood urea nitrogen (BUN) concentration ≤ 40 mg/dL and a serum creatinine concentration ≤ 1.5 mg/dL; and adequate coagulation status, defined as a platelet count $>75,000$ and a prothrombin time less than two times normal value.

All patients received one or more oral narcotic analgesics on a set, scheduled basis in dosages predetermined by their physicians on all nine days of the study. Patients received either five or six daily doses of narcotic on an every-four-hour dosing schedule; doses were given either 0400 through 2400 or 0800 through 2400. This flexibility in every-four-hour narcotic dosing was necessary, since some patients could sleep well for eight hours nightly and did not require an 0400 dose of narcotic. No changes were made in the narcotic regimen of any patient during the study period.

Using random number tables, patients were assigned by the hospital's investigational drug pharmacist to one of two ibuprofen treatment groups. Each patient received ibuprofen 400 mg or a look-alike placebo four times daily at 0800, 1200, 1800, and 2400 in one of two randomly assigned sequences[8,9]:

- Ibuprofen 400 mg q.i.d. on days 1–3, followed immediately by placebo q.i.d. on days 4–6, followed immediately by the initial regimen of ibuprofen on days 7–9; or
- Placebo q.i.d. on days 1–3, followed immediately by ibuprofen 400 mg q.i.d. on days 4–6, followed immediately by the initial regimen of placebo on days 7–9.

The study was conducted in a double-blind fashion with neither the investigators nor the patients knowing which ibuprofen regimen was used. No p.r.n. doses of narcotic or nonnarcotic analgesics were permitted during the nine days of the study.

Patients whose pain was controlled with nonnarcotic analgesics alone, patients who required only p.r.n. doses of narcotics, and patients who needed injectable narcotics for adequate pain control were excluded from the study. Patients who required doses of narcotics in addition to those provided in the study protocol were excluded from further participation. Also excluded were patients who were totally bedridden (as defined by Eastern Cooperative Oncology Group performance status of 4), since their cooperation in completing multiple pain assessments could not be assured. Additional exclusion criteria included the following: (1) active peptic ulcer disease or gastrointestinal bleeding; (2) concurrent cordotomy, transcutaneous nerve stimulation, alcohol hypophysectomy, local anesthetic injections or blocks, or palliative radiotherapy during the study period; and (3) concurrent therapy with antidepressants, benzodiazepines, sedative–hypnotics, amphetamines, tetrahydrocannabinol, hydroxyzine, anti-inflammatory agents, or nonnarcotic analgesics, any of which might have influenced analgesia.

The visual analogue method was used to evaluate five patient variables: pain relief, nausea, mood depression, daytime drowsiness, and nighttime sleeplessness. The visual analogue scale ranges from 0 to 100.[10-12] For each patient, the degree of pain relief, nausea, and mood depression was assessed six times daily at 0800, 1000, 1200, 1800, 2000, and 2400 on days 1, 3, 6, and 9 of the study. On those same days, an assessment of sleeplessness was made at 0800 and evaluations of drowsiness were performed at 1000, 1200, 1800, and 2000. All variables were also evaluated at baseline before each patient's initiation into the study. We determined that a rating of 35.0 out of 100.0 for nausea, mood depression, daytime drowsiness, and nighttime sleeplessness would be considered clinically important since this rating would indicate more than mild disturbance.

Medications for hospitalized patients were administered by the nurses or pharmacy technicians according to the policies and procedures of the UWHC unit dose system. Compliance was verified by a study investigator using tablet counts and appropriate charting of medication administration. At the time of each variable evaluation, an investigator blinded to the patient's group assignment distributed the appropriate evaluation form to the hospitalized patients, who completed the evaluation forms and returned them to the investigator.

Outpatient study participants were given one multiple-dose bottle containing a nine-day supply of the narcotic medication. They also received individual daily bottles of ibuprofen (nine bottles with four tablets in each bottle, labeled for days 1 through 9 of the study). Compliance was assessed by tablet counts throughout the study period; outpatients were also given "self-administration" schedules listing medication administration and evaluation times. Outpatients were given a full supply of evaluation sheets along with individual postage-paid return envelopes. They were instructed to fill out an evaluation sheet at each specified time, to enclose the individual evaluation form in an envelope immediately after it was completed, and to mail the form back to the investigators. This procedure minimized bias from comparison of pain ratings between consecutive evaluation times.

The 24-hour narcotic intake equated to injectable morphine was computed for each patient at baseline and during the study according to the Wisconsin Palliative Medication Profile (WPMP).[a] All data were collected on standardized data collection sheets and analyzed on the Sperry Univac 1100 Series Computer at the Wisconsin Clinical Cancer Center in Madison. The overall efficacy of the two therapeutic regimens was analyzed using the two-sample Wilcoxon Test.[b] The a priori level of significance was $p \leq 0.05$. The incidence of nausea, mood depression, daytime drowsiness, and nighttime sleeplessness for the two regimens was compared with baseline using the one-tailed chi-square test of proportions.

Results

Four of the 14 patients entered into the study failed to complete it. Patient 3 cited nausea as the reason for failing to complete the study. Patient 6 was unable to continue after day 3 because of an acute change in respiratory status requiring continuous oxygen and injectable morphine; this patient died the following day for reasons unrelated to study participation. Patient 7 withdrew from the study after day 1 because she "did not wish to continue at this time," and patient 1 resigned on day 1 without stating a reason. The four patients who resigned from the study were all women with solid tumors who ranged from 45 to 56 years of age (mean, 50.0 ± 4.1). Their baseline pain ratings and narcotic use were similar to those of the patients who completed the study.

Of the 10 patients who completed the study, five were men and five were women (Table 1). The study patients ranged in age from 39 to 67 years (mean 55.3 ± 8.5). The duration of their disease from initial diagnosis was 4–240 months (mean 55.3 ± 69.0). All the patients had metastatic disease, and six had bony involvement. Patient 8 and patient 10 were inpatients during the nine-day protocol; patient 2 and patient 12 were outpatients. The six remaining patients began the study while hospitalized and completed the evaluations at home upon discharge. A total of 177 of 180 evaluation forms were satisfactorily completed by the 10 study patients.

Table 1.
Description of Study Patients

Patient No.	Age (yr)	Sex	Diagnosis (Duration of Disease in Months)	Metastases Sites	Primary Pain Location
2	39	F	Adenocarcinoma breast (60)	Left humerus, femur, chest wall, skull	Left hip, skull
4	47	M	Adenocarcinoma colon (12)	Abdominal wall, presacrum	Lower back, hip
5	49	F	Infiltrating ductal carcinoma left breast (96)	Bone, chest wall	Left chest wall
8	46	F	Epidermoid squamous cell cervical carcinoma (240)	Pelvic sinus tract, pelvic bone	Gluteus, left hip
9	54	M	Leiomyosarcoma left pelvis (4)	Bone (L_3,L_4), left acetabulum, left iliac crest	Abdomen (lower left quadrant), left hip
10	67	F	Endometrial adenocanthoma (8)	Local extension, chest	Abdomen
11	63	M	Lung adenocarcinoma (72)	Bone, T_{10-11}	Lower back, left leg
12	56	F	Rectal adenocarcinoma (48)	Local extension, lung	Rectal area
13	59	M	Transitional cell bladder carcinoma (8)	Local extension, liver/spleen, iliac nodes	Lower back
14	63	M	Malignant melanoma (5)	Local extension, lymph nodes, scalp, lung	Right shoulder

All 10 patients had primary pain locations apparently related to the primary tumor or areas of metastases (Table 1). Thus, the investigators classified all of the patients in the first category of origin of pain described by Foley,[1] that of pain attributed to direct tumor involvement.

The patients' mean baseline pain rating just before entry into the study protocol was 44.4 ± 26.4 (range, 5.6–96.5) on a visual analogue scale from 0.0 through 100.0. The mean baseline 24-hour narcotic intake equated to injectable morphine according to the WPMP was 31 ± 17.6 mg (range, 12–60 mg) (Table 2). During the nine-day study period, the mean 24-hour narcotic intake equated to injectable morphine was 38.3 ± 18.8 mg (range, 12–70 mg).

Only three patients received chemotherapy during their study participation. No other medications implicated in influencing analgesia were administered to the patients during participation in the study.

For the 10 patients who completed the study, the randomization procedure resulted in an even distribution (5:5) between the two study sequences. The self-reported pain ratings on days 3, 6, and 9 of the study are presented in Table 3. Of the 10 patients, eight demonstrated a positive treatment effect with the active ibuprofen compared with the look-alike placebo.

The differences in overall median pain scores between the narcotic–ibuprofen phases and narcotic–placebo phases were analyzed using the two-sample Wilcoxon test.[b] The analgesic efficacy of the narcotic–ibuprofen combination was significantly greater than the analgesic efficacy of the narcotic–placebo combination. The extent of self-reported pain relief was further analyzed in the eight patients who responded positively to narcotic–ibuprofen; the overall improvement in analgesia averaged 39.1% (range, 3.1–76.2%).

The incidence of nausea, mood depression, daytime drowsiness, or nighttime sleeplessness did not increase significantly from baseline with the narcotic–ibuprofen regimen. During the narcotic–ibuprofen phase(s), two of 89 responses (2.2%) indicated clinically important nausea (visual analogue rating ≥35.0). Of 89 responses, 30 (33.7%) indicated mood depression, 17 of 60 responses (18.3%) indicated daytime drowsiness, and 3 of 15 responses (20%) indicated nighttime sleeplessness. During the narcotic–placebo phases, 14 of 89 responses (15.7%) indicated clinically important nausea. Of 89 responses, 44 (49.4%) indicated mood depression, 15

Table 2.
Comparison of Narcotic Intake at Baseline and During Study Period

Patient No.	Baseline: Oral Analgesic Regimen	Baseline: Narcotic Intake[a]	Study Period: Oral Analgesic Regimen[b]	Study Period: Narcotic Intake[a,c]
2	Levorphanol tartrate 2 mg q 4 h (0800–2400)	25	Levorphanol tartrate 2 mg q 4 h (0800–2400)	25
4[d]	Levorphanol tartrate 2 mg q 4 h (1200–2000)	15	Levorphanol tartrate 2 mg q 4 h (0800–2000) and 4 mg (2400)	30
5[d]	Levorphanol tartrate 2 mg q 6 h (0600–2400),	20	Percocet[f] 1 tab q 4 h (0800–2400)	12
8	Aspirin 650 mg q 4 h (0400–2400), Tylox[e] 2 caps q 4 h (0400–2400)	20	Percocet[f] 2 tabs q 4 h (0400–2400)	24
9	Levorphanol tartrate 4 mg q 4 h (0400–2400), zomepirac sodium 100 mg q.i.d.	60	Levorphanol tartrate 4 mg q 4 h (0400–2400)	60
10[d]	Percocet[f] 1 tab q 3 h (6 doses daily)	12	Percocet[f] 2 tabs q 4 h (0400–2400)	24
11	Levorphanol tartrate 2 mg q 4 h (0400–2400), zomepirac sodium 100 mg q 4 h (0400–2400)	30	Levorphanol tartrate 4 mg q 4 h (0400–2400)	60
12	Methadone hydrochloride 5 mg (0500, 0800, 1400) and 10 mg (2400), Ascriptin #3[g] (0800, 1200, 1600, 2000)	18.5	Codeine sulfate 60 mg q 4 h (0400–2400), methadone hydrochloride 5 mg (0800 & 1600) and 10 mg (2400)	28
13	Levorphanol tartrate 4 mg q 4 h (0400–2400)	60	Levorphanol tartrate 4 mg q 4 h (0400–1600) and 6 mg (2000 & 2400)	70
14	Levorphanol tartrate 4 mg q 4 h (0600–2200)	50	Levorphanol tartrate 4 mg q 4 h (0800–2400)	50

[a] This represents the 24-hour narcotic intake equated to injectable morphine (mg) according to the Wisconsin Palliative Medication Profile system.
[b] To this was added ibuprofen 400 q.i.d. during the ibuprofen phases of the study or look-alike placebo q.i.d. during the placebo phases.
[c] Patients remained on the same narcotic regimen during all phases of the study.
[d] Patient received antineoplastic drug during the study.
[e] Oxycodone hydrochloride 4.5 mg, oxycodone terephthalate 0.38 mg, acetaminophen 500 mg.
[f] Oxycodone hydrochloride 5 mg, acetaminophen 325 mg.
[g] Codeine phosphate 30 mg, aspirin 325 mg, and magnesium hydroxide and dried aluminum hydroxide, 150 mg.

Table 3.
Self-Reported Pain Ratings on Days 3, 6, and 9[a]

Time of Evaluation	Patient Number and Study Sequence[b] 2 (IPI)	4 (PIP)	5 (IPI)	8 (PIP)	9 (IPI)	10 (PIP)	11 (IPI)	12 (PIP)	13 (PIP)	14 (IPI)
Baseline	5.6	74.6	26.0	48.2	62.7	96.5	38.2	42.5	11.3	38.8
Day 3										
0800	13.0	3.5	29.3	78.6	65.8	95.2	42.3	25.6	3.4	17.3
1000	3.2	2.6	24.7	70.5	79.3	81.0	42.2	35.6	3.8	13.6
1200	6.9	2.4	60.0	64.8	38.9	99.5	46.3	71.2	4.4	16.7
1800	1.0	1.7	60.7	52.5	56.5	99.3	48.2	63.4	21.3	8.1
2000	3.8	2.4	59.4	43.3	35.1	99.3	46.9	31.8	18.0	8.4
2400	0.0	2.6	47.5	46.8	81.9	92.7	46.3	24.8	3.2	6.3
Mean ± S.D.	4.65 ± 4.33	2.53 ± 0.53	46.93 ± 14.84	59.42 ± 12.82	59.58 ± 18.08	94.5 ± 6.55	45.37 ± 2.29	42.07 ± 18.35	9.02 ± 7.59	11.73 ± 4.34
Median	3.5	2.5	53.5	58.7	61.2	97.3	46.3	33.7	4.1	11.0
Day 6										
0800	0.0	3.6	40.0	53.3	45.7	53.0	9.9	22.4	5.6	67.6
1000	0.5	1.4	42.0	41.0	45.9	30.6	24.4	26.2	11.0	67.2
1200	7.0	3.1	34.7	43.6	34.9	15.8	50.0	46.2	7.5	62.9
1800	12.7	1.4	41.1	39.2	40.0	26.2	50.6	65.3	10.5	43.5
2000	7.5	1.2	38.8	51.5	47.3	11.0	49.2	58.1	11.2	29.7
2400	NA[c]	1.2	28.7	44.8	42.5	12.7	13.2	46.2	13.7	33.7
Mean ± S.D.	5.54 ± 4.76	1.98 ± 0.98	37.55 ± 4.59	45.57 ± 5.18	42.72 ± 4.25	24.88 ± 14.43	32.88 ± 17.61	44.07 ± 15.52	9.92 ± 2.64	50.77 ± 15.75
Median	7.0	1.4	39.4	44.2	44.1	21.0	36.8	46.2	10.8	53.2
Day 9										
0800	3.1	8.0	29.3	39.4	39.0	97.7	49.1	11.9	12.8	8.7
1000	0.0	8.8	27.5	38.7	22.6	84.3	47.6	40.2	8.9	4.4
1200	0.6	7.5	41.0	58.2	29.7	58.3	40.2	50.3	11.2	22.7
1800	8.5	3.2	35.9	65.8	27.5	61.5	24.7	63.7	17.6	20.1
2000	1.8	9.0	34.4	74.9	13.7	68.5	66.6	63.0	20.6	16.2
2400	NA[c]	8.5	33.7	NA[c]	76.2	48.8	12.8	64.7	23.8	18.8
Mean ± S.D.	2.80 ± 3.04	7.5 ± 1.99	33.63 ± 4.4	55.4 ± 14.36	34.78 ± 20.02	69.85 ± 16.49	40.17 ± 17.43	48.97 ± 18.87	15.82 ± 5.29	15.15 ± 6.49
Median	1.8	8.3	34.1	58.2	28.6	65.0	43.9	56.7	15.2	17.5

[a] Self-reported pain rating measured on a visual analogue scale from 0 to 100.
[b] See the methods section for a complete description of the study sequence; IPI represents the sequence of ibuprofen, placebo, and ibuprofen, and PIP represents the sequence of placebo, ibuprofen, and placebo.
[c] Data not available.

of 60 responses (25%) indicated daytime drowsiness, and 5 of 15 responses (33.3%) indicated nighttime sleeplessness.

Discussion

This study was designed as a multiple-dose trial to analyze the efficacy of the analgesic regimens tested. To date, most other studies evaluating the analgesic efficacy of ibuprofen have been single-dose trials. Further, most of these studies have been conducted in acute pain conditions such as dysmenorrhea, postoperative hernia repair, and dental extractions.[13-19]

All 10 patients who completed this study had metastatic disease. Since eight of these patients experienced a positive treatment effect when ibuprofen was added to their narcotic regimens, we speculate that ibuprofen is beneficial as an analgesic treatment modality when added to a regimen of narcotic analgesics in patients with pain attributable to metastatic cancer. The nonsteroidal anti-inflammatory agents exert their analgesic action by inhibiting the biosynthesis of prostaglandins and the cycloendoperoxide precursors to prostaglandins.[20,21] The prostaglandins, in particular prostaglandin E_2, play a substantial role in pain mediation by triggering the release of two known pain mediators, bradykinin and histamine.[20] Additionally, osteolytic metastases induce the production of prostaglandins.[22] This in turn may cause osteolysis, sensitize free nerve endings, and augment pain perception.

The results of this study suggest that further investigation of the analgesic efficacy of ibuprofen in patients with pain associated with cancer is warranted. A larger sample of patients would allow subgrouping according to metastatic and nonmetastatic disease. Accrual of a larger patient sample would also allow categorization of patients according to pretreatment baseline pain estimates (mild, moderate, or severe pain). By studying patient subgroups such as these, practitioners might be able to predict which patients with pain from cancer would benefit the most from the addition of ibuprofen to their narcotic regimens.

Conclusion

In this preliminary study of 10 patients with metastatic disease, a treatment regimen of ibuprofen plus oral narcotic analgesics was more effective in relieving pain than was a regimen of oral narcotics alone. Further, the occurrence of nausea, mood depression, daytime drowsiness, and nighttime sleeplessness was not increased with the narcotic-ibuprofen regimen.

---

[a] Sorkness CA, Theisen JA, Cleeland CS et al. Development of the Wisconsin Palliative Medication Profile. Submitted for publication.

[b] Marascuilo LA, Serlin R. A common sense approach to theoretical statistics—a handbook for researchers and investigators. Submitted for publication.

References

1. Foley KM. Clinical assessment of cancer pain. *Acta Anaesth Scand.* 1982; 74(Suppl):91–6.
2. Daut RL, Cleeland CS. The prevalence and severity of pain in cancer. *Cancer.* 1982; 50:1913–8.
3. Bonica JJ. The total management of the patient with chronic pain. *Drug Ther.* 1973; 3:33–47.
4. Twycross RG. The use of narcotic analgesics in terminal illness. *J Med Ethics.* 1975; 1:10–7.
5. Grove WR, Fortner CL. Current concepts in the medical management of chronic pain. In: Oncology pharmacy practice. New York: Elsevier North Holland, Inc.; 1980:51–69.
6. Lewis BJ. The use of opiate analgesics in cancer patients. *Cancer Treat Rep.* 1979; 63:341–2.
7. Twycross RG. Bone pain in advanced cancer. *Top Ther.* 1978; 4:94.
8. Wang RI, Waite E. Crossover and parallel study of oral analgesics. *J Clin Pharmacol.* 1981; 21:162–8.
9. Koch GG. The use of non-parametric methods in the statistical analyses of the two-period change-over design. *Biometrics.* 1972; 28:577–84.
10. Littlejohns DW, Vere DW. The clinical assessment of analgesic drugs. *Br J Clin Pharmacol.* 1981; 11:319–32.
11. Quiding H, Oksala E, Happonen R et al. The visual analog scale in multiple-dose evaluations of analgesics. *J Clin Pharmacol.* 1981; 21:424–9.
12. Aitken RCB, Zealley AK. Measurement of moods. *Br J Hosp Med.* 1970; 4:215–24.
13. Cooper SA, Engel J, Ladov M et al. Analgesic efficacy of an ibuprofen-codeine combination. *Pharmacotherapy.* 1982; 2: 162–7.
14. Morrison JC, Ling FW, Forman EK et al. Analgesic efficacy of ibuprofen for treatment of primary dysmenorrhea. *South Med J.* 1980; 73:999–1002.
15. Larkin RM, Van Orden DE, Poulson AM et al. Dysmenorrhea: treatment with an antiprostaglandin. *Obstet Gynecol.* 1979; 54:456–9.
16. Hopkinson JH. Ibuprofen versus propoxyphene hydrochloride and placebo in the relief of postepisiotomy pain. *Curr Ther Res.* 1980; 27:55–63.
17. Iles JDH. Relief of postoperative pain by ibuprofen: a report of two studies. *Can J Surg.* 1980; 27:288–90.
18. Cooper SA, Needle SE, Kruger GO. Comparative analgesic potency of aspirin and ibuprofen. *J Oral Surg.* 1977; 35: 898–903.
19. Rondeau PL, Yeung E, Nelson P. Dental surgery pain analgesic. *Can Dent Assoc J.* 1980; 46:433–9.
20. Houde RW. Nonnarcotic alternatives for controlling cancer pain. *Drug Ther.* 1980; 47–50.
21. Gerbershagen HU. Nonnarcotic analgesics. In: Advances in pain research and therapy, Vol. 2, Bonica JJ, Ventafridda V, eds. New York: Raven Press; 1979:255–61.
22. Anon. Osteolytic metastases. *Lancet.* 1976; 2:1063–4.

“

Perioperative Prophylactic Use of Cephalosporins

We have examined all available reports where parenteral cephalosporins were compared in the prophylaxis of surgical infection. In none of the studies was a significant difference demonstrated between agents. However, many studies compared groups of patients that were too small to rule out significant differences. . . .

Caution is advised in the adoption of new, expensive antimicrobials for surgical prophylaxis. The newer cephalosporins present potential risks that were not as evident with older agents. Bleeding diathesis, GI side effects, and "disulfiramlike" reactions are frequently observed. We find no evidence that second-generation cephalosporins (such as cefamandole, cefoxitin, or ceforanide) or third-generation cephalosporins (such as cefotaxime, moxalactam, cefoperazone, and ceftizoxime) result in postoperative infection rates lower than with older agents such as cefazolin.

—DiPiro JT, Bowden TA, Hooks VH III. Prophylactic parenteral cephalosporins in surgery. *JAMA.* 1984; 252:3277–9.

”

Prediction of theophylline clearance using condition correction factors

MARK J. HAUMSCHILD AND JOHN E. MURPHY

Abstract: The predictive ability of different mathematical manipulations of condition correction factors in estimating total body clearance of theophylline in acutely ill hospitalized patients was evaluated.

Fifty acutely ill patients who were treated with constant aminophylline infusions were evaluated. Twenty-one patients were evaluated prospectively. Initial serum theophylline concentrations were ordered, and second concentrations were obtained at steady state. Twenty-nine patients were evaluated retrospectively and were included if two steady-state serum theophylline concentrations had been obtained. Each condition correction factor was determined by calculating the predicted normal clearance using a literature-derived clearance value and dividing it into the actual clearance obtained. The FDA condition correction factors were obtained by dividing the theophylline dose recommended for patients with a particular disease by the dose recommended for a normal patient. Pearson correlation coefficients for 15 mathematical manipulations were used to examine the relationship between the predicted clearance and actual clearance.

The predictability of theophylline clearance using the mathematical manipulations decreased as the number of condition correction factors increased. The mean actual clearance for four patients with no condition correction factors was only 2% greater than the mean standard clearance found in a previous study.

The use of 0.041 L/hr/kg as a standard clearance appears justified for calculating initial theophylline dosages in all patients. Patients with only one condition correction factor may use this factor to adjust dosage, but when more than one factor is present, the use of the other manipulations studied may result in either subtherapeutic or toxic serum concentrations.

Index terms: Aminophylline; Blood levels; Calculations; Dosage; Excretion; Metabolism; Methodology; Pharmacokinetics; Respiratory smooth muscle relaxants; Theophylline
Clin Pharm. 1985; 4:59–64

Although theophylline continues to be used extensively in the treatment of chronic obstructive pulmonary disease in the United States, its pharmacokinetics and pharmacodynamics are still poorly understood. It is well accepted that theophylline clearance, serum theophylline concentrations, and ultimately, therapeutic efficacy and drug toxicity are affected by multiple heterogeneous variables (diseases and drugs).[1,2] Conditions that have been reported to reduce theophylline clearance include severe pulmonary obstruction,[3,4] pulmonary edema,[5] and upper respiratory illnesses.[6] Although theophylline has a low hepatic extraction and clearance,[7] conditions such as congestive heart failure[8] and cirrhosis[9,10] can cause passive hepatic congestion and decrease theophylline clearance. Various drugs have also been reported to decrease theophylline clearance. These include allopurinol,[11] cimetidine,[12,13] erythromycin,[14–16] furosemide,[17] influenza virus vaccine,[18] oral contraceptive steroids,[19] propranolol hydrochloride,[20] triacetyloleandomycin (TAO),[21] and verapamil.[22] Cigarette smoking,[23,24] cystic fibrosis,[25] and phenobarbital[26] have been shown to increase theophylline clearance substantially through hepatic-enzyme induction.

The use of condition correction factors for these disease states and drugs to determine total body theophylline clearance and initial dosing has been advocated in previous publications.[3,24] This method simply requires that the clinician remember either the maintenance infusion rate or theophylline clearance value and then multiply it by the appropriate condition correction factor for various diseases and drugs. This method estimates the initial infusion rate or clearance for an individual patient. This method also has the advantage of allowing for the consideration of patients with multiple disease states and drug therapies.

In a recent publication, Gotz et al.[1] found that the condition correction-factor method of estimating theophylline clearance as proposed by Powell et al.[3] correlated poorly with actual clearance data obtained from acutely ill, hospitalized patients. In fact, they found no correlation.[1]

MARK J. HAUMSCHILD, M.S., PHARM.D., is Clinical Coordinator, Pharmacy Department, Morton F. Plant Hospital, Clearwater, FL. JOHN E. MURPHY, PHARM.D., is Associate Professor of Pharmacy, Mercer University Southern School of Pharmacy, and Director, Pharmacokinetics Service, Georgia Baptist Medical Center, Atlanta, GA.

Address reprint requests to Dr. Haumschild at the Pharmacy Department, Morton F. Plant Hospital, 323 Jeffords Street, P.O. Box 210, Clearwater, FL 33517.

Presented at the Clinical Research Forum at the 19th Annual ASHP Midyear Clinical Meeting, Dallas, TX, December 4, 1984.

We have also used the method of Powell et al.[3] and other condition correction factors presented throughout the literature to estimate clearance in our patients. By observing the predictability in a number of patients, we found that when the patients had multiple conditions and were receiving many drugs, the predicted clearance appeared to differ substantially from the actual clearance. We hypothesized that the condition correction-factor method may be valid in limited conditions, but that its use in patients with multiple conditions might be impracticable. Therefore, we examined these factors through various manipulations to determine if any clinical applications existed.

The purpose of this study was to evaluate the predictive ability of different mathematical manipulations of condition correction factors in estimating total body clearance of theophylline in acutely ill, hospitalized patients by correlating these predicted clearances with actual clearances.

Methods

Patient Population. Fifty acutely ill patients who were admitted to our hospital and treated with constant aminophylline infusion were evaluated. Twenty-one patients were evaluated prospectively. Initial theophylline serum concentrations were ordered by the patients' physicians, and second serum concentrations were obtained at steady state by the investigator. The other 29 patients were evaluated retrospectively and were included in this study if two theophylline serum concentrations had been ordered during the patient's hospitalization, and both serum concentrations were obtained at steady state.

Study Design. Patient records were reviewed (both prospectively and retrospectively) for pertinent information including age, sex, height, weight, blood gases, pulmonary-function tests, smoking history, disease states, and concurrent drug therapy. Medical conditions reported to influence theophylline disposition, such as smoking, congestive heart failure, pneumonia, and severe bronchial obstruction, were the same as those defined by Powell et al.[3] The diagnosis of pneumonia was based on clinical, bacteriological, and roentgenographic evidence. Patients were considered to be smokers if they smoked 10 or more cigarettes per day for at least the last two years. Congestive heart failure was defined as the presence of peripheral edema (without other causes of heart failure) with roentgenographic evidence of cardiac enlargement. Severe bronchial obstruction was considered to exist if the forced expiratory volume in one second ($FEV_{1.0}$) was less than 45% of the forced vital capacity, or if $FEV_{1.0}$ was less than one liter, or if the arterial partial pressure of carbon dioxide was greater than 45 mm Hg. Pulmonary edema was defined as diffuse bilateral chest rales on auscultation with roentgenographic evidence. The condition correction-factor values for the drugs affecting theophylline clearance were obtained from the studies previously listed.[11–22] In these studies, each condition correction factor was determined by calculating the predicted normal clearance for a patient and then dividing it into the actual clearance obtained in patients receiving a particular drug or in those with a particular disease state. For example:

$$\text{Pneumonia patient's CL/normal CL} = 0.0164\ \text{L/hr/kg}/0.0409\ \text{L/hr/kg} = 0.4$$

The FDA condition correction factors for theophylline dosing (young smoking adults, healthy nonsmoking adults, older patients, and patients with cor pulmonale, congestive heart failure, or liver disease)[27] were also used to determine predicted clearances and correlations. The FDA condition correction factors were obtained by dividing the theophylline dose recommended for patients with a particular disease by the dose recommended for a normal patient. For example:

$$\text{Dose for congestive heart failure patient/dose for normal patient} = 0.15\ \text{mg/kg/hr}/0.50\ \text{mg/kg/hr} = 0.3$$

No patients in our study had cor pulmonale or liver disease; therefore, the only FDA condition correction factors used were for older patients (>60 years), congestive heart failure patients, and young adult smokers (<40 years).

In the patients who were studied retrospectively, the condition correction factors were used in predicting clearance only if the clinician documented that the factors were present during this hospital admission.

Determination of Pharmacokinetic Variables. In all of the pharmacokinetic analyses, we assumed that theophylline pharmacokinetics were first order and constant in all subjects at all times.[3,24,28] The effects of dose-dependent pharmacokinetics and diurnal variation in theophylline clearance were not considered in the design of the study.[29] The patients' diets were not controlled.

Theophylline clearance determinations were made after the patients had received a constant aminophylline infusion without dosage alterations for a minimum of 24 hours. A constant-infusion pump was used for all patients throughout the study. Steady state was considered to exist when

- At least four to five estimated half-lives had elapsed,
- The infusion rate and its corresponding serum concentration were directly proportional to an increased or decreased infusion rate and its corresponding serum concentration, and
- Two serum theophylline concentrations obtained at least 12 hours apart were within 10% of one another.

The theophylline serum concentration that was determined to be at steady state was used to determine the patient's actual clearance.

Serum theophylline concentration assays were determined by fluorescent immunoassay (TDX, Abbott Laboratories) in our hospital laboratory. The average monthly coefficient of variation was approximately 2% at 12 μg/mL.

For each patient, actual total body theophylline clearance (CL) in L/hr was calculated using the following equation:

$$CL = SFR_o/C_{ss}$$

where S is the fraction of the labeled aminophylline dose that is theophylline (0.8), F is the fraction of theophylline absorbed (1.0), R_o is the aminophylline infusion rate in mg/hr, and C_{ss} is the serum theophylline concentration in mg/L at steady state.

Predicted normal clearance for each patient was estimated according to the patient's ideal body weight (IBW). The patient's IBW in kg was calculated by the following equations[30]:

Men: 50 kg + 2.3 kg (each inch > 5 feet)
Women: 45.5 kg + 2.3 kg (each inch >5 feet)

Theophylline half life ($t_{1/2}$) was estimated from each patient's volume of distribution (V) in liters, IBW in kg, and theophylline clearance using the following equation:

$$t_{1/2} = 0.693V/CL$$

where V = (0.48 L/kg)(IBW).

Data Analysis. "Predicted normal clearance" of theophylline in patients who did not have any conditions affecting theophylline clearance was estimated to be 0.0409 L/hr/kg of IBW.[3] Cigarette smoking was considered to increase standard theophylline clearance by a factor of 1.60.[23,24] The disease states, drugs, and the associated condition correction factors obtained from other studies as they relate to theophylline clearance are shown in Table 1. None of the patients in our study had cystic fibrosis or received allopurinol, influenza virus vaccine, or oral contraceptive steroids.

Independently, the effects of the condition correction factors on theophylline clearance were examined through 15 different mathematical manipulations. The numerical value resulting from each manipulation was multiplied by the predicted normal clearance to obtain each patient's predicted clearance. Mathematical manipulation 9 included the estimated predicted normal clearance values for all 50 patients (those with and without conditions affecting theophylline clearance), while mathematical manipulation 13 examined only those four patients with no factors present.

The Pearson correlation coefficient[31,32] was used to test for correlation between predicted and actual theophylline clearances. The predicted clearance values were determined using the mathematical manipulations involving the theophylline condition correction factors. The mean and standard deviation of the predicted and actual clearance for each mathematical manipulation were also determined to examine this relationship as it applied to toxic and subtherapeutic doses. A $p < 0.05$ was considered significant.

Results

There were 50 patients (19 men and 31 women) ranging in age from 29 to 91 years (mean ± S.D. = 63.2 ± 13.7) evaluated in this study. The patients were categorized according to the mathematical manipulations that resulted from their condition correction factors (Table 2). The Pearson correlation coefficient for each mathematical manipulation is listed in Table 3. These were used to examine the relationship between predicted clearance and actual clearance.

In the only manipulation that included all 50 patients (i.e., manipulation 9 or predicted normal clearance), the mean predicted clearance was 4% greater than the mean actual clearance, and a moderate positive correlation (0.411) was found. The "lowest factor only" manipulation included 46 patients and yielded a low correlation (0.278) and a mean predicted clearance that was 34% lower than the mean actual clearance.

Manipulations 1, 2, 5, and 6 each included 37 patients. Manipulation 1, or the "product of all factors" manipulation, resulted in a correlation of 0.196, while manipulation 2, or the "product of high and low factors" manipulation, yielded a correlation of 0.213. The "mean of all factors" and "mean of high and low factors" manipulations, or manipulations 5 and 6, respectively, resulted in correlations of 0.309

Table 1.
Disease States, Drugs, and Associated Condition Correction Factors

Conditions	Condition Correction Factor[a]
Disease States	
Congestive heart failure[7,8]	0.4
Pneumonia[5]	0.4
Pulmonary edema[8]	0.4
Severe bronchial obstruction[3,4]	0.8
Drugs	
Cimetidine[11,12]	0.6
Erythromycin[13–15]	0.7
Furosemide[16]	0.7
Phenobarbital[20]	1.2
Propranolol[17]	0.7
Triacetyloleandomycin[18]	0.7
Verapamil[19]	0.5
Conditions of FDA Guidelines[23]	
Young adult smokers (<40 yr)	1.6
Older patients (>60 yr)	0.6
Congestive heart failure	0.3

[a] This value is multiplied by the theophylline infusion rate or the patient's actual theophylline clearance to obtain an estimate of the initial theophylline infusion rate in an individual patient.

Table 2.
Patient Data and Their Condition Correction Factors

Patient Number (Sex)	Age (yr)	Actual Weight (kg)	IBW (kg)	Actual Clearance (L/hr)	Condition Correction Factors
1 (M)	71	52.2	66.1	2.00	Severe bronchial obstruction, smoking
2 (F)	68	72.7	59.3	2.53	Severe bronchial obstruction
3 (M)	55	88.2	60.5	2.15	Severe bronchial obstruction, smoking
4 (M)	63	77.2	75.3	2.80	Pneumonia
5 (M)	69	55.0	61.5	2.78	Congestive heart failure, severe bronchial obstruction
6 (M)	69	65.5	82.2	3.94	Severe bronchial obstruction
7 (F)	79	54.5	50.1	2.18	Severe bronchial obstruction, smoking
8 (F)	69	59.1	54.7	1.85	Congestive heart failure, severe bronchial obstruction, smoking
9 (M)	71	81.8	67.4	2.90	Severe bronchial obstruction, smoking
10 (F)	59	53.6	45.5	1.40	Severe bronchial obstruction, pneumonia, smoking
11 (F)	49	69.5	50.1	2.12	None
12 (F)	58	65.5	52.4	2.94	Severe bronchial obstruction, smoking
13 (M)	72	78.2	74.2	2.35	Severe bronchial obstruction, smoking
14 (F)	54	46.8	59.3	2.42	Congestive heart failure, severe bronchial obstruction, furosemide
15 (F)	73	81.8	59.3	2.08	Pneumonia
16 (F)	61	36.4	53.6	4.10	Congestive heart failure, severe bronchial obstruction, smoking
17 (F)	67	62.7	57.0	1.68	Furosemide, pneumonia
18 (M)	65	100.0	77.6	2.00	Furosemide, severe bronchial obstruction, smoking
19 (M)	71	71.7	68.4	2.80	Congestive heart failure, furosemide, pneumonia, smoking
20 (F)	69	64.9	57.0	2.19	Congestive heart failure, cimetidine, smoking
21 (F)	30	90.5	50.1	3.17	Pneumonia, smoking
22 (M)	83	60.0	66.1	0.90	Cimetidine, furosemide, severe bronchial obstruction, smoking
23 (F)	72	68.2	45.5	2.12	Severe bronchial obstruction
24 (M)	54	119.6	77.6	5.00	Severe bronchial obstruction, smoking
25 (F)	50	89.1	52.4	2.45	Erythromycin, severe bronchial obstruction, smoking
26 (M)	61	102.2	77.6	3.40	Severe bronchial obstruction, smoking
27 (F)	65	72.7	52.4	2.07	None
28 (F)	56	55.4	51.2	2.00	Cimetidine, severe bronchial obstruction, smoking
29 (M)	59	77.2	71.9	3.00	Congestive heart failure, severe bronchial obstruction, smoking
30 (F)	57	59.1	50.0	1.61	Severe bronchial obstruction, smoking
31 (F)	76	50.9	57.0	1.06	Severe bronchial obstruction, smoking
32 (F)	35	50.0	42.5	3.47	Smoking
33 (M)	36	71.4	63.8	2.72	Erythromycin, furosemide, smoking
34 (M)	78	48.0	68.4	1.82	Congestive heart failure, cimetidine, furosemide, severe bronchial obstruction
35 (F)	54	108.6	47.8	2.19	None
36 (F)	91	43.6	47.8	1.08	Cimetidine, erythromycin
37 (M)	79	65.0	74.2	2.64	Cimetidine, furosemide, severe bronchial obstruction, smoking
38 (F)	65	84.6	52.4	3.05	Furosemide, severe bronchial obstruction, smoking
39 (F)	55	70.5	45.5	1.45	Cimetidine
40 (F)	74	61.4	53.8	2.50	Erythromycin, propranolol hydrochloride, severe bronchial obstruction
41 (F)	86	62.7	57.0	2.11	Cimetidine
42 (F)	76	70.9	52.4	1.17	Severe bronchial obstruction
43 (F)	55	55.0	52.4	2.62	Cimetidine, severe bronchial obstruction, smoking
44 (M)	75	81.8	66.1	2.00	Severe bronchial obstruction, smoking
45 (M)	49	47.3	73.0	1.66	Severe bronchial obstruction, smoking
46 (F)	55	60.9	50.1	1.51	Cimetidine, furosemide, severe bronchial obstruction, smoking
47 (F)	42	52.0	45.5	1.79	None
48 (M)	74	72.3	68.4	3.48	Congestive heart failure, severe bronchial obstruction, smoking
49 (F)	29	54.5	61.6	2.31	Erythromycin, smoking
50 (F)	77	31.8	54.7	1.02	Congestive heart failure, severe bronchial obstruction, smoking

and 0.317, while their mean predicted clearances were greater (7% and 12%, respectively) than their actual clearances. The "FDA-one factor" manipulation, or manipulation 14, was used for 36 patients, and a positive correlation of 0.231 was determined. The mean predicted clearance in those patients was determined to be 34% less than the mean actual clearance. The "smoking alone" manipulation, or manipulation 10, was used in 33 patients and showed a correlation of 0.260. The mean predicted clearance for this factor exceeded the mean actual clearance by 62%. A low correlation resulted from manipulation 4, or the "product" or "mean" manipulations of three or more factors, in 21 patients. In the 16 patients who had only two factors present, manipulations 3 and 7 showed moderate positive correlations of 0.400 and 0.478, respectively, but resulted in a 21% overprediction in clearances. In nine patients where only a single condition correction factor was present (two patients were taking

Table 3.
Mathematical Manipulations of the Condition Correction Factors and the Resultant Correlations and Clearances

Mathematical Manipulations	Number of Patients	Pearson Correlation Coefficient	Clearance[a] (L/hr) Actual	Predicted
1. Product of all factors	37	0.196	2.34 ± 0.85	1.99 ± 1.11
2. Product of high and low factors	37	0.213	2.34 ± 0.85	2.31 ± 0.99
3. Product of patient with only two factors	16	0.400	2.34 ± 0.95	2.85 ± 1.06
4. Product of patient with three or more factors	21	0.050	2.35 ± 0.76	1.34 ± 0.57
5. Mean of all factors	37	0.309	2.34 ± 0.85	2.51 ± 0.67
6. Mean of high and low factors	37	0.317	2.34 ± 0.85	2.62 ± 0.67
7. Mean of patient with only two factors	16	0.478	2.34 ± 0.85	2.83 ± 0.77
8. Mean of patient with three or more factors	21	0.130	2.35 ± 0.76	2.27 ± 0.45
9. Predicted normal clearance	50	0.411	2.33 ± 0.82	2.43 ± 0.41
10. Smoking alone	33	0.260	2.45 ± 0.88	3.98 ± 0.62
11. Lowest factor only	46	0.278	2.36 ± 0.85	1.56 ± 0.59
12. Single factor only	9	0.699	2.41 ± 0.84	1.82 ± 0.73
13. No factors (predicted normal clearance)	4	0.588	2.04 ± 0.15	2.00 ± 0.10
14. FDA—one factor only	36	0.231	2.38 ± 0.79	1.58 ± 0.86
15. FDA—two factors	7	0.141	2.47 ± 0.98	0.44 ± 0.05

[a] Mean ± S.D.

cimetidine, four had severe bronchial obstruction, two had pneumonia, and one was a smoker), there was a moderate correlation of 0.699, in addition to a mean predicted clearance that was 25% less than the mean actual clearance. The "FDA-two factors" manipulation, or manipulation 15, was used in seven patients, and a low correlation (0.141) was found. There were only four patients with no factors present (predicted normal clearance), and they exhibited a moderate correlation of 0.588, and a mean predicted clearance that was within 2% of the mean actual clearance. There was no significant difference in the correlations for the patients evaluated prospectively versus those evaluated retrospectively.

Discussion

In this study we found that the predictability of the theophylline clearance using mathematical manipulations of condition correction factors decreased as the number of correction factors increased. Though the correlation between predicted and actual clearance using the single condition correction-factor manipulation was moderate, the mean predicted clearance was 25% less than the actual clearance. This could result in subtherapeutic serum concentrations, unless one calculated the dosage to yield a serum concentration in the upper end of the therapeutic range (20 μg/mL). The mean actual clearance for the four patients with no factors present was 0.0417 L/hr/kg, which was 2% greater than the mean standard clearance of 0.0409 L/hr/kg found in Powell's study.[3] Therefore, the use of 0.041 L/hr/kg may be a reliable predictor of clearance for patients with no factors, although the importance of this observation is limited by the low number of patients analyzed in this study using this manipulation.

The "predicted normal clearance" manipulation showed a moderate correlation and appears to be beneficial in determining theophylline clearance, since the mean predicted clearance was only 4% greater than the mean actual clearance. The possibility of a slowly developing toxicity exists, although monitoring serum concentrations periodically usually prevents this problem. There were moderate correlations for the "product" and "mean" manipulations in the patients with only two condition correction factors present, but because of the 21% overprediction in clearances, this manipulation would tend to promote toxicity. The "mean of high and low factors," "mean of all factors," and "smoking alone" manipulations showed a low correlation, and if they were used, they would probably result in toxic serum concentrations.

There were 33 patients who were classified as smokers, and of these, 26 showed an increased effect on actual clearance, while seven patients did not. Eighty percent of the patients with a history of smoking also had severe bronchial obstruction.

The "lowest factor only" and "FDA-one factor" manipulations also showed low correlations, but these manipulations would result in subtherapeutic serum concentrations if they were used. The FDA guidelines for theophylline dosing only apply to smokers who are young adults.[27] While many of the 36 patients included in the "FDA-one factor" manipulation were smokers, only four patients were young adult smokers. The remainder of the smokers in this study were therefore not accounted for in dosing through the FDA guidelines. This is part of the reason that the mean predicted clearance was so much lower than the mean actual clearance with this manipulation.

When multiplying all the various condition correction factors together, we found a low correlation in 37 patients with multiple factors. The "product" and "mean" of three or more factors, "product of high and low factors," and "FDA-two factors" manipulations also showed low correlations.

Conclusion

The use of 0.041 L/hr/kg as a standard clearance appears justified for calculating initial theophylline dosages in all patients. Patients with only one condition correction factor may use this factor to adjust dosage, but when more than one factor is present, the use of the other manipulations studied may result in either subtherapeutic or toxic serum concentrations. Therefore, close monitoring of theophylline concentrations in these patients is essential.

References

1. Gotz VP, Russell WL, Lopez LM. Evaluation of the "condition correction factor" method of estimating theophylline clearance. *Ther Drug Monit.* 1983; 5:103–7.
2. Hendeles L, Lyle B, Richardson RH. Frequent toxicity from iv aminophylline infusions in critically ill patients. *Drug Intell Clin Pharm.* 1977; 11:12–8.
3. Powell JR, Bozeh S, Hopewell P et al. Theophylline disposition in acutely ill hospitalized patients. *Am Rev Respir Dis.* 1978; 118:229–38.
4. Horai Y, Ishizaki T, Sasaki T et al. Individualized aminophylline therapy in patients with obstructive airway disease: oral dosage prediction from an intravenous test dose. *Eur J Clin Pharmacol.* 1982; 23:111–21.
5. Piafsky KM, Sitar DS, Rangno RE et al. Theophylline kinetics in acute pulmonary edema. *Clin Pharmacol Ther.* 1977; 21: 310–6.
6. Chang KC, Lauer BA, Bell TD et al. Altered theophylline pharmacokinetics during acute respiratory viral illness. *Lancet.* 1978; 1:1132–3.
7. Blaschke TF. Protein binding and kinetics of drugs in liver disease. *Clin Pharmacokinet.* 1977; 2:32–44.
8. Jenne JW, Chick TW, Miller BA et al. Apparent theophylline half-life fluctuations during treatment of acute left ventricular failure. *Am J Hosp Pharm.* 1977; 34:408–9.
9. Piafsky KM, Sitar DS, Rangno RE et al. Theophylline disposition in patients with hepatic cirrhosis. *N Engl J Med.* 1977; 296:1495–7.
10. Mangione A, Imhoff TE, Lee RV et al. Pharmacokinetics of theophylline in hepatic disease. *Chest.* 1978; 73:616–22.
11. Manfredi RL, Vessell ES. Inhibition of theophylline metabolism by long-term allopurinol administration. *Clin Pharmacol Ther.* 1981; 29:224–9.
12. Reitberg DP, Bernhard H, Schentag JJ. Alteration of theophylline clearance and half-life by cimetidine in normal volunteers. *Ann Intern Med.* 1981; 95:582–5.
13. Weinberger MM, Smith G, Milavety G et al. Decreased theophylline clearance due to cimetidine. *N Engl J Med.* 1981; 304:672.
14. May DC, Jarboe CH, Ellenburg DT et al. The effects of erythromycin on theophylline elimination in normal males. *J Clin Pharmacol.* 1982; 22:125–30.
15. Kozak PP, Cummins LH, Gillman SA. Administration of erythromycin to patients on theophylline. *J Allergy Clin Immunol.* 1977; 60:149–51.
16. Cummins LH, Kozak PP, Gillman SA. Erythromycin's effect on theophylline blood level. *Pediatrics.* 1977; 59:144.
17. Conlon PF, Grambau GR, Johnson CE et al. Effect of intravenous furosemide on serum theophylline concentration. *Am J Hosp Pharm.* 1981; 38:1345–7.
18. Renton KW, Gray JD, Hall RI. Decreased elimination of theophylline after influenza vaccination. *Can Med Assoc J.* 1980; 123:288–90.
19. Tornatore KM, Kanarkowski R, McCarthy TL et al. Effect of chronic oral contraceptive steroids on theophylline disposition. *Eur J Clin Pharmacol.* 1982; 23:129–34.
20. Conrad KA, Nyman DW. Effects of metoprolol and propranolol on theophylline elimination. *Clin Pharmacol Ther.* 1980; 28:463–7.
21. Weinberger M, Hudgel D, Specta S et al. Troleandomycin (TAO): an inhibitor of theophylline metabolism. *J Allergy Clin Immunol.* 1976; 57:262.
22. Burnakis TG, Seldon M, Czaplicki AD. Increased serum theophylline concentrations secondary to oral verapamil. *Clin Pharm.* 1983; 2:458–61.
23. Hunt SN, Jusko WJ, Yurchak AM. Effect of smoking on theophylline disposition. *Clin Pharmacol Ther.* 1976; 19: 546–51.
24. Powell JR, Thiercelin JF, Vozeh S et al. The influence of cigarette smoking and sex on theophylline disposition. *Am Rev Respir Dis.* 1977; 116:17–23.
25. Isles M, Spino E, Tabachnik H et al. Theophylline disposition in cystic fibrosis. *Am Rev Respir Dis.* 1983; 127:417–21.
26. Landay RA, Gonzalez MA, Taylor JC. Effect of phenobarbital on theophylline disposition. *J Allergy Clin Immunol.* 1978; 62:27–29.
27. Anon. IV dosage guidelines for theophylline products. *FDA Drug Bull.* 1980; 2:4–6.
28. Mitenko PA, Ogilvie RI. Rational intravenous doses of theophylline. *N Engl J Med.* 1973; 289:600–3.
29. Loughnan PM, Sitar DS, Ogilvie RI et al. Pharmacokinetic analysis of the disposition of intravenous theophylline in young children. *J Pediatr.* 1976; 88:874–9.
30. Devine BJ. Clinical pharmacy case studies. Case number 25: gentamicin therapy. *Drug Intell Clin Pharm.* 1974; 8:650–5.
31. Downie NM, Heath RW. Basic statistical methods. 5th ed. New York: Harper & Row Publishers, Inc.; 1983.
32. Jackson RA. Selected statistical procedures—research in pharmacy practice: principles and methods. Bethesda, MD: American Society of Hospital Pharmacists; 1981.

Research Notes

Managing hypertension with captopril and hydrochlorothiazide using two versus three daily doses

ARTHUR A. SCHUNA, GARY R. SCHMIDT, MICHAEL E. PITTERLE, THEODORE L. GOODFRIEND, GREGORY L. BEIRNE, AND A. VISHNU MOORTHY

Clin Pharm. 1985; 4:65–7

Captopril is an antihypertensive drug labeled for administration three times daily. Two previously published studies suggest that captopril is effective when given in a twice-daily dose.[1,2] Our study compared the antihypertensive effects of these two captopril dosing regimens in patients with essential hypertension who had failed to achieve adequate blood pressure control with hydrochlorothiazide alone.

Methods. This was a double-blind, crossover study in which each subject served as his own control. The study was conducted at the William S. Middleton Memorial Veterans Hospital following approval by the human subjects committee. The subjects were patients in the hypertension clinic who had failed to achieve adequate blood pressure control (defined as a reduction in diastolic blood pressure to less than 95 mm Hg) with hydrochlorothiazide therapy alone and were candidates for addition of a step-2 antihypertensive agent to their drug regimen. Exclusion criteria included recurrent dermatitis, malabsorption, current pregnancy or lactation, congestive heart failure, collagen vascular disease, recent febrile illness, known hypersensitivity to captopril or hydrochlorothiazide, serum creatinine concentration greater than 2.0 mg/dL, and end-organ damage other than mild cardiac hypertrophy or funduscopic changes greater than K–W Class II. All patients had initial white blood cell counts greater than 4500 per cu mm.

Informed consent was obtained from each patient who entered the study. After a drug-free washout period of two to four weeks, patients received hydrochlorothiazide 25 mg b.i.d. for four weeks. Patients who had a supine diastolic blood pressure between 95 and 120 mm Hg at the end of these four weeks were randomly assigned to one of two captopril treatment groups. Patients in both groups initially received a total daily captopril dose of 75 mg in addition to hydrochlorothiazide: group A patients received captopril 37.5 mg b.i.d., and group B patients received captopril 25 mg t.i.d. Patients in both groups took the same number of identical-appearing tablets each day throughout the study; a placebo tablet replaced the midday captopril dose in the twice-daily captopril schedule.

Each patient was evaluated two weeks after the initiation of captopril therapy. Patients whose supine diastolic blood pressure remained above 90 mm Hg at that time had their total daily dose of captopril increased to 150 mg; group A patients received captopril 75 mg b.i.d. and group B patients received captopril 50 mg t.i.d. Patients in each group were maintained on the respective dosing schedule for an additional eight weeks. After a total of 10 weeks, patients were crossed over to the alternate dosing schedule for another 10 weeks.

All tablets were taken on an empty stomach. The patients received no other vasoactive drugs during the study. No attempt was made to alter the patients' dietary sodium intake during the course of the study, but all patients reported that they followed a no-added-salt diet.

Patients were evaluated in the clinic every two weeks with measurements of supine and standing blood pressures. Patients were advised to withhold their drug dose on the morning of their clinic visit. Periodic hematologic analyses, blood chemistry determinations, and urinalyses were performed. Patients were questioned about adverse effects at

ARTHUR A. SCHUNA, M.S., is Clinical Pharmacy Coordinator and Clinical Associate Professor; GARY R. SCHMIDT is Hypertension Research Pharmacist and Clinical Instructor; MICHAEL E. PITTERLE, M.S., is Project Coordinator; THEODORE L. GOODFRIEND, M.D., is Associate Chief of Staff for Research and Professor of Internal Medicine and Pharmacology; GREGORY L. BEIRNE, M.D., is Chief, Renal Section, and Associate Professor of Internal Medicine; and A. VISHNU MOORTHY, M.D., is Nephrologist and Associate Professor of Internal Medicine, William S. Middleton Memorial Veterans Hospital and University of Wisconsin Schools of Pharmacy and Medicine, Madison, WI. At the time of this study, Pitterle was a pharmacy resident in ambulatory care, William S. Middleton Memorial Veterans Hospital.

Address reprint requests to Mr. Schuna at the Department of Pharmacy Service, William S. Middleton Memorial Veterans Hospital, 2500 Overlook Terrrace, Madison, WI 53705.

The assistance of Kathy Carver, M.S., Jan Hamielec, and the nursing personnel and clinic staff of the William S. Middleton Memorial Veterans Hospital is acknowledged.

Supported in part by a grant from the Squibb Institute for Medical Research, Princeton, NJ, and by the Veterans Administration.

Presented at the Clinical Research Forum at the 19th Annual ASHP Midyear Clinical Meeting, Dallas, TX, December 4, 1984.

each clinic visit. Compliance was evaluated by tablet counts of returned medication.

The captopril b.i.d. plus hydrochlorothiazide, captopril t.i.d. plus hydrochlorothiazide, and hydrochlorothiazide alone regimens were compared using the Scheffé multiple-comparison procedure.[3] The twice-daily captopril regimen was compared with the three-times-daily regimen using Student's *t* test. Hypotheses were tested at a level of significance of $p < 0.05$. For patients whose captopril dose was doubled, the blood pressure data for the lower-dose captopril regimen were excluded from the analysis. All data were reduced to machine-readable format. The Statistical Package for the Social Sciences was used to perform the *t* test and Scheffé test.[4] A sample size of 65 individual diastolic blood pressure measurements was calculated as necessary to determine significance at the 0.05 level, using a 5-mm-Hg blood pressure difference and a standard deviation of 10 mm Hg.[5]

Results. A total of 20 white men whose mean age was 57 years (range, 32–68 years) began the captopril regimen. The mean weight of the patients was 86 kg (range, 57.8–106.6). The mean blood pressure before initiation of captopril therapy was 152/99 mm Hg (range, 132–180/95–106).

One patient in group B was dropped from the study when he developed a rash 15 days after the initiation of captopril therapy. Two patients who were receiving a 75-mg daily dose of captopril (one in group A and one in group B) required a 150-mg daily dose after crossover. These three patients were excluded from statistical analysis. Data were evaluable for 17 patients, nine in group A and eight in group B.

One patient in group A developed profound hypotension after initiation of captopril therapy but continued in the study on a total daily dose of 37.5 mg. This patient's captopril dose was 12.5 mg t.i.d. before crossover and 18.75 mg b.i.d. after crossover. One patient achieved adequate blood pressure control with hydrochlorothiazide plus captopril 75 mg daily. The remaining 15 patients required hydrochlorothiazide plus captopril 150 mg daily to achieve adequate blood pressure control.

Our results are summarized in Table 1. Both captopril regimens resulted in significantly better blood pressure control than did hydrochlorothiazide therapy alone ($F = 38.02$, d.f. = 179). Thirteen patients (76%) achieved the treatment goal of supine diastolic blood pressure of less than 90 mm Hg. There was no significant difference in blood pressure control for the two captopril regimens. No hematologic or biochemical abnormalities were detected in any of the patients.

Discussion. The b.i.d. dosing regimen for captopril was as effective as the t.i.d. regimen in controlling blood pressure when captopril was used as a step-2 agent in the stepped-care approach to antihypertensive therapy. We found remarkable similarities in blood pressure control with the two treatment regimens.

Brunner et al.[6–8] reported that the maximum blood pressure response to captopril was seen with 25-mg doses, that higher doses of captopril increased the duration of that antihypertensive response in single-dose studies, and that captopril doses of 25–100 mg resulted in a return of blood pressure to baseline levels at six hours. For captopril given in a single dose of 200 mg, the duration of effect was greater than six hours. With long-term dosing of captopril, a b.i.d. regimen was effective for doses of 200–400 mg daily.

The Veterans Administration Cooperative Study Group performed a study using fixed doses of captopril ranging from 37.5 to 150 mg daily.[1] All doses were given in three divided doses, except the dose of 75 mg daily, which was given in a b.i.d. regimen. No significant differences in blood pressure or in the percentage of patients achieving goal blood pressure were evident at the end of seven weeks in any of the captopril-treated groups. More recently, this group studied the duration of antihypertensive effect for various doses of captopril. All patients had taken captopril for at least 26 weeks at the time of the study. The authors found no correlation between dose and extent or duration of therapeutic effect when doses of 25 mg or more were given.[9]

In an open-label study, Mimran and Jover[2] switched 12 patients who had been well controlled for an average period of seven months on a mean captopril dose of 85 mg t.i.d. to a b.i.d. regimen. The captopril dose was decreased to an average of 85 mg b.i.d. with no change in blood pressure control.

Our study, the Veterans Administration Cooperative Studies, and the study by Mimran and Jover all suggest that low doses of captopril are effective in a b.i.d. regimen. Brunner et al.[7] failed to demonstrate a prolonged antihypertensive effect from single doses of captopril in the range used in these studies. This suggests that there may be some cumulative effect from long-term captopril therapy that results

Table 1.
Blood Pressures Achieved with Captopril Therapy in Two Daily Doses and in Three Daily Doses

Drug Regimen	Blood Pressure[a] Supine	Standing
Hydrochlorothiazide 25 mg b.i.d.	153 (±16)/99 (±6)	149 (±16)/101 (±6)
Hydrochlorothiazide 25 mg b.i.d. plus captopril b.i.d.	134 (±15)/87 (±8)[b]	128 (±14)/87 (±9)[b]
Hydrochlorothiazide 25 mg b.i.d. plus captopril t.i.d.	134 (±15)/87 (±7)[b]	130 (±14)/89 (±9)[b]

[a] Mean ± S.D. for 17 patients.

[b] Significantly different from blood pressure achieved with hydrochlorothiazide alone.

in a prolongation of its action. Captopril is a thiol-containing compound that is metabolized to captopril disulfide and may also link with endogenous thiols such as cysteine and proteins. It has been demonstrated that these disulfides can be reconverted in vivo to active captopril.[10] Accumulation of these disulfides in the body may result in a depot delivery system that prolongs the drug's duration of activity.

Only one of 17 patients in our study responded to hydrochlorothiazide plus 75 mg of captopril daily. The VA Cooperative Study[1] reported that 80% of patients responded at seven weeks to the same treatment regimen. These differences in response rate may reflect differences in the patient populations tested. Another explanation is that the increased duration of effect from captopril that makes b.i.d. dosing possible may take several weeks to develop. The increased captopril dose was given to all of our patients who failed to achieve goal blood pressure at two weeks; two weeks may not have been a long enough time for observation of the prolonged duration of action noted with long-term dosing studies.

Lijnen et al.[11] were unable to demonstrate a suppression of plasma angiotensin converting enzyme (ACE) concentrations in plasma samples taken eight hours after the last dose of captopril in patients receiving the drug on a long-term basis. This suggests that the prolonged duration of captopril effect with long-term administration of the drug is achieved by a mechanism other than ACE inhibition.

Simplification of drug dosage regimens is an important factor in influencing patient compliance.[12,13] Most antihypertensive drugs may be given in a once-daily or twice-daily dosage regimen.[14] A regimen of captopril three times daily on an empty stomach may be more difficult to fit into a patient's daily routine than a b.i.d. schedule. We routinely use a twice-daily dosing regimen for captopril in our clinics, with good results. General use of the simpler regimen may improve compliance and success with this drug.

Conclusion. Step-2 antihypertensive therapy with captopril in a total daily dose of up to 150 mg was equally effective with two daily doses as with three daily doses.

References

1. Veterans Administration Cooperative Study Group on Antihypertensive Agents. Racial differences in response to low-dose captopril are abolished by the addition of hydrochlorothiazide. *Br J Clin Pharmacol.* 1982; 14:97S–101S.
2. Mimran A, Jover B. Maintenance of the antihypertensive efficacy of captopril despite consistent reduction in daily dosage. *Br J Clin Pharmacol.* 1982; 14:81S–85S.
3. Bohrnsteadt GW, Knoke D. Statistics for social data analysis. Itasca, IL: FE Peacock; 1982.
4. Nie HG, ed. SPSS^X user's guide. New York: McGraw–Hill; 1983.
5. Young MJ, Bresnitz EA, Strom BL. Sample size nomograms for interpreting negative clinical studies. *Ann Intern Med* 1983; 99:248–51.
6. Brunner HR, Waeber B, Wauters JP et al. Inappropriate renin secretion unmasked by captopril (SQ14 225) in hypertension of chronic renal failure. *Lancet.* 1978; 2:704–7.
7. Brunner HR, Gavras H, Waeber B et al. Oral angiotensin-converting enzyme inhibitor in long-term treatment of hypertensive patients. *Ann Intern Med.* 1979; 90:19–23.
8. Waeber B, Brunner HR, Brunner DB et al. Discrepancy between antihypertensive effect and angiotensin converting enzyme inhibition by captopril. *Hypertension.* 1980; 2:236–42.
9. Veterans Administration Cooperative Study Group on Antihypertensive Agents. Time course of antihypertensive effect on low-dose captopril in mild to moderate hypertension. *Clin Pharmacol Ther.* 1984; 36:307–14.
10. Migdalof BH, Wong KK, Lan SJ et al. Evidence for dynamic interconversion of captopril and its disulfide metabolite in vivo. *Fed Proc.* 1983; 39:757.
11. Lijnen P, Fagard R, Staessen J et al. Dose response in captopril therapy of hypertension. *Clin Pharmacol Ther.* 1980; 28: 310–5.
12. Porter AMW. Drug defaulting in a general practice. *Br Med J.* 1969; 1:218–22.
13. Eraker SA, Kirscht JP, Becker MH. Understanding and improving patient compliance. *Ann Intern Med.* 1984; 100: 258–68.
14. Joint National Committee on Detection, Evaluation, and Treatment of High Blood Pressure. The 1984 report of the Joint National Committee on Detection, Evaluation, and Treatment of High Blood Pressure. *Arch Intern Med.* 1984; 144:1045–57.

Salivary penetration of moxalactam

DANIEL T. CASTO, PETER GAL, JACK D. MCCUE, AND ALICIA A. ZUMWALT

Clin Pharm. 1985; 4:67–70

It is currently recommended that patients with *Haemophilus influenzae* type b (HIB) meningitis receive a four-day course of rifampin before discharge from the hospital to ensure eradication of the organism from the nasopharynx.[1,2] This recommen-

DANIEL T. CASTO, PHARM.D., is Assistant Professor of Pharmacy and Clinical Assistant Professor of Pediatrics, Schools of Pharmacy and Medicine, University of North Carolina (UNC), Chapel Hill; PETER GAL, PHARM.D., is AHEC Pharmacist and Director of Research, The Moses H. Cone Memorial Hospital, Greensboro, and Clinical Assistant Professor of Pharmacy, UNC; JACK D. MCCUE, M.D., is Associate Professor, School of Medicine, UNC, and Chief of the Internal Medicine Teaching Program, The Moses H. Cone Memorial Hospital; ALICIA A. ZUMWALT is an undergraduate student, School of Pharmacy, UNC.

Address reprint requests to Dr. Casto at the School of Pharmacy, Beard Hall 200H, The University of North Carolina, Chapel Hill, NC 27514.

Supported in part by a grant from Eli Lilly & Company, Indianapolis, IN.

dation is based on reports that ampicillin or chloramphenicol, the most commonly used agents for treating HIB meningitis, may not eradicate nasopharyngeal carriage even after they are administered at full therapeutic doses for 10 days or longer.[3,4] Hoeprich[5] showed that the degree of salivary penetration of an antimicrobial agent was useful as an indicator of its ability to eradicate nasopharyngeal carriage of *Neisseria meningitidis.* Similarly, studies have shown that HIB is most predictably eradicated from the nasopharynx by agents with good saliva penetrability.[6–11] We examined the diffusion of moxalactam into saliva as a means of assessing the drug's potential (1) for eradicating nasopharyngeal carriage when given as primary therapy to patients with HIB infections and (2) as a replacement for rifampin as a post-treatment eradicator of HIB, if rifampin resistance became a major problem.

Methods. Three men and five women volunteered for this study and were offered financial compensation for their participation. The mean age of the subjects was 28.6 years (range from 24 to 32 years), and the mean weight was 71.3 kg (range from 51.8 to 102.3 kg). All of the subjects were in good health, and none were taking any long-term medications. The study was approved by the Committee on the Protection of the Rights of Human Subjects, and written informed consent was obtained from each participant before enrollment.

On the day of the study, the subjects had a heparinized butterfly needle inserted into a forearm vein for the purpose of obtaining blood samples. Following reconstitution according to the manufacturer's recommendations, moxalactam disodium 1 g (Moxam, Eli Lilly & Co.) was added to 50 mL of 5% dextrose injection and administered intravenously into the opposite arm over a 10–15 minute interval. Following completion of the infusion, the i.v. line was flushed with 20 mL of 0.9% sodium chloride injection to ensure complete administration of the dose. Based on the reported penetration of moxalactam into a variety of body fluids,[12] we considered the 1-g dose sufficient for our test of salivary penetration.

Blood samples were obtained through the established heparin lock immediately before and 1, 2, 3, 4, and 6 hours after the initiation of drug administration. At each sampling, approximately 1.5 mL of blood was collected into a plastic syringe (Becton-Dickinson) and discarded to avoid including heparin in the sample. Using another plastic syringe, an additional 9 mL of blood was obtained, transferred to an unheparinized blood collection tube (SST Vacutainer, Becton-Dickinson), and allowed to clot. Following centrifugation, serum was harvested, placed in polyethylene storage vials (Serum Pro Vial, Fisher Scientific), and frozen at −40 °C until the time of analysis for moxalactam content. Saliva samples were obtained at the same times as blood samples. Subjects were asked to chew a piece of paraffin (Parafilm, American Can Co.) to stimulate saliva flow and facilitate collection of the samples. Saliva was collected in plastic medicine cups, immediately transferred into storage vials, and frozen at −40 °C until analysis.

Moxalactam concentrations in serum and saliva were determined by the high performance liquid chromatographic method of Divan.[11] The chromatographic equipment used included a 6000A solvent pump, U6K injector, 3.9 mm × 30 cm μBondapak/phenyl column, and 440 absorbance detector (all from Waters Associates, Inc.). The mobile phase consisted of one vial of tetrabutylammonium phosphate (PIC-A, Waters Associates, Inc.) added to one liter of a mixture of acetonitrile and distilled, deionized water in a ratio of 23:77. Detection was at 280 nm, and responses were recorded on a strip-chart recorder (Houston Instruments). Concentrations were determined by peak height measurement and use of a standard curve constructed by plotting the peak height versus known concentrations of moxalactam in spiked serum or saliva. The lower limit of sensitivity of the assay was 0.5 μg/mL, and the interday coefficient of variation was ≤ 9%.

Results. Peak serum concentrations of moxalactam occurred at the one-hour sampling time and ranged from 37.1 to 59.3 μg/mL. Mean serum concentration data are shown in Table 1.

Saliva concentrations were consistently below the assay's level of sensitivity (0.5 μg/mL). Only one sample (patient 6, 2-hr sampling time) had a quantifiable amount of moxalactam present (0.6 μg/mL). The corresponding serum concentration was 37.1 μg/mL. All remaining postdose saliva samples contained detectable, but not quantifiable, amounts of moxalactam.

Discussion. *Haemophilus influenzae* type b is the most common cause of bacterial meningitis and is especially important as a pathogen in pediatric patients.[2,13] The morbidity and mortality associated with HIB meningitis,[2,14] and the reported contagiousness of the disease among close contacts of the primary case[1,15,16] have prompted efforts to limit the spread of HIB infections through the prophylactic use of antimicrobial agents. To eradicate nasophar-

Table 1.
Serum Moxalactam Concentrations (μg/mL) Following a 1-g I.V. Dose

Time[a] (hr)	Mean Concentration	Range
1	48.0	37.1–59.3
2	31.3	25.9–38.3
3	21.5	18.4–26.6
4	15.4	11.4–19.9
6	7.8	6.0–10.3

[a] Time since infusion started.

yngeal carriage of HIB among close contacts of patients with HIB meningitis, both the Centers for Disease Control and the American Academy of Pediatrics now recommend the administration of rifampin as a prophtlactic measure among contacts.[1,2] They also suggest that the index meningitis patient receive a four-day course of rifampin before being discharged from the hospital because nasopharyngeal carriage of HIB can persist following a full treatment course of ampicillin[3] or chloramphenicol.[4] Failure to eradicate HIB carriage in the index patient may lead to reintroduction of the invasive organism to the high-risk population of close contacts, thereby negating any potential benefits of previous chemoprophylactic efforts. To our knowledge, information has not been published concerning nasopharyngeal carriage of HIB in patients treated with moxalactam, a third-generation cephalosporin with documented efficacy in HIB meningitis.[17]

The degree of salivary penetration of an antibacterial agent is useful as an indicator of its potential efficacy as a chemoprophylactic agent against *Neisseria meningitidis.*[5] Trisulfapyrimidines and rifampin, each of which were recognized as effective chemoprophylactic agents, achieved saliva concentrations greatly exceeding the minimum inhibitory concentration (MIC) for meningococcus. By contrast, the ineffective chemoprophylactic agents penicillin V, erythromycin estolate, and cephalexin penetrated saliva poorly and failed to achieve concentrations above the MIC for the pathogen. On this basis, it was proposed that the eradication of meningococcus from the nasopharynx was dependent on drug penetration into saliva, and that the measurement of salivary drug concentrations would be useful in screening agents for potential chemoprophylactic value. It is unknown whether the achievement of inhibitory salivary concentrations is predictive of an antibiotic agent's ability to eradicate the carriage of HIB. However, data concerning antimicrobial use to reduce HIB carriage indicate that the greatest efficacy is achieved with those agents that penetrate saliva well.[10]

As ampicillin and chloramphenicol resistance become more widespread, the newer agents, such as moxalactam, may be used more frequently for the treatment of HIB meningitis. Our results indicate that moxalactam does not penetrate saliva readily, even when serum concentrations are substantial. On this basis, it is questionable whether moxalactam can be expected to eliminate HIB from the nasopharynx of meningitis patients. The MIC for *H. influenzae* type b ranges from 0.03 to 0.78 μg/mL.[12] The saliva concentrations in our subjects could have been above the MIC for most strains of HIB, but below the sensitivity of our assay (0.5 μg/mL). It is also possible that the saliva concentrations in patients given multiple doses of moxalactam would be higher than what we observed in our subjects after single doses. However, in an unpublished study, HIB carriage persisted in one of four patients with meningitis who were treated with moxalactam (Piecoro JJ. Personal communication. 1984 May 4). On the basis of our findings, we recommend that HIB meningitis patients treated with moxalactam be given rifampin before discharge.

Based on our results, the use of moxalactam as a post-treatment eradicator of HIB cannot be advocated. However, with rifampin's history of developing resistance when used prophytactically against *N. meningitidis*,[18] and with reports of *H. influenzae* resistance beginning to appear,[19] other agents should be evaluated for their potential to eradicate nasopharyngeal carriage of HIB.

Conclusion. Moxalactam does not appear to penetrate saliva readily. Because of this apparently poor penetration, HIB meningitis patients treated with moxalactam should receive rifampin before discharge from the hospital to reduce the likelihood of persistent HIB colonization.

References

1. Report of the Committee on Infectious Diseases. 19th ed. Evanston, IL: American Academy of Pediatrics; 1982.
2. Centers for Disease Control. Prevention of secondary cases of *Haemophilus influenzae* type b disease. *MMWR.* 1982; 31: 672–80.
3. Michaels RH, Norden CW. Pharyngeal colonization with *Haemophilus influenzae* type b: a longitudinal study of families with a child with meningitis or epiglottitis due to *H. influenzae* type b. *J Infect Dis.* 1977; 136:222–8.
4. Shapiro ED. Persistent pharyngeal colonization with *Haemophilus influenzae* type b after intravenous chloramphenicol therapy. *Pediatrics.* 1981; 67:435–7.
5. Hoeprich PD. Prediction of antimeningococcic chemoprophylactic efficacy. *J Infect Dis.* 1971; 123:125–33.
6. Gessert C, Granoff DM, Gilsdorf J. Comparison of rifampin and ampicillin in day care center contacts of *Haemophilus influenzae* type b disease. *Pediatrics.* 1980; 66:1–4.
7. Ginsburg CM, McCracken GH, Rae S et al. *Haemophilus influenzae* type b disease: incidence in a day-care center. *JAMA.* 1977; 238:604–7.
8. Horner DB, McCracken GH, Ginsburg CM et al. Comparison of three antibiotic regimens for eradication of *Haemophilus influenzae* type b from the pharynx of infants and children. *Pediatrics.* 1980; 66:136–8.
9. Glode MP, Daum RS, Halsey NA et al. Rifampin alone and in combination with trimethoprim in chemoprophylaxis for infections due to *Haemophilus influenzae* type b. *Rev Infect Dis.* 1983; 5(Suppl):S549–55.
10. McCracken GH, Ginsburg CM, Zweighaft TC et al. Pharmacokinetics of rifampin in infants and children: relevance to prophylaxis against *Haemophilus influenzae* type b disease. *Pediatrics.* 1980; 66:17–21.
11. Divan WF, Obermeyer BD, Wolen RL et al. Measurement of serum and tissue concentrations of moxalactam using high pressure liquid chromatography. *Ther Drug Monit.* 1981; 3: 291–5.
12. Reed MD, Bertino JS, Aronoff SC et al. Evaluation of moxalactam. *Clin Pharm.* 1982; 1:124–34.
13. Dajani AS, Asmar BI, Thirumoorthi MC. Systemic *Haemophilus influenzae* disease: an overview. *J Pediatr.* 1979; 94:355–64.
14. Sell HW, Merrill RE, Doyne ED et al. Long-term sequellae of *Haemophilus influenzae* meningitis. *Pediatrics.* 1972; 49:206–11.
15. Ward JI, Fraser DW, Baraff LJ et al. *Haemophilus influenzae* meningitis—a national study of secondary spread in house-

hold contacts. *N Engl J Med.* 1979; 301:122–6.
16. Granoff DM, Daum RS. Spread of *Haemophilus influenzae* type b: recent epidemiologic and therapeutic considerations. *J Pediatr.* 1980; 97:854–60.
17. Kaplan SL, Mason EO, Mason SK et al. Prospective comparative trial of moxalactam versus ampicillin or chloramphenicol for treatment of *Haemophilus influenzae* type b meningitis in children. *J Pediatr.* 1984; 104:447–53.
18. Eickhoff TC. In vitro and in vivo studies of resistance to rifampin in meningococci. *J Infect Dis.* 1971; 123:414–20.
19. Murphy TV, McCracken GH, Zweighaft TC et al. Emergence of rifampin-resistant *Haemophilus influenzae* after prophylaxis. *J Pediatr.* 1981;406–9.

Amikacin pharmacokinetics in morbidly obese patients undergoing gastric-bypass surgery

ROBERT A. BLOUIN, KIM L. ROWSE BROUWER, KENNETH E. RECORD, WARD O. GRIFFEN, JR., PATRICIA M. PLEZIA, AND WILLIAM JOHN

Clin Pharm. 1985; 4:70–2

An increasing number of obese individuals are choosing gastric-bypass surgery for the treatment of morbid obesity. Complications during surgery or in the postoperative period may necessitate pharmacologic intervention, particularly with antibiotics such as the aminoglycosides.

Proper dosage adjustment for drugs that have a narrow therapeutic index is a challenge in this population. Earlier reports suggested that aminoglycoside dosages should be determined on the basis of ideal body weight (IBW) instead of total body weight (TBW).[1] However, recent studies suggest that physiologic changes in obesity may alter the pharmacokinetics of aminoglycoside antibiotics, necessitating larger total daily doses to maintain effective serum concentrations.[2–4] Similar conclusions have been reached in various studies, despite important differences in study populations and methods. Several studies in morbidly obese patients focused primarily on the postoperative gastric-bypass time period[2,3]; these studies did not differentiate between the pharmacokinetic consequences of physiologic changes caused by the surgery and those associated with morbid obesity.

We evaluated the effects of surgery on amikacin pharmacokinetics in morbidly obese patients and compared presurgical pharmacokinetic values in this population with values in a normal-weight control population.

Methods. The control population consisted of eight healthy women volunteers ranging from 24 to 39 years of age whose TBW was within 15% of IBW, and the study patients were five morbidly obese adults (three women and two men), age 24–50, undergoing gastric-bypass surgery (Table 1). Informed consent was obtained from all participants before the study. IBW was estimated by the method of Devine.[5] Body surface area (BSA) was determined by the method of DuBois and DuBois,[6] which has been shown to be accurate in estimating BSA in obese as well as lean individuals.[7]

Each patient in the control population received a single dose of amikacin 7.5 mg/kg TBW in the form of amikacin sulfate (Amikin, Bristol Laboratories, Syracuse, NY) through a peripheral intravenous line over approximately one minute. Blood samples were collected in nonheparinized tubes at 0, 5, 10, 15, 30, and 45 minutes and 1, 1.5, 2, 2.5, 3, 5, and 7 hours, either by venipuncture or through a venous catheter.

Each morbidly obese patient received amikacin 1200 mg in the form of amikacin sulfate through a peripheral intravenous line over one minute, 24 hours before surgery and 6–12 hours after surgery. Blood samples were collected in nonheparinized tubes at 0, 5, 10, 15, 30, and 45 minutes and 1, 1.5, 2, 2.5, 3, 4, 5, 6, 7, and 8 hours after each dose, through an arterial or venous catheter.

Serum amikacin concentrations were determined by a commercial radioimmunoassay (American Diagnostics, Newport Beach, CA). The lower limit of assay sensitivity was 2.5 μg/ml. Each sample was counted in duplicate. Standard curves (2.5 to 80 μg/ml) and controls were determined for each subject's set of data on each assay day and when a

Table 1.
Demographic Data (mean ± S.D.)

Variable	Control Group (*n* = 8)	Obese Patients (*n* = 5)
Age (yr)	28.5 ± 4.8	34.4 ± 10.5
Total body weight (kg)	58.5 ± 9.5	132.0 ± 21.5
Ideal body weight (kg)	56.7 ± 8.4	61.3 ± 11.2
Body surface area (sq m)	1.64 ± 0.18	2.35 ± 0.25

ROBERT A. BLOUIN, PHARM.D., is Associate Professor, College of Pharmacy; KIM L. ROWSE BROUWER, PH.D., is a Postdoctoral Fellow, College of Medicine; KENNETH E. RECORD, PHARM.D., is Associate Professor, College of Pharmacy; and WARD O. GRIFFEN, JR., M.D., is Professor, Department of Surgery, College of Medicine, University of Kentucky, Lexington. PATRICIA M. PLEZIA, PHARM.D., is Assistant Professor, College of Pharmacy, University of Arizona, Tucson. WILLIAM JOHN, M.D. is a Resident in Internal Medicine, College of Medicine, University of Kentucky.

Address reprint requests to Dr. Blouin at the College of Pharmacy, University of Kentucky, Washington and Gladstone Streets, Lexington, KY 40536-0053.

Supported in part by a grant from the University of Kentucky Research Foundation.

Presented at the 16th Annual ASHP Midyear Clinical Meeting, New Orleans, LA, December 10, 1981.

new assay kit was used. Samples in which the amikacin concentration exceeded 80 μg/ml were appropriately diluted to permit measurement within the standard curve range. Within-day and between-day coefficients of variation for the 7.5-, 15-, 30-, and 60-μg/ml controls were <3.5% and <7.6%, respectively.

NONLIN, a nonlinear least squares regression program, with a weight factor of $1/C_{obs}^2$ (observed concentration) was used to fit the individual serum data.[8] Pharmacokinetic values were calculated by methods previously described.[9]

Data were analyzed using Student's two-tailed *t* test. Unpaired statistical analysis was used in comparisons of control group data with presurgical data. Paired analysis was used for comparisons of presurgical and postsurgical data for the morbidly obese patients. A probability value of less than 0.05 was considered significant.

Results. Data for each subject were analyzed individually and, in each case, conformed to a two-compartment open model. The serum concentration–time profile for amikacin in all patients declined in a biexponential fashion. Pharmacokinetic values derived from these data are presented in Table 2.

Total body clearance (CL_T) of amikacin before surgery in the obese population was significantly increased compared with the control group. When the CL_T was standardized to a BSA of 1.73 sq m, the difference was not significant. In the control group, apparent volume of distribution V_{area} (estimated using areas under the curves) and volume of distribution at steady state V_{ss} differed significantly from the respective values before surgery in the obese population, uncorrected or corrected for either IBW or TBW. No significant differences in the terminal elimination rate constants (λ_2) were observed.

Total body clearance of amikacin was significantly increased after surgery compared with presurgical values (uncorrected and standardized to 1.73 sq m). V_{area} (corrected either for IBW or TBW) was significantly larger after surgery (0.43 liters/kg IBW and 0.20 liters/kg TBW, respectively). However, there was no significant difference between presurgical and postsurgical values for V_{ss} and λ_2.

Discussion. Aminoglycoside pharmacokinetics in the normal and diseased population has been well described.[10] Amikacin is a polar compound with a low molecular weight, eliminated principally by glomerular filtration and believed to distribute to extracellular fluid.[10]

Before surgery, the morbidly obese subjects had significantly larger clearances of amikacin (uncorrected) than the controls. Uncorrected values for V_{area} and V_{ss} were also larger. The actual distribution space of amikacin was larger in the morbidly obese population, but no change in λ_2 was observed. These differences are probably attributable to increases in extracellular water, total body water, and glomerular filtration, which are changes associated with obesity. Correlations between glomerular filtration rate and BSA are well established[11] and have served as a basis for standardizing renal clearance values to 1.73 sq m. Progressive increases in glomerular filtration rate within the extremes of the obese population have only recently been appreciated.[12]

The total body clearance of amikacin was elevated after surgery in the morbidly obese population. Uncorrected values of V_{area} were significantly increased after surgery. This change is probably attributable to a change in clearance, as previously described.[13] Although there was a trend toward an increase in V_{ss} after surgery, no significant difference from preoperative values was observed, possibly because of the relatively small sample of morbidly obese patients.

Numerous studies have documented changes in the pharmacokinetics of certain drugs as a result of surgery.[14,15] Surgical stress and endocrine changes can alter renal elimination and tissue distribution of compounds excreted by the kidney. Stokholm et al.[16] showed that in obesity, the glomerular filtration rate shows a significant positive correlation with the urinary excretion rate of free cortisol and the plasma level of cortisol. Maximum cortisol secretion occurs during major surgical stress.[14] Morbidly obese patients undergoing gastric-bypass surgery may have increased secretion of cortisol, which is associated with an increase in their glomerular filtration rate. Consequently, total body clearance of compounds primarily excreted by the kidney via glomerular

Table 2.
Pharmacokinetic Values (mean ± S.D.)

Variable	Control Group (n = 8)	Obese Patients (n = 5) Before Surgery	After Surgery
Total body clearance (ml/min)	83.2 ± 12.5	131.2 ± 19.6	159.2 ± 24.6
V_{area} (liters)	13.4 ± 2.3	22.1 ± 3.2	25.6 ± 3.2
V_{ss} (liters)	11.6 ± 2.0	20.0 ± 2.9	21.3 ± 2.5
λ_2 (hr^{-1})	0.378 ± 0.066	0.362 ± 0.066	0.375 ± 0.054
Terminal half-life (hr)[a]	1.83	1.91	1.84

[a] Harmonic mean.

filtration would be expected to increase in the postsurgical period.

In morbidly obese patients, the total daily dose of amikacin, and probably other aminoglycosides, needs to be dramatically increased both before and after surgery to maintain effective peak serum concentrations. To date, the safety of these large doses in morbidly obese patients has not been evaluated. Considerable controversy remains as to whether or not ototoxicity and nephrotoxicity associated with this class of drugs are related to serum concentration, total exposure, or multiple factors that may predispose the patient to tissue accumulation and organ damage.[10]

Conclusion. Larger total daily doses of amikacin must be given to morbidly obese patients to achieve effective peak serum drug concentrations. These patients should be monitored carefully.

References

1. Sarubbi FA, Hull JH. Amikacin serum concentrations: prediction of levels and dosage guidelines. *Ann Intern Med.* 1978; 89:612–8.
2. Bauer LA, Blouin RA, Griffen WO et al. Amikacin pharmacokinetics in morbidly obese patients. *Am J Hosp Pharm.* 1980; 3:519–22.
3. Blouin RA, Mann HJ, Griffen WO et al. Tobramycin pharmacokinetics in morbidly obese patients. *Clin Pharmacol Ther.* 1979; 26:508–12.
4. Korsager S. Administration of gentamicin to obese patients. *Int J Clin Pharmacol.* 1980; 18:549–53.
5. Devine BJ. Gentamicin therapy. *Drug Intell Clin Pharm.* 1974; 8:650–5.
6. DuBois D, BuBois ER. The measurement of the surface area of man. *Arch Intern Med.* 1915; 15:868–81.
7. Tucker GR, Alexander JK. Estimation of body surface area of extremely obese human subjects. *J Appl Physiol.* 1960; 15: 781–4.
8. Metzler CM, Elfring GL, McEwen AJ. A users manual for NONLIN and associated programs. Kalamazoo, MI: The Upjohn Company; 1974.
9. Gibaldi M, Perrier D. Pharmacokinetics. New York: Marcel Dekker; 1982.
10. Schentag JJ. Aminoglycosides. In: Evans WE, Schentag JJ, Jusko WJ, eds. Applied Pharmacokinetics. San Francisco: Applied Therapeutics; 1980.
11. McIntosh JF, Moler E, VanSlyke DD. Studies of urea excretion III: the influence of the body size on urea output. *J Clin Invest.* 1928; 6:467–483.
12. Dionne RE, Bauer LA, Gibson GA et al. Estimating creatinine clearance in morbidly obese patients. *Am J Hosp Pharm.* 1981; 38:841–4.
13. Jusko WJ, Gibaldi M. Effects of change in elimination on various parameters of the two-compartment open model. *J Pharm Sci.* 1972; 61:1270–3.
14. Kehlet H, Binder CHR. Alterations in distribution volume and biological half-life of cortisol during major surgery. *J Clin Endocrinol Metab.* 1973; 36:330–3.
15. Krasula RW, Yanagi R, Levitsky S et al. Pharmacokinetics of digoxin in children undergoing open heart surgery. *Circulation.* 1973; 48(Suppl IV):19.
16. Stokholm KH, Brochner-Mortensen J, Hoilund-Carlsen PF. Increased glomerular filtration rate and adreno-cortical function in obese women. *Int J Obes.* 1980; 4:57–63.

Lack of effect of ceftazidime on serum glucose in patients with liver disease

Thomas R. Beam, Jr., Mary T. Pasko, Jody A. Spooner, and Daniel S. Camara

Clin Pharm. 1985; 4:72–4

Ceftazidime is a new, β-lactamase-resistant cephalosporin antibiotic. Following intravenous or intramuscular administration, it is not metabolized and is excreted unchanged in the urine.[1] Glucose intolerance has not been previously described as a cephalosporin-related toxicity, and it was not evident during experiments with ceftazidime involving animals conducted by the manufacturer.[1]

During a premarketing evaluation of the pharmacokinetics and safety of ceftazidime in patients with severe hepatic dysfunction,[2] we noted elevations in randomly timed serum glucose values in the first four patients entered into the study. These observations prompted us to evaluate the possible relationship between ceftazidime administration and glucose intolerance.

Methods. Each of the 12 patients entered into the pharmacokinetics study was hospitalized for six days. A complete history and physical examination and baseline laboratory tests, including serum glucose determinations, were performed before patients received ceftazidime.

Each patient received 13 intravenous doses of ceftazidime 2 g (Glaxo, Inc., RTP, NC 27709, lot GCR 2337-E-1). Eleven of the doses were prepared in 50 mL of 5% dextrose injection and infused over 15 minutes every eight hours. Doses 4 and 13 were reconstituted to 10 mL with sterile water and administered over two to three minutes. Patients were monitored daily for clinical evidence of toxicity, and complete laboratory tests were performed again on days 3 and 6 of the study.

Thomas R. Beam, Jr., M.D., is Chief, Infectious Diseases, Buffalo VA Medical Center, and Associate Professor of Medicine and Clinical Assistant Professor of Pharmacy, SUNY at Buffalo. Mary T. Pasko, Pharm.D., is a pharmacist, Infectious Diseases Section, Buffalo VA Medical Center, and Clinical Assistant Professor of Pharmacy, SUNY at Buffalo. Jody A. Spooner is a research nurse, Buffalo VA Medical Center. Daniel S. Camara, M.D., is Chief, Gastroenterology, Buffalo VA Medical Center, and Assistant Professor of Medicine, SUNY at Buffalo.

Address reprint requests to Dr. Beam at the Buffalo VA Medical Center, 111F Infectious Diseases, 3495 Bailey Avenue, Buffalo, NY 14215.

The technical assistance of S. Gutman, M.D., and E. Gill is acknowledged.

Supported by the Veterans Administration and a grant from Glaxo, Inc.

After observing elevated glucose concentrations in four patients, we conducted several investigations to exclude certain explanations for these abnormalities. To eliminate the impact of untimed blood sampling, fasting and two-hour postprandial glucose determinations were obtained on days 1, 3, and 5 in all subsequent patients entered into the pharmacokinetics study. Fasting blood glucose values were also obtained on day 6 in these patients.

To evaluate the possibility of ceftazidime interference with the glucose assay, serum from three volunteers was mixed with laboratory-grade standard ceftazidime (Glaxo, lot UCBR-111) to yield concentrations of 1, 10, 100, and 200 μg/mL of ceftazidime. The drug was diluted in a solution of distilled deionized water and 10% (by weight) anhydrous sodium carbonate. A control sample was also prepared by adding 0.9% sodium chloride instead of the drug solution to the serum.

Glucose determinations were performed within one hour in a blinded fashion using the glucose oxidase[3] and hexokinase[4] methods. Aliquots of spiked serum refrigerated at 4 °C for 3 and 18 hours were also analyzed for glucose content.

Patients 4, 6, and 7 were readmitted for formal glucose-tolerance testing during rechallenge with ceftazidime. The purpose of the study and the risk of drug-induced glucose intolerance were reviewed with each participant. All signed an informed consent. Ceftazidime was administered according to the previously used protocol.

On days 1 and 5 of hospitalization, a fasting serum glucose was measured. Serum samples were then obtained 0.5, 1, 2, 3, and 5 hours following the ingestion of Glucola (100 g carbohydrate per 275 mL, Ames Division, Miles Laboratories, Elkhart, IN 46514). On days 2, 3, and 4, fasting and two-hour postprandial glucose determinations were made. Patients were given a standard hospital diet with no restrictions on total caloric intake or distribution among fats, carbohydrates, and protein.

Results. Follow-up fasting serum glucose determinations 7 to 21 days after completion of the study revealed normal values (<110 mg/dL) in two of the four patients with initial evidence of glucose intolerance. One patient, in whom elevations in serum glucose persisted, was given a diagnosis of maturity-onset diabetes. The fourth patient was lost to follow-up.

No glucose intolerance was observed in the remaining eight patients entered into the study. These patients all had similar mean ages as the first four patients (55.4 years versus 53.0 years), received a similar number of medications (4.0 versus 4.0), and had the same frequency of use of high-ceiling diuretics such as furosemide and ethacrynic acid (3 of 8 patients versus 2 of 4 patients).

In vitro analysis of the serum samples spiked with ceftazidime showed no correlation between drug content and serum glucose. The variability was 4% or less with the glucose-oxidase assay. Results with the hexokinase assay were also unaffected by ceftazidime content and deviated by 3% or less from glucose-oxidase determinations. Incubation for 3 or 18 hours had no effect on glucose concentrations by either method, excluding the possibility of a me-

Table 1.
Characteristics of Patients and Glucose-Tolerance Test Results at the Initiation and Completion of Rechallenge with Ceftazidime

Patient Number	Age (yr)	Liver Disease	Diuretics	Creatinine Clearance (mL/min)	Sampling Time[a] (hr)	Serum Glucose Determination (mg/dL) Day 1	Day 5
4	47	Chronic active hepatitis with esophageal varices	Spironolactone Furosemide	105	−0.5[b]	76	73
					0.5	157	155
					1.0	250	225
					2.0	205	193
					3.0	107	69
					5.0	59	61
6	59	Alcoholic cirrhosis with LaVeen shunt	Spironolactone Furosemide	65	−0.5[b]	97	93
					0.5	165	164
					1.0	192	241
					2.0	221	251
					3.0	215	202
					5.0	54	69
7	36	Alcoholic cirrhosis with LaVeen and mesocaval shunts	None	111	−0.5[b]	80	81
					0.5	225	198
					1.0	293	256
					2.0	237	183
					3.0	113	84
					5.0	75	89

[a] Time measured from administration of Glucola.
[b] Fasting determination.

tabolite causing colorimetric interference.

Clinical information and results of glucose-tolerance tests in the three patients readmitted for rechallenge with ceftazidime are shown in Table 1. Patient age,[5] degree of renal and hepatic dysfunction,[6] use of diuretics,[7] and previous outcome during the initial challenge with ceftazidime could have affected the results of the glucose-tolerance tests. There was no decline in glucose tolerance during the period of observation. Each of the clinical variables that could have produced abnormal glucose-tolerance results was inconsistently present except for severe hepatic dysfunction.

Discussion. We conducted this study to establish the likelihood of a previously undocumented adverse reaction to ceftazidime. During the study of safety and pharmacokinetics of ceftazidime, dechallenge resulted in a return of glucose values to normal except in one patient (patient 2), who remained a maturity-onset diabetic. Careful timing of sample collection in eight patients yielded no confirmation of the original observation. In vitro analysis did not confirm interference by either ceftazidime or possible metabolites with the automated chemistry equipment, an interaction previously documented for cefoxitin and creatinine.[8] The type of glucose intolerance observed in the patients rechallenged with ceftazidime led us to conclude that hepatic dysfunction was probably responsible for the original abnormalities noted.

Conclusion. In the patient population studied, ceftazidime had no effect on glucose tolerance or on laboratory assays for serum glucose.

References

1. Clinical investigator's manual. Ceftazidime (GR 20263). Research Triangle Park, NC: Glaxo, Inc.
2. Pasko MT, Beam TR, Camara DS. Safety and pharmacokinetics of ceftazidime in patients with chronic hepatic dysfunction. *J Antimicrob Chemother.* In press.
3. Trinder P. Determination of blood glucose using 4-amino phenazone as oxygen acceptor. *J Clin Pathol.* 1969; 22:158–61.
4. Richterich R, Dauwalder H. Determination of plasma glucose by hexokinase-glucose 6 phosphate dehydrogenase method. *Schweiz Med Wochenschr.* 1971; 101:615–8.
5. Davidson MB. The effect of aging on carbohydrate metabolism. A review of English literature and a practical approach to the diagnosis of diabetes mellitus in the elderly. *Metabolism.* 1979; 28:688–705.
6. Seltzer HS. Diagnosis of diabetes. In: Ellenberg M, Rifkin H, eds. Diabetes mellitus: theory and practice. New York: McGraw-Hill; 1970:436–507.
7. Dollery CT. Diabetogenic effect of long-term diuretic therapy. In: Lant AF, Wilson CM, eds. Modern diuretic therapy in the treatment of cardiovascular and renal disease. Amsterdam: Excerpta Medica; 1973:320–30.
8. Durham SR, Bignell AHC, Wise R. Interference of cefoxitin in the creatinine estimation and its clinical relevance. *J Clin Pathol.* 1979; 32:1148–51.

Predicting serum gentamicin concentrations in patients undergoing hemodialysis

MICHAEL J. MELBY, JOSEPH F. HEISSLER, EUGENE C. GROCHOWSKI, AND RICHARD A. STOCKMAR

Clin Pharm. 1985; 4:74–7

Several methods for the administration, serum concentration monitoring, and dosage adjustment of aminoglycosides in hemodialysis patients have been published.[1–5]

Goetz et al.[6] proposed a method using an average elimination rate constant (k_{dial}) for a given artificial kidney and applied that value to all patients who were receiving aminoglycoside therapy and undergoing dialysis with that artificial kidney. In this way, he proposed that hemodialysis patients receiving aminoglycoside therapy could be monitored accurately without obtaining multiple serum samples for drug assay.

The purpose of this study was to assess the accuracy of the predictive model proposed by Goetz to determine if gentamicin therapy in our hemodialysis patient population could be monitored more cost effectively by the implementation of this method and, if so, to replace our current method of serum gentamicin concentration monitoring (Figure 1) with this method.

Methods. *Patients.* The investigation was conducted in the renal unit of Bronson Methodist Hospital in Kalamazoo, Michigan. Candidates were those who were being treated for confirmed or suspected gram-negative bacillary infections and who (1) were men or women between 18 and 85 years of age, (2) had renal failure necessitating hemodialysis, (3) were undergoing dialysis for at least two hours, and (4) were not being treated with concomitant carbenicillin, ticarcillin, piperacillin, or any other drug or compound known to interfere with the in vivo activity, or in vitro assay, of gentamicin.

The protocol was approved by the Institutional Review Board. All patients gave informed consent.

MICHAEL J. MELBY is a pharmacy resident, Department of Pharmacy, University of Wisconsin Hospital, Madison. JOSEPH F. HEISSLER, PHARM.D., is Clinical Pharmacy Coordinator, Department of Pharmacy; EUGENE C. GROCHOWSKI, M.D., is a physician, Renal Medicine Department; and RICHARD A. STOCKMAR, PH.D., is Laboratory Clinical Chemist, Bronson Methodist Hospital, Kalamazoo, MI.

Address reprint requests to Mr. Melby at the Department of Pharmacy, University of Wisconsin Hospital, 600 Highland Avenue, Madison, WI 53792.

Presented at the Clinical Research Forum, 19th Annual ASHP Midyear Clinical Meeting, Dallas, TX, December 4, 1984.

Ten patients with end-stage renal disease (creatinine clearance values of less than 10 ml/min) were entered into the study.

Patients underwent dialysis for a minimum of two hours using an artificial kidney (CF 1211 Hollow-Fibre artificial kidney, Travenol Laboratories, Inc., Deerfield, IL). The membrane composition was cuprophane with a wall thickness of 11 μm and a surface area of 0.8 sq m. Vascular access allowed bidirectional inflow and outflow through the dialysis apparatus.

Sample Collection. Following the diagnosis of a documented or suspected gram-negative infection, a loading dose of 1.5–2.0 mg/kg of gentamicin sulfate was administered based on the patient's lean body weight and the site and severity of infection. Four equally spaced interdialysis blood samples were obtained for serum gentamicin concentrations between the loading dose and the next scheduled dialysis (see B in Figure 1). The last sample was drawn immediately before dialysis.

Three more intradialysis blood samples were obtained during the dialysis period, the final sample was obtained immediately after dialysis (see B in Figure 1).

After the initial dialysis, maintenance doses were recommended by the pharmacist commensurate with the goals of the physician for the serum gentamicin concentrations, which varied depending on the site and severity of infection. These were calculated using Goetz's predictive model with individual patient pharmacokinetic values. Subsequent interdialysis and intradialysis periods were monitored as shown in Figure 1.

Predictive Model. The predictive model used was based on standard aminoglycoside pharmacokinetic formulas described by Sawchuck and Zaske[7] and applied by Goetz and his co-workers (Appendix).

Blood Sample Analysis. All blood samples were frozen at −20 °C until analysis. Duplicate assays for serum gentamicin concentrations were performed by the enzyme-multiplied immunoassay technique (EMIT, Syva Corp., Palo Alto, CA). Samples were analyzed on the ABA 200 (Abbott Laboratories, North Chicago, IL). The coefficient of variance for the assay was less than 6.39%.

Pharmacokinetic Analysis. The serum concentration–time data were fitted to a single exponential expression by linear least-squares regression analysis to determine the elimination rate constant for the interdialysis (k_d) and intradialysis (k_{dial}) period. The half-life ($t_{1/2}$) was calculated from the following relationship:

$$t_{1/2} = 0.693/k_d$$

Predicted peak values were calculated using individual and group average k_{dial} and were compared with measured peak values for the same treatment periods for all patients.

Statistical Analysis. The Bartlett-Box procedure was used to test equality of variances across the predicted and measured group data. Analysis of variance was performed on the mean data.

Results. The individual pharmacokinetic data are presented in Table 1. The mean volume of distribution was 0.31 ± 0.05 L/kg, and the mean interdialysis half-life was 37.8 ± 15 hours. The intradialysis

Figure 1. Comparison of methods of gentamicin therapy monitoring: A represents the method employed before initiation of the study, B represents monitoring during the study period, and C represents the proposed monitoring method; where LD = loading dose, IDP = interdialysis period, HD = hemodialysis and D = dose.

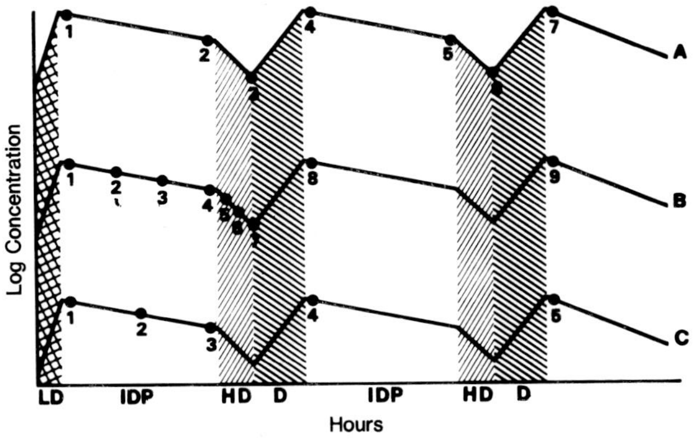

Table 1.
Individual Patient Pharmacokinetic Values

Patient Number	Interdialysis $t_{1/2}$ (hr)	Interdialysis k (hr^{-1})	Intradialysis $t_{1/2}$ (hr)	Intradialysis k (hr^{-1})	V (L/kg)	Blood Flow (mL/min)	Length of Dialysis (hr)
1	43.2	0.016	3.0	0.231	0.32	255	3.5
2	40.2	0.017	2.6	0.266	0.22	255	3.5
3	39.0	0.018	2.8	0.247	0.32	255	3.5
4	18.0	0.039	2.9	0.239	0.30	220	2.0
5	21.1	0.033	4.4	0.158	0.28	220	3.0
6	29.2	0.024	7.5	0.092	0.27	200	4.0
7	24.4	0.028	4.0	0.173	0.31	270	4.0
8	64.4	0.011	5.1	0.136	0.39	255	3.5
9	57.0	0.012	4.9	0.140	0.41	270	4.0
10	42.0	0.017	6.8	0.103	0.32	125	3.5
Mean	37.9	0.021	4.4	0.178	0.31	232	3.5
± S.D.	15.1	0.009	1.7	0.060	0.06	44.4	0.6

half-life for the artificial kidney averaged 4.4 ± 1.7 hours at a blood flow rate of 232 ± 44.4 mL/min. Dialysate flow rate was 500 mL/min in all cases.

The predicted peak serum gentamicin concentrations are presented in Table 2. The mean measured peak concentration was 5.7 μg/mL. The predicted peak concentration using individual patient-specific k_{dial} was 5.6 μg/mL, while that using group average k_{dial} was 5.5 μg/mL. The null hypothesis, that the means were not different across the groups, could not be rejected at an $\alpha = 0.05$ level of significance. No statistical difference could be shown between the means or the variances in either predictive group as compared with measured peak serum concentrations.

Discussion. An intradialysis elimination rate constant was established for the artificial kidney used in our dialysis unit. This value along with the patient-specific interdialysis elimination rate constant allowed us to dose prospectively and predict accurately serum gentamicin concentrations after a postdialysis infusion.

A 14-day course of antibiotic therapy using our institution's current method of monitoring (see A in Figure 1) would require obtaining 40 serum samples at a cost of $400. The same course of therapy, using the proposed predictive method (see C in Figure 1), would only require obtaining 16 samples for serum gentamicin concentrations at a cost of $160 resulting in a savings of $240 per patient. The amount of the savings at other institutions would depend on the method currently in use.

The predictive model relies heavily on the determination of k_d and k_{dial}. The number of monitorings required to characterize k_{dial} for a given artificial kidney is arbitrary, and consistently reproducible results should be the goal of this process. The k_d varies for each patient, regardless of patient similarities, and must be determined before application of the model. We recommend a three-point determination immediately following the initial dose and again anytime the patient's volume status or clinical condition changes.

Once these determinations can be ensured, the pharmacist can recommend prospectively a postdialysis dose knowing the length of time before the next dialysis and the length of that dialysis. The postdialysis peak concentration need only be checked for verification of the prediction or if the patient's clinical condition warrants it.

Our study was designed to avoid the well-known confounding effects of concomitant penicillin administration.[8] In practice, multiple characterizations of k_d may be required to assess fully the net effect. A single determination of k_d in a patient on concomitant penicillin therapy may not be sufficient because varying effects may be seen within the same patient during different monitoring periods.[9]

Conclusion. The predictive model for monitoring serum gentamicin concentrations in hemodialysis patients proposed by Goetz[6] was validated by this study. The method accurately predicts serum gentamicin concentrations while reducing the number of serum samples that must be assayed, which can reduce the cost of monitoring therapy.

References

1. Chan RA, Benner EJ, Hoeprich PD. Gentamicin therapy in renal failure: a nomogram for dosing. *Ann Intern Med.* 1972; 76:773–8.

Table 2.
Predicted versus Measured Peak Concentrations

Patient Number	Run Number	Predicted Concentration (μg/mL)		Measured Concentration (μg/mL)	Percent Error	
		Individual	Average		Individual	Average
1	1	6.41	6.65	5.85	9.6	13.7
	2	5.63	5.88	5.70	−1.2	3.2
2	1	6.33	6.92	6.30	0.5	9.8
3	1	5.45	5.66	4.90	11.2	15.5
	2	5.77	5.88	5.70	1.2	3.2
4	1	5.39	5.49	5.60	−3.8	−2.0
	2	6.26	6.48	7.00	−10.6	−7.4
	3	6.65	6.93	7.70	−13.6	−10.0
5	1	4.35	4.27	3.60	20.8	18.6
6	1	4.98	4.58	4.75	4.8	−3.6
	2	6.42	6.08	7.10	−9.6	−14.4
7	1	5.25	5.24	5.50	−4.5	−4.7
	2	5.36	5.35	6.20	−13.5	−13.7
	3	5.17	5.15	4.90	5.5	5.1
	4	5.35	5.35	6.20	−13.7	−13.7
8	1	4.25	4.07	4.80	−11.4	−15.2
9	1	4.44	4.36	3.80	16.8	14.7
10	1	5.95	5.54	6.70	−11.2	−17.3
	2	6.10	5.58	6.10	0.0	−8.5
	3	5.83	5.41	6.00	−2.8	−9.8
Mean		5.57	5.54	5.72	−1.3	−1.8
± S.D.		0.704	0.82	1.05	10.6	11.6

2. Halpren BA, Axline SG, Coplon NS et al. Clearance of gentamicin during hemodialysis: comparison of four artificial kidneys. *J Infect Dis.* 1976; 133:627–36.
3. Christopher TG, Blair AD, Forrey AW. Hemodialysis clearances of gentamicin, kanamicin, tobramycin, amikacin, ethambutol, procainamide and flucytosine, with a technique for planning therapy. *J Pharmacokinet Biopharm.* 1976; 4:427–31.
4. Christopher TG, Koran D, Blair AD. Gentamicin pharmacokinetics during hemodialysis. *Kidney Int.* 1974; 6:38–44.
5. Curter RE, Christopher TG, Forrey AW. Modifications of drug therapy in chronic dialysis patients. *Kidney Int.* 1975; Suppl 2:516–22.
6. Goetz DR, Pancorbo S, Hoag S. Prediction of serum gentamicin concentrations in patients undergoing hemodialysis. *Am J Hosp Pharm.* 1980; 37:1077–83.
7. Sawchuck RJ, Zaske DE, Cipolle RJ et al. Kinetic model for gentamicin dosing with the use of individual patient parameters. *Clin Pharmacol Ther.* 1977; 21:362–9.
8. Ervin FR, Bullock WE, Nuttall CE. Inactivation of gentamicin in patients with renal failure. *Antimicrob Agents Chemother.* 1976; 9:1004–11.
9. Lampasona V, Crass RE, Reines HD. Decreased serum tobramycin concentrations in patients with renal failure. *Clin Pharm.* 1983; 2:6–9.

Appendix—Pharmacokinetic Formulas Used for the Predictive Model

1. Calculation of postdialysis serum concentration:

$$C_{predial} = C_{peak}e^{-k_d t_{predial}}$$

$$C_{postdial} = C_{predial}e^{-k_{dial} t_{dial}}$$

$$C_{postdial} = C_{peak}(e^{-k_d t_{predial}})(e^{-k_{dial} t_{dial}}) \text{ [Combined]}$$

where C_{peak} = peak concentration after infusion (μg/mL), k_d = interdialysis elimination rate constant (hr^{-1}), $t_{predial}$ = time from infusion to dialysis (hr), $C_{predial}$ = concentration preceeding dialysis (μg/mL), k_{dial} = intradialysis elimination rate constant (hr^{-1}), and t_{dial} = time of dialysis (hr).

2. Calculation of volume of distribution:

$$V = D/(C_{peak} - C_{po})$$

where V = volume of distribution (L), D = dose (mg), and C_{po} = preinfusion concentration (μg/mL).

3. Calculation of predicted peak concentration:

$$C_{peak} \text{ predicted} = D/V + C_{postdial}$$

Evaluation of two methods for predicting initial lithium dosage without measuring serum concentrations

JOHN M. PATRIAS AND FRED H. MOORE

Clin Pharm. 1985; 4:77–9

The usefulness of lithium in treatment of acute mania and bipolar disorder is undisputed,[1-3] and its clinical applications are expanding.[4] Nevertheless, therapeutic benefits of lithium are bought at the cost of side effects and potential toxicity.[5] Lithium dosing is complicated because of lithium's narrow therapeutic range and the great interpatient variability in doses required to produce desired serum concentrations. An individualized approach to dosing and assessment is therefore necessary for safe and effective use of this drug.[6]

Currently, lithium dosage is most often calculated initially by empiric methods and then titrated on the basis of serum lithium determinations to achieve appropriate concentrations. Problems with this method may include errors in initial dosing with attendant risk of undertreatment or toxicity and a delay in reaching desired serum concentrations. To reduce these risks, methods for accurately predicting individual dosage requirements have been sought. Some have relied upon one or more serum lithium measurements.[7-9] These methods, though providing better tools for lithium dosing, have their drawbacks. Potential sources of error in these methods are related to the proper timing of dosing and sample collection and to the assay method itself. Inaccuracies in either factor could result in incorrect dosage recommendations.

Two methods have been proposed that do not rely on measuring serum lithium concentrations to make a prediction. Zetin et al.[10] proposed a prediction method based on patient age, sex, weight, lithium dosage form, and concomitant tricyclic antidepressant therapy. Pepin et al.[11] developed a method that predicts dosage based on an estimate of lithium body clearance. The objective of this study was to compare the accuracy of these two lithium dosage-prediction methods.

Methods. Laboratory records from our institution over a nine-month period (March–November 1983) were reviewed to identify patients who had serum lithium concentrations determined during this time. Patients' charts were then reviewed retrospectively and were included in the study if the following criteria were met:

1. All data necessary to calculate lithium dosage using each prediction method were available;
2. A steady-state lithium serum concentration, defined as a lithium concentration measured at least four days after the start of dosing or dosage change, was available; and
3. No diuretics were concurrently prescribed.

All patients received lithium carbonate or lithium carbonate slow-release tablets (Lithobid, Ciba)

JOHN M. PATRIAS, PHARM.D., is Assistant Professor of Pharmacy Practice, College of Pharmacy, University of Georgia, Athens, and Assistant Clinical Professor of Psychiatry, Medical College of Georgia, Augusta. FRED H. MOORE, PHARM.D., is Director of Pharmacy, Memorial Hospital of Adel, Adel, GA; at the time of this study, he was a Pharm.D. student, College of Pharmacy, University of Georgia.

Address reprint requests to Dr. Patrias at the Clinical Pharmacy Program, CJ-112, Medical College of Georgia, Augusta, GA 30912.

Presented at the Clinical Research Forum, 19th Annual ASHP Midyear Clinical Meeting, Dallas, TX, December 4, 1984.

as prescribed by their primary physician. Serum lithium concentrations ordered at the discretion of the primary physician were determined using atomic absorption spectrophotometry (Instrumentation Laboratory 551 Atomic Absorption Spectrophotometer, Instrumentation Laboratory, Inc., Wilmington, MA 01887).

The following equation for the Zetin method was derived from stepwise multiple linear regression analysis of data from 100 patients:

$$\text{Dose} = 6.215\,C_{li} - 1.926\text{form} - 2.844\text{TCA} - 0.070\text{age} + 1.885\text{sex} + 0.082\text{weight} + 5.143$$

where dose is expressed in hundreds of milligrams per day, C_{li} is the desired lithium concentration in meq/L, form = 0 for lithium carbonate or citrate or 1 for Lithobid, TCA = 1 for concomitant antidepressant use or 0 for no antidepressant use, age is in years, sex = 0 for female or 1 for male, and weight is in kg.

For the Pepin method, ideal body weight in kg was first estimated by the method of Devine,[12] and creatinine clearance (CL_{cr}) in mL/min was estimated by the Cockcroft–Gault method.[13] Lithium clearance (CL_{li}) in mL/min was then determined as $0.235CL_{cr}$. Lithium elimination half-life ($t_{1/2}$) in hours and elimination rate constant (k) in hr^{-1} were estimated using the following equations:

$$t_{1/2} = t_{1/2_{nl}}/1 - f_e[1 - (CL_{cr}/100)]$$

$$k = 0.693/t_{1/2}$$

where the "normal" lithium half-life ($t_{1/2_{nl}}$) = 24 hours and the fraction of the dose excreted unchanged (f_e) = 0.95. Lithium dose (D) in meq was calculated as follows:

$$D = C_{ss_{min}} V_{app}(1 - e^{-k\tau})/F(e^{-k\tau})$$

where $C_{ss_{min}}$ is the desired steady-state trough lithium concentration in meq/L, V_{app} is the apparent volume of distribution in liters (calculated as CL_{li}/k), τ is the dosage interval (24 hours), and F is the fraction absorbed (1.0). Lithium doses in meq were converted to mg for comparison of predicted and actual doses (300 mg lithium carbonate = 8.12 meq lithium).

Serum lithium concentrations produced by patients' actual doses (as recorded in the chart) were used as desired concentrations for each prediction method. Predicted doses were rounded to the nearest 300-mg increment. Comparison of predicted versus actual doses was made using Student's t test for paired data and linear regression analysis with a t statistic to test for differences between dependent correlations. Statistical significance was defined as $p < 0.05$.

Results. Chart reviews were completed on 42 patients; 23 met the inclusion criteria. The study sample consisted of 18 women and 5 men whose mean age was 41 years (range 14–76). Mean weight was 66 kg (range 50–101) with an estimated mean CL_{cr} of 76 mL/min (range 41–128). Table 1 shows actual and predicted lithium doses. While dose predictions using the Zetin method tended to be higher than actual doses and doses predicted by the Pepin method tended to be lower, neither was found to be significantly different from actual doses using Student's t test. Accurate predictions (rounded prediction equal to actual dose) occurred in 6 of 23 patients for the Zetin method and in 11 of 23 patients for the Pepin method. Neither method overpredicted by more than 600 mg/day.

Linear regression analysis of actual and predicted doses is shown in Figure 1 for the Zetin method and Figure 2 for the Pepin method. The tendencies of the Zetin and Pepin methods to overpredict and underpredict, respectively, are illustrated by each method's point scatter around the reference line. There was no significant difference between correlations.

Discussion. Both methods of lithium dosage prediction were easy to apply in the clinical setting, and statistically significant differences between them were not detected. However, differences that may be clinically important were found. Frequency of accurate prediction is important because delays in reaching target concentrations occur when dosage adjustments must be made. According to our findings, the Pepin method would require dosage adjustments in fewer patients.

The direction of prediction error is also important to consider. Overprediction carries the risk of producing toxicity, while underprediction may provide less than optimal therapy. Though neither method overpredicted by more than 600 mg/day, the Zetin method overpredicted almost three times as often

Table 1.
Actual and Predicted Lithium Doses and Serum Concentrations

Patient Group	Lithium Dose[a] (mg/day) Actual	Predicted: Zetin Method	Predicted: Pepin Method	Serum Lithium Concentration[b] (meq/L)
Women (n = 18)	950 ± 463	967 ± 243	733 ± 374	0.81 ± 0.26
Men (n = 5)	1320 ± 455	1500 ± 212	1320 ± 402	0.98 ± 0.30
All patients (n = 23)	1030 ± 477	1083 ± 323	861 ± 446	0.84 ± 0.27

[a] Mean ± S.D.
[b] Mean ± S.D. concentration produced by actual dose.

Figure 1. Relationship of predicted lithium dose to actual lithium dose for the Zetin method (O = single point and ● = multiple points).

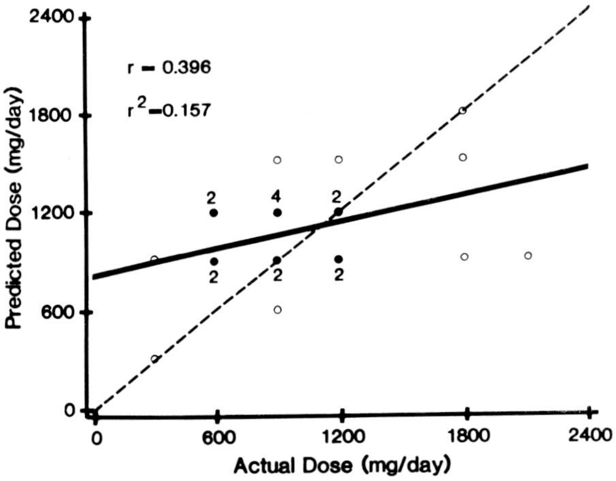

Figure 2. Relationship of predicted lithium dose to actual lithium dose for the Pepin method (O = single point and ●= multiple points).

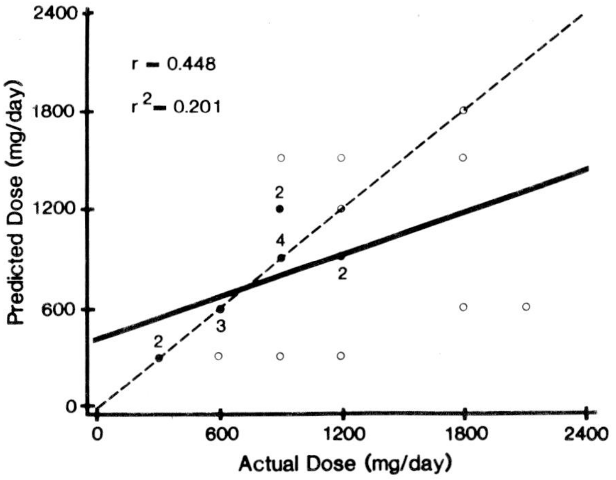

as the Pepin method. We believe that if error occurs, it is better to err on the side of underprediction since a delay in optimizing treatment in an acute-care setting is preferable to compounding a patient's illness with an adverse drug reaction. On that basis, the Pepin method may have greater potential for clinical application than the Zetin method. Statistical analysis revealed no significant difference between methods, yet our results indicate that the predictive tendencies of the tested methods are dissimilar enough to allow for clinical distinction.

No clear reasons for the relatively poor predictive ability of the Pepin method were found. Dugas and Feeney[14] proposed a compound effect of sex and weight correction factors in the equations. Substitution of actual weight for lean weight improved their prediction accuracy; similar substitution had no effect on our data. We found no clear relationship between patient weight and prediction error. Subsequent analysis of differences between correlations of predicted doses and CL_{cr} for both methods was also not significant in our sample.

Other implicated factors included noncompliance and greater dose requirements for certain manic patients. It was not possible to identify or control either of these factors in our retrospective study. We believe, however, that noncompliance was not an important factor in our hospitalized sample.

The small r^2 values for both methods compared with actual dose data indicate that substantial variation is unaccounted for. Neither method appears to have incorporated enough of the factors involved in lithium dosing.

Conclusion. The Pepin method appears to be a better predictor of lithium dosage than the Zetin method. However, larger prospective studies are needed to identify further the factors accounting for prediction errors in this method, especially its tendency to underestimate. Once identified, these factors may be assimilated into the equations to improve the predictive ability of this method for general application. Similar studies using the Zetin method may also be useful in clarifying the complicated pharmacokinetic relationships of lithium dosing.

References

1. Schou M. Lithium in psychiatric therapy and prophylaxis. *J Psychiatr Res.* 1968; 6:67–95.
2. Smulevitch AB, Zavidowskaya GI, Igonin AL et al. The effectiveness of lithium in affective and schizophrenic affective psychoses. *Br J Psychiatry.* 1974; 125:65–72.
3. Pokorny AD, Prien RF. Lithium in treatment and prevention of affective disorder. *Dis Nerv Syst.* 1974; 35:327–33.
4. Jefferson JW, Greist JH, Ackerman DL. Lithium encyclopedia for clinical practice. New York: American Psychiatric Press, Inc.; 1983.
5. Hansen HE, Amdisen A. Lithium intoxication: report of 23 cases and review of 100 cases from the literature. *Q J Med.* 1978; 47:123–44.
6. Amdisen A. Serum level monitoring and clinical pharmacokinetics of lithium. *Clin Pharmacokinet.* 1977; 2:73–92.
7. Cooper TB, Bergner PE, Simpson GM. The 24-hour serum lithium level as a prognosticator of dosage requirements. *Am J Psychiatry.* 1973; 130:601–3.
8. Cooper TB, Simpson GM. The 24-hour lithium level as a prognosticator of dosage requirements: a 2-year follow-up study. *Am J Psychiatry.* 1976; 133:440–3.
9. Marr MA, Djuric PE, Ritschel WA et al. Prediction of lithium carbonate dosage in psychiatric inpatients using the repeated one-point method. *Clin Pharm.* 1983; 2:243–8.
10. Zetin M, Garber D, Cramer M. A simple mathematical model for predicting lithium dose requirements. *J Clin Psychiatry.* 1983; 44:144–5.
11. Pepin SM, Baker DE, Nance KS et al. Lithium dosage calculation from age, sex, height, weight, and serum creatinine. Paper presented to 15th Annual ASHP Midyear Clinical Meeting. San Francisco, CA: 1980 Dec 9.
12. Devine BJ. Gentamicin therapy. *Drug Intell Clin Pharm.* 1974; 8:650–5.
13. Cockcroft DW, Gault MH. Prediction of creatinine clearance from serum creatinine. *Nephron.* 1976; 16:31–41.
14. Dugas JE, Feeney AM. Evaluation of a new lithium dosage-prediction technique. *Clin Pharm.* 1983; 2:249–52.

Editorials

Progress and problems with pain

Pain is the most common complaint that motivates patients to seek medical care. The literature is replete with essays, philosophical treatises, plays, and even novels centering on people in pain. Literary greats from Aristotle to Solzhenitsyn have written major tomes on the topic. Yet, most laymen and many health professionals still subscribe to serious and erroneous myths and misconceptions about pain.

During the past two decades, giant strides have been made in our understanding of pain. Most of this knowledge has come to light only in the past few years and is just now being integrated into curricula of schools of pharmacy, medicine, and nursing. Therefore, the vast majority of health professionals currently in practice were not exposed to these findings during their education and training. In 1979, the nomenclature committee of the International Association for the Study of Pain brought forth a well-accepted definition of this phenomenon: "An unpleasant sensory and emotional experience associated with actual or potential tissue damage, or described in terms of such damage."[1] Clinicians must recognize that pain has both physical and emotional components.

The traditional medical model of pain suggests that a one-to-one relationship exists between pain production at peripheral pain receptors (nociceptors) and pain integration on the cerebral level. But simple interruption of the anatomical pain pathways (e.g., with cordotomies) often fails to provide lasting pain relief. Clinical experience clearly demonstrates that anxiety, depression, and patients' previous pain experiences profoundly influence perception of pain.

The gate-control theory of pain, introduced in 1965,[2] provided a clinically useful but limited description of pain pathophysiology. This theory suggests that central control of pain integrates with physical stimuli to produce patients' response to pain. But it was not until the 1970s that the existence of human endorphins and stereospecific opioid receptors were demonstrated.[3] This endogenous pain-relieving system appears to provide better protection against acute pain than chronic pain. Therefore, only in the past few years have we had a scientific basis for differentiating between acute and chronic pain.

Today, knowledgeable pain clinicians recognize that the application of acute-pain management principles to chronic-pain patients is folly. Patients with severe, chronic pain are physiologically, psychologically, and pharmacologically different from persons experiencing acute pain. There are differences between acute and chronic pain in conduction pathways, autonomic response, biological value, mood and social effects, and appropriate treatments. While drugs are normally the treatments of choice for acute pain, they may or may not be useful in the management of chronic pain.[4] Indeed, in some chronic pain states, drugs might even be contraindicated.

In recent years, several new and efficacious methods of administering analgesics for severe pain have been developed. Spinal administration of narcotics via epidural and intrathecal routes allows profound, segmental analgesia with minimal systemic side effects when properly dosed.[5] Intraventricular administration of narcotics has also proven valuable in a limited patient population. New implantable devices such as the Ommaya reservoir for direct intrathecal administration of analgesics and the pumps for continuous administration of pain-relieving medications have been developed.[6] And patient-controlled analgesia (PCA) allows patients to control the frequency of their own analgesic injections by use of a programmable syringe pump that the patient activates by depressing a button.[7]

Progress has also been made in the relief of pain by nonpharmacologic methods. Myofascial trigger-point injections, electrical nerve stimulation, and physical procedures have been used with increasing success in appropriate patients. Pain management increasingly has become a multidisciplinary effort. Pain clinics and pain-management teams now include a variety of physician specialists, psychologists, nurses, pharmacists, social workers, physical therapists, and others, all of whom bring specific expertise to the activities. There is a very real need for more pharmacists to participate in such activities because drugs remain the cornerstone of most pain-management programs.

This issue of *Clinical Pharmacy* contains three research reports that address some of the new directions in pain management. Weingart et al.[8] have documented the efficacy of adding a nonsteroidal anti-inflammatory drug

(NSAID) to a narcotic in the management of cancer pain. Drugs that achieve the same outcome through different mechanisms are often supra-additive in their effects, but many clinicians assume incorrectly that the addition of "mild" analgesics such as NSAIDs to "potent" narcotic analgesics is useless. In fact, the desensitization of nociceptors by NSAIDs and the anti-inflammatory activity of these drugs may be more useful than narcotic analgesics if there is a major inflammatory component to the pain.

Bollish et al.[9] have demonstrated the usefulness of PCA in pain resulting from abdominal surgery. Of particular interest is the patients' strong preference for PCA over conventional postoperative analgesia. There are profound psychological implications to the patients being in control of their own analgesic regimens. Graves et al.[10] also demonstrated the usefulness of PCA. Their work further shows that serum concentrations of narcotics correlate with analgesia for a given patient, but narcotic requirements vary greatly among patients. Therefore, titration to response is essential for control of severe pain. Administration of "average" doses to all patients is totally unacceptable.

One pain question recently addressed in this country is the need for heroin as an analgesic. ASHP opposed the Compassionate Pain Relief Act, which was soundly defeated by the U.S. House of Representatives last September. This bill attempted to make heroin legal as an analgesic for patients with terminal cancer. I have previously discussed the folly of this attempt.[11] Heroin is simply diacetylmorphine. It is a prodrug for morphine and the active portion of heroin is morphine. There is no clinical advantage of heroin over morphine, and this has been well demonstrated in controlled studies.[12] Efforts by health professionals advocating the legalization of heroin simply demonstrates frustration over their own failure to control pain adequately.

Today we have the drugs, knowledge, and technology to allow effective management of severe pain in most patients. However, narcotics are still underdosed and given too infrequently in many patients. Physicians, nurses, and pharmacists harbor unrealistic fears of dependence induction[13] and unfounded fears about tolerance, which often lead to inappropriate dosing.

There is an acute need for major educational activities—directed at both health professionals and patients—on the appropriate use of analgesics. Practitioners often underestimate the intensity of patients' pain, and patients frequently underreport their complaints. Nonnarcotic analgesics or codeine analogs are often prescribed when morphine or other potent analgesics are needed. Analgesics are still ordered on an as-needed basis when time-contingent dosing is indicated for severe, chronic pain. Many patients and practitioners still believe that narcotics should be taken only "if absolutely necessary." In fact, if the drugs are taken on an appropriate time-contingent schedule, the total narcotic requirement is often less because anxiety, which results from recurring pain, is reduced. Noncompliance by patients is common because of the fear of addiction, but when there is severe, physical pain, dependence is extremely rare. Severe pain must be managed using several modalities. Failure to use appropriate nonanalgesic drugs and nondrug measures is a common problem, and lack of identification and alleviation of sources of the patients' anxiety is a common cause of failure to relieve pain.

There is a very real need for continuing research in pain management, but there is no reason for many patients to be experiencing the pain they suffer today. Pharmacists should be at the forefront of correcting misconceptions, assuring appropriate dosing, and integrating drug therapy into appropriate pain-treatment plans.

1. Merskey H. Pain terms. A list with definitions and notes on usage. IASP Subcommittee on Taxonomy. *Pain.* 1979; 6: 249–52.
2. Melzack R, Wall PD. Pain mechanisms: a new theory. *Science.* 1965; 150:971–9.
3. Basbaum AI, Fields HL. Endogenous pain control mechanisms: review of hypothesis. *Ann Neurol.* 1978; 4:451–62.
4. Reuler JB, Girard DE, Nardone DA. The chronic pain syndrome: misconceptions and management. *Ann Intern Med.* 1980; 93:588–96.
5. Magora F, Olshwang D, Eimerl D et al. Observations on extradural morphine analgesia in various pain conditions. *Br J Anaesth.* 1980; 52:247–52.
6. Coombs DW, Saunders RL, Gaylor MS et al. Relief of continuous chronic pain by intraspinal narcotics infusion via an implanted reservoir. *JAMA.* 1983; 250:2336–9.
7. Tamsen A, Hartvig P, Fagerlund C et al. Patient controlled analgesia: clinical experience. *Acta Anaesth Scand.* 1982; 74 (Suppl):157–60.
8. Weingart WA, Sorkness CA, Earhart RH. Analgesia with oral narcotics and added ibuprofen in cancer patients. *Clin Pharm.* 1985; 4:53–8.
9. Bollish SJ, Collins CL, Kirking DM et al. Efficacy of patient-controlled versus conventional analgesia for postoperative pain. *Clin Pharm.* 1985; 4:48–52.
10. Graves DA, Arrigo JM, Foster TS et al. Relationship between plasma morphine concentrations and pharmacologic effects in postoperative patients using patient-controlled analgesia. *Clin Pharm.* 1985; 4:41–7.
11. Lipman AG. The cruel hoax of heroin. *Hosp Formul.* 1984; 19:999. Editorial.
12. Kaiko RF, Wallenstein SL, Rogers AG et al. Analgesic and mood effects of heroin and morphine in cancer patients with postoperative pain. *N Engl J Med.* 1981; 304:1501–5.
13. Porter J, Jick H. Addiction rare in patients treated with narcotics. *N Engl J Med.* 1980; 302:123. Letter.

ARTHUR G. LIPMAN, PHARM.D.
Department of Pharmacy Practice
College of Pharmacy
University of Utah
Salt Lake City, UT 84112

How reliable are serum digoxin assays?

Over the years many questions have been raised regarding the relationship of serum digoxin concentrations (SDCs) to digoxin dose and to the therapeutic and toxic effects of digoxin. Several recent articles[1–5] have demonstrated the variable results obtained with different digoxin immunoassay kits and the unreliability of SDCs in certain patient populations.

Why do researchers suggest that the digoxin assay may be neither reliable nor specific? Since 1970, most SDC studies have used either a radioimmunoassay or an enzyme immunoassay.[1] The antibodies used in these assays may make the results of some of the studies questionable or at least difficult to interpret. Since each company can develop and use its own antibodies, measurements can vary greatly depending on the assay kit and supplier. It may not be possible to compare results from one study with those of another unless a kit from the same supplier was used in both. This problem was vividly demonstrated in a recent report describing a patient whose serum digoxin concentration measured on the same day using four different immunoassay kits varied by as much as 1 ng/mL, spanning the therapeutic to toxic serum concentration range.[3] Very different clinical decisions could have been made depending on the assay value reported.

It has also been shown that the antibodies in these assays react not only with digoxin, but also with digoxin metabolites.[1,4] Most patients do not metabolize digoxin to active and cross-reactive metabolites or accumulate these metabolites to a clinically important extent. However, a small subset of patients does metabolize the drug to cardioactive forms. This may explain why some patients experience toxicity when their serum digoxin concentrations are within the usual therapeutic range (generally designated as 0.8–2.0 ng/mL). In addition, patients with renal failure may accumulate cross-reactive metabolites, although evidence suggests that this accumulation is minimal.

Probably most important are the recent findings of endogenous substances that interfere with the digoxin assay, particularly in infants and patients with renal failure.[2,3,5] Graves et al.[2] detected a reactive, endogenous substance in 63% of patients who had serum creatinine concentrations greater than 2.0 mg/dL and were known *not* to be taking digoxin. Although the extent of the false-positive readings was variable depending on the supplier of the kit, the apparent SDCs were as high as 1.0 ng/mL.

Many studies have attempted to correlate digoxin dose with eventual blood concentration in an effort to minimize toxicity. However, most of these studies could not clearly demonstrate such an association and concluded that unexplained variables were at play. Better correlations between digoxin dose and SDC have been demonstrated when patients with renal failure are excluded, suggesting that endogenous substances in such patients account for a large part of the unexplained variability.

The evidence supporting a relationship between serum and myocardial digoxin concentrations and therapeutic effects has also been conflicting. When confounded by alterations in the volume of distribution and tissue binding in patients with renal failure and in those taking quinidine, accurate interpretation of SDCs is very difficult.[1,6]

Perhaps some of the lack of consistency in correlating SDCs with efficacy and toxicity rests with the assay. When new types of assays are commercially available, these relationships may become more clearly defined.

In light of these recent findings, what do we really know about digoxin's therapeutic window, particularly in patients with reduced renal function and in patients less than one and greater than 60 years old? These patients constitute a sizable portion of the population in whom relatively expensive SDCs are obtained and for whom important clinical decisions are being made based partly on the laboratory value. Adding to this concern is the evidence that the medical community does not order and interpret SDCs carefully and prudently.[6,7] SDCs are often performed for unjustifiable reasons and at inappropriate times, generating uninterpretable data at substantial expense.

Good indications for requesting an SDC are limited. When SDCs are drawn at appropriate times in carefully selected patients, they can assist in individualizing therapy, evaluating compliance, diagnosing toxicity, and assessing the effects of drug–drug or drug–disease interactions.[1] On the other hand, in the very young, the elderly, and particularly patients with renal failure, serum digoxin assays should be used with skepticism and only in addition to other clinical indicators for diagnosing toxicity or assessing compliance.

As summarized in one recent report, "There is a clear need for physicians to better identify the reasons for measuring plasma concentrations of digoxin and to request serum digoxin measurements only when there is a pertinent problem."[6] It is not that requests for digoxin measurements are wrong; it is just that justifiable requests are limited. We must carefully assess the patient's situation, history, clinical signs and symptoms, and potential for a subtherapeutic or toxic concentration before deciding to use the digoxin assay.

1. Aronson JK. Indications for the measurement of plasma digoxin concentrations. *Drugs.* 1983; 26:230–42.
2. Graves SW, Brown B, Valdes R. An endogenous digoxin-like substance in patients with renal impairment. *Ann Intern Med.* 1983;99:604–8.
3. Craver JL, Valdes R. Anomalous serum digoxin concentrations in uremia. *Ann Intern Med.* 1983; 98:483–4.
4. Wagner JG, Dick M, Behrendt DM et al. Determination of myocardial and serum digoxin concentrations in children by specific and nonspecific assay methods. *Clin Pharmacol Ther.* 1983;33:577–84.
5. Valdes R, Graves SW, Brown BA et al. Endogenous substances in newborn infants causing false-positive digoxin measurements. *J Pediatr.* 1983;102:947–50.
6. Clague HW, Twum-Barima Y, Carruthers SG. An audit of requests for therapeutic drug monitoring of digoxin: problems and pitfalls. *Ther Drug Monit.* 1983; 5:249–54.
7. Weintraub M. Interpretation of the serum digoxin concentration. *Clin Pharmacokinet.* 1977; 2:205–19.

MARTHA L. HYNECK, PHARM.D.
College of Pharmacy
The University of Michigan
Ann Arbor, MI 48109

Volume 4

Clinical Pharmacy has enjoyed considerable success during its first three years. Feedback from readers has been positive, and readership surveys have shown that *CP* is a well-read and highly respected journal. These successes have resulted directly from the dedication and allegiance of the pharmacists and physicians who have served as authors and reviewers of *CP* papers and from valuable advice by the journal's Editorial Board and Consulting Editors.

Some 7000 subscribers have supported *CP* since its first year; advertising support has developed more slowly but is increasing at an encouraging rate. These combined factors have assured that *CP* pays its own way at ASHP.

Although some types of *CP*'s editorial material had previously been published in the *American Journal of Hospital Pharmacy*, the realities of producing a journal devoted solely to drug therapy caused the editors to develop explicit criteria for various sections of the new journal. Readers may find useful the following synopses of *CP*'s major sections.

Drug Reviews. Most *CP* articles in this section are solicited; the goal is to publish timely, evaluative reviews of important new drugs near the time of their marketing in the United States. Drugs reviewed are those likely to be important therapeutic advances or to present dilemmas to hospital pharmacy and therapeutics committees. An extensive network of contacts at major pharmaceutical companies helps greatly in identifying new drugs and judging their importance.

Therapy Reviews. Many Therapy Reviews are unsolicited, although the editors encourage authors to contact the *CP* staff before preparing these articles. Within space limitations, most sound reviews of an adequate body of primary literature will find their way into the pages of *CP*.

Research. The editors and the Editorial Board believe that the long-term success of *CP* lies in articles that present original data, which are published in *CP*'s Research and Drug Experience sections. The number and quality of good research papers submitted to *CP* continue to grow. The Research section has been aided by the ASHP Midyear Clinical Meeting's Clinical Research Forum, which has now been expanded to the ASHP Annual Meeting. As more pharmacists become involved in clinical research, we hope that an increasing number of high-quality papers will be available for publication in *CP*.

Grand Rounds. Good material for this section, which is intended to be used as an educational tool, has not been plentiful. This is surprising in view of the number of Pharm.D. students who prepare such papers during clinical rotations. Young authors often seem inhibited about submitting papers for publication, but they shouldn't be; clinical faculty members have a role to play in encouraging their students to submit good case reports and literature reviews for publication.

Drug Experience. More articles are submitted for Drug Experience than for any other section. Very strict criteria are maintained for this section; only reports of drug effects that were previously unknown or not well established in humans are published.

Future plans call for monthly publication of *CP* in 1986. The issue size will decrease, but monthly publication will enable more timely publication of information as well as an increase in the overall number of pages published per year. The conversion to monthly publication is not expected to cause a substantial increase in *CP* subscription rates.

Gazing for a moment into the crystal ball, the editors see other changes in *CP*:

- The Research section will grow in importance within the journal, but review articles will continue to be an important component of *CP*.
- Articles on pharmacokinetics and pharmacodynamics will be published more frequently as the journal seeks to become a routine place for pharmacists practicing in these areas to publish their research.
- *CP* will continue to serve as "a bridge between the innovators in drug therapeutics and the large body of practitioners hungry for current, objective information on the safe and rational use of drugs."[1]

ASHP's young journal, *Clinical Pharmacy*, has a bright future based on a commitment to give pharmacists the drug therapy information they need to perform their clinical roles.

1. Zellmer WA. A journal for pharmacists. *Clin Pharm.* 1982;1:65. Editorial.

L. Michael Posey
William A. Zellmer

Pharmacokinetics IN DRUG THERAPY

The Pharmacokinetics in Drug Therapy column is edited by Gerald E. Schumacher, Pharm.D., Ph.D. This column is a forum for articles and other material that will assist practitioners in gaining a greater appreciation of the use of pharmacokinetic principles in (1) selecting, monitoring, and evaluating drug therapy, (2) interpreting and evaluating the drug literature, and (3) developing and evaluating dosage regimens.

Address all correspondence related to this column to: Gerald E. Schumacher, Dean, College of Pharmacy and Allied Health Professions, Northeastern University, 360 Huntington Avenue, Boston, MA 02115.

Choosing optimal sampling times for therapeutic drug monitoring

GERALD E. SCHUMACHER

Abstract: Recent advances linking pharmacokinetic theory with the selection of optimal sampling times and the influence of sampling times on the interpretation of serum drug concentrations are discussed.

For serum drug assay results to be interpreted easily, samples should be obtained during the postdistributive phase (for loading and maintenance doses) or at steady state (for maintenance doses). Beyond this, the choice of sampling times depends on whether peak, trough, or intermediate concentrations are being monitored. When intrapatient and interpatient variation in pharmacokinetic values are considered to be the principal components of variability, the best time for taking a single sample after a test dose in order to predict the average concentration during the steady-state dosage interval is when sample time equals 1.4 times the population half-life of the drug. Optimal sampling times to predict maximum or minimum steady-state concentrations may differ from those used to estimate the average concentration.

Efforts to decrease the number of samples needed to estimate accurately steady-state drug concentrations have led investigators to test "single-point" prediction methods following a test dose. However, for drugs administered by continuous infusion, it seems prudent to assay more than one serum sample obtained before steady state is achieved; a single sample obtained too early could contribute to inaccurate predictions.

Recommendations are presented for optimal sampling times for commonly monitored drugs.

Index terms: Blood levels; Dosage; Half-life; Pharmacokinetics; Time
Clin Pharm. 1985; 4:84–92

In only little more than a decade, clinical pharmacokinetics has spawned therapeutic drug monitoring, the use of serum drug concentrations has increased from sporadic to commonplace, and the correlation of these concentrations to response and outcome has been refined. Notwithstanding these advances, the quality of each interpretation of an assay still relies on the acumen of practitioners, the accuracy of assays, the appropriate use of pharmacokinetic models, and the correct selection of sampling times.

The timing of sample collection and its influence on the interpretation of serum drug assays is the focus of this paper. Pharmacokinetic theory has recently been linked with sampling-time selection to improve the reliability of estimating steady-state concentrations and dosage regimens. In this paper, I present a review of fundamental considerations in determining the timing of samples and newer, more sophisticated approaches to sample selection; recommendations are offered for optimal sampling times for commonly monitored drugs.

GERALD E. SCHUMACHER, PHARM.D., PH.D., is Dean, College of Pharmacy and Allied Health Professions, Northeastern University, Boston, MA.

Address reprint requests to Dr. Schumacher at the College of Pharmacy and Allied Health Professions, Northeastern University, 360 Huntington Avenue, Boston, MA 02115.

Sampling To Ensure Therapeutic Drug Concentrations

Monitoring of serum drug concentrations presumes that there is a documented relationship between drug concentrations and subtherapeutic, therapeutic, and toxic responses. It is then axiomatic that this relationship is best examined when two conditions for sampling are met:

1. Blood samples are drawn during the postdistributive phase for loading and maintenance doses.
2. Blood samples are drawn at steady state for maintenance doses.

Unfortunately, these principles are better known by many pharmacists than physicians and phlebotomists. Recent studies[1-4] of therapeutic drug monitoring practices in which pharmacists do not select sampling times show a high incidence of drug samples drawn before patients reach the postdistributive or steady-state phase.

The first consideration in sampling is to ensure that samples are obtained during the postdistributive phase. Only after distribution equilibrium is achieved are serum concentrations useful surrogates of tissue concentrations. Samples drawn too early after administration of a dose, while the bulk of the drug is still being absorbed or distributing throughout the body, are spurious and not reflective of the concentration of drug at its site of action.

After the postdistributive interval for sampling is determined, the number of doses to be administered before obtaining a sample must be estimated. It is these steady-state concentrations that are indicative of drug quantity in the patient upon continued dosing. A duration of three to five half-lives is used for predicting attainment of steady state. When a loading dose is administered to achieve a steady-state concentration rapidly and sustain it while maintenance doses are accumulating, it is not necessary to wait until accumulation is complete; the sampling interval may be selected during the postdistributive phase after the loading dose.

The choice of sampling time does depend on the decision to monitor concentrations near the peak, trough, or some intermediate time. This decision assumes that the sampling time correlates with documented reports of response and outcome. Aminoglycosides are frequently sampled for peak and trough concentrations; oral antiarrhythmics, lithium, and tricyclic antidepressants for trough concentrations; and digoxin near the midpoint of the dosage interval. Theophylline sampling is somewhat controversial; some clinicians recommend sampling for trough concentrations,[5] others recommend peak concentrations,[6,7] while others accept peak or trough measurements.[8,9] In general, peak concentrations are most difficult to characterize, vary with the type of dosage form administered, and may be achieved before reaching the postdistributive phase. Trough determinations are fixed, concentrations are more reproducible, and sampling is almost always assured to be in the postdistributive phase. For some drugs like digoxin, phenytoin, and phenobarbital, response has often been correlated with concentrations near the midpoint of the dosage interval.

Table 1 shows reasonable sampling times, taking into account the average interval for achieving postdistribution equilibrium, peak concentration, and steady state, for commonly monitored drugs in patients with average and normal clearance functions. A number of reference sources[7-9] provide guidelines for sampling times.

Sampling To Determine Drug Clearance

A number of investigators[10-12] have used intravenous bolus or infusion administration to individualize pharmacokinetic parameters to estimate more accurately serum drug concentrations and dosage regimens. Using these methods, two or more serum samples are obtained within the first few hours after administration to characterize individual patient values such as clearance (CL), half-life ($t_{1/2}$), and volume of distribution (V). These estimates are then used to modify dosage regimens, if necessary.

Dossing and coworkers[13] refined this approach by determining optimal sampling times for minimizing intrapatient and interpatient variance in clearance determination. On the basis of statistical considerations, they showed that the variance of the clearance has a minimum when the mean sampling time is equal to the reciprocal of the elimination rate constant, or 1.4 $t_{1/2}$, regardless of the number of samples obtained or the specific timing of sample collection. Sampling frequency determined in this way is optimal in the sense that the variance of the

Table 1.
Sampling and Steady-State Times for Commonly Monitored Drugs

Drug	Minimum Sampling Time (hr) During a Dosage Interval[a] i.v.	p.o.	Steady State (days)[b]
Aminoglycosides	1	. . .	0.5–1
Digoxin	6	8	5–7
Lithium	8	10,12[c]	4–6
Procainamide	1	2,3[c]	0.5–1
Quinidine	1	2,4[c]	1–1.5
Theophylline	1	2,5[c,d]	1–2

[a] Sampling is appropriate from this time on. Average time for achieving postdistribution equilibrium or peak drug concentration in patients with normal absorption, distribution, and clearance.

[b] Average time for achieving steady-state concentrations in patients with normal half-lives.

[c] First and second numbers refer to fast-release and slow-release dosage forms, respectively.

[d] About 70% of slow-release theophylline dosage forms reach peak drug concentrations in six hours or less.

clearance estimate will be larger for any alternative choice of the same number of sampling times. In practice, the optimal timing of samples can only be determined approximately, using the population $t_{1/2}$ as a reference, because the individual patient $t_{1/2}$ is unknown. For example, to individualize a clearance estimate in a patient taking a drug with a population $t_{1/2}$ of four hours, the optimal sampling time is approximately six hours after administering the bolus or starting the infusion. If three samples are going to be used to estimate clearance, samples obtained at 2, 6, and 10 hours, or 3, 6, and 9 hours, are appropriate because the mean time is six hours. An alternative sequence of times, such as 4, 8, and 12 hours, will lead to a greater confidence interval for the clearance estimate. If two levels are to be used, samples drawn at four and eight hours, for example, will minimize the variance in clearance.

Sampling To Estimate Steady-State Concentrations and Dosage Regimens from a Test Dose

In order to shorten the time required for estimating steady-state concentrations and dosage regimens and to decrease the number of samples required for these estimates, a number of investigators have studied the use of "single-point" prediction methods based upon administration of a test dose. Drugs studied in this manner include lithium,[14,15] tricyclic antidepressants,[16,17] chloramphenicol,[18] and theophylline.[19–21] Koup[22] provided a critical and comprehensive review of single-point prediction methods.

Slattery and coworkers[15,23–25] developed the theory and application of steady-state concentration and maintenance-dose prediction based on a single determination of drug concentration at some fixed time after administration of a single dose. The method was first applied to drugs amenable to one compartment analysis,[23,24] then extended to drugs yielding active metabolites,[25] and then to a drug such as lithium, for which the two-compartment model applies.[15]

Slattery showed that the relationship between the average steady-state concentration and a single concentration after a test dose depends on the function ψ as follows:

$$C_{av}/C_{t^*} = [(D_m/\tau)\psi]/D^* \quad (1)$$

where,

$$\psi = e^{kt^*}/k$$
$$= 1.44t_{1/2}e^{t^*/1.44t_{1/2}} \quad (2)$$

In these equations, C_{av} represents the average concentration during the dosage interval, τ, at steady state, C_{t^*} is the concentration at time t^* after the test dose, D_m and D^* are the maintenance and test doses, respectively, and k is the elimination rate constant.

Since $t_{1/2}$ varies among individuals, the true value of ψ varies throughout the population. Therefore, equations 1 and 2 demonstrate that the variation in C_{av} among patients who show the same C_{t^*}, and who are each given the same D^* and D_m/τ, is a function of interpatient variation in $t_{1/2}$. This would seem to confound the estimation of C_{av} and limit the application of the single-point prediction method. Fortunately, however, Slattery showed that ψ varies much less than $t_{1/2}$ over a finite range centered around the population $t_{1/2}$ and that the least variation occurs from an optimal sampling time, t^*, for the test dose that is equal to $1/k$, or 1.4 $t_{1/2}$. For a fourfold range in $t_{1/2}$ centered about the population value, which is a range not greater than the interpatient variation observed in many drugs commonly monitored using serum concentrations, the fluctuation of ψ is small enough to allow reasonably accurate predictions of C_{av} from knowledge of C_{t^*}. Accuracy declines markedly for patients with $t_{1/2}$ values outside this range. The method is not applicable for drugs demonstrating nonlinear behavior.

Table 2 presents optimal sampling times for commonly monitored drugs. Alternative times are not invalid, but they will result in a greater range in the confidence interval for estimation of C_{av}. Unadkat and Rowland[26] expanded the use of this method to include the relative variation in ψ for various sampling times and the percentage of the population included within various $t_{1/2}$ ranges selected.

Limitations in this approach for the single-point prediction of C_{av} include the following:

1. The steady-state value estimated is the average concentration during the dosage interval.

Table 2.
Optimal Sampling Times for Estimating Average Serum Drug Concentrations (C_{av})

Drug	Optimal Sampling Time (hr)[a]
Aminoglycosides	3
Digoxin	60
Lithium	32
Procainamide	
Arrhythmias[b]	7
No arrhythmias[b]	4
N-acetylprocainamide	
Arrhythmias[b]	16
No arrhythmias[b]	9
Quinidine	9
Theophylline	
Adult or geriatric nonsmokers	12
Adult or geriatric smokers	8
Children 6–17 years old	5
Cirrhosis or congestive heart failure[b]	24

[a] Time after a test dose to estimate C_{av} with minimum intrapatient and interpatient variation in patients with normal renal and hepatic function.
[b] Patients with the stated condition.

2. Maximum and minimum steady-state serum concentration ($C_{ss_{max}}$ and $C_{ss_{min}}$, respectively) estimates are not applicable.
3. Very rapid absorption and distribution of drug is assumed. This limits the approach to administration by intravenous bolus and those drugs whose absorption and distribution is completed considerably before sampling.
4. The approach is not model independent.

To overcome these limitations Love and coworkers[27] expanded the method to include variable sampling times that allow for monitoring $C_{ss_{max}}$ or $C_{ss_{min}}$, made the approach applicable to any route of administration, and developed equations that were model independent based on the function χ:

$$C_{ss_{t''}}/C_{t'} = (D_m \chi)/D^* \qquad (3)$$

where,

$$\chi = \{0.693[((t' - t'')/\tau)(\tau/t_{1/2})]\}/(1 - e^{-0.693(\tau/t_{1/2})}) \qquad (4)$$

In these equations, $C_{ss_{t''}}$ represents the steady-state drug concentration sampled at time t'' and the concentration $C_{t'}$ sampled at time t' from the test dose D^*.

This method provides for the option of choosing a sampling time during the steady-state interval (t'') that is different from the time selected for sampling after the test dose (t') and assumes that both t' and t'' are selected during the terminal linear phase of the concentration versus time profile, when the contribution of the other exponential terms becomes negligible; this stipulation allows for model independence and applicability to any route of administration. The method, however, does not apply to drugs exhibiting nonlinear behavior or when drug clearance changes markedly during the time from test dose sampling to steady state.

Using equation 4 and the approach of Love and coworkers,[27] I constructed a general family of curves for plots of χ versus $t_{1/2}/\tau$ ratios, as shown in Figure 1. Since these curves are normalized for τ intervals, they may be applied to any drug when selecting t', t'', and τ, given that the drug and sampling meet the general conditions stated above.

Oral theophylline administered to nonsmoking adults is presented as an example of using Figure 1 and equations 3 and 4. Assume a population $t_{1/2}$ of 8.1 hours, a standard deviation of 2.4 hours (leading to a 90% confidence interval for the $t_{1/2}$ of 4–12 hours), the use of a slow-release dosage form, and an eight-hour dosage interval. The following steps are used to determine the optimal sampling time for t':

1. Isolate the 90% confidence interval for $t_{1/2}/\tau$ on the horizontal axis. For this example the interval is 0.5–1.5 since $t_{1/2}/\tau$ is 4/8 to 12/8.
2. Identify the $(t' - t'')/\tau$ curve demonstrating the least variability on the vertical axis for the $t_{1/2}/\tau$ interval isolated. In this case, the least variability is shown by the curve representing $(t' - t'')/\tau$ of 0.5.
3. Select t'' for sampling at steady state. Assume in this case that a t'' of four hours is chosen to estimate a concentration close to the peak ($C_{ss_{max}}$) for most slow-release dosage forms of theophylline.
4. Calculate t' for sampling after administering the test dose. Since τ = 8 hours and t'' = 4 hours, and the optimal curve $(t' - t'')/\tau = 0.5$, then t' = 8 hours. The optimal sampling time for the test dose is at eight hours.
5. Estimate $C_{ss_{t''}}$ or D_m. Use equation 3 and a measured concentration at t' from the test dose to predict $C_{ss_{t''}}$ from a given D_m or, alternatively, predict D_m needed to yield a desired $C_{ss_{t''}}$. To do this, follow the selected $(t' - t'')/\tau$ curve until the midpoint of the chosen confidence interval on the horizontal axis is located. Then read the corresponding value of χ on the vertical axis. Use this value of χ, $C_{t'}$, D^*, and D_m to calculate $C_{ss_{t''}}$. Or, use χ, $C_{t'}$, the desired $C_{ss_{t''}}$, and D^* to calculate D_m.

This example shows that a t' of eight hours is optimal when monitoring at t'' of four hours during an eight-hour dosage interval at steady state. Other combinations of t' and t'' are optimal as long as $(t' - t'')/\tau$ is maintained at 0.5. For each optimal set of t' and t'' sampling times in this example, calculations show that the 90% confidence interval of 4–12 hours for $t_{1/2}$ will yield a range of steady-state concentrations at t'' of ± 12% from the mean concentration estimated using equation 3 and the assumed popu-

Figure 1. Relationship between $t_{1/2}/\tau$ and the function χ for various values of $(t' - t'')/\tau$.

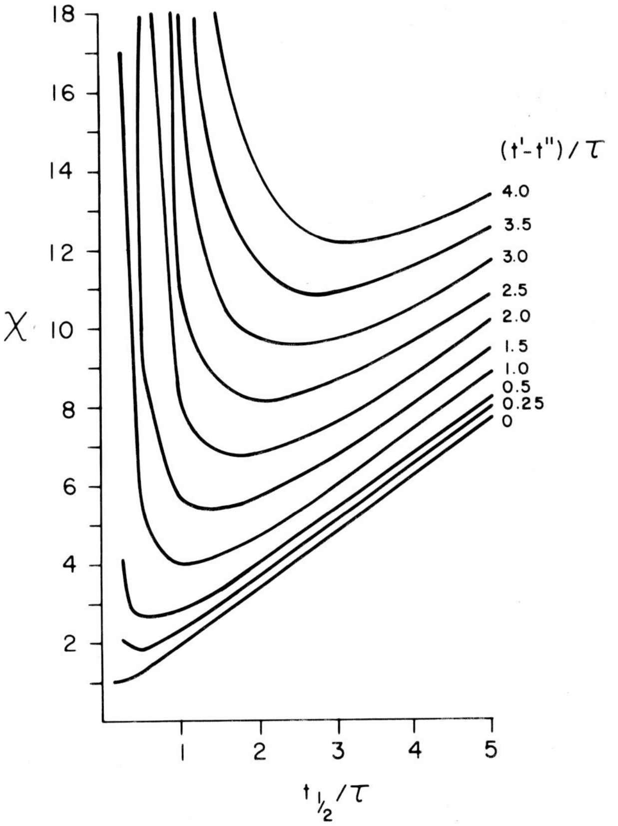

lation $t_{1/2}$ of 8.1 hours. In other words, although 90% of adult nonsmokers show a threefold interpatient range in $t_{1/2}$ values (4–12 hours), optimal sampling selection results in only a 12% variation about the mean steady-state concentration for the t'' and D_m chosen.

Alternatives to the optimal time may be selected by choosing a $(t' - t'')/\tau$ curve with more variability over the $t_{1/2}/\tau$ confidence interval than the optimal curve. In so doing, the confidence interval widens for the estimated steady-state concentration at t''. In this case, for example, choosing a t' of six or four hours, along with t'' of four hours as before, leads to a ±23% and ±35% variation, respectively, around the mean steady-state concentration. Less than optimal sampling thus leads to a doubling and tripling of the interpatient variability for peak monitoring of every eight-hour theophylline.

Using the above approach, I calculated appropriate sampling times corresponding to the usual steady-state monitoring times for drugs that are commonly monitored. Table 3 records the data for population $t_{1/2}$ and 90% confidence interval values used to calculate the sampling times from Figure 1. Table 4 shows the optimal sampling times for the various drugs. For some drugs, like digoxin, procainamide, and quinidine, optimal sampling times for the test dose may seem too long. In this case, the best alternative, shorter sampling time is reported, with a corresponding increase in the $C_{ss_{t''}}$ interpatient variability for 90% of patients. Although I have chosen the 90% confidence interval for $t_{1/2}$ to calculate sampling times, some practitioners may elect to use a larger or smaller interval. Using appropriate statistical techniques, an alternative confidence interval may be calculated, then converted to the corresponding $t_{1/2}/\tau$ interval for use in Figure 1, and the optimal t' may then be estimated.

In perusing Table 4, note that various sampling times are provided to meet differing needs and that these t' times are generally different from the t^* times to predict C_{av} shown in Table 2. This is because, in practice, monitoring at steady state for C_{av} is not common. For some drugs like procainamide, quinidine, and theophylline, both fast-release and slow-release dosage forms are available and this may result in varying sampling times. For some drugs like the aminoglycosides, multiple sampling times are used to meet monitoring goals. For drugs like the aminoglycosides, antiarrhythmics, and theophylline, varying dosage intervals may be selected, and this necessitates a varying selection of sampling times. For theophylline, data are provided in four categories of patients: adult nonsmokers, adult smokers, children, and adults with compromised liver function or congestive heart failure. Lastly, data are provided for both procainamide and *N*-acetylprocainamide (NAPA) in actively arrhythmic and nonarrhythmic patients. Since optimal sampling times for procainamide and NAPA are not congruent, an alternative time equivalent for both agents is provided for cases in which both are being monitored.

Table 3.
Population Half-lives[a] and 90% Confidence Intervals[b]

Drug	Mean (± S.D.) Half-life (hr)	90% Confidence Interval (hr)
Amikacin	2.3 ± 1	0.5–4
Digoxin	42 ± 19	11–73
Gentamicin	2.2 ± 1	0.5–4
Lithium	22 ± 8	9–35
Procainamide		
Arrhythmias[c]	5 ± 1.7	2–8
No arrhythmias[c]	3 ± 0.6	2–4
N-acetylprocainamide		
Arrhythmias[c]	10.9 ± 2.1	7–14
No arrhythmias[c]	6 ± 1.2	4–8
Quinidine	6.2 ± 1.8	3–9
Theophylline		
Adult or geriatric nonsmokers	8.1 ± 2.4	4–12
Adult or geriatric smokers	5.4 ± 1	4–7
Children 6–17 years old	3.7 ± 1.1	2–6
Cirrhosis or congestive heart failure[c]	16 ± 5	8–24
Tobramycin	2.2 ± 1	0.5–4

[a] Compiled from references 34–37 in patients with normal renal and hepatic function.
[b] Interval covering 90% of patients, based on the population half-life.
[c] Patients with the stated condition.

Sampling To Estimate Steady-State Concentrations and Dosage Regimens During a Continuous Infusion

During administration of a continuous intravenous infusion, the relationship between the steady-state concentration and a test concentration from a sample obtained before steady state for a one-compartment model is given by equation 5:

$$C_{ss_{inf}}/C_{t'} = 1/1 - e^{-t'/1.44t_{1/2}}$$
$$= 1/1 - e^{-(CL/V)t'} \qquad (5)$$

In this equation, $C_{ss_{inf}}$ denotes the steady-state concentration, $C_{t'}$ represents a sample drawn at time t' before reaching steady state, CL is the total drug clearance, and V the apparent volume of distribution.

The difficulty in selecting a single sampling time before steady state in order to estimate the steady-state concentration resulting from the continuous infusion is portrayed in Figure 2. Accumulation curves are presented for a one-compartment model, and expressed as the percent of $C_{ss_{inf}}$ for the population $t_{1/2}$ value, for seven different cases:

1. A normal curve: $t_{1/2}$, V, and CL represent population mean values.
2. A 0.5 $t_{1/2}$ curve: $t_{1/2}$ reduced to 50% of the population value, V unchanged, and CL therefore increased to 100% above the population value.
3. A 1.5 $t_{1/2}$ curve: $t_{1/2}$ increased to 50% above the

Table 4.
Optimal and Best Alternative Sampling Times for Estimating Various Steady-State Concentrations (C_{ss})

Drug	Dosing Interval (τ; hr)	Selected Monitoring Time at Steady State (t''; hr)	Optimal Sampling Time after a Test Dose: Sampling Time (t'; hr)[b]	Optimal Sampling Time after a Test Dose: Mean Variation (%)[b]	Best Alternative Sampling Time[c]: Sampling Time (t'; hr)[b]	Best Alternative Sampling Time[c]: Mean Variation (%)[b]
Amikacin	8	1	1	13		
	8	8	8	13		
	12	1	1	7		
	12	12	12	7		
Digoxin	24	8	32	20	24	34
Gentamicin	6	1	1	20		
	6	6	6	20		
	8	1	1	13		
	8	8	8	13		
Lithium	12	12	24	20	12	49
Procainamide[c]						
Arrhythmias[d]	4	4	8	14	4	43
	6	6	9	12	6	38
No arrhythmias[d]	4	4	6	4	4	18
	6	6	8	3	6	17
N-acetylprocainamide						
Arrhythmias[d]	4	4	16	3	4	30
	6	6	15	6	6	28
No arrhythmias[d]	4	4	10	3	4	26
	6	6	9	10	6	25
Quinidine	6	6	9	12	6	33
	8	8	12	10	8	29
	12	12	15	12	12	22
Theophylline						
Adult or geriatric nonsmokers	8	2	6	12		
	8	4	8	12		
	12	4	15	12	12	20
Adult or geriatric smokers	6	2	5	5		
	8	2	6	4		
	8	4	8	4		
	12	4	7	3		
Children 6–17 years old	6	2	4	12		
	8	4	6	6		
Cirrhosis or congestive heart failure[d]	8	2	20	8	8	26
	12	4	16	10	12	20
Tobramycin	6	1	1	20		
	6	6	6	20		
	8	1	1	13		
	8	8	8	13		

[a] Time after a test dose to estimate the corresponding C_{ss} at the t'' selected. This t' yields minimum intrapatient and interpatient variation in C_{ss} for optimal sampling. For best alternative sampling, t' yields a higher variation in C_{ss}.

[b] Percent variation in C_{ss} based on the 90% confidence interval.

[c] Alternative sampling time after a test dose. To be used, if desired, when the optimal sampling time after the first dose is longer than τ.

[d] Patients with the stated condition.

population value, V unchanged, and CL therefore decreased to 67% of the population value.

4. A 0.5 V curve: V reduced to 50% of the population value, $t_{1/2}$ unchanged, and CL therefore decreased to 50% of the population value.
5. A 1.5 V curve: V increased to 50% above the population value, $t_{1/2}$ unchanged, and CL therefore increased to 50% above the population value.
6. A 0.5 $t_{1/2}$, 0.5 V curve: Both $t_{1/2}$ and V decreased to 50% below the population values and clearance therefore unchanged.
7. A 1.5 $t_{1/2}$, 1.5 V curve: Both $t_{1/2}$ and V increased to 50% above the population values and clearance therefore unchanged.

As shown in Figure 2, single-point sampling too early in the infusion ($t'/t_{1/2}$ of 0.5 or 1.0 for example) can lead to misleading predictions of steady-state concentrations. Sampling at a time equal to one population $t_{1/2}$ ($t'/t_{1/2} = 1$) yields these misleading results:

1. The 1.5 $t_{1/2}$ curve is only about 10% greater than the normal curve for the population average, a difference that would not alarm most practitioners, yet the 1.5 $t_{1/2}$ curve will reach a steady-state concentration 50% greater than the population average.
2. Differences in the curves for 0.5 $t_{1/2}$ and 1.5 $t_{1/2}$ are not great enough to alert most practitioners, yet at

steady state the 1.5 $t_{1/2}$ curve will accumulate to a concentration 200% greater than the 0.5 $t_{1/2}$ curve.

3. The 0.5 $t_{1/2}$, 0.5 V curve is 50% greater than the normal curve, an observation that could suggest dosage revision by some practitioners, but at steady state the concentrations will be equal.
4. The curves for 0.5 $t_{1/2}$ and 1.5 $t_{1/2}$, 1.5 V are equal but the 0.5 $t_{1/2}$ curve will reach a steady-state concentration 50% less than the 1.5 V curve.

While sampling at a later time, perhaps at two times the population $t_{1/2}$ ($t'/t_{1/2} = 2$), does not resolve all of these problems, in each case the situation has become more clear, misperceptions are largely corrected, and the sampling results would lead most practitioners to appropriate action.

In some cases a bolus loading dose is administered in conjunction with the continuous infusion. This situation is portrayed in Figure 3 for the seven cases noted above. Here, the trends predicted by early sampling are more clear but some misleading results still emerge at $t'/t_{1/2} = 1$:

1. The 1.5 $t_{1/2}$ curve is nearly indistinguishable from the 0.5 $t_{1/2}$, 0.5 V curve, yet at steady state the 1.5 $t_{1/2}$ curve will accumulate to a concentration 50% greater than the 0.5 $t_{1/2}$, 0.5 V curve.
2. The 1.5 $t_{1/2}$ curve is only about 20% greater than the curve for the population average, but at steady state the 1.5 $t_{1/2}$ curve will accumulate to a concentration 50% above the normal curve.
3. The 1.5 $t_{1/2}$, 1.5 V curve is only about 25% greater than the 0.5 $t_{1/2}$ curve, yet at steady state the former will accumulate to a concentration 100% above the latter.

Once again, a single-point sample taken at two times the population $t_{1/2}$ ($t'/t_{1/2} = 2$) improves each case and clarifies the misperceptions.

The seven curves depicted in Figures 2 and 3 demonstrate the pitfalls practitioners face in therapeutic drug monitoring when using only one early sample to predict the eventual status at steady state. The range of cases presented, covering a threefold variation in $t_{1/2}$, V, and CL, is commonly encountered. Early sampling to detect marked variations from the normal clearance, at $t'/t_{1/2}$ of 1.0 or less, is most sensitive to alterations in V. When either $t_{1/2}$ or both $t_{1/2}$ and V are altered, misleading informa-

Figure 2. Relationship between $t'/t_{1/2}$ and the percent of $C_{ss_{inf}}$ for the population mean case in various cases of altered pharmacokinetic values during administration of a continuous intravenous infusion. Shown are the population mean case (·····), 0.5 $t_{1/2}$ (– – ·), 1.5 $t_{1/2}$ (–·–), 0.5 V(—), 1.5 V(——— ———), 0.5 $t_{1/2}$, 0.5 V (— — —), and 1.5 $t_{1/2}$, 1.5 V(— · ·).

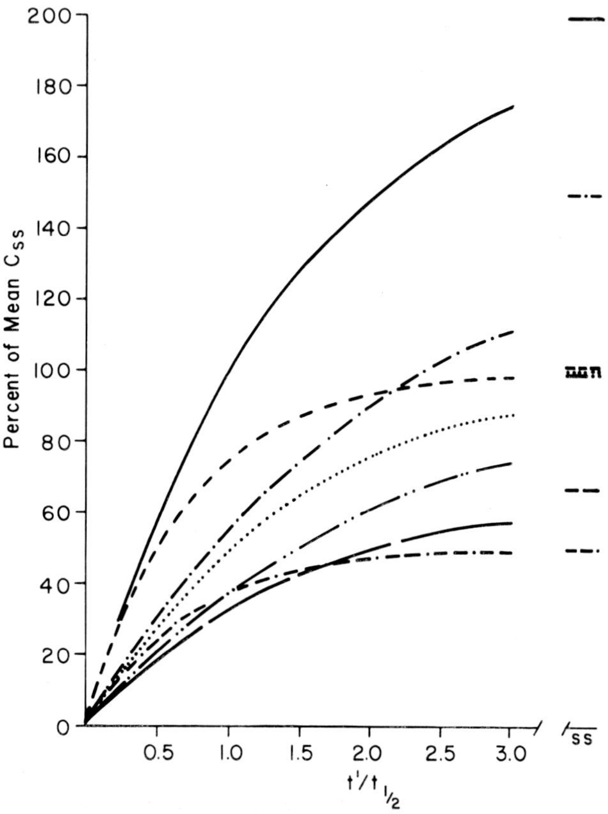

Figure 3. Relationship between $t'/t_{1/2}$ and the percent of $C_{ss_{inf}}$ for the population mean case in various cases of altered pharmacokinetic values during administration of an intravenous bolus plus a continuous infusion. Shown are the population mean case (·····), 0.5 $t_{1/2}$ (– – ·), 1.5 $t_{1/2}$ (–·–), 0.5 V(—), 1.5 V(——— ———), 0.5 $t_{1/2}$, 0.5 V(— — —), and 1.5 $t_{1/2}$, 1.5 V(— · ·).

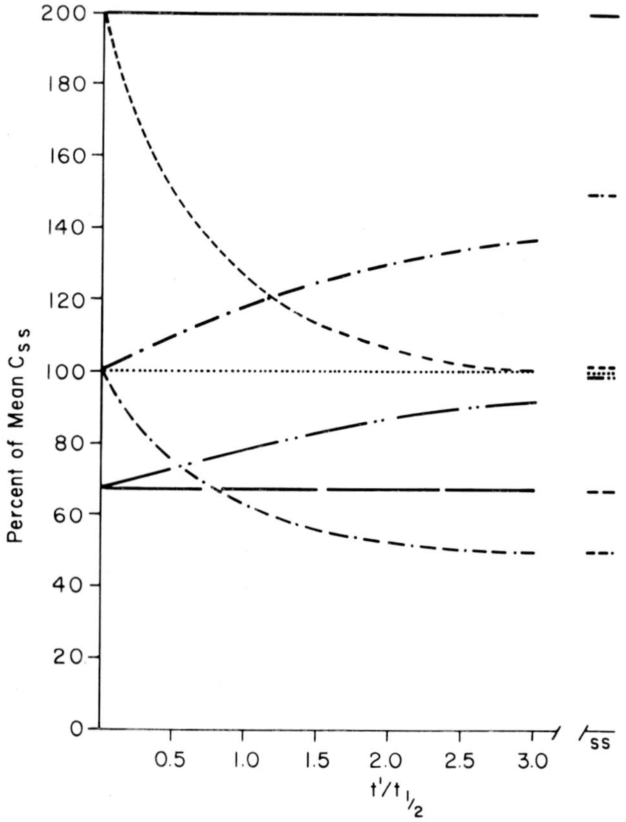

tion may be provided.

Therefore, even during this time of cost containment, it seems prudent to recommend that more than one sample be drawn before steady state for some drugs administered by continuous infusion. Practitioner curiosity and anxiety often dictate the frequency of sampling, but a single sample obtained too early could contribute to inaccurate perceptions in some situations. Sampling at $t'/t_{1/2} = 1$ and $t'/t_{1/2} = 2$–3 is generally appropriate. But if only one sample is to be obtained, it should be collected no earlier than $t'/t_{1/2} = 2$. For drugs with a very long $t_{1/2}$, impatience will probably mitigate against waiting until $t'/t_{1/2} = 1$ to obtain the first sample.

Future Directions in Sampling

Equations 1–5 and the above discussion centered on intrapatient and interpatient variations in CL, $t_{1/2}$, and V as the sole considerations responsible for deviations in $C_{t'}$ and C_{ss} from that expected. The accuracy and precision of pharmacokinetic estimates, the associated prediction of drug concentrations, and the actual measurement of concentrations are also dependent upon the errors associated with the time of sample collection, laboratory assay, and pharmacokinetic model specificity. In some cases these errors can contribute as much to intrapatient and interpatient variation as does the variation in pharmacokinetic values.

Some investigators[28–31] have begun to incorporate estimates of all these errors into calculations and have suggested that these considerations may sometimes alter the optimal sampling times presented in Tables 2 and 4. These investigations represent preliminary simulations, have yet to be applied prospectively in patients, and require additional study and evaluation. Nonetheless, errors in assay, sample collection time, and characterization of pharmacokinetic models undoubtedly contribute in some measure to the patient variations commonly observed. The use of Bayesian analysis[32] has recently been reported[33] as an approach to determine optimal sampling times. For the present, however, the use of the principles discussed above will improve the ability of practitioners to select sampling times and interpret the resulting concentrations during therapeutic drug monitoring.

References

1. Clague HW, Twum-Barima Y, Carruthers SG. An audit of requests for therapeutic drug monitoring of digoxin: problems and pitfalls. *Ther Drug Monit.* 1983; 5:249–54.
2. Bussey HI, Hoffman EW. A prospective evaluation of therapeutic drug monitoring. *Ther Drug Monit.* 1983; 5:245–8.
3. Guernsey BG, Hokanson JA, Ingrim NB et al. A utilization review of digoxin assays: sampling patterns and use. *Hosp Pharm.* 1984; 19:187–99.
4. Mason GD, Winter ME. Appropriateness of sampling times for therapeutic drug monitoring. *Am J Hosp Pharm.* 1984; 41:1796–801.
5. Winter ME, Katcher BS, Koda-Kimble MA. Basic clinical pharmacokinetics. San Francisco: Applied Therapeutics, Inc; 1980:145.
6. Hendeles L, Weinberger M, Johnson G. Theophylline. In: Evans WE, Schentag JJ, Jusko WJ, eds. Applied pharmacokinetics. San Francisco: Applied Therapeutics, Inc.; 1980:123.
7. Baer DM, Dito WR. Interpretations in therapeutic drug monitoring. Chicago: American Society of Clinical Pathologists; 1981.
8. Taylor WT, Finn AL, Gotcher S. Individualizing drug therapy: clinical notes on the application of drug monitoring. New York: Gross, Townsend, Frank, Inc; 1981.
9. Evans WE, Oellerich M. Therapeutic drug monitoring clinical guide. Irving, TX: Abbott Laboratories Diagnostics Division; 1984.
10. Sawchuck RJ, Zaske DE, Cipolle RJ et al. Kinetic models for gentamicin dosing with the use of individual patient parameters. *Clin Pharmacol Ther.* 1977; 21:362–9.
11. Chiou WL, Gadalla MAF, Peng GW. Method for rapid estimation of the total body drug clearance and adjustment of dosage regimens in patients during a constant-rate intravenous infusion. *J Pharmacokinet Biopharm.* 1978; 6:99–110.
12. Vozeh S, Kewitz G, Wenk M et al. Rapid prediction of steady-state serum theophylline concentration in patients treated with intravenous aminophylline. *Eur J Clin Pharmacol.* 1980; 18:473–7.
13. Dossing M, Volund A, Poulsen HE. Optimal sampling times for minimum variance of clearance determination. *Br J Clin Pharmacol.* 1983; 15:231–5.
14. Cooper TB, Simpson GM. The 24-hour lithium level as a prognosticator of dosage requirements: a 2-year follow-up study. *Am J Psychiatry.* 1976; 133:440–3.
15. Zimmerman CL, Slattery JT. Maintenance-dose prediction based on a single determination of concentration: general applicability to two-compartment drugs with reference to lithium. *J Pharm Sci.* 1983; 72:1262–6.
16. Montgomery SA, McAuley R, Montgomery DB et al. Dosage adjustment from simple nortriptyline spot level predictor tests in depressed patients. *Clin Pharmacokinet.* 1979; 4:129–36.
17. Brunswick DJ, Amsterdam JD, Mendels J et al. Prediction of steady-state imipramine and desmethylimipramine concentrations from single dose data. *Clin Pharmacol Ther.* 1979; 25:605–10.
18. Koup JR, Sack CM, Smith AL et al. Rapid estimation of chloramphenicol clearance in infants and children. *Clin Pharmacokinet.* 1981; 6:83–8.
19. Shapiro GG, Koup JR, Furukawa CT et al. Individualization of theophylline dosage using a single serum sample following a test dose. *Pediatrics.* 1982; 69:70–3.
20. Taylor DR, Kinney CD, McDevitt DG. Prediction of maintenance oral theophylline dosage using single oral doses in patients with obstructive airways disease. *Br J Clin Pharmacol.* 1983; 15:689–94.
21. Wilkens JH, Neuenkirchen H, Sybrecht GW et al. Individualizing theophylline dosage: evaluation of a single-point maintenance dose prediction method. *Eur J Clin Pharmacol.* 1984; 26:491–8.
22. Koup JR. Single-point prediction methods: a critical review. *Drug Intell Clin Pharm.* 1982; 16:855–62.
23. Slattery JT, Gibaldi M, Koup JR. Prediction of maintenance dose required to attain a desired drug concentration at steady-state from a single determination of concentration after an initial dose. *Clin Pharmacokinet.* 1980; 5:377–85.
24. Slattery JT. Single-point maintenance dose prediction: role of interindividual differences in clearance and volume of distribution in choice of sampling time. *J Pharm Sci.* 1981; 70:1174–6.
25. Wilson JM, Slattery JT. Maintenance-dose prediction based on a single determination of concentration: dose of parent drug required to give a desired steady-state concentration of metabolite. *J Pharm Sci.* 1983; 72:1174–8.
26. Unadkat JD, Rowland M. Further considerations of the sin-

gle-point single-dose method to estimate individual maintenance dosage requirements. *Ther Drug Monit.* 1982; 4: 201–8.

27. Love BL, Tsuei SE, Thomas J et al. The single-point method of dosage prediction: pharmacokinetic basis and method optimization. *Biopharm Drug Dispos.* 1982; 3:191–201.
28. D'Argenio DZ. Optimal sampling times for pharmacokinetic experiments. *J Pharmacokinet Biopharm.* 1981; 9:739–56.
29. D'Argenio DZ, Katz D. Sampling strategies for noncompartmental estimation of mean residence time. *J Pharmacokinet Biopharm.* 1983; 11:435–46.
30. D'Argenio DZ, Khakmahd K. Adaptive control of theophylline therapy: importance of blood sampling times. *J Pharmacokinet Biopharm.* 1983; 547–59.
31. Berg MJ, Lantz RK, Schoenwald RD et al. Optimization of pharmacokinetic monitoring: I. linear pharmacokinetics. *Ther Drug Monit.* 1983; 5:379–87.
32. Schumacher GE, Barr JT. Bayesian approaches in pharmacokinetic decision making. *Clin Pharm.* 1984; 3:525–30.
33. Peck CC, Perkins SW. Optimal sampling theory in a Bayesian context: a framework for choosing number and timing of clinical drug level measurements. *Clin Pharmacol Ther.* 1984; 35:266. Abstract.
34. Benet LZ, Sheiner LB. Design and optimization of dosage regimens: pharmacokinetic data. In: Gilman AG, Goodman LS, Gilman A, eds. The pharmacological basis of therapeutics. New York: Macmillan; 1980:1675–737.
35. Benet LZ, Massoud N, Gambertoglio JG. Pharmacokinetic basis for drug treatment. New York: Raven Press; 1984: 419–36.
36. Pechere JC, Dugal R. Clinical pharmacokinetics of aminoglycoside antibiotics. *Clin Pharmacokinet.* 1979; 4:170–99.
37. Penn DH. Procainamide. In: Mungall DR, ed. Applied clinical pharmacokinetics. New York: Raven Press: 1983:51–64.

Grand Rounds

Papers in the Grand Rounds section are patient case reports and literature review combined in a way that gives them high educational value. The papers lead off with a well-documented case report of an unusual drug experience (e.g., adverse drug reaction or other unexpected drug response, experimental use of a drug). The case generally deals with a difficult therapeutic problem or dilemma that is commonly encountered but may be overlooked or misunderstood. (Esoteric or rare occurrences of minor importance do not make good Grand Rounds material.) A literature review puts the case in perspective with previously reported similar cases and alternative treatments. The review is integrated with related discussions of the new case being reported.

CP readers are encouraged to use Grand Rounds for educational group discussions. For this purpose, discussion questions are printed at the end of Grand Rounds papers.

Treatment of trigeminal neuralgia: Use of baclofen in combination with carbamazepine

KAREN A. BAKER, JERRY W. TAYLOR, AND GILBERT E. LILLY

Abstract: A patient with trigeminal neuralgia who became refractory to carbamazepine but responded well to the addition of baclofen to his regimen is described, and the drug and surgical treatment of trigeminal neuralgia are discussed.

A 57-year-old white man sought medical help following a six-week history of paroxysmal pain in the right jaw. Rubbing the skin in the right third division of the trigeminal nerve produced a paroxysm of pain. Trigeminal neuralgia was diagnosed, and carbamazepine therapy was initiated with good results. Pain recurred upon discontinuation of the therapy, and carbamazepine was restarted. However, debilitating pain persisted despite continuous treatment that produced moderate postdose ataxia. Baclofen was added to the patient's regimen and increased to 60 mg daily with subsequent reductions in the carbamazepine dosages. The patient remained pain-free during the following 10 months.

Carbamazepine is considered the drug of choice and is initially very effective in treating trigeminal neuralgia. However, many patients are forced to discontinue drug therapy because of intolerance or ineffectiveness and are faced with surgery as their only option. Baclofen does not appear to be as effective as carbamazepine when used as a single agent. However, its apparent synergism with carbamazepine and phenytoin combined with its low incidence of serious side effects make baclofen a valuable adjunct in the treatment of refractory trigeminal neuralgia.

Index terms: Analgesics and antipyretics; Ataxia; Baclofen; Carbamazepine; Combined therapy; Dosage; Drug interactions; Trigeminal neuralgia; Toxicity
Clin Pharm. 1985; 4:93–6

Trigeminal neuralgia is a disorder of unknown cause characterized by brief paroxysms of intense facial pain. Carbamazepine is considered the drug of first choice and is initially effective in more than 80% of patients suffering from trigeminal neuralgia.[1] However, long-term treatment continues to be effective in only 56% of patients followed for up to 16 years.[2] Carbamazepine intolerance requires withdrawal of the drug in 5–19% of patients.[2,3] Until recently, those patients forced to discontinue drug therapy because of intolerance or ineffectiveness were faced with surgery as the only treatment option. This report describes a case of trigeminal neuralgia involving a patient who became refractory to

KAREN A. BAKER, M.S., is Clinical Assistant Professor, Division of Clinical and Hospital Pharmacy, College of Pharmacy, and Department of Pharmacy Administration, College of Dentistry, University of Iowa, Iowa City. JERRY W. TAYLOR, PHARM.D., is Associate Professor, Department of Clinical Pharmacy Practice, University of Mississippi, Jackson. GILBERT E. LILLY, D.D.S., is Professor and Head, Department of Oral Pathology and Diagnosis, College of Dentistry, University of Iowa, Iowa City.
Address reprint requests to Ms. Baker at the University of Iowa, S306 Dental Science Building, Iowa City, IA 52242.

carbamazepine but who responded well to the addition of baclofen to his regimen.

Case Report

A 57-year-old white man in good health came to the College of Dentistry Oral Pathology Department with a six-week history of paroxysmal pain in the right jaw beginning in January 1983. The pain was exacerbated by talking, eating, or swallowing and was not precipitated by heat, cold, or tooth movement. The patient had been apprehensive about tooth cleaning and was unshaven in the right jaw area. The paroxysmal pain was localized to the right third division of the trigeminal nerve. On physical examination no evidence of hypalgesia was found. However, rubbing of the skin in the third division produced a paroxysm of pain. The corneal reflexes were brisk, and the remaining cranial nerves intact. A panoramic radiograph failed to show organic pathology. Baseline hematologic values were within normal limits. A diagnosis of trigeminal neuralgia was made, and carbamazepine therapy was initiated (Table 1). The patient was initially well controlled with carbamazepine therapy at a dosage of 400 mg daily. Pain recurred two weeks following discontinuation of carbamazepine in July 1983. The carbamazepine therapy was restarted; however, debilitating pain persisted despite continuous treatment that produced moderate postdose ataxia (Table 1). The patient's hematologic values remained stable. In September 1983, a neurosurgeon was consulted. However, the patient declined surgery at that time. Baclofen was subsequently added to his regimen and titrated to a dose of 60 mg daily in three equally divided doses. Carbamazepine was continued as before and then gradually reduced from 1400 to 800 mg per day. In the following 10 months, the patient tolerated both medications well and was pain free except for two paroxysms, which occurred after another carbamazepine dosage reduction in June 1984 (Table 1).

Table 1.
Patient's Course of Therapy

Date	Carbamazepine Dose (mg/day)	Carbamazepine Serum Concentration (μg/mL)	Regimen or Dose Schedule	Comments
2/23/83	400	...	200 mg b. i. d.	Soft diet advised
3/1/83	400	5.9	200 mg b. i. d.	Pain free since 2/24, solids
3/8/83	400	5.3	200 mg b. i. d.	Drowsy, pain episode on 3/7
3/31/83	400	5.0	200 mg b. i. d.	Pain free, reduce to 200 mg/day
4/14/83	400	...	200 mg b. i. d.	Pain five days after reduction
4/28/83	400	4.3	200 mg b. i. d.	Pain free
6/13/83	400	4.1	200 mg b. i. d.	Pain free, try dose reduction
7/26/83	400	...	200 mg b. i. d.	Pain 14 days after discontinuation, resume therapy
8/11/83	800	7.6	400 mg b. i. d.	Dose increased 8/1, pain persists
8/16/83	1000	...	500 mg b. i. d.	Dose increased 8/11, pain free
8/25/83	1000	7.2	500 mg b. i. d.	Pain free, gait instability
8/30/83	1000	...	400-300-300 mg	Pain recurs, gait instability
9/3/83	1100	...	400-300-400 mg	Pain continues, no ataxia
9/6/83	1200	8.9	400-400-400 mg	Pain continues, increase to 1500 mg
9/8/83	1500	...	500-500-500 mg	Pain continues, increase to 1700 mg
9/11/83	1700	...	400-200-500-600 mg	Partial relief, periodic ataxia
9/14/83	1700	8.7	400-200-500-600 mg	Pain free one day, periodic ataxia
9/20/83	1700	...	400-200-500-600 mg	Pain free seven days, decrease to 1400 mg/day, advise neurosurgery consultation
9/27/83	1400	...	400-200-200-200-400 mg	Pain control inadequate, start baclofen 5 mg tid for five days then 10 mg tid for three days, decrease carbamazepine
10/4/83	1000	...	400-200-200-200 mg	Pain episodes twice, increase baclofen to 20 mg tid
10/11/83	1000	...	400-200-200-200 mg	Pain free since 10/4/83, reduce carbamazepine dosage
10/20/83	800	...	200 mg q. i. d.	Pain episode on 10/12 and 10/14, pain free from 10/15 on, all medication well tolerated
12/1/83	800	6.8	200 mg q. i. d.	Pain free
1/10/84	800	8.0	200 mg q. i. d.	Pain free
4/26/84	800	7.1	200 mg q. i. d.	Pain free
5/23/84	800	...	200 mg q. i. d.	Pain free, reduce carbamazepine, maintain baclofen at 20 mg tid
6/26/84	400	4.2	200 mg b. i. d.	Pain episode on 6/16 and 6/18, continue at present dosages
8/15/84	400	...	200 mg b. i. d.	Pain free, continue both medications

Discussion

Trigeminal neuralgia (tic douloureux) is an extremely painful affliction characterized by short paroxysms of high-intensity facial pain. The pain is confined to the distribution of the fifth cranial nerve and occurs most commonly in the lower jaw or cheek. The average age of onset is 55 years with 90% of cases diagnosed after age 40. Trigeminal neuralgia affects women more often than men and is more often right-sided than left-sided (1.7 to 1).[4] Most patients can identify stimuli that will reliably initiate the pain. The trigger zone is always within the fifth cranial nerve distribution and may change location with time. As in the case above, patients often take many precautions to avoid triggering stimuli and may be pain free for intervals lasting minutes, hours, days, months, or even years. Findings on neurological examination are normal, and the clinician must rule out causes of trigeminal irritation, such as tumor, and other kinds of facial pain, such as atypical facial pain. Trigeminal neuralgia is sometimes associated with multiple sclerosis, and in these patients the pain is more frequently bilateral and usually begins at a younger age.[5]

Many theories have evolved concerning the etiology of trigeminal neuralgia. These have included dental or jaw involvement, infected dental extraction sites, and viral infection of the gasserian ganglion of the trigeminal nerve. Evidence is now accumulating to support the theory that the majority of cases are caused by a compression-distortion phenomenon, usually attributable to an anomalous position of an arterial loop or venous channel.[6–9] However, tumors or arterial aneurysms have been identified in as many as 10% of cases and also cause this compression-distortion phenomenon.

Drug Treatment. Carbamazepine remains the drug of choice for trigeminal neuralgia even though patients often become refractory to treatment.[2] Optimal pain relief occurs at plasma carbamazepine concentrations ranging from 5.7 to 10.1 μg/mL. Therapeutic trials are difficult to evaluate because patients will typically experience complete remissions lasting several months or even years.[10,11] Pain relief in the patient described cannot be attributed to spontaneous remission since he experienced pain shortly after carbamazepine withdrawal. Carbamazepine-induced side effects on long-term therapy may result from plasma concentrations above 7.9 μg/mL[10] whereas serious idiosyncratic side effects appear unrelated to dose and require withdrawal of the drug.[3] Phenytoin is less effective in the treatment of trigeminal neuralgia than carbamazepine[12] and is commonly associated with dose-related side effects, such as nystagmus, ataxia, and drowsiness.

Surgical Treatment. If drug treatment fails to relieve the pain or side effects force discontinuation of treatment, surgery is usually considered. The ideal surgical procedure would allow for pain relief without producing any neurologic deficit, particularly numbness of the face. Microneurosurgical decompression of the fifth cranial nerve root entry zone as described by Jannetta[13] comes closest to achieving this ideal. The operation carries little risk of mortality or morbidity, and pain is relieved in more than 95% of patients. The absence of altered facial sensation, dysesthesia, and corneal anesthesia postoperatively give this operation a major advantage over all other procedures. The complications[6,7] of cerebellar dysfunction and fourth, sixth, seventh, or eighth cranial nerve dysfunction are uncommon. To avoid craniotomy in elderly or debilitated patients, controlled thermocoagulation of the gasserian ganglion is considered the most reliable destructive procedure available.[14] When compared with other destructive procedures, it offers the possibility of preserving touch sensation while destroying pain sensation. Complications include motor root impairment (24%), corneal anesthesia (4–13%), and others.[15] About 50% of patients will have pain recurrences within five years, and the procedure may be repeated.

Treatment with Baclofen. A less toxic yet more efficacious treatment for trigeminal neuralgia is needed. Baclofen resembles carbamazepine and phenytoin in depressing the response of spinal trigeminal neurons to maxillary nerve stimulation in cats.[16] This observation led to the administration of baclofen in the treatment of trigeminal neuralgia.

Fromm et al.[17] administered baclofen to 14 patients with trigeminal neuralgia who were intolerant of or refractory to carbamazepine. Initially, 10 patients experienced pain relief after receiving 60–80 mg/day of baclofen. Of these patients, two were taking carbamazepine, three were taking phenytoin, and five were receiving no concomitant medications. Seven patients (50%) remained pain free or almost pain free on baclofen therapy for 4–12 months.

Herring[18] reported a case involving a woman with multiple sclerosis and trigeminal neuralgia who did not respond to large doses of carbamazepine (1800 mg/day) in conjunction with other antispastic drugs. The addition of baclofen 80 mg/day resulted in adequate pain control.

Fromm et al.[19] conducted an open trial in another 50 patients with trigeminal neuralgia who were intolerant of or refractory to carbamazepine. If the frequency of attacks decreased after the addition of baclofen, the carbamazepine or phenytoin was gradually eliminated to determine whether baclofen alone would control the trigeminal neuralgia. The addition of baclofen provided pain relief in 37 (74%) of the patients, either alone (12 patients), or in combination with previously ineffective doses of carbamazepine or phenytoin (25 patients). In both Fromm studies,[17,19] long-term treatment with baclofen continued to be effective in 28 of 60 patients (47%), with 20 patients requiring concomitant therapy with previously ineffective doses of carbamazepine or phenytoin.

Baclofen appears to have a synergistic action with carbamazepine and phenytoin. In Fromm's open trial,[19] the addition of baclofen to regimens of carbamazepine or phenytoin that were previously ineffective produced pain control in twice as many neuralgia patients as the administration of baclofen alone. Drug intolerance manifest as drowsiness or nausea and vomiting was much more common when baclofen and carbamazepine were administered together than when baclofen was given alone.

Baclofen is an analog of the inhibitory neurotransmitter γ-aminobutyric acid (GABA) but may not resemble GABA in its mechanism of action. Baclofen has been shown to antagonize excitatory transmission, possibly by depressing the release of excitatory neurotransmitters.[20,21] Baclofen has also demonstrated a depressant effect on excitatory transmission in the spinal trigeminal nucleus of cats.[16,17] In all animal studies comparing *d* and *l* enantiomorphs, this effect has been attributed to *l*-baclofen.[22] As previously cited, both baclofen and carbamazepine have a similar depressant effect on excitatory synaptic transmission.[17] Crystallographic evaluation of carbamazepine and both enantiomorphs of baclofen show a surprisingly good fit of baclofen isomers to moieties of the carbamazepine molecule.[22] This may well be the reason that two structurally dissimilar drugs exert similar clinical and neurophysiologic effects. These results are consistent with the idea that *l*-baclofen and carbamazepine act at a common receptor site in the human trigeminal nucleus.[22]

Conclusion

Presently available clinical data suggest that baclofen is not as effective as carbamazepine in the treatment of trigeminal neuralgia. However, its synergistic effect with carbamazepine and phenytoin combined with its low incidence of serious side effects make baclofen a valuable adjunct in the treatment of refractory trigeminal neuralgia.

Discussion Questions

1. What are proposed mechanisms by which carbamazepine causes bone-marrow suppression? Is this effect dose or duration dependent?
2. Describe appropriate monitoring procedures to ensure the safe clinical use of carbamazepine.
3. What effect does carbamazepine enzyme induction have on control of disease states (e.g., seizure disorders or trigeminal neuralgia)? What serum concentrations are considered therapeutic when treating trigeminal neuralgia as opposed to seizure disorders?
4. What adverse effects have been documented after the sudden withdrawal of baclofen therapy?
5. Discuss the efficacy of phenytoin therapy in the treatment of trigeminal neuralgia. Under what circumstances should phenytoin be used to treat trigeminal neuralgia?

References

1. Rasmussen P, Riishede J. Facial pain treated with carbamazepine (Tegretol). *Acta Neurol Scand.* 1970; 46:385–90.
2. Taylor JC, Braver S, Espir MLE. Long-term treatment of trigeminal neuralgia with carbamazepine. *Postgrad Med J.* 1981; 57:16–8.
3. Crill WE. Carbamazepine. *Ann Intern Med.* 1973; 79:844–7.
4. Voorhies R, Patterson RH. Management of trigeminal neuralgia (tic douloureux). *JAMA.* 1981; 245:2521–3.
5. Penman J. Trigeminal neuralgia. In: Vinken PJ, Bruyn GW, eds. Handbook of clinical neurology. New York: American Elsevier Publishing Co., Inc.; 1968; 5:296.
6. Apfelbaum RI. A comparison of percutaneous radiofrequency trigeminal neurolysis and microvascular decompression of the trigeminal nerve for the treatment of trigeminal neuralgia. *Neurosurgery.* 1977; 1:16–20.
7. Lazar ML. Trigeminal neuralgia—recent advances in management. *Tex Med.* 1978; 74:45–8.
8. Lazar ML, Kirkpatrick JB. Trigeminal neuralgia and multiple sclerosis: demonstration of the plaque in an operative case. *Neurosurgery.* 1979; 5:711–7.
9. Loeser JD. What to do about tic douloureux. *JAMA.* 1978; 239:1153–5.
10. Tomson T, Tybring G, Bertilsson L et al. Carbamazepine therapy in trigeminal neuralgia: clinical effects in relation to plasma concentration. *Arch Neurol.* 1980; 37:699–703.
11. Henderson WR. Trigeminal neuralgia: the pain and its treatment. *Br Med J.* 1967; 1:7–15.
12. White JC, Sweet WH. Pain and the neurosurgeon: a forty-year experience. Springfield, IL: Charles C Thomas Publisher; 1969:173.
13. Jannetta PJ. Microsurgical approach to the trigeminal nerve for tic douloureux. *Prog Neurol Surg.* 1976; 7:170–4.
14. Sweet WH, Wespic JG. Controlled thermocoagulation of the trigeminal ganglion and rootlets for differential destruction of pain fibres. Part I. Trigeminal neuralgia. *J Neurosurg.* 1974; 39:143–8.
15. Bland JE, Lazar ML, Naarden AL. Treatment of pain syndromes. In: Rosenberg R, ed. The treatment of neurological diseases. Holliswood, NY: Spectrum Publishers; 1979.
16. Fromm GH, Terrence CF, Chattha AS et al. Role of inhibitory mechanisms in trigeminal neuralgia. *Neurology.* 1981; 31: 683–7.
17. Fromm GH, Terrence CF, Chattha AS et al. Baclofen in trigeminal neuralgia. Its effect on the spinal trigeminal nucleus: a pilot study. *Arch Neurol.* 1980; 37:768–71.
18. Herring R, Komizki A, Bachar M. Baclofen in trigeminal neuritis. *Harefuah.* 1982; 102:63–4.
19. Fromm GH, Terrence CF, Chattha AS. Baclofen in the treatment of trigeminal neuralgia: double-blind study and long-term follow-up. *Ann Neurol.* 1984; 15:240–4.
20. Potashner SJ. Baclofen: effects on amino acid release and metabolism in slices of guinea pig cerebral cortex. *J Neurochem.* 1979; 32:103–9.
21. Johnston GAR, Hailstone MH, Freeman CG. Baclofen: stereoselective inhibition of excitant amino acid release. *J Pharm Pharmacol.* 1981; 32:230–1.
22. Terrence CF, Sax M, Fromm GH et al. Effect of baclofen enantiomorphs on the spinal trigeminal nucleus and steric similarities of carbamazepine. *Pharmacology.* 1983; 27:85–94.

Drug Experience

Straightforward reports of unusual drug experiences are included in this section. These may be confirmations of previously reported drug experiences or brief apparent first reports. While selected references may be cited, the purpose of a Drug Experience report is not to present an extensive review of the literature.

A related section, Grand Rounds, includes papers that are well-documented patient case reports combined with a thorough review of the important literature to help put the case in perspective.

Toxicity and elimination of trazodone after overdose

ERKAN HASSAN AND DELWYN D. MILLER

Clin Pharm. 1985; 4:97–100

Since they were first introduced in the early 1960s, tricyclic antidepressants (TCAs) have been used extensively in the treatment of depression and in the management of enuresis in children. With the increased use of these agents, there has been a concomitant increase in TCA overdose.[1] The numerous reports of TCA overdose identify two major types of toxicity: (1) central and autonomic nervous system toxicity and (2) cardiovascular disturbances of rhythm and conduction.[2–5] Because of the large variation in individual susceptibility to the toxicity of TCAs, the outcome of an acute ingestion is difficult to predict. We report a case of trazodone overdose with very high serum concentrations without serious sequelae. This is the first report of serial determinations of serum concentrations obtained for the purpose of characterizing the elimination profile for trazodone after an overdose. We also review the available data on trazodone overdose, highlighting the differences between this structurally unique antidepressant and the TCAs in terms of toxicity and elimination after overdose.

Case Report. A 58-year-old, 60-kg white woman ingested approximately 60 100-mg trazodone hydrochloride tablets (Desyrel, Mead Johnson & Company, Evansville, IN 47721) and unknown quantities of lithium carbonate, theophylline, aspirin, and possibly other medications in a suicide attempt. Approximately one hour after ingestion, she was found drowsy but conscious and was taken by ambulance to the emergency room.

Physical examination showed that the patient was lethargic but arousable, with a blood pressure of 160/70 mm Hg, a regular pulse of 104 beats per minute, and a respiratory rate of 20 per minute. Her pupils were dilated to 8 mm bilaterally and were reactive to light. Findings of cardiovascular and abdominal examinations were within normal limits. Neurologically, the patient was lethargic, with intact reflexes. Results of all chemistry and hematologic studies were within normal limits. The initial electrocardiogram demonstrated a sinus tachycardia with a QRS duration of 80 msec, QT interval of 420 msec, PR interval of 100 msec, and nonspecific ST–T wave changes.

The initial trazodone serum concentration was 7453 ng/mL[a] 5.5 hours after ingestion. Subsequent serum trazodone concentrations are shown in Figure

ERKAN HASSAN, PHARM.D., is Assistant Professor, Department of Clinical Pharmacy, School of Pharmacy, University of Maryland, Baltimore, MD; at the time of this study, he was Clinical Pharmacist, Department of Pharmacy Services, University Hospitals of Cleveland, Cleveland, OH. DELWYN D. MILLER, PHARM.D., is Clinical Pharmacist, University Hospitals of Cleveland.

Address reprint requests to Dr. Hassan at the Department of Clinical Pharmacy, School of Pharmacy, University of Maryland, 20 North Pine Street, Baltimore, MD 21201.

The assistance of J. Green, Pharm.D., G. Oderda, Pharm.D., W. Klein-Schwartz, Pharm.D., and A. Forrest, Pharm.D., and the secretarial assistance of Renee Smith are acknowledged.

Supported in part by an educational grant from Mead Johnson Pharmaceutical Division.

Presented at the 18th Annual ASHP Midyear Clinical Meeting, Atlanta, GA, December 7, 1983.

1. Toxicological analyses of blood and urine were positive for lithium, salicylates, and theophylline; initial and subsequent serum concentrations of these agents are shown in Table 1.

Emergency treatment included gastric lavage and administration of activated charcoal 50 g plus oral magnesium citrate 17.5 g. No tablet fragments were seen in the gastric lavage fluid. The patient was admitted to the intensive-care unit. After approximately 10 hours, the patient's mental status cleared. Her vital signs remained stable during her intensive-care stay, with blood pressures of 140–160/60–80 mm Hg and regular pulse rates of 98–110. Subsequent electrocardiograms were within normal limits except for nonspecific ST–T wave changes. Telemetry monitoring throughout the patient's intensive-care stay demonstrated up to five unifocal ventricular premature depolarizations per minute; this was independent of the serum trazodone concentration. After approximately 30 hours of intensive monitoring, the patient was medically stable and was transferred to a psychiatric unit for continued monitoring.

Discussion. Central nervous system (CNS) toxicity usually begins within one to two hours after an acute overdose with TCAs. CNS stimulation consisting of agitation, hallucinations, and seizures may initially be present because of centrally mediated anticholinergic effects. CNS depression follows and may result in coma. Clonus, choreoathetosis, and hyperactive reflexes may also be present.[1]

Figure 1. Initial and subsequent serum trazodone concentrations.

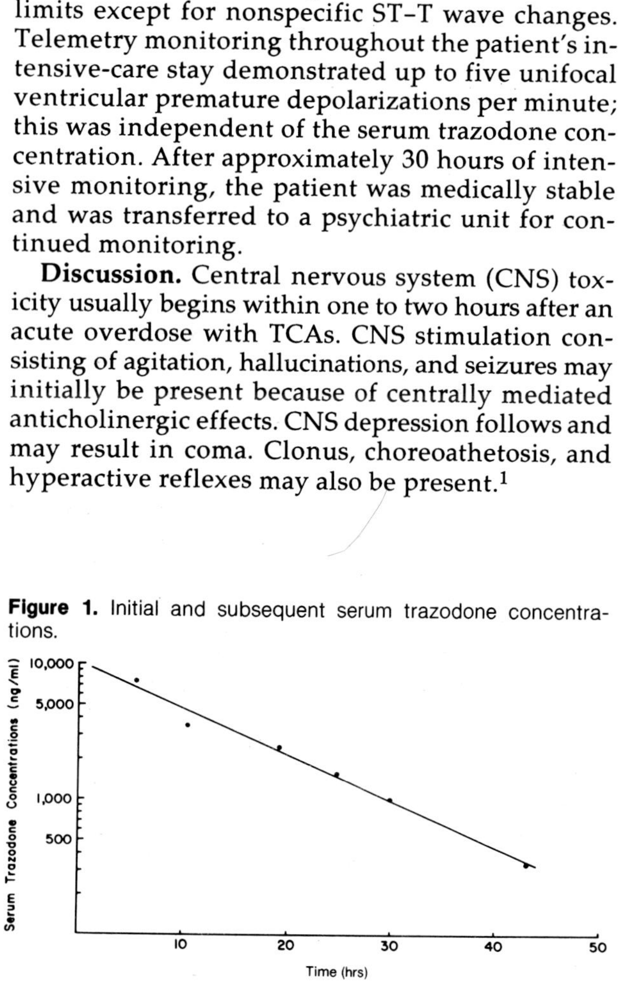

Table 1.
Results of Toxicological Analysis of Serum

Hours after Ingestion	Drug Concentration: Lithium (meq/L)	Salicylate (mg/dL)	Theophylline (mg/L)
5.5	1.12	27	25.8
10.5	0.73	19	30.8
19.25	0.45	7	29.5
43.0	0.26	2	2.5

The overall mortality rate for TCA overdose is 7–10%; the primary cause of death is cardiovascular toxicity.[6] The reported cardiac irregularities include conduction disturbances and various types of atrial and ventricular arrhythmias, the most common of which is sinus tachycardia.[6] The most reliable indicator of severity of a TCA overdose is a QRS interval ≥100 msec that corresponds with TCA plasma concentrations ≥1000 ng/mL.[7] A patient whose QRS interval is greater than 100 msec must be evaluated and treated as having ingested a potentially lethal dose of TCAs. There are at least four proposed pharmacologic mechanisms for TCA-induced cardiovascular toxicity: anticholinergic effects, blockade of norepinephrine reuptake at synaptic terminals, membrane-stabilizing effect, and α-adrenergic blocking properties.[5,6,8]

The correlations between toxic responses and TCA concentrations after overdose has been evaluated by only a few investigators. Spiker et al.[9] reported six patients with prolonged TCA elimination, while Pedersen et al.[10] were the first to characterize the elimination of TCAs after overdose. The latter authors indicated that nonlinear elimination of amitriptyline may occur with high serum concentrations. Gram et al.[11] and Bjerre et al.[12] indicated that a subgroup of patients may exist with saturable hydroxylation metabolism for desipramine and imipramine. Dose-dependent elimination of TCAs was also suggested by Spigelman et al.[13] These authors retrospectively reviewed patients treated with a low and a high dose of amitriptyline or desipramine. A predictable linear correlation in steady-state serum concentrations was not found with the two different dosages of desipramine; this was in contrast to the linear increase in steady-state serum concentrations from the low to high dose of amitriptyline. The current data indicate that TCAs may exhibit nonlinear pharmacokinetic properties because of hepatic enzyme saturation of metabolic pathways.

Trazodone is completely and rapidly absorbed from an oral dosage form.[14] Trazodone undergoes extensive liver metabolism into pharmacologically inactive products, with only a small amount excreted unchanged in the urine and feces. The normal terminal elimination half-life of radioactively labeled trazodone is reported to be between 6.3 and 13 hours.[15,16] The mean (± standard deviation) serum trazodone concentration following a 125-mg dose is reported to be 1460 (± 410) ng/mL two hours after the dose and 690 (± 360) ng/mL six hours after the dose.[17] Other studies have reported concentrations two hours after a 50-mg dose to be 550 to 600 ng/mL.[14] Clinical response to trazodone in ambulatory patients is usually seen with oral doses in the range of 150–400 mg per day, although some patients may require up to 600 mg per day. An association between serum trazodone concentration and therapeutic benefit or toxic effects is lacking; further investigation is required. There are no published data evaluating the elimination of trazodone after overdose.

In animal and human studies, trazodone has been found to have an anticholinergic profile similar to placebo because of trazodone's low affinity for muscarinic receptors.[18,19] Cardiac effects of trazodone in the dog model indicate minimal effects over a large dosage range when compared with imipramine.[20,21] Recently, trazodone has been implicated in (1) aggravating ventricular premature depolarizations in two patients with mitral-valve prolapse and documented couplets, (2) worsening arrhythmia status in a patient with stable nonsustained ventricular tachycardia, and (3) causing reversible first-degree atrioventricular block in one patient.[22-24] Because of the small number of patients reported with these complications, further clinical experience is needed to clarify the full impact of these cardiac effects of trazodone.

Published reports of trazodone overdose confirmed by biochemical measurement of the agent are rare.[25-28] Nine of the eleven patients in these reports were treated and discharged without complications. The remaining two patients died, one by drowning, the other from cardiopulmonary arrest. Both patients had also ingested one or more CNS depressants (confirmed at autopsy). Sufficient data were not obtained in any of the eleven patients for adequate calculation of trazodone elimination rates.

Review of unpublished reports to Mead Johnson & Company from the United States and the United Kingdom indicates that the incidence of serious toxicity from trazodone overdose alone, compared with TCA overdose, is low.[b] Of the 149 total overdose cases, only 10 deaths (6.7%) have been reported. In only one case was trazodone the sole agent reported to be ingested. In this case, death occurred after the patient was stable and had been transferred to a psychiatric ward for further therapy; autopsy findings revealed an acute myocardial infarction. The remaining nine patients also had histories of ingestion of unknown quantities of alcohol, benzodiazepines, or other sedative–hypnotics that may have contributed to their demise. In the surviving 139 patients, two cases of respiratory arrest, one case of priapism, one occurrence of seizure, two cases of right bundle-branch block, one case of atrioventricular block, and one T-wave inversion were reported. The remaining patients had minor CNS-depressant effects.

Our patient had a clinical course consistent with trazodone overdose. The minor CNS-depressant effect with uneventful recovery is similar to other reported cases of trazodone overdose. Although the patient at times had tachycardia and dilated pupils, these effects were most likely the result of other medications with anticholinergic properties that she may have ingested. There were no serious effects on intracardiac conduction, blood pressure, or ectopy from any of the agents ingested.

The initial trazodone serum concentration in our patient was 7453 ng/mL 5.5 hours after ingestion, by which time peak absorption had most likely occurred. Concentrations of the other drugs identified in the patient's blood were monitored for 43 hours. Serum theophylline concentrations continued to increase after hospitalization, probably because the patient ingested a sustained-release preparation. Repeated charcoal administration was not used since the patient was stable.

Serial serum trazodone concentrations were monitored for 43 hours after ingestion. The terminal elimination rate constant was 0.0786 hr^{-1} ($r = 0.99$). This corresponds to a terminal elimination half-life of approximately 8.8 hours. This patient's terminal elimination rate after overdose was the same as those reported following therapeutic doses.[6,16,29] Our patient ingested several other compounds, and it is not known if these agents affect trazodone metabolism, trazodone elimination, or both.

It is not known whether trazodone elimination is linear after overdose. In this patient we found a linear-decay curve throughout all concentrations measured. Our observation suggests that hepatic enzyme saturation did not occur. There may be a subpopulation of patients who manifest bimodal trazodone elimination, as suggested by Gram et al.,[11] for desipramine and its hydroxy metabolites. This can be determined by following the elimination of trazodone from high to low serum concentrations in a large number of patients.

Conclusion. In this case and others previously reported, limited clinical symptoms were observed following acute trazodone overdose. Overdoses of trazodone, unlike overdoses of the tricyclic or tetracyclic antidepressants, do not appear to cause serious cardiovascular or neurologic toxicity. This is the first report of serial serum trazodone concentrations obtained after overdose. An apparently linear elimination profile was observed as serum concentrations fell from approximately 7500 ng/mL to approximately 350 ng/mL, suggesting that appreciable saturation of metabolic enzymes and elimination mechanisms did not occur.

---

[a] Trazodone concentrations were determined by high-performance liquid chromatography, courtesy of National Psychopharmacology Laboratories, Inc., Knoxville, TN.

[b] Gamble DE, Mead Johnson Pharmaceutical Division. Written communication. 1984 Nov 1.

References

1. Hollister LE. Tricyclic antidepressants. *N Engl J Med.* 1978; 299:1106–9, 1168–72.
2. Burks JS, Walker JE, Rumack BH et al. Tricyclic antidepressant poisoning. Reversal of coma, choreoathetosis, and myoclonus by physostigmine. *JAMA.* 1974; 230:1405–7.
3. Noble J, Matthew H. Acute poisoning by tricyclic antidepressants: clinical features and management of 100 patients.

Clin Toxicol. 1969; 2:403–21.
4. Thorstrand C. Cardiovascular effects of poisoning with tricyclic antidepressants. *Acta Med Scand.* 1974; 195:505–14.
5. Vohra J, Burrows G, Hunt D et al. The effect of toxic and therapeutic doses of tricyclic antidepressant drugs on intracardiac conduction. *Eur J Cardiol.* 1975; 3(3):219–27.
6. Marshall JB, Forker AD. Cardiovascular effects of tricyclic antidepressant drugs: therapeutic usage, overdose, and management of complications. *Am Heart J.* 1982; 103:401–14.
7. Spiker DG, Weiss AN, Chang SS et al. Tricyclic antidepressant overdose: clinical presentation and plasma levels. *Clin Pharmacol Ther.* 1976; 18:539–46.
8. Vohra J, Hunt D, Burrows G et al. Intracardiac conduction defects following overdose of tricyclic antidepressant drugs. *Eur J Cardiol.* 1975; 2(4):453–8.
9. Spiker DG, Biggs JT. Tricyclic antidepressants prolonged plasma levels after overdose. *JAMA.* 1976; 236:1711–2.
10. Pedersen OL, Gram LF, Kirstensen CB et al. Overdosage of antidepressants: clinical and pharmacokinetic aspects. *Eur J Clin Pharmacol.* 1982; 23:513–21.
11. Gram LF, Bjerre M, Kragh-Sorensen P et al. Imipramine metabolites in blood of patients during therapy and after overdose. *Clin Pharmacol Ther.* 1983; 33:335–42.
12. Bjerre M, Gram LF, Kragh-Sorensen P et al. Dose-dependent kinetics of imipramine in elderly patients. *Psychopharmacology.* 1981; 75:354–7.
13. Spigelman AD, Jansen RL, Bruzek RJ. Apparent nonlinear kinetics of secondary-amine tricyclic antidepressants. *Clin Pharm.* 1983; 2:508–10. Letter.
14. Rawls WN. Trazodone. *Drug Intell Clin Pharm.* 1982; 16:7–13.
15. Brogden RN, Heel RC, Speight TM et al. Trazodone: a review of its pharmacological properties and therapeutic use in depression and anxiety. *Drugs.* 1981; 21:401–29.
16. Bryant SG, Ereshefsky L. Antidepressant properties of trazodone. *Clin Pharm.* 1982; 1:406–17.
17. Putzolu S, Pecknold JC, Baiocchi L et al. Trazodone: clinical and biochemical studies. II. Blood levels and therapeutic responsiveness. *Psychopharmacol Bull.* 1976; 12:40–1.
18. Gershon S, Newton R. Lack of anticholinergic side effects with a new antidepressant—trazodone. *J Clin Psychiatry.* 1980; 41:100–4.
19. Taylor DP, Hyslop DK, Riblet LA. Trazodone, a new nontricyclic antidepressant without anticholinergic activity. *Biochem Pharmacol.* 1980; 29:2149–50. Letter.
20. Byrne JE, Gomoll AW. Differential effects of trazodone and imipramine on intracardiac conduction in the anesthetized dog. *Arch Int Pharmacodyn Ther.* 1982; 259:259–70.
21. Gomoll AW, Byrne JE. Trazodone and imipramine: comparative effects on canine cardiac conduction. *Eur J Pharmacol.* 1979; 57:335–42.
22. Janowsky D, Curtis G, Zisook S et al. Ventricular arrhythmias possibly aggravated by trazodone. *Am J Psychiatry.* 1983; 140:796–7.
23. Vlay SC, Friedling S. Trazodone exacerbation of VT. *Am Heart J.* 1983; 106:604. Letter.
24. Irwin M, Spar JE. Reversible cardiac conduction abnormality associated with trazodone administration. *Am J Psychiatry.* 1983; 140:945–6. Letter.
25. Demorest D. Death involving trazodone. *J Anal Toxicol.* 1983; 7:63. Letter.
26. Lesar T, Kingston R, Dahms R et al. Trazodone overdose. *Ann Emerg Med.* 1983; 12:221–3.
27. Root I, Ohlson GB. Trazodone overdose: report of two cases. *J Anal Toxicol.* 1984; 8 (Mar–Apr):91–4.
28. Henry JA, Ali CJ, Caldwell R et al. Acute trazodone poisoning: clinical signs and plasma concentrations. *Psychopathology.* 1984; 17 (Suppl 2):77–81.
29. Jauch VR, Kopitar Z, Prox A et al. Pharmacokinetics and metabolism of trazodone in man. *Arzneim-Forsch.* 1976; 26: 2084–9.

Clonidine and naloxone in ultrashort opiate detoxification

PHILIP W. HOLMAN

Clin Pharm. 1985; 4:100–2

The severity of symptoms accompanying opiate withdrawal poses a dilemma for physicians anxious to help patients who want to break their opiate habit. However, clinicians' options have recently been widened by the addition of several innovative detoxification programs to their armamentarium.

Since Gold and his coworkers[1] reported that a single dose of clonidine hydrochloride could cause a reduction of opiate withdrawal symptoms, detoxification regimens using clonidine have been proposed. It was argued that decreasing the severity of withdrawal could increase the success rate of detoxification programs by enhancing patient acceptance. Subsequently, Gold et al.[2] found clonidine hydrochloride to be a safe and effective nonopiate treatment of opiate withdrawal. However, these detoxification programs required 14 days of hospitalization.

Following the success enjoyed by the early trials of rapid detoxification, Resnick et al.[3] suggested that naloxone hydrochloride be used to shorten the detoxification period of patients taking low doses of opiates. Resnick and Kastenbaum[4] demonstrated that detoxification with repeated doses of naloxone hydrochloride, precipitated withdrawal symptoms that decreased in severity allowing the ultrashort detoxification of 19 patients.

Riordan and Kleber[5] reported successful detoxification in four patients using clonidine and naloxone concomitantly. Their goal was to accomplish detoxification in a very short period of time while suppressing withdrawal symptoms. Their regimen involved only four days of hospitalized treatment.

While gradual detoxification is still in widespread use, the introduction of prospective payment systems will require the most rational and economic use of resources. We present a case of successful opiate detoxification that involved an ultrashort clonidine–naloxone regimen.

Case Report. A somewhat anxious 34-year-old white woman was admitted to our hospital with vomiting (not related to food), diarrhea, dehydration, hypokalemia (2.6 meq/L), and compliants of

PHILIP W. HOLMAN is a clinical pharmacist, Kenneth Norris Cancer Hospital, University of Southern California, 1441 Eastlake Avenue, Los Angeles, CA 90033.

The assistance of Donald G. Skinner, M.D., Professor and Division Chair of Surgery, Urology, University of Southern California School of Medicine, in reviewing this case report is acknowledged.

hallucinations. These symptoms, which resulted in a 4-kg weight loss, began shortly after she was discharged from our institution, five days before, following a successful bladder augmentation procedure (revision of a hemi-Kock pouch) to relieve chronic lower back pain.

The patient was gravida 13, para three, aborta 10, having undergone total abdominal hysterectomy, salpingo-ovariectomy, and multiple urinary-tract diversions culminating in the hemi-Kock procedure. She related an extensive history of polydrug use for the relief of chronic bladder and flank pain. The pain was thought to be caused by scarring and stricture of the urinary tract after multiple operations. She gave an unreliable drug history but admitted to using injectable meperidine hydrochloride, hydromorphone, diphenhydramine hydrochloride, prochlorperazine, and a narcotic pain cocktail extensively for several years. Upon the previous discharge from our institution, she was given morphine sulfate elixir 20 mg to be taken every four hours. She had subsequently entered a methadone rehabilitation program and was receiving 120 mg of methadone hydrochloride daily and was considered to be making progress in her rehabilitation. We believed that most of her symptoms were probably secondary to narcotic withdrawal and her chronic diarrhea was secondary to the hemi-Kock pouch procedure.

Intravenous replacement fluids with 5% Lactated Ringer's injection plus 40 meq/L of potassium at a rate of 150 mL/hr were started to hydrate the patient, with two additional 40-meq doses of oral potassium chloride given to correct the hypokalemia. No evidence of gastric or duodenal obstruction was found upon diagnostic upper-gastrointestinal tract studies.

On the day of admission, the patient continued to have nausea and vomiting and complained of flank pain. Meperidine hydrochloride 50 mg i.m. and hydroxyzine hydrochloride 50 mg i.m. were given every four hours for pain control. The second day she complained of nausea and vomiting about a half hour before each scheduled dose of meperidine and hydroxyzine. At this point, she expressed a sincere desire to abstain from narcotics. The meperidine and hydroxyzine were discontinued, and a clonidine–naloxone detoxification regimen[5] was initiated (Table 1).

On hospital day 2, the patient was placed on a regimen of clonidine hydrochloride 0.1 mg every eight hours. Within an hour after the initial dose, her blood pressure fell from 110/80 mm Hg to 94/60 mm Hg. This hypotension lasted throughout detoxification, with elevations during periods of intense anxiety. After premedication with clonidine, she had no complaint of pain or symptoms of withdrawal.

Shortly after the initial dose of naloxone, she demonstrated anxiety, hand and arm tremors, and nausea. The nausea was treated with prochlorperazine 25 mg rectally every four hours for a total of three doses. That afternoon and throughout the next two days, she became withdrawn and her behavior became more labile. Continued withdrawal was manifested by anxiety, tremors, and insomnia for the duration of the detoxification period. Flurazepam hydrochloride 30 mg was given nightly.

By hospital day 5, her behavior had stabilized and she engaged in activities and conversation. At this point, no withdrawal symptoms were precipitated by a 1.2-mg i.m. challenge dose of naloxone hydrochloride. She was discharged on a regimen of flurazepam hydrochloride 30 mg as needed for sleep and diphenoxylate hydrochloride 2.5 mg and atropine sulfate 0.025 mg with instructions to take one tablet after each loose stool for diarrhea secondary to short-bowel syndrome.

Discussion. Withdrawal from opiates has traditionally been accomplished by gradually decreasing the opiate dose. It is commonly believed that gradual detoxification causes a less severe period of withdrawal symptoms and is preferable to abrupt discontinuance of the drug. While this practice may appear desirable, it has not been shown to be more humane, and the success rates are actually lower than with abrupt withdrawal.[4–8]

Success in maintaining opiate abstinence using varying withdrawal regimens was studied by Chappell et al.[8] This group reported that those patients most rapidly withdrawn achieved the highest rate of opiate abstinence. Moreover, Resnick[3] found

Table 1.
Clonidine–Naloxone Opiate Detoxification Regimen

	Day of Regimen			
Drug	1	2	3	4
Naloxone hydrochloride	None	Start 0.4 mg i.m. every two hours for six doses 30 minutes after the second dose of clonidine	Start 0.8 mg i.m. every two hours for six doses 30 minutes after the second dose of clonidine	1.2 mg i.m.
Clonidine hydrochloride[a]	0.1 mg every eight hours	0.2 mg every eight hours	0.05 mg every 12 hours	None

[a] Clonidine hydrochloride (Catapres, Boehringer Ingelheim) is available in 0.1- and 0.2-mg scored tablets.

that given a choice, patients contemplating detoxification chose the shortest withdrawal period offered.

The extended period of somatic symptoms or secondary abstinence following the acute phase of opiate withdrawal is well known.[9] Anxiety, nausea, vomiting, and weakness are all manifestations of secondary abstinence.[9] Similar symptoms are frequently found among patients undergoing gradual methadone withdrawal and can be a cause of treatment failure. These symptoms eventually led to the hospitalization of our patient.

As reported by Gold,[10] the role of opiates in the prevention of acute panic states and as antidepressants by a subset of opiate users may contraindicate the use of clonidine. Therefore, careful screening and review of the patient's medical history is mandatory before initiating a clonidine regimen for opiate withdrawal.

Conclusion. Although we have reported our experience with only one patient, the results are consistent with those reported by Riordan and Kleber.[5] This regimen and similar programs may be suitable for rapid detoxification of patients undergoing withdrawal and seeking emergency treatment. Instead of reintroducing opiates, or continuing methadone maintenance or detoxification programs, the patient may choose ultrashort detoxification. As long as the inadequacies of conventional treatment of opiate dependence remain an issue, continued use and further study of alternative therapies are warranted.

References

1. Gold MS, Redmond DE, Kleber HD. Clonidine blocks acute opiate withdrawal symptoms. *Lancet.* 1978; 2:599–602.
2. Gold MS, Pottash AC, Sweeney DR et al. Opiate withdrawal using clonidine. *JAMA.* 1980; 243:343–6.
3. Resnick R, Kastenbaum R, Washton A et al. Naloxone precipitated withdrawal: a method for rapid induction onto naltrexone. *Clin Pharmacol Ther.* 1977; 21:409–3.
4. Resnick R, Kastenbaum R, Gastanaga P et al. Experimental techniques for rapid withdrawal from methadone maintenance: results of pilot trials. In: Seray E, Shorty V, Alkaense H, eds. Developments in the field of drug abuse. Cambridge, MA: Schenkman Publishing; 1975:321–7.
5. Riordan CE, Kleber HD. Rapid opiate detoxification with clonidine and naloxone. *Lancet.* 1980; 5:1079–80.
6. Blachly PH, Casey D, Marcel LJ et al. Titration of the opiate abstinence syndrome with naloxone. Paper presented at the First National Drug Abuse Conference. Chicago, IL: 1974 Mar 30.
7. Report to the Mayor's Committee on Drug Addiction to the Honorable Richard C. Patterson, Jr., Commissioner of Correction, New York City. *Am J Psychiatry.* 1930; 87:433–8.
8. Kurland AA, McCabe L. Rapid detoxification of the narcotic addict with naloxone hydrochloride. A preliminary report. *Clin Pharmacol.* 1976; 16:66–75.
9. Martin WR, Jasinski DR. Physiological parameters of morphine dependence in man: tolerance, early abstinence, protracted abstinence. *J Psychiatr Res.* 1969; 7:9–17.
10. Gold MS, Pottash AL, Sweeney DR et al. Rapid opiate detoxification: clinical evidence of antidepressant and antipanic effects of opiates. *Am J Psychiatry.* 1979; 7:982–3.

Metoclopramide-induced tetanus-like dystonic reaction

ROBERT DELLAVALLE, JAMES L. WIELENGA, AND OWEN TAYLOR

Clin Pharm. 1985; 4:102–3

Recently, intravenous metoclopramide was approved for the prevention of vomiting associated with cisplatin administration. Side effects associated with its use include sedation, diarrhea, fatigue, insomnia, dizziness, and various extrapyramidal symptoms. The extrapyramidal symptoms reportedly occur in up to 27% of patients treated with i.v. metoclopramide.[1] The symptoms can range from mild restlessness to severe dystonic reactions resembling tetanus. These tetanus-like extrapyramidal reactions, although rare, may occur with greater frequency in young adults, and when higher doses of metoclopramide are used.[1,2] This report describes a severe tetanus-like extrapyramidal reaction induced by a single dose of metoclopramide in a middle-aged patient previously tolerant to its repeated use.

Case Report. A 50-year-old white woman was given a diagnosis of invasive ductal carcinoma of the right breast. Clinically it was staged as follows: lymph-node involvement 0, metastatic spread 0, and tumor size 1.5 cm. Two of 16 nodes in the axillary region were found to be positive for tumor. An excisional biopsy was performed in May 1982. The metastatic survey was negative. She received a 5000-rad tumor dose in 25 fractions over a five-week period. At that time, her tolerance to the therapy was considered good. She was subsequently placed on a biweekly cyclic chemotherapy regimen consisting of methotrexate 70 mg and fluorouracil 850 mg, alternating with methotrexate 70 mg, fluorouracil 850 mg, cyclophosphamide 850 mg, and vincristine sulfate 2.0 mg. All medications were administered by i.v. piggyback except for vincristine, which was given i.v. push over two minutes.

Because the patient's chemotherapy-induced emesis was unresponsive to aggressive conventional antiemetic therapy, a modified i.v. metoclopramide hydrochloride regimen was instituted. One dose (1.5

ROBERT DELLAVALLE, PHARM.D., and JAMES L. WIELENGA, PHARM.D., are Clinical Assistant Professors, College of Pharmacy, University of Tennessee Center for Health Sciences, and Associate Director and Director of Pharmacy Services, respectively, Bradley County Memorial Hospital, Cleveland, TN. OWEN TAYLOR, M.D., is a physician, Department of Internal Medicine, Bradley County Memorial Hospital.

Address reprint requests to Dr. DellaValle at the Department of Clinical Pharmacy, Bradley County Memorial Hospital, North Chambliss Avenue, Cleveland, TN 37311.

mg/kg) infused over 15 minutes was administered 35 minutes before chemotherapy. This single-dose regimen was successfully employed for 14 consecutive biweekly treatment periods. Reported side effects were occasional insomnia and mild restlessness. To ensure therapy reproducibility, all medications, including metoclopramide, were administered via an infusion pump and supervised by a member of the i.v. therapy team. All medications were prepared in the pharmacy under the direct supervision of a pharmacist.

Forty-five minutes after the 15th dose of metoclopramide, the patient reported increasing tightness of the mouth, chest, right shoulder, and right arm. This "tightness" progressively increased, and within 10 minutes of onset, substantial nuchal rigidity was present. Respirations were stertorous in nature. Although the patient's airway was patent, she complained of difficulty breathing. Her vital signs at this time were blood pressure 160/100 mm Hg, pulse 108 beats/min, and respirations 26 breaths/min.

The symptoms gradually abated, and within 35 minutes of the initial complaint, the patient was asymptomatic.

Discussion. The use of high-dose i.v. metoclopramide hydrochloride (1.0–2.0 mg/kg) as an antiemetic agent has been reported to be safe and effective.[3] While mild extrapyramidal reactions such as anxiety and restlessness are common, there have been few reports of torticollis, trismus, and dystonia.[2–4]

The tetanus-like reaction we observed was unusual because of the patient's age and previous tolerance to high-dose i.v. metoclopramide therapy. Other reports describing undesirable effects with metoclopramide use have evaluated multiple-dose, short-term therapy.[2,4,5] The patient described in this report received metoclopramide hydrochloride (1.5 mg/kg) in a single-dose regimen for 14 consecutive biweekly treatment periods. The extrapyramidal symptoms of mild restlessness and insomnia were sporadic and did not require therapeutic intervention. Accidental overdosing was not likely since drug preparation and administration were closely supervised by the pharmacy and i.v. therapy team. Altered drug distribution and elimination were also unlikely since no changes occurred in either renal or hepatic function study results.

Recent published reports have supported a possible relationship between age and the occurrence of metoclopramide-induced extrapyramidal reactions. Bui et al.[2] reported a 36.3% occurrence rate of undesirable side effects in association with high-dose metoclopramide therapy. Of 69 patients enrolled in their study (median age 55 years), 13 demonstrated trismus and eight had dyskinesia. When age was taken into account, toxic effects were observed in eight of nine patients younger than 30 years. Kris et al.[1] also described an age-related occurrence in 14 of 452 patients given high-dose metoclopramide therapy. Of 22 patients between 15 and 29 years of age, six experienced acute dystonic reactions (27.3%). Among those patients between 30 and 70 years of age (n = 430), eight experienced acute dystonic reactions (1.8%).

Intravenous diphenhydramine is effective in prevention of metoclopramide-induced extrapyramidal reactions. Its concomitant use with the initial dose of metoclopramide has been advocated for patients under 30 years of age and for individuals with a history of extrapyramidal reactions.[1] We support these recommendations and emphasize the need for routine diphenhydramine prophylaxis in individuals who demonstrate only mild, intermittent extrapyramidal symptoms.

Conclusion. In general, extrapyramidal reactions to high-dose i.v. metoclopramide have been reported to occur more frequently after short-term therapy in patients under 30 years of age. The extrapyramidal reaction described in this patient was unique because of the patient's age and previously demonstrated tolerance to repeated administration of the drug, and because of the severity of the reaction. We suggest that routine prophylaxis with diphenhydramine be considered in patients exhibiting mild, intermittent extrapyramidal symptoms regardless of patient age or previous tolerance.

References

1. Kris MG, Tyson LB, Gralla RJ et al. Extrapyramidal reactions with high-dose metoclopramide. *N Engl J Med.* 1983; 309:433. Letter.
2. Bui NB, Marit G, Hoerni B. High dose metoclopramide in cancer chemotherapy-induced nausea and vomiting. *Cancer Treat Rep.* 1982; 66:2107–8.
3. Gralla RJ. Metoclopramide: a review of antiemetic trials. *Drugs.* 1983; 25 (Suppl 1):63–73.
4. Strum SB, McDermed JE, Opfell RW et al. Intravenous metoclopramide: an effective antiemetic in cancer chemotherapy. *JAMA.* 1982; 247:2683–6.
5. Gralla RJ, Itri LM, Pisko SE et al. Antiemetic efficacy of high-dose metoclopramide: randomized trials with placebo and prochlorperazine in patients with chemotherapy-induced nausea and vomiting. *N Engl J Med.* 1981; 305:905–9.

CP Continuing Education

The ASHP Continuing Education system gives readers a self-assessment mechanism for selected articles in Clinical Pharmacy *and the* American Journal of Hospital Pharmacy. *It also allows readers to obtain continuing education credit for these articles.*

For the purpose of CE-credit enrollment, a blank answer sheet is published at the end of each installment of the column for the CE articles in that issue. An enrollee accumulates these answer sheets until the enrollment is submitted, using the form that is published in the May–June and November–December issues of Clinical Pharmacy *and in the June and December issues of the* American Journal of Hospital Pharmacy. *Any combination of tests within a 12-month period, from both* Clinical Pharmacy *and* American Journal of Hospital Pharmacy, *may be included in an enrollment. More complete details about enrollment in the system will appear in the semiannual enrollment form.*

All education aspects of the program are directed by Warren E. McConnell, Ph.D., Special Assistant in the ASHP Executive Office.

Article 680-204-8502 (see page 27)
Qualifies for 1.0 hour of CE credit

Enalapril, a nonsulfhydryl angiotensin-converting enzyme inhibitor

Learning Objectives

After studying this article, the reader should be able to

1. Compare the antihypertensive efficacy, pharmacokinetics, and adverse effects of enalapril and captopril.
2. List three beneficial hemodynamic effects of enalapril in patients with congestive heart failure.
3. Identify patients with hypertension or congestive heart failure who are most likely to benefit from enalapril therapy.
4. List a class of drugs that may interact with enalapril.
5. Recommend an initial dosage regimen for enalapril in patients with normal and impaired renal function.

Self-assessment Questions

For each question there is one best answer only.

1. The sulfhydryl moiety found in captopril and other drugs such as D-penicillamine but not in enalapril has been associated with which of the following side effects of captopril?
   a. Thrombocytopenia.
   b. Proteinuria.
   c. Loss of hair.
   d. None of the above alternatives is correct.
2. Which of the following statements concerning enalaprilat is *not* true?
   a. It is formed by ester hydrolysis of enalapril.
   b. It is a more potent inhibitor of angiotensin-converting enzyme than enalapril and captopril.
   c. It is the lysine conjugate of enalapril.
   d. It is the only known metabolite of enalapril.
3. In patients with congestive heart failure, enalapril produces all of the following effects *except*
   a. An increase in cardiac index.
   b. An increase in pulmonary-capillary wedge pressure.
   c. An increase in stroke volume.
   d. An increase in renal blood flow.
4. When given alone for hypertension, enalapril has efficacy comparable to that of
   a. Hydrochlorothiazide.
   b. Captopril.
   c. Beta blockers.
   d. All of the above alternatives are correct.
5. Some patients receiving enalapril for hypertension secondary to bilateral renal artery stenosis may be at risk for developing
   a. Congestive heart failure.
   b. Hypokalemia.
   c. Severe hypotension.
   d. Renal failure.
6. Enalapril should be used with caution in patients concurrently receiving

a. Digoxin.
b. Spironolactone.
c. Both of the above alternatives are correct.
d. None of the above alternatives is correct.

7. The usual starting dosage of enalapril maleate in patients with abnormal renal function is

a. 250 mg b.i.d.
b. 25 mg q.d.
c. 40 mg b.i.d.
d. 5 mg q.d.

8. Based on the side effect experience with captopril, enalapril treatment should be monitored carefully, especially in patients with

a. Lupus erythematosis.
b. Diabetes mellitus.
c. Psychiatric disorders.
d. Hyperthyroidism.

9. The hypotensive effect of enalapril

a. Correlates with the magnitude of the serum concentration of enalaprilat during acute and chronic treatment.
b. Results primarily from a decrease in peripheral vascular resistance.
c. Is usually accompanied by an increase in heart rate.
d. Alternatives b and c are both correct.

10. Based on current experience, which of the following patients would be the *most* suitable candidate for enalapril therapy?

a. A 26-year-old black woman with pre-eclampsia.
b. A 7-year-old child with hypertension and insulin-dependent diabetes mellitus.
c. A 44-year-old hypertensive white man with severe chronic obstructive lung disease.
d. A 70-year-old black woman with systolic hypertension.

Answer sheet

January–February 1985 ***Clinical Pharmacy***

Note: An enrollment form for the ASHP Continuing Education System appears in the May–June and November–December issues. Please accumulate all the answer sheets you wish to use in one enrollment and submit them at one time with a completed enrollment form.

Place an X in the box(es) at the top of the column(s) corresponding to the test(s) you are taking. Darken the boxes corresponding to the correct answers.

☐
680-204-8502
1.0 hour

	a	b	c	d
1.	☐	☐	☐	☐
2.	☐	☐	☐	☐
3.	☐	☐	☐	☐
4.	☐	☐	☐	☐
5.	☐	☐	☐	☐
6.	☐	☐	☐	☐
7.	☐	☐	☐	☐
8.	☐	☐	☐	☐
9.	☐	☐	☐	☐
10.	☐	☐	☐	☐

ASHP Use Only
(1.0)8502______(3)

Current Literature

Book Reviews

Antacids and Other Drugs in Gastrointestinal Diseases

By W. A. Ritschel.

Published by Drug Intelligence Publications, Inc., 1241 Broadway, Hamilton, IL 63241, 1984. viii + 189 p. Price $24.50.

The stated purpose of this book is to "help physicians or other health professionals make intelligent choices in the treatment of gastrointestinal disorders." This six-by-nine-inch softbound book is intended to serve as a source of documented quick information on the treatment of upper gastrointestinal-tract diseases, primarily those associated with gastric-acid secretion.

The book is divided into four chapters. The first chapter provides a very brief review of the anatomy and physiology of the esophagus, stomach, and duodenum. Although the author attempts to present the most pertinent information, topics such as gastrointestinal motility, gastric emptying, and gastrointestinal absorption are much too complex to be handled well in such a brief format.

The second chapter includes an overview of the etiology, pathology, symptoms, and treatment of gastritis and peptic ulcers as well as a discussion of stress ulcers, drug-induced ulcers, reflux esophagitis, and acid pulmonary aspiration syndrome. Unfortunately much of the information in this chapter is either common knowledge to most practicing physicians and clinical pharmacists or is covered too superficially to be of value. This is especially true of the sections on stress ulcers, drug-induced ulcers, and reflux esophagitis.

The third chapter on antacids is the major thrust of the book, as one would expect from the book's title. This comprehensive chapter reviews information on antacid pharmacology, side effects, pharmacokinetic drug interactions, product formulations, and guidelines for the selection of antacids. Although much of this material is similar to what appears in the seventh edition of the *Handbook of Nonprescription Drugs*, the smaller size of this book enables better use as a quick reference. In addition, the author has broadened the scope of this chapter by including a concise but thorough discussion of both in vivo and in vitro testing of antacids.

The last chapter provides information on the anticholinergic agents and cimetidine, with very brief overviews of ranitidine, sucralfate, and some of the investigational antiulcer agents. When included, the material on indications, dosages, side effects, pharmacokinetics, and drug interactions is generally accurate and up-to-date.

The book contains a number of helpful tables, graphs, and figures. The tables are well organized and facilitate quick information retrieval. Overall, each chapter and most of the tables contain numerous accurate, current, and appropriate literature citations.

The most informative chapter in the book is the one that deals with antacids. Most of the information in the other chapters offers little that cannot be found in medical texts or in more complete drug reviews. Consequently, the book's usefulness as a reference for pharmacists engaged in clinical practice is somewhat limited. Despite these problems, physicians and pharmacists looking for a quick overview of antacids and other drugs used in the treatment of selected upper gastrointestinal disorders may find this book useful.

Reviewed by Rosemary R. Berardi, Pharm.D., Veterans Administration Medical Center and College of Pharmacy, The University of Michigan, Ann Arbor, MI 48109.

Antimicrobial Prescribing, Second Edition

By Burt R. Meyers.

Published by Antimicrobial Prescribing, Inc., P.O. Box 3153, Princeton, NJ 08540, 1983. 147 p. Price $14.95.

The stated purpose of this text is to serve as a guide and quick reference to aid in the selection of antimicrobial agents. The book begins with a brief, sound review of the principles of antibiotic therapy, bacterial resistance patterns, and interpretation of antimicrobial susceptibility tests. The author also included a special section on the newer β-lactam antibiotics; he promotes use of these agents for infections in which the causative organism is not known and as potential substitutes for combination antibiotic therapy.

The text is divided into seven sections covering the antibiotics; antimicrobial therapy by pathogen; therapy by site of infection; antibiotic dosage by age, disease, and renal function; antibiotic interactions and side effects; antimicrobial prophylaxis; and investigational antibiotics.

The majority of the information is provided in tabular form. References are not listed.

The antibiotic section has general comments on the pharmacology, indications, and adverse reactions common to each class of antimicrobials, and specific comments on individual drugs. Tables furnish data on general antibacterial activity, usual dosages in adults and children, protein binding, serum half-life during normal renal function and oliguria, common side effects, and comments. The information is concise, accurate, and relevant to clinical practice.

The therapy by pathogen section indicates empiric antibiotic choice, alternative drug choices, and whether supplemental therapy is necessary. The therapy by site of infection section covers all the usual areas of infection with general symptomatology, contributing factors to the infection, probable pathogens, empiric and alternative antibiotic selection, duration of treatment, and measures other than antibiotics necessary to resolve the infection.

The dosage section provides the usual adult and pediatric antimicrobial dosages, special dosages by site of infection, and neonatal antibiotic dosages. There is also a section that covers antibiotic dosage in renal dysfunction and the effect of dialysis on serum antibiotic concentrations. Adjustments in aminoglycoside dosage are recommended by use of either the rule of eights (dosage interval of 8 times the serum creatinine) or the Sarubbi and Hull nomogram.

The prophylaxis section covers medical situations (e.g., otitis media, meningitis, newborns), surgical situations, dental procedures, and instrumentation. The immunization section reviews prophylaxis and treatment of the usual diseases, plus tetanus, rabies, and hepatitis. The text concludes with information on five new antibiotics in the clinical trials stage of research.

Pharmacists will find that this text meets its goal of providing a guide and quick reference for antibiotic selection. The text could have been improved by the addition of information on inhibitory antibiotic concentrations, pharmacokinetic principles of dosing, and references to facilitate further research.

Reviewed by Marc H. Stranz, Pharm.D., Methodist Hospital, Lubbock, TX 79414.

A Clinical Companion to Biochemical Studies, Second Edition

By Victor Schwarz.

Published by W. H. Freeman and Company, 41 Madison Ave., New York, NY 10010, 1984. xiv + 162 p. Price $14.95.

This text attempts to present clinical correlations to the study of biochemistry. A total of 22 brief chapters on a wide range of diseases are provided. Each chapter opens with a short description of a patient case, including presenting signs, symptoms, and laboratory evaluations of the particular disease. The case is followed by a two-to-three page discussion of the biochemical mechanisms of the disease process. This discussion makes liberal use of figures, tables, and photographs to illustrate the disease mechanisms, particularly the underlying biochemical explanations. Each chapter closes with a series of questions to "stimulate" the reader to pursue the topic further.

On initial cursory examination of the text, I thought I had found a much-needed mechanism to review the biochemical background on a number of common diseases, background I had not retained from undergraduate studies. Unfortunately, this text is not a "Biochemical Companion to Clinical Studies" and is therefore of very limited value to clinical pharmacists. The author's intent is to provide a clinical correlate for students concurrently studying biochemistry, and the text is meant to be used in conjunction with traditional biochemistry texts. For its stated purpose, the text is clearly valuable.

The style of the text is direct, and certainly it is more easily read than biochemistry textbooks with which I am familiar. There are a number of aspects, though, that will limit the usefulness of the text in any setting. First, of the large number of disease entities one can find described in any textbook of internal medicine, only 22 are discussed here. The topics range from lactose deficiency and phenylketonuria to myocardial infarction and alcoholism. The reason for the choice of topics is not apparent (there are chapters on homocysteinuria and orotic aciduria), and the organization of topics (hereditary spherocytosis is followed by ketoacidosis in diabetes then by lead poisoning) is random. There are numerous diseases not discussed.

The case presentations are purposely very brief, and the information provided often has questionable clinical relevance. For example, in the chapter on myocardial infarction, the only "laboratory data" presented are postmortem myocardial concentrations of glycogen, lactate, ATP, and creatine phosphate. Another problem is that units of concentration are often given that differ from traditional units of reporting in the United States (e.g., glucose reported in mmol/L).

Overall, I cannot recommend this textbook for purchase by clinical pharmacists and drug information centers. Perhaps, with the above limitations noted, it would be appropriate for inclusion in a school of pharmacy library and could be recommended to students in the early phase of pharmacy education who desire clinical correlations to their biochemical studies.

Reviewed by Joseph T. DiPiro, Pharm.D., Department of Pharmacy Practice, University of Georgia, Room CJ-112, Medical College of Georgia, Augusta, GA 30912.

Manual of Antibiotics and Infectious Diseases, Fifth Edition

By John E. Conte, Jr., and Steven L. Barriere.

Published by Lea & Febiger, 600 Washington Square, Philadelphia, PA 19106, 1984. xiv + 351 p. Price $18.50 (U.S.), $23.25 (Canada).

Many new antibiotics have been introduced to the U.S. market over the last few years, thereby making it difficult for the clinician to keep abreast of the major advances in the treatment of many infectious diseases. Furthermore, prospective pricing has complicated the therapeutic decision process; the increasing emergence of resistant organisms has also contributed to increased complexity of treating hospital-acquired infections. Conte and Barriere's *Manual of Antibiotics and Infectious Diseases*, now in its fifth edition, provides the clinician with a brief but compre-

Continued on page 116

Current Literature *Continued from page 114*

hensive review of specific antibiotics and a discussion of the current management of empiric and established infections.

The text is divided into eight sections: Antibiotics, Empiric Antibiotic Therapy, Therapy of Established Infections, Antibiotic Sensitivities, Prophylactic Antibiotics, Availability and Clinical Use of Immunobiologic Agents and Antiparasitic Drugs, Viral Hepatitis: Clinical and Serological Summary, and Sexually Transmitted Diseases. An index has been included in this version of the manual; this is a welcome aid.

"Antibiotics" commences with a limited discussion of pharmacokinetic principles (these were in a separate chapter in the fourth edition); the kinetics information is sufficient for the practitioner to comprehend the pharmacology information that follows. Over 75 individual antimicrobial agents are subsequently reviewed including acylovir, new and investigational third-generation cephalosporins, aztreonam, ketoconazole, netilmicin, and cinoxacin. One prominent investigational agent omitted is imipenem–cilastatin. The authors summarize the potential clinical uses of each agent, based on in vitro activity and results of clinical trials. Most important, they emphasize the major differences among the newer β lactams. Recommendations for dosage adjustment in renal disease including dialysis are valuable; one improvement is the inclusion of the Hull–Sarubbi nomogram for the aminoglycosides.

"Empiric Antibiotic Therapy" has been updated to include sexually transmitted diseases (STDs); one minor addition are guidelines for the empiric treatment of hospital-acquired adult pneumonias. As the authors forewarn, the use of one or more antibiotics in the empiric treatment of an infection is not meant to replace culture and sensitivity tests. "Therapy of Established Infection" (section 4) must be consulted once infecting organisms are identified. Major changes within this section include the recommendations of cefotaxime and moxalactam as drugs of choice for gram-negative meningitis; single-dose therapy for uncomplicated urinary-tract infections is also mentioned. When reading this section the clinician is made aware of several alternative therapies, although the authors emphasize the antibiotics of choice.

"Antibiotic Sensitivities" contains very complete comparisons of bacterial in vitro activity among the major antibiotics; aztreonam has been included when gram-negative bacteria are contrasted. The authors have created a separate table to outline the minimum inhibitory concentrations for susceptible organisms of the newer cephalosporins, which should prove valuable to the practitioner.

"Prophylactic Antibiotics" provides the classical recommendations for surgical and medical prophylaxis. Justifiably, the authors have suggested that second- and third-generation cephalosporins provide no added benefit over older agents in this setting. A major addition to this section is a discussion of chemoprophylaxis for secondary cases of *Haemophilus influenzae* type B disease; increased risk of disease among day-care center children exposed to invasive disease is unknown.

The uses and availability of immunobiologic agents and antiparasitic drugs are outlined and discussed in detail (approximately one third of the book) in section 6. The authors have added to this edition a discussion of the diphtheria/pertussis/tetanus, measles, and mumps vaccines. Updates on the pneumococcal, polio, and rabies immunizations and the varicella-zoster immune globulin are provided. The reader can readily find dosage schedules, toxicity information, and distribution centers for these agents from the well-organized tables. This section is very well referenced compared with other sections of the manual.

"Viral Hepatitis" has been greatly expanded in this edition to include a complete discussion of all three types of hepatitis from serologic markers to clinical management. Figures and tables effectively summarize major features and serve as useful guidelines for making therapeutic decisions. The recommended uses of immune globulins and the controversial hepatitis B virus vaccine are also discussed.

"Sexually Transmitted Diseases" outlines the treatment guidelines (e.g., CDC recommendations) for the major STD syndromes, excluding the acquired immunodeficiency syndrome.

The *Manual of Antibiotics and Infectious Diseases* is a well-organized text that may best be used as a reference source for obtaining information quickly. Although the text could be used in a "cookbook" fashion, the authors have included alternative treatment modalities and controversies in their discussions, which should enable the practitioner to make individualized yet rational decisions. This manual should be a valuable tool for the inexperienced clinician or pharmacy student who is expected to provide information on the management of a variety of infectious diseases.

Reviewed by Teresa A. Tartaglione, Pharm.D., Department of Pharmacy and Pharmaceutics, Medical College of Virginia/ Virginia Commonwealth University, Richmond, VA 23298.

Side Effects of Drugs, Annual 8, 1984

Edited by M.N.G Dukes.

Published by Excerpta Medica, Amsterdam, 1984. Available from Elsevier Science Publishing Co., P.O. Box 1663, New York, NY 10163. xxiii + 476 p. Price $67.25.

This annual of side effects has been published in January of each year since 1977. Its purpose is to provide a critical and up-to-date review of new information concerning adverse drug reactions and drug interactions from the clinician's point of view. The book can be used separately or as a supplement to the comprehensive encyclopedic text in the field, Meyler's *Side Effects of Drugs*, 10th edition, which was published in June 1984.

Annual 8 reviews all reports providing important new information on adverse reactions to drugs from July 1, 1982, to June 30, 1983. References cited are those providing new information or those clarifying previously reported drug-induced illness.

The book was edited by M.N.G. Dukes, who serves as Vice Chairman of the Netherlands Committee for the Evaluation of Medicine. He has selected 61 contributors from all over the world including 16 from the Netherlands, 5 from the U.S.S.R. and 3 from the U.S. The international selection of authors provides reviews of many drugs not generally available in the United States.

Side Effects of Drugs, Annual 8 contains 51 chapters dealing with reactions to individual drugs such as lithium, or to closely related drug groups, such as antihypertensives. Dukes begins the book with an editorial entitled "The seven pillars of foolishness" in which he recounts the recent disasters that have occurred with the nonsteroidal anti-inflammatory analgesics. He calls for a reassessment of drug promotional policies within the pharmaceutical industry.

Several chapters in the *Annual* deserve special comment. "Dermatologicals and Cosmetics" contains a table listing information concerning contact sensitivity to topical drugs and occupational contact with drugs causing contact allergy. An additional table summarizes contact allergy reported to cosmetic ingredients. "Antihypertensive Drugs" reviews important newer agents including captopril and minoxidil. The chapter on intravenous infusions provides an excellent summary of several specific problems of total intravenous nutrition including cholestasis, infections and complications, and drug incompatibilities with intravenous fluids. The chapter (47) reviewing cytostatic and immunosuppressive drugs is quite comprehensive, containing 30 pages and 175 references. Several chapters are quite brief (Social Drugs, Diuretic Drugs, and Immunomodulating Agents), containing only four pages each, but this may only reflect the lack of new information about these agents. Most chapters in the book are excellent and accomplish the stated purpose of the text.

Annual 8 is a valuable reference source that provides an update on the rapidly expanding subject of drug-induced diseases. The authors have again done an excellent job of summarizing the recent literature on the subject of adverse drug reactions and organizing the material in a format to meet the needs of the clinician.

Annual 8 and its companion text, Meyler's *Side Effects of Drugs*, 10th edition, should be available for easy access to every practicing physician and pharmacist. Although their cost will prevent most practitioners from owning a personal copy, it should be available in all medical libraries and drug information centers.

Reviewed by Ronald B. Stewart, M.S., College of Pharmacy (Box J-4), University of Florida, Gainesville, FL 32610.

Books Received

Books are listed as received; selected books may be reviewed in Book Reviews in subsequent issues.

Alcohol and the Fetus: A Clinical Perspective, by Henry L. Rosett and Lyn Weiner. Published by Oxford University Press, Inc., 200 Madison Ave., New York, NY 10016, 1984, xiii + 220 p. Price $24.95.

The Alkaloids: Chemistry and Pharmacology (Volume XXIII), edited by Arnold Brossi. Published by Academic Press, Inc., Orlando, FL 32887 and 24/28 Oval Road, London NW1 7DX, England, 1984. xix + 399 p. Price $85.00, £59.50.

Antimicrobial Therapy, edited by Angela M. Ristuccia and Burke A. Cunha. Published by Raven Press, 1140 Avenue of the Americas, New York, NY 10036, 1984. xvi + 618 p. Price $98.50.

Applied Therapeutic Drug Monitoring. Volume I: Fundamentals; Volume II: Review and Case Studies, edited by Thomas P. Moyer and Roger L. Boeckx. Published by the American Association for Clinical Chemistry, 1725 K St., N.W., Washington, DC 20006, 1982 (Vol. I), 1984 (Vol. II). Vol. 1 xii + 241 p.; price $15.00. Vol. II xi + 387 p.; price $19.50 (members), $22.00 (nonmembers). Bound set $30.00 (members), $35.00 (nonmembers).

Azides and Nitrenes: Reactivity and Utility, edited by Eric F. V. Scriven. Published by Academic Press, Inc., Orlando, FL 32887 and 24/28 Oval Road, London NW1 7DX, England, 1984. xii + 542 p. Price $99.50, £70.00.

Bedside Clinical Pharmacokinetics: Simple Techniques for Individualizing Drug Therapy, by Carl C. Peck. Published by Pharmacometrics Press, 6219 Poindexter Lane, Rockville, MD 20852, 1984. 98 p. Price $5.00, students $4.00; 5% tax for Maryland residents.

Beta-Adrenoceptors in Asthma, edited by J. Morley. Published by Academic Press Inc., Orlando, FL 32887 and 24/28 Oval Road, London NW1, England, 1984. x + 283 p. Price $21.50, £14.00.

Boyd's Introduction to the Study of Disease (Ninth Edition), by Huntington Sheldon. Published by Lea & Febiger, 600 Washington Square, Philadelphia, PA 19106-4198, 1984. vii + 702 p. Price $28.50, Canada $35.75.

Experimental and Clinical Toxicokinetics, edited by Avraham Yacobi and Herbert Barry III. Published by the American Pharmaceutical Assn., 2215 Constitution Ave., N.W., Washington, DC 20037, 1984. xvi + 188 p. Price $39.00 ($26.00 for APhA members); add $7.80 for postage and handling on foreign orders.

Guide to Clinical Studies and Developing Protocols, by Bert Spilker. Published by Raven Press, 1140 Avenue of the Americas, New York, NY 10036, 1984. xvii + 302 p. Price $45.00.

Mechanism of Drug Action, edited by Thomas P. Singer, Tag E. Mansour, and Raul N. Ondarza. Published by Academic Press, Inc., Orlando, FL 32887, and 24/28 Oval Road, London NW1 7DX, England, 1983. xvii + 405 p. Price $39.00, £30.50.

Pharmaceutical Statistics: Practical and Clinical Applications, by Sanford Bolton. Published by Marcel Dekker, Inc., 270 Madison Ave., New York, NY 10016, 1984. xiv + 526 p. Price $75.00.

Phosphorus-31 NMR: Principles and Applications, edited by David G. Gorenstein. Published by Academic Press, Inc., Orlando, FL 32887, and 24/28 Oval Road, London NW1 7DX, England, 1984. xiv + 604 p. Price $79.00, £61.00.

Practical Aspects of Intravenous Drug Therapy Techniques for the Practicing: Nurse, Pharmacist, Physician, written and published by Richard D. Leff and Robert J. Roberts, 1984. Available from Pediatric Clinical Pharmacology, The University of Iowa, Iowa City, IA 52242. 112 p. Price $10.00.

Advertising Index

American Society of Hospital Pharmacists
American Hospital Formulary Service—Drug Information 85, inside back cover
Clinical Pharmacy, 26, 26A, 26B
Position Available, 92
Bristol Laboratories, Division of Bristol-Myers Company
Cefadyl, 115–116
Precef, 16–18
Cambridge University Press
Publications, 25
International Pharmaceutical Federation
45th International Congress, 104
Lederle Laboratories, A Division of American Cyanamid Company
Maxzide, 9–10
Smith Kline & French Laboratories
Ancef, 15
Cefizox, inside front cover, 107–110
Monocid, 6–8
E. R. Squibb & Sons, Inc.
Institutional, 4–5
Stuart Pharmaceuticals, Division of ICI Americas, Inc.
Institutional, outside back cover
The Upjohn Company
Cleocin, 20–22
Micronase, 12–14
University of Massachusetts Medical Center
Position Available, 117

News

Dietary modifications recommended for reducing heart disease

Persons with blood cholesterol concentrations above the 75th percentile for the population require some form of treatment to lower blood cholesterol, according to an expert panel at the National Institutes of Health Consensus Development Conference on Lowering Blood Cholesterol to Prevent Heart Disease, December 10–12, 1984. The panel recommended that all Americans over the age of two years adopt a diet low in fat and cholesterol to reduce the risks of coronary heart disease.

After considering evidence from genetic, pathologic, epidemiologic, and clinical intervention trials, the panel concluded that the relationship between elevated blood cholesterol levels and coronary heart disease is established "beyond a reasonable doubt" and that "appropriate changes in . . . diet will reduce blood cholesterol levels." In making its recommendations, the panel frequently cited the results of the recently completed Lipid Research Clinics Coronary Primary Prevention Trial, which demonstrated substantial reductions in heart attack rates in patients whose elevated cholesterol concentrations were reduced by therapy with diet plus cholestyramine (Questran, Mead Johnson).

Antonio M. Gotto, Jr., M.D., of the Baylor College of Medicine and President of the American Heart Association, recommended a massive screening program to identify high-risk individuals. He suggested using a total blood cholesterol concentration of 240–250 mg/dL in persons older than 40 years old as an "alert" value requiring some type of intervention. Acknowledging the need to adjust target levels of blood cholesterol for age, sex, and other factors, Gotto said, "It is imperative that we simplify [the screening process] as much as possible for the practitioner if we're going to expect him or her to carry it out."

The panel defined two levels of hypercholesterolemia needing treatment. Persons with blood cholesterol values above the 90th percentile for the population should be treated intensively by dietary means and, if necessary, drug therapy. Individuals with cholesterol levels between the 75th and 90th percentiles should receive diet therapy; few will require drug treatment, according to the panel. Specific cholesterol values at various ages for which treatment should be initiated are shown in the table. The goal of therapy would be to reduce total cholesterol concentrations to about 180 mg/dL for adults under 30 and to about 200 mg/dL for persons 30 and older. According to Gotto, it may be necessary to aim for a cholesterol concentration of 140 mg/dL in children if the 180–200 mg/dL target levels for adults are to be achieved. Although most studies have been conducted in men at high risk for coronary heart disease, the panel recommended that women with hypercholesterolemia be treated similarly to men, stating that coronary heart disease is also the leading cause of death in women and that blood cholesterol is a risk factor.

Cholesterol Values for Selecting Men and Women at Moderate and High Risk (Requiring Treatment)

	Serum Cholesterol Concentrations (mg/dL)	
Age (years)	Moderate Risk	High Risk
2–19	>170	>185
20–29	>200	>220
30–39	>220	>240
≥40	>240	>260

Noting the continuous relationship between blood cholesterol and coronary heart disease, the panel extended its recommendations for lowering blood cholesterol to the entire U.S. population. Specifically, the panel advocated lowering total dietary fat intake from 40% to 30% of total calories, limiting saturated and polysaturated fat intake to 10% of total calories each, and reducing daily cholesterol intake to 250–300 mg. Such a diet should be implemented early in life, the panel noted, when lifestyle patterns are being developed.

Speaking on drug therapy of hypercholesterolemia, W. Virgil Brown, M.D., of the Mount Sinai School of Medicine in New York, said that two experimental drugs, compactin and mevinolin, produced marked reductions in cholesterol concentrations in patients with familial hypercholesterolemia when used in combination with colestipol, a bile-acid sequestrant. Compactin and mevinolin inhibit the rate-limiting enzyme in cholesterol biosynthesis and have been relatively free of serious side

Continued on page 131

900 mg q8h

efficacy plus convenience

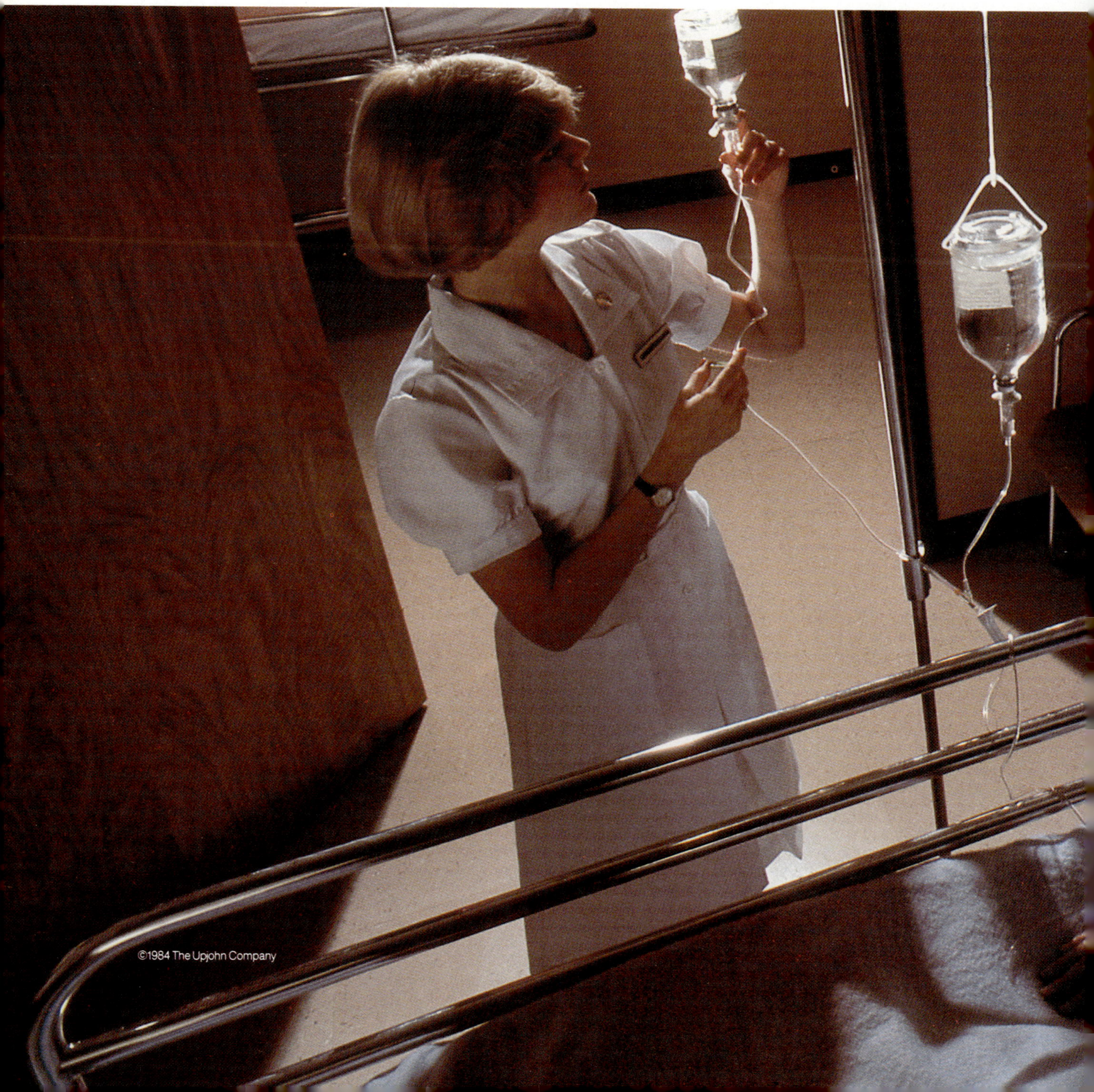

Continued from page 123

effects in the few trials reported thus far, Brown added. The consensus panel noted that only the bile-acid sequestrants and nicotinic acid had been shown to reduce the incidence of coronary heart disease and that the long-term safety of any cholesterol-lowering drug "when given over decades" was not known. The decision to use drug therapy must be made on a case-by-case basis, the panel stated, and should only be used after maximum dietary modification has been tried.

OLIN H. WELSH, JR.

Drug-induced blood disorders very rare

A study of more than 200,000 people by the Boston Collaborative Drug Surveillance Program has shown that drugs are very rarely associated with blood disorders.[1] Only quinidine/quinine and sulfa-containing drugs were associated with blood disorders in more than one patient during the 10-year study period.

Using computerized pharmacy records of the Group Health Cooperative of Puget Sound in Seattle, researchers recorded drug ingestion by patients who had been discharged between 1972 and 1981 with diagnoses of pancytopenia, granulocytopenia, hemolytic anemia, thrombocytopenia, or other unspecified blood diseases. Prescription drugs obtained at the cooperative's pharmacies were correlated with occurrences of blood disorders.

A total of 391 patients were identified with blood-cell deficiencies; in only 26 cases could drug therapy not be ruled out. Of these, 11 patients appeared to have quinidine/quinine-induced thrombocytopenia, and sulfa-containing drugs were likely responsible for eight cases of blood disorders. Even though large numbers of patients received certain drugs often reported to cause blood disorders—such as phenylbutazone, indomethacin, ibuprofen, and allopurinol—no cases were identified in this study.

The authors commented that their results are consistent with reports from Sweden, both in incidence of drug-induced blood disorders[2-4] and in increased risk for persons older than 49 years.[4] The increased risk with age was not entirely explainable by increased drug use in that population; sulfa-containing products were used more often in younger people, but six of the eight cases of sulfa-associated problems occurred in people older than 65 years.

1. Danielson DA, Douglas SW III, Herzog P et al. Drug-induced blood disorders. *JAMA*. 1984; 252:3257–60.
2. Böttiger LE, Furhoff AK, Holmberg L. Fatal reactions to drugs: a ten-year material from the Swedish Adverse Drug Reaction Committee. *Acta Med Scand*. 1979; 205:451–6.
3. Böttiger LE, Furhoff AK, Holmberg L. Drug-induced blood dyscrasias: a ten-year material from the Swedish Adverse Drug Reaction Committee. *Acta Med Scand*. 1979; 205:457–61.
4. Böttiger LE, Westerholm B. Drug-induced blood dyscrasias in Sweden. *Br Med J*. 1973; 3:339–43.

Continued on page 134

When a type II diabetic patient needs more than diet, unique MICRONASE® Tablets (glyburide) are a logical first choice.

Choosing antidiabetic

1. Micronase—a rational choice in type II diabetes

Insulin levels are normal or elevated in most patients with type II diabetes, although insulin action is markedly impaired. MICRONASE helps normalize the tissue response to endogenous insulin.

Initially, MICRONASE helps lower serum glucose in responsive patients by stimulating the release of additional insulin. As therapy continues, MICRONASE is believed to promote peripheral glucose metabolism by helping to correct defects at the cellular receptor and postreceptor levels.

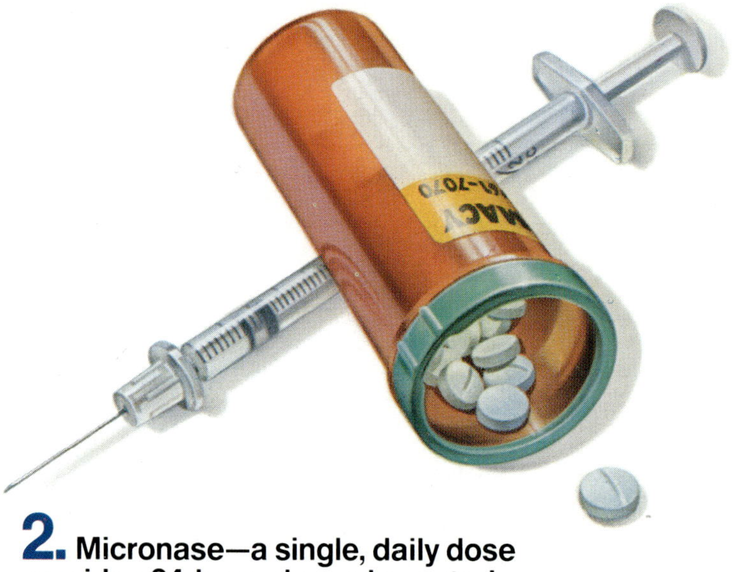

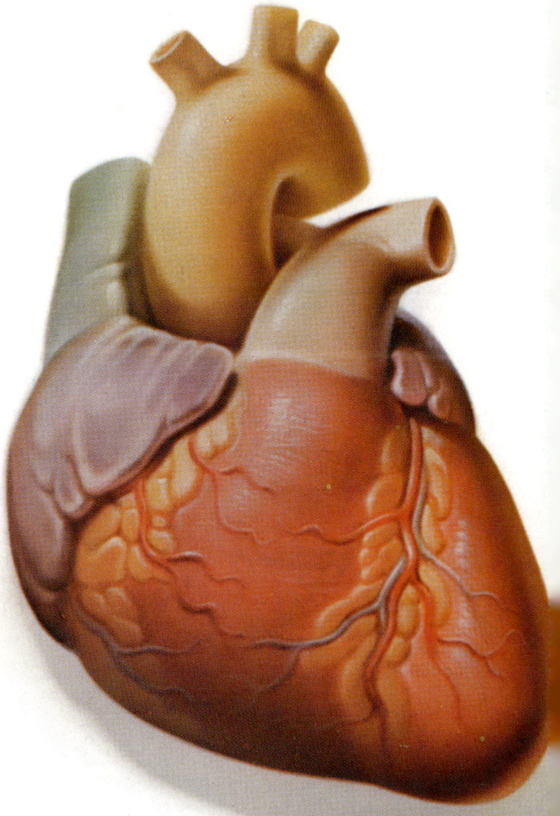

2. Micronase—a single, daily dose provides 24-hour glycemic control

MICRONASE provides 24-hour control of blood glucose with a single, daily, low-milligram dose. MICRONASE may be taken with food, since food intake does not appear to affect its bioavailability.

3. Micronase—for the type II diabetic patient who is also hypertensive: Control without risk of water retention

This may also be significant for the type II diabetic pati
with congestive heart failure. MICRONASE actually caus
mild diuresis.

:herapy today

I. Micronase—for the diabetic patient ith moderate renal impairment: ontrol plus unique dual excretion... 0% urine, 50% bile

limination of MICRONASE equally in bile and urine reduces the sk of drug accumulation, which may result in hypoglycemia. asma clearance of MICRONASE is prolonged only in patients ith severe renal impairment.

5. Micronase—for the patient who fails on other diabetic therapy: Potency and dosage flexibility

MICRONASE may prove effective when other drugs fail. Five mg of MICRONASE is approximately equivalent to 250 mg of chlorpropamide or 500 mg of acetohexamide in its ability to lower blood glucose. The dosage range of MICRONASE allows for greater dosage flexibility than other agents.

Overdosage of sulfonylureas, including MICRONASE, can cause hypoglycemia. Although the interpretations are controversial, the UGDP study reported in 1970 that the use of tolbutamide, an oral hypoglycemic drug, was associated with increased cardiovascular mortality.

Upjohn The Upjohn Company
Kalamazoo, MI 49001

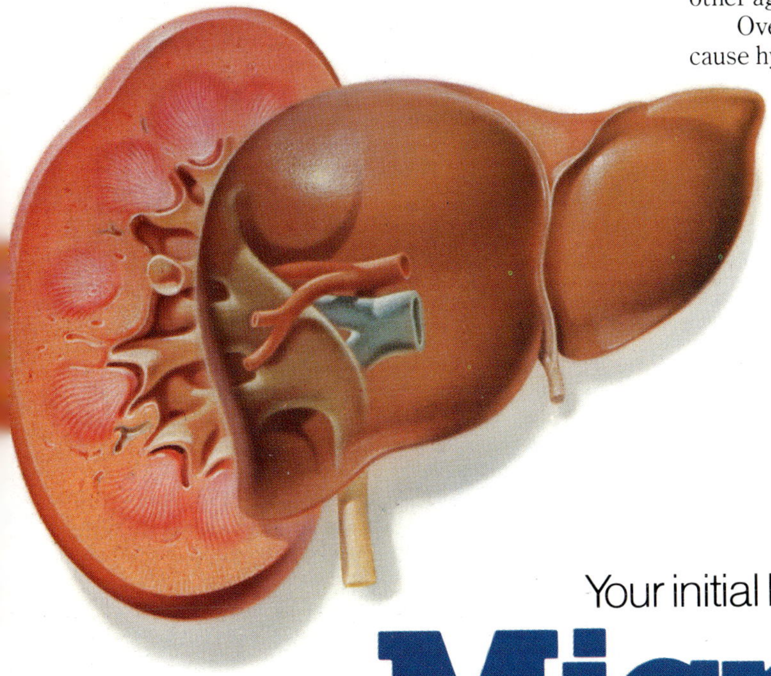

Your initial Rx in type II diabetes

Micronase®

glyburide, **5 mg** Tablets

For brief summary of prescribing information, please turn page.

News *Continued from page 131*

Long-acting third-generation cephalosporin ceftriaxone reaches U.S. market

Ceftriaxone sodium (Rocephin, Roche Laboratories), a third-generation cephalosporin with a half-life of eight hours, was approved by FDA on December 21 for treatment of a variety of systemic infections. The drug, which has received favorable reviews based on investigational data, is expected to have a major impact on the use of third-generation cephalosporins in hospitals.

Ceftriaxone can be administered intravenously or intramuscularly. The drug's time to peak concentration after i.v. injection is 20–30 minutes, and the time to peak concentration after i.m. injection is two to three hours. The peak serum concentration of 140 $\mu g/mL$ achieved with ceftriaxone exceeds those of other available third-generation cephlosporins.[1]

Overall, ceftriaxone's spectrum of activity is similar to those of other third-generation cephalosporins, and its chief utility lies in its longer half-life. Ceftriaxone is indicated for treatment of certain infections of the lower respiratory tract, skin and skin structures, urinary tract, and bones and joints. The drug is also labeled for treatment of uncomplicated gonorrhea, bacterial septicemia, pelvic inflammatory disease, and meningitis.

The wholesale price of ceftriaxone is $22.95 per 1-g vial and $12.50 per 500-mg vial.

1. Barriere SL, Flaherty JF. Third-generation cephalosporins: a critical evaluation. *Clin Pharm.* 1984; 3:351–66.

Nomifensine, a second-generation antidepressant, approved by FDA

Nomifensine maleate (Merital, Hoechst-Roussel), a second-generation antidepressant, was approved by FDA on December 31. The drug has been under investigation in the U.S. since 1973.

Nomifensine is a dopaminergic agonist that shares properties common to both apomorphine and amphetamine. In contrast to the sedation caused by most antidepressants, restlessness and agitation are common side effects of nomifensine; the drug is therefore not generally recommended for use in agitated depression.

Nomifensine should be taken twice a day—in the morning and early afternoon—on an empty stomach. The usual dose is 50 mg b.i.d., although doses as high as 300 mg per day have been administered.

The drug will be available as 50-mg capsules in bottles of 100. Marketing is not expected until May–June. A detailed review of nomifensine is scheduled for a mid-1985 issue of *CP*.

Naltrexone approved by FDA

Naltrexone (Trexan, DuPont Pharmaceuticals), a long-acting opiate antagonist approved recently by FDA, is the first agent marketed solely for the treatment of opiate

Continued on page 141

Continued from page 134

dependence. The drug was reviewed by Crabtree[1] in the May–June 1984 issue of *CP*.

Naltrexone was approved for adjunctive treatment of opiate addiction. Patients must be detoxified or opiate-free for 7–10 days before naltrexone therapy can begin; the drug lacks agonist effects and therefore causes no dependence.

Naltrexone is rapidly and completely absorbed in the gastrointestinal tract; extensive "first-pass" metabolism converts 95% of an oral dose to several metabolites. One metabolite—6-β-naltrexol—is believed to exert much of naltrexone's pharmacologic effect.

Because naltrexone's duration of effect can be increased by elevating the dose, the patient can use one of two dosing regimens: one 50-mg tablet per day or 350 mg per week in three divided doses. DuPont's direct list price to hospitals for the 50-mg tablets is $84 per bottle of 50.

1. Crabree BL. Review of naltrexone, a long-acting antagonist. *Clin Pharm.* 1984; 3:273–80.

Panel considers treatment of travelers' diarrhea

Antibiotic prophylaxis against travelers' diarrhea is not needed, but anti-infective agents can be used appropriately in treating moderate to severe cases of this condition, according to an NIH Consensus Development Conference held January 28–30 in Bethesda, MD. An expert panel considered epidemiology, causes, prevention, treatment, and needed research on travelers' diarrhea, which affects 16 million people worldwide annually, including 8 million Americans.

Travelers' diarrhea is characterized by a twofold or greater increase in the frequency of bowel movements. Commonly associated symptoms include abdominal cramps, nausea, bloating, urgency, and malaise. Episodes usually begin abruptly (most often on third day after arrival in the country being visited), result in four to five loose or watery stools per day, and resolve in three to four days. Travelers' diarrhea is acquired through ingestion of fecally contaminated food or water; especially risky foods include raw meat, raw vegetables, and raw seafood. Enterotoxigenic *Escherichia coli* is the organism most often implicated.

The panel concluded that the only prophylactic measure supported by published data is proper instruction of travelers in sensible dietary practices. Prophylactic antimicrobial agents, immunization, and the use of nonantimicrobial medications were not recommended.

Therapy of travelers' diarrhea is optional since most cases are self-limiting. The panel recommended the following if treatment is desired:

1. If rapid relief of symptoms is desired after one or two unformed stools accompanied by cramps, nausea, or malaise, diphenoxylate hydrochloride (with atropine sulfate, Lomotil) or loperamide hydrochloride (Imodium) may be taken. An alternative is to start bismuth subsalicylate (Pepto-Bismol and other products) 30 mL every 30 minutes for eight doses. Although this regimen decreases the number of stools and increases their consistency, it does not improve symptoms during the first four hours of treatment.
2. If it is important to shorten the course or decrease the severity of moderate to severe travelers' diarrhea, antimicrobial agents may be taken. After three or more loose stools with symptoms, consideration can be given to a short course of trimethoprim–sulfamethoxazole (Bactrim; Septra), trimethoprim (Trimpex; Proloprim) alone, or doxycycline (Vibramycin).
3. A small percentage of travelers have persisting diarrhea with fever and blood or mucus in the stools. This suggests that a more serious colitis is involved, and such individuals should seek medical attention.

The panel also recommended that travelers to areas of high risk (Latin America, Africa, the Middle East, and Asia) obtain (in advance) an antimotility drug or bismuth subsalicylate for milder forms of travelers' diarrhea, and an antimicrobial agent trimethoprim–sulfamethoxazole, trimethoprim alone, or doxycycline for more severe travelers' diarrhea. Advice concerning side effects of these drugs and various aspects of hygiene and dietary precautions should be obtained.

Copies of the panel's final statement are available at no cost from the NIH Office of Medical Applications of Research, Building 1, Room 216, NIH, Bethesda, MD 20205.

Oral acyclovir approved for treatment of genital herpes

Oral acyclovir (Zovirax, Burroughs Wellcome), the first oral medication for the treatment of genital herpes simplex virus (HSV) infections, was approved for marketing in the United States by FDA. Acyclovir has been available in ointment and intravenous formulations since 1982. While oral acyclovir is a more convenient formulation, it is considered the most effective formulation available, especially for treatment of initial episodes of HSV infections.

Oral acyclovir, which was the subject of a review by True and Carter[1] and an editorial by Barriere[2] in the November-December 1984 issue of *Clinical Pharmacy*, was approved (1) for the treatment of initial or recurrent genital HSV infections, (2) as suppressive therapy to prevent recurrences of genital infections, and (3) for prophylaxis in immunocompromised patients with disseminated herpetic infections. The drug lacks curative properties but reduces viral shedding and increases the rate of healing that may be important in reducing spread of the genital herpes.

For treating genital infections, patients should take one 200-mg capsule every four hours while awake for a total of five capsules daily for 10 days during initial episodes and for five days during recurrences. For prophylactic therapy, patients should take one 200-mg capsule three times daily for up to six months. Prophylactic therapy should be used only for patients experiencing six or more recurrences of genital herpes per year.

Patients have reported minimal adverse effects with oral acyclovir. The most common adverse effects reported are nausea and vomiting and headache. Oral acyclovir should not be taken during pregnancy.

The drug became available February 11 in 200-mg capsules. The cost to the patient for a five-day course of treatment is about $16.

1. True BL, Carter BL. Update on acyclovir: oral therapy for herpesvirus infections. *Clin Pharm.* 1984; 3:607–13.
2. Barriere SL. Oral acyclovir: a pill too easy to swallow? *Clin Pharm.* 1984; 3:655. Editorial.

Combination product approved for deep-vein thrombosis

Embolex (dihydroergotamine mesylate [DHE] and heparin sodium; with lidocaine HCl, Sandoz, Inc.) has been approved for prevention of postopertive deep-vein thrombosis (DVT). The product, which should decrease DVT-related deaths from pulmonary embolism (PE), can be used in patients undergoing major pelvic, thoracic, or abdominal surgery.

Embolex should be administered by deep subcutaneous injection two hours preoperatively and every 12 hours postoperatively for five to seven days. FDA approved two formulations: DHE 0.5 mg/2500 IU heparin and DHE 0.5 mg/5000 IU heparin, but only the latter will be available intially. Heparin prevents hypercoagulability; DHE, which increases venous tone, prevents DVT by accelerating venous return. Lidocaine hydrochloride 7.46 mg is added for its local anesthetic properties.

A clinical study demonstrated that Embolex with 5000 IU of heparin is significantly more effective than the same dose of heparin alone in preventing DVT. Patients treated with Embolex given twice a day had only a 9.4% incidence of DVT, compared with a 16.8% rate for the same dose of heparin alone.[1]

Embolex became available February 11 in 0.7-ml ampuls. The wholesale price to hospitals is $54.00 per box of 20 ampuls and $260.04 per box of 100 ampuls.

1. The Multicenter Trial Committee. Dihydroergotamine–heparin prophylaxis of postoperative deep vein thrombosis: a multicenter trial. *JAMA*. 1984; 251:2960–6.

Long-acting bronchodilator marketed

Bitolterol mesylate (Tornalate, Winthrop–Breon Laboratories), a bronchodilator with a duration of effect of up to eight hours, was approved by FDA on December 28. The drug is similar to other available β agonists in its therapeutic uses and side effects.

Bitolterol, a prodrug, is converted by ester hydrolysis in tissues and blood to the active drug colterol. The drug exerts its bronchodilating effects three to four minutes after it is inhaled. In clinical studies, the duration of bronchodilator activity was at least five hours in most patients and eight hours or more in 25–35% of patients.

Bitolterol is available in a 15-ml metered-dose inhaler containing 16.4 g of drug. The usual dose for relief of bronchospasm is one or two inhalations at an interval of at least one to three minutes followed by a third inhalation if needed. For prevention of bronchospasm, bitolterol is usually taken in two inhalations every eight hours.

Isotretinoin associated with new adverse effects

In addition to the continuing problems with the teratogenicity of isotretinoin (Accutane, Roche Laboratories) in women who become pregnant while taking the drug, new problems have been associated with use of the product. These problems include minimal skeletal hyperostosis in patients on short-term therapy for severe recalcitrant acne, problems in controlling blood glucose in known or suspected diabetics, and persistence of some adverse effects after cessation of therapy.

The skeletal hyperostosis problem has occurred before but only in patients using isotretinoin for long-term, high-dose therapy of disorders of keratinization. A new study shows that 7 of 32 patients studied prospectively had bony spur formation along one or more vertebrae; the problems were only detected on roentgenograms taken one year after therapy with isotretinoin 1–2 mg/kg/day taken for four months for severe, recalcitrant acne. Roche reports that the hyperostosis has been asymptomatic, and the patients are being followed to learn more about the long-term implications of the problem.

Some patients have experienced problems in the control of their blood sugar while taking isotretinoin, and the company now recommends periodic blood glucose determinations for known or suspected diabetics taking Accutane.

Some adverse effects of isotretinoin seem to persist even after discontinuation of the drug; this has been observed with the hyperostosis effect and also with dry eyes. These new findings underscore the need for careful patient selection and use of isotretinoin for only its labeled indication—severe recalcitrant acne unresponsive to conventional therapies, including systemic antibiotics.

Cardioselective β blocker acebutolol approved by FDA

Acebutolol hydrochloride (Sectral, Ives Laboratories) has been approved by FDA for the management of both hypertension and ventricular arrhythmias. In therapeutic doses acebutolol is a cardioselective β-adrenoreceptor blocking agent with mild intrinsic sympathomimetic activity.

The antihypertensive affect of acebutolol is similar to that of combination antihypertensive therapy with propranolol and hydrochlorothiazide. The antiarrhythmic effect is comparable with that achieved with combinations of propranolol and quinidine.

The drug is absorbed from the gastrointestinal tract and is subject to extensive first-pass hepatic metabolism. Acebutolol has a half-life of three to four hours, but an equicardioselective active metabolite has a half-life of 8–13 hours. The drug can be taken once or twice daily.

The product will be available March 20 in 200- and 400-mg capsules in bottles of 100 and unit dose packages of 100.

Injectable agent approved for urinary-tract infections

Amdinocillin (Coactin, Roche Laboratories), the first penicillin that binds to penicillin-binding protein-2 (PBP-2), was approved recently by FDA for treatment of urinary-tract infections (UTIs). All other marketed penicillins inhibit cell-wall synthesis by binding to PBP-1 and PBP-3, and amdinocillin is sometimes active against certain multiresistant strains commonly resistant to other β-lactam antibiotics.

Continued on page 144

See next page for brief summary of prescribing information.

News *Continued from page 142*

Amdinocillin is highly active against gram-negative bacteria and is slightly active against gram-positive bacteria. The drug is indicated alone or in combination with other β-lactam antibiotics for the treatment of UTIs caused by *Escherichia coli*, *Klebsiella pneumoniae*, *Klebsiella* species, and *Enterobacter* species.

FDA classified amdinocillin a drug of little or no therapeutic gain, although its mechanism of action may prove important for the treatment of some complicated UTIs. The drug is synergistic with other β-lactam antibiotics, and, with combination antibiotic therapy, resistance is less likely. Its wholesale price is $6.00 and $3.50 per 1-g and 500-mg vial, respectively.

News Briefs

- **Iodohippurate sodium I 123 injection (Nephroflow, Medi-Physics)** has been approved by FDA for diagnostic evaluation of kidney function.

- Twice-a-day oral dosing of **cimetidine 400 mg (Tagamet, Smith Kline & French)** has been approved for the short-term treatment of duodenal ulcers.

- A new agent for treatment of Cushing's syndrome will soon be available from Winthrop-Breon Laboratories; **trilostane (Modrastane)** inhibits an enzyme in the adrenal glands necessary for production of some steroid hormones and is under investigation for use in metastatic breast cancer.

- **Calcitonin (Calcimar, USV Pharmaceutical)** is now approved for treatment of postmenopausal osteoporosis.

- A **$15,000 grant** is available from the Parenteral Drug Association Foundation for Pharmaceutical Sciences for **research in parenteral nutrition;** the deadline for application is July 15, and more information is available from the Foundation at P.O. Box 242, Garden City, NY 11530; 516-248-6713.

- A new home-study course on the **treatment of hemostatic disorders** is available for health professionals from the Sales Office, American Association of Blood Banks, 1117 North 19th Street, Arlington, VA 22209; "Treating Hemostatic Disorders: A Problem Oriented Approach" costs $8.

- The American College of Physicians has launched a campaign to assure that adults are properly immunized; ***Guide for Adult Immunization,*** a handbook that discusses clinical issues related to specific vaccines, is available from ACP, 4200 Pine Street, Philadelphia, PA 19104, for $10 (Pennsylvania residents add 6% sales tax).

- **Quinacrine hydrochloride,** an unapproved drug being studied by LyphoMed for treating recurrent pneumothorax, has been designated an orphan drug by FDA.

- The clinical and economic impact of **cefonicid (Monocid, Smith Kline & French)** is the subject of a special supplement to *Reviews of Infectious Diseases;* single copies are available for $15.00 to institutions and $9.50 to individuals from the journal at P.O. Box 37005, Chicago, IL 60637.

Letters

The Letters *column is a forum for rapid exchange of ideas among readers of* CP. *Liberal criteria are applied in the review of submissions to encourage contributions to this column.*

The Letters *column includes the following types of contributions: (1) comments, addenda, and minor updates on previously published work, (2) alerts on potential problems related to drug therapy or clinical research, (3) observations or comments on trends in drug therapy or clinical research, and (4) brief expressions of opinion about controversies in drug therapy or clinical research.*

Letters need not be submitted with the journal's manuscript checklist. The following conditions, however, must be adhered to: (1) the body of the letter must be no longer than two typewritten pages, (2) the use of references, tables, and illustrations should be minimized, (3) the authors' names, affiliations, and mailing addresses must be typed at the end of the letter in the format used by CP, *and (4) the entire letter (including references, tables, and authors' names) must be typed double spaced on plain white paper (not letterhead). Following acceptance of a letter, the authors are required to sign an exclusive publication statement and a copyright-transferral form.*

Cimetidine-induced alopecia

Only two case reports of alopecia associated with the use of cimetidine (Tagamet, Smith Kline & French) have been reported in the literature.[1,2] In both instances, the problem was reversed upon discontinuation of the medication; upon rechallenge, one patient again began losing hair.[1] The FDA Division of Drug Experience has received more than 60 case reports of alopecia associated with cimetidine use.[3] Alopecia has occurred in men and women (27 to 76 years of age) taking cimetidine for a time period ranging from two days to two years.

We would like to report another case of cimetidine-associated alopecia. Our patient was a 64-year-old white man treated for a duodenal ulcer with cimetidine 300 mg four times daily. After two weeks of therapy, the patient noticed that he had larger than normal amounts of hair on his hairbrush. At a follow-up appointment, approximately three weeks after beginning cimetidine, the alopecia was noted to be moderately severe, affecting the entire scalp but no other parts of the body. At that time the cimetidine was discontinued, and ranitidine (Zantac, Glaxo) was started.

An extensive search of causative factors revealed none other than the cimetidine. The patient had not taken any medications reported to cause hair loss, nor did he have any history of alopecia or any history of disease states known to be associated with alopecia. At the latest follow-up visit, his hair was almost back to pretreatment fullness.

1. Ahmad S. Cimetidine and alopecia. *Ann Intern Med.* 1979; 91:930.
2. Virchburger MI, Prelevic GM, Brkic S et al. Transitory alopecia and hypergonadotropic hypergonadism during cimetidine treatment. *Lancet.* 1981; 1:1160–1.
3. Khalsa JH, Graham CF, Jones JK. Cimetidine-associated alopecia. *Int J Dermatol.* 1983; 22:202–4.

Carl J. Tullio, M.S.
Mark A. Roberts, M.D.

U.S. Air Force Regional Hospital Maxwell
Maxwell AFB, AL 36112

Putting amoxicillin–potassium clavulanate in perspective

The one consolation for pharmacy and therapeutics committees in the antibiotic field over the past few years has been the oral anti-infective area. Even though several new products have been marketed, they have been chiefly for outpatient therapy and have generally not been added to the formulary. Amoxicillin–potassium clavulanate is the latest oral product, and it appears to fall in the outpatient category.

Why then do Stein and Gurwith[1] recommend strong consideration of this product to formularies? Reed and Blumer[2] and Neu[3] defer a recommendation until more data are available.

When reviewing new medications one must keep a proper perspective. Many hospitals are entering the community pharmacy market. When time comes to stock these pharmacies, I am sure many will be surprised at the number of medications that must be available. But this is the outpatient market, and, as hospital pharmacy directors, our formularies are written for inpatients.

I especially appreciate the Formulary Recommendation section of *Clinical Pharmacy*'s reviews. Yet I think that this section should be in the perspective of "inpatient" hospital pharmacy. All new medications must still be reviewed. Amoxicillin–potassium clavulanate may be ideal for pediatric hospitals or institutions with large outpatient clinics, but each institution must evaluate new products in light of their specific patient population and antibiotic-resistance patterns. General recommendations can be made, but including patient selection as a factor in the Formulary Recommendation section would be extremely valuable.

1. Stein GE, Gurwith MJ. Amoxicillin–potassium clavulanate, a β-lactamase-resistant antibiotic combination. *Clin Pharm.* 1984;3:591–9.

2. Reed MD, Blumer JL. Amoxicillin–potassium clavulanate: rational pharmacology meets clinical infectious disease. *Clin Pharm.* 1984;3:653–4. Editorial.
3. Neu HC. Amoxicillin and potassium clavulanate: an antibiotic combination. *Pharmacotherapy.* 1984; 4:133–4. Commentary.

ALLEN J. VAIDA, PHARM.D., Director of Pharmacy Services
Suburban General Hospital.
2701 DeKalb Pike
Norristown, PA 19401

Editor's note: The Formulary Recommendation section of CP *Drug Reviews is designed to provide general advice to a large number of hospitals of all sizes and types. An outpatient drug product such as amoxicillin–potassium clavulanate would obviously have limited utility in a hospital with few outpatient services. Hospitals must consider their individual characteristics in making formulary decisions based on all available evidence and advice, including published advice such as that in* CP *Drug Reviews.*

I.V. amantidine sulfate for extrapyramidal crisis

Of the numerous drugs commonly used in Parkinson's disease, only biperiden (Akineton, Knoll Pharmaceutical) and benztropine mesylate (Cogentin, Merck Sharp & Dohme) are available in injectable dosage forms. In Europe oral amantadine sulfate has been shown to be an effective and safe antiparkinsonian drug[1] with effectiveness equal to that of amantadine hydrochloride (Symmetrel, Du Pont).[2]

In 1973, injectable amantidine sulfate was shown to be safe and effective in patients with Parkinson's disease with akinetic crisis, insufficient response, or overly severe side effects from oral therapy.[3] Additional later reports established the indications, efficacy, and safety of this mode of treatment in 137 patients with various forms of Parkinson's disease.[4,5] The limited value of the previously mentioned injectable drugs in akinetic crisis, and the European experience encouraged us to try i.v. amantidine sulfate for extrapyramidal crisis.

We have used daily i.v. infusions of amanthidine sulfate (Adamanntyl-amine sulphate) 200 mg in specially prepared bottles of 5% fructose 500 mL (donated by Merz & Company, Frankfurt, Germany) in 10 patients with long-standing Parkinson's disease. These patients were admitted with severe akinetic crisis, inability to swallow, and disorientation. In all patients, L-dopa was discontinued abruptly because of minor trauma; upper-respiratory or urinary-tract infection with fever; nausea and vomiting; or terrifying visual hallucinations. Previous drug regimens were initiated when possible, but if no improvement occurred after three to five days, i.v. amantidine infusion was begun for at least three days.

The clinical response was dramatic in all patients. In one, reinstitution of oral amantidine sulfate and previous medications was followed by a relapse of akinetic crisis. He responded promptly to a second course of amantidine sulfate infusions. No side effects were observed, and we were able to discharge the patients after a short hospitalization. Only mild and reversible side effects of intravenous amantidine sulfate were usually reported, such as restlessness or insomnia; 1 of 53 patients had seizures.[5]

The dose should be determined by the clinical response in each case. In severe cases, up to three infusions can be given daily as continuous drips; therapy can be continued for as long as 10–12 days. When possible, oral amantidine sulfate 100 mg q.i.d. should be started.

1. Funfgold EW. Adamantyl aminosulphate—a drug with a new mechanism of action for the treatment of Parkinson's disease. *Med Klin.* 1970; 39:1703–6.
2. Schwab RS, England AC, Poskanzer DC et al. Amantadine in treatment of Parkinson's disease. *JAMA.* 1969; 208:1168–70.
3. Danielczyk W. Rehabilitation of akinetic crises. *Med Welt.* 1973; 24:1278–82.
4. Muschard F, Voller GW. Activity of amantadine sulphate as an infusion solution in the treatment of Parkinson's disease. *Med Welt.* 1973; 24:183–4.
5. Oppel F, Klaes H. Die amantadinsulfat infusion in der akutbehandlung des morbus Parkinson. *Kilnkarzt.* 1981; 10:559–65.

N. GADOTH, M.D.
H. SROKA, M.D.
G. GOLDHAMMER, M.D.
J. ALCALAY, M.D.
M. BECHAR, M.D.

Department of Neurology
Beilinson Medical Center
Sackler School of Medicine
Tel-Aviv University
Petah-Tiqva, Israel

Therapy Reviews

Allogeneic bone marrow transplantation in the treatment of hematologic diseases

GARY C. YEE AND TIMOTHY R. MCGUIRE

Abstract: The current use of allogeneic bone marrow transplantation in various hematologic diseases is reviewed.

Bone marrow transplantation (BMT) involves infusion of bone marrow from a suitable donor into a properly conditioned recipient. Most BMT is allogeneic, in which the donor is genetically dissimilar but shares some common tissue antigens with the recipient. Almost all patients undergoing allogeneic BMT must be "prepared" with high-dose cyclophosphamide to prevent graft rejection. Most patients with hematologic malignancy also receive total body irradiation to eradicate malignant cells located in areas inaccessible to the systemic circulation.

Bone marrow transplantation is the treatment of choice for severe aplastic anemia. In acute myelogenous leukemia, the best results are observed in young patients undergoing BMT in first remission. In acute lymphoblastic leukemia, BMT is usually reserved for patients in second or subsequent remission. Early results are promising in patients with chronic myelogenous leukemia who receive BMT before the accelerated phase or blast crisis of this disease. Allogeneic BMT offers an opportunity for cure in some patients with relapses of Hodgkin's disease or those with certain subtypes of non-Hodgkin's lymphoma. Other diseases for which BMT has been used include severe combined immune deficiency disease, Fanconi's anemia, and multiple myeloma.

Complications of BMT include graft failure or rejection, acute and chronic graft-versus-host disease, and infectious complications; late complications, such as restrictive and obstructive pulmonary disease, cataracts, sterility, and secondary malignancies, may also occur.

Bone marrow transplantation has become an important treatment for many hematologic diseases, but it will probably remain a treatment reserved for only a few highly specialized centers. If morbidity and mortality caused by transplant-related complications can be reduced, BMT may be offered to older patients and those without HLA-identical sibling donors.

Index terms: Combined therapy; Cyclophosphamide; Dosage; Hematologic diseases; Immunosuppressive agents; Radiation; Toxicity; Transplantation
Clin Pharm. 1985; 4:149–60

Bone marrow transplantation (BMT) is a process that involves infusion of marrow from a suitable donor into a properly conditioned recipient with serious disease. In the past 20 years, BMT has become an important treatment modality for a variety of malignant and nonmalignant diseases. Between 1939 and 1969, 203 patients had received BMT.[1] In the United States alone, there are now at least 35 active BMT units, involving over 1000 patients per year.[2] BMT has been extensively reviewed in the medical[3–5] but not the pharmacy literature. This review will summarize the current use of BMT in the treatment of aplastic anemia, acute and chronic leukemia, lymphoma, and certain other hematologic diseases, with an emphasis on the drugs used in BMT patients.

Selection of Donors

Three types of donors are used in bone marrow transplantation.[3] In autologous BMT, patients receive their own bone marrow that was procurred

GARY C. YEE, PHARM.D., is Associate in Medical Oncology, Division of Clinical Research, Fred Hutchinson Cancer Research Center, and Clinical Assistant Professor, Department of Pharmacy Practice, University of Washington School of Pharmacy, Seattle, WA. TIMOTHY R. MCGUIRE is a Pharm.D. candidate, Philadelphia College of Pharmacy and Science, Philadelphia, PA.

Address reprint requests to Dr. Yee at the Fred Hutchinson Cancer Research Center, 1124 Columbia Street, Seattle, WA 98104.

The assistance of Drs. H. Joachim Deeg, Anthony Shields, and Michael S. Kennedy is acknowledged.

Supported in part by grant CA 33252 awarded by the National Cancer Institute, Department of Health and Human Services.

This is **article 680-204-8506** in the **ASHP Continuing Education System.** See page 224 for learning objectives and test questions.

before intensive drug and radiation therapy. In syngeneic or isogeneic BMT, an identical monozygous twin serves as the donor. Most BMT is allogeneic, however, in which the donor is genetically dissimilar but shares some common tissue antigens. Immunologic compatibility is evaluated with studies of antigens determined by the major histocompatibility complex. In man, this complex is referred to as the HLA (human leukocyte antigen) complex.[6] Four major loci, located on the sixth chromosome, have been defined and are designated HLA-A, HLA-B, HLA-C, and HLA-D. HLA-D matching is performed with a mixed lymphocyte culture (MLC) response.

The most common donor for allogeneic BMT is an HLA-identical sibling. In patients with at least one sibling, about 40% have one who is HLA-identical.[3] For those patients with no HLA-identical sibling, siblings or relatives who are matched at some but not all loci can also serve as donors.[7] Occasionally, unrelated HLA-identical persons have served as donors,[8] but the chance of any one person being a match for a nonrelative is small.

This review will focus on allogeneic BMT between HLA-identical siblings. When appropriate, results with other types of donors will also be discussed.

Preparative Regimens for Bone Marrow Transplantation

Nearly all patients undergoing allogeneic BMT must be conditioned (or "prepared") before marrow infusion.[9] The purpose of the preparative regimen is to suppress the immune system of the recipient so that the graft is not rejected. In patients with malignant disease, another goal of the preparative regimen is to kill as many malignant cells as possible. Table 1 shows commonly used preparative regimens.

The standard drug included in most preparative regimens is cyclophosphamide, a drug with both immunosuppressive and cytotoxic effects. At the Fred Hutchinson Cancer Research Center in Seattle (hereafter referred to as the Seattle group), patients with aplastic anemia are given a total of four 50-mg/kg doses of cyclophosphamide on days −5 to −2, where day 0 is designated as the day of transplant.[3] In patients with hematologic malignancy, two 60-mg/kg doses of cyclophosphamide are given several days before total body irradiation begins.[3]

The side effects of high-dose cyclophosphamide can be severe.[3,10] Nausea and vomiting occur in all patients but can usually be controlled with standard antiemetic therapy. Alopecia begins by day 7 or 8 and progresses to total or almost total alopecia by day 21. About 25% of BMT patients have clinically evident hemorrhagic cystitis, but only about 1% of patients have life-threatening hemorrhagic cystitis. Specific treatment is usually unnecessary. It is important to maintain a brisk urine flow to minimize local contact of the bladder mucosa to irritating cyclophosphamide metabolites. Preliminary studies in Europe show that 2-mercaptoethane sulfonate (MESNA) can ameliorate cyclophosphamide-induced cystitis.[11,12]

Other rare but potentially serious side effects of high-dose cyclophosphamide therapy include cardiotoxicity[13] and syndrome of inappropriate antidiuretic hormone secretion.[14]

Because of the high incidence of leukemic relapse in some leukemia patients and graft rejection in

Table 1.
Preparative Regimens Used by Major Marrow Transplant Teams in the United States

Transplant Team	Regimen: Drug	Regimen: Total Body Irradiation
Aplastic Anemia		
Seattle[34,37,38]	Cyclophosphamide 50 mg/kg for four doses	None
UCLA[17]	Cyclophosphamide 50 mg/kg for four doses	300 rads as a single dose
Minnesota[36]	Cyclophosphamide 50 mg/kg for four doses	750 rads as a single dose[a]
Acute Leukemia[b]		
Seattle[20,39,51,53]	Cyclophosphamide 60 mg/kg for two doses	920–1000 rads as a single dose
Seattle[20–23]	Cyclophosphamide 60 mg/kg for two doses	200 rads for six or seven doses
	Cyclophosphamide 60 mg/kg for two doses	225 or 250 rads for seven doses
Johns Hopkins[44]	Cyclophosphamide 50 mg/kg for four doses Busulfan 4 mg/kg for four doses	None
Minnesota[52]	Cyclophosphamide 60 mg/kg for two doses	750 rads as a single dose
Memorial[54]	Cyclophosphamide 60 mg/kg for two doses	120 rads for 11 doses
City of Hope[41,55,56]	Cyclophosphamide 80–100 mg/kg as a single dose Cytarabine 5 mg/kg for two doses	1000 rads as a single dose
Chronic Myelogenous Leukemia		
Seattle[61,65] and UCLA[63]	Cyclophosphamide 60 mg/kg for two doses	1000 rads as a single dose
Seattle[61,65]	Cyclophosphamide 60 mg/kg for two doses	200 rads for six doses
Minnesota[62]	Cyclophosphamide 60 mg/kg for two doses	280 rads for three doses

[a] Total lymphoid irradiation, not total body irradiation.

[b] Selection of conditioning regimen may depend on type of acute leukemia (myelogenous versus lymphoblastic) and disease status (remission versus relapse).

aplastic anemia patients, other drugs, such as busulfan or cytarabine, are sometimes added to the basic cyclophosphamide regimen (Table 1).[9,15,16]

Most BMT patients also receive total body irradiation. In patients with malignant disease, the rationale is to eradicate malignant cells located in areas inaccessible to the systemic circulation. In some patients with aplastic anemia, low-dose total body irradiation is added to the standard cyclophosphamide regimen in an effort to decrease the risk of graft rejection.[17] However, as discussed later in the section on infection, the dose of total body irradiation appears to correlate with the risk of interstitial pneumonitis.[18,19] The standard total body irradiation regimen involves the administration of a 1000-rad midline tissue dose, which is more than twice the lethal dose of radiation for a normal person. Most centers give fractionated rather than single-dose irradiation to patients with malignant disease.[20–23] The rationale for this approach is an improved therapeutic ratio—to destroy more leukemic cells and marrow stem cells while sparing other normal tissues.[24]

The nonmarrow acute toxicities of total body irradiation are generally mild, consisting of low-grade fever, nausea, vomiting, diarrhea, and tender swelling of the parotid gland.[25] Hepatic venocclusive disease, defined as an obliteration of the small intrahepatic central venules, is the most severe complication of the preparative regimen.[26] The incidence of venocclusive disease is related to the intensity of the preparative regimen, with leukemic patients having a higher incidence (21%) than patients with aplastic anemia (5%).[27] Clinical signs of venocclusive disease include sudden weight gain, ascites, hepatomegaly, and increased serum bilirubin concentrations occurring within the first three weeks after transplant. Many patients with venocclusive disease develop renal failure and encephalopathy.

Most patients receiving cyclophosphamide and total body irradiation develop severe oral complications that are manifested as mucositis, ulceration, hemorrhage, infection, and xerostomia. These complications are most severe 7–14 days after transplantation, with gradual healing by three to four weeks. Oral pain associated with mucosal toxicity can be severe; many patients require continuous intravenous infusions of morphine. Since oral intake is compromised, parenteral nutrition is also required.

Technique of Bone Marrow Aspiration

Bone marrow from the donor is obtained by aspirations from the anterior and posterior iliac crests.[28] The procedure takes less than two hours and yields 200–1200 ml depending on the size of the donor. The marrow is transferred into tissue culture medium containing preservative-free heparin. The pooled marrow is then passed through a series of stainless-steel screens to break up aggregated particles, resulting essentially in a single-cell suspension. This last step is important to avoid potentially lethal marrow emboli. The marrow is then given to the recipient intravenously like a blood transfusion over several hours (Figure 1). After the infused cells enter the systemic circulation, they reseed and grow in the bone marrow cavity of the recipient. Although the donor experiences local soreness for a few days, the procedure is usually well tolerated, with no delayed complications resulting from the marrow aspiration.[29]

Clinical Results of Bone Marrow Transplantation

Aplastic Anemia. Aplastic anemia is a disease characterized by peripheral blood pancytopenia and marrow hypoplasia.[30] BMT is generally considered to be the treatment of choice for severe aplastic anemia. The prognosis for these patients is poor when treated with supportive care with or without androgen therapy; about 50% die within three to four months, and about 70% are dead by 12 months.[31] Antithymocyte globulin, given either alone[32] or in combination with androgens,[33] is currently the most effective immunosuppressive treatment for severe aplastic anemia. Although about 50% show improvement in hematopoiesis, most of these responses are partial, with complete resolution of anemia, granulocytopenia, and thrombocytopenia.

The opportunity for long-term survival after BMT is lower in patients who receive multiple transfusions than in those who are untransfused.[34] Initially, only about half of patients who received multiple transfusions became long-term survivors after BMT.[34,35] Several approaches have been used to reduce graft rejection in this high-risk group. Additional drugs,[15,34] low-dose total body irradiation,[17]

Figure 1. Scheme for allogeneic bone marrow transplantation in the treatment of hematologic malignancies. Most preparative regimens include cyclophosphamide and total body irradiation; patients with aplastic anemia are usually prepared with cyclophosphamide alone. (From *Cancer Treat Rep.* 1984; 68:145–161. Reproduced with permission.)

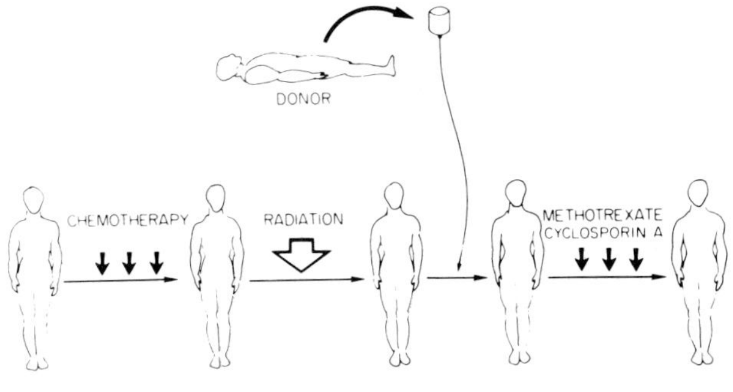

or total lymphoid irradiation[36] have been added to the standard cyclophosphamide regimen. Another approach is to give donor buffy-coat cells to the recipient.[37] These cells provide an additional source of donor cells, reducing the risk of graft rejection and improving long-term survival to about 70% (Table 2).

About 80% of patients who have not received any prior transfusions experience long-term survival after BMT (Table 2).[34,38] The improved results compared with transfused patients are related to a reduced incidence of graft rejection in untransfused patients.

Acute Leukemia. Initially, for ethical reasons, only patients with end-stage acute leukemia received BMT. Of the first 100 patients, 12 are alive in unmaintained remission 8–14 years after BMT.[39] It is important to note that these patients were not curable with any other treatment at the time they received BMT. Ninety percent were in relapse at the time of BMT and many had experienced multiple relapses. Based on these promising results, it was considered reasonable to offer BMT to patients at an earlier stage of their disease. Thus, in 1976, a series of studies were begun to treat selected patients who were in remission but considered to have a poor prognosis.

Response rates and median survival have steadily improved in patients with acute myelogenous leukemia treated with antineoplastic drug therapy. About 20% of these patients survive for more than five years and are possibly cured of their disease.[40] For patients with acute myelogenous leukemia in first remission (Figure 2) treated with allogeneic BMT, long-term survival is observed in 50–60% (Table 2).[20,41–43]

The standard conditioning regimen in patients with acute myelogenous leukemia is cyclophosphamide and total body irradiation (Table 1).[9] Fractionated irradiation appears to be superior to single-dose irradiation.[20] Other drugs have been added to cyclophosphamide in the preparative regimen, but they have not substantially decreased the leukemic relapse rate (20%).[9,16,39] One marrow-transplant team has reported that busulfan and cyclophosphamide (without total body irradiation) can also produce long-term survival.[44]

Since BMT-related complications are more common and more severe in older patients, survival is related to age.[45] In patients with acute myelogenous leukemia receiving transplants while in first remission, about 75% of patients less than 20 years old have experienced long-term survival. For those 20–29 years old, the long-term survival rate decreases to about 40%, and only about 25% of patients 30–50 years old become long-term survivors.

The proportion of long-term survivors after BMT decreases when patients with acute myelogenous leukemia undergo transplantation while in relapse or in second or subsequent remission (Table 2).[21,39,43,44,46] One study suggests that patients should receive transplants as soon as possible after the first relapse.[46] Thus, it appears that long-term survival is not superior in patients receiving transplants while in second remission compared with those receiving transplants while in first relapse.

Patients with acute lymphoblastic leukemia were initially not treated with BMT while in first remission because many of these patients, particularly children, experience prolonged disease-free survival after antineoplastic drug therapy and central nervous system prophylaxis.[47] Therefore, patients in second or subsequent remission (Figure 2) were selected for BMT because these remissions were usually short, and long-term survivors after leukemic relapse were extremely rare.[48,49] About 25% of patients prepared with cyclophosphamide and 1000 rads of total body irradiation become long-term survivors.[50–53] When fractionated total body irradiation is given instead of single-dose total body

Table 2.
Current Results with Allogeneic Bone Marrow Transplantation[a]

Disease	Status	% of Patients with Long-Term Survival
Aplastic anemia	Untransfused	80–85
	Transfused	65–70
Acute myelogenous leukemia	First remission[b]	40–70
	Second remission	20–25
	First relapse	25–30
	Multiple relapses	10–15
Acute lymphoblastic leukemia	First remission[c]	30–50
	Second or third remission	25–35
	Multiple relapses	10–15
Chronic myelogenous leukemia	Chronic phase	50–60
	Accelerated or blastic phase	15–30

[a] See text for references.
[b] Results dependent on patient age.
[c] Refers to high-risk or poor-prognosis patients.

Figure 2. Current application of allogeneic bone marrow transplantation in the treatment of acute myelogenous leukemia (AML) and acute lymphoblastic leukemia (ALL).

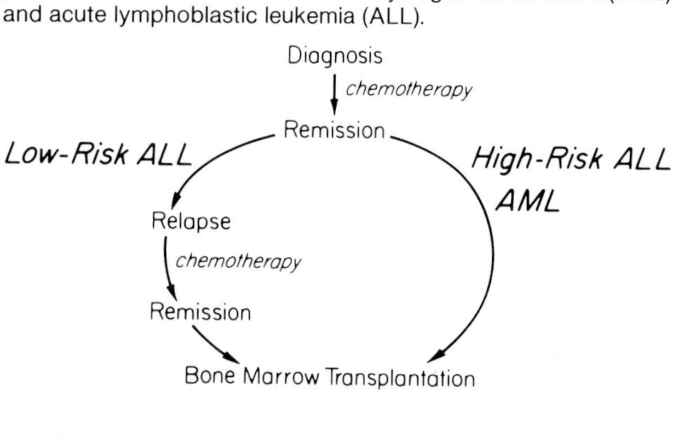

irradiation, results are slightly improved, with about one-third of patients experiencing long-term survival (Table 2).[23,54] Since leukemic relapse is a cause of death in about one-half of these patients, some transplant groups have added other antileukemic drugs to the standard cyclophosphamide regimen.[50,55,56] Preliminary studies suggest that regimens including high-dose cytarabine appear to reduce the relapse rate.[57] Another approach is to administer low-dose maintenance therapy after BMT to eradicate residual leukemic cells.[52]

In the past few years, clinical and laboratory data have been used to identify patients with acute lymphoblastic leukemia who are at high risk for leukemic relapse.[47] Although over 50% of low-risk or good-prognosis patients are cured of their disease with combination chemotherapy and central nervous system prophylaxis, long-term survival is uncommon for patients with high-risk or poor-prognosis acute lymphoblastic leukemia. Several BMT groups are currently exploring the benefit of performing BMT in these high-risk patients while in first remission (Figure 2).[50,56,58]

Chronic Myelogenous Leukemia. Chronic myelogenous leukemia is a myeloproliferative disease of middle-aged adults. This neoplastic disease probably arises from malignant transformation of a single hematopoietic stem cell and is associated with a cytogenetic marker, the Philadelphia chromosome.[59] Patients usually respond well to therapy with a single antineoplastic agent during the chronic phase, but all eventually enter blast crisis and die of their disease (median survival 36–44 months after initial diagnosis).[59]

Initially, BMT was offered to patients with chronic myelogenous leukemia in accelerated phase or blast crisis.[60] As with patients with acute leukemia transplanted while in relapse, only 15–30% become long-term survivors free of the Philadelphia chromosome.[60–63] Encouraged by these results, the Seattle group and other groups began to perform BMT on patients during the chronic phase of the disease. All patients are prepared with cyclophosphamide and total body irradiation and many also receive other antineoplastic drugs, such as dimethylbusulfan, daunorubicin, or cytarabine. Longer follow-up will be needed, but early results suggest that 50–60% of these patients can be cured with BMT (Table 2).[60,63–66] Most of the treatment failures result from transplant-related complications rather than leukemic relapse.

Lymphoma. Although most patients with Hodgkin's disease and some with non-Hodgkin's lymphoma are cured with combination chemotherapy, the prognosis for patients who relapse is poor. Early results, primarily with syngeneic BMT, show that some of these relapsed patients can be cured with BMT.[67,68] In addition, very few patients with some histologic subtypes of non-Hodgkin's lymphoma, including all nodular lymphomas and diffuse poorly differentiated lymphocytic lymphoma, are cured with chemotherapy. Allogeneic BMT appears to offer an opportunity for cure in about 10–20% of these patients.[67,68] Various preparative regimens have been used, but all have included cyclophosphamide and total body irradiation.

Other Diseases. Severe combined immune deficiency disease is characterized by impaired humoral and cellular immunity, resulting in death from infection, usually in the first year or two of life. BMT is beneficial in about 50% of these infants, producing partial or complete return of lymphocyte function and serum immunoglobulin levels.[69–71] Since these infants are unable to reject foreign tissue, preparation of the recipient is usually not required for successful engraftment.

Fanconi's anemia is an inherited disorder associated with progressive pancytopenia and congenital abnormalities. These patients are prepared for BMT with the identical regimen used in patients with aplastic anemia, but they experience more severe complications than patients with aplastic anemia.[72] The reasons for the increased sensitivity to the preparative regimen is unclear, but may be related to defective DNA repair. Some patients have been successfully treated with BMT and have experienced reversal of chromosomal abnormalities and restored hematopoiesis.

Other diseases that have been treated with BMT include multiple myeloma, osteopetrosis, Wiskott–Aldrich Syndrome, thalassemia, sickle cell anemia, and inherited storage diseases.[69–71]

Complications of Bone Marrow Transplantation

Graft Failure or Rejection. Initial engraftment usually occurs in the first three weeks after transplantation and is evidenced by rising peripheral blood counts and the presence of hematopoietic precursor cells in the marrow.[3] The presence of donor cells is confirmed with genetic markers.[73]

Graft rejection after initial engraftment is uncommon in patients with leukemia but not in patients with aplastic anemia. Patients with aplastic anemia who reject their graft have a high mortality rate, with only about 25% experiencing long-term survival.[74] Storb et al.[74] have identified five factors that are associated with graft rejection in patients with aplastic anemia: (1) previous blood transfusions, (2) a positive relative response in mixed leukocyte culture, (3) a low number of infused marrow cells, (4) marrow grafts from male donors, and (5) lack of infusion of viable donor buffy-coat cells in addition to the marrow for transfused patients. These data emphasize the importance of performing transplants early in patients with aplastic anemia, before the patient has been immunized against "minor" histocompatibility antigens of the donor. This is presumably caused by preceding blood transfusions and is expressed as a positive relative response in mixed leukocyte culture.

Graft-Versus-Host Disease. Graft-versus-host disease (GVHD) is caused by immunocompetent donor T lymphocytes reacting against antigens on host tissues. The onset of GVHD can occur early (acute) or late (chronic) in the posttransplant course.[75–77]

Acute Graft-Versus-Host Disease. Acute GVHD usually becomes clinically evident during the first four weeks of BMT.[78] The overall incidence of moderate to severe (grades II–IV) GVHD is 40–60% after allogeneic BMT[75–79] and increases with increasing age of the recipient.[80] The principal target organs for acute GVHD are the skin, liver, and gastrointestinal tract.[78] Acute GVHD is classified into four grades, depending on the degree of involvement of these three organs.[3] Grade I disease involves only the skin while grades II–IV involve the skin and either the liver or gastrointestinal tract, or both. The initial sign of acute GVHD is usually a generalized maculopapular rash. Acute GVHD usually progresses, involving the liver, gastrointestinal tract, or both. Intestinal GVHD is manifested as diarrhea but may progress to abdominal pain and ileus. Hepatic GVHD is usually asymptomatic, consisting of increases in serum bilirubin, serum glutamic–oxalacetic transaminase (SGOT), and alkaline phosphatase. Acute GVHD is associated with infection, which is frequently the cause of death. For example, the incidence of cytomegaloviral pneumonia is 13%, 16%, 23%, and 32% in patients with grade 0 or I, II, III, and IV GVHD, respectively.[18]

Treatment of established acute GVHD is unsatisfactory, therefore aggressive preventive treatment is usually given. Based on studies in dogs receiving marrow grafts, the standard regimen for prophylaxis of acute GVHD is "long" methotrexate, given for about 100 days after transplantation.[81] Similar studies in dogs also showed that severe GVHD usually developed when no immunosuppression is given after transplantation.[82] Although no randomized, controlled studies have been done in humans, one nonrandomized study in young patients who received transplants for a variety of diseases shows that the incidence and severity of acute GVHD is not different in BMT patients given methotrexate prophylaxis compared with those given no GVHD prophylaxis.[83] However, in that study, the incidence of grades II–IV acute GVHD in methotrexate-treated patients less than 20 years old (70%) was higher than that reported in several large studies (20–45%).[35,50,84]

Many transplant groups are exploring the efficacy of combinations of immunosuppressive agents. The use of combination therapy in animals is particularly promising; the combination of cyclosporine and "short" methotrexate (given on days 1, 3, 6, and 11 days posttransplant) is one of the most effective regimens ever tested by the Seattle group.[82] One randomized study showed that antithymocyte globulin, methotrexate, and prednisone were superior to methotrexate alone in reducing the incidence of GVHD.[80] However, Weiden and co-workers reported no difference in the incidence of GVHD between patients treated with antithymocyte globulin plus methotrexate and those treated with methotrexate alone.[85]

The dosages, schedule, routes of administration, and major side effects of immunosuppressive agents are listed in Table 3. The immunosuppressive doses of methotrexate and cyclophosphamide are generally lower than those used for anticancer therapy, but they can still cause mild to moderate toxicity. This is particularly true in BMT patients since they frequently develop hepatic or renal dysfunction, which may alter the pharmacokinetics of these agents. BMT patients are especially susceptible to the marrow-suppressive effects during the period before engraftment. We currently monitor methotrexate concentrations after both intravenous and intrathecal administration. If the 24-hour concentration is greater than 0.5 μM (or $>0.01\ \mu M$ at 48 hours), we consider these patients "high-risk" and usually recommend leucovorin rescue. Patients with renal dysfunction, severe hepatic dysfunction, or "third spaces" (e.g., ascites) are also at higher risk of developing toxicity.

Cyclosporine (formerly called cyclosporin A) is a cyclic endecapeptide with selective immunosuppressive activity. Cyclosporine is extensively metabolized and subject to biliary elimination. Patients with hepatic dysfunction[86] or diarrhea[87] may have altered cyclosporine pharmacokinetics. Monitoring of serum or whole-blood cyclosporine concentrations is necessary in most patients. The precise therapeutic range of cyclosporine is unknown, but we currently attempt to maintain trough serum concentrations (as measured by radioimmunoassay) between 100 and 250 ng/ml.

One major advantage of cyclosporine is its lack of bone marrow toxicity.[88] Cyclosporine-treated patients engraft more rapidly than methotrexate-treated patients, as measured by recovery of granulocytes and a reduced requirement for platelet transfusions, and they also are discharged earlier from the hospital.[89] Furthermore, after hospital discharge, cyclosporine-treated patients experience less nausea, vomiting, and mucositis than methotrexate-treated patients. Although nearly all patients develop reversible renal dysfunction while receiving the drug, the toxic effect of cyclosporine is difficult to assess because most patients also receive nephrotoxic antibiotics such as aminoglycosides, vancomycin, and amphotericin B during the period of severe granulocytopenia.[90]

Antithymocyte globulin is an important drug in the treatment or prevention of acute GVHD. The initial source of antithymocyte globulin was rabbits or goats,[91,92] but it is now obtained from

Table 3.
Immunosuppressive Agents Used for Prevention or Treatment of Acute Graft-Versus-Host Disease

Drug	Route	Daily Dose	Schedule	Major Toxicities
Methotrexate (as the sodium salt)	Intravenous	15 mg/sq m on day 1, then 10 mg/sq m thereafter	Once daily on days 1, 3, 6, and 11, then weekly to day 102	Marrow suppression and mucositis
Antithymocyte globulin	Intravenous	7 mg/kg	Once every other day for six doses	Fever and chills, rash, nausea, serum sickness, and marrow suppression
		15 mg/kg	Once every other day for seven doses	
Corticosteroids (prednisone, methylprednisolone)	Oral or Intravenous	1–2 mg/kg	Divided doses	Gastritis, cataracts, adrenal suppression, glucose intolerance, hypertension, and central nervous system effects
Cyclosporine	Intravenous	3–5 mg/kg	Every 12 hours until about day 14	Renal dysfunction, hepatotoxicity, tremors, nausea, hypertension, hirsutism, and hypomagnesemia
	Oral	7.5–12.5 mg/kg	Every 12 hours until day 180	
Cyclophosphamide	Intravenous	7.5 mg/kg	Once daily on days 1, 3, 5, 7, and 9, then weekly to day 100	Marrow suppression, hemorrhagic cystitis, nausea

horses.[80,84,92] Although the drug is as effective as steroids in the treatment of established GVHD,[92] its role in preventive therapy is unclear.[80,84] Most of the side effects are mild and are related to administration of a foreign protein.

Corticosteroids are effective immunosuppressive agents but they have many chronic toxicities. The most commonly used corticosteroids are prednisone or methylprednisolone, given at dosages of 1–2 mg/kg.[80,92] Although higher daily doses have been used, there is no evidence that they are more effective than standard dosages.[93,94]

Monoclonal antibodies are used in two ways to prevent or treat GVHD. First, in an attempt to eliminate donor T lymphocytes capable of initiating GVHD, donor marrow is pretreated with monoclonal antibodies before marrow infusion.[95,96] Second, monoclonal antibodies directed at T cells are given systemically to treat established acute GVHD refractory to conventional therapy.[97]

Chronic Graft-Versus-Host Disease. Chronic GVHD usually occurs after day 100.[98] It is more common in patients with aplastic anemia who receive donor buffy-coat cells, which may account for the more frequent incidence in patients with aplastic anemia (42%) compared with those with acute leukemia (20%).[99] As with acute GVHD, the risk of developing chronic GVHD increases with age. Most patients who develop chronic GVHD have a previous history of acute GVHD, although 20–30% develop the disease de novo. Chronic GVHD is classified as limited or extensive, depending on pathologic findings and the extent of systemic involvement.[98] Nearly all (90%) patients have extensive disease, with involvement of the skin, liver, eyes, mouth, esophagus, or other organs. If no functional impairment is present, patients with limited disease are not treated. Extensive chronic GVHD must be treated, because if left untreated, many patients will die of infections or become disabled from severe contractures.

Chronic GVHD is treated with corticosteroids, sometimes with antithymocyte globulin, cyclophosphamide, or azathioprine. Treatment is continued until signs and symptoms of the disease have resolved, usually over a period of several months. As chronic GVHD improves, the cytotoxic drug is discontinued, followed by gradual tapering of corticosteroid therapy. Since patients are usually leading fairly normal lives at this stage, it is important to minimize unnecessary side effects of therapy.

Acute and chronic GVHD may also have beneficial effects. Immunocompetent donor cells that are responsible for GVHD can also exert their cytotoxic effects on residual leukemic cells. The probability of leukemic relapse after day 150 is highest in patients with no GVHD, lowest in patients with acute GVHD who subsequently develop chronic GVHD, and intermediate in patients with either acute or chronic GVHD alone.[100,101] However, because of the detrimental effect of acute GVHD on mortality, survival is superior in patients with chronic GVHD alone, intermediate in patients with acute GVHD with or without chronic GVHD, and poorest in patients with neither acute nor chronic GVHD.

Infection. Infectious complications of the post-transplant course can be divided into three major phases: (1) an early granulocytopenic phase lasting 20–30 days after transplantation, (2) an intermediate phase between recovery of circulating granulocytes and day 100, and (3) a late phase after day 100.[102–104]

Early Phase. Nearly all BMT patients develop fever

shortly after transplantation, corresponding with a fall in circulating granulocytes.[105,106] Often fever is the only sign of infection; other signs or symptoms of infection may be absent because of suppressed inflammatory responses. Most patients have at least one positive blood culture during the period of granulocytopenia. At the Fred Hutchinson Cancer Research Center in Seattle, about one-half of the isolated organisms are aerobic gram-negative bacteria, primarily *Escherichia coli, Klebsiella* spp. and *Pseudomonas* spp.[102] Gram-positive organisms constitute most of the remaining isolated organisms, which may be related to the use of indwelling right atrial catheters (e.g., Hickman catheters),[107,108] or widespread use of broad-spectrum antibiotics.[109] The regimen currently used in Seattle for preventive or empiric treatment consists of tobramycin, ticarcillin, and vancomycin. In some clinical situations, third-generation cephalosporins are also added. If fever persists and the patient is colonized with fungi, amphotericin B is added for empiric antifungal coverage. Trimethoprim–sulfamethoxazole is given pretransplant and after granulocytes have recovered for prophylaxis against *Pneumocystis carinii* pneumonia.[102]

Laminar-airflow room isolation (with skin cleansing, topical and oral nonabsorbable antibiotics, and sterile food) and granulocyte transfusions are also used in some BMT centers to prevent infection. Both modalities have been shown to decrease infection significantly in BMT patients,[110,111] but some investigators feel that the added expense and potential complications outweigh these benefits.[103] The use of a protective environment may have additional benefits.[79,106] For reasons that are unclear, patients with aplastic anemia in laminar-airflow rooms have a reduced incidence or a delay in onset (or both) of acute GVHD.[79,106] This benefit is not observed in patients with acute leukemia,[105] which may be related to more severe mucositis and thus poorer compliance with oral antibiotic administration in these patients.

In many patients, mucocutaneous herpes-simplex infection begins during the period of mucositis and can persist for weeks.[102] Lesions begin to heal in most patients as circulating granulocytes increase but in some patients lesions can spread and cause pneumonia.[112] Treatment is symptomatic and involves antiviral drug therapy and meticulous oral care. Since acyclovir has been shown to hasten healing of lesions, decrease the period of viral shedding, and reduce the oral pain,[113,114] it is now used as prophylactic treatment in patients at high risk (high pretransplant titers of antibody against herpes-simplex virus) for developing infection.[115,116]

Intermediate Phase. From day 30 to day 100 after transplantation, interstitial pneumonia is a frequent complication in BMT patients, occurring in about 40% of allogeneic marrow recipients.[18,117] Patients with leukemia have a higher incidence (48%) than patients with aplastic anemia (27%), which is probably related to the additional toxicity of total body irradiation.[18,19] Increasing age and GVHD are also associated with a higher risk of interstitial pneumonia. The incidence of interstitial pneumonia is about 17% in syngeneic BMT patients, which shows the association with GVHD.[118] Interstitial pneumonia usually occurs in the first three months after transplantation, with the median day of onset being about day 50. The clinical syndrome is characterized by fever, cough, tachypnea, hypoxia, and interstitial pulmonary infiltrates on chest roentgenograms.

The most common cause of interstitial pneumonia in allogeneic BMT patients is cytomegalovirus, comprising about 45% of all cases.[18] In contrast, no cases of cytomegaloviral pneumonia occurred in syngeneic BMT patients.[118] *Pneumocystis carinii*, herpes simplex, varicella-zoster, or other viruses can be isolated in about 25% of cases. A causative organism cannot be isolated in the remaining 30% of cases. The mortality from all forms of interstitial pneumonia is high, ranging from about 60% for patients with idiopathic pneumonia to 90% for patients with cytomegaloviral pneumonia.

Results of treatment of interstitial pneumonia have been uniformly poor. Although acyclovir is of proven value in patients with mucocutaneous herpes-simplex lesions, it has not reduced the mortality rate of cytomegaloviral pneumonia, even when used in high doses.[119] Other antiviral agents, such as vidarabine,[120] interferon,[121,122] or both[123] are also ineffective. Most transplant centers are studying ways to prevent the disease. The most promising preventive treatment is cytomegalovirus immune or hyperimmune globulin.[124,125] In patients seronegative for cytomegalovirus, it is also important to minimize the use of granulocyte transfusions from seropositive donors.[126]

Late Phase. After day 100, infection is related to residual immunodeficiency, usually caused by chronic GVHD or the immunosuppressive therapy (i.e., steroids) of chronic GVHD.[127] Nearly half of all BMT patients eventually develop varicella-zoster infections.[128] About 80% of these patients have localized herpes zoster, with the remainder developing disseminated varicella infection. The median time of onset is about five months, with the majority of cases occurring within the first year. Because 12% of patients who develop varicella-zoster infections during the first four months die, they are treated aggressively with antiviral therapy.[129,130] Patients who develop infection after day 150 are treated at the first sign of visceral spread. Many late survivors also develop infections with gram-positive cocci, particularly *Streptococcus pneumoniae*.[131] Immunization with pneumococcal vaccine has been tried, but BMT patients are unable to develop an adequate immune response.[132] The approach used by the Seattle group is to give prophylactic trimethoprim–sulfamethoxazole to patients at high-risk for developing late infections.[102]

Late Complications. Both restrictive and obstructive pulmonary disease can occur as a late complication of BMT.[25,133,134] Restrictive disease is observed in about 20% of patients by one year, with gradual return of pulmonary function to pretransplant levels. Although the incidence of obstructive disease increases as follow-up time increases, most cases are mild and severe airflow obstruction is rare.

The use of total body irradiation or corticosteroids is associated with cataract formation.[25,133–135] Cataracts have been observed as early as one year after BMT, with 75% of the patients treated with single-dose total body irradiation involved by the sixth year. Fractionated total body irradiation appears to decrease the incidence of cataracts to about 20%.[135] Nearly all patients with cataracts are successfully treated with surgery.

The combination of high-dose cyclophosphamide and total body irradiation causes sterility in most postpubertal patients and delayed or absent onset of secondary sex characteristics in prepubertal patients.[133,134,136] The incidence of gonadal dysfunction may be reduced in patients prepared with fractionated total body irradiation as compared to those prepared with single-dose total body irradiation. Most patients receiving cyclophosphamide alone recover but some older women patients experience premature menopause. Similarly, some men prepared with cyclophosphamide alone have prolonged azoospermia. However, men or women prepared with cyclophosphamide alone have fathered or given birth to normal children.

Secondary malignancies have been reported in BMT patients prepared with cyclophosphamide and total body irradiation.[25,133,134,137] Of 1549 consecutive patients who have undergone transplantation at the Fred Hutchinson Cancer Research Center in Seattle, 20 patients have developed secondary malignancies after BMT.[137] Six patients had recurrence of leukemia in cells of donor origin, eight patients developed lymphoproliferative disorders, and six patients developed solid tumors. In the Seattle series, only one of the 257 patients with aplastic anemia prepared without total body irradiation developed a secondary malignancy (acute lymphoblastic leukemia). Nine additional cases have also been reported from other BMT centers.[137]

Conclusion

In the past 20 years, the status of allogeneic BMT has changed from experimental therapy to an important treatment modality for many hematologic diseases. Although BMT offers the hope for cure for many patients, it will probably remain a treatment reserved only for a select number of highly specialized centers. If morbidity and mortality caused by transplant-related complications can be reduced, BMT may be offered to more patients, such as patients older than 45–50 years of age or those without HLA-identical sibling donors.

References

1. Bortin MM. A compendium of reported human bone marrow transplants. *Transplantation.* 1970; 9:571–87.
2. Report from the International Bone Marrow Transplant Registry (IBMTR), 1983. *Exp Hematol.* 1984; 12:199–204.
3. Thomas ED, Storb R, Clift RA et al. Bone-marrow transplantation. *N Engl J Med.* 1975; 292:832–43, 895–902.
4. O'Reilly RJ. Allogeneic bone marrow transplantation: current status and future directions. *Blood.* 1983; 62:941–64.
5. Thomas ED. Marrow transplantation for malignant diseases. *J Clin Oncol.* 1983; 1:517–31.
6. van Rood JJ, deJongh B, Claas FHJ et al. New facts on HLA genetics: are they relevant in bone marrow transplantation. *Semin Hematol.* 1984; 21:65–80.
7. Clift RA, Hansen JA, Thomas ED et al. Marrow transplantation from donors other than HLA identical siblings. *Transplantation.* 1979; 28:235–42.
8. Hansen JA, Clift RA, Thomas ED et al. Transplantation of marrow from an unrelated donor to a patient with acute leukemia. *N Engl J Med.* 1980; 303:565–7.
9. van Bekkum DW. Conditioning regimens for marrow grafting. *Semin Hematol.* 1984; 21:81–90.
10. Buckner CD, Rudolph RH, Fefer A et al. High-dose cyclophosphamide therapy for malignant disease. *Cancer.* 1972; 29:357–65.
11. Berrigan MJ, Marinello AJ, Pavelic Z et al. Protective role of thiols in cyclophosphamide induced urotoxicity and depression of hepatic drug metabolism. *Cancer Res.* 1982; 42:3688–93.
12. Scheef W, Klein HO, Burkert H et al. Controlled clinical studies with an antidote against the urotoxicity of oxazaphosphorines: preliminary results. *Cancer Treat Rep.* 1979; 63:501–5.
13. Gottdiener JS, Appelbaum FR, Ferrans VJ et al. Cardiotoxicity associated with high dose cyclophosphamide therapy. *Arch Intern Med.* 1981; 141:758–63.
14. Defronzo RA, Braine H, Colvin M et al. Water intoxication in man after cyclophosphamide therapy. *Ann Intern Med.* 1973; 78:861–9.
15. Storb R, Thomas ED, Weiden PL et al. Aplastic anemia treated by allogeneic bone marrow transplantation: a report on 49 new cases from Seattle. *Blood.* 1976; 48:817–41.
16. Thomas ED, Buckner CD, Fefer A et al. Efforts to prevent recurrence of leukemia in marrow graft recipients. *Transplant Proc.* 1978; 10:163–5.
17. Gale RP, Ho W, Feig S et al. Prevention of graft rejection following bone marrow transplantation. *Blood.* 1981; 57: 9–12.
18. Meyers JD, Flournoy N, Thomas ED. Nonbacterial pneumonia after allogeneic marrow transplantation: a review of ten years' experience. *Rev Infect Dis.* 1982; 4:1119–32.
19. Keane TJ, Van Dyk J, Rider WD. Idiopathic interstitial pneumonia following bone marrow transplantation: the relationship with total body irradiation. *Int J Radiat Oncol Biol Phys.* 1981; 7:1365–9.
20. Thomas ED, Clift RA, Hersman J et al. Marrow transplantation for acute nonlymphoblastic leukemia in first remission using fractionated or single dose irradiation. *Int J Radiat Oncol Biol Phys.* 1982; 8:817–21.
21. Buckner CD, Clift RA, Thomas ED et al. Allogeneic marrow transplantation for acute non-lymphoblastic leukemia in relapse using fractionated total body irradiation. *Leuk Res.* 1982; 6:389–94.
22. Clift RA, Buckner CD, Thomas ED et al. Allogeneic marrow transplantation using fractionated total body irradiation in

patients with acute lymphoblastic leukemia in relapse. *Leuk Res.* 1982; 6:401–7.
23. Clift RA, Buckner CD, Thomas ED et al. Allogeneic marrow transplantation for acute lymphoblastic leukemia in remission using fractionated total body irradiation. *Leuk Res.* 1982; 6:409–12.
24. Peters LJ, Withers HR, Cundiff JH et al. Radiobiological considerations in the use of total-body irradiation for bone-marrow transplantation. *Radiology.* 1979; 131:243–7.
25. Deeg HJ. Acute and delayed toxicities of total body irradiation. *Int J Radiat Oncol Biol Phys.* 1983; 9:1933–9.
26. Shulman HM, McDonald GB, Matthews D et al. An analysis of hepatic venocclusive disease and centrilobular hepatic degeneration following bone marrow transplantation. *Gastroenterology.* 1980; 79:1178–91.
27. McDonald GB, Sharma P, Matthews DE et al. Venocclusive disease of the liver after bone marrow transplantation: diagnosis, incidence, and predisposing factors. *Hepatology.* 1984; 4:116–22.
28. Thomas ED, Storb R. Technique for human marrow grafting. *Blood.* 1970; 36:507–15.
29. Bortin MM, Buckner CD. Major complications of marrow harvesting for transplantation. *Exp Hematol.* 1983; 11: 916–21.
30. Camitta BM, Storb R, Thomas ED. Aplastic anemia. *N Engl J Med.* 1982; 306:645–52.
31. Camitta BM, Thomas ED, Nathan DG et al. A prospective study of androgens and bone marrow transplantation for treatment of severe aplastic anemia. *Blood.* 1979; 53:504–14.
32. Champlin R, Ho W, Gale RP. Antithymocyte globulin treatment in patients with aplastic anemia. *N Engl J Med.* 1983; 308:113–8.
33. Doney K, Dahlberg SJ, Monroe D et al. Therapy of severe aplastic anemia with anti-human thymocyte globulin and androgens: the effect of HLA-haploidentical marrow infusion. *Blood.* 1984; 63:842–8.
34. Storb R, Thomas ED, Buckner CD et al. Marrow transplantation for aplastic anemia. *Semin Hematol.* 1984; 21:27–35.
35. Bortin MM, Gale RP, Rimm AA. Allogeneic bone marrow transplantation for 144 patients with severe aplastic anemia. *JAMA.* 1981; 245:1132–9.
36. Ramsay NKC, Kim T, Nesbit ME et al. Total lymphoid irradiation and cyclophosphamide as preparation for bone marrow transplantation in severe aplastic anemia. *Blood.* 1980; 55:344–6.
37. Storb R, Doney KC, Thomas ED et al. Marrow transplantation with or without donor buffy coat cells for 65 transfused aplastic anemia patients. *Blood.* 1982; 59:236–46.
38. Storb R, Thomas ED, Buckner CD et al. Marrow transplantation in thirty "untransfused" patients with severe aplastic anemia. *Ann Intern Med.* 1980; 92:30–6.
39. Thomas ED, Buckner CD, Banaji M et al. One hundred patients with acute leukemia treated by chemotherapy, total body irradiation and allogeneic marrow transplantation. *Blood.* 1977; 49:511–33.
40. Keating MJ, McCredie KB, Bodey GP et al. Improved prospects for long-term survival in adults with acute myelogenous leukemia. *JAMA.* 1982; 248:2481–6.
41. Forman SJ, Spruce WE, Farbstein MJ et al. Bone marrow ablation followed by allogeneic marrow grafting during first complete remission of acute nonlymphocytic leukemia. *Blood.* 1983; 61:439–41.
42. Thomas ED, Buckner CD, Clift RA et al. Marrow transplantation for acute nonlymphoblastic leukemia in first remission. *N Engl J Med.* 1979; 301:597–9.
43. Zwaan FE, Jansen J. Bone marrow transplantation in acute nonlymphoblastic leukemia. *Semin Hematol.* 1984; 21:36–42.
44. Santos GW, Tutschka PJ, Brookmeyer R et al. Marrow transplantation for acute nonlymphocytic leukemia after treatment with busulfan and cyclophosphamide. *N Engl J Med.* 1983; 309:1347–53.
45. Thomas ED, Clift RA, Buckner CD. Marrow transplantation for patients with acute nonlymphoblastic leukemia who achieve a first remission. *Cancer Treat Rep.* 1982; 66: 1463–6.
46. Appelbaum FR, Clift RA, Buckner CD et al. Allogeneic marrow transplantation for acute nonlymphoblastic leukemia after first relapse. *Blood.* 1983; 61:949–53.
47. Mauer AM. Therapy of acute lymphoblastic leukemia in childhood. *Blood.* 1980; 56:1–10.
48. Rivera G, Aur RJ, Dahl GV et al. Combined VM-16 and cytosine arabinoside in treatment of refractory childhood lymphocytic leukemia. *Cancer.* 1980; 45:1284–8.
49. Reaman GH, Ladisch S, Echelberger C et al. Improved treatment results in the management of single and multiple relapses of acute lymphoblastic leukemia. *Cancer.* 1980; 45:3090–4.
50. Buckner CD, Clift RA. Marrow transplantation for acute lymphoblastic leukemia. *Semin Hematol.* 1984; 21:43–47.
51. Thomas ED, Sanders JE, Flournoy N et al. Marrow transplantation for patients with acute lymphoblastic leukemia: a long-term follow-up. *Blood.* 1983; 62:1139–41.
52. Woods WG, Nesbit ME, Ramsay NK et al. Intensive therapy followed by bone marrow transplantation for patients with acute lymphocytic leukemia in second or subsequent remission: determination of prognostic factors. *Blood.* 1983; 61:1182–9.
53. Johnson LF, Thomas ED, Clark BS et al. A comparison of marrow transplantation with chemotherapy for children with acute lymphoblastic leukemia in second or subsequent remission. *N Engl J Med.* 1981; 305:846–51.
54. Dinsmore R, Kirkpatrick D, Flomenberg N et al. Allogeneic bone marrow transplantation for patients with acute lymphoblastic leukemia. *Blood.* 1983; 62:381–8.
55. Blume KG, Beutler E, Bross KJ et al. Bone marrow ablation and allogeneic marrow transplantation in acute leukemia. *N Engl J Med.* 1980; 302:1041–6.
56. Scott EP, Forman SJ, Spruce WE et al. Bone marrow ablation followed by allogeneic bone marrow transplantation for patients with high risk acute lymphoblastic leukemia during complete remission. *Transplant Proc.* 1983; 15:1395–6.
57. Coccia PF, Strandjord SE, Gordon EM et al. High-dose cytosine arabinoside and fractionated total body irradiation as preparation for bone marrow transplantation for childhood acute leukemia in remission—a preliminary report. *Proc Am Soc Clin Oncol.* 1983; 2:175. Abstract.
58. Gale RP, Kersey JH, Bortin MM et al. Bone marrow transplantation for acute lymphoblastic leukaemia. *Lancet.* 1983; 2:663–7.
59. Koeffler HP, Golde DW. Chronic myelogenous leukemia—new concepts. *N Engl J Med.* 1981; 304:1201–9, 1269–74.
60. Speck B, Gratwohl A, Osterwalder B et al. Bone marrow transplantation for chronic myeloid leukemia. *Semin Hematol.* 1984; 21:48–52.
61. Doney KC, Buckner CD, Thomas ED et al. Allogeneic bone marrow transplantation for chronic granulocytic leukemia. *Exp Hematol.* 1981; 9:966–71.
62. McGlave PB, Arthur DC, Kim TH et al. Successful allogeneic bone marrow transplantation for patients in the accelerated phase of chronic granulocytic leukaemia. *Lancet.* 1982; 2: 625–7.
63. Champlin R, Ho W, Arenson E et al. Allogeneic bone marrow transplantation for chronic myelogenous leukemia in chronic or accelerated phase. *Blood.* 1982; 60:1038–41.
64. Goldman JM, Baughan AS, McCarthy DM. Marrow transplantation for patients in the chronic phase of chronic granulocytic leukaemia. *Lancet.* 1982; 2:623–5.
65. Clift RA, Buckner CD, Thomas ED et al. Treatment of chronic granulocytic leukaemia in chronic phase by allogeneic marrow transplantation. *Lancet.* 1982; 2:621–2.
66. Speck B, Bortin MM, Champlin R et al. Allogeneic bone marrow transplantation for chronic myelogenous leukaemia. *Lancet.* 1984; 1:665–8.

67. Appelbaum FR, Thomas ED. Review of the use of marrow transplantation in the treatment of non-Hodgkin's lymphoma. *J Clin Oncol.* 1983; 1:440–7.
68. O'Leary M, Ramsay NK, Nesbit ME et al. Bone marrow transplantation for non-Hodgkin's lymphoma in children and young adults. *Am J Med.* 1983; 74:497–501.
69. Kadota RP. Bone marrow transplantation for diseases of childhood. *Mayo Clin Proc.* 1984; 59:171–84.
70. Rappeport JM, Smith BR, Parkman R et al. Application of bone marrow transplantation in genetic diseases. *Clin Hematol.* 1983; 12:755–73.
71. O'Reilly RJ, Brochstein J, Dinsmore R et al. Marrow transplantation for congenital disorders. *Semin Hematol.* 1984; 21:188–221.
72. Deeg HJ, Storb R, Thomas ED et al. Fanconi's anemia treated by allogeneic marrow transplantation. *Blood.* 1983; 61: 954–9.
73. Sparkes RS. Cytogenetic analysis in human bone marrow transplantation. *Cancer Genet Cytogenet.* 1981; 4:345–52.
74. Storb R, Prentice RL, Thomas ED et al. Factors associated with graft rejection after HLA identical marrow transplantation for aplastic anemia. *Br J Haematol.* 1983; 55:573–85.
75. Neudorf S, Filipovich A, Ramsay N et al. Prevention and treatment of acute graft-versus-host disease. *Semin Hematol.* 1984; 21:91–100.
76. Storb R. Pathophysiology and prevention of graft-versus-host disease. In: Advances in immunobiology: blood cell antigens and bone marrow transplantation. New York: Alan R. Liss; 1984:337–66.
77. Sullivan KM, Parkman R. The pathophysiology and treatment of graft-versus-host disease. *Clin Hematol.* 1983; 12: 775–89.
78. Glucksberg H, Storb R, Fefer A et al. Clinical manifestations of graft versus host disease in human recipients of marrow from HLA matched sibling donors. *Transplantation.* 1974; 18:295–303.
79. Storb R, Prentice RL, Buckner CD et al. Graft-versus-host disease and survival in patients with aplastic anemia treated by marrow grafts from HLA identical siblings. *N Engl J Med.* 1983; 308:302–7.
80. Ramsay NK, Kersey JH, Robison LL et al. A randomized study of the prevention of acute graft versus host disease. *N Engl J Med.* 1982; 306:392–7.
81. Storb R, Epstein B, Graham TC et al. Methotrexate regimens for control of graft versus host disease in dogs with allogeneic marrow grafts. *Transplantation.* 1970; 9:240–6.
82. Deeg HJ, Storb R. Experimental marrow transplantation. In: White DJG, ed. Cyclosporin A: proceedings of an international conference on cyclosporin A. New York: Elsevier; 1982:121–34.
83. Lazarus HM, Coccia PF, Herzig RH et al. Incidence of acute graft-versus-host disease with and without methotrexate prophylaxis in allogeneic bone marrow transplant patients. *Blood.* 1984; 64:215–20.
84. Bortin MM, Gale RP, Day HEM et al. Bone marrow transplantation for acute myelogenous leukemia: factors associated with early mortality. *JAMA.* 1983; 249:1166–75.
85. Weiden PL, Doney D, Storb R et al. Antihuman thymocyte globulin for prophylaxis of graft versus host disease. *Transplantation.* 1979; 27:227–30.
86. Yee GC, Kennedy MS, Storb R et al. Effect of hepatic dysfunction on cyclosporine pharmacokinetics in marrow transplant patients. *Blood.* In press.
87. Atkinson K, Biggs JC, Britton K et al. Oral administration of cyclosporin A for recipients of allogeneic marrow transplants: implications of clinical gut dysfunction. *Br J Haematol.* 1984; 56:223–31.
88. Hellmann A, Goldman JM. Effects of cyclosporin A on human granulopoiesis in vitro. *Transplantation.* 1980; 30: 386–7.
89. Deeg HJ, Storb R, Thomas ED et al. Marrow transplantation for acute nonlymphoblastic leukemia in first remission: preliminary results of a randomized trial comparing cyclosporine and methotrexate for the prophylaxis of graft-versus-host disease. *Transplant Proc.* 1983; 15:1385–8.
90. Kennedy MS, Deeg HJ, Siegel M et al. Acute renal toxicity with combined use of amphotericin B and cyclosporine after marrow transplantation. *Transplantation.* 1983; 35:211–5.
91. Storb R, Gluckman E, Thomas ED et al. Treatment of established human graft versus host disease by antithymocyte globulin. *Blood.* 1974; 44:57–75.
92. Doney KC, Weiden PL, Storb R et al. Treatment of graft-versus-host disease in human allogeneic marrow graft recipients: a randomized trial comparing antithymocyte globulin and corticosteroids. *Am J Hematol.* 1981; 11:1–8.
93. Bacigalupo A, Lint MT, Frassoni F et al. High dose bolus methylprednisolone for the treatment of acute graft versus host disease. *Blut.* 1983; 46:125–32.
94. Kanojia MD, Anagnostou AA, Zander AR et al. High-dose methylprednisolone treatment for acute graft-versus-host disease after bone marrow transplantation in adults. *Transplantation.* 1984; 37:246–9.
95. Prentice HG, Blacklock HA, Janossy G et al. Depletion of T-lymphocytes in donor marrow prevents significant graft-versus-host disease in matched allogeneic leukemic marrow transplant recipients. *Lancet.* 1984; 1:472–5.
96. Filipovich AH, Vallera DA, Youle RJ et al. Ex-vivo treatment of donor bone marrow with anti-T-cell immunotoxins for prevention of graft-versus-host disease. *Lancet.* 1984; 1: 469–71.
97. Martin PJ, Hansen JA, Remlinger K et al. Murine monoclonal anti-human T cell antibodies for the prevention and treatment of graft-versus-host disease. In: Recent advances in bone marrow transplantation. New York: Alan R. Liss; 1984:313–29.
98. Sullivan KM, Shulman HM, Storb R et al. Chronic graft versus host disease in 52 patients: adverse natural course and successful treatment with combination immunosuppression. *Blood.* 1981; 57:267–76.
99. Storb R, Prentice RL, Sullivan K et al. Predictive factors in chronic graft versus host disease in patients with aplastic anemia treated by marrow transplantation from HLA identical siblings. *Ann Intern Med.* 1983; 98:461–6.
100. Weiden PL, Flournoy N, Thomas ED et al. Antileukemic effect of graft versus host disease in human recipients of allogeneic marrow grafts. *N Engl J Med.* 1979; 300:1068–73.
101. Weiden PL, Sullivan KM, Flournoy N et al. Antileukemic effect of chronic graft versus host disease. *N Engl J Med.* 1981; 304:1529–33.
102. Meyers JD, Thomas ED. Infection complicating bone marrow transplantation. In: Young LS, Rubin RH, eds. Clinical approach to infection in the immunocompromised host. New York: Plenum; 1982:507–51.
103. Winston DJ, Ho WG, Champlin RE et al. Infectious complications of bone marrow transplantation. *Exp Hematol.* 1984; 12:205–15.
104. van der Meer JWM, Guiot HFL, van den Broek PJ et al. Infections in bone marrow transplant recipients. *Semin Hematol.* 1984; 21:123–40.
105. Buckner CD, Clift RA, Thomas ED et al. Early infectious complications in allogeneic marrow transplant recipients with acute leukemia: effects of prophylactic measures. *Infection.* 1983; 11:243–50.
106. Navari RM, Buckner CD, Clift RA et al. Prophylaxis of infection in patients with aplastic anemia receiving allogeneic marrow transplants. *Am J Med.* 1984; 76:564–72.
107. Hickman RO, Buckner CD, Clift RA et al. A modified right atrial catheter for access to the venous system in marrow transplant recipients. *Surg Gynecol Obstet.* 1979; 148:871–5.
108. Sanders JE, Hickman RO, Aker S et al. Experience with double lumen right atrial catheters. *J Parenter Enter Nutr.* 1982; 6:95–9.
109. Wade JC, Schimpff SC, Newman KA et al. *Staphylococcus epidermidis:* an increasing cause of infection in patients with

granulocytopenia. *Ann Intern Med.* 1982; 97:503–8.
110. Buckner CD, Clift RA, Sanders JE et al. Protective environment for marrow transplant recipients: a prospective study. *Ann Intern Med.* 1978; 89:893–901.
111. Clift RA, Sanders JE, Thomas ED et al. Granulocyte transfusions for the prevention of infection in patients receiving bone-marrow transplants. *N Engl J Med.* 1978; 298:1052–7.
112. Ramsey PG, Fife KH, Hackman RC et al. Herpes simplex virus pneumonia. *Ann Intern Med.* 1982; 97:813–20.
113. Mitchell CD, Bean B, Gentry SR et al. Acyclovir therapy for mucocutaneous herpes simplex infections in immunocompromised patients. *Lancet.* 1981; 1:1389–92.
114. Wade JC, Newton B, McLaren C et al. Intravenous acyclovir to treat mucocutaneous herpes simplex virus infection after marrow transplantation. *Ann Intern Med.* 1982; 96:265–9.
115. Rein S, Burns WH, Laskin OL et al. Acyclovir prophylaxis of herpes-simplex-virus infections. *N Engl J Med.* 1981; 305:63–7.
116. Wade JC, Newton B, Flournoy N et al. Oral acyclovir for prevention of herpes simplex virus reactivation after marrow transplantation. *Ann Intern Med.* 1984; 100:823–8.
117. Bortin MM, Kay HE, Gale RP et al. Factors associated with interstitial pneumonitis after bone marrow transplantation for acute leukaemia. *Lancet.* 1982; 1:437–9.
118. Appelbaum FR, Meyers JD, Fefer A et al. Nonbacterial nonfungal pneumonia following marrow transplantation in 100 identical twins. *Transplantation.* 1982; 33:265–8.
119. Wade JC, Hintz M, McGuffin RW et al. Treatment of cytomegalovirus pneumonia with high dose acyclovir. *Am J Med.* 1982; 73 (Suppl 1):249–56.
120. Kraemer KG, Neiman PE, Reeves WC et al. Prophylactic adenine arabinoside following marrow transplantation. *Transplant Proc.* 1978; 10:37–40.
121. Meyers JD, Day LM, Lum LG et al. Recombinant leukocyte A interferon for the treatment of serious viral infections after marrow transplant: a phase I study. *J Infect Dis.* 1983; 148:551–5.
122. Meyers JD, McGuffin RW, Neiman PE et al. Toxicity and efficacy of human leukocyte interferon for treatment of cytomegalovirus pneumonia after marrow transplantation. *J Infect Dis.* 1980; 5:555–62.
123. Meyers JD, McGuffin RW, Bryson YJ et al. Treatment of cytomegalovirus pneumonia after marrow transplant with combined vidarabine and human leukocyte interferon. *J Infect Dis.* 1982; 146:80–4.
124. Meyers JD, Leszczynski J, Zaia J et al. Prevention of cytomegalovirus infection by cytomegalovirus immune globulin after marrow transplantation. *Ann Intern Med.* 1983; 98: 442–6.
125. O'Reilly RJ, Reich L, Gold J et al. A randomized trial of intravenous hyperimmune globulin for the prevention of cytomegalovirus (CMV) infections following marrow transplantation: preliminary results. *Transplant Proc.* 1983; 15:1405–11.
126. Hersman J, Meyers JD, Thomas ED, et al. The effect of granulocyte transfusions on the incidence of cytomegalovirus infection after allogeneic marrow transplantation. *Ann Intern Med.* 1982; 96:149–52.
127. Atkinson K. Storb R, Prentice RL et al. Analysis of late infections in 89 long-term survivors of bone marrow transplantation. *Blood.* 1979; 53:720–31.
128. Atkinson K, Meyers JD, Storb R et al. Varicella zoster virus infection after marrow transplantation for aplastic anemia or leukemia. *Transplantation.* 1980; 29:47–50.
129. Balfour HH, Bean B, Laskin OL et al. Acyclovir halts progression of herpes zoster in immunocompromised patients. *N Engl J Med.* 1983; 308:1448–53.
130. Whitley RJ, Soong SJ, Dolin R et al. Early vidarabine therapy to control the complications of herpes zoster in immunosuppressed patients. *N Engl J Med.* 1982; 307:971–5.
131. Winston DJ, Schiffman G, Wang DC et al. Pneumococcal infections after human bone-marrow transplantation. *Ann Intern Med.* 1979; 91:835–41.
132. Winston DJ, Winston GH, Schiffman G et al. Pneumococcal vaccination of recipients of bone marrow transplants. *Arch Intern Med.* 1983; 143:1735–7.
133. Sullivan KM, Deeg JD, Sanders JE et al. Late complications after marrow transplant. *Semin Hematol.* 1984; 21:53–63.
134. Deeg HJ, Storb R. Thomas ED. Bone marrow transplantation: a review of delayed complications. *Br J Haematol.* 1984; 57: 185–208.
135. Deeg HJ, Flournoy N, Sullivan KM et al. Cataracts after total body irradiation and marrow transplantation: a sparing effect of dose fractionation. *Int J Radiat Oncol Biol Phys.* In press.
136. Sanders JE, Buckner CD, Leonard JM et al. Late effects of gonadal function of cyclophosphamide, TBI, and marrow transplantation. *Transplantation.* 1983; 36:252–5.
137. Deeg HJ, Sanders J, Martin P et al. Secondary malignancies after marrow transplantation. *Exp Hematol.* In press.

Management of maldigestion associated with pancreatic insufficiency

RICHARD S. PERRY AND JEFF GALLAGHER

Abstract: The etiology, pathophysiology, clinical presentation, dietary management, and drug therapy of maldigestion associated with pancreatic insufficiency are reviewed.

Maldigestion can occur in a number of conditions that lead to pancreatic insufficiency but is seen most frequently in patients with alcohol-related chronic pancreatitis or cystic fibrosis. Destruction of pancreatic tissue and obstruction of the ducts that lead into the small intestine prevent pancreatic secretions from reaching the small intestine and result in weight loss, anorexia, abdominal distention, and changes in the appearance and frequency of stools.

The goal of dietary intervention in patients with maldigestion is to provide sufficient calories and protein to maintain weight while limiting fat intake to an amount that the patient can tolerate. Medium-chain triglycerides can be substituted for dietary fat in patients whose symptoms continue despite dietary fat restriction. Drug therapy involves supplementing deficient pancreatic enzymes with pancreatin or pancrelipase. Regimens must be individualized for each patient because of problems with gastric inactivation of orally administered enzymes, lack of standardization of commercially available preparations, and large interpatient variation in response. In selecting an enzyme supplement preparation, the amount of available enzyme activity, dosage form, number of dosage units needed per dose, dosage schedule, and product cost must be considered. When enzyme supplementation alone does not adequately control the symptoms of maldigestion, a histamine H_2-receptor antagonist or antacids may be added to the therapeutic regimen.

Although complete resolution of the symptoms of maldigestion is difficult to achieve, a regimen of dietary modification and pancreatic-enzyme replacement can improve patients' quality of life.

Index terms: Gastrointestinal drugs; Maldigestion; Nutrition; Pancreatic insufficiency
Clin Pharm. 1985; 4:161–9

Pancreatic insufficiency results in an inadequate amount of pancreatic enzymes in the proximal duodenum, where they are needed for adequate digestion of food substrates.[1] The resulting malabsorption of substrates causes loss of fat, protein, and carbohydrate in the stool and associated symptoms of weight loss, diarrhea, and steatorrhea. Pancreatic insufficiency has three general etiologies: (1) a reduction in the quantity of enzymes released from the pancreas, (2) specific isolated enzyme deficiencies in which only one enzyme is deficient, and (3) loss of enzyme-activation capabilities throughout the small intestine.[1,2] Specific disease states associated with each of these etiologies are listed in Table 1.

The treatment of maldigestion resulting from pancreatic insufficiency includes dietary management and pancreatic-enzyme supplementation. Unfortunately, problems are often encountered in managing patients with maldigestion because of poor patient compliance, alterations in patients' dietary habits, or changes in disease activity. These problems may be compounded by factors inherent in the commercially available pancreatic-enzyme-replacement products. First, the enzyme content of pancreatic-enzyme products and the methods of labeling these products vary greatly among manufacturers.[3-6] Other difficulties arise because in vitro assay techniques for pancreatic-enzyme products also vary among manufacturers and do not correlate consistently with in vivo activity or patient re-

Table 1.
Etiologies of Pancreatic Insufficiency

Reduced Enzyme Secretion
Chronic pancreatitis
Cystic fibrosis
Pancreatic cancer
Pancreatectomy
Specific Enzyme Deficiency
Amylase deficiency
Lipase deficiency
Trypsin deficiency
Colipase deficiency
Loss of Enzyme-Activation Ability
Deficiency of enterokinase

RICHARD S. PERRY, PHARM.D., is Assistant Professor of Clinical Pharmacy, College of Pharmacy, North Dakota State University, and Clinical Pharmacist, St. Luke's Hospital, Fargo, ND. JEFF GALLAGHER is Staff Pharmacist, Scott and White Clinic, Temple, TX.

Address reprint requests to Dr. Perry at the Department of Pharmacy Practice, College of Pharmacy, North Dakota State University, Fargo, ND 58105.

This is **article 680-204-8507** in the **ASHP Continuing Education System.** See page 225 for learning objectives and test questions.

sponse.[6] Other pertinent factors include the poor bioavailability of various dosage forms, the effect of gastric secretions on enzyme activity, cost (may hinder compliance), and other more poorly defined causes of interpatient variability.

Unfortunately, much of the available literature concerning the treatment of maldigestion is based upon studies in small numbers of patients. Because populations in these studies are frequently heterogeneous and the study methods differ, divergent conclusions are often obtained. It is therefore difficult to reach sound therapeutic decisions about the management of maldigestion.

This article will review the normal physiology of pancreatic secretions and briefly describe the disease states that can lead to maldigestion and altered pancreatic function. The management of maldigestion and problems with therapy will be discussed, and recommendations will be made for the optimal use of pancreatic extracts and adjunctive therapy.

Physiology of Normal Pancreatic Function

The pancreas plays an important role in the digestion and absorption process. A major function of the pancreas is the secretion of a number of proteolytic enzymes, including trypsin (protease), chymotrypsin, lipase, and amylase, that are responsible for most of the digestion that occurs in the small intestine. These enzymes are secreted as a protein-rich juice that also contains bicarbonate, chloride, sodium, potassium, and various trace elements. Lipase, amylase, colipase, and ribonuclease are secreted in activated form. Trypsin is secreted as a proenzyme (trypsinogen) that is activated in the lumen of the small intestine by enterokinase; trypsin then activates other proteases and phospholipase, which are also secreted in their inactive forms.

Each component of the normal pancreatic secretion has a specific function. Because pancreatic enzymes are inactivated at a pH less than 4, bicarbonate is present in pancreatic fluid to neutralize the gastric acid that is delivered to the duodenum with each meal and thus protect the enzymes from inactivation. Amylase splits straight-chain polysaccharides into disaccharides and monosaccharides, while proteases (trypsin, chymotrypsin, and elastase) cleave peptide bonds in protein substrates. Lipase acts on dietary triglycerides in the presence of colipase and bile acids to form fatty acids and monoglycerides, which are then available for micelle formation and absorption. Colipase, which is secreted in pancreatic fluids, binds to triglycerides in the presence of bile acids and forms a complex with lipase. This results in hydrolysis of the triglyceride molecules to monoglycerides and long-chain fatty acids. Bile salts then combine with the monoglycerides and long-chain fatty acids to form soluble micelles that are absorbed from the intestinal lumen. In the absence of colipase, fat maldigestion may occur.[7] It is important to note that an abnormality involving any aspect of normal gastrointestinal (GI) physiology can result in maldigestion of food substrates.

Pancreatic secretions are controlled by several different GI hormones, the most important of which are secretin and cholecystokinin (CCK). Secretin stimulates secretion of a high-volume pancreatic fluid that is rich in bicarbonate. CCK stimulates secretion of a low-volume pancreatic fluid that has a low bicarbonate concentration but is rich in enzyme content. When both hormones are secreted the action of each is potentiated, although bicarbonate output is maximal while enzyme output is only 70% of maximum. Vasoactive intestinal peptide (VIP) has a minor effect on pancreatic response to secretin and CCK; it increases the stimulatory effect of CCK on bicarbonate secretion but produces only a mild increase in protein secretion.

Secretin and CCK exert their effects during the secretory phases of the digestive process (Table 2).

Table 2.
Physiology of Normal Pancreatic Secretion

Phase	Characteristics of Pancreatic Output
Basal	Low volume Bicarbonate output 2% of maximal Enzyme output 15% of maximal
Cephalic (secretion mediated by sight and smell of food)	Moderate volume Low bicarbonate concentration High enzyme concentration
Gastric (secretion mediated by gastric distention, rate of gastric emptying, and possible vagal stimulation)	Moderate volume Low bicarbonate concentration High enzyme concentration
Intestinal (secretion mediated by presence of food in the duodenum, secretin, cholecystokinin, and vasoactive intestinal peptide[a])	High volume pH-dependent increase in bicarbonate Enzyme output 70% of maximal

[a] Potentiates cholecystokinin effect on bicarbonate.

During the basal phase, both bicarbonate and enzyme outputs are low. The sight or smell of food initiates the cephalic phase, during which bicarbonate output remains low but enzyme output is high. During the gastric phase, distention of the stomach by food maintains the output of bicarbonate and enzymes. With gastric emptying and passage of food into the small intestine, enzyme output increases to 70% of maximum. Enzyme output during this intestinal phase is four to five times that of the basal phase and continues as long as food is present in the duodenum.[8,9] Bicarbonate output increases inversely with the pH of food entering the small intestine. All these responses are mediated by GI hormones and the concentration of nutrient substrate entering the proximal small intestine. A more detailed discussion of this process may be found in several excellent reviews.[7,10,11]

Pancreatic enzymes function best at pH 7–9, and rapid inactivation of the enzymes occurs as gastric or duodenal pH decreases. Heizer et al.[12] studied the effect of gastric juice on pancreatic enzyme activity. They found that lipase was inactivated by gastric acid or pepsin at a pH less than 4.5 and trypsin was inactivated by pepsin at a pH less than 3.5. In a study of six patients with pancreatic insufficiency, DiMagno et al.[13] found that only 22% of trypsin activity and 8% of lipase activity remained when duodenal pH fell below 4. Normal subjects, studied in the same manner, consistently maintained a duodenal pH greater than 4 and demonstrated a high level of enzyme activity.

Fortunately, the pancreas maintains a large reserve of pancreatic enzymes and secretes far greater quantities than are actually needed for normal digestion.[14,15] Fat maldigestion, as evidenced by the presence of more than 7% of ingested fat in the stool per 24 hours, is only apparent when lipase output has been reduced to less than 10% of normal.[14,15] Kalser et al.[16] reported that patients with as much as 95% of their pancreas removed had the ability to absorb 80% of dietary fat. DiMagno and colleagues[14] concluded that 90% of maximal trypsin output must be lost before azotorrhea (defined as more than 2.5 g of nitrogen in the stool per 24 hours) is apparent. These results highlight the fact that pancreatic insufficiency and maldigestion are not synonymous; maldigestion usually occurs only when pancreatic insufficiency is advanced.[14]

Other factors that can affect enzyme activity include the availability and binding of colipase to lipase and a reduction in the intraluminal amount of bile acids available for fat digestion.[15,17–20] A reduction in the amount of bile acid is most easily explained by acid precipitation in the duodenum and excretion of the bile acids.[20] Many factors can affect the activity of pancreatic enzymes and contribute to the problems encountered in the management of maldigestion.

Pathophysiology and Clinical Presentation

Maldigestion syndromes can be caused by a variety of conditions, but in the United States the most common cause of pancreatic-enzyme deficiency is chronic pancreatitis resulting from alcohol ingestion.[21] Other less frequent causes include idiopathic pancreatitis and metabolic disorders such as hyperlipidemia.[21] In children, cystic fibrosis is the most common cause of maldigestion.[7,22] Maldigestion is characterized by symptoms of weight loss, anorexia, abdominal distention, and changes in the appearance and frequency of stools. Pain resulting from both maldigestion and the underlying disease process is also a major symptom in patients with acute and chronic pancreatitis.[21]

Maldigestion associated with pancreatitis or cystic fibrosis results from the failure of pancreatic enzymes to reach the proximal duodenum.[21] In cystic fibrosis, maldigestion develops after precipitation or coagulation of pancreatic secretions causes obstruction of the ducts that empty into the duodenum.[7,22] In chronic pancreatitis, permanent destruction of tissue and variable obstruction of the pancreatic ducts lead to a decrease in the amount of enzymes produced and an impairment in the ability of the pancreas to release enzymes into the duodenum.[21] Because it is not possible to restore normal secretory function to the pancreas, the major goal of treatment is replacement of pancreatic enzymes through dietary supplementation.

Dietary Management of Maldigestion

Pancreatic insufficiency with maldigestion is managed with replacement therapy using pancreatic enzymes. However, an important adjunct to enzyme replacement therapy is dietary modification. Most patients with maldigestion experience minimal symptoms from a normal dietary load of protein or carbohydrate because alternate digestive mechanisms (e.g., enzymes in saliva and gut mucosa) are available for those substrates.[10,23,24] Therefore, dietary management is focused on the adjustment of fat intake.[24] The goals of therapy are to provide adequate calories and protein to maintain weight while limiting fat intake to an amount that can be tolerated by the patient.[23] A high-protein, high-carbohydrate diet that provides 100–150 g of protein and 400 g or more of carbohydrate is recommended initially.[23] Fat intake should be limited to 30–60 g daily at the beginning of treatment.[23,24] If steatorrhea is controlled with this amount, dietary fat intake may be increased as tolerated by the patient.[23]

Medium-chain triglycerides (MCTs) can be a useful substitute for dietary fat in patients who continue to experience steatorrhea despite dietary fat restriction and pancreatic-enzyme replacement. About 30% of MCTs can be absorbed directly, and the remaining portion is easily hydrolyzed by intestinal lipase and does not require bile acids for absorption.[23,25] Unfortunately, many patients find MCT preparations to be unpalatable and may experience diarrhea, nausea, or bloating when beginning therapy with MCTs.[1,23,24] MCTs have been most useful in children with cystic fibrosis, because they tend to accept dietary modifications more readily than adults.[26]

Drug Therapy of Maldigestion

Despite careful attention to the dietary management of maldigestion, most patients continue to experience steatorrhea and require therapy with pancreatic-enzyme supplements. The goal of drug therapy is to correct the deficiencies in pancreatic-enzyme secretions by administering commercially prepared enzyme supplements in quantities sufficient to reduce the symptoms of maldigestion and improve the patient's quality of life. Although accomplishing this goal would seem to be a relatively simple task, numerous difficulties are encountered with pancreatic-enzyme therapy.

Steatorrhea has been shown to occur only when pancreatic-lipase output is less than 10% of normal.[14] Accordingly, treatment should merely involve replacing enough lipase to raise duodenal lipase concentrations to greater than 10% of normal. However, even when treatment with an apparently adequate quantity of pancreatic enzymes is instituted, complete correction of steatorrhea seldom occurs.[13] Despite this less than optimal response, most patients experience a decrease in fecal weight, fecal fat content, and fecal nitrogen with improvement in clinical symptoms.[13]

There are several explanations for the inconsistencies in patient response to enzyme therapy. The disease process is extremely variable and large interpatient variation in the onset and course of pancreatic insufficiency is common.[21,27] Factors that can affect patient response to therapy include altered gastric emptying, hypersecretion or hyposecretion of gastric acid, decreased pancreatic-bicarbonate secretion, and altered bile-salt kinetics.[13,17–19,28–34] Considerable differences exist between the available enzyme products; the products of many manufacturers do not comply with established USP standards.[35] There may also be considerable deviation from the labeled enzyme activity, as evidenced by the results of in vitro assays (Table 3). Patient response may be affected by frequent formulation changes, the presence of ineffective additives in product formulation, and use of different delivery systems.

Considerations in Product Selection. One of the first decisions that must be made when initiating enzyme-replacement therapy is which product to use. Pancreatin is an official enzyme preparation that is extracted from the pancreases of swine or oxen. According to USP standards, pancreatin preparations must contain at least 25 units of amylase activity, 25 units of trypsin activity, and 2 units of lipase activity per milligram.[35] Although some products contain higher ratios of lipase to either trypsin or amylase than required by USP standards, this is appropriate because lipase activity contributes most to relief of the symptoms of malabsorption. Pancreatin is the least potent of the enzyme preparations, and patients usually must take a large number of dosage units each day to relieve symptoms.

Pancrelipase is the other official enzyme formulation; each milligram must contain 24 units of lipase activity, 190 units of amylase activity, and 100 units of trypsin activity.[35] Because it is more potent, patients can take fewer dosage units per day to obtain symptom relief. However, it is also more expensive.

Much of the confusion surrounding enzyme content in commercial formulations is the result of inconsistent labeling practices. Products may be labeled to indicate units of activity, milligrams of activity, or a combination of both, making product comparisons difficult (Table 4). It should be noted

Table 3.
Comparison of In Vitro Assays of Pancreatic Lipase Activity

Product (Dosage Form)	Manufacturer	Labeled Lipase Content (units)	Tested Lipase Content (units)		
			Graham[3]	Guilean[4]	Parient[5]
Convertin (enteric-coated tablet)[a]	Ascher	...	28	456	78
Cotazym (capsule)	Organon	8,000	2,014	2,296	4,630
Dactilase (tablet)[a]	Lakeside	...	...	501	376
Enzypan (enteric-coated tablet)	Norgine	...	297	1,350	830
Festal (enteric-coated tablet)	Hoechst	6,000	2,073	1,090	1,270
Ilozyme (tablet)	Adria	11,000	3,600	...	...
Kanulase (tablet)	Dorsey	1,000	11	395	94
Ku-Zyme (capsule)	Kremers–Urban	150	170	58	94
Pancreatin (tablet)	Lilly	650	507	570	...
Viokase (tablet)	Viobin	6,500	1,636	1,960	2,230

[a] Product no longer commercially available.

that British and European products are generally higher in lipase activity than trypsin or amylase activity; this can be especially important when interpreting the results of clinical investigations.[36]

A major factor in choosing a product is the amount of enzyme activity that is actually delivered to the proximal duodenum. Products with the largest amount of lipase activity generally produce the greatest improvement in patients with maldigestion syndromes.[3,13,30] Under optimal conditions in which no inactivation of enzyme occurs, an estimated 30,000 units of lipase must be taken with each meal to abolish steatorrhea.[37,38] This is difficult to achieve with standard formulations because only 8% of ingested lipase (providing less than 1% of normal pancreatic output) reaches the lumen of the small intestine and is available for digestion.[13] Trypsin activity is important to a lesser extent. Trypsin is more resistant to gastric secretions than lipase, and as much as 22% of an administered dose reaches the duodenum intact.[12,13]

Pancreatic enzymes are formulated as powders, granules, tablets, enteric-coated tablets, enteric-coated encapsulated microspheres, and capsules. Each dosage form has some advantages in bioavailability, patient acceptance, cost, or clinical effectiveness.

Powder formulations of pancreatic enzymes are mixed with food to provide a greater dispersion of the enzymes and to create conditions that are nearly physiologic. However, increased dispersion of the enzymes can have the disadvantage of making the enzymes more available for inactivation by gastric secretions. Some patients experience nausea with powder formulations, which can decrease patient acceptance.[39] Hypersensitivity reactions have been reported in the parents of children with cystic fibrosis who use powdered enzyme replacements.[40,41] The reaction appears to be mediated by IgE and is characterized by an acute onset of wheezing, choking, shortness of breath, and rhinorrhea several months after the initial exposure. For these reasons, powder formulations are used infrequently.

Granules that have been enteric-coated or pH-protected are reported to be superior to conventional and enteric-coated tablet formulations. Ihse et al.[42] compared a pancreatic granule formulation with three conventional formulations and found that the granules produced an increase in enzyme activity in the proximal segment of the small intestine. However, granule formulations have not gained widespread use in the U.S. because of poor patient acceptance. Tablet and capsule formulations have become the mainstay of therapy in this country because of good patient acceptance, reasonable cost, and satisfactory response in many patients.

Problems with gastric inactivation of the enzymes have prompted the development of enteric-coated preparations. These preparations can be divided into two groups: enteric-coated tablets and enteric-coated encapsulated microspheres (ECEM). By using a pH-sensitive coating that dissolves at a pH greater than 5, enteric-coated preparations protect the enzymes from inactivation by gastric acid. The coating dissolves in the more alkaline environment of the duodenum, and the enzymes are released.

Unfortunately, enteric-coated tablets sometimes do not deliver enough enzyme to the duodenum for a clinical response.[3,28] Most patients with pancreatic insufficiency do not secrete adequate amounts of bicarbonate into the proximal duodenum and have a lower pH than is normally present,[13,20,43] and the coating does not dissolve.[3,28] Some patients also experience a transient period during a meal in which gastric pH increases above 6 and then decreases below 4 just before gastric emptying.[38] Such a fluctuation in gastric pH results in premature release and subsequent inactivation of enzymes in the stomach.[38]

Studies that reported gastric inactivation or poor

Table 4.
Currently Available Pancreatic Enzyme Products

Product (Dosage Form)	Manufacturer	Ingredients: Amylase (units)	Lipase (units)	Protease (units)	Other
Cotazym (capsule)	Organon	30,000	8,000	30,000	25 mg calcium carbonate
Cotazym-S (enteric-coated capsule)	Organon	20,000	5,000	20,000	
Festal II (enteric-coated tablet)	Hoechst	30,000	6,000	20,000	25 mg bile constituents, 50 mg hemicellulose
Festalan (enteric-coated tablet)	Hoechst	30,000	6,000	20,000	25 mg bile constituents, 50 mg hemicellulose, 1 mg atropine
Ilozyme (tablet)	Adria	30,000	11,000	30,000	
Ku-Zyme-HP (capsule)	Kremers–Urban	30,000	8,000	30,000	
Pancrease (enteric-coated capsule)	Johnson & Johnson	20,000	4,000	25,000	
Pancreatin (plain tablet)	Lilly	8,125	650	8,125	
Pancreatin (enteric-coated tablet)	Lilly	25,000	2,000	25,000	
Phazyme (enteric-coated tablet)	Reed & Carnrick	2,000	240	3,000	60 mg simethicone
Phazyme-95 (enteric-coated tablet)	Reed & Carnrick	4,000	480	6,000	95 mg simethicone
Viokase (tablet)	Viobin	48,000	6,500	32,000	

bioavailability of enzymes with standard formulations prompted a search for a formulation that would protect the enzymes from inactivation and have improved bioavailability. Enteric-coated encapsulated microspheres were designed to move through the pyloris and disperse more rapidly than enteric-coated tablets yet still be protected from gastric inactivation.[44] Several clinical studies have evaluated the efficacy of ECEM versus conventional formulations in patients with pancreatic insufficiency, with conflicting results.[28-30,45-49] Three clinical studies involving a total of 43 patients compared ECEM with conventional enzyme preparations and found a significant improvement in symptoms of maldigestion.[29,45,46] The results of these studies contrast with the results of four other studies that compared the response of 29 patients to ECEM versus conventional enzyme formulations and found no difference in response.[28,30,47,48]

These studies may be criticized on several accounts. Each included a small sample size (ranging from 6 to 23 patients per study). Patient populations were frequently heterogeneous and included patients with cystic fibrosis and patients with exocrine pancreatic insufficiency. The order of treatment was randomized in all studies, but only one used a double-blind design.[28] The studies compared many different conventional enzyme formulations at different dosages, and the endpoints of therapy were different in each report. For these reasons, it is difficult to conclude that the ECEM formulation is superior to more conventional dosage forms.

It is, however, possible to draw some conclusions about ECEM. They are probably as efficacious as conventional tablet and capsule products. They may require fewer dosage units per day to produce an adequate patient response, particularly if substituted for less potent conventional products.[29,47,48] Patient acceptance of ECEM may be great because of the need for fewer dosage units and a less frequent incidence of such side effects as cramping and bloating.[30,45-47] Unfortunately, the formulation available in the U.S. is considerably more expensive than other products that produce comparable results.

An important consideration in terms of patient acceptance of enzyme-replacement therapy is a convenient dosage schedule. Administration of enzyme replacements with meals and snacks should encourage patient compliance because of the convenience of prandial dosing. An early study reported that the continuous presence of pancreatin in the duodenum during digestion was of utmost importance.[50] The authors reported that hourly doses of pancreatin were more effective in reducing steatorrhea than doses given with each meal. This finding was disputed by two studies that found no difference between hourly administration and a prandial dosing schedule.[13,16] The discrepancy between these conclusions probably relates to differences in fat malabsorption between the study populations.

Dosing of pancreatic enzymes is determined by patient response to therapy. Gastric inactivation of the enzymes may be substantial and large doses of enzymes are frequently required to obtain the desired improvement in maldigestion. Because the doses recommended by the manufacturers are usually inadequate to produce a reasonable response, each patient's dose must be titrated to achieve the maximal therapeutic effect with minimal side effects. It is possible to make some estimation of the required dose: since a person normally secretes 100,000 units of lipase per hour, and maldigestion occurs when secretion is reduced to less than 10% of normal, a minimum of 30,000 IU of lipase would have to be taken by the patient at each meal (assuming that all ingested lipase reached the duodenum in active form).[37,38] The enzyme contents of commercially available enzyme-replacement preparations are reported in Table 4.

Adjuncts to Enzyme Therapy. Pancreatic-enzyme supplementation alone may not completely control the symptoms of maldigestion. Despite the development of innovative dosage forms for pancreatic enzymes, rapid gastric inactivation of the enzymes continues to hinder therapy. The addition of antacids or histamine H_2-receptor antagonists to a regimen of enzyme supplements has been advocated as a means by which to prevent gastric inactivation of enzymes. The results of clinical studies that examined the use of these drugs as adjuncts to enzyme-replacement therapy are summarized in Table 5.

Histamine H_2-Receptor Antagonists. Nine clinical studies have examined the use of H_2-receptor antagonists as adjuncts to pancreatic-enzyme therapy in patients with maldigestion.[17,28,29,31-33,51-53] Virtually all these studies used cimetidine as adjunctive therapy. However, similar results should be obtainable with ranitidine. Comparison of study results is difficult because study designs and procedures varied, endpoints of therapy differed, and several enzyme preparations and dosage schedules were used.

Some general conclusions about the use of H_2-receptor antagonists as adjuncts to enzyme-replacement therapy can be drawn from these studies. H_2-receptor antagonists can increase patient response to pancreatic enzymes when used as adjuncts to enzyme therapy, but interpatient response is quite variable. The beneficial effects of H_2-receptor antagonists appear to result from an increase in both gastric and duodenal pH and a corresponding decrease in the inactivation of administered pancreatic enzymes.[53] Intragastric volume is also decreased, which limits the dilution of enzyme concentrations and increases enzyme activity.[53] H_2-receptor antagonists may be less effective in patients with cystic fibrosis who secrete large amounts of gastric acid.[29,31,33,51] Conversely, patients who secrete low or normal amounts of acid are more likely to respond well to H_2-receptor antagonists.[28,38,54] An improvement in steatorrhea is most likely if H_2-receptor antagonists are administered with high doses of lipase with each meal.[37]

Antacids. Nine studies have reported the results of adjunctive antacid therapy in patients with pancreatic insufficiency and cystic fibrosis.[17,28,29,32,47,51,55–57] Comparison of study results is again confounded by the problems noted for H_2-receptor blocker studies, but some general conclusions regarding the use of antacids as adjuncts to enzyme therapy can be drawn. Patient response to adjunctive antacid therapy is quite variable and depends on the type of antacid used, the frequency of administration, and the quantity given. To be effective, antacids must raise gastric pH above the level that inactivates enzymes (i.e., above 4). Antacids must be given before or during meals to produce a beneficial effect.[19,55,56] Two studies in which antacids were given after meals showed no benefit.[17,28]

Results of most studies indicate that antacids containing aluminum hydroxide or sodium bicarbonate are the only agents that produce an improvement in digestion of dietary fat and symptoms of malabsorption.[51,55–57] Antacids containing magnesium or calcium increase gastric pH but can cause increased steatorrhea.[55] The deleterious effects of magnesium and calcium are thought to result from precipitation of bile acids in the duodenum and formation of calcium soaps.[55,58] Intragastric volume is increased by the administration of any antacid[28]; this may be a disadvantge of antacid use because an increased volume would result in a decrease in pancreatic-enzyme concentration and a corresponding decrease in enzymatic effect.

Adverse Effects of Enzyme-Replacement Therapy. Although therapy with pancreatic enzymes usually does not cause severe side effects, certain adverse effects are associated with pancreatic-enzyme replacements. Hyperuricosuria has been reported in patients with cystic fibrosis receiving high-dose enzyme-replacement therapy,[59,60] possibly because of the high purine content of most pancreatic-enzyme preparations.[59,60] An older group of patients with cystic fibrosis who experienced hyperuricemia on high-dose enzyme therapy had age-related hyperuricemia possibly caused by a decrease in renal clearance of uric acid or renal damage from previous hyperuricosuria.[59,61] Of major concern is the potential for hyperuricosuria to lead to permanent kidney damage from crystal deposition.[59,60] Dietary modification to limit fat intake in conjunction with a modest reduction in enzyme dose may be necessary to control hyperuricosuria.[60]

Pancreatic enzymes have also been reported to form insoluble complexes with folic acid, which can lead to folic acid deficiency.[62] Although the clinical importance of this effect is unclear, careful monitoring and supplementation of folic acid may be necessary.[62] Problems with GI intolerance and pulmonary hypersensitivity reactions in parents of patients with cystic fibrosis were mentioned earlier. The frequency of hyperuricosuria and GI intolerance appear to be dose related and occur more frequently at higher doses. Other adverse effects from the use of pancreatic extracts are uncommon.

Recommendations for Initiating Therapy

Because of the large variability in patient response to therapy and in the therapeutic agents themselves, therapy must be individualized. Educating patients about their disease and including them in the deci-

Table 5.
H_2-Receptor Blockers and Antacids as Adjunctive Therapy in Pancreatic Insufficiency

Reference No.	Diagnosis (No. Patients)	Conclusions
28	Chronic pancreatitis (6)	Addition of antacid to enzymes no more effective than enzymes alone; cimetidine useful as an adjunct in patients who fail on enzymes.
29	Cystic fibrosis (11)	No significant difference between enzymes alone and antacids; in three patients, the H_2-receptor blocker further reduced steatorrhea compared with enzymes alone.
31	Cystic fibrosis (10)	Addition of H_2-receptor blocker to enzyme-replacement-therapy regimen significantly reduced fecal fat and nitrogen.
32	Chronic pancreatitis (2)	Addition of antacid H_2-receptor blocker resulted in an increase in duodenal pH and an increase in enzyme activity.
47	Cystic fibrosis (11)	Improved fat absorption in nine patients when antacid was added to enzyme therapy, but antacids added to cost of therapy and decreased patient acceptance.
51	Cystic fibrosis (15)	Addition of H_2-receptor blocker or bicarbonate to enzyme replacement therapy regimen resulted in significant improvement in fat and nitrogen absorption, but combination showed no additive effect.
56	Unknown (6)	In one patient addition of antacid improved fat absorption after enzymes alone failed.
57	Chronic pancreatitis (2)	Marked reduction in diarrhea when antacid was added to enzyme therapy.

sions about their therapy will increase patient acceptance and compliance. Management of maldigestion should begin with a standardized low-fat diet. When drug therapy is initiated, a product should be chosen based on its potential for improving steatorrhea and weight loss, its cost, and convenience of its dosing schedule. A trial of several products at similar therapeutic doses, each given for a three-day period, might be helpful in identifying the most effective preparation. The patient should be instructed to record his dietary intake and monitor stool number, stool description, and other symptoms as a means of evaluating each product. At the end of the trials the patient and physician should determine which product provided the best results at the most reasonable cost. Therapy with that product could then be adjusted to assure an adequate response. If an inadequate response occurs with a product, a change to a different product formulation might improve the response.

In patients who cannot be controlled adequately on enzyme therapy alone, addition of a histamine H_2-receptor antagonist to the therapeutic regimen may enhance enzyme activity. If antacids are to be used, sodium bicarbonate or aluminum hydroxide is the antacid of choice because these appear to be more efficacious. The inconvenience and cost of antacids must be weighed against the cost of the H_2-receptor antagonist when deciding on adjunctive therapy.

Conclusion

Pancreatic insufficiency frequently leads to maldigestion, necessitating dietary and sometimes drug interventions. Provision of adequate quantities of pancreatic enzyme to control symptoms is the major goal of drug therapy. Complete resolution of the symptoms of maldigestion is difficult to achieve, but the symptoms can be controlled to the extent that the patient's quality of life is improved. The clinical response to therapy, patient compliance with and acceptance of therapy, cost of therapy, and knowledge of the disease process are all important factors in determining appropriate management of maldigestion caused by pancreatic insufficiency.

References

1. Grendell JH. Nutrition and absorption in diseases of the pancreas. *Clin Gastroenterol.* 1983; 12:551–62.
2. Ghishan FK, Lee PC, Lebenthal E et al. Isolated congenital enterokinase deficiency. *Gastroenterology.* 1983; 85:727–31.
3. Graham DY. Enzyme replacement therapy of exocrine pancreatic insufficiency in man. *N Engl J Med.* 1977; 296:1314.
4. Giulian BB, Singh LM, Mansfield AO et al. Treatment of pancreatic exocrine insufficiency: I. In vitro lipolytic activities of pancreatic lipase and fifteen commercial pancreatic supplements. *Ann Surg.* 1967; 165:564–70.
5. Pairent FW, Howard JM. Pancreatic exocrine insufficiency: IV. The enzyme content of commercial pancreatic supplements. *Arch Surg.* 1978; 110:739–41.
6. Yeh TL, Rubin ML. Potency of pancreatic enzyme preparations. *N Engl J Med.* 1977; 297:615–6.
7. Gray GM. Maldigestion and malabsorption: clinical manifestations and specific diagnosis. In: Sleisenger MH, Fordtran JS, eds. Gastrointestinal disease. Philadelphia: W. B. Saunders Company; 1983:228–56.
8. MacGregor I, Parent J, Meyer JH. Gastric emptying of liquid meals and pancreatic and biliary secretion after subtotal gastrectomy or truncal vagotomy and pyloroplasty in man. *Gastroenterology.* 1977; 72:195–205.
9. Brunner H, Northfield TC, Hofmann AF et al. Gastric emptying and secretion of bile acids, cholesterol, and pancreatic enzymes during digestion. *Mayo Clin Proc.* 1974; 49: 851–60.
10. Sleisenger MH. Pathophysiology of the gastrointestinal tract. In: Smith LH, Thier SO, eds. Pathophysiology: the biological principles of disease. Philadelphia: W. B. Saunders Company; 1981:1506–689.
11. Meyer JM. Pancreatic physiology. In: Sleisenger MH, Fordtran JS, eds. Gastrointestinal disease. Philadelphia: W. B. Saunders Company; 1983:1426–36.
12. Heizer WD, Cleaveland CR, Iber FL. Gastric inactivation of pancreatic supplements. *Bull Johns Hopkins Hosp.* 1965; 116: 261–70.
13. DiMagno EP, Malagelada JR, Go VLW et al. Fate of orally ingested enzymes in pancreatic insufficiency. *N Engl J Med.* 1977; 296:1318–22.
14. DiMagno EP, Go VL, Summerskill WHJ. Relations between pancreatic enzyme outputs and malabsorption in severe pancreatic insufficiency. *N Engl J Med.* 1973; 288:813.
15. Gaskin KJ, Durie PR, Lee L et al. Colipase and lipase secretion in childhood-onset pancreatic insufficiency. *Gastroenterology.* 1984; 86:1–7.
16. Kalser MH, Leite CA, Warren WD. Fat assimilation after massive distal pancreatectomy. *N Engl J Med.* 1968; 279: 570–6.
17. Regan PT, Malagelada JR, DiMagno EP et al. Reduced intraluminal bile acid concentrations and fat maldigestion in pancreatic insufficiency: correction by treatment. *Gastroenterology.* 1979; 77:285–9.
18. Regan PT, Malagelada JR, Go VLW et al. The effect of treatment on abnormalities of intraluminal bile acid metabolism in pancreatic insufficiency. *Gastroenterology.* 1978; 74:1084. Abstract.
19. Weber AM, Roy CC, Chartrand L et al. Relationship between bile acid malabsorption and pancreatic insufficiency in cystic fibrosis. *Gut.* 1976; 17:295–9.
20. Go VLW, Poley JR, Hofmann AF et al. Disturbances in fat digestion induced by acidic jejunal pH due to gastric hypersecretion in man. *Gastroenterology.* 1970; 58:638–46.
21. Grendell JH. Chronic pancreatitis. In: Sleisenger MH, Fordtran JS, eds. Gastrointestinal disease. Philadelphia: W. B. Saunders Company; 1983:1485–514.
22. Stafford RJ, Grand RJ. Hereditary disease of the exocrine pancreas. *Clin Gastroenterol.* 1982; 11:141–65.
23. Taubin EL, Spiro HM. Nutritional aspects of chronic pancreatitis. *Am J Clin Nutr.* 1973; 26:367–73.
24. Regan PT, DiMagno EP. The medical management of malabsorption. *Mayo Clin Proc.* 1979; 54:267–74.
25. Greenberger NJ, Summerskill TG. Medium-chain triglycerides: physiologic considerations and clinical implications. *N Engl J Med.* 1969; 280:1045–58.
26. Kuo PT, Huang NN. The effect of medium-chain triglycerides upon fat absorption and plasma lipid and depot fat of children with cystic fibrosis of the pancreas. *J Clin Invest.* 1965; 44:1924–33.
27. Perez MM, Newcomer AD, Moertel CG et al. Assessment of weight loss, food intake, fat metabolism, malabsorption, and treatment of pancreatic insufficiency in pancreatic cancer. *Cancer.* 1983; 52:346–52.
28. Regan PT, Malagelada JR, DiMagno EP et al. Comparative effects of antacids, cimetidine and enteric coating on the therapeutic response to oral enzymes in severe pancreatic

insufficiency. *N Engl J Med.* 1977; 297:854–8.
29. Gow R, Francis P, Bradbear R et al. Comparative study of varying regimens to improve steatorrhoea and creatorrhoea in cystic fibrosis: effectiveness of an enteric-coated preparation with and without antacids and cimetidine. *Lancet.* 1981; 2:1071–4.
30. Graham DY. An enteric-coated pancreatic enzyme preparation that works. *Dig Dis Sci.* 1979; 24:906–9.
31. Cox KL, Isenberg JN, Osher AB et al. The effect of cimetidine on maldigestion in cystic fibrosis. *J Pediatr.* 1979; 94:488–92.
32. Saunders JHB, Drummond S, Wormsley KG. Inhibition of gastric secretion in treatment of pancreatic insufficiency. *Br Med J.* 1977; 1:418–9.
33. Boyle BJ, Long WB, Balistreri WF et al. Effect of cimetidine and pancreatic enzymes on serum and fecal bile acids and fat absorption in cystic fibrosis. *Gastroenterology.* 1980; 78: 950–3.
34. Saunders JHB, Cargill JM, Wormsley KG. Gastric secretion of acid in patients with pancreatic disease. *Digestion.* 1978; 17:365–9.
35. Pancrelipase and pancreatin. In: The United States pharmacopeia, 20th rev., and The national formulary, 15th ed. Rockville, MD: The United States Pharmacopeial Convention; 1980:580–4.
36. Cho YW, Aviado DM. Clinical pharmacology for pediatricians. I. Pancreatic enzyme preparations with special reference to enterically coated microspheres of pancrelipase. *J Clin Pharmacol.* 1981; 21:224–37.
37. DiMagno EP. Controversies in the treatment of exocrine pancreatic insufficiency. *Dig Dis Sci.* 1982; 27:481–4. Editorial.
38. DiMagno EP. Medical treatment of pancreatic insufficiency. *Mayo Clin Proc.* 1979; 54:435–42.
39. Anon. Pancreatic extracts. *Lancet.* 1977; 2:73–4. Editorial.
40. Bergner A, Berner RK. Pulmonary hypersensitivity with pancreatin powder exposure. *Pediatrics.* 1975; 55:814–7.
41. Twarog FJ, Weinstein SF, Khaw KT et al. Hypersensitivity to pancreatic extracts in parents of patients with cystic fibrosis. *J Allergy Clin Immunol.* 1977; 59:35–40.
42. Ihse I, Lilja P, Lundquist I. Intestinal concentrations of pancreatic enzymes following pancreatic replacement therapy. *Scand J Gastroenterol.* 1980; 15:137–44.
43. Dutta SK, Russell RM, Iber FL. Influence of exocrine pancreatic insufficiency on the intraluminal pH of the proximal small intestine. *Dig Dis Sci.* 1979; 24:529–34.
44. Green DM. Tablets of coated aspirin microspherules—a new dosage form. *J New Drugs.* 1966; 6:294–304.
45. Valerio D, Whyte EHA, Schlamm HT et al. Clinical effectiveness of a pancreatic enzyme supplement. *J Parenter Enter Nutr.* 1981; 5:110–4.
46. Mischler EH, Parrell S, Farrell PM et al. Comparison of effectiveness of pancreatic enzyme preparations in cystic fibrosis. *Am J Dis Child.* 1982; 136:1060–3.
47. Nassif EG, Younoszai MK, Weinberger MM et al. Comparative effects of antacids, enteric coating, and bile salts on the efficacy of oral pancreatic enzyme therapy in cystic fibrosis. *J Pediatr.* 1981; 98:320–3.
48. Dutta SK, Rubin J, Harvey J. Comparative evaluation of therapeutic efficacy of pH-sensitive enteric coated pancreatic enzyme preparation with conventional pancreatic enzyme therapy in the treatment of exocrine pancreatic insufficiency. *Gastroenterology.* 1983; 84:476–82.
49. Warwick WJ, Budd JR. Comparison of two forms of enteric-coated pancrelipase in six teenagers with cystic fibrosis. *Clin Ther.* 1982; 5:15–20.
50. Jordan PH, Grossman MI. Effect of dosage schedule on the efficacy of substitution therapy in pancreatic insufficiency. *Gastroenterology.* 1959; 36:447–51.
51. Durie PR, Bell L, Linton W et al. Effect of cimetidine and sodium bicarbonate on pancreatic replacement therapy in cystic fibrosis. *Gut.* 1980; 21:778–86.
52. Staub JL, Sarles H, Soule JC et al. No effect of cimetidine on the therapeutic response to oral enzymes in severe pancreatic insufficiency. *N Engl J Med.* 1981; 304:1364–5. Letter.
53. Regan PT, Malagelada JR, DiMagno EP et al. Rationale for the use of cimetidine in pancreatic insufficiency. *Mayo Clin Proc.* 1978; 53:79–83.
54. Regan PT, Malagelada JR, DiMagno EP et al. Postprandial gastric function in pancreatic insufficiency. *Gut.* 1979; 20: 249–54.
55. Graham DY. Pancreatic enzyme replacement: the effect of antacids on cimetidine. *Dig Dis Sci.* 1982; 27:485–90.
56. Veeger W, Abels J, Hellemans N et al. Effect of sodium bicarbonate and pancreatin on the absorption of vitamin B-12 and fat in pancreatic insufficiency. *N Engl J Med.* 1962; 267: 1341–4.
57. Haro EN, Faloon WW. The effect of bicarbonate on pancreatic enzyme activity. *Clin Res.* 1964; 12:207. Abstract.
58. Graham DY, Sackman JW. Mechanism of enhanced steatorrhea by Ca^{+2} and Mg^{+2} in pancreatic insufficiency. *Gastroenterology.* 1981; 80:1161. Abstract.
59. Nousia-Arvanitakis S, Stapleton FB, Linshaw MA et al. Therapeutic approach to pancreatic extract-induced hyperuricosuria in cystic fibrosis. *J Pediatr.* 1977; 90:302–5.
60. Stapleton FB, Kennedy J, Nousia-Arvanitakis S et al. Hyperuricosuria due to high dose pancreatic extract therapy in cystic fibrosis. *N Engl J Med.* 1976; 295:246–8.
61. Davidson GP, Hassel FM, Crozier D et al. Iatrogenic hyperuricemia in children with cystic fibrosis. *J Pediatr.* 1978; 93: 976–8.
62. Russell RM, Dutta SK, Oaks EV et al. Impairment of folic acid absorption by oral pancreatic extracts. *Dig Dis Sci.* 1980; 25: 369–73.

Nontraditional analgesics for the management of postherpetic neuralgia

MICHAEL THOMPSON AND MICHELLE BONES

Abstract: The pathogenesis and clinical manifestations of herpes zoster and postherpetic neuralgia and the use of nontraditional analgesics in the management of postherpetic neuralgia are reviewed.

Herpes zoster represents the reactivation in an immunocompromised host of dormant varicella-zoster virus (*Herpesvirus varicellae*) contracted during a previous episode of chickenpox. Fever, neuralgia, and paresthesia occur four to five days before skin lesions develop. Acute herpes zoster pain usually does not last more than two weeks after all skin lesions have healed. Postherpetic neuralgia is defined as pain that persists in the affected dermatomes after the disappearance of all skin crusts. The neuralgia can vary from "lightninglike" stabbing pain to constant, burning pain with hyperesthesia; it can persist for years and is often refractory to traditional analgesic therapy.

A number of nontraditional analgesic agents have been used in the management of postherpetic neuralgia. Tricyclic antidepressants, especially amitriptyline, have been used alone and in combination with phenothiazines or anticonvulsants (carbamazepine, phenytoin, valproate sodium), with good results. The effectiveness of phenothiazines or anticonvulsants as sole therapeutic agents has not been demonstrated. Although the intralesional administration of corticosteroids appears to be beneficial, considerable fear about the potential for these agents to precipitate widespread viral dissemination exists. Positive results have been reported with levodopa, amantadine, and interferon, but the role of these agents in the prevention of postherpetic neuralgia remains unclear.

Nontraditional analgesic agents are useful in the management of postherpetic neuralgia, but patients must be selected and monitored appropriately. A tricyclic antidepressant (especially amitriptyline) is a reasonable first choice.

Index terms: Amitriptyline; Analgesics and antipyretics; Anticonvulsants; Antidepressants; Carbamazepine; Herpes zoster; Neuralgia; Phenothiazines; Phenytoin; Valproate sodium
Clin Pharm. 1985; 4:170–6

Herpes zoster (shingles) is one manifestation of infection with *Herpesvirus varicellae*, commonly known as the varicella-zoster virus. Varicella-zoster virus also causes chickenpox, and herpes zoster represents the reactivation of latent virus contracted from an earlier episode of chickenpox. Neoplasms, immunosuppressant drugs, and radiation therapy are among the many factors known to convert this virus from a latent state to an infectious state.[1,2]

The early clinical presentation of herpes zoster is characterized by exanthematous eruptions, sensory neuronal damage, and pain in the corresponding dermatome. Pain that persists after the disappearance of skin lesions is defined as postherpetic neuralgia.[1] Although self-limiting, the pain can be extremely severe and debilitating and can persist for years, especially in elderly and immunocompromised individuals. The administration of traditional analgesic and narcotic agents usually offers little relief. Thus, a variety of nontraditional analgesic drug therapies have emerged in recent decades to provide relief from this distressing complication.

This article describes the pathology, pathogenesis, and clinical manifestations of herpes zoster and postherpetic neuralgia, reviews the use of various nontraditional agents for management of postherpetic neuralgia, and evaluates published case reports and studies in which these agents have been used.

Pathology and Pathogenesis

In a patient with chickenpox, varicella-zoster virus moves from the skin and mucosal lesions into the endings of sensory nerves and travels along the nerve to the corresponding sensory ganglia. While in the sensory ganglia, the virus does not multiply. Although the virus retains the ability to revert to an infectious state, it lies dormant in the ganglia and poses no problem clinically in patients with adequate, well-functioning immune systems.[1,2] If small amounts of virus do revert to an infectious state, they are neutralized by antibodies or destroyed by cellular immune responses before replication and widespread dissemination of the virus can occur.[1]

Varicella-zoster virus remains in a dormant state until the host becomes immunocompromised.

MICHAEL THOMPSON, PHARM.D., is Assistant Professor of Clinical Pharmacy, College of Pharmacy, Florida Agricultural and Mechanical University, and Clinical Pharmacist Preceptor, Family Practice Medicine Service, Tallahassee Memorial Regional Medical Center, Tallahassee, FL. MICHELLE BONES is a Doctor of Pharmacy candidate, College of Pharmacy, Florida Agricultural and Mechanical University, Tallahassee.

Address reprint requests to Dr. Thompson at the College of Pharmacy, Florida Agricultural and Mechanical University, Tallahassee, FL 32307.

Malignancies (e.g., Hodgkin's disease), immunosuppressive drugs, and radiation therapy are among the many factors that can suppress the immune system and predispose patients to herpes zoster. A list of factors known to suppress the immune system and thereby precipitate this disorder is presented in Table 1.

Once the host has become immunocompromised, the virus multiplies and spreads within the ganglion, causing neuronal necrosis and inflammation that lead to neuralgia.[1] Pathologic changes in the ganglion include intense lymphocytic infiltration, necrosis of nerve cells and fibers, endothelial proliferation and lymphocytic cuffing of small vessels, focal hemorrhage, and inflammation of the ganglion sheath. After the virus has spread within the ganglion, it moves downward through the sensory nerve, causing neuritis, and is released around the nerve endings. Release of the virus produces the characteristic herpes zoster rash.[1] The cutaneous lesions associated with herpes zoster are histologically identical to those of chickenpox; in both disorders, there is ballooning of infected skin cells, formation of multinucleated giant cells, and accumulation of cutaneous edema fluid in vesicles.[3]

Individuals who have never been exposed to varicella-zoster virus usually develop chickenpox upon first infection with the virus. The pathogenic model presented in this paper assumes that herpes zoster develops only in adults who have previously had chickenpox. In contradiction to this generally accepted hypothesis are anecdotal reports of herpes zoster cases that developed following an individual's initial exposure to varicella-zoster virus. At present, however, the importance of these findings is not clear.[4]

Clinical Manifestations

Herpes Zoster. Herpes zoster most commonly affects the thoracic, cervical, lumbar, and sacral nerves and the ophthalmic division of the trigeminal nerve (in decreasing order of occurrence).[2] Fever, neuralgia, and paresthesia typically occur four or five days before skin lesions develop. The neuralgia is localized in the areas served by the specific sensory nerves that were affected during a previous episode of chickenpox and is caused by pathologic changes in the sensory ganglia.[1,2] The pain can be constant or intermittent and varies from superficial itching, tingling, or burning to severe deep pain.[1] Depending upon the location of the affected dermatome, the neuralgia that occurs before skin lesions develop can resemble the pain associated with myocardial infarction, duodenal ulcer, pleurisy, or biliary colic and can make the initial diagnosis of herpes zoster difficult.

Table 1.
Known Precipitating Factors for Herpes Zoster

Age (greater than 60 years old)
Drugs
Cancer chemotherapeutic agents
Other immunosuppressant agents (e.g., corticosteroids)
Heavy metal therapy or poisoning
Irradiation of spinal column
Neoplasms
Hodgkin's disease and other lymphomas
Tumor involvement of spinal cord, dorsal root ganglion, or adjacent structures
Renal transplants

Skin lesions in herpes zoster resemble those seen in chickenpox.[1–4] They begin as maculopapular eruptions and develop into vesicles filled with clear fluid. The lesions progress to cloudy pustules and end in crust and scab formation.[4] Once crusts have formed, the patient is no longer infectious. New lesions usually continue to develop for three or four days, while crusts can persist for several weeks.

Herpes zoster lesions usually are arranged unilaterally on a dermatome in bandlike clusters that follow radicular lines.[2] The high concentration of lesions on skin areas that contained the greatest density of chickenpox rash[1] is believed to result from transmission of larger quantities of varicella-zoster virus into the corresponding sensory ganglia in those areas.

Approximately 10–15% of reported cases of herpes zoster involve the ophthalmic division of the trigeminal nerve. The rash in ophthalmic zoster can extend from eye level to the vertex of the skull but usually does not cross the midline of the forehead.[1] According to Oxman,[1] if the supratrochlear and supraorbital branches only are involved, the eye is usually spared. However, conjunctivitis, scleritis, iridocyclitis, extraocular muscle palsies, ptosis, and mydriasis can occur if the nasociliary branch is involved. Involvement of the second and third divisions of the trigeminal nerve can produce symptoms and lesions in the mouth, ears, pharynx, or larynx.[4]

Infrequently, neuralgia occurs without skin eruption; this condition is known as zoster sine eruptione. Leptomeningitis, spinal fluid pleocytosis, and myelitis can occur if the virus spreads proximally along the posterior nerve root. If motor neurons in the anterior horn become involved and the anterior nerve root becomes inflamed, palsies can develop.[2] On rare occasions, widespread dissemination of the virus results in meningoencephalitis.[4]

Postherpetic Neuralgia. In general, the pain associated with herpes zoster persists for one to two weeks after all skin lesions have healed, although hypoesthesia or hyperesthesia may remain.[2] Pain that persists in the affected dermatomes after the disappearance of all skin crusts is considered to be postherpetic neuralgia.[1] The character of the pain varies from patient to patient and ranges from "lightninglike" jabs of pain to a constant, burning pain that can be exacerbated by gentle contact with the skin (i.e., hyperesthesia).[5] In patients with hyperesthetic areas of the skin, contact with clothing can result in unbearable pain.[3] Although this neuralgia is self-limiting, pain duration is longer in elderly and immunocompromised individuals.[6]

Investigators vary greatly in their opinions of when acute herpes zoster pain becomes postherpetic neuralgia. For example, some investigators define postherpetic neuralgia as pain that persists more than two months from its onset.[7,8] Others have defined postherpetic neuralgia as pain that persists for 24 months after the disappearance of lesions.[9] Regardless of the official definition, this persistent, exhausting, and intractable pain often does not respond adequately to traditional analgesic agents.

Treatment of Postherpetic Neuralgia

Acute herpes zoster pain can usually be treated with anti-inflammatory drugs, analgesics, narcotics, continuous epidural analgesia with a local anesthetic, or a combination of all of these.[3] Fortunately, pain experienced during this acute phase generally disappears within 7 to 10 days.

Throughout the past several decades, a wide variety of methods have been explored for providing sustained analgesic relief to patients with postherpetic neuralgia. These methods have included the administration of posterior pituitary hormones, procaine, thiamine, cyanocobalamin, aspirin, and cobra venom; autohemotherapy (reinjection of the individual's own blood); repeated spraying with ethyl chloride; skeletal traction; procaine ionization; and local vibration.[6] More radical procedures, such as the subarachnoid injection of alcohol, avulsion of the involved nerve, injection of alcohol and local anesthetics into the nerve root, rhizotomy, cordotomy, prefrontal leukotomy, and stereotaxic procedures have also been used in severe cases. A list of drugs that have been used in the management of postherpetic neuralgia in recent years is presented in Table 2. Table 3 summarizes the available studies in patients receiving various nontraditional analgesics for postherpetic neuralgia.

Tricyclic Antidepressants. In 1965, Woodforde and associates[6] reported that 11 of 14 patients receiving amitriptyline for postherpetic neuralgia experienced good to complete relief from pain. Analgesic response was usually achieved within one to two weeks following initiation of therapy, although four weeks was required for maximum effects. Because this was an uncontrolled trial and other analgesics were freely administered, a reduction in pain or complete resolution of pain could not be attributed to amitriptyline administration alone.

In 1973, Taub[10] reported that amitriptyline provided little analgesic effect when given alone for postherpetic neuralgia, but that better analgesic response was obtained when amitriptyline was combined with a phenothiazine (perphenazine, fluphenazine, or thioridazine). This finding is reinforced by another report of the effects of psychotropic drugs in the management of chronic pain disorders,[11] in which a marked dimunition in postherpetic neuralgia occurred within one to two weeks in the absence of all narcotic analgesics. One patient who had received nortriptyline for two years without noticeable relief from pain did experience pain relief when this combination regimen was started. Weis and associates[12] reported successful results in nine patients treated with a fixed combination of amitriptyline hydrochloride 25 mg and perphenazine 2 mg. All patients except one experienced pain relief at the end of one week.

Recognizing that previous studies involving the administration of tricyclic antidepressants were uncontrolled or complicated by the use of other drugs and nerve blocks, Watson et al.[13] conducted a double-blind, placebo-controlled, crossover study using amitriptyline in patients with postherpetic neuralgia. In this trial, 16 of 24 patients had good to excellent relief of pain on a median amitriptyline dose of 75 mg daily. Pain was assessed by a verbal subjective pain score and visual analog scale. Personality and depression were also assessed by the Minnesota Multiphasic Personality Inventory and the Beck depression inventory. Interestingly, pain relief in nine patients with diagnoses of clinical depression was not associated with a notable amitriptyline-induced antidepressant effect. In patients who experienced pain relief, serum concentrations of amitriptyline were below or at the low end of the acceptable therapeutic range for treating depression.

Table 2.
Nontraditional Analgesics Used in Postherpetic Neuralgia

Reference	Drug	Dosage (mg/day)	Side Effects or Adverse Effects
13	Amitriptyline	50–75	Sedation, anticholinergic side effects (e.g., dry mouth, urinary retention, blurred vision)
16, 17	Chlorprothixene[a]	50–100	Extrapyramidal effects, sedation, anticholinergic effects
20	Phenytoin[a]	300–400	Acute signs of toxicity: drowsiness, nystagmus, ataxia
	Carbamazepine	600–800	Blood dyscrasias, skin and liver-function abnormalities
25, 26	Triamcinolone	≤ 60[b]	Abscess formation, cutaneous atrophy, signs of systemic toxicity (e.g., "moon face")

[a] Best used in combination with a tricyclic antidepressant.

[b] Recommended concentration is triamcinolone 2 mg/mL in 0.9% sodium chloride injection.

Thus, the investigators concluded that amitriptyline's analgesic effect was probably not related to its antidepressant properties alone.

The mechanism of analgesic action of the tricyclic antidepressants may be related to their ability to inhibit the reuptake of such biogenic amines as serotonin and norepinephrine, or to their ability to potentiate the effects of other analgesics.[3,14] Specific interrelationships between tricyclic antidepressants and morphine have been discussed.[14] For example, both morphine and tricyclic antidepressants may interfere with the reuptake of catecholamines into brain synaptosomes.[15] Lee and Spencer[14] demonstrated that the analgesic action of morphine could be abolished when biogenic amines were depleted from neuronal storage sites with reserpine and then restored when small amounts of serotonin were injected directly into the brain ventricles of the affected animals.

Phenothiazines. Although the phenothiazines are usually used in combination with tricyclic antidepressants for the management of postherpetic neuralgia, phenothiazines have also been studied as sole therapeutic agents for postherpetic pain.[16,17] In 1974, Farber and Burks[16] reported that 27 of 30 patients receiving chlorprothixene 50 mg every six hours orally for herpes zoster neuralgia experienced total relief within 72 hours of beginning therapy. How-

Table 3.
Controlled and Noncontrolled Trials Using Nontraditional Analgesics for Postherpetic Neuralgia

Reference	Study Design	No. Subjects	Ages (yr)	Pain Duration (mo) before Therapy	Drugs Used	Comments
6	Uncontrolled	14	60–89	1–168	Amitriptyline	Complete to good pain relief in 11 patients
10	Uncontrolled	5	56–74	0.5–12	Amitriptyline with a phenothiazine	Poor response with amitriptyline alone, better response when combined with a phenothiazine
12	Uncontrolled	9	40–79	2–30	Amitriptyline with perphenazine	Pain relief in all subjects within one week
13	Controlled	24	49–81	4–108	Amitriptyline versus placebo	Good to excellent relief in 16 patients on median dose of 75 mg, poor response at lower median dose of 50 mg
17	Controlled	13	Not stated	Not stated	Chlorprothixene versus placebo	Only four patients reported pain relief; two of these were eliminated because of side effects, and relief lasted less than five months in remaining two
	Uncontrolled	19	Not stated	Not stated	Chlorprothixene	Only one patient had lasting relief
20	Uncontrolled	34	40–88	3–180	Carbamazepine or phenytoin with nortriptyline; nerve blocks	Complete to good relief in 79% of patients
22	Controlled	29	Not stated	≥30	Clomipramine plus carbamazepine versus electrical stimulation	Final study group small with only 9 of 16 patients completing study; marked pain relief by eight weeks
23	Uncontrolled	25	50–90	1–10	Valproate sodium with amitriptyline	Marked improvement in 17 patients during study period
25	Uncontrolled	53[a]	Not stated	Not stated	Triamcinolone injected subcutaneously	Excellent response in 41% of patients; 32% had improved relief
26	Controlled	128[b]	50–90	6–144	Triamcinolone versus 0.9% sodium chloride injected subcutaneously	Complete cure in 35.2% of patients; 28.9% still had occasional pain
27	Uncontrolled	21	30–90	1.5–72	Triamcinolone with bupivacaine	Nine patients reported good to excellent relief; four others had significant relief
28	Uncontrolled	5	67–80	3–48	Bupivacaine plus methylprednisolone acetate injected epidurally	Immediate pain relief but no more than 50% pain relief apparent at follow-up

[a] An additional 58 patients with acute herpes zoster pain were also studied.

[b] The control group consisted of four patients who received 0.9% sodium chloride injection; an additional 272 patients with acute herpes zoster pain were also studied.

ever, these patients' neuralgia did not appear to be postherpetic in nature.

In the first of two trials by Nathan,[17] 4 of 13 patients reported pain relief on a regimen of chlorprothixene 50 mg daily for one week followed by 50 mg twice daily for an additional week. Two patients were forced to discontinue therapy when side effects developed, and the effectiveness of the regimen diminished after five months in the two patients who continued therapy. In the second trial, only 1 of 19 patients receiving a regimen of chlorprothixene 50 mg every six hours reported lasting pain relief.

The exact mechanism of analgesic effect from phenothiazines is unknown. It is not clear whether the analgesic effects are related to the anxiolytic properties or dopamine-antagonist effects of the phenothiazines, or whether the analgesic effects are caused by some other unknown mechanism.

Anticonvulsants. Tricyclic antidepressants have also been used in combination with anticonvulsant agents. The use of anticonvulsant drugs for neuralgia of other etiologies is not uncommon.[18,19] Hatgandi and associates[20] reported that 79% of the patients they studied had good or complete pain relief from combination therapy with nortriptyline and carbamazepine or phenytoin. However, care must be taken when administering carbamazepine because of its adverse effects on the bone marrow, skin, and liver.[21]

Gerson and colleagues[22] found combination therapy with carbamazepine and clomipramine to be superior to transcutaneous electrical nerve stimulation for the management of postherpetic pain. Since plasma concentrations of clomipramine and its primary metabolite were elevated during carbamazepine administration, the authors concluded that carbamazepine might interfere with the hepatic metabolism of clomipramine. Further research is needed to substantiate this claim.

Raftery[23] reported that 17 of 25 patients had substantial pain relief when treated with a combination of valproate sodium and amitriptyline for 3 to 18 months. This is the only trial that looked at the use of valproate sodium in postherpetic neuralgia.

Anticonvulsants are thought to produce analgesia by raising the threshold for repetitive firing of neurons involved in nociperception.[3] Results from some animal studies have suggested that these drugs may also activate certain pathways for pain suppression in the central nervous system.[24] Since controlled investigations of the use of anticonvulsants as sole therapy for postherpetic neuralgia are lacking, these agents should be used only in combination with a tricyclic antidepressant until their effectiveness as single agents is proved.

Corticosteroids. The use of corticosteroids in the treatment of postherpetic neuralgia is controversial.[1,25,26] Opponents of the use of corticosteroids cite the potential for these drugs to precipitate widespread viral dissemination as a primary disadvantage to their use.[1] This is especially important because most patients with herpes zoster are already immunosuppressed and corticosteroids can cause further immunosuppression.

Epstein[25] noted that approximately 41% of patients with postherpetic neuralgia reported excellent pain relief from daily subcutaneous injections of triamcinolone 2 mg/mL in 0.9% sodium chloride into areas of burning pain or pruritis. An additional 32% of patients experienced enough pain relief to improve their quality of life. Unfortunately, the ages and concurrent disease states of these patients were not provided; these are important factors to consider because immunosuppressed and elderly patients have pain of a longer duration and greater severity than do other patients. The location of these patients' pain also was not documented. According to Crue and associates,[5] postherpetic neuralgia in the ophthalmic division of the trigeminal nerve is often very difficult to manage successfully. Thus, a patient population of relatively young, immunocompetent patients, only a few of whom complain of ophthalmic involvement, is likely to respond better to therapeutic interventions than are more seriously ill patients.

In a 1981 study, Epstein[26] corrected many of the deficiencies of his earlier study[25] by providing information about each subject's age, duration of neuralgia, and complications from steroid therapy. Complete pain relief was achieved in 35.2% of patients and good results (i.e., occasional pain) were achieved in 28.9% of patients with postherpetic neuralgia who received triamcinolone 2 mg/mL in 0.9% sodium chloride subcutaneously. In some patients, subcutaneous administration of triamcinolone caused tenderness in the injected area and other complications (Table 2). In a control group of four patients who had been treated previously with triamcinolone and then received injections of 0.9% sodium chloride instead, all four patients reported increased pain after two to three days and requested a return to the previous injection (triamcinolone).

Ditton[27] reported that nine patients achieved good to excellent pain relief from intralesional injections of triamcinolone 10–20 mg mixed with bupivacaine, while four patients received relief that contributed substantially to their overall management. Interestingly, when burning and hyperesthesia were prominent features of the neuralgia, good to excellent results could be obtained from this procedure. However, when pain was localized, deeply situated, and characterized by a dull ache, intralesional injections of steroids were not successful in providing analgesia.

Perkins et al.[28] studied the analgesic effects of methylprednisolone acetate 80 mg mixed with 8–12 mL of bupivacaine 0.25% and administered epidurally to five patients with postherpetic neuralgia. Although some patients experienced immediate pain relief, none of the patients reported more than 50% relief of pain on follow-up. It is possible that these patients might have required additional injections to sustain the initial analgesic effects.

Although corticosteroids have been used without causing apparent viral dissemination, this finding could be a reflection of patient selection. For example, if patients with leukemias, lymphomas, or other major immunodeficiencies are excluded from a study, then corticosteroid administration might not lead to widespread viral dissemination.

Prevention of Postherpetic Neuralgia

It is important to note that the administration of certain agents during the acute phase of herpes zoster may reduce a patient's chance of developing postherpetic neuralgia. In 1970, Eaglestein et al.[8] reported that the administration of corticosteroids during the early phase of herpes zoster infections prevented postherpetic neuralgia or shortened its duration. Only 30% of patients who received varying dosages of oral triamcinolone during a three-year period developed postherpetic neuralgia, compared with 73% of patients who received a placebo. Patients in each group were comparable in terms of age, sex, race, duration of disease, general health, and healing time of skin lesions. However, patients with hypertension, tuberculosis, lymphomas, leukemia, bleeding peptic ulcers, diabetes, cardiac disease, or bacterial infections were specifically excluded, so the potential for any patient to develop widespread viral dissemination was greatly reduced.

In 1980, Keczkes and Basheer[7] studied the occurrence of postherpetic neuralgia in patients receiving prednisolone 40 mg daily for 10 days with a gradual reduction in dosage over three weeks versus patients receiving carbamazepine. Postherpetic neuralgia developed in 65% of patients receiving carbamazepine but in only 15% of patients treated with prednisolone. Widespread skin eruption and viral dissemination did not occur, but patients at risk for these complications were excluded. The investigators recommended that patients over 50 years of age, especially those with trigeminal nerve involvement, be given systemic glucocorticoid therapy within seven days from the onset of herpes zoster. Other investigators have reported similar findings when glucocorticoids were administered intralesionally.[26,29]

The administration of various other drugs during the early phases of herpes zoster has been reported to reduce either the incidence or duration of postherpetic neuralgia. Examples of these different agents are levodopa,[30] amantadine,[31] and human leukocyte interferon.[32] However, no significant effects on the development of postherpetic neuralgia were seen in studies when acyclovir,[33] varicella-zoster immune globulin,[34] or bupivacaine[35] was administered during the early stages of herpes zoster. A recently published report[36] suggested that oral acyclovir could reduce the incidence of chronic neuralgia if given early in the infection, but the total number of patients studied was small.

Conclusion

Although well-designed, evaluable clinical trials are limited, the available literature on the use of nontraditional analgesics in postherpetic neuralgia suggests that these agents can be used effectively for control of postherpetic pain when patients are carefully selected and monitored.

A tricyclic antidepressant, especially amitriptyline, seems a reasonable first choice for analgesia when therapy with traditional analgesics has failed. Phenothiazine derivatives (e.g., perphenazine) or anticonvulsants (e.g., phenytoin) can be used in conjunction with a tricyclic antidepressant. Corticosteroids should be used only in patients who do not have neoplasms or other disorders that predispose them to increased immunosuppression and the possibility of dissemination of the virus to other areas of the body.

References

1. Oxman MN. Herpes zoster. In: Braude AI, Davis CE, Fierer J, eds. Medical microbiology and infectious diseases. Philadelphia: WB Saunders; 1981:1663–71.
2. Ray CG. Chickenpox (varicella) and herpes zoster. In: Harrison's principles of internal medicine. 10th ed. Petersdorf RG, Adams RD, Braunwald E et al., eds. New York: McGraw-Hill Book Co.; 1983:1121–4.
3. Stein JM, Warfield CA. Herpes zoster and postherpetic neuralgia. *Hosp Pract.* 1982; 17:96A–96O.
4. Dolin R, Reichman RC, Mazur MH et al. Herpes zoster-varicella infections in immunosuppressed patients. *Ann Intern Med.* 1978; 89:375–88.
5. Crue BL, Todd EM, Maline DB. Postherpetic neuralgia—conservative treatment regimen. In: Pain research and treatment. Los Angeles: Academic Press; 1975:289–92.
6. Woodforde JM, Dwyer B, McEwen BW et al. Treatment of postherpetic neuralgia. *Med J Aust.* 1965; 2:869–72.
7. Keczkes K, Basheer AM. Do corticosteroids prevent postherpetic neuralgia? *Br J Dermatol.* 1980; 102:551–5.
8. Eaglestein WH, Katz R, Brown JA. The effects of corticosteroid therapy on the skin eruption and pain of herpes zoster. *JAMA.* 1970; 211:1681–3.
9. Yardley DE, Schwartz RA, Adams HG. Herpes zoster. *Am Fam Phys.* 1983; 28:138–44.
10. Taub AT. Relief of postherpetic neuralgia with psychotropic drugs. *J Neurosurg.* 1973; 39:235–9.
11. Merskey H, Hester RA. The treatment of chronic pain with psychotropic drugs. *Postgrad Med J.* 1972; 48:594–8.
12. Weis O, Sriwatanakul K, Weintraub M. Treatment of postherpetic neuralgia and acute herpetic pain with amitriptyline and perphenazine. *S Afr Med J.* 1982; 62:274–5.
13. Watson PC, Evans RJ, Reed K et al. Amitriptyline versus placebo in postherpetic neuralgia. *Neurology.* 1982; 32: 671–3.
14. Lee R, Spencer PSJ. Antidepressants and pain: a review of the pharmacological data supporting the use of certain tricyclics in chronic pain. *J Int Med Res.* 1977; 5 (Suppl 1):146–56.
15. Clouet DH, Williams N. The effect of narcotic analgesic drugs on the uptake and release of neurotransmitters in isolated synaptosomes. *J Pharmacol Exp Ther.* 1973; 188:419.

16. Farber GA, Burks JW. Chlorprothixene therapy for herpes zoster neuralgia. *South Med J.* 1974; 67:808–12.
17. Nathan PW. Chlorprothixene in post-herpetic neuralgia and other severe chronic pains. *Pain.* 1978; 5:367–71.
18. Rall TW, Schleifer LS. Drugs effective in the therapy of the epilepsies. In: Goodman and Gilman's the pharmacological basis of therapeutics. Gilman AG, Goodman LS, Gilman A, eds. New York: Macmillan Publishing Co., Inc.; 1980:460.
19. Ibid. p 455.
20. Hatgandi VS, Boas RA, Richards EG. Postherpetic neuralgia: management with antiepileptic and tricyclic drugs. In: Bonica JJ, ed. Advances in pain research and therapy. Vol. 1. New York: Raven Press; 1976:583–7.
21. American hospital formulary service—drug information 84. McEvoy GK, ed. Carbamazepine. Bethesda, MD: American Society of Hospital Pharmacists; 1984:691–4.
22. Gerson GR, Jones BB, Luscombe DK. Studies on the concomitant use of carbamazepine and clomipramine for the relief of postherpetic neuralgia. *Postgrad Med J.* 1977; 53(Suppl 4):104–9.
23. Raftery H. The management of postherpetic pain using sodium valproate and amitriptyline. *Ir Med J.* 1979; 72:399–401.
24. Hitchcock E, Teixeira M. Anticonvulsant activation of pain suppressive systems. *Appl Neurophysiol.* 1982; 45:582–93.
25. Epstein E. Intralesional triamcinolone therapy in herpes zoster and postzoster neuralgia. *Eye Ear Nose Throat Mon.* 1973; 52:416–7.
26. Epstein E. Treatment of herpes zoster and postzoster neuralgia by subcutaneous injection of triamcinolone. *Int J Dermatol.* 1981; 20:65–8.
27. Ditton JN. Intralesional triamcinolone–bupivacaine in the treatment of post-herpetic neuralgia. In: Peck C, Wallace M, eds. Problems in pain: proceedings of the 1st Australia–New Zealand conference. Pergamon Press; 1980:262–6.
28. Perkins HM, Hanlon PR. Epidural injection of local anesthetic and steroids for relief of pain secondary to herpes zoster. *Arch Surg.* 1978; 113:253–4.
29. Shreuder M. Pain relief in herpes zoster. *S Afr Med J.* 1983; 63:820–1.
30. Kernbaum S, Hauchecorne J. Administration of levodopa for relief of herpes zoster pain. *JAMA.* 1981; 246:132–4.
31. Gailbraith AW. Prevention of post-herpetic neuralgia by amantadine hydrochloride. *Br J Clin Pract.* 1983; 37:304–6.
32. Merigan TC, Rand KH, Pollard RB et al. Human leukocyte interferon for the treatment of herpes zoster in patients with cancer. *N Engl J Med.* 1978; 298:981–7.
33. Balfour HH, Bean B, Laskin O et al. Acyclovir halts the progression of herpes zoster in immunocompromised patients. *N Engl J Med.* 1983; 308:1448–53.
34. Stevens DA, Merigan TC. Zoster immune globulin prophylaxis of disseminated zoster in compromised hosts. *Arch Intern Med.* 1980; 140:52–4.
35. Riopelle JM, Naraghi M, Grush KP. Chronic neuralgia incidence following local anesthetic therapy for herpes zoster. *Arch Dermatol.* 1984; 120:747–50.
36. Finn R, Smith MA. Oral acyclovir for herpes zoster. *Lancet.* 1984; 2:575.

“

A Strategy for *Hemophilus influenzae* Type b Vaccination

It has been known for many years that antibody to the capsular polysaccharide of [*Hemophilus influenzae* type b] HIB, polyribosylribitol-phosphate (PRP), is protective against HIB disease. Although purified PRP administered as a vaccine is relatively free of severe side effects, it is not immunogenic or protective when administered to infants younger then 1 year of age, and its protective efficacy is questionable in those 12 to 23 months of age. . . .

. . . After reviewing the information gathered thus far, I believe that the PRP vaccine should be licensed and recommended for use. I would exercise caution, however, and recommend it initially for children 24 months of age and older, especially those attending day-care centers. This recommendation is supported by available epidemiologic, immunogenicity, and efficacy data and avoids taking the substantial risk that with the universal immunization of 18-month-old children the vaccine could prove to have little, if any, protective benefit. With this strategy there may be increased costs for immunization and concerns about lower immunization rates, but the reassurance about PRP efficacy at 24 months of age should be paramount. At this time, there are simply insufficient data for a definitive recommendation for universal PRP use in 18-month-old children. There are also other concerns about the duration of immunity, the acceptance of the vaccine, and, in the near future, the prospects of having much better vaccines.

—Ward JI. Is *Hemophilus influenzae* type b disease preventable? *JAMA.* 1985; 253: 554–6. Editorial.

”

Research

Pharmacokinetics of ceftriaxone in subjects with renal insufficiency

STEVEN F. KOWALSKY, ROGER M. ECHOLS, AND MARIE A. PARKER

Abstract: The pharmacokinetics of ceftriaxone was studied in 14 men and women volunteers with renal insufficiency.

Subjects were grouped by renal function: those with end-stage renal disease (CL_{cr} < 15 mL/min/1.73 sq m) but not receiving dialysis, those with severe renal insufficiency (CL_{cr} 16–30 mL/min/1.73 sq m), and those with moderate renal insufficiency (CL_{cr} 31–60 mL/min/1.73 sq m). Ceftriaxone 1 g as the sodium salt was administered by i.v. infusion over 30 minutes, and blood and urine samples were collected before and up to 48 hours after drug administration. The pharmacokinetic data were described using a nonlinear least-squares computer program.

For volunteers with a creatinine clearance of <15 mL/min/1.73 sq m, the mean half-life was 15.6 hours. For subjects with a creatinine clearance of 31–60 mL/min/1.73 sq m, the mean half-life was 11.9 hours. Plasma ceftriaxone concentrations measured at the conclusion of the infusion (mean peak concentration 122 ± 53.1 μg/mL) or 24 hours after the infusion (mean concentration 20.2 ± 6.14 μg/mL) were similar in each study group.

A dose of ceftriaxone 1 g every 24 hours in patients with renal insufficiency is probably adequate for inhibiting most susceptible gram-positive and gram-negative microorganisms.

Index terms: Blood levels; Ceftriaxone; Ceftriaxone sodium; Cephalosporins; Dosage; Half-life; Pharmacokinetics

Clin Pharm. 1985; 4:177–81

Ceftriaxone is a new aminothiazolyl-methoxy-imino-acetamidocephalosporin with broad-spectrum antimicrobial activity.[1–5] Substitution at the 7 position of the cephalosporin nucleus with an α-methoxamino group provides stability against β-lactamase inactivation, while chemical modification of the 3-heterocyclic-thiomethyl moiety affects the plasma half-life and renders ceftriaxone metabolically stable. Biliary clearance accounts for the elimination of approximately 40% of an administered dose.[6] Studies done in anephric patients support an extrarenal route of elimination, since elimination half-lives were increased only slightly ($t_{1/2}$ = 8.6 hours for normal subjects and 11.9 hours for anephric subjects).[7] A prolonged serum half-life,[8] the ability to penetrate the cerebrospinal fluid,[9–12] and broad-spectrum antibacterial activity make ceftriaxone a promising and unique cephalosporin antibiotic.

The purpose of our study was to describe the pharmacokinetics of ceftriaxone in adult volunteers with varying degrees of renal insufficiency and to determine an appropriate dosage regimen based on renal function.

STEVEN F. KOWALSKY, PHARM.D., is Associate Professor of Clinical Pharmacy, Department of Clinical Science and Practice, Albany College of Pharmacy, Albany, NY. ROGER M. ECHOLS, M.D., is Associate Professor of Medicine and MARIE A. PARKER, R.N., is Coordinator of Research Protocols, Division of Infectious Diseases, Albany Medical College, Albany, NY.

Address reprint requests to Dr. Kowalsky at the Department of Clinical Science and Practice, Albany College of Pharmacy, 106 New Scotland Avenue, Albany, NY 12208.

The assistance of William R. Stoll, Ph.D., Albany College of Pharmacy, with statistical analysis, and the secretarial assistance of Mary Jo Paley are acknowledged.

Plasma and urine ceftriaxone assays were performed by Robert Weinfeld, Assistant Research Group Chief, Department of Pharmacokinetics and Biopharmaceutics, Hoffmann-La Roche, Inc.

Presented in part at the 22nd Interscience Conference on Antimicrobial Agents and Chemotherapy, Miami, FL, October 5, 1982.

Methods

Ceftriaxone (as the sodium salt, lot numbers C 11253-01 and C 116871-01) was supplied by Hoffmann-La Roche Inc., Nutley, NJ, as a dry, sterile powder for reconstitution and intravenous administration.

Study Population. Fourteen adult men and women volunteers with no known allergies to penicillin or cephalosporin antibiotics were studied. Written informed consent, approved by the Human Research Committee of Albany Medical College, was obtained from each study subject. No volunteers had taken antibiotics for at least 72 hours before the time of evaluation. Each subject was selected on the basis of a prestudy 24-hour creatinine clearance (CL_{cr}) and assigned to one of three groups: group A (n = 5), CL_{cr} < 15 mL/min per 1.73 sq m but not on dialysis; group B (n = 6), 15–30 mL/min per 1.73 sq m; and group C (n = 3), 31–60 mL/min per 1.73 sq m. Table 1 lists mean age, body surface area, and creatinine clearance for each group. Subjects ranged in age from 19 to 69 years, in body surface area from 1.57 to 2.21 sq m, and in creatinine clearance from 4 to 52 mL/min per 1.73 sq m.

Each subject had a physical examination and laboratory evaluation before inclusion in the study. Laboratory tests obtained before and after the study protocol included a complete blood count with differential, platelet count, Coombs' test (direct and indirect), SMA-18, 24-hour creatinine clearance, urinalysis, and serum pregnancy test. Each subject over 40 years of age had a prestudy electrocardiogram and chest roentgenogram if none was recorded within the past one or two years, respectively. Concomitant disease states seen in this study population were hypertension (n = 2), diabetes mellitus (n = 1), glomerulonephritis (n = 5), chronic pyelonephritis (n = 3), gout (n = 1), and nephrolithiasis (n = 1). There was no laboratory or clinical evidence of hepatic disease in any study subject. Prestudy pregnancy tests revealed that none of the six women participating in the protocol was pregnant.

Specimen Collection. Each subject fasted from midnight until two hours after drug administration. After baseline serum and urine samples were taken, each subject was placed in the supine position and given ceftriaxone 1 g (as the sodium salt) by drip infusion over 30 minutes, using an infusion pump (IMED, San Diego, CA). Ceftriaxone was reconstituted with sterile water for injection 9.6 mL and mixed with 0.9% sodium chloride injection 50 mL.

Blood samples for plasma antibiotic concentration determinations were obtained in all subjects at 5, 10, 20, 30, 35, 40, and 45 minutes and 1, 1.5, 2, 3, 4, 6, 8, 12, 24, 36, and 48 hours after the infusion. The first 14 plasma samples were taken from a 0.2-mL-capacity intermittent infusion set. The first 0.5–1.0 mL was discarded, and a 3.0-mL blood sample was collected for analysis. The remaining samples were obtained by separate venipunctures. Blood specimens were collected in sterile heparinized tubes and centrifuged, and the plasma was pipetted and immediately frozen at −70 °C.

Urine samples were collected 0–2 hours before drug infusion and at intervals of 0–2, 2–4, 4–6, 6–8, 8–12, 12–18, 18–24, and 24–48 hours thereafter. The total urine volume was recorded, and a 15-mL portion was frozen at −70 °C.

All samples were assayed within six months of collection. According to plasma and urine ceftriaxone stability studies conducted by Hoffmann-La Roche Inc., the drug has a decomposition rate in plasma of approximately 1% per month and in urine of approximately 2% per month if samples are stored at −20 °C.

Assay Technique. Plasma and urine samples were assayed for ceftriaxone by Hoffmann-La Roche Inc., using an automated, reverse-phase, ion-pairing high-performance liquid chromatography method previously described.[8] The assay sensitivity limits were 5 μg/mL for plasma and 10 μg/mL for urine. The interassay precision was, on the average, 5% over a concentration range of 5–400 μg/mL.

Pharmacokinetic Analysis. After the 30-minute drip infusion of ceftriaxone, the drug concentration–time data (Figure 1) were fitted individually to the following biexponential equation:

$$C = \sum_{i=1}^{n} Y_i \, e^{-\lambda_i t}$$

using a nonlinear least-squares computer program,[13] where λ_i is the disposition rate constant for Y_i and Y_i is the coefficient corresponding to R and S (initial estimates of A and B) at the zero-time intercept. To take into consideration the drip infusion method of drug administration, thus minimizing the

Table 1.
Description of Study Groups

Characteristic[a]	Group A (n = 5)	Group B (n = 6)	Group C (n = 3)	Variance Ratio (F)
Age (yr)	41.4 ± 20.6	42.0 ± 11.9	41.7 ± 20.8	0.002
Body surface area (sq m)	1.68 ± 0.174	1.89 ± 0.092	1.85 ± 0.412	1.301
Creatinine clearance (mL/min/1.73 sq m)[b]	9.10 ± 5.54	22.4 ± 5.16	45.9 ± 9.70	31.494

[a] Mean ± S.D.
[b] Significant difference among the groups.

Figure 1. Mean (± S.D.) ceftriaxone concentration–time profile after a single i.v. dose in patients with renal insufficiency; ● = CL_{cr} <15 mL/min/1.73 sq m (n = 5), ○ = CL_{cr} 15–30 mL/min/1.73 sq m (n = 6), △ = CL_{cr} 31–60 mL/min/1.73 sq m (n = 3).

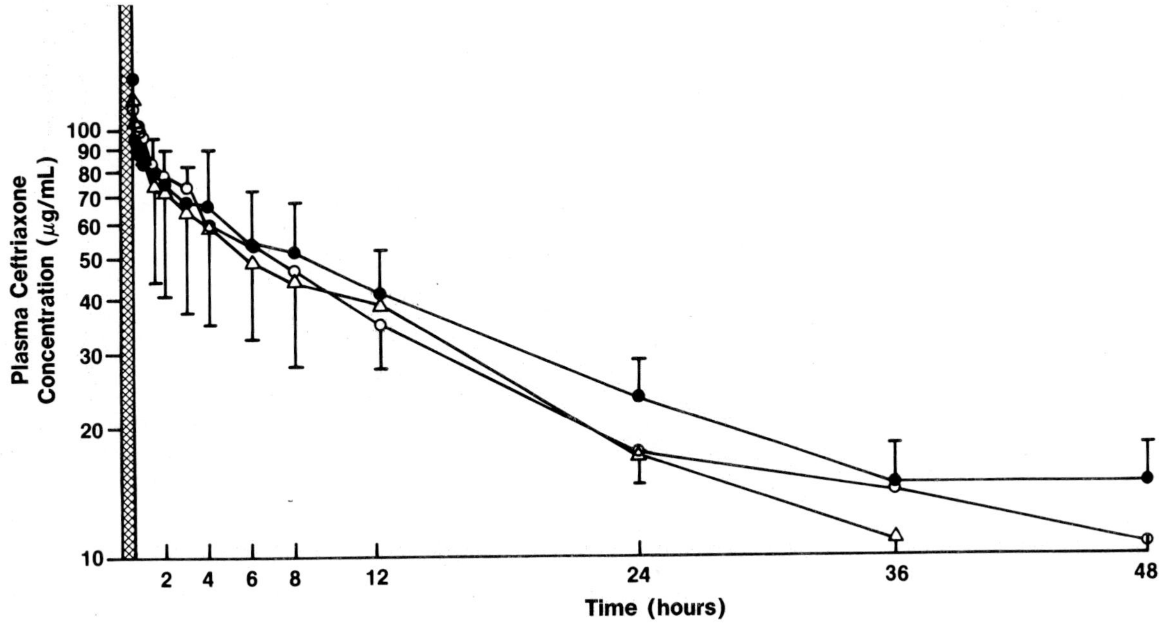

error in describing the pharmacokinetic values, the biexponential equation was modified accordingly.[14] A weighting factor of 1/the square of the observed concentration of ceftriaxone was used. The pharmacokinetic values were subsequently calculated by the following equations:

$$V_{ss} = D \sum_{i=1}^{n} C_i/\lambda_i^2 \Big/ \left[\left(\sum_{i=1}^{n} C_i/\lambda_i\right)^2\right]$$

$$CL = D \Big/ \sum_{i=1}^{n} C_i/\lambda_i$$

where D is the intravenous dose of ceftriaxone, C_i is the coefficient corresponding to A and B (the final coefficients) at the zero-time intercept, V_{ss} is the steady-state volume of distribution, and CL is the total body clearance of ceftriaxone. The area under the curve (AUC) was calculated as follows:

$$AUC = \sum_{i=1}^{n} C_i/\lambda_i$$

The average renal clearance of ceftriaxone was calculated from the slope of the line plotting the cumulative amount of drug excreted unchanged in the urine versus the area under the plasma concentration–time curve as determined by the trapezoidal rule. To take into consideration the concentration-dependent plasma protein binding of ceftriaxone that can result in a concentration dependence (and thus a time dependence) of the renal clearance, an alternate method of calculating the renal clearance of ceftriaxone was used. The renal clearance for each patient was calculated according to the following equation:

$$CL_R = Ae_{t1}^{t2}/AUC_{t1}^{t2}$$

where CL_R is the renal clearance of ceftriaxone, Ae_{t1}^{t2} is the amount of drug excreted during the time interval t_1–t_2, and AUC_{t1}^{t2} is the area under the drug concentration–time curve for the same interval as determined by the trapezoidal rule.

Statistical Analysis. Group data and pharmacokinetic values were evaluated by one-way analysis of variance (ANOVA) to detect differences among groups A, B, and C. The a priori level of significance was set at $p \leq 0.05$.

Results

The intravenous administration of ceftriaxone resulted in no local pain or phlebitis in any of the study subjects. No important systemic toxicities occurred during or after drug administration. One patient complained of a transient metallic taste, two patients experienced mild diarrhea for one day, and one patient had one episode of vomiting immediately after the infusion. Poststudy laboratory test values were not substantially different from prestudy tests.

Plasma concentrations of ceftriaxone at the conclusion of the infusion (peak concentration) were similar in the three study groups (mean ± S.D. plasma concentration 122 ± 53.1 μg/mL). Likewise, the plasma concentrations of ceftriaxone measured 24 hours after drug administration (mean ± S.D. 20.2 ± 6.14 μg/mL) were similar for the three groups. Table 2 lists the mean pharmacokinetic values calculated for each group. Except for renal clearance, there were no significant differences among the

Table 2.
Ceftriaxone Pharmacokinetic Variables by Study Group

Variable	Mean (± S.D.) Value by Group			Variance Ratio (*F*)
	A ($n = 5$)	B ($n = 6$)	C ($n = 3$)	
Zero-time intercept A (μg/mL)	57.5 ± 68.4	36.8 ± 12.8	39.4 ± 15.0	0.350
Zero-time intercept B (μg/mL)	71.8 ± 23.9	71.0 ± 11.3	71.3 ± 30.1	0.002
Elimination rate constant α (hr^{-1})	51.0 ± 109	0.813 ± 0.387	1.66 ± 0.191	0.926
Elimination rate constant β (hr^{-1})	0.044 ± 0.013	0.059 ± 0.017	0.058 ± 0.019	1.290
AUC (μg·hr/mL)[a]	1672 ± 347	1348 ± 364	1251 ± 296	1.784
V_{ss} (L/kg)[b]	0.240 ± 0.106	0.168 ± 0.031	0.195 ± 0.038	1.509
CL (mL/min/1.73 sq m)[c]	10.6 ± 1.77	12.1 ± 3.31	12.9 ± 1.25	0.940
CL_R (mL/min/1.73 sq m)[d]	1.24 ± 0.371	1.13 ± 0.239	2.60 ± 0.598	6.449

[a] Area under plasma concentration–time curve.
[b] Steady-state volume of distribution.
[c] Total body clearance of ceftriaxone.
[d] Renal clearance of ceftriaxone; significantly different among the groups.

Table 3.
Ceftriaxone Excretion in Urine during 48 Hours after Dose

Collection Interval (hr)	Amount (mg) of Ceftriaxone in Urine[a]		
	Group A	Group B	Group C
0–2	14.1 ± 8.15[b]	15.4 ± 5.02	29.9 ± 22.5
2–4	9.71 ± 5.53	10.6 ± 5.78[c]	28.7 ± 24.4[d]
4–6	7.67 ± 5.32[b]	10.4 ± 4.78	21.9 ± 9.57
6–8	12.4 ± 7.10	9.26 ± 2.74[b]	17.6 ± 9.27
8–12	11.2 ± 6.16	9.98 ± 3.45	21.6 ± 7.96
12–18	16.6 ± 7.46	16.8 ± 4.92[b]	20.0 ± 1.57
18–24	11.8 ± 5.90[b]	10.1 ± 3.36[b]	21.9 ± 17.3
24–48	24.2 ± 8.70[e]	28.1 ± 6.94[e]	34.5 ± 1.48[d]
0–48[f]	108	111	196

[a] Mean ± S.D.; $n = 5$ for group A, 6 for group B, 3 for group C unless otherwise indicated.
[b] Computed from four samples.
[c] Computed from five samples.
[d] Computed from two samples.
[e] Computed from three samples.
[f] Total amount excreted unchanged; this represents 10.8%, 11.1%, and 19.6% of the total dose for Groups A, B, and C, respectively.

groups. Table 3 gives the amounts of ceftriaxone excreted in the urine for groups A, B, and C. Approximately 10.8%, 11.1%, and 19.6%, respectively of ceftriaxone was excreted unchanged in the urine in the first 48 hours after drug administration in groups A, B, and C, respectively. Percentages excreted within the first 24 hours were 8.35%, 7.25%, and 16.2%, respectively, for the three groups. No evidence of concentration dependence for renal clearance of ceftriaxone was noted, since no trend was observed when the renal clearance of ceftriaxone was calculated for each urine-collection interval. When plotting the cumulative amount of ceftriaxone excreted unchanged in the urine versus the area under the plasma concentration–time curve, the correlation coefficient was ≥0.97.

Discussion

Ceftriaxone is an expanded-spectrum cephalosporin antibiotic with in vitro antibacterial activity against gram-positive and gram-negative organisms. Pharmacokinetic studies in humans with normal renal function[8] and in anephric patients[7] have shown plasma half-life for intravenously administered ceftriaxone to be 6.5–8.6 hours and 12 hours, respectively.

In this evaluation of the pharmacokinetics of ceftriaxone in patients with impaired renal function, nonlinear, two-compartment pharmacokinetic analysis was used to show that the half-life of ceftriaxone, in subjects with normal liver function, was not significantly different between the groups studied and was only slightly greater than that observed in normal adult volunteers. The renal clearance of ceftriaxone, expressed as a percentage of total body clearance, ranges from 35 to 60% in subjects with normal renal function.[8,15–18] In our subjects the renal clearance of ceftriaxone was 12%, 9%, and 20% of the total body clearance for groups A, B, and C, respectively; these results emphasize the nonrenal route of drug elimination. The difference in renal clearance of ceftriaxone probably reflects Type I error and should not be considered clinically important. Other authors have observed the concentration dependence of the renal clearance of ceftriaxone,[19] but this was not our experience. Possible explanations might be that plasma concentrations of ceftriaxone in our study (Figure 1) were not as high as those in Figure 2 of reference number 19 and that our infusion time was 30 minutes compared with the 5 minutes used in the previous study.[19]

The slight variability in the pharmacokinetics of ceftriaxone in our study subjects suggests that if substantial changes in serum concentrations are observed, renal function is unlikely to be the cause. Hemodialysis[20] and peritoneal dialysis[18] have little effect on the clearance of ceftriaxone; therefore, substantial changes in elimination might be the result of hepatic disease affecting the nonrenal elimination of ceftriaxone. Although it was not within the scope of this study to evaluate the biliary elimination of ceftriaxone, the drug may accumulate in patients with both hepatic and renal insufficiency. In such patients, monitoring plasma concentrations might be appropriate.

Conclusion

Our results suggest that a ceftriaxone dose of 1 g every 24 hours in patients with renal insufficiency would be more than adequate to inhibit the majority of susceptible gram-positive and gram-negative microorganisms. Such patients have elimination rates for ceftriaxone similar to those of normal patients, so dosage adjustment is not needed.

References

1. Angehrn P, Probst PJ, Reiner R et al. Ro 13-9904, a long-acting broad-spectrum cephalosporin: In vitro and in vivo studies. *Antimicrob Agents Chemother.* 1980; 18:913–21.
2. Eickhoff TC, Ehert J. Comparative in vitro studies of Ro 13-9904, a new cephalosporin derivative. *Antimicrob Agents Chemother.* 1981; 19:435–42.
3. Hall MJ, Westmacott D, Wong-Kai-In P. Comparative in vitro activity and mode of action of ceftriaxone (Ro 13-9904), a new highly potent cephalosporin. *J Antimicrob Chemother.* 1981; 8:193–203.
4. Hinkle AM, Bodey GP. In vitro evaluation of Ro 13-9904. *Antimicrob Agents Chemother.* 1980; 18:574–8.
5. Neu HC, Metropol NJ, Fu KP. Antibacterial activity of ceftriaxone (Ro 13-9904), a B-lactamase-stable cephalosporin. *Antimicrob Agents Chemother.* 1981; 19:414–23.
6. Seddon M, Wise R, Gillett AP et al. Pharmacokinetics of Ro 13-9904, a broad-spectrum cephalosporin. *Antimicrob Agents Chemother.* 1980; 18:240–2.
7. Stoeckel K, McNamara PJ, Hoppe-Seyler G et al. Single-dose ceftriaxone kinetics in functionally anephric patients. *Clin Pharmacol Ther.* 1983; 33:633–41.
8. Patel IH, Chen S, Parsonnet M et al. Pharmacokinetics of ceftriaxone in humans. *Antimicrob Agents Chemother.* 1981; 20:634–41.
9. Cadoz M, Denis F, Felix H et al. Treatment of purulent meningitis with a new caphalosporin—Rocephin (Ro 13-9904). *Chemotherapy.* 1981; 27:57–61.
10. Del Rio M, Chrane D, Shelton S et al. Ceftriaxone versus ampicillin and chloramphenicol for treatment of bacterial meningitis in children. *Lancet.* 1983; 1:1241–4.
11. Latif R, Dajani AS. Ceftriaxone diffusion into cerebrospinal fluid of children with meningitis. *Antimicrob Agents Chemother.* 1983; 23:46–8.
12. Reed MD, Rekate HL, Arnoff SC et al. Single-dose plasma and cerebrospinal fluid pharmacokinetics of ceftriaxone in infants and children. *Clin Pharm.* 1983; 2:558–63.
13. Ray AA, ed. SAS User's Guide. Cary, NC: SAS Institute Inc.; 1982.
14. Wagner JG et al. Pharmacokinetic parameters estimated from intravenous data by uniform methods and some of their uses. *J Pharmacokinet Biopharm.* 1977; 5:161–82.
15. Luderer JR, Patel IH, Durkin J et al. Age and ceftriaxone kinetics. *Clin Pharmacol Ther.* 1984; 35:19–25.
16. Patel IH, Weinfeld RE, Konikoff J et al. Pharmacokinetics and tolerance of ceftriaxone in humans after single-dose intramuscular administration in water and lidocaine diluent. *Antimicrob Agents Chemother.* 1982; 21:957–62.
17. Pollock AA, Tee PE, Patel IH et al. Pharmacokinetic characteristics of intravenous ceftriaxone in normal adults. *Antimicrob Agents Chemother.* 1982; 22:816–23.
18. Ti T, Fortin L, Kreet JH et al. Kinetic disposition of intravenous ceftriaxone in normal subjects and patients with renal failure on hemodialysis or peritoneal dialysis. *Antimicrob Agents Chemother.* 1984; 25:83–7.
19. Stoeckel K, McNamara PJ, Brandt R et al. Effects of concentration-dependent plasma protein binding on ceftriaxone kinetics. *Clin Pharmacol Ther.* 1981; 29:650–7.
20. Cohen D, Appel GB, Scully B et al. Pharmacokinetics of ceftriaxone in patients with renal failure and in those undergoing hemodialysis. *Antimicrob Agents Chemother.* 1983; 24:529–32.

"

An Ounce of Prevention Is Worth . . .

Human liver transplantation has ceased to be an experimental technique and now offers the potential for prolonged survival of good quality to a substantial number of individuals. The best results with hepatic transplantation have been obtained in children, the main indications being biliary atresia and metabolic defects such as Wilson's disease and alpha-1-antitrypsin deficiency. . . .

As experience and success with liver transplantation improves and physicians and surgeons become more adventurous, we should begin to look at potential needs and costs. Evans [Evans RW. Issues in liver transplantation. *Lancet.* 1983; 2:1306.] has estimated that the cost of a liver transplant is somewhere between $70,000 and $240,000, the former being nearer the realistic cost of a child transplant, the latter that in an adult. In American terms these costs are about those of a heart transplant and five times those of a renal transplant. The limited statistical data on the incidence of end-stage liver disease indicate that there may be at least 2000 potential liver recipients a year in the United States alone. . . .

The . . . most searching question concerns what priority should be given to liver transplantation, in relation not only to transplantation of other organs, but also to the less spectacular aspects of prevention and early detection of liver disease.

—Anon. Liver transplantation 1985 and beyond. *Lancet.* 1985; 1:27–8. Editorial.

"

Altered gentamicin pharmacokinetics during the perioperative period

DWIGHT D. KLOTH, BERNARD R. TEGTMEIER, CLIFFORD KONG, MICHAEL P. AKAHOSHI, STACIE HAYASE LEACH, J. DAVID BEATTY, AND JOHN A. ZAIA

Abstract: The effect of surgery on the pharmacokinetics of gentamicin sulfate in hospitalized patients was studied.

Patients with cancer undergoing surgery of the head and neck were given gentamicin sulfate in doses calculated to achieve peak serum concentrations of 6–8 μg/mL and trough concentrations of 1–2 μg/mL. Each patient received a loading dose at the time of surgical incision, followed by five maintenance doses at eight-hour intervals. Steady-state peak and trough serum gentamicin concentrations were predicted using a one-compartment open pharmacokinetic model and literature values for volume of distribution (*V*) and first-order elimination rate constant (*k*). Serum gentamicin concentrations were measured 0.25 hours before and at 0.5, 3.5, and 6.5 hours after completion of infusion of the second maintenance dose. Peak and trough serum concentrations were obtained by extrapolation from these measured concentrations using weighted, nonlinear least squares regression. Predicted versus measured serum gentamicin concentrations and estimated versus observed values for *V* and *k* were compared.

Eight men and seven women had evaluable serum gentamicin concentrations. Patients received a mean calculated maintenance dose of 4.4 ± 0.7 mg/kg/day. Mean extrapolated peak and trough serum gentamicin concentrations were significantly lower than predicted, and observed values of *V* and *k* were significantly greater than estimated values.

Gentamicin dosages calculated using standard pharmacokinetic variable values may not produce therapeutic concentrations in patients undergoing surgery. Monitoring of serum concentrations with dosage adjustment when indicated is necessary for optimal therapy in these patients.

Index terms: Aminoglycosides; Blood levels; Dosage; Drugs, body distribution; Excretion; Gentamicin; Gentamicin sulfate; Pharmacokinetics; Rate constants; Surgery
Clin Pharm. 1985; 4:182–5

In addition to the treatment of serious gram-negative infections, gentamicin or other aminoglycosides are sometimes used along with other injectable antibiotics for perioperative prophylaxis in surgical procedures.[1] Because of the relatively narrow margin between therapeutic and toxic gentamicin serum concentrations, a number of investigators have studied the relationship of gentamicin dose to serum concentration in order to develop pharmacokinetic models[2–4] and dosing nomograms[5] for the calculation of optimal dosing regimens. These pharmacokinetic models and dosing nomograms are generally based on "average" patient values for pharmacokinetic variables.

The pharmacokinetics of gentamicin are known to be affected by factors such as fever,[2] obesity,[6] age,[7] and ascites.[8] While the metabolism of hepatically cleared drugs has been studied,[9] the effect of surgery on the pharmacokinetics of renally excreted drugs has not been as well examined.[10]

We conducted this study to determine whether there were any consistent deviations between expected and actual gentamicin concentrations in a group of cancer patients receiving prophylactic gentamicin and cefoxitin for complex surgical resections of head and neck tumors, when a priori gentamicin dosing was determined with a pharmacokinetic model.

Methods

Written informed consent was obtained from each patient before enrollment in the study; institutional review board approval was also obtained. All patients received a loading dose of gentamicin sulfate in the operating room at the time of the first operative incision, followed by five maintenance doses at eight-hour intervals. Loading and maintenance doses were calculated to achieve peak serum concentrations of 6–8 μg/mL and trough concentrations

DWIGHT D. KLOTH, PHARM.D., is Clinical Pharmacist, Department of Pharmacy Services; BERNARD R. TEGTMEIER, PH.D., is Medical Microbiologist, Department of Infectious Diseases; and CLIFFORD KONG, PHARM.D., is Clinical Pharmacist, Department of Pharmacy Services, City of Hope National Medical Center, Duarte, CA. MICHAEL P. AKAHOSHI, PHARM.D., is Clinical Pharmacist, Hoag Memorial Hospital Presbyterian, Newport Beach, CA; at the time of this study, he was Clinical Pharmacist, Department of Pharmacy Services, City of Hope National Medical Center; STACIE HAYASE LEACH, PHARM.D., is Clinical Pharmacist, Department of Pharmacy Services; J. DAVID BEATTY, M.D., is Surgeon, Department of General Oncologic Surgery; and JOHN A. ZAIA, M.D., is Director of Virology and Infectious Diseases, Division of Pediatrics, City of Hope National Medical Center.

Address reprint requests to Dr. Kloth at the City of Hope National Medical Center, 1500 East Duarte Road, Duarte, CA 91010.

The assistance of Robert J. Hayashi, Pharm.D., in conducting this study, Roger W. Jelliffe, M.D., for donation of computer time for pharmacokinetic analysis, and Karen Moss and Dian De Sha for secretarial support is acknowledged.

of 1–2 μg/mL. For patients considered obese, i.e., actual body weight (ABW) more than 10% greater than ideal body weight (IBW), the dosing weight for gentamicin was calculated as follows[6]:

$$\text{Dosing weight} = \text{IBW} + 0.4(\text{ABW} - \text{IBW})$$

Loading doses were infused over 30 minutes; maintenance doses were administered over a 60-minute period. A Hewlett-Packard HP 85 programmable calculator was used to calculate loading and maintenance doses and to predict steady-state peak and trough serum gentamicin concentrations ($C_{ss_{max}}$ and $C_{ss_{min}}$, respectively) using the one-compartment open pharmacokinetic model described by Sawchuk and Zaske.[2] The following equations were used in these calculations:

$$D_L = C_{max}kVT/(1 - e^{-kT})$$

$$D_M = C_{max}kVT(1 - e^{-k\tau})/(1 - e^{-kT})$$

$$C_{ss_{max}} = R_o(1 - e^{-kT})/kV(1 - e^{-k\tau})$$

$$C_{ss_{min}} = R_o(e^{kT} - 1)/kV(e^{k\tau} - 1)$$

where D_L is the loading dose in mg, C_{max} is the desired peak serum gentamicin concentration in μg/mL, k is the first-order elimination rate constant in hours^{-1}, V is the volume of distribution in L/kg, T is the infusion time in hours, D_M is the maintenance dose in mg, τ is the dosing interval in hours, and R_o is the infusion rate of gentamicin in mg/hr.

The a priori model assumed a volume of distribution of 0.25 L/kg.[2] Creatinine clearance (CL_{cr}) was estimated by the method of Jelliffe.[11] The first-order elimination rate constant for gentamicin was calculated using the following equation[3,12]:

$$k = 0.0032CL_{cr} + 0.00693$$

Gentamicin clearance (CL) was calculated using the following equation:

$$CL = kV$$

Serum gentamicin concentrations were measured 0.25 hours before the second maintenance dose and at 0.5, 3.5, and 6.5 hours following the completion of infusion of the second maintenance dose. Gentamicin concentrations were determined using an enzyme immunoassay, EMIT (Syva, Palo Alto, CA). Peak and trough serum gentamicin concentrations were extrapolated from measured concentrations using a weighted, nonlinear least-squares regression program assuming a one-compartment pharmacokinetic model.[13]

The differences between predicted and extrapolated serum gentamicin concentrations and between estimated and observed k values were analyzed with the Student's t test for paired data. The difference between the observed volume of distribution and the a priori volume of distribution was analyzed with the Student's t test for the comparison of a sample mean with a population parameter. The degree of association between variables was analyzed with the Kendall coefficient of rank correlation. All differences with a $p < 0.05$ were considered to be significant.

Results

Of 17 patients with cancer of the head and neck who received perioperative gentamicin and cefoxitin, two were not evaluable because of missed serum gentamicin concentrations.

The 15 evaluable patients ranged in age from 52 to 75 years, with a mean ± S.D. age of 66 ± 5.7 years. The group consisted of eight men and seven women. Measured serum creatinine concentrations in these patients ranged from 0.6 to 1.7 mg/dL, with a mean of 1.0 ± 0.2 mg/dL. Estimated creatinine clearance ranged from 39 to 80 mL/min/1.73 sq m, with a mean of 57 ± 11 mL/min/1.73 sq m. Patient weight ranged from 46 to 88.6 kg, with a mean of 62.5 ± 13.3 kg. After correction for obesity, dosing weights ranged from 46 to 88.6 kg, with a mean of 62.5 ± 13.0 kg. With the possible exception of obesity, no factors known to alter gentamicin pharmacokinetics were present in the study population.

Calculated maintenance doses of gentamicin ranged from 60 to 130 mg every eight hours, with a mean dose of 91 ± 19 mg every eight hours (3.0–5.8 mg/kg/day, mean 4.4 ± 0.7 mg/kg/day). The differences between predicted and extrapolated peak and trough serum gentamicin concentrations are presented in Table 1. The extrapolated peak concentrations were markedly lower than predicted concentrations in 14 (93%) of the 15 patients studied. Also, the mean extrapolated peak and trough concentrations were both significantly lower than predicted concentrations for this group of patients.

The estimated and observed values of pharmacokinetic variables for this group of patients are summarized in Table 2. The observed elimination rate constants were significantly greater than those that were based on preoperative estimates of creatinine clearance and used to calculate gentamicin doses. Analysis of the serum concentration data also revealed that the observed volumes of distribution for this group of patients were significantly greater than the a priori value (0.25 L/kg). As a direct result of the higher values for elimination rate constant and volume of distribution in these patients, values for total body clearance of gentamicin were higher than predicted.

In an attempt to explain these findings, the medical records of the study patients were reviewed. Complete data on fluid intake and output for the day of surgery were available on 14 of the 15 patients studied. All 14 patients were in positive fluid balance (not corrected for insensible loss), which ranged from 0.8 to 5.5 liters (0.009–0.073 L/kg); mean ± S.D. excess fluid per patient was 2.4 ± 1.3 liters (0.039 ± 0.02 L/kg). The degree of fluid overload, on

Table 1.
Predicted versus Extrapolated[a] Serum Gentamicin Concentrations in Study Patients

Patient No.	Age (yr)	Sex	Dosing Weight (kg)	Peak Concentrations (μg/mL) Predicted	Extrapolated	Difference	Trough Concentrations (μg/mL) Predicted	Extrapolated	Difference
1	68	M	55.0	7.8	3.4	4.4	1.9	0.6	1.3
2	70	F	59.5	7.0	4.6	2.4	1.9	1.0	0.9
3	52	M	46.0	7.0	3.5	3.5	1.1	0.8	0.3
4	64	F	60.2	6.4	3.7	2.7	1.8	0.3	1.5
5	64	M	88.6	7.0	4.7	2.3	1.6	0.9	0.7
6	75	F	59.1	4.9	2.3	2.6	1.4	0.6	0.8
7	68	F	47.0	6.5	4.7	1.8	2.1	1.0	1.1
8	72	M	60.0	7.8	6.0	1.8	2.1	1.6	0.5
9	57	F	56.8	8.4	5.9	2.5	1.8	1.1	0.7
10	70	M	80.6	6.3	3.8	2.5	1.7	0.5	1.2
11	68	F	56.7	6.4	5.3	1.1	1.6	0.8	0.8
12	67	M	60.2	6.8	4.4	2.4	1.7	1.0	0.7
13	67	M	78.9	6.1	4.2	1.9	1.7	0.5	1.2
14	64	F	52.5	6.8	6.6	0.2	1.6	0.9	0.7
15[b]	65	M	69.5	7.9	5.8	2.1	3.4	1.1	2.3
Mean ± S.D.	66.1 ± 5.7		62.0 ± 12.2	6.9 ± 0.9	4.6 ± 1.2	2.3 ± 1.0	1.8 ± 0.5	0.8 ± 0.3	1.0 ± 0.5

[a] Extrapolated from measured serum concentrations using linear regression analysis.
[b] The a priori serum concentration goals were more aggressive in this patient.

Table 2.
Estimated versus Observed Values for Pharmacokinetic Variables in Study Patients

Patient No.	Dose (mg/kg/day)	*k* (hours^{-1}) Estimated	Observed	*V* (L/kg) Estimated	Observed	CL (L/hr/kg) Estimated	Observed
1	5.2	0.20	0.25	0.25	0.52	0.05	0.13
2	4.5	0.19	0.22	0.25	0.35	0.05	0.08
3	5.2	0.26	0.20	0.25	0.56	0.06	0.11
4	4.0	0.18	0.36	0.25	0.32	0.04	0.11
5	4.4	0.17	0.22	0.25	0.35	0.04	0.08
6	3.0	0.18	0.18	0.25	0.50	0.04	0.09
7	3.8	0.13	0.23	0.25	0.29	0.03	0.07
8	5.0	0.17	0.18	0.25	0.32	0.04	0.06
9	5.8	0.25	0.24	0.25	0.33	0.06	0.08
10	4.5	0.19	0.29	0.25	0.35	0.05	0.11
11	4.2	0.20	0.27	0.25	0.26	0.05	0.07
12	4.5	0.20	0.21	0.25	0.37	0.05	0.08
13	3.8	0.20	0.29	0.25	0.31	0.05	0.09
14	4.6	0.16	0.28	0.25	0.22	0.04	0.06
15	3.9	0.15	0.24	0.25	0.24	0.04	0.06
Mean ± S.D.	4.4 ± 0.7	0.19 ± 0.03	0.24 ± 0.05	0.25 ± 0.00	0.35 ± 0.10	0.05 ± 0.01	0.09 ± 0.02

a weight basis, appeared to be associated with the differences noted between predicted and extrapolated gentamicin serum concentrations, although statistical significance was not demonstrated (Kendall coefficient of rank correlation = 0.3889, $p < 0.06$).

Discussion

In the present study, the use of an a priori pharmacokinetic model resulted in dosages higher than the often used "80 mg q 8 hours" regimen. Nevertheless, extrapolated serum concentrations were significantly lower than those predicted by the pharmacokinetic model, suggesting that the pharmacokinetic behavior of gentamicin is markedly altered during the perioperative period. Pharmacokinetic analysis of the serum concentration data revealed higher values for *k*, *V*, and CL than those estimated by the a priori model.[2,3,12]

The reason for these changes in gentamicin pharmacokinetics is not entirely clear. None of the patients had characteristics known to influence gentamicin pharmacokinetics, such as fever, ascites, or concomitant use of carbenicillin or ticarcillin. While not significant, the apparent association between degree of fluid overload and the difference between predicted and extrapolated serum concentrations suggests that the altered pharmacokinetics noted in the present study may be partly related to the altered hydration state of the patient during the perioperative period.

In a study of 242 surgical patients, Zaske et al.[3] noted alterations in volume of distribution as a result of pathophysiological changes. Those patients with peritonitis or congestive heart failure had larger volumes of distribution and thus required larger doses to achieve therapeutic concentrations. Conversely, patients thought to be clinically dehydrated had low distribution volumes and required less drug to reach optimal concentrations. Although these investigators did not indicate whether gentamicin half-life was influenced by the hydration state of the patients in their study, it seems reasonable that the administration of large volumes of crystalloid, colloid, and blood products during complex surgery could result in increased renal clearance as the kidneys respond to this fluid challenge.

From the results of our study, it would appear that gentamicin dosing based on standard pharmacokinetic values can often result in subtherapeutic serum concentrations in the surgical patient receiving large volumes of fluids during surgery. While it is not known what effect "subtherapeutic" serum concentrations may have on the outcome of surgical prophylaxis, these observations may have even more important implications for the perioperative management of surgical patients with serious gram-negative infection. The management of these patients may be further complicated by the possibility of changing pharmacokinetic behavior during the immediate postoperative period. Additional studies will need to examine this possibility by identifying the pharmacokinetic behavior during the preoperative, intraoperative, and postoperative periods. Studies of this nature will be necessary before the effects of surgery on gentamicin pharmacokinetics are fully understood.

Conclusion

Until the pharmacokinetic behavior of gentamicin during the perioperative period is more completely understood, gentamicin dosages calculated preoperatively using standard pharmacokinetic variable values cannot be relied on to produce therapeutic concentrations during the perioperative period. Appropriate monitoring and analysis of serum gentamicin concentrations, with appropriate dosage adjustment where needed, remains the definitive method of achieving optimal dosing regimens in this patient population.

References

1. Guglielmo BJ, Hohn DC, Koo PJ. Antibiotic prophylaxis in surgical procedures: a critical analysis of the literature. *Arch Surg.* 1983; 118:943–55.
2. Sawchuk RJ, Zaske DE. Pharmacokinetics of dosing regimens which utilize multiple intravenous infusions: gentamicin in burn patients. *J Pharmacokinet Biopharm.* 1976; 4:183–95.
3. Zaske DE, Cipolle RJ, Strate RJ. Gentamicin dosage requirements: wide interpatient variations in 242 surgery patients with normal renal function. *Surgery.* 1980; 87:164–9.
4. Sawchuck RJ, Zaske DE, Cipolle RJ et al. Kinetic model for gentamicin dosing with the use of individual patient parameters. *Clin Pharmacol Ther.* 1977; 21:362–9.
5. Sarubbi FA, Hull JH. Amikacin serum concentrations: predictions of levels and dosage guidelines. *Ann Intern Med.* 1978; 89 (Part I): 612–8.
6. Schwartz SN, Pazin GJ, Lyon JA et al. A controlled investigation of the pharmacokinetics of gentamicin and tobramycin in obese subjects. *J Infect Dis.* 1978; 138:499–505.
7. Zaske DE, Sawchuk RJ, Strate RG. The necessity of increased doses of amikacin in burn patients. *Surgery.* 1978; 84:603–8.
8. Gill MA, Kern JW. Altered gentamicin distribution in ascitic patients. *Am J Hosp Pharm.* 1979; 36:1704–6.
9. Elfstrom J. Drug pharmacokinetics in the postoperative period. *Clin Pharmacokinet.* 1979; 4:16–22.
10. Lucas CE. The renal response to acute injury and sepsis. *Surg Clin North Am.* 1976; 56:953–75.
11. Jelliffe RW. Creatinine clearance: bedside estimate. *Ann Intern Med.* 1973; 79:604–5.
12. Jelliffe RW, Knight R, Buell J et al. Computer assistance for gentamicin therapy (USC*PACK). *Clin Res.* 1970; 18:441.
13. Forrest A, Gilman T, Rodman J et al. A time-shared computer program for adaptive control of aminoglycoside therapy. *Clin Pharmacol Ther.* 1980; 27:254.

Predicting plasma procainamide concentrations resulting from a sustained-release preparation

DAVID M. DIPERSIO AND MOSES S.S. CHOW

Abstract: Two methods of predicting plasma procainamide concentrations (PPCs) for a sustained-release procainamide (SRP) dosage form were compared using previously published data on 12 healthy subjects.

Methods A and B were both based on a one-compartment pharmacokinetic model requiring an elimination rate constant and area under the concentration–time curve from an immediate-release oral procainamide dosage form and in vitro dissolution data from the SRP product. Method A also used an absorption rate constant. The predicted versus measured PPCs for two sets of peak and trough concentrations in each subject were evaluated using linear regression.

The mean predicted PPCs by both methods followed the measured PPCs closely; however, the time of peak concentration was predicted more accurately by method A. The evaluation of predictive performance showed good precision and a small but statistically significant bias with either method; peak values were overpredicted and trough values were underpredicted.

These two methods adequately predicted plasma procainamide concentrations in healthy subjects following a sustained-release procainamide preparation.

Index terms: Absorption; Blood levels; Cardiac drugs; Dosage forms; Excretion; Methodology; Models; Pharmacokinetics; Procainamide; Procainamide hydrochloride; Rate constants; Sustained-action medications
Clin Pharm. 1985; 4:186–91

The use of pharmacokinetic methods to predict in vivo serum or plasma concentrations of drugs on the basis of in vitro dissolution rate has been described.[1–7] Good correlations between predicted and measured serum concentrations following the administration of sustained-release theophylline have been shown in human subjects.[2,3,6–8] Whether these methods are useful for predicting plasma concentrations of other sustained-release preparations is unknown. The purpose of this study was to evaluate two of these methods in predicting the plasma procainamide concentrations at steady-state following a sustained-release procainamide (SRP) preparation.

Methods

Data from a study published by Smith and Kinkel[9] on SRP were used for the present study. In the previous study, plasma procainamide concentrations (PPCs) were determined in 12 healthy volunteers in a crossover study using either 250-mg capsules of procainamide hydrochloride (Pronestyl hydrochloride, E. R. Squibb & Sons lot 43151), an immediate-release procainamide (IRP) given every three hours for 18 doses, or a 500-mg SRP tablet (Procan-SR, Parke-Davis and Company, lot RX-43021) given every six hours for a total of nine doses. PPCs were determined hourly from 0 to 6 hours and from 24 to 30 hours following the initial administration of each formulation. Additionally, PPCs were determined before and 1, 2, 3, 4, 5, 6, 9, 12, and 15 hours after the last dose of each formulation. PPCs were determined in duplicate using a high-pressure liquid chromatography (HPLC) assay. The coefficient of variation of this assay was 2.5% at procainamide concentrations of 2.5 mg/L and 5.6% at concentrations of 1.0 mg/L.

Before predicting PPCs, individual pharmacokinetic values were determined following the administration of IRP. The slope of the log-linear portion of the plasma procainamide concentration–time curve for the IRP ($-k$) was calculated for each subject using least-squares regression. The area under the concentration–time curve (AUC) for the IRP was calculated using a summation of linear trapezoidal measurements.[10] The steady-state AUC for a six-hour dosing interval was calculated for IRP as the mean of two six-hour dosing intervals, 24–30 hours and 48–54 hours for each subject. (No difference was observed between the AUCs of these dosing intervals.) The determination of the apparent volume of distribution (V) and fraction of procainamide absorbed orally (F) was not possible because the information following i.v. administration was not known.[10] Therefore, the composite term V/F

DAVID M. DIPERSIO, PHARM.D., is Clinical Pharmacy Fellow, Hartford Hospital, Hartford, CT, and Assistant Clinical Professor, School of Pharmacy, University of Connecticut, Storrs. MOSES S. S. CHOW, PHARM.D., is Director, Drug Information Services, Department of Pharmacy, Hartford Hospital, and Associate Clinical Professor, School of Pharmacy, University of Connecticut.

Address reprint requests to Dr. Chow at the Drug Information Center, Hartford Hospital, 80 Seymour Street, Hartford, CT 06115.

The assistance of Parke–Davis and Company, Division of Warner-Lambert Co., Detroit, MI, in supplying raw data used in this study is acknowledged.

Presented at the 19th Annual ASHP Midyear Clinical Meeting, Dallas, TX, December 4, 1984.

was determined from the following equation:

$V/F = \text{Dose}/[(\text{AUC})(k)]$

In addition to the pharmacokinetic values, the in vitro dissolution rate and fraction of sustained-release for SRP were determined. The in vitro dissolution data of the SRP product used were obtained from the manufacturer. The dissolution test was performed using six SRP tablets dissolved in water at 37 °C with the USP rotating basket apparatus set at 100 revolutions/minute. Based on the dissolution data, a plot was made of log (1 − cumulative fraction dissolved) versus time (Figure 1). The apparent dissolution rate constant (k_d) was calculated as the negative slope of the log-linear portion of the curve,[1,11] and the sustained-release fraction of procainamide available was determined as the y-intercept of the line. The immediate-release fraction was calculated as 1 − sustained-release fraction (Figure 1).

Prediction Methods. Two methods were used to predict the PPCs reported in the study by Smith and Kinkel.[9]

Method A is a modification of a method proposed by Wiegand and Taylor (Appendix A).[1] This method predicts PPC at any time after a single dose when the immediate- and sustained-release fraction, in vitro

Figure 1. Semilogarithmic plot of (1 − cumulative fraction dissolved) versus time.

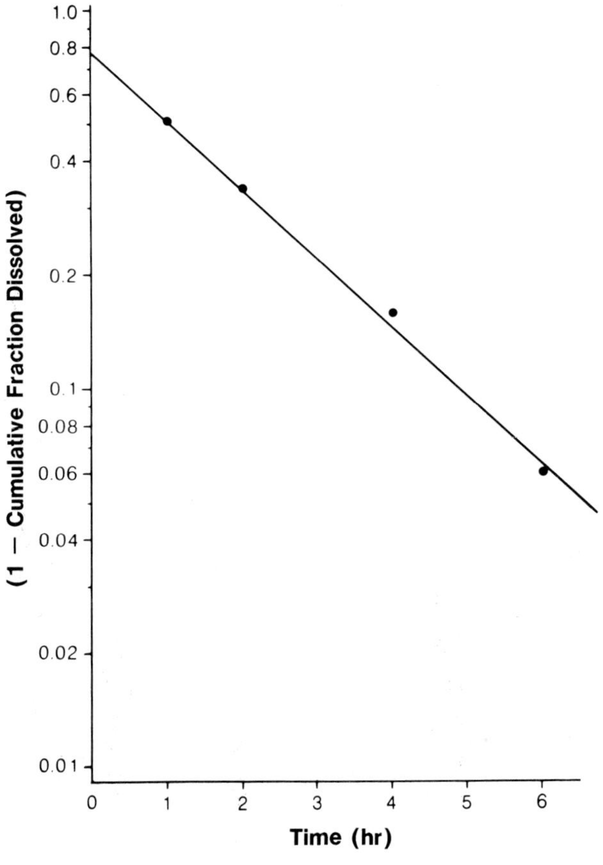

apparent dissolution rate (k_d) of the SRP, and the absorption rate (k_{01}), elimination rate (k), and AUC of the IRP are known. The specific dissolution data and pharmacokinetic values were obtained as described. A mean literature value of 2 hr^{-1} was used as the k_{01} for procainamide[12] since insufficient blood samples were available in the study by Smith and Kinkel[9] to determine absorption rate accurately.

Method B is a modification of a Wagner–Nelson pharmacokinetic model[13] originally proposed by Heimlich et al.[7] Detailed equations for the original method[7,8] are shown in Appendix B. This method estimates PPC following a single oral dose when the AUC and k of the immediate-release product and cumulative fraction of the sustained-release product dissolved in vitro are known. The individual values of AUC and k for the IRP were obtained from the data as described previously. The fraction of dose dissolved at any time was estimated from the linear interpolation of dissolution data. Since the in vitro dissolution data for the SRP used in this study was only known up to six hours (a time when 94% of the procainamide was released in vitro), the fraction of procainamide dissolved after six hours was estimated using the apparent first-order release rate (k_d) as determined from Figure 1. Dissolution was considered complete at 11 hours, when greater than 99% of the procainamide was predicted to be in solution. The prediction of PPCs for doses other than the first dose was done by using the method of superposition.[10]

Determination of Prediction Performance. In each subject, peak and trough PPCs (two and six hours, respectively) were predicted using data after the fifth and ninth SRP doses. In addition, PPCs during the washout phase following the administration of SRP were predicted.

The predictive performance in determination of peak and trough PPCs for each method was evaluated in the manner described by Sheiner and Beal.[14] Precision, as measured by the mean-squared prediction error (MSE), and bias, as measured by the mean prediction error (ME), and 95% confidence intervals for these values were determined. The difference in prediction performance between the two methods (change in MSE and change in ME and 95% confidence intervals) was calculated.

The relationship between predicted and measured peak and trough PPCs of SRP for each method was also evaluated by linear-regression analysis.

Results

The time course of the mean measured and predicted PPCs for both methods following the final SRP dose is shown in Figure 2. The mean predicted PPC by both methods followed the measured PPC closely. However, the time of peak concentration was predicted more accurately by method A than method B.

The predicted versus measured peak and trough PPCs for methods A and B are shown in Figures 3 and 4, respectively. Linear-regression analysis of all data points demonstrated good correlation between predicted and measured PPCs for both methods.

Precision as measured by MSE (95% confidence interval) and bias as measured by ME (95% confidence interval) for peak and trough PPCs and the predictive performance for method A relative to method B (change in MSE and change in ME) are shown in Table 1. Good precision was produced using either method; however, a small but statistically significant bias was evident in both peak and trough procainamide predictions (95% of peak PPC values being overpredicted and 95% of trough PPC values being underpredicted). Based on calculations of the changes in MSE and ME, method B was found

Figure 2. Mean plasma procainamide concentrations versus time following the final dose of sustained-release procainamide. Data points represent the mean values for 12 subjects for the measured (— X —) and predicted concentrations by both methods A (- - ● - -) and B (· · · O · · ·).

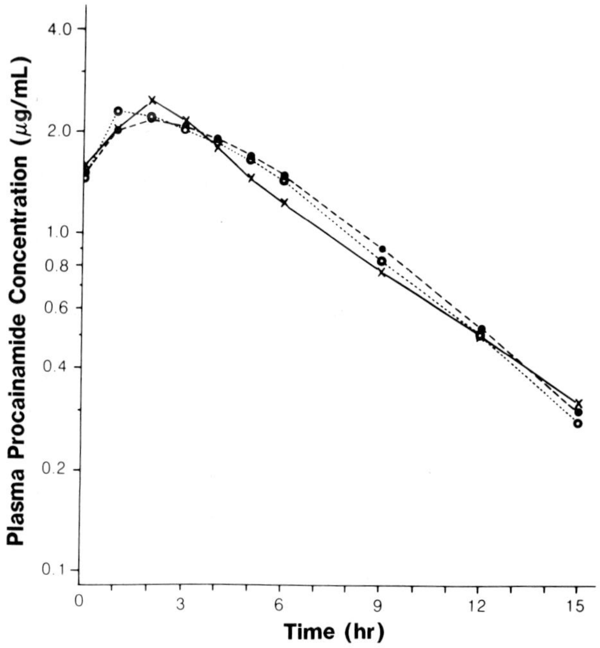

Figure 3. Measured versus predicted procainamide concentrations for two sets of peak (●) and trough (O) samples using method A.

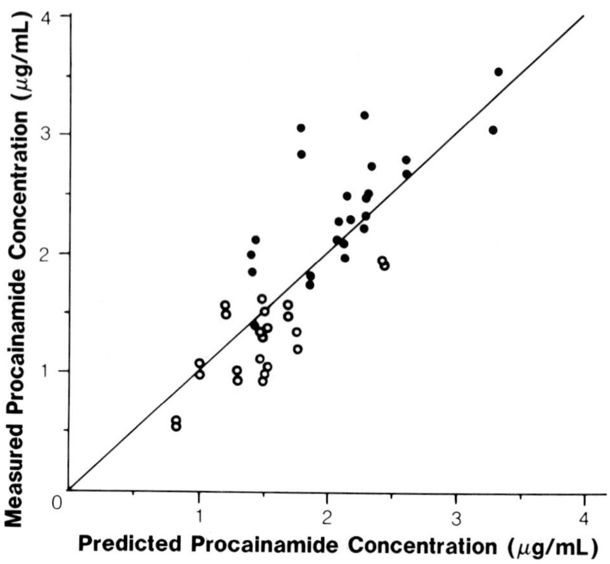

Figure 4. Measured versus predicted procainamide concentrations for two sets of peak (●) and trough (O) samples using method B.

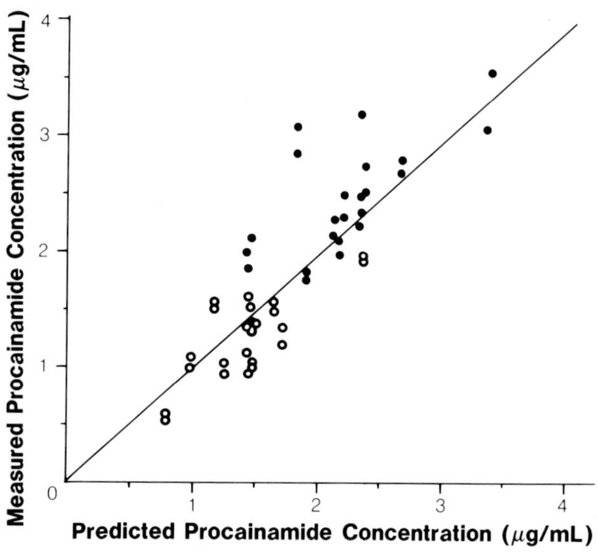

Table 1.
Performance Evaluation of Methods A and B Based on the Precision and Bias for the Peak and Trough Concentrations and the Predictive Performance of Method A Relative to Method B

Method	Precision		Bias	
	Peak	Trough	Peak	Trough
A[a]	0.223 (0.044, 0.402)	0.124 (0.078, 0.146)	−0.276 (−0.442, −0.111)	0.207 (0.093, 0.322)
B[a]	0.207 (−0.034, 0.380)	0.093 (0.056, 0.131)	−0.223 (−0.394, −0.051)	0.169 (0.056, 0.281)
A versus B[b]	0.016 (−0.004, 0.036)	0.027 (0.003, 0.052)	−0.054 (−0.043, 0.065)	0.036 (0.028, 0.044)

[a] Represents mean-squared prediction error for precision and mean prediction error for bias.
[b] Precision or bias of method A relative to method B.

to be more precise and less biased than method A in predicting trough PPC, but the magnitude of the difference between the two methods was quite small.

Discussion

We found that peak and trough PPCs following the administration of a SRP product (Procan SR) can be predicted by two methods that use in vitro dissolution and individual variables obtained from measured PPCs following oral IRP dosing. Although a small but statistically significant degree of bias was observed with both methods, the low MSE indicated that both methods A and B are relatively precise.

When using these two methods to predict PPCs, several assumptions are made. For method A, a one-compartment pharmacokinetic model is used to describe procainamide.[1,10] While this is too simplistic in describing procainamide pharmacokinetics, a one-compartment model with first-order absorption and elimination has been shown to be generally adequate for describing oral procainamide.[12,15,16] In using method A, it is assumed that a first-order dissolution rate follows an SRP dosage form. Examination of in vitro dissolution data for the SRP dosage form in our study (Figure 1) showed good approximation of first-order release. Thus, the pharmacokinetic and dissolution characteristics of SRP fit the theoretical considerations assumed in the use of this model, and this may account for the ability of method A to predict PPC.

In method A, we used an average absorption rate constant (k_{01}) reported in the literature for predicting individual PPCs. This may represent a potential source of prediction error. However, in a situation where a single rate is large relative to other rate constants used in the model, the smaller rate constants predominantly affect the shape of the plasma concentration–time curve.[17] The mean value of k_{01} (2 hr^{-1}) in our study was large in comparison with the k_d (0.42 hr^{-1}) and k (0.21 hr^{-1}). Thus, the literature value of k_{01} used in method A would not be expected to produce substantial error.

A major assumption made in using method B is that in vitro dissolution can adequately describe in vivo absorption. A good correlation (r = 0.98) between in vitro dissolution and in vivo absorption was observed for the SRP product (Figure 5). This may account for the relatively good results obtained by method B in predicting PPC.

Since both methods A and B have been shown to be adequate in predicting procainamide concentrations in healthy subjects, these methods may be applied in certain clinical settings. A specific example would be the transfer from IRP preparations to an individualized dose of SRP. Caution must be observed, however, in using these methods in the clinical setting. In certain disease states, changes in absorption may occur.[18] For example, in patients with severe diarrhea, much of the procainamide in the sustained-release product can pass through the gastrointestinal tract without being released.[19] Other factors that preclude the use of these predictive methods include changes in hepatic and renal function, and the addition or modification in concomitant drugs known to interfere with procainamide pharmacokinetics such as cimetidine.[20] Further studies are needed to verify the accuracy and usefulness of these two methods in the clinical setting.

Another potential application of methods A and B could be in the initial evaluation of different sustained-release formulations. Once the in vitro dissolution characteristics of the SRP formulation are determined, mean pharmacokinetic values for the patient group could be used to simulate the in vivo PPC–time curve with either method A or B. This approach could provide a means of selecting a desirable sustained-release preparation before conducting initial bioavailability studies. Further research is necessary to verify the applicability of such an approach.

Conclusion

Peak and trough PPCs could be accurately predicted following the administration of a SRP product to healthy volunteers using two methods, each based on in vitro dissolution data and pharmacokinetic values from IRP. These methods may be useful in individualizing procainamide therapy for certain patients, but further studies are needed to verify their accuracy and practicality in a clinical setting.

Figure 5. Average fraction of procainamide absorbed in vivo versus fraction of the sustained-release procainamide product dissolved in vitro; where (——) represents the line of best fit from the least-squares regression and (- - -) represents the line of identity.

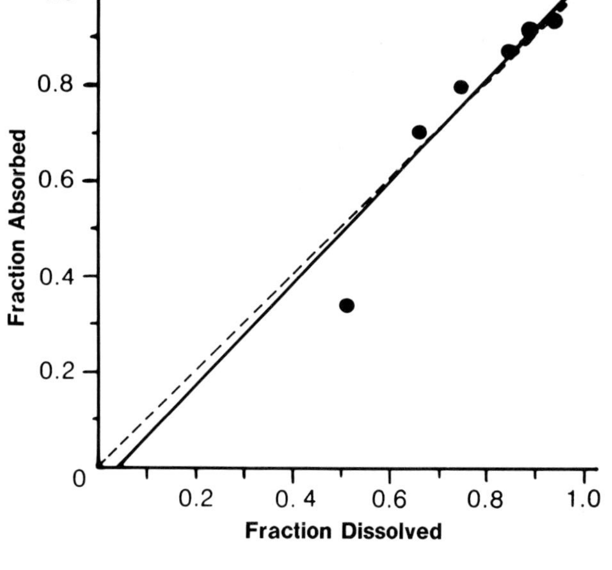

References

1. Wiegand RG, Taylor JD. Kinetics of plasma drug levels after sustained release dosage. *Biochem Pharmacol.* 1960; 3:256–63.
2. Weinberger M, Hendeles L, Wong L et al. Relationship of formulation and dosing interval to fluctuation of serum theophylline concentration in children with chronic asthma. *J Pediatr.* 1981; 99:145–52.
3. Weinberger M, Hendeles L, Bighey L. The relation of product formulation to absorption of oral theophylline. *N Engl J Med.* 1978; 299:852–7.
4. Wagner JG. Biopharmaceutics: absorption aspects. *J Pharm Sci.* 1961; 50:359–92.
5. Levy G, Leonards JR, Procknal JA. Development of in vitro dissolution tests which correlate quantitatively with dissolution rate-limited drug absorption in man. *J Pharm Sci.* 1965; 54:1719–22.
6. Weinberger M, Hendeles L. Slow-release theophylline: rationale and basis for product selection. *N Engl J Med* 1983; 308:760–4.
7. Heimlich BN, Golub A, Cohen DM. Pharmacokinetic analysis and correlation of bioavailability and dissolution data for a sustained-release theophylline tablet. Paper presented at the 25th National Meeting of the Academy of Pharmaceutical Sciences, American Pharmaceutical Association. Hollywood, FL: 1978 Nov 13.
8. Gonzalez MA, Golub AL. Theo-Dur and Theo-Dur Sprinkle: controlled-release systems for theophylline. *Drug Dev Ind Pharm.* 1983; 9:1379–96.
9. Smith TC, Kinkel AW. Plasma levels of procainamide after administration of conventional and sustained-release preparations. *Curr Ther Res.* 1980; 27:217–28.
10. Gibaldi M, Perrier D. Pharmacokinetics. New York: Marcel Dekker, Inc; 1975.
11. Wagner JG. Interpretation of percent dissolved–time plots derived from *in vitro* testing of conventional tablets and capsules. *J Pharm Sci.* 1969; 58:1253–7.
12. Manion CV, Lalka D, Baer DT et al. Absorption kinetics of procainamide in humans. *J Pharm Sci.* 1977; 66:981–4.
13. Wagner JG. Fundamentals of clinical pharmacokinetics. Hamilton, IL: Drug Intelligence Publications, Inc: 1975.
14. Sheiner LB, Beal SL. Some suggestions for measuring predictive performance. *J Pharmacokinet Biopharm.* 1981; 9: 503–12.
15. Koch-Weser J, Klein SW. Procainamide dosage schedules, plasma concentrations, and clinical effects. *JAMA.* 1971; 215:1451–60.
16. Lima J. Procainamide. In: Evans WE, Schentag JJ, Jusko WJ, eds. Applied pharmacokinetics: principles of therapeutic drug monitoring. San Francisco: Applied Therapeutics; 1980:404–10.
17. Taylor JD, Wiegand RG. The analog computer and plasma drug kinetics. *Clin Pharmacol Ther.* 1971; 3:464–72.
18. Boxenbaum HG. Physiological and pharmacokinetic factors affecting performance of sustained-release dosage forms. *Drug Dev Ind Pharm.* 1982; 8:1–25.
19. Woosley RL, Cerskus I, Roden, D. Antiarrhythmic therapy: clinical pharmacology update. *J Clin Pharmacol.* 1984; 24: 295–305.
20. Christian CD, Meridith CG, Speeg KV. Cimetidine inhibits renal procainamide clearance. *Clin Pharmacol Ther.* 1984; 36:221–7.

Appendix A

Method A, originally proposed by Wiegand and Taylor,[1] is a one-compartment pharmacokinetic model that incorporates variables of first-order release, absorption, and elimination:

$$C = \{[FDf_s(k_{01}k_d)]/[V(k_{01} - k_d)(k - k_d)]\}(e^{-k_d t} - e^{-kt}) + \{(FDf_i k_{01}) - [(FDk_{01}k_d/k_{01} - k_d)]/[V(k - k_{01})][(e^{-k_{01}t} - e^{-kt})]\}$$

where C is the concentration of the drug in the plasma, V is the apparent volume of distribution of the drug, F is the fraction of drug absorbed from the dosage form, D is the dose administered, f_i is the immediate-release fraction as a decimal, f_s is the sustained-release fraction as a decimal, k is the first-order elimination rate of the drug from the body, k_{01} is the first-order absorption rate constant for the drug, k_d is the first-order rate of drug release from the dosage form, and t is the time of determination of the plasma concentration.

In using Method A for this study, the values of dissolution rate constant (k_d), the immediate-release fraction (f_i), and the sustained-release fraction (f_s) are determined from least-squares exponential curve fitting of the plot of log (1 − cumulative fraction dissolved) verus time (Figure 1). The observed first-order elimination rate constant (k) is derived from concentrations measured in vivo following administration of an immediate-release preparation. V/F is determined as Dose/(AUC) k, where AUC is the mean area under the time curve at steady state for the subject. An average value of 2 hr^{-1} obtained from the literature was used for the absorption rate constant, k_{01}.

Appendix B

Method B is a rearrangement of an equation derived by Wagner and Nelson[13] to determine the amount of drug absorbed from an extravascular site at any time period. The original Wagner-Nelson equation is described mathematically as

$$A_t/V = C_t + k \int_0^t C\,dt \qquad (1)$$

where A_t is the amount of drug absorbed at time t, V is the apparent volume of distribution for the drug, C_t is the plasma concentration at time t, k is the apparent first-order rate constant of elimination (derived from the negative slope of the terminal log-linear portion of the immediate-release product), and $\int_0^t Cdt$ is the area under the concentration–time curve (AUC) from time 0 to time t, which is calculated using the linear trapezoidal method.

When 100% of the dose of drug is absorbed (when time = ∞), the equation simplifies to the form

$$A_\infty/V = k \int_0^\infty C\,dt = (FD)/V \qquad (2)$$

where $\int_0^\infty Cdt$ is the total AUC following a single dose, D is the dose given, and F is the fraction of the D that is absorbed.

The fraction of a dose absorbed at any time can then be determined by dividing equation 1 by equation 2

$$f_t = \left(C_t + k \int_0^t C\,dt\right) \Big/ \left(k \int_0^\infty C\,dt\right) \qquad (3)$$

where f_t is the fraction of dose absorbed from time 0 to time t.

Rearranging the equation to solve for C_t results in equation 4

$$C_t = \left(f_t k \int_0^\infty C\,dt\right) - \left(k \int_0^t C\,dt\right) \qquad (4)$$

Defining the integral from time 0 to time t in terms of the trapezoidal rule results in the relationship

$$C_t = f_t k \int_0^\infty C\,dt - k[\Delta t/2](C_t + C_{t-1}) - k \int_0^{t-1} C\,dt \qquad (5)$$

where Δt is the time interval from the previous time point, t-1, to time t, C_{t-1} and C_t are the respective concentrations to calculate the AUC for the time interval, and $\int_0^{t-1} C\,dt$ is the area under the concentration–time curve from time 0 to the time before the measurement at time t.

The final relationship is obtained by rearranging and solving for C

$$C_t = f_t \int_0^{\infty} C\,dt - \int_0^{t-1} C\,dt - (\Delta t/2)C_{t-1} \Big/ \Delta t/2 + 1/k \quad (6)$$

Method B assumes that the fraction of drug released in vitro at any time is equivalent to f_t, the fraction of total drug absorbed in vivo at that time.[6,7] Therefore, the f_t values calculated in equation 3 can then be substituted in equation 6 to generate C values at any time after a single dose.

Phenytoin therapy and immune response to influenza vaccine

MARC LEVINE, B. LYNN BEATTIE, DONALD M. MCLEAN, AND DAVID CORMAN

Abstract: The effect of long-term phenytoin therapy on the immune response to inactivated influenza vaccine was evaluated.

The patients were 31 white men who were receiving long-term phenytoin therapy for seizure disorders and 31 age-matched controls. Prevaccination blood samples were collected, and the patients were vaccinated subcutaneously with 0.5-mL inactivated whole-virion trivalent influenza vaccine. Venous blood samples were collected at 2, 4, 6, 9, 12, and 24 weeks after vaccination and stored at −20 °C until analysis. Total serum phenytoin concentrations were measured by fluorescence polarization immunoassay. Immune response was measured by assaying the sera for hemagglutinin-inhibiting antibody to each of the three antigenic strains. Seroconversion was defined as a fourfold or greater increase in serum antibody titer following vaccination.

In the phenytoin-treated patients, the mean (± S.D.) serum phenytoin concentration before vaccination was 9.9 ± 6.1 μg/mL. Prevaccination geometric mean titers were high enough in both groups to indicate that these patients had been exposed to these or related antigens, and medical records confirmed that some of the patients had been vaccinated the year before. The percent of patients demonstrating seroconversion to each antigen at week 4 was low in both groups, and there were no significant differences between the two groups. The cumulative seroconversion responses observed up to week 24 were also not significantly different.

Long-term phenytoin therapy should not affect the efficacy of influenza vaccine in patients who have been previously exposed to infection or vaccination with identical or related strains.

Index terms: Antibodies; Anticonvulsants; Blood levels; Dosage schedules; Drug interactions; Immunization; Influenza vaccines; Phenytoin; Vaccines
Clin Pharm. 1985; 4:191–4

Immune stimulation in animal models has been shown to decrease the hepatic metabolism of certain drugs.[1] This appears to be caused by a decrease in the cytochrome P-450 fraction of liver microsomes. Respiratory infections in humans caused by Influenzavirus and other viruses have been associated with temporary reductions in the elimination of theophylline[1,2] and phenytoin.[3] Influenza vaccination has been used experimentally to assess the effects of immune stimulation on drug metabolism. Now there is evidence to suggest that influenza vaccination can decrease the hepatic metabolism of theophylline[4] and aminopyrine,[5] although conflicting data exist.[6,7] In a recent study, Levine et al.[8] found no effect of influenza vaccination on mean steady-state serum phenytoin concentrations in 15 elderly subjects. However, two of these subjects experienced temporary increases in serum phenytoin concentrations that were possibly caused by vaccination.

MARC LEVINE, PH.D., is Assistant Professor, Faculty of Pharmaceutical Sciences, The University of British Columbia (UBC) and Head, Division of Clinical Pharmacy, Shaughnessy Hospital; B. LYNN BEATTIE, M.D., is Associate Professor and Head, Division of Geriatric Medicine, Department of Medicine, UBC, and Head, Department of Geriatrics and Continuing Care, Shaughnessy Hospital; DONALD M. MCLEAN, M.D., is Professor, Division of Medical Microbiology, Faculty of Medicine, UBC; and DAVID CORMAN is Clinical Pharmacist, Department of Pharmacy Shaughnessy Hospital and Clinical Instructor, Faculty of Pharmaceutical Sciences, UBC, Vancouver, British Columbia, Canada.

Address reprint requests to Dr. Levine at the University of British Columbia, 2146 East Mall, Vancouver, British Columbia, Canada V6T 1W5.

The assistance of the medical and nursing staffs of the Department of Geriatrics and Continuing Care, Shaughnessy Hospital, is acknowledged.

Supported by a grant from the British Columbia Medical Services Foundation.

In general, the studies that have investigated the effects of influenza vaccination on drug metabolism have not measured the immune responses to the vaccine. The immune response to influenza vaccine is known to be affected by factors, such as patient age, previous exposure to vaccines or active virus, and prevaccination antibody titre,[9-11] which may partly account for the conflicting results that have been obtained in these studies. Long-term phenytoin therapy has been reported to impair both humoral and cell-mediated immunity,[12-14] although its effects on immune response to influenza vaccine have not been investigated. If phenytoin inhibits the immune response to influenza vaccination, this might partly explain why vaccination apparently does not decrease phenytoin metabolism in most patients receiving long-term therapy. This study was undertaken to determine whether long-term phenytoin therapy would alter the immune response to inactivated influenza vaccine.

Methods

The patients were 31 white men (mean age 74.3 years, range 58 to 91 years) who were receiving long-term phenytoin therapy for seizure disorders, and 31 age-matched white men not receiving phenytoin who served as controls. Two of the control patients were being treated with other antiepileptic drugs for seizure disorders. The study was reviewed and approved by the Committee on Research and Other Studies Involving Human Subjects of the University of British Columbia and by the research committee of Shaughnessy Hospital. Informed consent was obtained from all participants.

There were no documented immunodeficiency states in either patient group, and none of the patients was receiving systemic steroids or cytotoxic agents. There were three malignancies diagnosed in the phenytoin-treated group versus two in the control group. All patients were long-term care residents of Shaughnessy Hospital. The Department of Geriatrics and Continuing Care of the hospital primarily serves elderly male veterans because of a long-standing affiliation with the Department of Veterans' Affairs.

Prevaccination venous blood samples were collected from all of the patients, and within the next two weeks, the patients were vaccinated subcutaneously with 0.5-mL inactivated whole-virion trivalent influenza vaccine (Fluviral, Institut Armand-Frappier, Quebec, Canada, lot 3-60011, expiration date Mar 8, 1985). The 1983–84 vaccine consisted of 15 μg/0.5 mL each of the following Influenzavirus strains—A/Philippines/2/82 (H3N2), A/Brazil/11/78 (H1N1), and B/Singapore/222/79. Venous blood samples for analysis of antibody titers and serum phenytoin concentrations were collected at 2, 4, 6, 9, 12, and 24 weeks after vaccination, and sera were stored at −20 °C until analysis. The patients and other long-term care residents were monitored throughout the study for signs or symptoms of influenza infection. When influenza infection was suspected, sputum samples or throat swabs were taken for microbiologic analysis. No cases of influenza were detected during the study period.

Total serum phenytoin concentrations were measured using a commercial fluorescence polarization immunoassay (TDX System, Abbott Laboratories) with a between-day coefficient of variation of < 5%. Immune response to the influenza vaccine was measured by assaying the patients' sera for hemagglutinin-inhibiting (HI) antibody to each of the three antigenic strains according to the method described by McLean.[15] Homologous antigens were obtained from the Laboratory Centre for Disease Control, National Health and Welfare, Ottawa, Canada. The assay used measured serum antibody titer in the range from 1:10 to 1:1280. According to convention, serologic response (seroconversion) was defined as a fourfold or greater increase in serum antibody titer relative to baseline (e.g., patients with initial titers < 1:10 were deemed to have seroconverted when their postvaccination titers were ≥ 1:40). Seroconversion could not be detected in subjects with initial titers ≥ 1:640 since the upper limit of the assay was 1:1280 so data from these individuals were not included in the analysis. Cumulative seroconversion was defined as the percentage of patients with a fourfold or greater increase in antibody titer relative to baseline at any time after vaccination. For calculating geometric mean reciprocal titers, serum antibody titers < 1:10 were arbitrarily set at 1:5. The responses of the phenytoin-treated patients were compared with the control group by chi-square analysis using Yates' correction for continuity, and statistical significance was defined as $p < 0.05$.

Results

In the phenytoin-treated patients, the mean (± S.D.) serum phenytoin concentration before vaccination was 9.9 ± 6.1 μg/mL (range 1.8 to 22.8 μg/mL).

Although several changes in phenytoin dosage were made, the mean serum phenytoin concentration remained in the range of 9.9–10.7 μg/mL throughout the study. Five of the 31 phenytoin-treated patients had serum phenytoin concentrations ≤5 μg/mL throughout the study period.

The trivalent influenza vaccine used in 1982–83, the year before this study, contained Influenzavirus strain A/Bangkok/79 as the H3N2 subtype instead of A/Philippines/2/82. The other two strains were the same as those subsequently included in the 1983–84 vaccine. The medical records of our phenytoin-treated group showed that 15 patients were vaccinated in 1982–83, eight were not vaccinated, and vaccination status could not be determined in eight cases. In the control group, five patients were vaccinated in 1982–83, 10 were not vaccinated, and vaccination status was unknown in 16 patients.

Prevaccination geometric mean antibody titers were high enough to indicate that the patients had been exposed to these or related antigens, and these titers were similar in the phenytoin-treated and control groups (Table 1). A reciprocal antibody titer of ≥ 40 is considered necessary for minimum protection against Influenzavirus. More than half the patients were unprotected against each antigen, and no significant differences were detected between the phenytoin-treated and control groups before vaccination.

The data in Table 2 show that the percent of patients demonstrating seroconversion to each antigen at week 4 was low in both the phenytoin-treated and control groups, and that there were no significant differences between the two groups. The cumulative seroconversion responses observed up to week 24 were also not significantly different in the phenytoin-treated and control groups (Table 2), although these were considerably greater than those measured at week 4. These same findings were true of all other single time determinations for which data were available. This was explained by our observations that 16–26% of seroconversion responses occurred after four weeks following vaccination and that 68–77% of the responders experienced a fourfold or greater decline in peak antibody titer during the study period.

Figure 1 illustrates the effect of the vaccine on geometric mean titers against Influenzavirus A/Philippines. The magnitude and pattern of the change in the geometric mean titer were similar in the phenytoin-treated and control groups. Geometric mean titers were maximal by weeks 2–4 and began to decline 9–12 weeks after vaccination. A similar pattern was observed for geometric mean titers against Influenzavirus A/Brazil and B/Singapore.

Table 1.
Prevaccination Serology of Phenytoin-Treated and Control Patients

Antigen	Geometric Mean Reciprocal Antibody Titer ($n = 31$): Phenytoin	Control	% Patients with Reciprocal Titers < 40 ($n = 31$)[a]: Phenytoin	Control
A/Philippines	28	34	48	61
A/Brazil	19	13	68	81
B/Singapore	34	20	48	65

[a] No significant differences were detected between the phenytoin-treated and control groups by chi-square analysis.

Table 2.
Percentage of Phenytoin-Treated and Control Patients with Seroconversion after Influenza Vaccination[a]

Antigen	Week 4: Phenytoin	Control	Cumulative to Week 24[c]: Phenytoin	Control
A/Philippines	45 (n[b] = 29)	56 ($n = 27$)	76 ($n = 29$)	88 ($n = 25$)
A/Brazil	30 ($n = 30$)	55 ($n = 31$)	66 ($n = 29$)	74 ($n = 27$)
B/Singapore	24 ($n = 29$)	42 ($n = 31$)	66 ($n = 29$)	75 ($n = 28$)

[a] No significant differences were detected between the phenytoin-treated and control groups by chi-square analysis.
[b] Total number of subjects.
[c] Total numbers of patients differ from those at week 4 because of individuals who did not seroconvert and who either died or refused to provide one or more blood samples before week 24.

Discussion

Vaccination with influenza vaccine induces both humoral and cell-mediated immune responses. Most evidence, however, suggests that it is the serum IgG HI antibody produced in response to the vaccination that is most directly involved in conferring immunity to subsequent infection. An HI serum antibody titer of approximately 1:40 is required for minimum (50%) protection. The response of a vaccinated population is thought to be greatest four weeks after vaccination, but the duration of the response is quite variable.[10,11]

In the 1970s, several reports appeared suggesting that long-term phenytoin therapy can cause humoral and cell-mediated immunodeficiencies.[12–14] In one study, phenytoin-treated patients were unable to mount a primary antibody response to *Salmonella typhi* vaccine.[12] In the present study, prevaccination serology was similar in the phenytoin-treated and control groups, and it indicated that these patients had been exposed to these or related

Figure 1. Effect of influenza vaccine on the geometric mean titers against Influenzavirus A/Philippines/2/82/(H3N2); ● represent the control patients and O represent the phenytoin-treated patients.

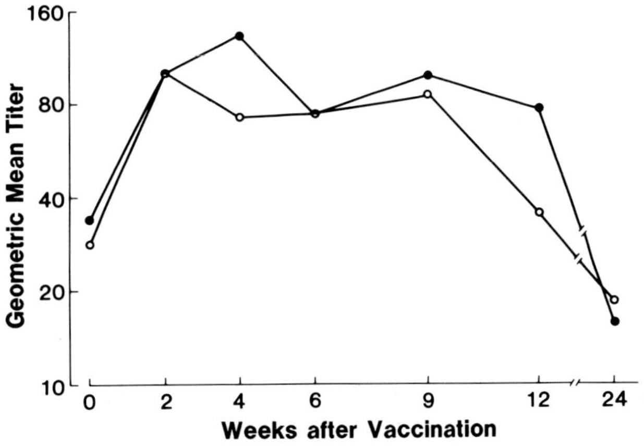

antigens previously (Table 1). We observed no significant differences between the groups in percent seroconversion measured at four weeks after vaccination or cumulatively (Table 2). Cumulative seroconversion frequencies were consistently greater than those measured at single times because some patients responded later than four weeks after vaccination and peak antibody titers frequently declined rapidly after seroconversion. This was reflected in the geometric mean titers against Influenzavirus A/Philippines (Figure 1), which was the new viral strain in the 1983–84 vaccine. Geometric mean titers, which were similar in both groups, peaked by weeks 2–4 and began to decline 9–12 weeks after vaccination. By week 24 after vaccination, a clinically important decrease in geometric mean titer had occurred in both groups. These observations suggest that a single dose of the vaccine may not ensure minimal protection against infection throughout the influenza season.

Our results suggest that long-term phenytoin therapy has no effect on humoral immune response in this population. Since our patients had antibodies against these or related strains of influenza, it is possible that phenytoin therapy could alter primary but not secondary antibody responses. This could be determined by investigating humoral responses to influenza vaccine in previously unexposed children or adults receiving long-term phenytoin therapy. The most consistently observed effect of phenytoin has been a deficiency in the IgA class of serum antibody,[16,17] and this would not have been detected by our assay.

The elimination of drugs metabolized by the cytochrome P-450 enzyme system can be decreased by influenza vaccination, although not all studies have agreed.[6,7]

Our results suggest that these differences may be partly related to incomplete seroconversion in vaccinated groups and variability in the onset and duration of the immune response to the vaccine.

Conclusion

Long-term phenytoin therapy should not affect the efficacy of influenza vaccine in patients who have been previously exposed to infection or vaccination with identical or related strains.

References

1. Renton KW. Effects of infection and immune stimulation on theophylline metabolism. *Semin Perinatol.* 1981; 5:378–82.
2. Chang KC, Lauer BA, Bell TD et al. Altered theophylline pharmacokinetics during acute respiratory viral illness. *Lancet.* 1978; 1:1132–3.
3. Levine M, Jones MW. Toxic reaction to phenytoin following a viral infection. *Can Med Assoc J.* 1983; 128:1270–1. Letter.
4. Renton KW, Gray JD, Hall RI. Decreased elimination of theophylline after influenza vaccination. *Can Med Assoc J.* 1980; 123:288–90.
5. Kramer P, McClain CJ. Deprression of aminopyrine metabolism by influenza vaccination. *N Engl J Med.* 1981; 305: 1262–4.
6. Hansten PD. Vaccine–drug interactions. *Drug Interact Newsl.* 1984; 4:21–4.
7. D'Arcy PF. Vaccine–drug interactions. *Drug Intell Clin Pharm.* 1984; 18:697–700.
8. Levine M, Jones MW, Gribble M. Increased serum phenytoin concentration following influenza vaccination. *Clin Pharm.* 1984; 3:505–9.
9. Ruben FL. Prevention of influenza in the elderly. *J Am Geriatr Soc.* 1982; 30:577–80.
10. Office of Technology Assessment. Cost effectiveness of influenza vaccination. Washington, DC: United States Government Printing Office; 1981:Dec.
11. Potter C, Oxford JS. Determinants of immunity to influenza infection in man. *Br Med Bull.* 1979; 35:69–75.
12. Sorrell TC, Forbes IJ, Burness FR et al. Depression of immunological function in patients treated with phenytoin sodium (sodium diphenylhydantoin). *Lancet.* 1971; 2:1233–5.
13. Grob PJ, Herold GE. Immunological abnormalities and hydantoins. *Br Med J.* 1972; 2:561–3.
14. Masi M, Paalucci P, Perrocco P et al. Immunosuppression by phenytoin. *Lancet.* 1976; 1:860. Letter.
15. McLean DM. Immunological investigation of human virus diseases. New York: Churchill Livingstone Inc.; 1982.
16. Kanoh T, Uchino H. Immunodeficiency and epilepsy. *Lancet.* 1976; 1:860–1. Letter.
17. Fontana A, Sauter R, Grob PJ et al. IgA deficiency, epilepsy and hydantoin medication. *Lancet.* 1976; 2:228–31.

Intermittent dobutamine hydrochloride infusions in outpatients with chronic congestive heart failure

DAVID S. ROFFMAN, MARK M. APPLEFELD, WILLIAM R. GROVE, BARRY S. TALESNICK, FREDERICK J. SUTTON, KATHRYN A. NEWMAN, AND WILLIAM P. REED

Abstract: Patients with severe chronic congestive heart failure were treated with intermittent dobutamine hydrochloride infusions administered on an outpatient basis with a portable infusion device.

Eleven patients (eight women and three men), ages 28–71 years, were given initial dobutamine hydrochloride infusions at a rate of 1–2 μg/kg/min, and the dose was gradually increased to a maximum dose of 15 μg/kg/min. Patients were considered dobutamine responders if their cardiac output increased by at least 30% and pulmonary-capillary wedge pressure did not rise. After a sustained hemodynamic response was demonstrated, the infusion was discontinued to assess the patients' symptoms during drug-free intervals. The patients were instructed and trained in proper catheter care after a venous-access catheter was surgically implanted. Patients were also shown how to use the ambulatory infusion pump.

The patients were treated with long-term intermittent dobutamine hydrochloride infusions for 3–24 months. All patients adjusted easily to the routine of catheter and pump care and drug administration. The mean dose of dobutamine hydrochloride resulting in the maximum improvement in cardiac index was 9.4 μg/kg/min. All patients observed an improvement in their symptoms of congestive heart failure during the drug infusions and the intervals between the infusions. There was a mean reduction of 1.2 in New York Heart Association functional class. There were 18 congestive heart failure-related hospital readmissions among the 11 patients during 108 cumulative months of long-term dobutamine therapy.

The intermittent administration of dobutamine hydrochloride via a portable infusion system appears to have improved the functional capacity of the 11 patients studied. This may be a viable treatment alternative for selected ambulatory patients with severe heart failure who demonstrate hemodynamic improvement with dobutamine.

Index terms: Ambulatory care; Devices; Dobutamine hydrochloride; Dosage; Drug administration; Heart failure; Patient education; Surgical supplies; Sympathomimetic agents
Clin Pharm. 1985; 4:195–9

Chronic congestive heart failure is a comon disease affecting three to four million Americans annually.[1] With a growing geriatric population and rapidly developing critical-care technology, the number of patients surviving with advanced forms of heart failure may well increase. Patients with more severe disease usually require repeated hospital admissions to control their symptoms. The cost of hospitalization for these patients approaches $3 billion annually in the United States.[a]

Drug therapy for congestive heart failure has traditionally depended on the use of cardiac glycosides and diuretics. During the past decade, the addition of preload- and afterload-reducing agents has gained widespread appeal in the treatment of patients with moderate or severe heart failure. However, it is now clear that the initial salutory response to vasodilator therapy did not confer long-term benefit.[2–4] The development of tolerance and the failure of some patients to respond to vasodilator agents have dampened the initial enthusiasm.

Dobutamine is an effective inotropic agent with additional β_2 adrenergic and competitive α-antagonist properties that increase myocardial contractility while reducing systemic vascular resistance.[5,6] Although short-term hemodynamic improvement with dobutamine has been well documented, its effects on cardiac output and functional capacity during prolonged infusions are unclear. To investigate further data suggesting that sympathetic tolerance may be of clinical importance and symptomatic improvement may persist for days to weeks after an infusion has been discontinued, we administered dobutamine on a long-term intermittent

DAVID S. ROFFMAN, PHARM.D., is Associate Professor of Clinical Pharmacy, School of Pharmacy, University of Maryland (UMD) and Therapeutic Consultant, Coronary Care Unit, University of Maryland Hospital; MARK M. APPLEFELD, M.D., is Associate Professor of Medicine, School of Medicine, UMD and Cardiologist, Division of Cardiology, University of Maryland Hospital; and WILLIAM R. GROVE, M.S., is Director, Clinical Research Pharmacy Services, University of Maryland Cancer Center. BARRY S. TALESNICK, M.D., is a Cardiology Fellow, Division of Cardiology; FREDERICK J. SUTTON, M.D., is Associate Professor of Medicine, School of Medicine, UMD and Director, Coronary Care Unit; KATHRYN A. NEWMAN, M.S., is Infection Research Coordinator, University of Maryland Cancer Center; and WILLIAM P. REED, M.D., is Associate Professor of Surgery, Surgical Oncology, School of Medicine, UMD and University of Maryland Hospital, Baltimore.

Address reprint requests to Dr. Roffman at the School of Pharmacy, UMD, Baltimore, MD 21201.

The secretarial assistance of Renee T. Smith is acknowledged.

Supported in part by Cormed, Inc., Medina, NY.

basis (i.e., 48 hours each week) to outpatients with intractable congestive heart failure.[7,8]

Methods

We studied 11 congestive heart failure patients (eight women and three men), ages 28–71 (mean 52.2) years from January 1982 to April 1984. The study was approved by the Human Volunteers Research Committee of the University of Maryland at Baltimore. All patients gave informed consent. Patients were eligible for this study if they

1. Failed to demonstrate hemodynamic improvement in cardiac output, pulmonary artery pressure, or pulmonary capillary wedge pressure with vasodilator therapy (i.e., hydralazine, nitrates, captopril, or prazosin),
2. Showed improvement in the hemodynamic measurements listed above during inpatient dobutamine or dopamine infusions,
3. Were not suitable candidates for heart surgery, and
4. Were able to understand, accept, and demonstrate appropriate catheter and infusion pump care.

Patients were admitted to the coronary-care unit, and their response to vasodilator and inotropic therapy was assessed with the use of a flow-directed balloon-tipped catheter. Dobutamine hydrochloride infusions were initiated at a rate of 1–2 μg/kg/min, and the dose was gradually increased in 2-μg/kg/min increments at 2–3 hour intervals to a maximum dose of 15 μg/kg/min. If the systolic pressure increased more than 10 mm Hg, heart rate increased more than 10 beats/min, ventricular ectopic beats exceeded six beats/min, or angina pectoris appeared, the dose of dobutamine hydrochloride was decreased. Hemodynamic measurements were obtained at each dose level. Patients were considered dobutamine responders if their cardiac output increased at least 30% and pulmonary capillary wedge pressure did not rise. In two patients, dopamine hydrochloride (1–5 μg/kg/min) was added to the regimen because of its ability to mediate an increased renal blood flow independent of dobutamine.

After a sustained hemodynamic response was demonstrated during the 48-hour infusion, the infusion was discontinued and the patients' symptoms were assessed during a drug-free three- to five-day period. (This was done to ensure that the patients would not become severely symptomatic during the intervals without medication.) A venous-access catheter (Hickman, six patients; Cormed Mediport, five patients) was surgically implanted under local anesthesia. The patient and a responsible family member were instructed and trained in the proper catheter care to minimize the incidence of complications. An ambulatory infusion pump (Cormed model ML-6-6, Medina, NY 14103) was used in all patients.

The ambulatory infusion pump is a portable rotary pump that operates at an adjustable flow rate of approximately 10–50 mL/24 hours. Each pump is accompanied by a flow-rate meter that is used to set the desired infusion rate. The power source is a rechargeable nickel-cadmium battery pack. A fully charged battery pack can operate the pump for a maximum of seven days. For our application, a battery pack was used for two 48-hour infusions before being replaced with a freshly charged battery. A sterile, disposable 50-mL reservoir bag with tubing set (Cormed) was used to contain the drug solution. A soft-lined pouch was provided that allowed the patient to wear the pump using adjustable shoulder straps.

The amount of dobutamine in solution in the reservoir was calculated on the basis of the dose that produced the most beneficial hemodynamic response during inpatient treatment and was adjusted to accommodate the solubility of the drug and the flow rate. Stability studies were conducted by Eli Lilly and Company to allow use of dobutamine hydrochloride solution in Bacteriostatic Water for Injection, USP, for 48 hours at room temperature. Solutions of dobutamine hydrochloride exceeding 25 mg/mL may not be used because of the tendency to precipitate. Two patients received a combination of dobutamine and dopamine hydrochloride in the same solution that was administered through the infusion device. The compatibility of this combination was verified by the manufacturer.[b]

The contents of the reservoir bags contained approximately a 2–4 hour additional supply of dobutamine hydrochloride to allow for priming the tubing (requires approximately 1 mL) and to ensure that the bag would not empty completely during a 48-hour infusion. In some cases, the amount of additional drug and solution placed in the reservoir bag was calculated to allow ease of drug measurement. For example:

> A 65-kg patient requires 6 μg/kg/min of dobutamine hydrochloride for a 48-hr infusion.
>
> Total amount of drug to be infused in 48 hours = 1123 mg.
>
> 1123 mg of dobutamine hydrochloride divided by 25 mg/mL = 44.9 mL of concentrated dobutamine hydrochloride solution.
>
> If 1250 mg/50 mL of concentrated dobutamine hydrochloride solution were placed in a reservoir bag at a flow rate of 22.5 mL/24 hours, then 1125 mg would actually be infused in 48 hours. After the infusion, about a five-hour supply of solution would remain in the bag and tubing.

If the patient's weight and dosage required more than 1500 mg of dobutamine hydrochloride in 48 hours, a 24-hour drug supply was prepared, and the pump refilled after the initial 24-hour infusion period. At the beginning of the study period, patients returned to the pharmacy weekly to have their pump filled. Starting in 1983, patients were trained to prepare their own infusions at home or were supplied the prepared solution by a home health-care agency. Patients accepted this responsibility readily. Training was started during the initial hospitalization and continued as necessary on an outpatient basis. Patients were shown the proper procedures for drug reconstitution, filling the reservoir, inserting the reservoir and tubing into pump, and battery exchange and recharge. Individuals were available 24 hours a day for pump-related problems or questions. An individualized patient-information sheet, containing step-by-step instructions was given to patients who prepared their own doses.

Results and Discussion

The 11 patients were treated with long-term intermittent dobutamine hydrochloride infusions for 3–24 (mean 9.8) months. The etiologies of congestive heart failure in these patients were idiopathic cardiomyopathy (four patients), ischemic cardiomyopathy (three patients), valvular heart disease (two patients), radiation-induced cardiomyopathy (one patient), and doxorubicin cardiomyopathy (one patient). Seven patients were initially New York Heart Association (NYHA) functional class 4, while four were classified as NYHA class 3.

Initial hemodynamic measurements in nine patients showed an average cardiac index of 1.7 (in a range from 0.9 to 2.7) L/min/sq m (Table 1). The mean dose of dobutamine hydrochloride resulting in the maximum improvement in cardiac index in these patients was 9.4 (in a range from 1.5 to 15) μg/kg/min, with an average cardiac index of 2.9 (in a range from 1.7 to 4.0) L/min/sq m, an increase over baseline of 59%.

All patients adjusted easily to the routine of catheter and pump care and drug administration. Congestive symptoms improved in each during the drug infusions and in the intervals between drug infusions. During drug infusions, there was mean reduction of patient NYHA class of 1.2 (Table 2).

Table 1.
Acute Hemodynamic Response to Dobutamine Hydrochloride

		Baseline and Peak Dobutamine Measurements[a]											
Patient Number	Dobutamine (μg/kg/min)	Blood Pressure (mm Hg)		Heart Rate (beats/min)		Pulmonary Artery Pressure (mm H_2O)		Pulmonary Capillary Wedge Pressure (mm H_2O)		Cardiac Index (L/min/sq m)		Left Ventricular Ejection Fraction (%)	
1	1.5	107/76	110/74	70	76	35/10	34/12	8	9	2.3	3.5	13	27
2	15	96/58	108/66	96	116	27/13	31/14	13	...	2.7	4.0	15	...
4	15	88/56	92/52	85	90	46/30	35/23	...	...	0.9	1.7	6	...
6[b]	5	120/80	120/70	88	86	68/28	61/21	24	21	1.7	2.6	20	...
7	10	...	...	...	...	50/38	...	28	15	1.6	2.3	20	...
8	9	120/80	122/80	137	134	45/29	39/20	26	...	2.4	3.9	...	...
9	15	96/80	98/46	100	121	69/30	70/13	22	22	1.2	2.6	20	29
10	5	102/70	130/60	88	100	33/15	30/10	12	7	2.4	2.5	30	48
11	9	130/70	...	115	116	46/26	40/17	18	8	2.2	3.1	22	29

[a] The number on the left in each column represents the baseline value, and the number on the right the peak value.
[b] Received dobutamine hydrochloride 5 μg/kg/min and dopamine hydrochloride 1 μg/kg/min.

Table 2.
Clinical Response of Patients Receiving Long-Term Intermittent Dobutamine Hydrochloride Infusions

Patient Number	Duration of Dobutamine Therapy (months)	NYHA Functional Class: Before Dobutamine	NYHA Functional Class: After Dobutamine	Drugs Failed	Number of Hospital Readmissions
1	13	4	2	Digoxin, hydralazine, captopril, prazosin	3
2	10	3	2	Digoxin, hydralazine	0
3	24	4	2	Digoxin, hydralazine, captopril	5
4	3	4	4	Digoxin, hydralazine, captopril, prazosin	0
5	20	4	3	Digoxin, hydralazine, captopril, prazosin	5
6	6	4	3	Digoxin, captopril, prazosin	1
7	3	4	3	Digoxin, hydralazine, captopril, prazosin	1
8	3	3	2	Digoxin, hydralazine, prazosin	1
9	8	3	2	Digoxin, hydralazine, captopril, prazosin	1
10	9	4	2	Digoxin, hydralazine, captopril	0
11	9	4	3	Digoxin, captopril, prazosin	1
Mean	9.8	3.7	2.5	...	1.5

The major objective in the use of long-term ambulatory dobutamine infusions was to improve the quality of life for these patients. To date, no form of drug therapy has been shown to improve the survival rate among patients with chronic heart failure. Thus, an improvement in functional capacity that permits patients to ambulate when they were previously disabled by their congestive symptoms should be considered a worthwhile therapeutic goal. Achieving this goal may only be a temporary necessity. For example, one of our patients and a subsequently reported patient[9] were maintained on intermittent dobutamine hydrochloride infusions until suitable donor hearts could be obtained for transplantation.

Medical complications that developed in our patients consisted of nine infectious episodes. Three infections involved Mediport sites and were thought to be caused by the inability of the patients to anchor the access needle (Huber point) properly to the Mediport site. The Mediport had to be removed to treat the infection adequately in one patient. In the other two patients, oral antibiotic therapy resolved the infections, and it was not necessary to remove the access system.

There were six instances of local cellulitis at the exit site of the Hickman catheter. Each case was promptly recognized by the patient and physician. All were treated with 7–10 day courses of appropriate oral antibiotic therapy. No patient had to be hospitalized for these events, and the dobutamine infusions were not interrupted. These infections were thought to be caused by the difficulty in maintaining skin hygiene when the Hickman catheter exited at the midline cleavage plane in women. With improved attention to skin hygiene, these events have not recurred during the past 14 months. Furthermore, it is now our policy to have the Hickman catheter exit more laterally. In addition, we no longer use the Mediport access system in our patients. The only bacteremic episode occurred in a patient who knowingly violated the protocol for Hickman catheter care. This patient required hospitalization and ultimately died from a pulmonary embolism.

There were 18 congestive heart failure related hospital readmissions among the 11 patients during 108 cumulative months of long-term dobutamine therapy. Of 18 readmissions, 10 were for two patients who received dobutamine intermittently for 20 and 24 months (Table 2). Three of these episodes occurred during the last four months of life in one patient whose heart failure was truly intractable to medical therapy.

It is uncertain whether survival is enhanced by this form of therapy. Eight of our 11 patients died 3–24 months after starting long-term dobutamine therapy. One patient (patient 6) died several months after undergoing cardiac transplantation. This patient's dobutamine therapy had been discontinued immediately after transplantation. One patient (patient 1) died suddenly, presumably because of a fatal ventricular arrhythmia, which is a common cause of death among patients with severe congestive heart failure. Four other patients died of complications directly related to their low cardiac output. One patient died of a malignant tumor recurrence and another of a pulmonary embolism. Three patients remain on therapy at eight to nine months after initiation.

The ambulatory infusion pump was found to be quite reliable for this application. In six instances, patients returned to the pharmacy for a refill of their reservoir bag only to find that it had not emptied properly. Four of these failures were caused by inadvertent pinching of the tubing that remains inside the pump housing as the pump was closed. This was remedied by changing the location of the tubing inside the pump housing before closure, and there has been only one similar event during the past 14 months.

On two occasions the rechargeable battery pack apparently failed to hold a charge and required replacement. On two other occasions, the solution was reported to have leaked inside the pump—once because of inadequate tightening of the tubing connection and once because of a defect in the reservoir bag.

On another occasion, a patient discontinued therapy after only a few hours duration and returned the pump to the pharmacy two days later. Upon inspection of the reservoir bag, an obvious precipitate was present. This problem did not occur in any other patient's drug reservoir and probably was caused by preparing the dobutamine hydrochloride in Bacteriostatic Sodium Chloride for Injection, USP. Since this occurrence, only bacteriostatic water for injection has been used as the diluent. (Because of a common-ion effect, concentrated solutions of dobutamine hydrochloride are more stable in water than in sodium chloride.) There were no hemodynamic complications from any of these events. However, the pumps were refilled promptly in each instance, and second 48-hour drug infusions were given.

Conclusion

Patients with advanced heart failure or those who are unable to tolerate conservative drug therapy may require alternative methods of treatment, such as dobutamine or dopamine therapy. The intermittent administration of dobutamine hydrochloride via a portable infusion system appears to have improved the functional capacity of the 11 patients we studied. Although this report is not a placebo-controlled trial, it suggests that there are ambulatory treatment alternatives for a select number of patients with severe heart failure who demonstrate hemodynamic improvement with dobutamine. Further investigation of the effect of long-term dobutamine on survival is warranted.

[a] Extrapolated from 1982 data for the State of Maryland obtained from the Maryland Health Services Cost Review Commission, assuming $3000 per admission for Medicare patients with congestive heart failure.

[b] Eli Lilly and Company. Internal memorandum. 1983 May 31.

References

1. Braunwald E, Mock MM, Watson JT. Congestive heart failure: a propitious time for intensified research. *Am J Cardiol.* 1983; 51:603–5.
2. Franciosa JA, Weber KT, Levine TB et al. Hydralazine in the long term treatment of chronic heart failure: lack of difference from placebo. *Am Heart J.* 1982; 104:587–94.
3. Packer M, Medina N, Yushak M. Hemodynamic and clinical tolerance to long-term captopril therapy for severe chronic heart failure. *Clin Res.* 1983; 31:211. Abstract.
4. Markham RV Jr, Corbett JR, Gilmore A et al. Efficacy of prazosin in the management of chronic congestive heart failure: a 6 month randomized, double blind, placebo-controlled study. *Am J Cardiol.* 1983; 51:1346–52.
5. Goldstein RA, Passamini ER, Roberts R. A comparison of digoxin and dobutamine in patients with acute infarction and cardiac failure. *N Engl J Med.* 1980; 303:846–50.
6. Ruffolo RR, Spradlin TA, Pollock, GD et al. Alpha and beta adrenergic effects of the stereoisomers of dobutamine. *J Pharmacol Exp Ther.* 1981; 219:447–52.
7. Applefeld MM, Newman KA, Grove WR et al. Intermittent, continuous outpatient dobutamine infusion in the management of congestive heart failure. *Am J Cardiol.* 1983; 51:455–8.
8. Ramkumar V, El-Fakahany EE, Roffman DS et al. The effect of intermittent dobutamine infusions on beta adrenergic receptors in human lymphocytes. *Fed Proc.* 1984; 43:355. Abstract.
9. Hodgson JM, Aja M, Sorkin RP. Intermittent ambulatory dobutamine for patients awaiting cardiac transplantation. *Am J Cardiol.* 1984; 53:375–6.

Bioavailability assessment of a new liquid controlled-release pseudoephedrine product

DAVID A. GRAVES, KEITH S. ROTENBERG, JAMES R. WOODWORTH, LEWIS P. AMSEL, AND ORVILLE N. HINSVARK

Abstract: Development of a liquid controlled-release pseudoephedrine product is described.

Two bioequivalence studies were conducted. In a single-dose study involving 20 subjects, the bioavailabilities of five controlled-release suspensions with a broad range of drug-release rates were compared with an immediate-release form of pseudoephedrine hydrochloride in a four-way crossover, incomplete block, sequence-randomized study. Serial blood sampling up to 36 hours after drug ingestion provided area-under-the-curve (AUC), maximum plasma concentration (C_{max}), and time to peak (t_{max}). In the multiple-dose study, involving 18 subjects, the bioavailability of the optimal formulation determined from the single-dose study was compared with a reference pseudoephedrine hydrochloride syrup. Serial blood sampling up to 12 hours after drug ingestion was performed to determine AUC, C_{max}, and t_{max}.

The single-dose investigation showed that all formulations were bioequivalent except the product with the slowest release rate, which had lower AUC and C_{max} values. The results of the multiple-dose study confirmed these findings with the reference syrup.

The use of a series of drug formulations with a wide range of release rates permitted selection of an optimal product in addition to providing the information needed to ensure continuous production of bioequivalent products.

Index terms: Blood levels; Dosage forms; Drugs, availability; Equivalency; Formulations; Release; Pharmacokinetics; Pseudoephedrine hydrochloride; Suspensions; Sustained-action medications; Sympathomimetic agents

Clin Pharm. 1985; 4:199–203

DAVID A. GRAVES, PHARM.D., is Clinical Pharmacist, KEITH S. ROTENBERG, PH.D., is Associate Director, and JAMES R. WOODWORTH, PH.D., is Clinical Pharmacokineticist, Clinical Pharmacology, Medical Research Division; LEWIS P. AMSEL, PH.D., is Director, Analytical and Pharmaceutical Sciences; and ORVILLE N. HINSVARK, PH.D., is Director, Analytical Chemistry Department, Pennwalt Pharmaceutical Division, Rochester, NY.

Address reprint requests to Dr. Graves at the Medical Research Division, Pennwalt Pharmaceutical Division, P.O. Box 1710, Rochester, NY 14623.

The analytic-support assistance of Bruce D. Shepardson is acknowledged.

Presented at the Clinical Research Forum, 19th Annual ASHP Midyear Clinical Meeting, Dallas, TX, December 4, 1984.

Pseudoephedrine, a sympathomimetic amine and an orally effective nasal decongestant, is an isomer of ephedrine with similar actions. Although pseudoephedrine is less potent as a central nervous system and cardiovascular stimulant than epinephrine, it has almost equivalent nasopharyngeal vasoconstrictor activities.[1] The Pennkinetic System (Pennwalt Pharmaceutical Division, Rochester, NY) uses a coated drug-resin complex to permit the controlled-release of drugs in solid or liquid formulations.[2] The rate of drug release can be varied by changing the thickness of the coating. Clinical studies in humans are performed to ensure that the studied formulations are bioequivalent and will not dissolve precipitously (dose dump). Batches of manufactured drugs sold to the general public do not undergo bioequivalence testing. Therefore, bioequivalence studies must also provide mechanisms for prospectively identifying batches of manufactured drug formulations that may dose dump or not be bioequivalent.

The results from investigations we conducted to develop a liquid controlled-release pseudoephedrine product with the Pennkinetic System are presented with descriptions of the study methods. Two basic studies were necessary. A single-dose bioequivalence study was conducted to establish in vitro and in vivo correlations and permit the selection of an ideal controlled-release formulation. This optimal formulation was then tested in a multiple-dose trial. Additionally, the in vitro and in vivo correlations derived from the single-dose investigation were used to propose manufacturing specifications.

Methods

Single-Dose Study. Twenty healthy men ranging from 18 to 38 years of age gave written consent to participate in the single-dose phase. The bioavailability and bioequivalence of five controlled-release (coated pseudoephedrine-resin complex) suspensions were evaluated and compared with an immediate-release syrup of pseudoephedrine hydrochloride in a four-way crossover, incomplete block, sequence-randomized study with a one-week washout interval between treatments. Each subject received the immediate-release reference solution (formulation A) in addition to three of the five controlled-release suspensions (formulations B, C, D, E, and F [listed in order of lightest to heaviest coating], resulting from separately manufactured lots). One half (60 mg/10 mL) of the immediate-release dose was given at time 0 and again at 6 hours, while the controlled-release products (equivalent to 120 mg of pseudoephedrine hydrochloride per 10 mL) were administered at time 0 only. The total dose for all treatments was equivalent to 120 mg of pseudoephedrine hydrochloride.

The study participants reported to the test facility the evening before receiving the medication to ensure a fasting state. Subjects were served identical lunch and dinner meals at 4 and 10 hours following drug administration during each phase of the crossover study. Blood samples were drawn from subjects into heparinized tubes before dosing and again at 0.5, 1, 2, 4, 6, 6.5, 7, 8, 10, 12, 15, 24, and 36 hours. Plasma samples were frozen and analyzed for pseudoephedrine content using gas chromatography.

Multiple-Dose Study. The bioavailability and bioequivalence of the optimal formulation determined from the single-dose study (formulation D) was compared with a reference pseudoephedrine hydrochloride syrup (Sudafed, Burroughs Wellcome, lot 1J1805) in the multiple-dose, crossover study. Eighteen healthy men provided written informed consent and were randomly assigned one of the two treatment groups and took the dose around-the-clock for one week. One treatment group took a 10-mL immediate-release dose at 0700, 1300, 1900, and 0100 (60 mg of pseudoephedrine hydrochloride), and the other treatment group took a dose equivalent to 120 mg of pseudoephedrine hydrochloride in the controlled-release preparation (10 mL) at 0700 and 1900. A one-week washout interval separated crossover treatments.

Plasma samples were collected before the administration of the 0700 dose each day for both treatment weeks. Blood samples were also drawn on the last day of each dosing week at 0700 (0 hour) and at 0.5, 1, 2, 4, 6, 6.5, 7, 8, 10, and 12 hours. On these intensive blood-sampling days, meals were standardized. The plasma samples were then analyzed for pseudoephedrine concentration as in the single-dose study.

Sample Analysis. Pseudoephedrine was extracted from 1-mL samples after 520 ng of methylaminomethylbenzyl alcohol (MAMBA) was added to each sample as an internal standard (using siliconized glassware). Initially, 200 μL of 1.0 *N* hydrochloric acid was added to each sample, vortexed briefly, and then 4 mL of hexane was added. Each sample was vortexed for five seconds and centrifuged for five minutes. The hexane layer was discarded, and 2 mL of methylene chloride and 0.5 mL of 25% sodium hydroxide (*w/w*) were added to each sample. The samples were extracted by shaking for 15 minutes and then centrifuged. The aqueous layer was discarded, and the methylene chloride was transferred to a siliconized vial. The samples were derivatized with 100 μL of trifluoroacetic anhydride at room temperature for one hour. Samples were dried under a gentle stream of nitrogen, reconstituted with 350 μL of methylene chloride, and dried again. The samples were then reconstituted with 110 μL of hexane, vortexed briefly, and the vials were capped until injection. Three microliters of each reconstituted sample were analyzed by gas chromatography.

A Hewlett-Packard model 5840A gas chromatograph equipped with a nitrogen-phosphorus detector was used for the analysis. A two-meter glass column (internal diameter 2 mm) packed with 2% OV-101 on 80–100 mesh Chromasorb-W-HP was used, with helium as the carrier gas at a rate of 30 mL/min. Detector gas flows were set as follows; air 50 mL/min, 8% hydrogen in helium 40 mL/min. An isothermal system was used with the injection port temperature set at 250 °C, oven temperature of 130 °C, and detector temperature of 250 °C. Retention times for pseudoephedrine and MAMBA were 3.0 and 2.3 minutes, respectively.

This assay was linear up to 1000 ng/mL, using peak area ratios, with a calculated correlation coefficient of 0.999 between 40 and 1000 ng/mL. The coefficient of variation at 50 and 500 ng/mL was 7.6 and 3.3%, respectively. The minimum quantifiable limit was 40 ng/mL as defined by 95% confidence limits. All samples analyzed were within this linear range.

Bioavailability Assessment. In the single-dose study, partial area-under-the-curve (AUC) was calculated for the first 12 hours (AUC_{12}) (the intended dosing interval) and to the last data point (36 hours, AUC_{36}) using the trapezoidal method. AUC_{12} and AUC_{36} were used since previous experience supported the use of AUC_{12} as a predictor of steady-state performance giving better intertreatment resolution than AUC_{36}.[3] The observed maximum plasma concentrations (C_{max}) and the times at which they occurred (t_{max}) for each treatment were tabulated. In the case of formulation A, where two separate doses were given, the highest (absolute) C_{max} was used. For the multiple-dose study, the steady-state AUC (AUC_{ss}), C_{max}, and t_{max} were determined as in the single-dose investigation. AUC_{ss}, the AUC from 0 to 12 hours in the multiple-dose investigation, was analogous to AUC_{36} in the single-dose study.

These variables were subjected to an analysis of variance (ANOVA) accounting for formulation, period, and subject effects (repeated measures). Posthoc comparisons were performed using Scheffé's test and the least-squares estimates of treatment means. A p value less than 0.05 was considered statistically significant. The power for each analysis was that of a t statistic calculated using estimates of formulation effects and the ANOVA mean-squared error.[4,5]

In Vitro and In Vivo Correlations. In vitro dissolution data were collected according to a method described in the *United States Pharmacopeia* in 1000 mL of 0.08 *M* potassium chloride at 37 °C.[6–8] The mean percent of drug dissolved at 0.5, 1, 3, and 6 hours was calculated from five different samples. In vitro and in vivo correlations considered this percent amount as an independent variable, and AUC_{12}, AUC_{36}, and C_{max} were considered dependent variables. Simple linear regressions were applied accordingly. A Student's t test for paired data was applied to the slope estimate to detect whether it was significantly different from zero. A significant ($p < 0.05$) slope term implied a significant overall relationship.

Results

Single-Dose Study. Concentration versus time curves from each treatment are illustrated in Figure 1. There was no drug detectable in the plasma samples drawn 36 hours following the dose. Mean AUC_{12} values were 2301, 2542, 2394, 2229, 2195, and 1426 ng·hr/mL for formulations A, B, C, D, E, and F, respectively. Corresponding mean AUC_{36} values were 3837, 3462, 3421, 3390, 3243, and 2381 ng·hr/mL. On an individual basis, at least 75% of the AUC ratios for each formulation were above 0.75 (using formulation A as the reference) except formulation F. Corresponding mean C_{max} values were 297, 321, 280, 261, 250, and 175 ng/mL. Formulation D appeared in all cases to have optimal release characteristics in vivo, having median pharmacokinetic values (B and C releasing faster, E and F releasing slower). ANOVA indicated significant variation among subject and treatment means for all derived pharmacokinetic variables. Significant treatment effects were discerned with Scheffé's test, which indicated that formulation F was significantly different from formulations A through E for AUC_{12}, AUC_{36}, and C_{max}. The powers to detect a difference of 20% was 0.96, 0.84, and 0.89 for AUC_{12}, AUC_{36}, and C_{max}, respectively. The t_{max} values were statistically longer for the controlled-release formulations since they have been designed for a longer dosing

Figure 1. Mean plasma concentrations in the single-dose study. For formulation A, n = 20; for formulations B through F, n = 12.

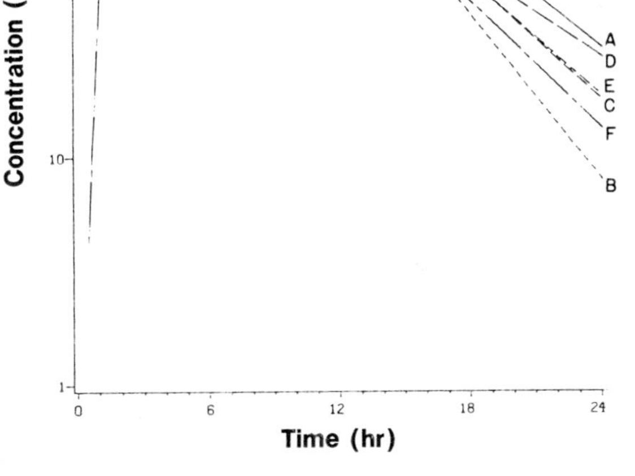

interval. Therefore, formulation F was not considered bioequivalent, and formulations B through E were considered bioequivalent, releasing an adequate amount of drug at an acceptable rate.

A slower dissolution rate was evident in those formulations with a greater amount of coating, as shown in Table 1, which contains the results of all in vitro dissolution testing with the controlled-release preparations. Using these values as independent variables, and AUC_{12}, AUC_{36}, and C_{max} as dependent variables, correlations were developed (Table 2). Significant relationships were found for AUC_{12} and C_{max}, while AUC_{36} was independent of the percent of drug dissolved. This was not surprising, since all formulations except F were found to be bioequivalent to the reference with ANOVA, resulting in a correlation slope that was not significantly different from zero. Generally, the correlations were better for the samples removed early in the dissolution testing, and the six-hour samples were the least useful. An illustration of C_{max} versus the percent drug dissolved at 0.5 hour is provided (Figure 2).

Based on its release characteristics in vivo and in vitro, formulation D was selected as the optimal controlled-release preparation and was studied after the administration of multiple doses at steady-state conditions.

Multiple-Dose Study. Steady-state concentrations were achieved in all subjects in the multiple-dose study by day 3 or 4 based on mean morning predose pseudoephedrine concentrations from samples drawn on days 1 through 6 (Table 3). The resulting AUC_{ss}, C_{max}, and t_{max} values from the last day of each dosing week are shown in Table 4. Plasma concentrations are depicted in Figure 3. No significant treatment effects were found except for the expected difference with t_{max}. The power to detect a 20% difference was 0.93 and > 0.99 for AUC_{ss} and C_{max}, respectively. On an individual basis, more than 75% of subjects had an AUC_{ss} for formulation D that was greater than 75% of the AUC_{ss} for the reference formulation. The multiple-dose investigation thus supported the bioequivalence conclusions made for formulation D following the single-dose study. Formulation D was found to be a bioequivalent controlled-release product that did not dose dump under the conditions of this study.

Discussion

The single-dose study results indicated that the Pennkinetic System gave complete release, except formulation F (AUC_{12}, AUC_{36}), and no preparation dose dumped (C_{max}). The multiple-dose study supported these findings for formulation D with a marketed reference (Sudafed, Burroughs Wellcome) establishing bioequivalence. These studies were prospectively designed to establish an ideal rate of

Table 1.
Mean Dissolution Data

Formulation	Mean (±S.D.) Percent Dissolved In Vitro			
	0.5 hr	1 hr	3 hr	6 hr
B	68.3 ± 1.1	76.8 ± 1.2	90.3 ± 2.1	94.3 ± 1.2
C	56.1 ± 1.0	66.1 ± 0.9	82.9 ± 1.1	92.7 ± 1.6
D	49.9 ± 1.0	53.4 ± 1.2	66.5 ± 0.9	73.9 ± 1.9
E	43.1 ± 0.5	46.0 ± 0.5	58.2 ± 1.0	67.1 ± 3.2
F	26.3 ± 1.0	31.5 ± 1.2	44.2 ± 1.3	54.8 ± 1.8

Figure 2. Maximum concentration (C_{max}) from the single-dose study versus percent dissolved at 0.5 hours in vitro. Mean C_{max} (in vivo) and percent drug dissolved (in vitro) values are shown with the resultant line of regression.

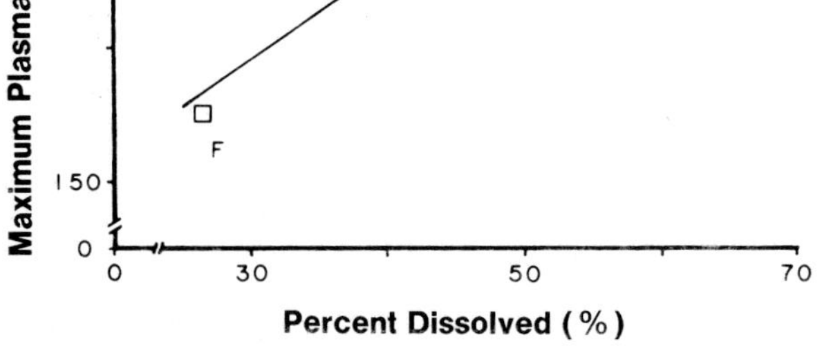

Table 2.
In Vitro and In Vivo Correlation Results

Variable	Time during In Vitro Testing			
	0.5 hr	1 hr	3 hr	6 hr
AUC_{12} R^{2a}	0.965	0.916	0.870	0.801
Slope	36.0	31.1	28.7	30.1
AUC_{36} R^2	0.786	0.701	0.686	0.669
Slope	25.8	21.6	20.2	22.0
C_{max} R^{2a}	0.984	0.939	0.908	0.858
Slope	3.40	2.95	2.74	2.93

[a] $p < 0.05$ at all time points.

Table 3.
Mean (±S.D.) Morning Predose Plasma Concentrations (ng/mL) During the Multiple-Dose Study

Day	Formulation	
	Reference	D
1	0	0
2	140 ± 47	131 ± 47
3	149 ± 69	141 ± 46
4	139 ± 57	144 ± 57
5	157 ± 59	146 ± 64
6	155 ± 53	140 ± 44

Table 4.
Mean (±S.D.) Pharmacokinetic Variables Determined in the Multiple-Dose Study

Formulation	AUC_{ss} (ng·hr/mL)	Ratio[a] (AUC_{ss})	95% Confidence Interval[b] Lower	Upper	C_{max} (ng/mL)	Ratio[a] (C_{max})	95% Confidence Interval[b] Lower	Upper	t_{max} (hr)
Reference	3186 ± 1057	...	...	...	360 ± 114	...	...	...	1.7 ± 1.0
D	3088 ± 707	1.030 ± 0.237	0.878	1.105	347 ± 87	0.996 ± 0.197	0.883	1.057	5.2 ± 1.8

[a] Ratio of AUC_{ss} and C_{max} for formulation D divided by that of the reference formulation.
[b] Confidence interval of ratios.

Figure 3. Mean plasma concentrations in the multiple-dose study (n = 12). The curve labeled D represents the concentrations following ingestion of formulation D; curve REF represents concentrations following ingestion of the reference formulation.

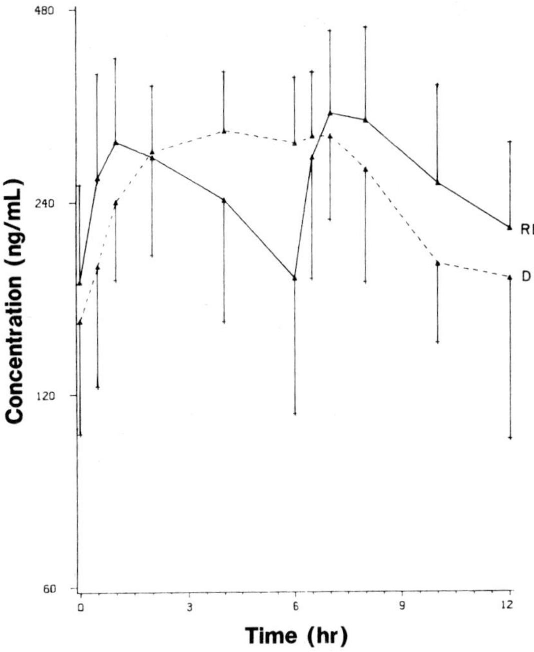

drug release as well as in vitro and in vivo correlations. The use of a series of drug formulations with an intentionally broad range of release rates permitted selection of an optimal formulation in addition to contributing information about pharmacokinetic factors that are affected by varying pseudoephedrine release rates.

It was not surprising that total AUC_{36} was not significantly related to release rates and coating level with in vitro and in vivo correlations because previous work with the Pennkinetic System suggested that complete release occurs even with heavily coated particles. The only limiting factor appears to be gastrointestinal transit time. Apparently with pseudoephedrine, a coating level somewhere between formulations E and F causes the drug to be released too slowly, and hence a portion of the dose is not absorbed, as seen with formulation F.

We did not attempt to characterize in vitro release rates, as suggested by others.[9] Since the release of drug from the Pennkinetic System is not first- or zero-order, it is not appropriate to define percent drug dissolved versus time plots using linear rate constants. Similarly, we did not use in vivo terms other than AUC, C_{max}, and t_{max} with pharmacokinetic analyses, as other derived variables (e.g., terminal elimination half-life, area under the first product–moment curve), while being model independent, are dependent on absorption and elimination linearity.

Conclusion

The methods described in these studies have permitted us to establish in vitro dissolution specifications for controlled-release pseudoephedrine; this ensures the continuous production of a bioavailable drug product. These types of studies have been exceedingly useful to us with other drugs and potentially could be applied to other drug-delivery systems.

References

1. Goodman and Gilman's the pharmacologic basis of therapeutics. 6th ed. Gilman AG, Goodman LS, Gilman A, eds. New York: Macmillan Publishing Co., Inc.; 1980:168–9.
2. Amsel L. Pennkinetic: a flexible drug delivery system. In: Controlled-release drug delivery and Pennkinetic. Springfield, NJ: Omega Communications, Inc; 1983.
3. Amsel LP, Hinsvark ON, Rotenberg KS et al. Recent advances in sustained-release technology using ion-exchange polymers. *Pharm Tech.* 1984; 8:28–48.
4. Owen DB. Handbook of statistical tables. Reading, MA: Addison-Wesley Publishing Co.; 1962.
5. Pearson ES, Hartley HO. Biometrika tables for statisticians. Volume 1. London: Biometrika Trust; 1976:141.
6. Cox DC, Douglas CC, Furman WB et al. Guidelines for dissolution testing. *Pharm Tech.* 1978; 2:41–53.
7. Cox DC, Furman WB, Moore TW et al. Guidelines for dissolution testing: an addendum. *Pharm Tech.* 1984; 8:42–6.
8. The United States Pharmacopeia, 20th rev., and the national formulary, 15th ed. Rockville, MD: The United States Pharmacopeial Convention; 1982:310–1.
9. Chambliss WG, Cleary RW, Fischer R et al. Effect of docusate sodium on drug release from a controlled-release dosage form. *J Pharm Sci.* 1981; 70:1248–51.

Research Note

Treatment of cancer-associated hypercalcemia with mithramycin and oral etidronate disodium

DANIEL H. SHEVRIN, LINDA R. BRESSLER, WILLIAM P. MCGUIRE, SUBHASH C. KUKREJA, LAWRENCE J. KUKLA, AND THOMAS E. LAD

Clin Pharm. 1985; 4:204–5

The management of cancer-associated hypercalcemia is often difficult because of the lack of an effective oral agent and the transient effects of available injectable drugs. Mithramycin is the most effective drug currently available[1]; its mechanism of action is thought to be inhibition of bone resorption.[2] It has a short duration of action (usually 3–5 days) and can have substantial cumulative toxicity.[2,3] The diphosphonates are a group of compounds that inhibit bone resorption in vitro and in vivo.[4] Etidronate disodium is the only diphosphonate currently available for clinical use in the United States, and it is used most frequently in the treatment of Paget's disease of bone.[5] Because oral etidronate disodium appears to have little activity when used alone in the treatment of cancer-associated hypercalcemia,[1,6] we designed this study to determine whether oral etidronate disodium would be useful as an adjunct to mithramycin in the treatment of hypercalcemia of malignancy.

Methods. This study was approved by the Institutional Review Boards at the West Side Veterans Administration Hospital and the University of Illinois Hospital. Patients were eligible to enter the study if they met the following criteria: a malignancy other than multiple myeloma or lymphoma, severe hypercalcemia (>11.5 mg/dL after hydration), adequate renal function (urea nitrogen <20 mg/dL after hydration), normal platelet count (>100,000/cu mm), and no calcium-lowering or antineoplastic treatment during the study period. Patients with hypercalcemia received 0.9% sodium chloride injection i.v. at a rate of 125–165 mL/hour for 24 hours. The total serum calcium concentration was determined after 24 hours of fluid administration; if the patient's serum calcium concentration exceeded 11.5 mg/dL (normal range 8.5–10.2 mg/dL), the patient was enrolled in the study after informed consent was obtained.

Each patient received an i.v. bolus dose of mithramycin 25 μg/kg. Patients were then randomly assigned to receive either adjunctive therapy with oral etidronate disodium (10 mg/kg/day) or no adjunctive therapy.

Once patients were admitted into the study, total serum calcium concentrations were determined daily while patients were hospitalized and twice weekly when patients were monitored in the outpatient clinic. Additional mithramycin was given to patients in either group if the serum calcium concentration obtained 24 hours after the initial dose of mithramycin had not decreased or if the serum calcium concentration exceeded 11.5 mg/dL after an initial reduction. The number of days between doses of mithramycin was recorded for each patient and considered a separate data point for statistical analysis. A two-tailed Student's t test was used to evaluate any differences in serum calcium concentrations or mithramycin dosing intervals for the two treatment groups. A p value less than or equal to 0.05 was considered significant.

Results. Eight patients entered the study, and four patients were assigned to each treatment group. All patients had advanced non-small-cell lung cancer (seven squamous and one large cell). The mean number of days between mithramycin doses was significantly greater for the group that received etidronate disodium than for the group that did not receive etidronate disodium (Table 1). The other variables measured were not significantly different between the two groups (Table 1).

Table 2 shows that the mean numbers of study days spent as outpatients and as inpatients were not significantly different between the two treatment groups. Similarly, the mean numbers of calcium concentration determinations done for outpatients and for inpatients were not significantly different between the two groups.

Both regimens were well tolerated. No patients receiving etidronate disodium developed diarrhea,

DANIEL H. SHEVRIN, M.D., is Instructor in Medicine, University of Illinois at Chicago (UIC), and Staff Physician, Section of Medical Oncology, University of Illinois Hospital (UIH), Chicago. LINDA R. BRESSLER, PHARM.D., is Clinical Assistant Professor, College of Pharmacy, UIC. WILLIAM P. MCGUIRE, M.D., is Associate Professor of Clinical Medicine, UIC, and Chief, Section of Medical Oncology, UIH. SUBHASH C. KUKREJA, M.D., is Associate Professor of Medicine, UIC, and Staff Physician, West Side Veterans Administration Medical Center (WSVAMC), Chicago, IL. LAWRENCE J. KUKLA, M.D., is Assistant Professor of Medicine, UIC, and Staff Physician, WSVAMC. THOMAS E. LAD, M.D., is Associate Professor of Clinical Medicine, UIC, and Chief of Medical Oncology Services, WSVAMC.

Address reprint requests to Dr. Shevrin at the Medical Oncology Section, Department of Medicine, University of Illinois Hospital, P.O. Box 6998, Chicago, IL 60680.

Table 1.
Serum Calcium Concentrations and Mithramycin Dosing Schedules for Patients Receiving and Not Receiving Etidronate Disodium

	Mithramycin plus Etidronate Disodium		Mithramycin Only	
Variable	No. Observations	Mean ± S.D.	No. Observations	Mean ± S.D.
Initial serum calcium concentration (mg/dL)[a]	4	14.3 ± 1.7	4	14.3 ± 0.5
Serum calcium (mg/dL) after hydration[a]	4	13.6 ± 2.0	4	13.5 ± 0.9
Serum calcium (mg/dL) during therapy[a]	86	12.0 ± 1.3	54	12.3 ± 0.9
Number of mithramycin doses	29	7.3 ± 5.3	27	6.8 ± 4.9
Days between mithramycin doses[b]	25	9.2 ± 5.5	23	5.1 ± 2.6

[a] Normal range = 8.6–10.2 mg/dL.
[b] Significantly different for the two treatment regimens.

Table 2.
Number of Hospital Days and Serum Calcium Concentration Determinations during Inpatient and Outpatient Periods

	Inpatient		Outpatient	
Patient	No. Hospital Days	No. Calcium Levels	No. Hospital Days	No. Calcium Levels
Treated with Mithramycin plus Etidronate Disodium				
1	69	41	130	36
2	20	8	23	6
3	8	8	13	4
4	21	14	10	2
Mean ± S.D.	29.5 ± 27	17.8 ± 16	44 ± 58	12 ± 16
Treated with Mithramycin Only				
5	20	10	0	0
6	30	25	6	2
7	6	6	0	0
8	4	3	107	22
Mean ± S.D.	15 ± 12	11 ± 10	28.3 ± 53	6 ± 10.7

the most commonly reported adverse reaction.[4] One patient receiving mithramycin developed mild renal insufficiency (creatinine 2.3 mg/dL). Deaths were attributed to progression of lung cancer and hypercalcemia. Median survival of the two groups was similar (37 and 40 days).

Discussion. Since the literature suggests that etidronate disodium alone would not be likely to control cancer-associated hypercalcemia, we decided to evaluate the calcium-lowering effect of etidronate disodium on the basis of its ability to prolong the interval between doses of mithramycin. The use of etidronate disodium increased this interval by an average of four days. Clinically, such a prolongation might allow administration of mithramycin only once instead of twice weekly. Theoretically, fewer doses of mithramycin would be required and the risk of cumulative toxicity would be decreased. Because there were no significant differences between the two treatment groups in the numbers of inpatient and outpatient days or in the numbers of inpatient and outpatient serum calcium concentration determinations, we believe that the prolongation in the mithramycin dosing interval reflects improved control of hypercalcemia in the group receiving etidronate disodium.

The dose of etidronate disodium used in this study (10 mg/kg/day) was chosen to avoid the possible development of osteomalacia. However, since osteomalacia should not be a major concern in patients with a short life expectancy, a higher dose of etidronate disodium could be used.

Conclusion. The addition of etidronate disodium to standard intermittent mithramycin therapy might improve the quality of life for patients with hypercalcemia of malignancy by permitting less frequent mithramycin dosing.

References

1. Mundy GR, Wilkinson R, Heath DA. Comparative study of available medical therapy for hypercalcemia of malignancy. *Am J Med.* 1983; 74:421–32.
2. Kiang DT, Loken MK, Kennedy BJ. Mechanism of the hypocalcemic effect of mithramycin. *J Clin Endocrinol Metab.* 1979; 48:341–4.
3. Slayton RE, Shnider BI, Elias E et al. New approach to the treatment of hypercalcemia: the effect of short-term treatment with mithramycin. *Clin Pharmacol Ther.* 1971; 12:833–7.
4. Russel RGG, Smith R. Diphosphonates. Experimental and clinical aspects. *J Bone Joint Surg.* 1973; 55B:66–86.
5. Khairi MRA, Altman RD, DeRose GP et al. Sodium etidronate in the treatment of Paget's disease of bone. *Ann Intern Med.* 1977; 87:656–63.
6. Jung A. Comparison of two parenteral diphosphonates in hypercalcemia of malignancy. *Am J Med.* 1982; 72:221–6.

Grand Rounds

Papers in the Grand Rounds section are patient case reports and literature review combined in a way that gives them high educational value. The papers lead off with a well-documented case report of an unusual drug experience (e.g., adverse drug reaction or other unexpected drug response, experimental use of a drug). The case generally deals with a difficult therapeutic problem or dilemma that is commonly encountered but may be overlooked or misunderstood. (Esoteric or rare occurrences of minor importance do not make good Grand Rounds material.) A literature review puts the case in perspective with previously reported similar cases and alternative treatments. The review is integrated with related discussions of the new case being reported.

CP readers are encouraged to use Grand Rounds for educational group discussions. For this purpose, discussion questions are printed at the end of Grand Rounds papers.

Immune globulin in the treatment of autoimmune thrombocytopenic purpura

CINDY J. WORDELL, ELIZABETH A. STUBITS, KAREN J. TIETZE, JANICE A. GASKA, AND ELLEN M. COSGROVE

Abstract: Two patients with autoimmune thrombocytopenic purpura (ATP) who received high-dose intravenous immune globulin before undergoing splenectomy are described, and the pathogenesis, clinical presentation, diagnosis, and treatment of chronic ATP are reviewed.

One patient was a 62-year-old white man who was admitted to the hospital with a history of thrombocytopenia and probable steroid-induced diabetes mellitus. The second patient was a 24-year-old black woman who was admitted for recurrent bleeding episodes and splenectomy. In both patients, immune globulin 1.5 g/kg administered over four to six days resulted in marked elevations of platelet counts.

ATP is a platelet disorder of unknown etiology. Platelets with surface-bound antiplatelet antibody are destroyed by the reticuloendothelial system. As the platelet count falls below 30,000–50,000/cu mm, the patient may manifest signs of bleeding such as petechiae, purpura, ecchymosis, menorrhagia, epistaxis, and bleeding from other mucosal surfaces. Corticosteroids are the initial treatment of choice. Splenectomy is considered for children with life-threatening hemorrhage and for patients who do not respond to corticosteroids. Patients who are refractory to steroid therapy and splenectomy may respond to immunosuppressant agents. Approximately, 80% of patients treated with immune globulin have responded with an increase in platelet count, although this increase is sometimes transient.

Immune globulin therapy is recommended for emergency treatment of ATP, as preoperative medication before splenectomy, and for young children in order to postpone splenectomy. Despite a good response to treatment, immune globulin therapy should not be considered a cure for ATP.

Index terms: Dosage; Globulin immune; Purpura
Clin Pharm. 1985; 4:206–13

CINDY J. WORDELL, PHARM.D., is Advanced Resident in Drug Information, Thomas Jefferson University Hospital, Philadelphia. ELIZABETH A. STUBITS, PHARM.D., is Pharmacy Resident in Pharmacokinetics, University of California at San Francisco, San Francisco. KAREN J. TIETZE, PHARM.D., AND JANICE A. GASKA, PHARM.D., are Assistant Professors of Clinical Pharmacy, Philadelphia College of Pharmacy and Science, Philadelphia. ELLEN M. COSGROVE, M.D., is Associate Professor of Medicine, Hahnemann University, Philadelphia.

Address reprint requests to Dr. Tietze at the Department of Pharmacy, Philadelphia College of Pharmacy and Science, 43rd and Kingsessing Mall, Philadelphia, PA 19104.

The assistance of Diana L. Esbin in the preparation of this manuscript is acknowledged.

Presented in part at the poster session of the 18th Annual ASHP Midyear Clinical Meeting, Atlanta, GA, December 7, 1983.

Autoimmune thrombocytopenic purpura (ATP) is a platelet disorder of unknown etiology.[1-4] Three clinical presentations have been identified. These include acute, recurrent, and chronic ATP (Table 1). The acute form, which may follow a viral infection, occurs most frequently in children between the ages of two and six years. The female to male ratio is approximately 1 to 1. Overall, the mortality rate of acute ATP is approximately 1%. Recurrent ATP usually occurs in young adult women between 20 and 40 years of age. This form is characterized by an insidious onset and self-limited intermittent episodes of thrombocytopenia. Chronic ATP, a disease of adults, is characterized by persistent thrombocytopenia lasting more than six months, and the female to male ratio is approximately 3 to 1.

ATP is considered a diagnosis of exclusion. Other potential causes of thrombocytopenia, such as transfusions, diseases (e.g., systemic lupus erythematosus and lymphoreticular disorders), and drugs[5] (e.g., quinidine), must be considered and excluded.

In this paper, the pathogenesis, clinical presentation, diagnosis, and treatment of chronic ATP are reviewed, with an in-depth discussion of the use of immune globulin therapy. Two case reports are also presented that illustrate the use of high-dose intravenous immune globulin in the presplenectomy treatment of patients with ATP.

Case Reports

Case 1. A 62-year-old white man was admitted with a history of thrombocytopenia. The patient's thrombocytopenia was first documented three months before this admission. At that time, a bone-marrow biopsy showed adequate megakaryocytes and platelet-associated IgG antibodies were identified. No splenomegaly was noted on physical examination. A diagnosis of ATP was made. The patient was started on a regimen of prednisone 60 mg every morning, which was decreased to 20 mg every other day to minimize fluid retention.

On admission the patient complained of recurrent nose bleeds and gingival bleeding. He denied any nausea, vomiting, hematuria, hematemesis, abdominal pain, headaches, trauma, or toxin exposure.

Pertinent medical history findings included a diagnosis of a non-Hodgkin's lymphoma in 1972, which was treated with nitrogen mustard and methotrexate; angina; adenocarcinoma of the prostate (stage II B), which was treated with radiation; peripheral vascular disease; hypertension; and a right upper-lobe infiltrate with a positive purified protein derivative of tuberculin (PPD) history. He had a family history of leukemia but no history of bleeding abnormalities. He had a 40-pack-year smoking history (equivalent to one pack of cigarettes per day for 40 years).

On admission, the vital signs were within normal limits. The patient was a well-developed, well-nourished man in no apparent distress. Pertinent physical findings were petechiae over the anterior and posterior trunk. The stool was heme-positive. No masses or hepatosplenomegaly were found in an abdominal examination.

Laboratory findings on admission were within normal ranges with the exceptions of a serum glucose determination of 404 mg/dL (normal 70–115 mg/dL) and a platelet count of 6000/cu mm (normal 150,000–500,000/cu mm).

The patient had been taking prednisone 20 mg orally every other day for three months, furosemide 40 mg orally every morning for six years, isoniazid 300 mg orally every morning for three months, and diazepam 5 mg orally as needed for anxiety. He had also received several vincristine sulfate doses in the past three months.

The patient was admitted to the hospital with thrombocytopenia and probable steroid-induced diabetes mellitus. Prednisone therapy was continued at a dose of 20 mg every other day. Seven days into the hospitalization, the prednisone dose was increased to 100 mg daily. After two weeks of high-dose prednisone therapy, high-dose intravenous immune globulin therapy of 1.5 g/kg over six days was initiated. The day following the last dose of immune globulin, the platelet count was 98,000/cu mm, and a splenectomy was performed. The platelet count following surgery was 7000/cu mm on the second postoperative day (Figure 1). Corticosteroids were continued, and mercaptopurine and androgens were started one week following surgery. Findings upon bone-marrow examination remained unchanged following surgery.

The patient was hospitalized for several weeks following surgery with numerous complications involving infections. During the year following splenectomy, the patient had multiple hospital admissions for the management of thrombocytopenia. Treatment included prednisone and a course of slow vinblastine infusions.[9] Platelet counts remained less than 50,000/cu mm during the year following surgery.

Case 2. A 24-year-old black woman was admitted for recurrent bleeding episodes and splenectomy. Three weeks before this admission, ATP was diagnosed following a nine-month history of spontaneous bruising, occasional epistaxis, intermittent spontaneous gingival bleeding, and an episode of near syncope for which she was brought to the emergency room. The patient had no history of drug or toxin exposure. A platelet count of 5000/cu mm and megakaryocyte hyperplasia on bone-marrow biopsy confirmed the diagnosis of ATP. Other hematologic disorders were ruled out because of a normal hemoglobin electrophoresis pattern and negative anti-

Table 1.
Clinical Presentations of Autoimmune Thrombocytopenic Purpura

Clinical Presentation	Age Group Prevalence	Female: Male Ratio	Duration of Disease
Acute	Children	1:1	One to two months (usually less than six months)
Recurrent	Children and adults	Not described	Initial episode lasts less than six months with recurrences
Chronic	Adults	3:1	Greater than six months to years

Figure 1. Platelet count during the hospitalization of patient 1; where IG = immune globulin and VC = vincristine sulfate.

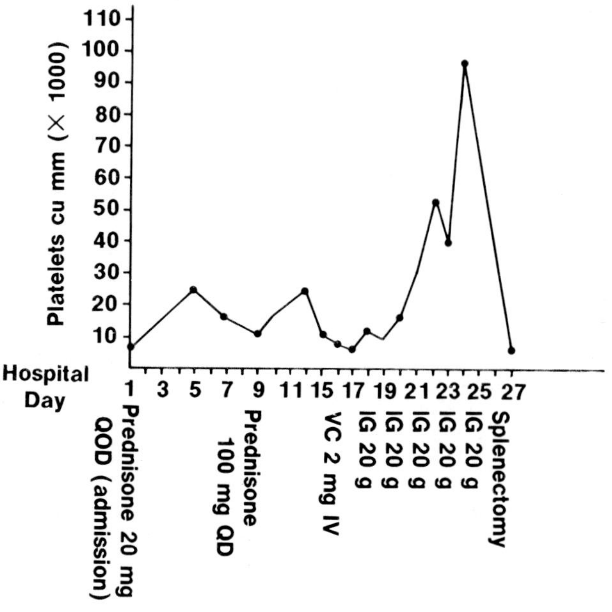

Figure 2. Platelet count during the hospitalization of patient 2; where IG = immune globulin, HC = hydrocortisone succinate, and COR = cortisone acetate.

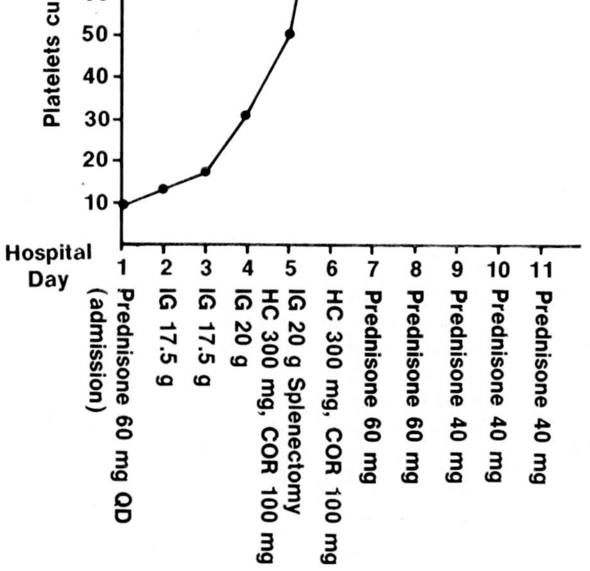

nuclear antibody titer, lupus erythematosus preparation, rheumatoid factor, and Coombs' tests. She was treated with prednisone 120 mg daily (2 mg/kg/day) for one week and was discharged on day 10 with a platelet count of 23,000/cu mm on an oral dose of 60 mg of prednisone daily. Three days after discharge, she noted the onset of gingival oozing, spontaneous development of ecchymosis on her left thigh, one occurrence of spontaneous epistaxis, and the development of petechiae on her extremities. She denied hematuria, hematemesis, bright red blood in her stools, menorrhagia, joint pain or swelling, abdominal pain, headache, syncope, and visual changes. Her family history was negative for sickle-cell disease and other bleeding abnormalities. The patient denied smoking, the use of nonprescription or recreational drugs, and the use of alcohol.

The patient had been taking prednisone 60 mg daily (1 mg/kg/day) for two weeks, ferrous sulfate 325 mg orally twice daily for three weeks, and a combination tablet of pseudoephedrine hydrochloride 60 mg and triprolidine hydrochloride 2.5 mg, three times daily for two days before admission.

On admission, the vital signs were within normal limits. The physical examination confirmed petechiae and ecchymoses on the left upper arm and the mucous membranes of the mouth. Abdominal examination failed to reveal masses or hepatosplenomegaly.

Laboratory findings on admission were within normal ranges except for a hematocrit of 39.6% (normal 42–52%), white blood cell count of 13,600/cu mm (normal 4,800–10,800/cu mm) with a normal differential, and a platelet count of 9000/cu mm (normal 150,000–500,000/cu mm). Urinalysis showed a pH within normal limits, 2+ hemoglobin, 2+ bacteria, and 0–2 red blood cells per high-power field.

Splenectomy was scheduled for hospital day 5. The patient received immune globulin in an effort to elevate the platelet count before splenectomy. She received a total of 1.5 g/kg over a four-day period. The platelet count rose from 13,000/cu mm before the administration of the first dose to 50,000/cu mm on the day of surgery, when 75% of the total dose had been received. The patient's gingival oozing ceased at this time. The fourth dose was administered the morning of surgery, and on postoperative day 1 the patient had a platelet count of 96,000/cu mm (Figure 2). The patient's recovery was uneventful, and she was discharged six days after splenectomy with a platelet count of 97,000/cu mm. The prednisone therapy was slowly tapered and discontinued.

Discussion

Clinical Features. The clinical presentation of a patient with ATP depends upon the degree of thrombocytopenia. A platelet count greater than 50,000/cu mm will usually support hemostasis. As the platelet count falls below 30,000–50,000/cu mm, the patient may manifest signs of bleeding such as petechiae, purpura, ecchymoses, menorrhagia, epistaxis, and bleeding from other mucosal surfaces. Platelet counts less than 10,000/cu mm may result in severe, spontaneous episodes of bleeding. Bleeding abnormalities will not usually be severe enough to result in central nervous system hemorrhage.[2,3] Trauma, fever, infection, azotemia, and antiplatelet drugs may enhance the bleeding tendency.[4]

Both patients discussed here manifested clinical signs and symptoms of ATP including thrombocytopenia, petechiae, ecchymoses, and spontaneous bleeding (nasal and gingival).

Diagnosis. ATP is diagnosed based on the following[2]:

1. Increased platelet destruction shown by thrombocytopenia or shortened platelet survival.
2. Increased number of megakaryocytes in the bone marrow.
3. The presence of bound antiplatelet antibodies without concurrent conditions known to cause their production such as septicemia or hypergammaglobulinemia.
4. Exclusion of other primary clinical disorders that are capable of causing the above criteria, such as systemic lupus erythematosus, lymphoma, and drug-induced thrombocytopenia.
5. The absence of splenomegaly, except in children (in whom a palpable spleen may be normal).

Pathogenesis. A serum antiplatelet factor was identified in the 1950s. Subsequently the serum antiplatelet factor was demonstrated to be an immunoglobulin of the IgG type either alone or in combination with IgM or IgA.[1-3] Though disease severity does not correlate with the presence of antiplatelet antibody, it is associated with the presence of platelet-bound antiplatelet antibody.[2] The antiplatelet antibody may bind to megakaryocytes in the bone marrow, but the importance of this antimegakaryocyte antibody is not known.

In addition to the serum- and bone-marrow-bound antiplatelet antibodies, patients with ATP also may have circulating immune complexes. The role of circulating immune complexes in this disorder is not well established. Some investigators have hypothesized that decreased platelet survival results from the deficient immune response to the adherence of infectious antigens or small immune complexes to the platelets.[6]

Since the identification of antiplatelet antibody in patients with ATP, the term "idiopathic" is no longer used.[2] Bound antiplatelet antibody has been identified in 90–95% of the cases of ATP. In the 5–10% of the cases where this cannot be found, the term idiopathic thrombocytopenic purpura is used.

Platelets with surface-bound antiplatelet antibody are destroyed by the reticuloendothelial system (RES), which includes the spleen, liver, and bone marrow. The spleen is a site of antiplatelet antibody production and the primary site of platelet destruction. The liver is not capable of major antibody production and has a small collection of platelets. The phagocytic cells in the liver are more efficient than those of the spleen and may contribute to platelet destruction after splenectomy or when there is a very high level of antiplatelet antibody.[2,3]

Treatment. The primary goal of treatment is to obtain a complete remission, which is possible in 80–90% of patients. In cases where a complete remission is not achievable, the therapeutic goal is to maintain the platelet count above 30,000–50,000/cu mm. All drugs (e.g., aspirin, dipyridamole, sulfinpyrazone, nonsteroidal anti-inflammatory agents) that affect the production or function of platelets should be avoided in these patients.

Corticosteroids are the initial treatment of choice for ATP. Therapy is usually initiated with oral prednisone 1 mg/kg/day or an equivalent corticosteroid. A response can be expected after three to seven days with the maximal response within two to three weeks. The dose of prednisone may be increased to 1.2–2 mg/kg/day. Once platelet counts are within the normal range, the prednisone dose should be tapered by 10–20 mg per week to a maintenance dose of less than 10 mg/day. Remission in 40–60% of cases has been reported with steroid therapy.[1-3]

Splenectomy should be considered for children with life-threatening hemorrhage and for patients who do not achieve a satisfactory response to corticosteroids within a two- to six-month period of time.[1,2] Approximately 80% of the patients refractory to corticosteroids will respond to splenectomy. The response is secondary to the removal of the primary site of antibody production and platelet destruction. Patients who do not respond well to splenectomy may benefit from the postsplenectomy administration of steroids.[3] Ten percent of the patients who have had a splenectomy may relapse within one to five years.[1,3]

Patients who are refractory to steroid therapy and splenectomy may respond to immunosuppressant agents, such as azathioprine, cyclophosphamide, or vincristine sulfate.[1-3] Azathioprine, in doses of 1–2 mg/kg/day, either alone or in combination with corticosteroids infrequently results in complete remission, but adequate platelet levels may be achieved with prolonged maintenance therapy.[3] Complete remissions have been reported using cyclophosphamide in doses of 2–3 mg/kg/day orally or 300–600 mg/sq m intravenously every three weeks. Remissions have occurred within two to eight weeks in 30–40% of refractory ATP patients. Cyclophosphamide therapy is continued for four to six weeks after adequate platelet counts are achieved.[3] Vincristine sulfate (0.025 mg/kg, maximum dose of 2 mg) or vinblastine sulfate (0.125 mg/kg, maximum dose of 10 mg) may be given intravenously every 7–10 days. Response is rapid but transient, and long-term remission is unusual.[2,3]

Experimental treatment modalities have included plasmapheresis,[2,3] danazol,[7] in vitro[8] and in vivo[9] vinca alkaloids, and until the recent approval of Sandoglobulin (Sandoz Pharmaceuticals) for this indication, high-dose intravenous immune globulin.[10–38]

Immune Globulin Therapy. The beneficial effect of high-dose immune globulin was first reported by Imbach et al.[10,11] in a group of 13 children. All of the children had an increase in platelet count following the administration of 0.4 g/kg/day of immune globulin for five consecutive days. Seven of the children had chronic idiopathic thrombocytopenic purpura, and all but one could be maintained in remission on a dose of 0.4 g/kg administered intravenously every one to six weeks. Since this original report, there have been additional reports[12–35] of 171 patients treated with high-dose immune globulin for either acute or chronic ATP. These included 42 children and 129 adults (Table 2), and of the 171 total, 138 (81%) had at least a transient elevation in their platelet count. Total induction doses ranged from 1 to 5 g/kg administered over 3–10 consecutive days. Some patients received additional "maintenance" doses.

The mechanism of action of intravenous immune globulin in ATP is not well established. The increased platelet destruction seems to be related to the IgG-bound platelet antibody. Consistent with this, the level of platelet-bound IgG is inversely correlated with the platelet count and platelet survival.[3] Several mechanisms have been suggested.[13,24,26,36–39]

Jungi et al.[39] recently summarized three hypothetical models of action of immune globulin in ATP therapy. These are as follows:

1. Infusion of exogenous IgG provides the antibodies against circulating infectious antigens or small immune complexes that the patient cannot produce endogenously. The antigens and small immune complexes are converted into larger aggregates by the infused IgG. These are then eliminated by the RES leaving the platelets intact.
2. By exogenously increasing the levels of monomeric IgG (single-constituent IgG), the platelets may be protected from being coated by circulating immune complexes. This probably occurs via competitive binding between monomeric IgG and circulating immune complexes to the platelet Fc receptors.
3. Monomeric IgG may nonspecifically bind to the Fc receptors of platelets (coat the platelet) and thereby

Table 2.
Summary of Literature Reports of Patients Treated with Immune Globulin

Reference Number	Number of Patients	Age (yr)	Total Cumulative Induction Dose (g)	Duration of Therapy (days)	Response[a]	
					Effective	Not Effective
10, 11	13[b]	0.5–14	2	5	13	0
12	4	Adults	2	5	2	2
13	4	Adults	1–1.5	4–5	4	0
14	1	6	2	5	0	1
15	1[c]	Adults	2.45	5	1	0
16	12[c]	Adults	1.6–2.3	4–5	4	8[d]
17	13	2 Children 11 Adults	2	5	11	2
18	4	2 Children 11 Adults	2	5	2	2
19	8	6 Children 2 Adults	0.5 g/kg/day	4–10	7	1
20	25	1 Child 24 Adults	2	5	25	0
21	9	Adults	0.25–0.4 g/kg/day	5–7	8	1
22	1	Adults	2	5	0	1
23	1	13	2	5	0	1
24	4	Adults	2	5	3	1
25	1[e]	Adults	2	5	1	0
26	12	8 Children 4 Adults	2	5	12	0
27	5	Adults	2	5	5	0
28	1	Neonate	2	5	1	0
29	16	12–86	2	3–5	11	5
30	18	Adults	2	5	12	6
31	1[e]	Adult	2.25	7	1	0
32	1[e]	Adult	2	5	1	0
33	2[e]	1 Neonate 1 Adult	1.2	3	2	0
34	8	Adults	2	5	8	0
35	6	Children	2	5	3	3

[a] Response defined by each author.
[b] Four ATP patients in reference 10 were reported in reference 11.
[c] Four of the ATP patients reported in reference 15 were reported in reference 16; therefore, in this table they are only included with reference 16.
[d] Three patients who required discontinuation of therapy secondary to adverse effects are classified as treatment failures.
[e] ATP in pregnant patients.

inhibit the phagocytosis of platelets by macrophages in the RES.

Other postulated mechanisms of action include (1) an inhibition of the production of antiplatelet antibodies by the large exogenous source of IgG, (2) preferential binding of IgG-coated erythrocytes to RES macrophages resulting in competitive inhibition of the binding of IgG-coated platelets, and (3) release of platelets from the spleen into the circulation following IgG infusion.

Five classes of immunoglobulins (IgM, IgD, IgE, IgG, and IgA) are found in man. Immunoglobulins are responsible for providing the humoral immunity necessary for defense against bacterial infections. Other functions of immunoglobulins include harnessing the vasoactive chemicals in mast cells and basophils, B cell class switching, and protection of mucous membrane surfaces. The major immunoglobulin class is IgG, which has a mean normal serum concentration of 1200 mg/dL. IgG can be further divided into four subclasses. These subclasses, their concentration, and functions are listed in Table 3.[40]

The IgG fraction is obtained from donor plasma that has been previously screened for hepatitis B surface antigen. The Cohn cold-ethanol fractionation method is used to separate the IgG as precipitate GG (fraction II).[41] This preparation of IgG is acceptable for intramuscular administration. Anticomplementary aggregates (ACA) of IgG are formed during this plasma fractionation process. These anticomplementary aggregates are capable of activating complement without an antigen being present. Intravenous administration of the intramuscular preparation may result in ACA-induced anaphylactic or anaphlactoid reactions.[42] The intramuscular preparation also contains prekallikrein activator (PKA). Circulatory collapse may result from intravenous PKA administration.[43]

Several different methods have been used in an effort to develop an IgG preparation that can be given safely by i.v. infusion.[43]

1. *Enzymatic degradation* of the IgG molecule with pepsin or plasmin is used to remove the Fc portion of the molecule. This eliminates ACA, but unfortunately the molecule lacks important Fc-functions, such as interacting with cell-surface receptors.[43]
2. *Chemical modification* of the IgG molecule through cleavage of the interchain disulfide bridges by sulfonation or reduction, and then alkylation removes ACA.[43] This is the method used by Cutter Laboratories to produce its immune globulin product.[44]
3. *Mild acid treatment* at pH 4 in the presence of trace amounts of pepsin during fractionation prevents the formation of IgG aggregates preventing ACA. These preparations contain primarily intact IgG molecules; therefore, the full range of activities are maintained.[43] This is the method used by Sandoz Pharmaceuticals in preparing its immune globulin product.[45]

IgG prepared for intravenous administration is compared for IgG subclass content to the World Health Organization 67/97 reference plasma (Table 4).[41,42]

Side effects of high-dose immune globulin are infrequent in ATP patients. Anaphylactoid reactions rarely occur following the administration of the intravenous immune globulin preparation. Patients may complain of flushing, chest tightness, dyspnea, abdominal and back pains, nausea, vomiting, and diarrhea.[43,46] These adverse effects do not usually occur in patients with intact immune systems. Other side effects include hypersensitivity reactions secondary to antigens (such as IgA) in the immune globulin preparation. If inappropriate processing or handling of the immune globulin occurs, patients may also have complications because of the presence of prekallikrein activator, kallikrein, or pyrogens.

Of the 171 patients reported in the literature, only three required discontinuation of therapy because of side effects. Side effects included chills, hyperthermia, cutaneous rash, and laryngeal edema. We did not see any adverse effects during treatment of our two patients.

Our review of the literature indicated that approximately 80% of patients treated with high-dose intravenous immune globulin responded with an increase in platelet count. The increased platelet count is often transient.

Table 3.
Subclasses of Immunoglobulin G[40]

Subclass	Mean Normal Serum Concentration (mg/dL)	Biological Functions
IgG1	840	Tissue protection; complement fixation
IgG2	240	Activity against polysaccharide containing bacteria
IgG3	80	Complement fixation
IgG4	40	Protects respiratory tract; harnesses mast cells and basophils
Total IgG	1200	Tissue protection from bacteria

Table 4.
Immunoglobulin G Subclass Distribution by Method of Preparation[41,42]

Method of Preparation	Percent of IgG Subclass 1	2	3	4
World Health Organization reference plasma	60.0	29.4	6.5	4.1
Mild acid treatment[a]	60.5	30.2	6.6	2.6
Reduction and alkylation[b]	70.2	28.2	0	1.6

[a] Sandoglobulin (Sandoz Pharmaceuticals) is prepared by this method.

[b] Gamimune (Cutter Laboratories) is prepared by this method.

Immune globulin therapy is recommended for the emergency treatment of ATP, as preoperative medication before splenectomy, and for young children in order to postpone splenectomy. Experience to date does not support the long-term treatment of chronic ATP with immune globulin. Despite a good response to treatment, immune globulin therapy should not be considered a cure for ATP.[47] Only immune globulin intravenous (Sandoglobulin, Sandoz Pharmaceuticals) is approved for the treatment of ATP. The recommended dose for the treatment of ATP is 0.4 g/kg/day for five consecutive days.

One important consideration is the cost of a course of therapy of high-dose intravenous immune globulin. A total dose of 2 g/kg for a 70-kg patient costs an average of $5,900. This expense will have to be weighed against the potential benefit of elevating the platelet count to an acceptable range.

Conclusion

Corticosteroids are the initial treatment of choice in ATP. Treatment of corticosteroid-resistant ATP includes other immunosuppressants, splenectomy, and therapies such as plasmapheresis and high-dose intravenous immune globulin.

Both of our patients received high-dose i.v. immune globulin before splenectomy in an effort to minimize bleeding complications secondary to surgery. In both cases, the platelet counts rose to greater than 50,000/cu mm, and a splenectomy was performed without complications.

Discussion Questions

1. In case 1, the patient failed to respond to splenectomy. What postoperative drug treatment could be recommended for this patient's ATP?
2. Would long-term use of i.v. immune globulin in a patient with corticosteroid-resistant ATP be advisable? Discuss the advantages and disadvantages of high-dose immune globulin.
3. Would a patient who fails to respond to a treatment course of Sandoz's immune globulin (Sandoglobulin) benefit from a trial of Cutter's product (Gamimune)?
4. Discuss the benefits versus the costs for a typical course of therapy with high-dose i.v. immune globulin in a patient with ATP.
5. A patient with ATP responsive to high-dose i.v. immune globulin experiences flushing, chest tightness, and nausea. Should immune globulin therapy be stopped?

References

1. Burns TR, Saleem A. Idiopathic thrombocytopenic purpura. *Am J Med.* 1983; 75:1001–7.
2. Karpatkin S. Autoimmune thrombocytopenic purpura. *Blood.* 1980; 56:329–43.
3. McMillan R. Chronic idiopathic thrombocytopenic purpura. *N Engl J Med.* 1981; 304:1135–47.
4. Baldini M. Idiopathic thrombocytopenic purpura. *N Engl J Med.* 1966; 274:1245–51, 1301–6, 1360–7.
5. Hackett T, Kelton JG, Powers P. Drug-induced platelet destruction. *Semin Thromb Hemostas.* 1982; 8:116–37.
6. Lurhuma AZ, Riccomi H, Masson PL. The occurrence of circulating immune complexes and viral antigens in idiopathic thrombocytopenic purpura. *Clin Exp Immunol.* 1977; 28:49–55.
7. Ahn YS, Harrington WJ, Simon SR et al. Danazol for the treatment of idiopathic thrombocytopenic purpura. *N Engl J Med.* 1983; 308:1396–9.
8. Ahn YS, Byrnes JJ, Harrington WJ et al. The treatment of idiopathic thrombocytopenia with vinblastine-loaded platelets. *N Engl J Med.* 1978; 298:1101–7.
9. Ahn YS, Harrington WJ, Mylvaganam R et al. Slow infusion of vinca alkaloids in the treatment of idiopathic thrombocytopenic purpura. *Ann Intern Med.* 1984; 100:192–6.
10. Imbach P, d'Apuzzo V, Hirt A et al. High-dose intravenous gammaglobulin for idiopathic thrombocytopenic purpura in childhood. *Lancet.* 1981; 1:1228–31.
11. Imbach P, Barandun S, Baumgartner C et al. High-dose intravenous gammaglobulin therapy of refractory, in particular, idiopathic thrombocytopenia in childhood. *Helv Paediatr Acta.* 1981; 46:81–6.
12. Schmidt RE, Budde U, Schafer G et al. High-dose intravenous gamma globulin for idiopathic thrombocytopenic purpura. *Lancet.* 1981; 2:475–6.
13. Fehr J, Hofmann V, Kappeler U. Transient reversal of thrombocytopenia in idiopathic thrombocytopenic purpura by high-dose intravenous gamma globulin. *N Engl J Med.* 1982; 306:1254–8.
14. Schmidt B, Forster J. Increased platelet-associated IgG in child on high-dose gammaglobulin for idiopathic thrombocytopenic purpura. *Lancet.* 1982; 2:39–40.
15. Bierling P, Farcet JP, Dvedari N et al. Increased platelet-associated IgG in patient on high-dose gammaglobulin for autoimmune thrombocytopenic purpura. *Lancet.* 1982; 2:388.
16. Bierling P, Farcet JP, Dvedari N et al. Gamma globulin for idiopathic thrombocytopenic purpura. *N Engl J Med.* 1982; 307:1150.
17. Faradji A, Lang JM, Boilletot A et al. Purpura thrombocytopenique idiopathique: traitement par transfusion d'immunoglobulines polyvalentes intraveineuses. *Nouv Presse Med.* 1982; 11:3107–10.
18. Blanchette VS, Luke D, Heubsch L et al. Immune thrombocytopenic purpura (ITP): correlation of reticuloendothelial system (RES) activity and platelet response to high-dose intravenous gammaglobulin therapy. *Blood.* 1982; 60(Suppl 1):184a.
19. Wahlen W, Graf N, Nienhaus KH et al. Untersuchungen zur thrombozytenmorphologie und funktion unter hochdosierter immunglobulin-therapie bei akuter und chronischer idiopathisch thrombozytopenischer purpura (ITP). 1 Mitteilung. *Klin Paediatr.* 1983; 195:17–23.
20. Newland AC, Minchinton RM, Treleaven JG et al. High-dose intravenous IgG in adults with autoimmune thrombocytopenia. *Lancet.* 1983; 1:84–7.
21. Abe T, Matsuda J, Kawasugi K et al. Clinical effect of intravenous immunoglobulin on chronic idiopathic thrombocytopenic purpura. *Blut.* 1983; 47:69–75.
22. Rowbotham B, Brearley RL. High-dose intravenous IgG in adults with autoimmune thrombocytopenia. *Lancet.* 1983; 1:410.
23. Hamasaki T, Sakano T, Tanaka Y et al. Idiopathic thrombocytopenic purpura treated with high doses of intravenous gammaglobulin and prednisolone: a case report. *Hiroshima J Med.Sci.* 1983; 32:79–81.
24. Carroll RR, Noyes WD, Kitchens CS. High-dose intravenous immunoglobulin therapy in patients with immune thrombocytopenic purpura. *JAMA.* 1983; 249:1748–50.
25. Morgenstern GR, Measday B, Hegde UM. Autoimmune thrombocytopenia in pregnancy: new approach to manage-

ment. *Br Med J.* 1983; 287:584.
26. Bussel JB, Kimberly RP, Inman RD et al. Intravenous gammaglobulin treatment of chronic idiopathic thrombocytopenic purpura. *Blood.* 1983; 62:480–6.
27. Budde U, Schafer G, Niese D et al. Intravenous immunoglobulin in immune thrombocytopenia. *Lancet.* 1983; 2: 578.
28. Chirico G, Duse M, Ugazio AG et al. High-dose intravenous gammaglobulin therapy for passive immune thrombocytopenia in the neonate. *J Pediatr.* 1983; 103:654–5.
29. Brearley RL, Rowbotham B. Gammaglobulin in the management of immune thrombocytopenia. *Br J Haematol.* 1983; 55:558–9.
30. Schmidt RE, Budde U, Broschen-Zywietz C et al. High-dose gammaglobulin therapy in adults with idiopathic thrombocytopenic purpura (ITP) clinical effects. *Blut.* 1984; 48:19–25.
31. Mizunuma H, Takahashi Y, Taguchi H et al. A new approach to idiopathic thrombocytopenic purpura during pregnancy by high-dose immunoglobulin G infusion. *Am J Obstet Gynecol.* 1984; 148:218–9.
32. Tchernia G, Dreyfus M, Laurian Y et al. Management of immune thrombocytopenia in pregnancy: response to infusions of immunoglobulins. *Am J Obstet Gynecol.* 1984; 148:225–6.
33. Newland AC, Boots MA, Patterson KG. Intravenous IgG for autoimmune thrombocytopenia in pregnancy. *N Engl J Med.* 1984; 310:261–2.
34. Oral A, Nusbacher J, Hill JB et al. Intravenous gamma globulin in the treatment of chronic idiopathic thrombocytopenic purpura in adults. *Am J Med.* 1984; 76(3A):187–92.
35. Warrier I, Lusher JM. Intravenous gamma globulin treatment in chronic idiopathic thrombocytopenic purpura in children. *Am J Med.* 1984; 76(3A):193–8.
36. Salama A, Mueller-Eckhardt C, Kiefel V. Effect of intravenous immunoglobulin in immune thrombocytopenia. *Lancet.* 1983; 2:193–5.
37. Schmidt KG, Rasmussen JW, Diederichsen H et al. Release of platelets into the circulation induced by gamma globulin treatment in a case of idiopathic thrombocytopenic purpura. *Blut.* 1984; 48:27–31.
38. Imbach P, Jungi TW. Possible mechanisms of intravenous immunoglobulin treatment in childhood idiopathic thrombocytopenic purpura (ITP). *Blut.* 1983; 46:117–24.
39. Jungi TW, Imbach P, Barandun S. Specific and nonspecific mechanisms of action of immunoglobulin G in therapy of idiopathic thrombocytopenic purpura (ITP). *Blut.* 1984; 48: 345–51.
40. Dwyer JM. Thirty years of supplying the missing link: history of gamma globulin therapy for immunodeficient states. *Am J Med.* 1984; 76:46–52.
41. Skvaril F. Qualitative and quantitative aspects of IgG subclasses in i.v. immunoglobulin preparations. In: Nydegger UE, ed. Immunohemotherapy: a guide to immunoglobulin prophylaxis and therapy. New York: Academic Press; 1981: 113–22.
42. Romer J, Morgenthaler JJ, Scherz R et al. Characterization of various immunoglobulin preparations for intravenous application. I. Protein composition and antibody content. *Vox Sang.* 1982; 42:62–73.
43. Romer J, Spath PJ. Molecular composition of immunoglobulin preparations and its relation to complement activation. In: Nydegger UE, ed. Immunohemotherapy: a guide to immunoglobulin prophylaxis and therapy. New York: Academic Press; 1981:123–30.
44. Cutter Biologicals. Immune globulin intravenous, 5% (in 10% maltose). Gamimune product literature. Berkeley, CA; 1984 Jun.
45. Sandoz Inc. Immune globulin intravenous. Sandoglobulin product literature. East Hanover, NJ; 1984 Feb.
46. Barandun S, Morell A. Adverse reactions to immunoglobulin preparations. In: Nydegger UE, ed. Immunohemotherapy. A guide to immunoglobulin prophylaxis and therapy. New York: Academic Press; 1981:223–7.
47. Gaedicke G, Imbach P, Kleihauer E. The place of intravenous immunoglobulin (IgG i.v.) therapy in thrombocytopenia. *Blut.* 1984; 48:409–13.

"

Inappropriate Use of Plasma Volume Expanders

Over the past decade hospitals throughout the United States have experienced a dramatic increase in utilization of fresh-frozen plasma (FFP). Since this has paralleled a corresponding increase in transfusion of packed red blood cells in relation to whole blood, it may be inferred that much of the FFP is being transfused as a volume expander, rather than as a source of clotting factors or plasma proteins. Use of plasma in this manner not only increases the cost of transfusion, but also increases the risk of transfusion-transmitted disease.

. . . The requirement for routine use of FFP for management of patients receiving a massive transfusion cannot be supported on scientific grounds. A bleeding tendency in these patients should be evaluated through appropriate studies. Most often this is due to platelet deficiency; therefore, such patients may require platelet concentrates as specific supplemental treatment. It must be recognized that each platelet concentrate contains approximately 50 mL of relatively fresh plasma with labile clotting factors. Since deficiency of labile plasma clotting factors to levels that would interfere with hemostasis is uncommon in these patients, [single-donor plasma] can be transfused interchangeably with FFP in most instances.

Unfortunately, strict guidelines for use of FFP based on currently available studies necessarily are vague. Without doubt, since most of this product currently is used for volume replacement, its use generally should be replaced by less dangerous colloid or crystalloid solutions.

—Oberman HA. Inappropriate use of fresh-frozen plasma. *JAMA.* 1985; 253: 556–7. Editorial.

"

Propranolol-induced depression and psychosis

WILLIAM A. PARKER

Abstract: Episodes of depression and acute psychosis in two patients receiving propranolol hydrochloride are described, and the literature on propranolol-induced depression and psychosis is reviewed.

A 42-year-old woman developed severe depression, marked apathy, social withdrawal, and anorexia after taking propranolol hydrochloride (80 mg/day) for three months to control her hypertension. Five days after the dose was reduced to 40 mg/day, there was a major improvement in her depressive symptoms, with a complete resolution in eight days. Upon rechallenge with 80 mg/day of propranolol, she again experienced depressive symptoms. Atenolol 50 mg/day was substituted for the propranolol therapy, and she exhibited a complete remission of her depression. The second patient was a 63-year-old man who had been taking propranolol hydrochloride 160 mg/day for three months without incident. Because of an increased frequency of anginal attacks, the dosage was increased to 240 mg/day. Within two days, he demonstrated such agitation, excitement, and combativeness that he had to be controlled with a 25-mg dose of methotrimeprazine. When the propranolol dose was reduced to 160 mg/day, his psychotic symptoms rapidly cleared. However, when the dose was subsequently increased to 200 mg/day, he again showed increased agitation. After substituting atenolol 100 mg/day for propranolol, the patient's mental status returned to normal.

Both of these patients experienced symptoms that were temporally associated with propranolol. Both patients were subsequently controlled without symptoms with atenolol therapy. Propranolol is a highly lipophilic β blocker that achieves high concentrations in the brain.

When continued β-blocking therapy is necessary or β blockade is indicated, a weakly lipophilic agent such as atenolol is indicated.

Index terms: Depression; Hypotensive agents; Propranolol hydrochloride; Psychotic disorders; Toxicity

Clin Pharm. 1985; 4:214–8

The Boston Collaborative Drug Surveillance Program reported that adverse reactions to propranolol occurred in nearly 10% of hospitalized patients treated with this β-adrenergic blocking agent.[1] The reported neurologic and psychiatric side effects of propranolol have included lassitude, fatigue, insomnia, vivid nightmares, hypnagogic hallucinations, confusional states, schizophrenic psychoses, and depression.[2–5] Although depression is regularly mentioned as a possible side effect of propranolol therapy, clinical reports of depression have been infrequent,[5–9] and one author has estimated that the risk of this side effect is less than 0.1%.[10] Others have confirmed this low incidence.[11,12] Considering that an estimated 15% of the population will experience at least one severe depressive episode during their lifetime, it is surprising there are not more reports of patients with depression who are taking β blockers.[12] Similarly, propranolol has been implicated infrequently in the induction of acute psychotic reactions and organic brain syndrome.[8,13–36] In fact, there has been more interest in the use of propranolol and other β blockers in the treatment of psychiatric illness than in their psychiatric side effects.[37–39]

The following cases describe episodes of depression and acute psychosis in two patients receiving propranolol hydrochloride. The cases also demonstrate the beneficial response obtained by substituting a nonlipophilic β-blocking agent (atenolol), which has a very low affinity for the central nervous system (CNS), for propranolol.

Case Reports

Case 1. A 60-kg, 42-year-old white woman without a history of psychiatric illness was given a prescription for propranolol hydrochloride to control her essential hypertension. For the past six months, she had been taking hydrochlorothiazide 50 mg daily. The dose of propranolol hydrochloride was maintained at 80 mg/day for two months, during which time she noted symptoms of fatigue, lack of concentration, and insomnia developing about a month after beginning the therapy. Her symptoms became progressively worse over the next month. She experienced increased difficulty in falling asleep with profound insomnia at night, daytime hypersomnia, episodic crying spells, apathy and lack of energy, sharply decreased libido, and diminished desire for social interactions. She demonstrated severe mood depression consisting of marked apathy, social withdrawal, loss of energy

WILLIAM A. PARKER, PHARM.D., M.B.A., is Associate Professor and Coordinator, Clinical Pharmacy, Dalhousie University and Clinical Pharmacist, Halifax Infirmary, Halifax, Nova Scotia.

Address reprint requests to Dr. Parker at the College of Pharmacy, Dalhousie University, Halifax, Nova Scotia, Canada B3H 3J5.

The assistance of Murray Nixon, M.D., and Beverly Atkinson is acknowledged.

and interest in daily activities, and a 5-kg weight loss attributed to anorexia over the two months. Although she was not actively suicidal, she did relate feelings of worthlessness and hopelessness on occasions.

She exhibited no illnesses other than seasonal rhinitis and hypertension, which was well controlled by the hydrochlorothiazide and propranolol therapy. She was receiving no other medications and was a nonsmoker and nondrinker. Results of a routine complete blood count, urinalysis, serum electrolytes, blood chemistries, and thyroid-function tests were within normal limits. Her blood pressure was well controlled at 122/84 mm Hg.

The propranolol hydrochloride dose was reduced to 40 mg daily, and there was a major improvement in her depressive symptoms five days later with a complete resolution in eight days. Her sleep patterns returned to normal, her energy and appetite returned, and she began to interact freely with other patients on the hospital ward. The diuretic dose was left unchanged, but since her hypertension was incompletely controlled (blood pressure 136/94 mm Hg), the dose of propranolol hydrochloride was gradually increased back to 80 mg daily over the next two weeks. Within five days of reaching 80 mg/day, she again experienced insomnia and mild depressive symptoms consisting of a loss of energy, apathy, and anorexia. At this point, the propranolol therapy was stopped and atenolol 50 mg daily was substituted. There was no decrease in blood pressure control. Over the next week, there was once again a rapid and complete remission of her anorexia, decreased energy, and apathy, and she remained euthymic and socially active for six months while taking the atenolol.

Case 2. A 75-kg, 63-year-old retired white man with no history of psychiatric illness was given a prescription for propranolol hydrochloride to control essential hypertension and angina pectoris. He had been receiving propranolol hydrochloride 160 mg/day for three months, without incident, along with sublingual nitroglycerin 0.6 mg as needed, and triamterene 50 mg plus hydrochlorothiazide 25 mg twice daily for several years. His blood pressure was well controlled at 136/84 mm Hg, and findings upon physical examination were noncontributory except for mild obesity. There was a history of mild maturity-onset diabetes mellitus controlled by diet. Blood glucose test results showed a concentration of 7.0 mmol/L (normal range from 3.6 to 5.8 mmol/L).

Because of a recent increase in the frequency of anginal attacks, the patient's propranolol hydrocloride dose was increased to 240 mg/day. Within two days he started to complain of difficulty concentrating. He also became agitated with excitement and showed occasional confusion and disorientation. He related vivid nightmares and auditory hallucinations, which prompted his admission to the hospital. Over the next two days, he became irritable and difficult for the nursing staff to manage. The hallucinations continued and were accompanied by delusions of persecution and paranoia. A single intramuscular dose of methotrimeprazine 25 mg (as the hydrochloride salt) was administered to control his agitation, excitement, and combativeness.

During the period of mental confusion, there were no important alterations in the test results for serum electrolytes, complete blood count, blood chemistries, arterial blood gases, or urinalysis. Brain scan and lumbar puncture yielded normal results, and blood cultures were negative.

Because of the rapid onset of symptoms following the increase in propranolol dosage, the dose was reduced to 160 mg/day again. The patient's psychotic symptoms cleared completely over the next 48 hours. Since there was still a need for better anginal control, the propranolol dose was slowly increased to 200 mg/day, at which point, the patient again began complaining of concentration difficulties and increased agitation. At this time, the propranolol dose was tapered off over a week while introducing atenolol 100 mg/day. The patient's mental status again cleared quickly and remained normal following stabilization on atenolol. His blood pressure remained controlled at 124/83 mm Hg. At a six-month follow-up examination, the patient remained free of psychiatric symptoms while taking atenolol 100 mg/day, nitroglycerin 0.6 mg sublingual as needed, and triamterene 50 mg plus hydrochlorothiazide 25 mg twice daily; nitroglycerin ointment 4 cm at bedtime had been added for improved control of nocturnal angina.

Discussion

The psychiatric syndromes (depression and psychosis) that these two patients experienced were temporally associated with the initiation of propranolol therapy. Although neither case was blinded or controlled by placebo, the fact that the symptoms of these patients were dose related and temporally associated with propranolol withdrawal and rechallenge strongly indicates a direct relationship.

Psychopharmacologic Effects. Neurochemical findings suggest several theories that could explain the psychiatric side effects of propranolol.

Propranolol blocks postsynaptic β-adrenergic receptors and inhibits the release of norepinephrine from adrenergic nerve endings, a mechanism consistent with the catecholaminergic hypothesis of affective disorders relating depression to decreased central norepinephrine activity.[40,41] The decreased interaction of norepinephrine with neural adrenergic receptors may also be responsible for propranolol-induced psychosis.[16] Animal studies have also shown that propranolol can produce a reversible, dose-dependent increase in brain tyrosine hydroxylase, a rate-limiting enzyme in catecholamine synthesis.[42] The administration of drugs interfering with norepinephrine synthesis has been associated with psychosis in some individuals.[16] Propranolol is also a potent antagonist of serotonin binding, which could explain propranolol-induced psychosis.[16]

Another theory relates depression to a postsynaptic noradrenergic receptor hypersensitivity resulting from chronic β-blockade rather than altered availability of neurotransmitters.[43] This theory is supported by the following three findings: (1) an increased number and density of β-adrenergic receptor cells after long-term propranolol therapy,[44,45] (2) a reduced β-adrenergic receptor sensitivity following long-term antidepressant therapy,[8,46] and (3) a reduced β-adrenergic receptor sensitivity with subsequent antidepressant activity from β-adrenergic agonists.[47–50] Gershon et al.[16] reported a case involving a patient with propranolol-induced psychosis who experienced euphoria immediately after the propranolol therapy was discontinued. They attributed the euphoria to the unmasking of β-adrenergic receptor hypersensitivity that developed during the blockade with propranolol.

Oppenheim[5] suggested that propranolol may produce two types of depressive syndrome: (1) a drug-dependent form that is rapidly reversible with stopping the drug, and (2) a classical major depressive form that is nonresponsive to drug stoppage, which most likely occurs in patients who are biologically predisposed to depressive illness. The same may be said for propranolol-induced psychosis, as shown by the induction of acute psychotic reactions and organic brain syndromes, with some patients requiring antipsychotic drug therapy to reverse the psychotic effects.[7,17]

Clinical Characteristics. Most reports of propranolol-induced depression have involved women, and a family history of depression or previous treatment for depression is common. The woman in this case who developed depression while taking propranolol did not have a family or personal history of depression. Reports of propranolol-induced psychoses have involved a more equal sex distribution of patients. Just as with depression, there has often been a family or personal history of mental illness, but this has not been a consistent finding, and it is not helpful in confirming or refuting a drug-induced relationship in any particular patient. Both propranolol-induced depression and psychosis have occurred in adults of all ages (20–70 years). Rechallenges with β blockers have been infrequently reported, but those reported have usually been positive.[23,25,28] Both of our patients' symptoms recurred following an increase in their propranolol dose.

Reported cases of propranolol-induced depression have most often suggested a dose–response relationship, with most depressive symptoms occurring at or above 80 mg/day following at least a month of therapy. This was the case in our first patient, with symptoms disappearing when the dose was reduced from 80 to 40 mg/day and recurring when the dose was again increased to 80 mg/day.

Propranolol-induced psychoses have usually been reported following high doses (>500 mg/day) or in the treatment of patients with active major psychiatric illness, although Gershon et al.[16] and Koehler and Guth[13] reported cases of psychoses at or below dosage levels ordinarily used to treat many common disorders (less than 160 mg/day). In another study, a single 40-mg dose was reported to produce visual hallucinations; however, the patient had acute schizophrenia and the propranolol was being administered to assess its antipsychotic potential.[26]

Both propranolol-induced depression and psychosis have usually been readily reversible following the discontinuation of propranolol or a reduction in dose. Depressive symptoms have usually cleared within five to eight days while acute psychosis has usually cleared within a couple days. Our patient's depressive symptoms completely cleared by day 8 in the first instance and by day 7 in the second instance following a reduction in the propranolol dosage. The psychosis we observed in our second patient resolved within two days. Occasionally, patients have a more protracted recovery that requires concomitant antidepressant or antipsychotic drug therapy; however, these symptoms have also been reversible. Patients with a history of cardiac arrhythmias or angina should be given an alternative therapy for these conditions before withdrawing propranolol. The propranolol therapy should be tapered over several days to avoid cardiovascular complications.[23]

Lipophilicity and Psychiatric Side Effects. Propranolol, which has well-documented CNS activity, is quite lipophilic, achieving high drug concentrations in the brain (Table 1).[51–53] Psychotic symptoms such as hallucinations have been reported with other lipophilic β blockers including practolol,[54] oxprenolol hydrochloride,[15,54] and pindolol,[55] and the intraocular administration of the more hydrophilic timolol maleate.[56] On the other hand, atenolol, which has a low incidence of CNS side effects, has a much lower lipid solubility and a lower transport into the brain.[51–53,57,58] Cruickshank[51] found that atenolol attained brain concentrations 20 times lower than propranolol after long-term oral dosing, which could account for the difference in CNS effects. Nonetheless, Sklar and Huck[31] reported a case of propranolol-induced psychosis that did not respond to either atenolol or timolol maleate, which are both more hydrophilic.

The clinical utility of substituting atenolol for propranolol when psychiatric side effects are present has been reported.[5,7,9,21,30,33,36,58] Fraser and Carr[21] reported two cases of patients with hyper-

Table 1.
Comparison of β-Blocker Lipophilicity and Transport into the Central Nervous System[51–53]

β-Blocker	Mean Ratio[a] Plasma:CSF	Brain:Plasma	Brain:CSF
Atenolol	7–15	0.1–0.2	1.3–2
Metoprolol[b]	1–3	12–14	16–17
Oxprenolol[b]	13	50	36
Pindolol[b]	3.3	. . .	. . .
Propranolol[b]	10–21.5	17–26	171–273

[a] Ratios dependent upon β-blocker dosage.
[b] Cerebrospinal fluid (CSF) concentrations of the lipophilic β-blockers (all except atenolol) approximate the concentration of unbound, free drug in the plasma.

tension who experienced propranolol-induced psychoses that disappeared when propranolol was replaced by atenolol. Oppenheim[5] described one patient with hypertension and one with angina, and McNeil et al.[7] described a patient who was recovering from a myocardial infarction who all recovered from propranolol-induced depression following atenolol substitution. Finally, Mattiasson and Henningsen[9] found that 97 (14%) of 705 hypertensive patients receiving lipid-soluble β blockers experienced CNS side effects (including nightmares, insomnia, or hallucinations in 50 patients, and fatigue or depression in 42 patients). Overall, 75 (77%) of these patients responded favorably to the substitution of atenolol for propranolol. Of these 75 patients, 50 (91%) with predominantly centrally mediated CNS side effects (nightmares, insomnia, or hallucinations) responded favorably, while only 25 (60%) with fatigue or depression responded. Since no information was provided on the number of patients with fatigue versus the number with depression, it is difficult to speculate on the less favorable outcome with atenolol; however, continued fatigue after the cessation of propranolol therapy may be related to the peripheral β-blocking effects of atenolol. In a subsequent report, Henningsen and Mattiasson[58] reported that 24 of 33 patients experiencing CNS side effects with noncardioselective β blockers improved after switching to atenolol.

Conclusion

Clinicians should be aware that propranolol may induce dose-dependent, centrally mediated mood disturbances and psychoses typical of psychiatric illnesses. These symptoms, which warrant tapering and discontinuing treatment, should be distinguished from nonspecific symptoms, such as lassitude and fatigue, that are caused by peripheral β blockade. When continued β-blocking therapy is necessary to control hypertension or when it is indicated in a patient with a history of psychiatric illness, a weakly lipophilic agent such as atenolol would be a rational choice.

Discussion Questions

1. When evaluating a patient for suspected propranolol-induced depression or psychosis, what factors help to establish a causal relationship between the drug and the clinical symptoms? What criteria are used to decide whether or not to rechallenge the patient with propranolol?
2. What symptoms and tests would help to establish diagnoses of depression and psychosis? What drugs besides β blockers may precipitate or aggravate a depressive or psychotic syndrome?
3. Propranolol-induced depression and psychosis generally exhibit a dose-response relationship. What drugs and conditions may produce an increase in serum propranolol concentrations?
4. What considerations should be made in switching a patient with cardiovascular disease from propranolol to a hydrophilic β blocker, and how might this type of switch be accomplished?

References

1. Greenblatt DJ, Koch-Weser J. Adverse reactions to propranolol in hospitalized medical patients: a report from the Boston Collaborative Drug Surveillance Program. *Am Heart J*. 1973; 86:478–84.
2. Stephens SA. Unwanted effects of propranolol. *Am J Cardiol*. 1966; 18:463–8.
3. Greenblatt DJ, Shader RI. On the psychopharmacology of beta-adrenergic blockade. *Curr Ther Res*. 1972; 14:615–25.
4. Peters ND, Anderson KC, Reid PR et al. Acute mental status changes caused by propranolol. *Johns Hopkins Med J*. 1978; 143:163–4.
5. Oppenheim G. Propranolol-induced depression: mechanism and management. *Aust NZ J Psychiatry*. 1983; 17:400–2.
6. Waal HJ. Propranolol-induced depression. *Br Med J*. 1967; 2:50.
7. McNeil GN, Shaw PK, Dock DS. Substitution of atenolol for propranolol in a case of propranolol-related depression. *Am J Psychiatry*. 1982; 139:1187–8.
8. Petrie WM, Maffucci RJ, Woosley RL. Propranolol and depression. *Am J Psychiatry*. 1982; 139:92–3.
9. Mattiasson I, Henningsen NC. Side effects during treatment with lipid-soluble beta adrenergic blocking substances. In: Proceedings of the 8th World Congress of Cardiology. Tokyo, Japan: 1978 Sep. Abstract.
10. Fitzgerald JD. Propranolol-induced depression. *Br Med J*. 1967; 11:372–3.
11. Salem RB, Stewart RB. Depression from beta-adrenergic-blocking drugs. *Drug Intell Clin Pharm*. 1984; 18:741–2.
12. Berger PA. Medical treatment of mental illness. *Science*. 1978; 200:974.
13. Koehler K, Guth W. Schizophrenic-ahnliche psychose nach einnahme von propranolol. *Munch Med Wschr*. 1977; 119:443–4.
14. Whitlock FA, Bonfield AR. Propranolol psychosis. *Med J Aust*. 1980; 1:184–5.
15. Steinert J, Pugh CR. Two patients with schizophrenic-like psychosis after treatment with beta-adrenergic blockers. *Br Med J*. 1979; 1:790.
16. Gershon ES, Goldstein RE, Moss AT et al. Psychosis with ordinary doses of propranolol. *Ann Intern Med*. 1979; 90: 938–9.
17. Prakash R, Campbell TW, Petrie WM. Psychoses with propranolol: a case report. *Can J Psychiatry*. 1983; 28:657–8.
18. Voltolina EJ, Thompson SI, Tisue J. Acute organic brain syndrome with propranolol. *Clin Toxicol*. 1971; 4:357–9.
19. Atsmon A, Blum I. The discovery. In: Roberts E, Amacher P, eds. Propranolol and schizophrenia. New York: Alan R Liss; 1978:5–38.
20. Topliss D, Bond R. Acute brain syndrome after propranolol treatment. *Lancet*. 1977; 2:1133–4.
21. Fraser HS, Carr AC. Propranolol psychosis. *Br J Psychiatry*. 1976; 129:508–9.
22. Kurland ML. Organic brain syndrome with propranolol. *N Engl J Med*. 1979; 300:366.
23. Horn JR, Rylander ML, Hicks HM. Propranolol-induced hallucinations. *Clin Pharm*. 1982; 1:464–8.
24. Arensberg D, Wenger NK. Psychosis: a probable result of propranolol therapy. *Int J Addict*. 1979; 14:785–7.
25. Hinshelwood RD. Hallucinations and propranolol. *Br Med J*. 1969; 2:445.
26. Shopsin B, Hirsch J, Gershon S. Visual hallucinations and propranolol. *Biol Psychiatry*. 1975; 10:105–7.
27. Judd F, Mass A. Propranolol psychosis. *Med J Aust*. 1982; 1: 370.

28. Remick RA, O'Kane J, Sparling TG. A case report of toxic psychosis with low-dose propranolol therapy. *Am J Psychiatry.* 1981; 138:850–1.
29. Fleming PD, Drachman DA. Propranolol, hallucinations, and sleep disturbances. *Am J Psychiatry.* 1982; 139:540–1.
30. Westerlund A. Atenolol and timolol. *N Engl J Med.* 1982; 307:1343–4.
31. Sklar SJ, Huck LA. Possible association of nonlipophilic β-blockers and acute psychosis. *Clin Pharm.* 1983; 2:274–7.
32. Gomolin IH. Psychosis with oral doses of propranolol. *Ann Intern Med.* 1979; 91:496.
33. Fleminger R. Visual hallucinations and illusions with propranolol. *Br Med J.* 1978; 1:1182.
34. Lieberman A, Kronzon I, Colvin S et al. Propranolol: an unrecognized cause of central nervous system dysfunction in patients undergoing cardiopulmonary bypass. *Ann Thorac Surg.* 1980; 29:378–80.
35. Yorkston NJ, Zaki SA, Themen FA et al. Safeguards in the treatment of schizophrenia with propranolol. *Postgrad Med J.* 1976; 52 (Suppl 4):175–80.
36. McGahan DJ, Wojslaw A, Prasad V et al. Propranolol-induced psychosis. *Drug Intell Clin Pharm.* 1984; 18:601–3.
37. Middlemiss DN, Buxton DA, Greenwood DT. Beta-adrenoceptor antagonists in psychiatry and neurology. *Pharmacol Ther.* 1981; 12:419–37.
38. Jefferson JW. Beta-adrenergic receptor blocking drugs. *Arch Gen Psychiatry.* 1974; 31:681–91.
39. Suzman MM. Use of beta-adrenergic receptor blocking agents in psychiatry. In: Palmer GC, ed. Neuropharmacology of central nervous system and behavioral disorders. New York: Academic Press; 1980:358.
40. Schildkraut JJ. The catecholamine hypothesis of affective disorders: a review of supporting evidence. *Am J Psychiatry.* 1965; 122:509–22.
41. Schildkraut JJ, Davis JM, Klerman GL. Biochemistry of depression. In: Efron DH, ed. Psychopharmacology: a review of progress. Washington, DC: US Public Health Services; 1968.
42. Sullivan JL, Segal DS, Kuczenski RT et al. Propranolol-induced rapid activation of rat striatal tyrosine hydroxylase concomitant with behavioral depression. *Biol Psychiatry.* 1972; 4:193–203.
43. Segal DS, Kuczenski RT, Mandell AJ. Theoretical implications of drug-induced adaptive regulation for a biogenic amine hypothesis of affective disorder. *Biol Psychiatry.* 1974; 9: 147–59.
44. Sulser F, Mobley PL. Regulation of central nonadrenergic receptor function: new vistas of the mode of action of antidepressant treatments. In: Usdin E, Bunney WE Jr, Davis JM, eds. Neuroreceptors—basic and clinical aspects. New York: John Wiley & Sons; 1981.
45. Glaubiger G, Lefkowitz RJ. Elevated beta adrenergic receptor number after chronic propranolol treatment. *Biochem Biophys Res Commun.* 1977; 78:720–5.
46. Charney DS, Menkes DB, Henigar GR. Receptor sensitivity and the mechanism of action of antidepressant treatment. *Arch Gen Psychiatry.* 1981; 38:1160–80.
47. Belmaker RH. Receptors, adenylate cyclase, depression and lithium. *Biol Psychiatry.* 1981; 16:333–50.
48. Lerer B, Ebstein RP, Belmaker RH. Subsensitivity of human beta adrenergic adenylate cyclase after salbutamol treatment of depression. *Psychopharmacology.* 1981; 75:169–72.
49. Lecrubier Y, Puech AJ, Jouvent R et al. A beta adrenergic stimulant (salbutamol) versus clomipramine in depression: a controlled study. *Br J Psychiatry.* 1980; 136:354–8.
50. Simon P, Lecrubier Y, Jouvent R et al. Experimental and clinical evidence of antidepressant effects of beta-adrenergic stimulants. *Psychol Med.* 1978; 8:335–8.
51. Cruickshank JM. The clinical importance of cardioselectivity and lipophilicity in beta blockers. *Am Heart J.* 1980; 100: 160–78.
52. Taylor EA, Jefferson D, Carroll JD et al. Cerebrospinal fluid concentrations of propranolol, pindolol and atenolol in man: evidence for central actions of beta-adrenoceptor antagonists. *Br J Clin Pharmacol.* 1981; 12:549–59.
53. Neil-Dwyer G, Bartlett J, McAinsh J et al. Beta-adrenoceptor blockers and the blood brain barrier. *Br J Clin Pharmacol.* 1981; 11:549–53.
54. Petrie JC, Galloway DB, Jeffers TA et al. Adverse reactions to beta-blocking drugs: a review. *Postgrad Med J.* 1976; 52 (Suppl 4):63–9.
55. Waal-Manning HJ. Hypertension: which beta-blocker? *Drugs.* 1976; 12:412–41.
56. Yates D. Syncope and visual hallucinations, apparently from timolol. *JAMA.* 1980; 244:768–9.
57. VanZwieten PA, Timmermans PB. Comparison between the acute hemodynamic effects and brain penetration of atenolol and metoprolol. *J Cardiovasc Pharmacol.* 1979; 1:85–96.
58. Henningsen NC, Mattiasson I. Long-term clinical experience with atenolol—a new selective beta-1-blocker with few side effects from the central nervous system. *Acta Med Scand.* 1979; 205:61–6.

Drug Experience

Straightforward reports of unusual drug experiences are included in this section. These may be confirmations of previously reported drug experiences or brief apparent first reports. While selected references may be cited, the purpose of a Drug Experience report is not to present an extensive review of the literature.

A related section, Grand Rounds, includes papers that are well-documented patient case reports with a thorough review of the important literature to help put the case in perspective.

Life-threatening anaphylaxis following subcutaneous administration of isosulfan blue 1%

STEPHEN M. LONGNECKER, MICHAEL M. GUZZARDO, AND LEE P. VAN VORIS

Clin Pharm. 1985; 4:219–21

Historically, the injection of vital or patent blue dyes for visualizing the lymph vessels before their cannulization has been a relatively benign procedure when compared with the risks of radiocontrast media injection. Various dyes such as methylene blue have been used for this purpose since the 1930s but never have received formal approval by the Food and Drug Administration because they have not been systematically studied for efficacy and safety. Recently, isosulfan blue 1% (Lymphazurin 1%, Hirsch Industries) has been approved for use for the visualization of the lymphatics during bipedal lymphography. In manufacturer-sponsored clinical trials the dye has received a favorable safety record.[1] There have been no reports of life-threatening toxicity associated with this compound, and the reported adverse effects have not been serious.[1,2] The following case report describes an episode of severe, immediate, life-threatening anaphylaxis occurring after the subcutaneous administration of isosulfan blue 1%. Intensive resuscitative measures and subsequent short-term hospitalization were necessary.

Case Report. A 51-year-old woman was found to have squamous cell carcinoma of the cervix stage IIIB. She had a six-year history of hypertension for which she had been taking metroprolol tartrate 50 mg twice daily, although she had not taken any for the last month. No other findings in her medical history were notable. She denied allergies to foods, medications, and dyes, and reported no previous exposure to radiocontrast media.

As part of an evaluation before radiotherapy, a bipedal lymphangiogram was ordered. To visualize the lymphatics of the feet, the patient received a subcutaneous injection of approximately 0.5 mL of 1% isosulfan blue (Lymphazurin 1%, Lot 023049, Hirsch Industries, 4912 Broad Street, Richmond, VA 23230) between the first, second, and third toes of both feet. A few minutes later, she began to notice a tingling sensation that advanced up her legs to her back. After this she noted difficulty swallowing and then lost consciousness. There was a two-centimeter wide pinkish streak from the injection sites cephalad along the course of the lymph vessels to approximately the midcalf. Her blood pressure dropped to undetectable levels, and she quickly manifested generalized urticaria and angioedema. The lungs were found clear to auscultation, and the heart rhythm was found to be regular at a rapid rate between 120 and 130 beats per minute. At this time she received 50 mg i.v. diphenhydramine hydrochloride, and a cardiopulmonary arrest team was summoned.

Resuscitation was begun with intravenous fluids, military antishock trousers, 50 mg of intramuscular diphenhydramine hydrochloride, 1 mg of intravenous epinephrine hydrochloride, 250 mg of intravenous hydrocortisone sodium succinate, and titrated intravenous dopamine hydrochloride. At no time was she without spontaneous respirations or normal sinus rhythm. Within 8 to 10 minutes of the initial loss of consciousness, the patient was alert and responding appropriately, with a minimum systolic blood pressure of 100 mm Hg; she was slowly weaned from the dopamine over a two-hour period.

STEPHEN M. LONGNECKER, PHARM.D., is an ASHP Foundation–Bristol Oncology Fellow, The Johns Hopkins Medical Center, Baltimore, MD. At the time of this study, he was a clinical pharmacist in oncology, Hamot Medical Center, Erie, PA. MICHAEL M. GUZZARDO, M.D., and LEE P. VAN VORIS, M.D., are with the Departments of Medicine and Family Practice, Hamot Medical Center.

Address reprint requests to Dr. Longnecker at the Oncology Center, The Johns Hopkins Medical Center, 600 Wolfe Street, Baltimore, MD 21205.

She had no further local reaction at the dye injection site but she did continue to have generalized urticaria and edema in her hands and feet. She was admitted to the hospital overnight for observation and was given 50 mg of intramuscular diphenhydramine hydrochloride as necessary. Laboratory studies showed a total white blood count of 14,100/cu mm (band neutrophils 39%, polymorphonuclear leukocytes 40%, lymphocytes 19%, monocytes 2%), a hematocrit of 45%, and a platelet count of 557,000/cu mm. Urinalysis, electrolyte, and blood sugar determinations were within normal limits. The patient was discharged from the hospital 24 hours after the reaction feeling well, with normal findings upon physical examination. A follow-up examination two weeks later confirmed that she continued to feel well.

Discussion. Isosulfan blue, a 2,5-disulfonated patent blue dye of the triphenylmethane family, is the first dye of its type to be approved by the FDA for the selective localization of the lymphatic system before lymphangiography. Although this compound is not considered a radiocontrast material, it is widely used before radiographic procedures involving the lymphatic vessels. The subcutaneous administration of isosulfan blue between the web spaces of the toes provides visual identification of the distal lymphatic vessels minutes after its injection. After the administration of isosulfan blue, a pair of small incisions are made for the cannulization of the lymph vessel, and radiocontrast material can be injected. The 1% concentration of isosulfan blue was chosen during initial studies because of the low incidence of local inflammatory reactions.[3]

Reports on the safety of isosulfan blue have shown that it is capable of producing severe reactions in patients before lymphangiography, but these studies have used unstandardized concentrations and dosages of the dye or used the dye with other drugs.[4,5] From a large survey of workers using the patent blue dyes, Koehler et al.[6] found an 0.18% (57/32,000) overall incidence of hypersensitivity reactions with varying degrees of severity. In many of these instances, unusually high concentrations of the dyes were used and they were used with local anesthetics. Early reports of severe anaphylaxis to 2,5-disulfonated triphenylmethane dyes (Alphazurine 2G, Allied Chemical Corp., Morristown, NJ) were published by Kopp[4] and Mortazave,[5] but again it was not clear whether these incidents were attributable to the dye concentration or concomitant local anesthetic use. During phase III trials of isosulfan blue dye, the use of a concentration of 1% without local anesthetic was associated with no instances of serious reaction in 543 adults.[6] It is clear that when isosulfan blue is used in the proper 1% concentration without local anesthetics the possibility of a severe reaction occurring is quite low.

The largest risks to patients undergoing lymphangiography are those posed by the radiocontrast agents. Reports of serious reactions to radiocontrast media have documented appreciable morbidity and mortality.[7,8] The use of injectable radiocontrast media can result in serious life-threatening allergic side effects in a small number of patients. Additionally, 5 to 8% of these tests result in less serious urticarial reactions.[9] The current risk of mortality has been estimated to be between 1 in 40,000 to 1 in 50,000 deaths per procedure[10,11] or 500 deaths per year.[12]

It is well documented that these adverse reactions can occur without having had previous exposure to radiocontrast media.[11] In addition, a history of an adverse reaction may lead to serious reactions upon repeat exposure.[13] In most instances of serious "allergic-like" medication reactions without a history of previous sensitizing exposure, it is generally concluded that the mechanism involved is a direct release of histamine or the activation of the alternate complement pathway. Many instances of unpredictable life-threatening drug allergies have been shown to be caused by these mechanisms as in the case of opiates, polymixin B, and curare, and these types of reactions may not require previous exposure to the sensitizing agent or hapten formation.[12,14–17] It appears that these reactions, including those induced by radiocontrast media, can produce this effect by directly causing the degranulation of mast cells and basophils resulting in massive histamine release[8,12,14,15,17] or by producing alternate complement pathway anaphylaxotoxins.[14,15,17,18] Since histamine is the primary mediator of the effects that follow a reaction of this type, it is improbable that such an event could be distinguished from an immunologically induced event. These types of reactions have been called nonimmunologically mediated drug allergies and idiopathic anaphylactic episodes.[8,12,14–18] Although idiopathic anaphylactic reactions have not been reported subsequent to the use of isosulfan blue 1%, it is not unreasonable to assume a nonimmunological mechanism is involved. The absence of a history of previous exposure to this or similar compounds in this patient supports the possibility of such a mechanism, although the patient could have been exposed to a number of unrelated compounds that could have sensitized her to triphenylmethane dyes.

Isosulfan blue 1% may become a widely used agent in preparing patients for lymphangiograpy, and it appears that the injection of this compound can result in severe anaphylactic reactions in patients without previous exposure. One way to deal with this potential problem might be to use a single oral dose of antihistaminic premedication before administering the injectable dye compounds, using antihistaminic agents such as diphenhydramine hydrochloride 50 mg, cimetidine 200–300 mg, or ranitidine 200 mg. Similar approaches were recently suggested at a NIH-sponsored symposium on drug allergy[19] based upon clinical experience.[20] This type of pretreatment regimen might help decrease the incidence and severity of anaphylactic episodes caused by injectable radiocontrast agents.

Conclusion. This case represents the first published report of a severe life-threatening toxic episode following the subcutaneous administration of isosulfan blue in a patient with no apparent history of allergy. With the well-established mortality rate of 500 deaths per year attributable to the administration of radiocontrast media and related agents, it is clear that these procedures must be examined closely to reduce the number of adverse reactions, especially those of an allergic preventable nature. Emergency treatment must be readily available during procedures involving isosulfan blue and other injectable radiocontrast media, and the health-care personnel working with these agents should be aware that a negative history of drug allergy before exposure does not preclude the possible occurrence of life-threatening anaphylactic reactions.

References

1. Hirsch JI, Tisnado J, Cho S et al. Use of isosulfan blue for identification of lymphatic vessels: experimental and clinical evaluation. *Am J Roentgenol.* 1982; 139:1061–4.
2. Castellino RA, Bergiron C, Markovits P. Experience with 659 consecutive lymphograms in children. *Cancer.* 1977; 40: 1097–101.
3. Gangolli SD, Grasso P, Golberg L. Physical factors determining the early local tissue reactions produced by food colorings and other compounds injected subcutaneously. *Food Cosmet Toxicol.* 1967; 5:601–21.
4. Kopp WL. Anaphylaxis from alphazurine 2G during lymphography. *JAMA.* 1966; 198: 200–1.
5. Mortazavi SH, Burrown BD. Allergic reaction to patent blue dye in lymphangiography. *Clin Radiol.* 1971; 22:389–90.
6. Koehler PR. Complications and accidents. In: Ruttman A, ed. Progress in lymphology: proceedings of the international symposium on lymphography. Zurich: Stuttgart: 1966.
7. Witten DW, Hirsch FD, Hartman GW. Acute reactions to urographic medium. *Am J Roentgenol.* 1973; 119:832–40.
8. Lasser EC. Basic mechanisms of contrast media reactions. *Radiology.* 1968; 91:63–5.
9. Soter NA. Immediate type hypersensitivity disease: urticaria and angioedema. In: Cecil R, Wyngaarden JB, Smith LH, eds. Textbook of medicine. Philadelphia: WB Saunders Co.: 1982; 1796–800.
10. Ansel G. Adverse reactions to contrast agents: scope of problem. *Invest Radiol.* 1970; 5: 374–91.
11. Fischer HW, Doust VL. An evaluation of pretesting in the problem of serious and fatal reactions to excretory urography. *Radiology.* 1972; 103:497–501.
12. DeSwarte RD. Drug allergy. In: Patterson R, ed. Allergic diseases. Philadelphia: JB Lippincott; 1980:452–583.
13. Egwang TG, Befus AD. The role of complement in the induction and regulation of immune responses. *Immunology.* 1984; 51:207–24.
14. Van Arsdel PP. Adverse drug reactions. In: Middleton E, Reed CE, Ellis EF, eds. Allergies: principles and practice. St. Louis: CV Mosby; 1978:1389–414.
15. Sheffer AL. Idiopathic anaphylaxis. In: Lichtenstein LM, Fauci AS, eds. Current therapy in allergy and immunology 1983–1984. Burlington, Ontario: BC Decker; 1983:84–7.
16. Parker CW. Drug allergy (part 1). *N Engl J Med.* 1973; 292: 511–4.
17. Bhat KN, Arroyave CM, Crown R. Reaction to radiographic contrast agents: new developments in etiology. *Ann Allergy.* 1976; 37:169–73.
18. Simon RA, Schatz M, Stevenson DD et al. Radiographic contrast media infusions: measurement of histamine, complement, and fibrin split products and correlation with clinical parameters. *J Allergy Clin Immunol.* 1979; 63:281–8.
19. Goldstein RA, Patterson R. Drug allergy: prevention, diagnosis, and treatment. *Ann Intern Med.* 1984; 100:302–3.
20. Greenberger PA, Patterson RA, Simon R et al. Pretreatment of high risk patients requiring radiocontrast media studies. *J Allergy Clin Immunol.* 1981. 67:185–7.

Carbamazepine-induced thrombocytopenia in a young child

JOAN MARIE BRADLEY, ROSALIE SAGRAVES, AND ANTHONY C. KIMBROUGH

Clin Pharm. 1985; 4:221–3

Carbamazepine has been used as an anticonvulsant since 1962 in Europe and 1974 in the United States; previously, it had been used for trigeminal neuralgia. It is effective against generalized tonic-clonic, simple partial, and complex partial seizures.[1] Carbamazepine is less sedating than phenobarbital and phenytoin, making it an attractive anticonvulsant for use in children.[2–4] Carbamazepine has FDA approval for use only in children older than 6 years, although it is being used in general practice in younger children also.[3,4]

Initial reports of carbamazepine-induced adverse hematologic events have made some practitioners apprehensive about using this agent. Transient leukopenia that improves despite continued use of the drug is the most common complication, but aplastic anemia, pancytopenia, eosinophilia, and thrombocytopenia have all been reported.[5] Thrombocytopenia is very rare. The following report is believed to be the first report of a profound isolated carbamazepine-induced thrombocytopenia in a young child.

JOAN MARIE BRADLEY, PHARM.D., is Assistant Professor, Faculty of Pharmacy and Pharmaceutical Sciences, University of Alberta, Edmonton, Canada. ROSALIE SAGRAVES, PHARM.D., is Associate Professor, College of Pharmacy, The University of Texas at Austin, Austin. ANTHONY C. KIMBROUGH, M.D., is Director of Ambulatory Care, Austin Pediatric Education Program, Austin, TX.

Address reprint requests to Dr. Sagraves at Room 5.110, College of Pharmacy, The University of Texas at Austin, Austin, TX 78712-1074.

Presented at the 19th Annual ASHP Midyear Clinical Meeting, Dallas, TX, December 3, 1984.

Case Report. The patient was a Latin American girl aged 4 years, 11 months, who was admitted to an Austin, TX, hospital with a chief complaint of scattered petechiae. She has had a generalized tonic-clonic seizure disorder following *Haemophilus influenzae* type B meningitis at age 1 year, 6 months. The disorder was well controlled with phenobarbital, but excessive hyperactivity that interfered with school work required discontinuation of the drug.

Two weeks before admission to the hospital, carbamazepine was started at 100 mg three times daily, while the phenobarbital was being tapered. A complete blood cell count with platelets, performed using an automated method using an Ortho ELT8, was within normal limits when carbamazepine therapy was started. The child had been in good health before admission. In particular, her history was negative for viral illness that may precede idiopathic thrombocytopenia purpura.

On admission, the child was found to be a normal, well-developed girl, with no clinically relevant findings other than scattered petechiae. Initial laboratory studies were all within normal limits except for a platelet count of 14,000/cu mm performed by phase microscopy. The carbamazepine was withdrawn; no other drugs were discontinued or initiated at that time. Bone-marrow aspiration was not performed. Platelet counts, obtained using phase microscopy, were 23,000 and 30,000/cu mm on day 2; 174,000/cu mm on day 4; and 239,000/cu mm on day 5. Platelet counts obtained one month later were 216,000/cu mm.

Because of the severe thrombocytopenia and the availability of alternative anticonvulsants, it was deemed unethical to rechallenge the patient.[6] Using the criteria of Naranjo,[7] this adverse reaction is a probable drug reaction, lacking in rechallenge to confirm the correlation. The child's seizures are currently well controlled with phenytoin and sodium valproate.

Discussion. Thrombocytopenia caused by carbamazepine is very rare despite early series reporting an incidence of 1–2%.[8,9] Large series, involving hundreds of patients followed with regular platelet counts have not shown any cases of thrombocytopenia.[2–4,10,11] Previous cases reported have been single case reports of adults[8,9,12,13] or adolescents.[14,15] One study showed a statistically significant decrease in mean platelet counts of an adult patient population, but the study did not report individual decreases.[1] The platelet counts reported, although decreased, were still within normal limits.

Evaluation of the previously published reports by Naranjo's criteria gives probabilities of carbamazepine causing thrombocytopenia of possible to probable. No case is considered a definite adverse drug reaction since patients were not rechallenged with the drug. The onset of the thrombocytopenia in the previously reported cases ranged from one week to two months after the drug was initiated. The degree of thrombocytopenia, when noted in the reports, ranged from mild (platelet counts of 80,000/cu mm) to severe (platelet counts of 2,000–11,000/cu mm).[8,12–15] Following carbamazepine withdrawal, platelet counts returned to normal within four to seven days in all previously reported cases. Patients demonstrated either no symptoms at all,[8] purpura,[12–15] or epistaxis.[15]

Bone-marrow examination, when performed, showed a variety of changes, ranging from none at all[13] to increased numbers of immature megakaryocytes[15] or adequate numbers but inactive megakaryocytes.[12] Positive immunological response by the patients' sera to carbamazepine was demonstrated by several investigators.[12,13,15] The mechanism of thrombocytopenia appears to be increased platelet destruction by splenic and hepatic macrophages because of drug–plasma protein-antibody complexes adsorbing onto the surface of the platelets.[16]

Recommendations for monitoring for hematologic adverse reactions vary.[2,3,5,17,18] Excessive monitoring would be expensive and uncomfortable for the patient. Inadequate monitoring would expose the patient to dangerous consequences of decreased blood cell components. After reviewing the cases of carbamazepine-induced thrombocytopenia, we recommend that complete blood and platelet counts be obtained before starting the drug. Initially, these tests should be repeated at least biweekly or monthly for three months. All reported cases of this reaction occurred within three months of starting the drug. Subsequently, hematologic monitoring could be repeated every three to six months.

Conclusion. Although hematologic reactions to carbamazepine are rare, they may occur. The young child reported here experienced thrombocytopenia consistent with other reported cases of carbamazepine-induced thrombocytopenia. Patients and parents should be counseled about the signs of thrombocytopenia, and adequate hematologic monitoring should be performed before and during carbamazepine administration.

References

1. Cereghino JJ, Brock JT, Van Meter JC et al. Carbamazepine for epilepsy. *Neurology*. 1974; 24:401–10.
2. Gamstorp I. Nine years' experience with Tegretol in epileptic children. In: Wink CAS, ed. Tegretol in epilepsy. Macclesfield: Geigy Pharmaceuticals; 1973:6–11.
3. Huf R, Schain RJ. Long-term experiences with carbamazepine (Tegretol) in children with seizures. *J Pediatr*. 1980; 97: 310–2.
4. Schain RJ, Ward JW, Guthrie D. Carbamazepine as an anticonvulsant in children. *Neurology*. 1977; 27:476–80.
5. Killian JM, Tegretol in trigeminal neuralgia with special reference to hematopoietic side effects. *Headache*. 1969; 9: 58–63.
6. Hoigné R. Drug induced immune-thrombocytopenia. *Acta Haematol*. 1982; 68–70. Editorial.

7. Naranjo CA, Busto U, Sellers EM et al. A method for estimating the probability of adverse drug reactions. *Clin Pharmacol Ther.* 1981; 30:239–45.
8. Davis EH. Clinical trials of Tegretol in trigeminal neuralgia. *Headache.* 1969; 9:77–82.
9. Sturman RH, O'Brien FH. Non-surgical treatment of tic douloureux with carbamazepine (#G32883). *Headache.* 1969; 9:88–91.
10. Livingston S, Pauli LL, Berman W. Carbamazepine (Tegretol) in epilepsy: nine year follow-up study with special emphasis on untoward reactions. *Dis Nerv Sys.* 1974; 35:103–7.
11. Hanke NFJ. Clinical tolerance of Tegretol. In: Wink CAS, ed. Tegretol in epilepsy. Macclesfield: Geigy Pharmaceuticals; 1973:11–3.
12. Shoenfeld Y, Ben Baruch N, Livni E, et al. Carbamazepine (Tegretol)-induced thrombocytopenia. *Acta Haematol.* 1982; 68:74. Letter.
13. Karpatkin S. Drug-induced thrombocytopenia. *Am J Med Sci.* 1971; 262:68–78.
14. Rutman JY. Effect of carbamazepine on blood elements. *Ann Neurol.* 1978; 3:373. Letter.
15. Kornberg A, Kobrin I. IgG antiplatelet antibodies due to carbamazepine. *Acta Haematol.* 1982; 68:70–2.
16. Moake JL, Funicella T. Common bleeding problems. *Clin Symp.* 1983; 35:1–32.
17. Hart RG, Easton JD. Carbamazepine and hematological monitoring. *Ann Neurol.* 1982; 11:309–12.
18. Lorgé M. Some aspects of clinical tolerance of Tegretol. In: Wink CAS, ed. Tegretol in epilepsy. Macclesfield: Geigy Pharmaceuticals; 1973:113–5.

CP Continuing Education

The ASHP Continuing-Education System gives readers a self-assessment mechanism for selected articles in Clinical Pharmacy *and the* American Journal of Hospital Pharmacy. *It also allows readers to obtain continuing-education credit for these articles.*

For the purpose of CE-credit enrollment, a blank answer sheet is published at the end of each installment of the column for the CE articles in that issue. An enrollee accumulates these answer sheets until the enrollment is submitted, using the form that is published in the May–June and November–December issues of Clinical Pharmacy *and in the June and December issues of the* American Journal of Hospital Pharmacy. *Any combination of tests within a 12-month period, from both* Clinical Pharmacy *and* American Journal of Hospital Pharmacy, *may be included in an enrollment. More complete details about enrollment in the system will appear in the semiannual enrollment form.*

All education aspects of the program are directed by Warren E. McConnell, Ph.D., Special Assistant in the ASHP Executive Office.

Article 680-204-8506 (see page 149)
Qualifies for 1.0 hour of CE credit

Allogeneic bone marrow transplantation in the treatment of hematologic diseases

Learning Objectives

As a result of studying this article, the reader should be able to

1. Compare autologous, syngeneic, and allogeneic bone marrow transplantation.
2. Identify the major diseases for which bone marrow transplantation is useful.
3. List the purpose of and the major drugs included in the preparative regimen.
4. Describe the major complications occurring after bone marrow transplantation.
5. List the major immunosuppressive drugs used to treat acute and chronic graft-versus-host disease.

Self-assessment Questions

For each question there is one best answer only.

1. The most common donor for allogeneic bone marrow transplantation is
   a. An identical twin.
   b. The patient himself or herself.
   c. An HLA-identical sibling.
   d. A partially HLA-matched family member.
2. Allogeneic marrow transplantation has been used to treat all but which one of the following diseases?
   a. Familial erythroblastic anemia.
   b. Acute leukemia.
   c. Chronic myelogenous leukemia.
   d. Multiple myeloma.
3. Which one of the following statements about hematologic diseases is true?
   a. Patients with severe aplastic anemia usually respond poorly to drug therapy.
   b. Acute lymphocytic leukemia has a uniformly poor prognosis in both children and adults treated with chemotherapy and central nervous system prophylaxis.
   c. Acute myelogenous leukemia in adults is usually responsive to cancer chemotherapy, and bone marrow transplantation should be reserved for only the most resistant cases.
   d. Bone marrow transplantation should not be considered early in chronic myelogenous leukemia because the disease progresses slowly and has a good prognosis.
4. In which one of the following patients is bone marrow transplantation most likely to be used (assuming a suitable donor is available)?
   a. A 6-year-old child with newly diagnosed, standard-risk, acute lymphoblastic leukemia.
   b. A 40-year-old with chronic lymphocytic leukemia.
   c. A 20-year-old with newly diagnosed acute myelogenous leukemia.
   d. A 12-year-old child with mild aplastic anemia.
5. Which one of the following posttransplant complications is most common in patients receiving bone marrow transplantation for aplastic anemia compared with patients receiving it for leukemia?
   a. Infection.
   b. Interstitial pneumonitis.
   c. Graft rejection.
   d. Graft-versus-host disease.
6. Which one of the following drugs is *not* used in preparative regimens for bone marrow transplant?
   a. Cyclophosphamide.
   b. Busulfan.
   c. Methotrexate.
   d. Cytarabine.

7. Which one of the following statements concerning acute graft-versus-host disease is correct?

   a. Acute graft-versus-host disease is probably caused by donor B-lymphocytes reacting against the recipient.
   b. Acute graft-versus-host disease usually occurs in the first week after transplantation.
   c. Features of acute graft-versus-host disease resemble those of autoimmune diseases.
   d. None of the above alternatives is true.

8. Which one of the following drugs is *not* used to prevent or treat acute graft-versus-host disease?

   a. Cyclosporine.
   b. Methotrexate.
   c. Antithymocyte globulin.
   d. Chlorambucil.

9. Which of the following statements concerning interstitial pneumonia is not true?

   a. The incidence of interstitial pneumonia is higher in leukemia patients receiving total body irradiation.
   b. The incidence of interstitial pneumonia is higher in patients with moderate to severe graft-versus-host disease.
   c. Cytomegalovirus is the most common infectious cause of interstitial pneumonia.
   d. Patients with cytomegaloviral pneumonia respond well to high-dose antiviral chemotherapy.

10. Which one of the following is *not* a common late complication of bone marrow transplantation in acute leukemia?

    a. Cataracts.
    b. Sterility.
    c. Restrictive lung disease.
    d. Graft rejection.

Article 680-204-8507 (see page 161)
Qualifies for 1.0 hour of CE credit

Management of maldigestion associated with pancreatic insufficiency

Learning Objectives

After studying this article, the reader should be able to

1. Describe the function of pancreatic enzymes and the role of GI hormones in regulating the secretion of those enzymes.
2. Identify three general etiologies of pancreatic insufficiency and one specific disease state associated with each etiology.
3. List four factors that can affect a patient's response to therapy with pancreatic enzyme supplements.
4. Discuss the benefits and limitations of adjunctive therapy with histamine H_2-receptor antagonists or antacids in patients with maldigestion.
5. Describe the appropriate treatment components for the initial management of a patient with maldigestion.

Self-assessment Questions

For each question there is one best answer only.

1. The leading cause of maldigestion in the U.S. adult population is

   a. Alcoholic pancreatitis.
   b. Cystic fibrosis.
   c. Cancer.
   d. Idiopathic pancreatitis.

2. The GI hormone responsible for stimulating the largest output of pancreatic enzyme is

   a. Secretin.
   b. Vasoactive intestinal peptide.
   c. Cholecystokinin.
   d. Alternatives b and c are both correct.

3. The factor that is most important in determining patient response to therapy with pancreatic enzyme supplements is the

   a. Acid secretory status of the patient.
   b. Amount of lipase present in a given pancreatic enzyme supplement.
   c. Underlying cause of maldigestion.
   d. Amount of lipase that is actually delivered to the duodenum by a given pancreatic enzyme supplement.

4. The dosage form of pancreatic enzyme that is least effective in correcting steatorrhea is

   a. Powders.
   b. Enteric-coated tablets.
   c. Capsules.
   d. Enteric-coated encapsulated microspheres.

5. Which of the following statements is true concerning the use of antacids in the treatment of maldigestion?

   a. Antacids have no effect on intragastric volume.
   b. Antacids are most effective when taken after a meal.
   c. Antacids are effective when used as single agents for the treatment of maldigestion.
   d. Antacids that contain aluminum hydroxide or sodium bicarbonate are more effective than other antacids.

6. Adverse effects associated with the use of pancreatic enzyme supplements include all of the following except

   a. Hyperuricosuria.
   b. GI intolerance.
   c. Pulmonary hypersensitivity.
   d. Hepatotoxicity.

7. The beneficial effects of histamine H_2-receptor antagonists result from all of the following except

a. An increase in gastric pH.
b. A decrease in intragastric volume.
c. A decrease in enzyme inactivation.
d. Stimulation of pancreatic enzyme secretion.

8. Which of the following patients would derive the least benefit from adjunctive therapy with histamine H_2-receptor antagonists?

a. A patient with cystic fibrosis.
b. A patient receiving high doses of lipase.
c. A patient who secretes subnormal amounts of gastric acid.
d. All of the above patients would derive equal benefit.

9. Which of the following dosage schedules for pancreatic enzyme supplementation would produce the most beneficial response?

a. Frequent administration of supplements, both before and after meals.
b. Hourly administration of supplements during waking hours.
c. Administration of supplements with meals and snacks.
d. Administration of supplements one hour after each meal and at bedtime.

10. In designing an initial treatment regimen for a patient with maldigestion, which of the following would be most appropriate?

a. An increase in dietary fat to 100 g per day and administration of high-potency pancreatic enzyme supplements.
b. Restriction of dietary fat to 40 g per day and administration of high-potency pancreatic enzyme supplements.
c. Restriction of dietary fat to 40 g per day, administration of enzyme supplements, and adjunctive therapy with cimetidine.
d. No dietary restrictions, administration of enteric-coated encapsulated microspheres, and adjunctive therapy with an aluminum hydroxide-containing antacid to increase gastric pH above 4.

Answer sheet

March–April 1985 *Clinical Pharmacy*

Note: An enrollment form for the ASHP Continuing-Education System appears in the May–June and November–December issues. Please accumulate all the answer sheets you wish to use in one enrollment and submit them at one time with a completed enrollment form.

Place an X in the box(es) at the top of the column(s) corresponding to the test(s) you are taking. Darken the boxes corresponding to the correct answers.

☐ 680-204-8506 1.0 hour	a b c d	☐ 680-204-8507 1.0 hour	a b c d
1.	☐☐☐☐	1.	☐☐☐☐
2.	☐☐☐☐	2.	☐☐☐☐
3.	☐☐☐☐	3.	☐☐☐☐
4.	☐☐☐☐	4.	☐☐☐☐
5.	☐☐☐☐	5.	☐☐☐☐
6.	☐☐☐☐	6.	☐☐☐☐
7.	☐☐☐☐	7.	☐☐☐☐
8.	☐☐☐☐	8.	☐☐☐☐
9.	☐☐☐☐	9.	☐☐☐☐
10.	☐☐☐☐	10.	☐☐☐☐

ASHP Use Only
(1.0)8506______(3)
(1.0)8507______(3)

Current Literature

Book Reviews

Clinical Pharmacy and Therapeutics, Third Edition

Edited by Eric T. Herfindal and Joseph L. Hirschman. Published by Williams & Wilkins, 428 East Preston Street, Baltimore, MD 21202, 1984. xvi + 977 p. Price $39.95.

Evolving practices in contemporary pharmacy have increased the practitioner's responsibilities, and the need for an expanded clinical therapeutics knowledge base has thus increased as well. In the forword, Herfindal and Hirschman indicate that this text is an "... attempt to meet the information needs of pharmacy students," and, as the preface suggests, this edition of *Clinical Pharmacy and Therapeutics* can "... serve as a starting point" for those pharmacists and pharmacy students wishing to expand their clinical data base."

This book is very similar to the second edition in style and format. All the chapters are written by contributors with extensive clinical experience in the subjects discussed, and most portions are well written and referenced. There are a number of new topics covered, such as mycotic and parasitic infections, diarrhea and constipation, fluid and electrolytes, and pain management, as well as revisions of other subjects such as parenteral nutrition and thyroid and parathyroid disorders. Additionally, some subjects have been dropped, including myasthenia gravis.

The book is divided into 13 sections. Section 1, entitled "General," comprises five chapters. The chapter on clinical toxicology gives a general overview on the treatment of poisonings and is useful for those persons not familiar with toxicology. The chapter on parenteral nutrition gives a concise overview of nutritional support. The chapter on pediatrics has a number of useful tables (e.g., pediatric definitions, age-dependent half-lives of antibiotics in serum, drugs excreted in breast milk). It is very well written and exceptionally well referenced.

The chapter on alcoholism contains a very informative table on complications of this problem. Under drug therapy of acute alcohol abstinence syndrome, however, the author states that the only benzodiazepine with no active metabolites is oxazepam; of note is the conspicuous lack of reference to lorazepam, which also has no active metabolites and is marketed in a dosage form that can be given either intravenously or intramuscularly. References for the use of lithium in the treatment of acute alcohol withdrawal would be helpful. Some subject material in this chapter is presented in a confusing fashion, requiring a second reading of the section. The table on alcohol content of nonprescription and prescription agents is useful.

Section 2 discusses a variety of infectious disease processes. Respiratory, urinary-tract, enteric, mycotic, parasitic, and central nervous system infections; infective endocarditis; tuberculosis; and sexually transmitted diseases are covered. Sexually transmitted diseases in homosexual men, a frequently overlooked problem, is adequately discussed. Succinct tables are included on the treatment of mycotic, helminthic, protozoal, and ectoparasitic infections, but more information on ketoconazole would be useful.

Section 3 (gastrointestinal diseases) discusses peptic-ulcer disease (including a short but adequate discussion of ranitidine), ulcerative colitis, hepatitis, cirrhosis, and diarrhea and constipation.

Section 4 includes basic discussions of cardiovascular disorders, such as angina pectoris, congestive heart failure (a concise discussion of pathogenesis is included), thromboembolic disease, cardiac arrhythmias, and a comprehensive discussion of hypertension. The chapter on angina pectoris includes a thorough discussion of the effects of nitrates and β blockers on the major determinants of myocardial oxygen consumption and a short discussion of calcium-channel blockers.

Section 5 (respiratory diseases) presents information on asthma and chronic obstructive pulmonary disease. Some statements in this section are not adequately referenced and there is a paucity of current literature citations.

The remainder of the book, sections 6 through 13, cover endocrine, metabolic, renal, rheumatic, hematologic, neurologic, psychiatric, ophthalmologic, dermatologic, and neoplastic diseases. The chapter on renal disease gives a number of pharmacokinetic equations on dosing drugs in patients with various degrees of renal failure. The complexities of the pharmacokinetics discussed might make this section difficult to understand for the inexperienced clinician, and many of the tables in this chapter are simply lists of drugs that may cause various types of renal dysfunction without assigning clinical importance.

The chapter on rheumatoid arthritis gives a very cursory overview of this disease and its treatment; the investiga-

Continued on page 235

Continued from page 228

tional agent auranofin, an oral gold product expected to be marketed soon, is not mentioned. Anemias are discussed thoroughly. The chapter on insomnia and anxiety (chapter 35) doesn't mention that methaqualone is no longer available. Also, use of other benzodiazepines for insomnia might have been stressed more.

In the affective-disorders chapter, the author's discussion of the dexamethasone-suppression test does not reflect the controversy over this test's true usefulness. A well-referenced and complete discussion of schizophrenia and psychosis misstates that "piperazine phenothiazines yield higher blood concentrations than chlorpromazine. . ." and thus appear to be more suitable for clinical studies. Although the author is correct in stating that no proven treatment exists for the neuroleptic malignant syndrome, no mention is made of dantrolene or bromocriptine, which show promise in selected cases. The chapter on breast cancer is concisely written, and the chapter discussing headache is extensively referenced.

While pharmacokinetics of specific drugs are discussed when appropriate, a chapter reviewing basic pharmacokinetic principles would be very helpful. This book is very much improved over the earlier editions, but it is too general and at times superficial (e.g., many chapters lack adequate discussions of pathophysiology), to be of substantial use to pharmacists already routinely involved in patient care. In spite of these shortcomings, this textbook will be a worthwhile purchase for its intended audience—pharmacy students and pharmacists with little clinical training.

Reviewed by Michael E. Ward, Pharm.D., Psychiatric Pharmacy Practice Program, University of Texas Health Science Center, San Antonio, TX 78284.

Guide to Clinical Studies and Developing Protocols

By Bert Spilker.
Published by Raven Press, 1140 Avenue of the Americas, New York, NY 10036, 1984. xvii + 302 p. Price $45.00.

This text addresses the major issues associated with the design, conduct, and reporting of clinical studies. It provides an excellent resource for pharmacists who are interested in becoming involved in clinical study work as well as a resource for pharmacy students in their curricula.

The first section of the book provides a background and discussion of the elements necessary to develop a study design. It reviews such key features as how to establish study objectives, what types of blind are available, how to determine what sample size will be necessary to answer the study objectives, procedures for randomization, as well as how to develop a dosing schedule based on pharmacokinetic parameters. In addition, the author reviews the phases of clinical trials as seen by the FDA. Phase I are preclinical studies that are done in normal volunteers in which safety evaluations are the primary objective; Phase II are initial studies related to efficacy in selective patient populations initially and then the pivotal studies in larger well-controlled studies; Phase III studies are conducted in patient populations for which the drug is intended in which both safety and efficacy are evaluated in relatively large numbers of patients; and Phase IV are studies that are conducted once the drug is marketed that should provide additional information on the drugs efficacy and safety profile usually in different populations, new age groups, new durations of treatment as well as drug interactions.

Section 2 provides a step-by-step approach to developing and writing the protocol that will be followed to answer the stated study objectives. Tables and checklists assure that the reader (investigator) has included and addressed such important factors as characteristics of the patient to be included in the study, characteristics of the disease and its treatment, environmental and other factors to be used as inclusion or exclusion criteria, as well as procedures for screening examinations.

Chapter 16—on identifying, choosing, and evaluating efficacy indicators—is perhaps the key chapter in the text; these indicators will be used to evaluate whether the study objective has been achieved or not. Table 16.16 contains an example of grading systems that may be used in some clinical conditions. Chapter 17 on safety indicators provides an exhaustive check list for lab examinations and tests that might be necessary to evaluate the safety of a compound. The chapter on ensuring compliance and the chapter on preparing and packaging of drugs are obviously written by a person who has had practical experience in this area.

The chapters on preparing and polishing the boilerplate of the protocol provide an excellent initial approach for

Continued on page 238

Please turn page for brief sum

One-dose protection that lasts longer than the surgery*

12-hour protection eliminates the need for intraoperative dosing

Precef should usually be administered 1 hour before the operation to achieve an effective concentration in the wound tissues

One-dose protection against the most common surgical pathogens

Excellent coverage of both gram-negative and gram-positive pathogens*

Well tolerated IM or IV

- Excellent safety record, less than 2% incidence of adverse reactions in 1,534 patients treated with Precef†
- No cases of drug-related pseudomembranous colitis have been reported; however, this condition has been reported with the use of other cephalosporins and other broad-spectrum antibiotics, and its occurrence should be borne in mind

One-dose economy

Lower drug acquisition costs than with multi-dose regimens

Lower costs for infusion sets and diluents

One-dose simplicity

Simplest possible dosage for most general surgical prophylactic procedures – one gram, one dose – which means fewer IVs

Gives you more control; eliminates potential problems with follow-up doses and helps prevent inappropriate use

Reduces chance of administration errors

*Against possible infections due to susceptible pathogens.
†Refer to Official Package Circular for complete information on side effects.

BRISTOL®

Division of Bristol-Myers Company
Syracuse, New York 13221-4755

l prescribing information.

Current Literature *Continued from page 235*

pharmacy investigators who have not previously had experience in clinical research as well as for those who have. It ensures that every step is completed. The chapter on designing data-collection forms or case-report forms provides both a pro and con discussion of the various formats that may be used. For example, Spilker discusses the advantages of a case-report form that is chronologic versus segmented by type of data collected (i.e., laboratory data are separated from clinical data). The chronologic format is easier to complete by the investigator, but the data-collection form that is segmented by type of data requested allows easy review for trends.

The author completes the book by reviewing the process that should be involved in selection of investigators, in prestudy meetings, and in monitoring and troubleshooting a study once it is underway.

Overall, the text is an excellent practical guide to conducting a clinical studies program. This book is a useful reference for pharmacists conducting research, for students, and researchers in the pharmaceutical industry.

Reviewed by Catherine Angell Sohn, Pharm.D., Medical Affairs Department, Smith Kline & French Laboratories, 1900 Market Street, Philadelphia, PA 19101.

New Drugs Annual: Cardiovascular Drugs (Volume 2)

Edited by Alexander Scriabine.
Published by Raven Press, 1140 Avenue of the Americas, New York, NY 10036, 1984. x + 273 p. Price $41.50.

This text is the second volume of a series containing comprehensive reviews of new cardiovascular drugs. Of 13 cardiovascular agents reviewed, two have been approved previously for use in the U.S. by the Food and Drug Administration; the remaining 11 are in various stages of clinical evaluation.

This book uses six classifications based on the most likely major clinical use of each drug: antihypertensives, antiarrhythmics, antianginals, vasodilators, cardiac stimulants, and cerebral antihypoxic and antimigraine drugs. Since most drugs will have more than one indication, this scheme is somewhat arbitrary.

The vast majority of contributors to this text are from the pharmaceutical industry and are involved in the research and development of new drugs. The other contributors are from academic centers in the United States and Europe and are apparently involved in the animal or human trials of the investigational agents they discuss.

Each compound is intensively reviewed, and both published and unpublished data are presented in the areas of pharmacology, toxicology, biochemistry, pharmacokinetics, and clinical use. To have a full appreciation for this book, the reader should have some background in basic science research; otherwise the animal and human data presented will be difficult to understand. Most contributors present little information on clinical use of the drugs. Only the chapters on verapamil and diltiazem have detailed discussions on clinical use, since these—the only marketed agents—have been used widely.

This book is well written. The use of graphs and tables facilitates comprehension of the material. This book will

Continued on page 240

Continued from page 238

be a welcome addition to the personal library of pharmacists with a strong interest in cardiology and research. Practically speaking, this book would be well-suited for drug information centers and medical libraries. In the future, this series of texts may be a valuable reference to pharmacists, pharmacologists, and physicians involved in cardiology and cardiovascular research.

Reviewed by Bradley G. Wulf, Pharm.D., Department of Pharmacy Practice, College of Pharmacy, University of Nebraska Medical Center, 42nd and Dewey Avenue, Omaha, NE 68105.

Books Received

Books are listed as received; selected books may be reviewed in Book Reviews in subsequent issues.

Applied Therapeutic Drug Monitoring. Volume I: Fundamentals; Volume II: Review and Case Studies, edited by Thomas P. Moyer and Roger L. Boeckx. Published by the American Association for Clinical Chemistry, 1725 K St., N.W., Washington, DC 20006, 1982 (Vol. I), 1984 (Vol. II). Vol. I xii + 241 p.; price $15.00. Vol. II xi + 387 p.; price $19.50 (members), $22.00 (nonmembers). Bound set $30.00 (members), $35.00 (nonmembers).

Bedside Clinical Pharmacokinetics: Simple Techniques for Individualizing Drug Therapy, by Carl C. Peck. Published by Pharmacometrics Press, 6219 Poindexter Lane, Rockville, MD 20852, 1984. 98 p. Price $5.00, students $4.00; 5% tax for Maryland residents.

Chemical Toxicology and Clinical Chemistry of Metals, edited by Stanley S. Brown and John Savory. Published by Academic Press Inc., 111 Fifth Avenue, New York, NY 10003, 1983. xiv + 416 p. Price $35.00, £20.00.

Diuretics: Chemistry, Pharmacology, and Clinical Applications, edited by Jules B. Puschett and Arthur Greenberg. Published by Elsevier Science Publishing Co., Inc., 52 Vanderbilt Ave., New York, NY 10017, 1984. 569 p. Price $88.00; dfl-300.00.

Dispensing of Medication, 9th Edition, edited by Robert E. King. Published by Mack Printing Company, Easton, PA 18042, 1984. 536 p. Price $28.95.

Hepatitis A, edited by Robert J. Gerety. Published by Academic Press, Inc., Orlando, FL 32887, 1984. xiii + 282 p. Price $49.00.

The History of Lithium Therapy, by F. Neil Johnson. Published by Oxford University Press, 200 Madison Ave., New York, NY 10016, 1984. xvii + 198 p. Price $49.00.

Human Tumour Drug Sensitivity Testing *In Vitro*, edited by Philip P. Dendy and Bridget T. Hill. Published by Academic Press Inc., 111 Fifth Ave., New York, NY 10003, 1983. x + 333 p. Price $60.00, £35.00.

Immunotoxicology, edited by G. Gordon Gibson, Ronald Hubbard, and Dennis V. Parke. Published by Academic Press Inc., 111 Fifth Ave., New York, NY 10003, 1983. xxv + 505 p. Price $32.00, £19.60.

Learning to Live with Diabetes (Noninsulin-Dependent). Published by Medicine in the Public Interest, Inc., Suite 304, 65 Franklin St., Boston, MA 02110, 1984. Copies available from PIP, P.O. Box 3852, Grand Central Station, New York, NY 10163. iv + 87 p.

Learning to Live with Osteoarthritis. Published by Medicine in the Public Interest, Inc., Suite 304, 65 Franklin St., Boston, MA 02110, 1984. Copies available from PIP, P.O. Box 3852, Grand Central Station, New York, NY 10163. 62 p.

Medical Abbreviations: 2300 Conveniences at the Expense of Communications and Safety, Second Edition, by Neil M. Davis. Published by Neil M. Davis Associates, 1143 Wright Drive, Huntingdon Valley, PA 19006, 1985. ii + 62 p. Price $3.25 ($2.35 each for 20 or more copies).

Medicinal Chemistry: A Biochemical Approach, by Thomas Nogrady. Published by Oxford University Press, 200 Madison Ave., New York, NY 10016, 1985. xiv + 449 p. Price $47.50 (cloth), $27.95 (paperback).

Practice of Critical Care Pharmacy, edited by Thomas C. Majerus and Joseph F. Dasta. Published by Aspen Systems Corporation, 1600 Research Boulevard, Rockville, MD 20850, 1985. xvi + 315 p. Price $36.00.

The Psychopharmacology of Lithium, by F. Neil Johnson. Published by Oxford University Press, 200 Madison Ave., New York, NY 10016, 1984. ix + 327 p. Price $69.00.

Advertising Index

American Cancer Society
Institutional, 235
American Society of Hospital Pharmacists
Clinical Pharmacy, 148, 148A, 148B
Clinical Research Forum, 239
Position Available, 131
Biotrack, Inc.
Warfcalc, 147
Bristol Laboratories, Division of Bristol-Myers Company
Cefadyl, 143–144
Precef, 236–238
International Pharmaceutical Federation
45th International Congress, 227
National Council on Patient Information and Education
Institutional, 223
Lederle Laboratories, A Division of American Cyanamid Company
Maxzide, 139–140
Pfipharmecs, Division of Pfizer Corporation
Institutional, inside back cover
Roche Laboratories, Division of Hoffmann-La Roche Inc.
Coactin, 121, 127–130
Rocephin, 229–234
Smith Kline & French Laboratories
Ancef, inside front cover
Monocid, 135–138
Stuart Pharmaceuticals, Division of ICI Americas, Inc.
Institutional, outside back cover
The University of Florida
Fellowship Program, 146
The Upjohn Company
Cleocin, 124–126
Micronase, 132–134

News

Phospholipids may hold key to allergic and immunologic reactions

A new class of potent phospholipid molecules that has been implicated in many aspects of allergy and inflammation may explain the cellular and subcellular events involved in diverse pathologic events such as myocardial infarction and anaphylaxis. Originally termed platelet-activating factor (based on the bioassay used for its detection), these unique, ether-linked phospholipids, 1-*O*-alkyl-2-acetyl-*sn*-glycero-3-phosphocholine (or acetyl glyceryl ether phosphorylcholine, AGEPC) are now recognized to be among the most potent of mediators of allergic and inflammatory events.

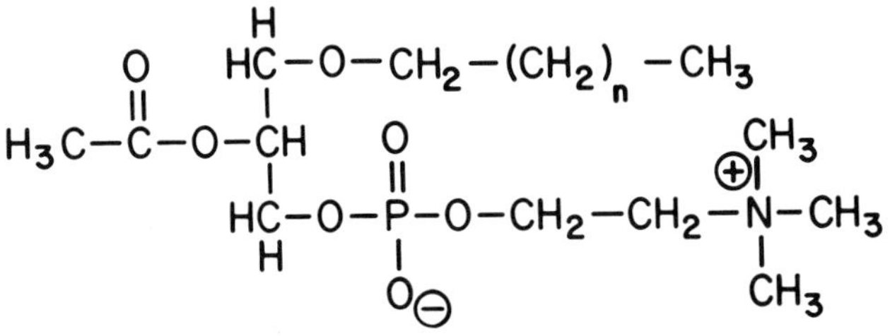

Chemical structure of 1-*O*-alkyl-2-acetyl-*sn*-glycero-3-phosphocholine. The length of the carbon chain denoted by *n* may be 14 or 16.

Recently developed instruments have enabled investigators to isolate and identify these compounds. Current studies to evaluate these new mediators likely will revolutionize our understanding of the treatment—and possibly prevention—of allergic and inflammatory tissue injury in many diverse diseases.

Compound Induces Anaphylactic Symptoms. Platelet-activating factor (PAF) was initially described in 1972 as a soluble material released from antigen-stimulated leukocytes; it caused platelets to undergo both aggregation and secretion of granular contents (e.g., serotonin, histamine). These pioneering studies involved only small amounts of PAF, and structural elucidation of the molecules required eight additional years of investigations and technological advances. As a result, the PAF released from antigen-stimulated, IgE-sensitized basophils is now known to be the phospholipid AGEPC.

PAF is released into the bloodstream during IgE-mediated anaphylaxis; similarly, intravascular infusion of AGEPC evokes virtually identical physiologic events as occur during the anaphylactic response (i.e., acute thrombocytopenia, neutropenia, basopenia, intravascular platelet release and thromboxane production, hematocrit increases with concomitant increased pulmonary resistance, decreased pulmonary compliance, pulmonary hypertension, and systemic hypotension potentially leading to respiratory arrest and death). These severe biological events occur within 30 seconds after the administration of AGEPC (0.5 μg/kg) and are largely reversed within 60 minutes. In short, this single phospholipid appears capable of promoting all the biological consequences that follow the IgE-triggered allergic response. Therefore, a variety of more recent studies have been addressed towards characterization of the pathobiological potential of this unique new mediator.

Other Effects of AGEPC. This compound has a spectrum of potent biological activities as assessed in diverse in vitro assays: (1) platelet aggregation, granule release, and thromboxane production (0.1–1 n*M*); (2) neutrophil chemotaxis, aggregation, granule release, and superoxide and leukotriene production; (3) smooth-muscle contraction; (4) monocyte chemotaxis, aggregation, and superoxide production; (5) hepatic glycogenolysis; and (6) decreased myocardial contractility with negative inotropic effects on the myocardium. AGEPC in vivo has been shown to induce (1) decreased cardiac output; (2) increased cutaneous vascular permeability in humans and animals with neutrophil accumulation (demonstrated in animals only); (3) decreased coronary artery flow; (4) decreased myocardial contractility; and (5) increased urinary protein excretion in association with loss of glomerular anionic charge.

The effects of various antihistamines, nonsteroidal anti-inflammatory agents, calcium-channel blockers, and α-adrenergic antagonists on many of these in vitro and in vivo effects have been or are being evaluated; in brief, AGEPC appears to have *direct* actions in most of these bioassays. Thus, because of these profound biological activities associated with many aspects of allergy and inflammation, the search for specific antagonists to block these effects is currently under intense investigation.

Speculation that PAF (or AGEPC) is involved in promoting tissue injury in inflammatory disease is prompted by the observation that PAFs are produced by a variety of cells associated with allergy and inflammation, including basophils, mast cells, eosinophils, neutrophils, monocytes, macrophages, platelets, and endothelial cells. In addition, it is present in amniotic fluid during labor, in cardiac tissues after myocardial infarction, and in normal human urine and saliva. It does not exist preformed within cells; rather,it is rapidly synthesized following cell stimulation. Thus, studies are under way to characterize structurally these PAFs and to identify

Continued on page 248

Continued from page 245

PAF precursors and metabolic enzymes; this information undoubtedly will lead to the development of inhibitors of PAF biosynthesis.

A related fact of equal importance is that PAF-producing cells can also generate a multitude of other mediators associated with allergy and inflammation (e.g., histamine, serotonin, and arachidonic acid metabolites, including leukotrienes or the slow-reacting substance of anaphylaxis, prostaglandins, thromboxane, and prostacyclin). Possible synergistic effects of the multiple potent mediators may serve to enhance the biologic consequences of cell activation. This complex series of possible reactivity by stimulated cells only serves to complicate efforts to develop inhibitors or antagonists of these events.

Although an attractive candidate for mediating similar events in humans, future studies on this new class of phospholipids remain to be performed to prove conclusively that these unique molecules are involved in human disease. Nevertheless, that such biological compounds exist prompts the current investigations to characterize their role in normal as well as exaggerated physiological events. New types of treatments for inflammatory and allergic reactions may well result.

1. Vargaftig BB, Chignard M, Mencia-Huerta JM et al. Pharmacology of arachidonic metabolites and of platelet-activating factor. In: Gordon JL, ed. Platelets in biology and pathology. New York: Elsevier; 1981:373–406.
2. O'Flaherty JT. Biology of disease. Lipid mediators of inflammation and allergy. *Lab Invest.* 1982; 47:314–29.
3. McManus LM, Pinckard RN, Hanahan DJ. Acetyl glyceryl ether phosphorylcholine (AGEPC) in allergy and inflammation. In: Boström H, Ljungstedt N, eds. Stockholm: Almqvist and Wiksell International; 1983:165–84.
4. Ludwig JC, McManus LM, Pinckard RN. Synthesis-release coupling of platelet-activating factors (PAF) from stimulated human neutrophils. *Adv Inflam Res.* 1985. In press.

Linda M. McManus, Ph.D., Associate Professor of Pathology
The University of Texas Health Science Center
7703 Floyd Curl Drive
San Antonio, TX 78284

AIDS tests reach market as cases increase

Two tests for detecting serum antibodies to the virus responsible for the acquired immunodeficiency syndrome (AIDS) have now been marketed. The AIDS tests are being used voluntarily by blood banks to screen potential donors; people with positive results are referred to physicians for further evaluation.

The two tests both use the enzyme-linked immunosorbent assay (ELISA) technique for detecting antibody to the human T-cell leukemia virus-III (HTLV-III). Abbott Laboratories and Electro-Nucleonics have marketed tests, and three other companies have similar tests under consideration at FDA, which will mandate testing of blood and blood products in the near future.

Meanwhile, a recent *JAMA* report has underscored concern among health officials in the U.S. about spread of the disease among heterosexuals.[1] Seven women whose husbands had AIDS or AIDS-related complex were studied; three had AIDS-related complex and four had antibodies to HTLV-III. Two of the husbands were i.v. drug abusers, and four others were promiscuous heterosexually. One had no known risk factor. Heterosexual promiscuity is becoming recognized as a risk factor, especially among men who frequent prostitutes. An epidemic of AIDS in central Africa is apparently spreading through heterosexual contacts.

1. Redfield RR, Markham PD, Salahuddin SZ et al. Frequent transmission of HTLV-III among spouses of patients with AIDS-related complex and AIDS. *JAMA.* 1985; 253:1571–3.

I.V. indomethacin marketed for patent ductus arteriosus

An intravenous formulation of indomethacin (Indocin, Merck Sharp & Dohme) was approved February 19 for treatment of patent ductus arteriosus (PDA) in premature infants. FDA approved labeling for the product, specifying that premature neonates weighing between 500 and 1750 grams may receive the i.v. drug if 48 hours of usual medical management has not cleared a "hemodynamically significant" PDA.

As shown in the figure, the ductus arteriosus normally closes within 15 hours after a normal full-term delivery, but premature neonates often retain the open ductus and thereby compromise their circulatory functions. Indo-

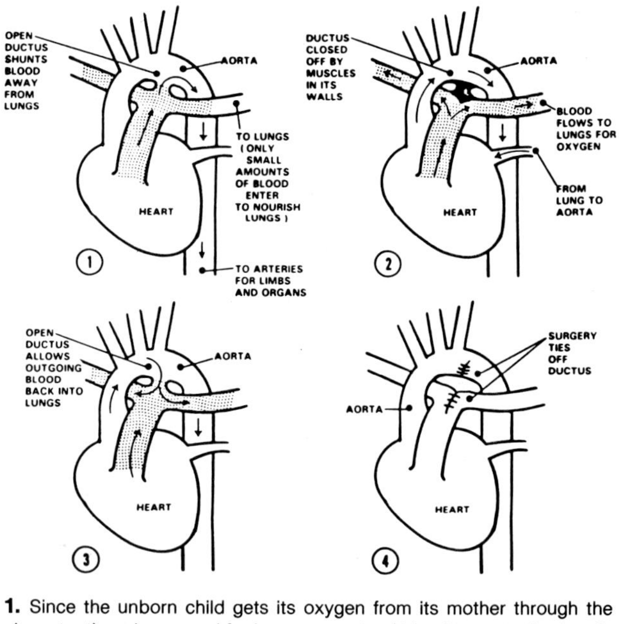

1. Since the unborn child gets its oxygen from its mother through the placenta, there is no need for large amounts of blood to go to the fetus's lungs to obtain oxygen. Indeed, the fetus's lungs are semicollapsed. Thus, a "bypass" called the ductus arteriosus diverts the major blood flow from the lungs until the infant is born. **2.** After the infant is born, the baby's lungs inflate with air and blood moves freely in the lungs, taking up oxygen. No longer needed, the bypass closes—that is, the muscles in the walls of the ductus arteriosus close it within about 15 hours following birth. **3.** Sometimes, especially in premature infants, the ductus remains "patent" or open. This allows some of the already oxygenated blood in the aorta to flow back into the lungs, rather than to the body, where it is needed. **4.** In surgery, the "patent" or open bypass is tied off. With the intravenous drug, the muscles act to close the ductus as in illustration 2.

Continued on page 252

News *Continued from page 248*

methacin is thought to close the duct by inhibiting the action of prostaglandin E1, which has been shown to dilate the ductus arteriosus in patients with some types of congenital abnormalities. PDAs that did not respond to medical management (fluid restriction, diuretics, digitalis, respiratory support) previously were closed surgically. The results of a trial of i.v. indomethacin versus placebo in 421 infants was reported in 1983 in the *Journal of Pediatrics.*[1]

1. Gersony WM, Peckham GJ, Ellison RC et al. Effects of indomethacin in premature infants with patent ductus arteriosus: results of a national collaborative study. *J Pediatr.* 1983; 102:895–906.

Patients, professionals good guessers in double-blind trial

Almost 80% of patients correctly guessed that they were receiving active drug, and about 70% of health professionals surmised whether patients were receiving placebo or β blockers in a double-blind trial of 3837 patients.[1] Of the patients in the placebo group, 57% believed they were receiving active therapy.

The assessment was made as part of the β-Blocker Heart Attack Trial (BHAT), which tested the efficacy of propranolol versus placebo in reducing mortality in postmyocardial infarction patients. The authors speculated that the side effects of propranolol may have enabled patients and professionals to determine who was receiving active drug; they called the belief of patients receiving placebo that they were getting propranolol "wishful thinking." Professionals tended to predict accurately which patients were in each group, apparently because of heart rate and other indicators of β-blocker activity.

1. Byington RP, Curb JD, Mattson ME. Assessment of double-blindness at the conclusion of the β-blocker heart attack trial. *JAMA.* 1985; 253:1733–6.

News Briefs

• **Metoclopramide hydrochloride** (Reglan, A. H. Robins) has been approved by FDA for treatment of gastroesophageal reflux in oral doses of 10–15 mg taken up to four times daily (30 minutes before meals and at bedtime). This is the only prescription drug approved for this indication.

• **"Thromboembolic Disease"** is a 56-minute videotape available from Norwich Eaton Pharmaceuticals that covers medical treatment and prevention, diagnosis, filter placement, and catheter embolectomy. To arrange a showing of the tape, contact a Norwich Eaton representative or the company's Professional Services Department, 17 Eaton Avenue, Norwich, NY 13815. Also available from the company is the third in a series of monographs on **"Current Concepts in Nutritional Support"**; this one covers vitamin and mineral requirements in the stressed patient and essential and unessential amino acids.

Letters

The Letters *column is a forum for rapid exchange of ideas among readers of* CP. *Liberal criteria are applied in the review of submissions to encourage contributions to this column.*

The Letters *column includes the following types of contributions: (1) comments, addenda, and minor updates on previously published work, (2) alerts on potential problems related to drug therapy or clinical research, (3) observations or comments on trends in drug therapy or clinical research, and (4) brief expressions of opinion about controversies in drug therapy or clinical research.*

Letters need not be submitted with the journal's manuscript checklist. The following conditions, however, must be adhered to: (1) the body of the letter must be no longer than two typewritten pages, (2) the use of references, tables, and illustrations should be minimized, (3) the authors' names, affiliations, and mailing addresses must be typed at the end of the letter in the format used by CP, *and (4) the entire letter (including references, tables, and authors' names) must be typed double spaced on plain white paper (not letterhead). Following acceptance of a letter, the authors are required to sign an exclusive publication statement and a copyright-transferral form.*

Acetylcysteine for severe atelectasis in premature infants

Acetylcysteine is a potent mucolytic agent used to reduce the viscosity of secretions containing mucoproteins. In patients with cystic fibrosis, acetylcysteine helps in clearing the upper respiratory tract,[1,2] and it has also been used for the prevention of obstruction of endotracheal tubes during mechanical ventilation in infants.[3] We report our experience with the use of acetylcysteine in premature infants suffering from recurrent atelectasis during assisted ventilation.

Five premature infants with pulmonary disease were treated with acetylcysteine (Mucomyst, Mead Johnson & Co., Evansville, IN 42721) to relieve severe recurrent pulmonary atelectasis (see table). Acetylcysteine was used only when at least four days of chest physiotherapy treatment, consisting of postural drainage, vibration, percussion, saline lavage, and selective intubation of the atelectatic lung, had failed to relieve the atelectasis. A 5% solution of acetylcysteine was prepared by diluting 20% acetylcysteine with 0.9% sodium chloride, and 2 mL of this solution was then administered by nebulization through the endotracheal tube every six hours for two to four days. In all five patients, the atelectasis was relieved after one to two days of treatment; three infants were extubated, while the other two showed substantial improvement. No side effects were recorded in our patients during or after the treatment.

We believe the use of acetylcysteine should be considered in infants with recurrent or severe atelectasis during mechanical ventilation when other types of therapy fail.

1. Denton R, Kwart H, Litt M. *N*-acetylcysteine in cystic fibrosis. *Annu Rev Resp Dis.* 1967; 95:643–51.
2. Rease HW. The use of *N*-acetylcysteine in the treatment of cystic fibrosis. *J Pediatr.* 1964; 65:542–57.
3. King R. Acetylcysteine in airway maintenance. *Lancet.* 1967; 1:900–1.

Jacob Amir, M.D.
Eliahu Wilunsky, M.D.
Israel Zelikovic, M.D.
Salomon H. Reisner, M.B., Ch.B.

Department of Neonatology
Beilinson Medical Center
Petah Tiqva, Israel 49 100

Demographic Information for Patients Treated with Acetylcysteine

Patient No.	Gestational Age (weeks)	Birth Weight (g)	Age at Treatment (days)	Type of Pulmonary Disease
1	29	980	26	Pneumonia
2	29	1430	24	Pneumonia
3	34	1650	38	Bronchopulmonary dysplasia
4	26	800	184	Bronchopulmonary dysplasia
5	23	730	28	Bronchopulmonary dysplasia

Continued on page 258

When a type II diabetic patient needs more than diet, unique MICRONASE® Tablets (glyburide) are a logical first choice.

Choosing antidiabetic

1. Micronase—a rational choice in type II diabetes

Insulin levels are normal or elevated in most patients with type II diabetes, although insulin action is markedly impaired. MICRONASE helps normalize the tissue response to endogenous insulin.

Initially, MICRONASE helps lower serum glucose in responsive patients by stimulating the release of additional insulin. As therapy continues, MICRONASE is believed to promote peripheral glucose metabolism by helping to correct defects at the cellular receptor and postreceptor levels.

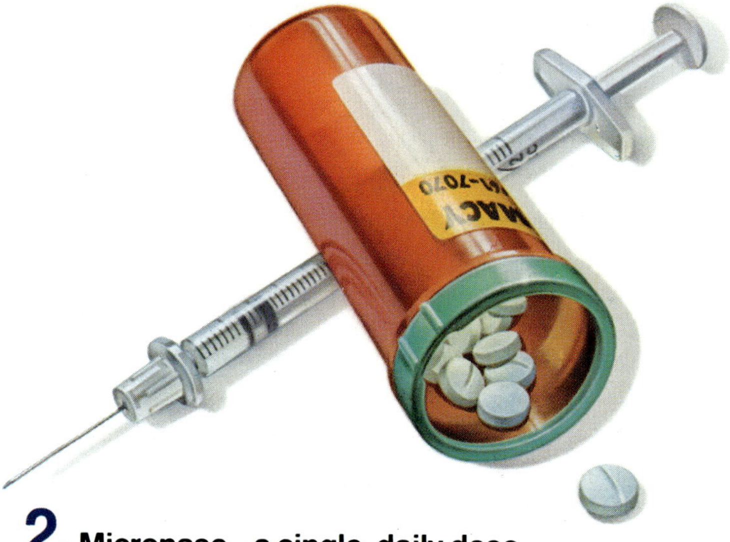

2. Micronase—a single, daily dose provides 24-hour glycemic control

MICRONASE provides 24-hour control of blood glucose with a single, daily, low-milligram dose. MICRONASE may be taken with food, since food intake does not appear to affect its bioavailability.

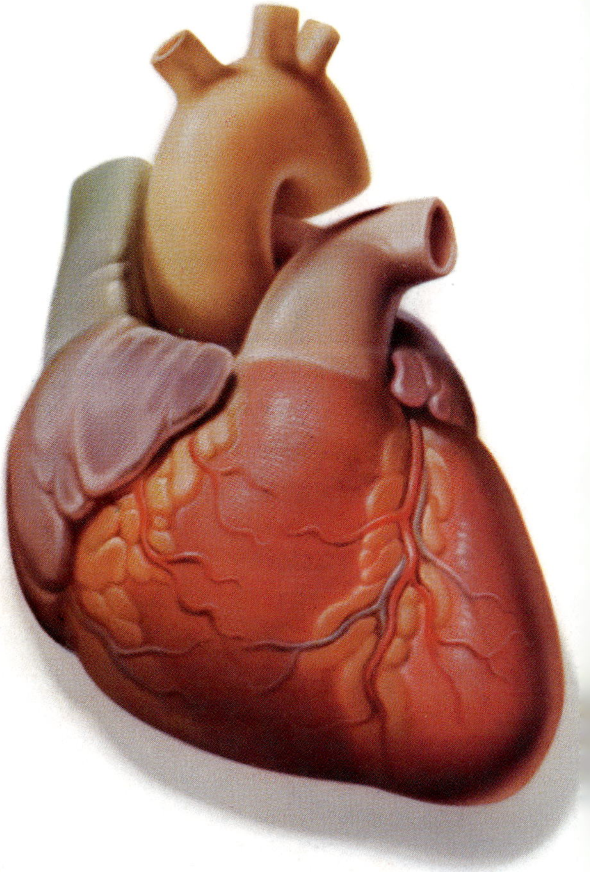

3. Micronase—for the type II diabetic patient who is also hypertensive: Control without risk of water retention

This may also be significant for the type II diabetic patient with congestive heart failure. MICRONASE actually causes mild diuresis.

therapy today

4. Micronase—an important consideration in the type II diabetic patient with renal impairment: Control plus unique dual excretion... 50% urine, 50% bile

Elimination of MICRONASE equally in bile and urine reduces the risk of drug accumulation, which may result in hypoglycemia. MICRONASE should be used with caution in patients with renal impairment; however, in a single-dose study, plasma clearance of MICRONASE was prolonged only in patients with severe renal impairment.

5. Micronase—for the patient who fails on other diabetic therapy: Potency and dosage flexibility

MICRONASE may prove effective when other drugs fail. Five mg of MICRONASE is approximately equivalent to 250 mg of chlorpropamide or 500 mg of acetohexamide in its ability to lower blood glucose. The dosage range of MICRONASE allows for greater dosage flexibility than other agents.

Overdosage of sulfonylureas, including MICRONASE, can cause hypoglycemia. Although the interpretations are controversial, the UGDP study reported in 1970 that the use of tolbutamide, an oral hypoglycemic drug, was associated with increased cardiovascular mortality.

Upjohn The Upjohn Company
Kalamazoo, MI 49001

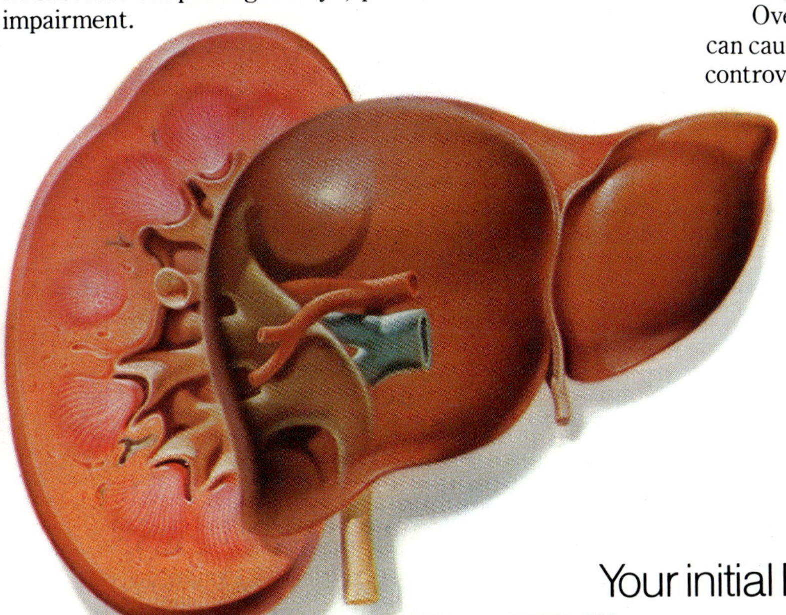

Your initial Rx in type II diabetes

Micronase®

glyburide, **5 mg** Tablets

For brief summary of prescribing information, please turn page.

Letters *Continued from page 255*

Pharmacologic effects of the triazolo group

Triazolam and alprazolam have, in addition to the classic benzodiazepine nucleus, a heterocyclic ring with three nitrogens called the triazolo group (see figure). If triazolam or alprazolam have pharmacologic properties different from those of the traditional benzodiazepines, one might hypothesize a unique structure–activity relationship based on the presence of the triazolo group. Two possible distinctive properties—the Van der Kroef adverse reaction to triazolam and an antidepressant action of alprazolam—are of note.

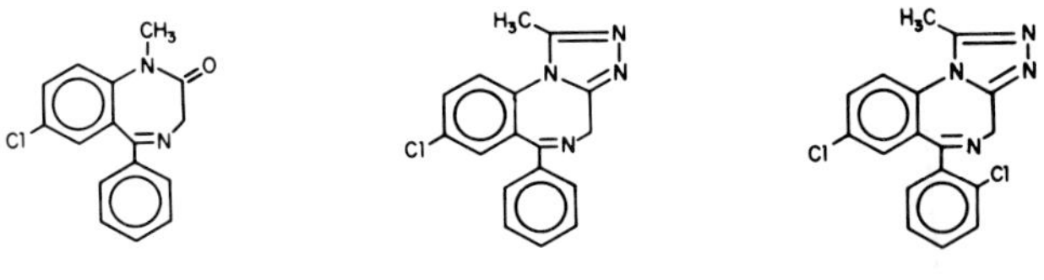

Chemical structures of diazepam (left), alprazolam (middle), and triazolam. Note the triazolo group in alprazolam and triazolam consisting of a heterocyclic ring with three nitrogens.

The Van der Kroef reaction is named for a Dutch psychiatrist who reported 25 cases of a "cluster syndrome" of adverse behavioral reactions to triazolam.[1] Some of the symptoms were severe malaise, depersonalization, derealization, paranoid reactions, depression, nightmares, severe suicidal tendencies, and acute and chronic anxiety; there were 20 other psychiatric, sensory, and neurologic symptoms. The existence of this syndrome, which has not been reported by clinicians in other countries, was hotly debated in the literature.

Several theories may be put forth to explain the Van der Kroef reaction (assuming it exists). First, the triazolo group may impart distinctive properties to triazolam. Second, a 1-mg dose was used, which allows a rapid decrease in blood concentrations that could result in a withdrawal reaction. The onset of withdrawal syndromes to benzodiazepines may parallel their durations of action.[2] Both rebound anxiety[2] and rebound insomnia[3] have been reported with triazolam. (To test the hypothesis that shorter-acting benzodiazepines may result in withdrawal syndromes of rapid onset, one might consider midazolam, an ultrashort-acting benzodiazepine. Apparently withdrawal reactions have not occurred with this investigational intravenous agent when given in brief courses.)

A third theory is that the formulation used at the time of the reports may have differed in some way from the current formulation and contributed to the reactions. Data on the formulation used in Holland in 1979 are not available.

The proposed antidepressant action of alprazolam is similarly controversial, although early reports suggested an antidepressant action. A study comparing the anti-

Continued on page 266

Letters *Continued from page 258*

depressant effects of diazepam, alprazolam, imipramine, and placebo showed that alprazolam was not significantly more efficacious than diazepam.[4] The currently accepted caveat is that alprazolam has more antidepressant action than diazepam, an earlier onset of activity than tricyclic antidepressants, but no more effectiveness than imipramine in the long run. (Alprazolam's purported antipanic effect is probably an extension of its antianxiety effect.) Alprazolam has no known side effects that distinguish it from traditional benzodiazepines,[5] suggesting that the triazolo group does not impart a special side-effect profile.

While the possibility of a unique pharmacologic action of the triazolo group is intriguing, the existing data by no means conclusively support this theory. It remains simply an interesting possibility.

1. Van der Kroef C. Reactions to triazolam. *Lancet.* 1979; 2:526. Letter.
2. Morgan K, Oswald I. Anxiety caused by a short-life hypnotic. *Br Med J.* 1982; 284:942.
3. Kales A, Schart MB, Kales JD et al. Rebound insomnia. *JAMA.* 1979; 241:1692–5.
4. Weissman MM, Prusuff BA, Klaber HD et al. Alprazolam (Xanax) in the treatment of major depression. Paper presented to the Annual Congress of the Collegian Internale Neuropsychopharmacologicum. Florence, Italy: 1984 Jun 20–22.
5. Fawcett JA, Kravita HM. Alprazolam: pharmacokinetics, clinical efficacy, and mechanism of action. *Pharmacotherapy.* 1982; 2:243–53.

GEORGE TANIGUCHI, PHARM.D., Resident in Mental Health
University of Tennessee Center for the Health Sciences
874 Union Avenue
Memphis, TN 38163

Venoconstriction by angiotensin II

In a review of enalapril, a new angiotensin-converting enzyme (ACE) inhibitor, Vlasses et al.[1] presented the hypothesis that enalapril has effects beyond those associated with inhibition of serum ACE. The effectiveness of the drug in reducing preload in patients with congestive heart failure (CHF) is seen by the authors as evidence of this since "...angiotensin II has not been shown to have venoconstrictive effects...."

Although it seems certain that enalapril has actions other than ACE inhibition, angiotensin II does in fact cause mild venoconstriction. This is clearly stated by Guyton,[2] who pointed out that the effect is substantial enough to cause a 20% increase in mean circulatory filling pressure. Thus, the beneficial effects of enalapril in CHF may partially result from antagonism of venoconstriction caused by angiotensin II.

1. Vlasses PH, Larijani GE, Conner DP et al. Enalapril, a nonsulfhydryl angiotensin-converting enzyme inhibitor. *Clin Pharm.* 1985; 4:27–40.
2. Guyton AC. Short-term regulation of mean arterial pressure: nervous reflex and hormonal mechanisms for rapid pressure control. In: Textbook of medical physiology. Philadelphia, PA: W.B. Saunders Company; 1981:256.

JOSEPH T. RACKSON, Staff Pharmacist
Saint Joseph Hospital
7620 York Road
Baltimore, MD 21204

Therapy Reviews

Pathophysiology and treatment of deep-vein thrombosis and pulmonary embolism

Barry L. Carter, Mark E. Jones, and L. Anthony Waickman

Abstract: The pathophysiology of deep-vein thrombosis (DVT) and pulmonary embolism (PE) is briefly discussed, and the efficacy, dosage and administration, laboratory monitoring, and adverse effects of thrombolytic agents, heparin, and warfarin are reviewed.

Acute therapy of DVT and PE is usually initiated with intravenous heparin; however, thrombolytic agents such as streptokinase and urokinase may be preferred in patients with massive PE or severe DVT when clot lysis rather than clot stabilization is deemed necessary. For DVT or PE, an intravenous loading dose of streptokinase or urokinase is given, followed by a continuous infusion of the drug. Therapy with streptokinase is continued for 24 hours in patients with PE and for 72 hours in those with DVT; urokinase is continued for 12 hours in patients with PE. Monitoring of blood coagulation tests during thrombolytic therapy is recommended primarily for ensuring that a lytic state is achieved.

Intravenous heparin is preferred for acute treatment of DVT or PE; controversy exists regarding whether administration by continuous infusion or intermittent bolus injection is superior. Heparin dosage is usually adjusted to maintain the activated partial-thromboplastin time (APTT) ratio between 1.5 and 2.5; however, the ideal therapeutic range has never been firmly established. After acute treatment with heparin, most patients should continue to receive either warfarin or subcutaneous heparin for several months to prevent recurrent thromboembolism.

Bleeding is the major adverse effect of thrombolytic agents and anticoagulants. The risk of bleeding with heparin and warfarin therapy increases with excessive prolongation of the APTT and prothrombin time (PT), respectively.

Future clinical trials should further define the role of thrombolytic agents in the treatment of DVT and PE and the efficacy of less-intense warfarin therapy for pulmonary embolism or arterial thromboembolic events.

Index terms: Anticoagulants; Dosage; Heparin; Pulmonary embolism; Streptokinase; Thrombolytic agents; Thrombophlebitis; Toxicity; Urokinase; Warfarin
Clin Pharm. 1985; 4:279–96

Heparin was first described in 1916 and became available for clinical use in 1935.[1] By 1960, several papers had reported the efficacy of heparin in thromboembolic disorders.[2–4] However, as early as 1942, Allen et al.[5] described the disadvantages of heparin as being (1) the cost of therapy (about $10 per day), (2) the need for continuous infusion or repeated injections, and (3) the difficulty in maintaining a constant therapeutic effect on coagulation time. Thus, a long-acting oral anticoagulant drug was sought.

It had been well known that cattle frequently died from severe bleeding disorders. Link and associates[6,7] identified the responsible agent in spoiled sweet clover. The clinical use of dicoumarol was described in the early 1940s, and warfarin was synthesized at the University of Wisconsin in 1948 (the name warfarin being derived from the *W*isconsin *A*lumni *R*esearch *F*oundation).[5,8]

Although anticoagulants have been used clinically for almost 50 years, our knowledge about these drugs remains incomplete. For instance, clinicians disagree on how heparin should be administered and monitored, what the appropriate treatment length with heparin and warfarin should be, and what degree of anticoagulation should be

Barry L. Carter, Pharm.D., is Assistant Professor, College of Pharmacy, University of Iowa, Iowa City. Mark E. Jones, Pharm.D., is Clinical Pharmacist, Davenport Medical Education Foundation, Davenport, IA. L. Anthony Waickman, M.D., is Assistant Director of Housestaff Education, and Associate, Divisions of General Medicine and Cardiology, Department of Internal Medicine, University of Iowa.

Address reprint requests to Dr. Carter at the College of Pharmacy, University of Iowa, Iowa City, IA 52242.

This is **article 680-204-8508** in the **ASHP Continuing Education System.** See page 336 for learning objectives and test questions.

used. Many of these topics have only recently been addressed in controlled trials.

In this paper we will briefly review the pathophysiology of thromboembolism and suggest guidelines for the clinical use of anticoagulants and thrombolytic agents in the therapy of acute deep-vein thrombosis (DVT) and pulmonary embolism (PE).

Pathophysiology of DVT and PE

The validity of the three mechanisms responsible for thromboembolism proposed by Virchow[9]—vascular injury, venous stasis, and hypercoagulability—has stood the test of time. Arterial thrombi are generally associated with vascular injury and result from platelet adherence to collagen within the subendothelium of the damaged vessel wall.[10,11] Additional platelets are recruited after the release of adenosine diphosphate (ADP), epinephrine, and other platelet components. This results in platelet aggregation and initiation of the intrinsic clotting cascade, which eventually causes the formation of a fibrin plug.[11]

Venous thrombi may form following injury or venous stasis. Vascular injury is important in the genesis of venous thrombi following surgery and trauma. Venous stasis may also contribute to vascular injury. Hamer et al.[12] demonstrated that even short periods of stasis can cause hypoxia and endothelial damage to venous valves with subsequent thrombus formation on the valve cusp. In addition, stasis promotes fibrin formation, and locally sluggish flow protects the activated clotting factors from hepatic clearance and protects fibrin from the fibrinolytic system.[11,13]

The release of tissue thromboplastin or collagen may result in activation of coagulation during surgery, trauma, childbirth, or malignancy.[11,14] Other conditions associated with hypercoagulable states include pregnancy, antithrombin III deficiency, and protein C deficiency. Factors that may predispose to the formation of DVT are listed in Table 1.

Typically, venous thrombi form at valves or bifurcations in the veins of the lower extremities. Thrombi may develop in any of the major veins, but most originate in the calf.[13] The major dangers DVT poses to the patient include compromised blood flow to the lower extremity, destruction of venous architecture, and embolization. Distortion and destruction of venous valves occurs when valvular endothelium becomes involved in the thrombus organization and recanalization process. Thrombus organization results in a recanalized vein devoid of valves or a vein with severely displaced, rigid valves.[15] Partially obstructing thrombi reorganize, leaving varying degrees of venous valvular destruction; in addition, penetrating vein valves are damaged. The result is an abnormal venous circulation and venous hypertension. These hemodynamic abnormalities leave patients prone to develop dependent edema, stasis dermatitis, pain, and chronic ulcers—commonly known as the postphlebitic syndrome. Bauer[16] reported in 1942 that 99% of patients with DVT who were not treated with anticoagulants had edema after one year, and 79% had leg ulcers 20 years after the acute episode. Anticoagulation has reduced the incidence of postphlebitic syndrome, but it still occurs in up to 50% of patients with femoral or iliac vein thrombosis after four-year follow-up.[17] However, the incidence approaches zero if venous architecture returns to normal after thrombolytic therapy, although incomplete clot lysis is still associated with abnormal venous hemodynamics.[17–24]

About 15–20% of known venous thrombi in the legs embolize to the lungs. These emboli may be small and asymptomatic or massive and life threatening. Platelets bind to thrombin within the emboli, and a coating of aggregated platelets forms around the embolus.[25] This platelet aggregation causes release of serotonin and thromboxane A_2, which results in intense vasoconstriction.[26–29] The pulmonary arteriolar vasoconstriction can then lead to pulmonary hypertension and right-sided heart failure, which may be fatal.[14,30–32] Pretreatment with high doses of heparin has been shown to inhibit the pulmonary vasoconstriction in dogs[28] and rabbits[25,29] if given before the release of emboli. However, the clinical applicability of these findings for treatment of PE may be limited since heparin was given before the emboli were released.

Emboli originate more commonly from proximal veins in the leg (i.e., above the knee) than from the calf. Many clinicians believe that calf-vein thrombi rarely embolize, and when they do, the clinical consequences are minor. Therefore, controversy exists concerning whether calf-vein thrombosis should be aggressively treated.[14,33,34] However, recent evidence suggests that calf-vein thrombosis can be a source for serious pulmonary embolism.[35–37] In addition, up to 30% of calf-vein thrombi propagate to sites above the knee where they are more likely to embolize.[36,37] Therefore,

Table 1.
Factors Associated with Increased Risk of Thromboembolism.[11–14]

Obesity
Immobilization
Congestive heart failure
Trauma
Surgery
Neoplasm
Pregnancy
Antithrombin III deficiency
Protein C deficiency
Protein S deficiency
Oral contraceptive therapy

some authors have recommended aggressive treatment of thrombosis located below the knee. This issue has not been resolved.

Before the routine use of anticoagulants, the mortality from PE was reported to be 20–50%.[3,38] Barritt and Jordan[3] reported five nonfatal recurrences of PE and five deaths in 19 patients with PE who did not receive heparin treatment. In contrast, there were no deaths or recurrences in 16 patients treated with heparin plus an oral anticoagulant for at least 14 days. These results were thought to be so convincing that treatment of PE with heparin was considered essential in an additional 38 patients, and no deaths occurred in these patients. Subsequent studies have demonstrated that the mortality from PE is less than 2% when treated with anticoagulants.[39-41]

A discussion of the diagnosis of DVT and PE and of primary prophylaxis of these disorders with dihydroergotamine–heparin, dextran, or antiplatelet drugs is beyond the scope of this paper. Many excellent references on these topics are available.[11,13,14,33,34,42-50]

Once a presumptive diagnosis of acute DVT or PE has been made, the treatment goals are as follows:

- To prevent further thrombus propagation,
- To prevent embolization,
- To promote thrombus resolution,
- To restore normal venous hemodynamics, and
- To prevent the postphlebitic syndrome.

Additional management for serious or life-threatening PE or proximal-vein DVT may include clot lysis with thrombolytics or surgical removal of the clot (i.e., embolectomy).

Acute Treatment of DVT and PE

Acute management of DVT includes bedrest, elevation of the leg(s), and administration of analgesics for pain. For acute PE, oxygen should be given and, if necessary, respiration should be supported. Intravenous fluids, vasopressors, or antiarrhythmic agents may be required in some patients.

Acute therapy of DVT and PE is usually initiated with heparin. However, if diagnostic tests confirm massive PE or proximal-vein DVT, it may be necessary to discontinue heparin and begin thrombolytic therapy. Figure 1 shows a suggested algorithm for acute therapy of DVT and PE.

Thrombolytic Agents. In 1948, Tillett and Sherry[51] performed the first clinical studies using streptokinase to lyse organized pleural effusions. In 1954, Tillett et al.[52] used streptokinase intravenously "to determine whether or not clots occurring within the vascular system as the result of disease may be subject to streptococcal fibrinolysis." Intense research since that time has clearly answered this question in the affirmative.

A number of thrombolytic agents have been developed, including streptokinase, urokinase, activated human and porcine plasmin, extrinsic plasminogen activators (including human tissue-type plasminogen activator), and an acylated streptokinase–plasminogen complex. We will limit our discussion to streptokinase and urokinase because of their current clinical availability and proven worth.

Mechanism of Action. Streptokinase is an antigenic, nonenzymatic protein excreted by Group C β-hemolytic streptococci that combines with plasminogen in vivo to form an active streptokinase–plasminogen complex (Figure 2). This complex converts both free and fibrin–fibrinogen absorbed plasminogen to the active proteolytic enzyme, plasmin.

Urokinase is a nonantigenic, active enzyme recovered from human fetal-kidney tissue culture or urine. Urokinase directly converts plasminogen to plasmin without requiring active intermediates. Theoretically, this mechanistic difference could have important clinical implications. The plasminogen bound into the streptokinase-plasminogen complex is not available for conversion to plasmin. Only small quantities of plasminogen are complexed at low streptokinase doses, leaving large quantities of plasminogen available for conversion to plasmin. At high streptokinase doses, most plasminogen will be complexed with streptokinase, leaving little free plasminogen available for conversion to plasmin. Theoretically, thrombolytic intensity and bleeding risk should be greater with low-dose streptokinase and, conversely, thrombolysis may be limited with high-dose streptokinase because of limited plasminogen availability. Although this effect can be demonstrated in vitro,[53] it has never been shown to be clinically important.

Plasmin produced by streptokinase or urokinase can then cause lysis of the fibrin clot. Because free circulating plasminogen is activated, both pathologic clots and hemostatic plugs are exposed to active plasmin. In addition, plasmin degrades fibrinogen and coagulation factors V, VIII, and XIII. It also liberates fibrin split products, which possess anticoagulant properties. This total effect is known as the lytic state.

Efficacy in DVT. The ideal treatment for formed clots would be to rapidly lyse the clot, restore the venous circulation, prevent venous valvular damage, and prevent the postphlebitic syndrome. Numerous early studies have shown that streptokinase and urokinase can achieve these goals in selected patients.[17-24,54-69] Complete clot lysis occurs in 30–65% of patients if clinical symptoms are present for less than three days, and a substantial but variable frequency of lysis occurs if symptoms are present for up to seven days.[22,57,59,62,69] Clot lysis has been documented with symptoms present for as long as 28 days, but this is an uncommon finding.[57]

Streptokinase has proved to be no better than

Figure 1. Algorithm for the acute management of pulmonary embolism (PE) and deep-vein thrombosis (DVT). *Note*: If heparin was initiated before the diagnosis of massive PE or proximal-vein DVT was confirmed, it should be discontinued before initiating thrombolytic therapy.

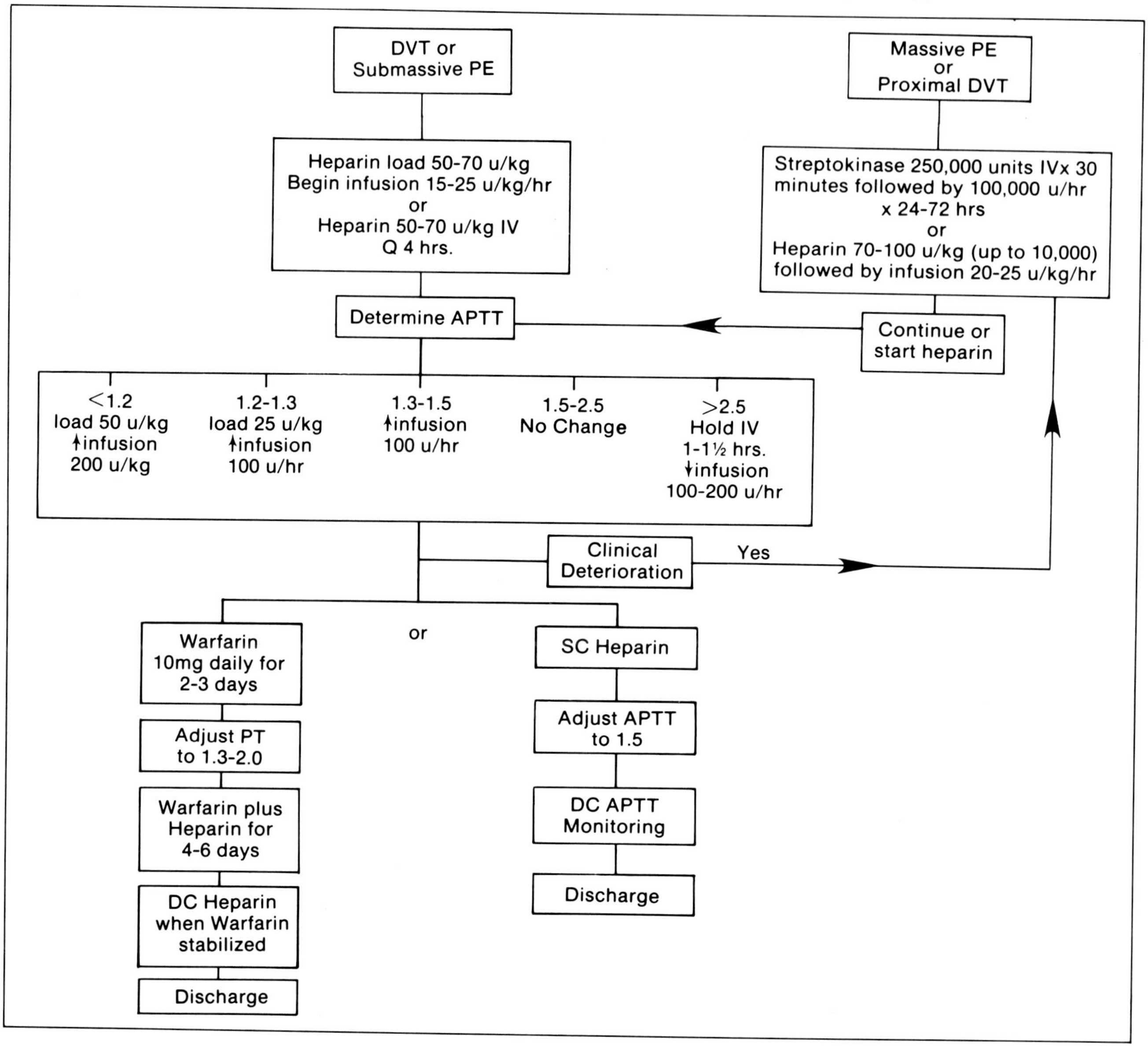

Figure 2. Diagram of the fibrinolytic system showing the points at which urokinase (UK) and streptokinase (SK) act.

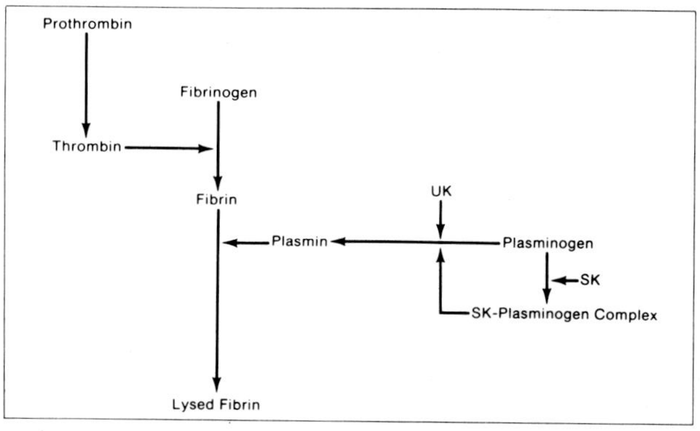

heparin for promoting clot lysis when given for 12 hours.[64] Streptokinase was reported to be superior to heparin when given for 24 hours, but substantial quantities of residual clot remained.[63] Although continuous thrombolytic therapy has been administered for as long as 26 days, benefit begins to wane after three days.[57] The standard length of treatment for DVT is now 72 hours.[59,70,71]

One concern about lysing peripheral-vein clots with thrombolytic agents relates to the possibility that the clot may embolize to the lung with greater frequency than that seen with heparin. However, emboli occur with equal frequency in patients treated with heparin or streptokinase.[21,55,62,69] This is a reassuring finding considering that the goal of heparin therapy is clot stabilization while that of streptokinase is clot lysis.

Efficacy in PE. Both streptokinase and urokinase have been shown to be superior to heparin with regard to angiographically proven pulmonary-artery thrombus clearance.[72-76] However, thrombolytic therapy plays a relatively small role in the overall treatment of PE.

The two largest studies of thrombolytic therapy for PE to date were done by the Urokinase Pulmonary Embolism Trial Study Group.[72,73] Comparing a 12-hour intravenous infusion of urokinase with conventional heparin anticoagulation, urokinase produced significantly greater improvement in the pulmonary arteriogram and in lung-scan abnormalities at 24 hours than did heparin. However, there was no significant difference between the two groups from post-treatment day 5 through a follow-up of one year. There was also no difference between groups receiving a 12-hour and 24-hour urokinase infusion and a 24-hour streptokinase infusion. Thus, thrombolytic therapy would need to be reserved for clinical situations where immediate clinical benefit is needed, i.e., cases of "pulmonary emboli with significant hemodynamic disturbances or where there has been obstruction of blood flow to a lobe or multiple segments. . . ."[77] Although survival has not been shown to increase with thrombolytic therapy, these recommendations are reasonable in these uncommon but clearly high-risk cases.

Sharma et al.[78] demonstrated that pulmonary-capillary blood volume returns to normal in patients with PE after treatment with either streptokinase or urokinase; however, it remains abnormal for up to a year in patients treated with heparin. In addition, pulmonary diffusing capacity approaches normal at one year in the thrombolytic-treated group but remains clearly below normal in the heparin group. This information in the heparin-treated group may be important in our understanding of persistent postembolic pulmonary hypertension.[79] These positive results with thrombolytic therapy have caused some authors to suggest broadening the indications for thrombolytic therapy of PE to include patients with pre-existing severe pulmonary vascular disease who would not tolerate further chronic pulmonary-microcirculation dysfunction (e.g., patients with emphysema, interstitial lung disease, and recurrent nonlife-threatening pulmonary emboli).[80] However, benefit in these patient populations remains to be proven.

Patient Selection. Patients being considered for thrombolytic therapy must be carefully selected and managed. The diagnosis of life-threatening PE or proximal-vein DVT must be clearly documented radiographically. Diagnosis based on any criteria other than the gold standard (pulmonary angiography or venography) must be suspect if thrombolytic therapy is contemplated. Pulmonary arteriograms should be done using an upper-extremity approach because the basilic vein is easily observed and compressed to prevent bleeding. The inguinal approach should be avoided because the femoral vein is not easily compressed and the potential risk of bleeding is great.

Contraindications to thrombolytic therapy[81-83] are listed in Table 2. Product labeling does not define what level of blood pressure constitutes severe hypertension, but one author has recommended avoiding thrombolytics in patients with diastolic blood pressures over 125 mm Hg.[71]

Although pregnancy is listed as a relative contraindication, streptokinase has been used successfully as early as the ninth week of pregnancy without fetal injury.[20,84,85] Data from two patients receiving radiolabeled streptokinase suggest that it does not cross the placenta.[84] Thrombolytic agents are not recommended during pregnancy because safety has not been proven; therefore, the clinical benefit of therapy must be weighed against the potential risk. Thrombolytic therapy should not be considered if delivery could occur during the treatment course.

Normal menses has not been considered a contraindication to thrombolytic therapy, and one case report has described no increase in menstrual bleeding during streptokinase infusion.[86] These authors suggest that thrombolytic therapy may be contraindicated during the first 20 hours of the menstrual period when hemostasis is critically de-

Table 2.
Contraindications to Thrombolytic Agents[70,71,77,81,83]

Absolute Contraindications
- Cerebrovascular accident or intracranial or intraspinal surgery within the past two months
- Active internal bleeding
- Intracranial neoplasm

Relative Contraindications
- Major surgery, obstetrical delivery, organ biopsy, puncture of a noncompressible vessel, or serious gastrointestinal bleeding within the previous 10 days
- Recent trauma, including cardiopulmonary resuscitation
- Severe uncontrolled hypertension
- Suspected left-heart thrombus (i.e., mitral stenosis and atrial fibrillation)
- Subacute bacterial endocarditis
- Hemostatic defects,including those caused by severe renal or hepatic disease
- Pregnancy
- Cerebrovascular disease
- Diabetic hemorrhagic retinopathy
- Previous severe allergic reaction
- Septic thrombophlebitis
- Partially or totally occluded arteriovenous or intravenous cannula at a seriously infected site
- Active and progressive cavitating lung disease
- Ulcerative cutaneous or mucous-membrane lesions
- Any condition in which bleeding constitutes a serious hazard or would be particularly difficult to control because of its location

pendent upon clot formation and hemostatic plugs. They also suggest that thrombolytic therapy is safe later during the course of menstrual bleeding when hemostasis is dependent upon arteriolar constriction.

Dosage and Administration. Bell and Meek[71] outlined several general guidelines for patient care during thrombolytic therapy:

1. A complete history and physical examination and complete laboratory testing must be done to exclude contraindications such as pre-existing hemostatic defects.
2. All invasive procedures should be avoided except for careful venipunctures with a 22-gauge or smaller-gauge needle.[71,77] If arterial puncture is necessary, the radial or brachial artery should be used and the artery compressed afterwards for a minimum of 15 but preferably 30 minutes. Blood pressures should be taken only in the arms.
3. The patient should be handled carefully to avoid bruising from lifting or pulling while in bed.
4. Antiplatelet agents and other anticoagulants should not be given concurrently with thrombolytic agents. However, in the absence of contraindications and before the use of thrombolytic therapy, patients should be treated with heparin to avoid thrombus propagation. Heparin therapy should be stopped before thrombolytic therapy is begun, and the activated partial thromboplastin time (APTT) or the thrombin time should be less than two times the control value.

Both streptokinase and urokinase have been proven to lyse thrombi in vivo. However, there is greater clinical experience with streptokinase and it costs considerably less than urokinase.

Treatment with streptokinase begins with a loading dose to neutralize pre-existing streptococcal antibodies. Loading doses generally range from 200,000 to 600,000 International Units (IU) in 0.9% sodium chloride injection or 5% dextrose injection given over 30 minutes. A standard loading dose of 250,000 IU has been used in the United States since 1980.[77] The loading dose is followed by a continuous infusion at 100,000 IU/hour. The thrombin time, APTT, or the whole-blood euglobulin clot-lysis time should be repeated four hours after initiating therapy to ensure that the lytic state is achieved[70,71,77]; further laboratory monitoring during thrombolytic therapy is not necessary. If the chosen laboratory test is less than 1½ times the control value four hours after initiating therapy, streptokinase should be stopped and the use of urokinase should be considered.

The constant infusion of streptokinase should continue for 24 hours in patients with PE and 72 hours in patients with DVT. Selected patients with DVT may benefit from longer treatment if a venogram shows residual thrombus, the clinical course is stable, and the clinical estimate for eventual complete clot lysis is high. Practitioners must realize that the shorter treatment courses for PE are inadequate for the treatment of most cases of coexisting proximal-vein DVT.[59,70-71] The benefits of streptokinase therapy for DVT would not be realized with courses shorter than 72 hours, and the potential risks of incompletely lysed venous thrombi would continue to exist.

Urokinase therapy for PE begins with a loading dose of 4400 IU/kg given over 10 minutes, followed by a constant infusion of 4400 IU/kg/hr for a total of 12 hours. Because urokinase is a human protein and does not evoke an antigenic response, laboratory monitoring is not as important during urokinase therapy as it is during streptokinase therapy.[70] However, it is reassuring to know that a lytic state has been achieved, and for this reason laboratory monitoring is recommended.

Most authors agree that no test predicts efficacy or risk of bleeding during thrombolytic therapy. Some authors believe that a fibrinogen level greater than 0.8 g/L is associated with a poor rate of clot lysis with streptokinase.[69]

When the thrombolytic infusion is finished, the APTT should be monitored closely until it is two times the control value. At that point, a continuous infusion of heparin should be started (without a loading dose) and adjusted to maintain the APTT at twice the control value.

Heparin. *Mechanism of Action.* Heparin is a heterogenous substance composed of polymers of variable molecular weight. This heterogeneity results in binding reactions to antithrombin III that are not uniform and may explain some of the variability in response seen clinically. Heparin catalyzes the reaction between antithrombin III and serine proteases in the clotting cascade (activated clotting factors IX, X, XI, XII, and thrombin).[87,88] The reaction with antithrombin III almost instantaneously neutralizes the activated clotting factors and prevents them from activating their respective substrates, thus halting further coagulation.

Heparin does not alter a formed thrombus; it only prevents further coagulation and propagation of the thrombus. This allows the natural thrombolytic components in blood to lyse the clot slowly.

After intravenous administration, the half-life of heparin ranges between 0.5 and 2.5 hours (mean 1.5 hours).[89,90] Some investigators have found that heparin clearance is increased in patients with PE[91,92] while others have not.[90] Average heparin dosage requirements are similar in patients with PE and DVT, but considerable variability exists among patients.[41,90,93]

Clinical Efficacy. Intravenous administration of heparin is preferred to other routes of administration for treatment of DVT and PE. Heparin may be given either by continuous i.v. infusion via infusion pump or by intermittent i.v. bolus injection. Whether infusion is superior to bolus therapy continues to be debated. Evaluation of administration methods focuses upon the incidence of bleeding and the risk of recurrent thromboembolism with each method. Table 3 summarizes the studies that have compared these two methods of heparin administration.

In a randomized, prospective study using monitoring with the partial thromboplastin time, Salzman et al.[40] found that the incidence of major bleeding episodes was 8% with intermittent bolus injection versus 1% with continuous infusion. Patients in the continuous infusion group required less heparin (mean 24,480 units/day) than those receiving intermittent bolus injections (31,740 units/day). There was one recurrence of thromboembolism (PE) in each group. These results were supported by others.[94] It was suggested that the lower incidence of bleeding with continuous infusion of heparin might be secondary to the elimination of excessive peak heparin concentrations seen with intermittent bolus injection. Other studies have found that the two methods are associated with similar bleeding frequencies, with the infusion method slightly favored.[95–97] Wilson et al.[97] noted that the incidence of bleeding was similar with both methods in patients with a low risk of bleeding. The incidence of bleeding associated with the intermittent bolus injection method was significantly higher than that of the continuous infusion method in patients at risk for bleeding (e.g., those with recent surgery or trauma, a history of gastrointestinal bleeding, age over 60, or severe hypertension).

Earlier studies indicated that the efficacy of both administration methods was similar, as determined by the incidence of recurrent thromboembolism during heparin treatment.[40,94,96] However, it has been argued that these studies were based upon imprecise clinical diagnosis.[97] Wilson et al.[97] used follow-up lung scans in 29 patients receiving intermittent bolus heparin and 36 receiving heparin by continuous infusion in a randomized, prospective study. These investigators found significantly fewer recurrences in the group receiving intermittent bolus therapy (28% versus 3%). However, this study used numerous dosing and monitoring methods, and many PE recurrences were detected by lung scan, a test that lacks specificity. Also, the majority of patients with recurrences had two consecutive APTT values below 1.5 times the control value, indicating that the infusion rates were not well controlled.

The controversy concerning which method is more acceptable continues. Some clinicians prefer intermittent bolus injection[97,98] while continuous infusion is used by others.[40,41]

Dosage and Administration. Heparin has traditionally been initiated with an i.v. bolus injection of 5,000–10,000 units followed by infusion of the drug at a rate of 1,000 units per hour. These large loading doses were advocated based upon data in dogs[28] and rabbits[25,29] demonstrating that heparin could prevent the vasoconstriction that occurs after pulmonary embolism. However, these studies may have limited clinical applicability since the animals were pretreated with heparin before the embolus was released into the pulmonary circulation. An alternative method of initiating therapy is to begin with a loading dose of 50–70 units/kg of heparin followed by a constant infusion of 15–25 units/kg/hr (Figure 1).[40] Patients at risk for bleeding (Table 4) should be started at the low end of the recommended dosage ranges. The infusion is then adjusted based upon appropriate coagulation studies (discussed later).

If the intermittent-injection method is preferred, injections should be given every four to six hours. Suggested initial dosage regimens include administration of 60–100 units/kg of heparin every four hours or 100–150 units/kg every six hours.

Table 3.
Comparison of Bleeding and Recurrent Pulmonary Embolism (PE) in Studies Using Intermittent Bolus (IB) Injection and Continuous Infusion (CI) of Heparin

Study	Heparin Administration Method	*n*	% Major Bleeding	No. Patients with Recurrent PE
Salzman[40] 1975[a]	IB	72	8	1/72
	CI	69	1	1/69
Glazier[94] 1976	IB	21	33	0
	CI	20	0	1/20
Mant[95] 1977	IB[b]	36	11	ND[c]
	CI	40	15	ND
Wilson[96] 1979	IB	40	10	ND
	CI	40	5	ND
Wilson[97] 1981	IB	29	17	1/29
	CI	36	8	10/36

[a] Only data in patients whose dosage was monitored and adjusted based on coagulation studies are reported.

[b] Patients receiving intermittent i.v. bolus heparin all received 5000 units every four hours (unadjusted by APTT); patients on continuous-infusion heparin received doses adjusted to an APTT of 60–100 seconds. This is the only study in which patients on continuous-infusion heparin received higher daily dosages than those on intermittent i.v. bolus heparin.

[c] Not done.

Table 4.
Risk Factors for Hemorrhage in Patients Receiving Anticoagulants[143–145]

Recent surgery
Trauma (or risk of trauma)
Intramuscular injections
Severe hypertension
Malignancy
Age over 60
Peptic ulcer disease (or history of peptic ulcers)
Polypharmacy
Presence of any potential bleeding site (lumbar puncture, intra-arterial puncture, aneurysm, biopsy site)
Congenital or acquired hemostatic defect

Heparin should not be given intramuscularly because of pain and the increased potential for bleeding. Heparin can be administered subcutaneously in patients without venous access. An initial i.v. bolus of 50–70 units/kg is followed by 125–200 units/kg given subcutaneously every eight hours. If single injections do not exceed 20,000 units, 175–300 units/kg of heparin can be given every 12 hours.

Pharmacokinetic methods have been used to aid in the determination of heparin dosage when given by infusion or intermittent injection.[90,99,100] Chenella et al.[99] described a method for determining initial heparin infusion rates based upon an estimate of the patients' volume of distribution and rate of elimination. The authors reported that there was less variance in the APTT with this method than with an infusion method based on body weight alone.

Cipolle et al.[90] described an interesting approach to evaluating heparin pharmacokinetics. Before heparin therapy, they mixed each patient's blood with heparin to produce six concentrations of heparin (units/ml); the patients' APTT for each concentration of heparin was then determined. Patients were then given a bolus injection of heparin, and serial APTTs were determined. By comparing the in vivo and in vitro results, a heparin concentration–time curve, pharmacokinetic variables, and dosage predictions could be derived for each patient. While the method appeared reliable, the authors did not recommend its use because of time requirements and expense.

Laboratory Monitoring. The coagulation study most commonly used to monitor heparin therapy is the APTT, but some have reported good results with the activated clotting time of whole blood (ACT) or the thrombin time.[41,101,102] The accepted therapeutic range for the APTT is 1.5–2.5 times the control value; for the ACT, it is 150–190 seconds.[4,103] It should be realized that these ranges have been established based upon limited information; the ideal range has never been firmly established. Clinical studies have indicated that thromboembolic recurrence was more frequent when the APTT remained below a ratio of 1.5.[97,104] Basu et al.[104] treated 234 patients with continuous heparin infusion and reported recurrent thromboembolism in five patients; all five had APTTs less than 1.5 times the control value. Patients with recurrences had significantly more APTT ratios less than 1.5 (71%) during therapy than patients who did not have recurrences (28%).

The APTT ratio of 1.5–2.5 is generally based upon comparison of the patient's APTT with a normal laboratory control of pooled plasma. Some authors have suggested that it may be more appropriate to generate a ratio based upon the patient's pretreatment APTT.[102] It should also be noted that APTT sensitivities vary substantially with different reagents and instruments, making comparisons between laboratories difficult.[102,105,106]

With these limitations in mind, the following monitoring should be performed. Before initiating heparin therapy, baseline values of patient weight, prothrombin time (PT), APTT (or ACT), and an estimation of the platelet count should be obtained. The APTT should be obtained three to four times on the first day of heparin administration, after dosage increases, and at least daily throughout treatment. An advantage of administering heparin by continuous infusion is that the APTT can be obtained at any time during therapy as long as it is four hours after a dosage increase or a loading dose. However, i.v. infusion pumps are not free from error and the APTT should be interpreted accordingly.[40,107] Unexpected results might be obtained because of incorrect infusion rate, pump error, incorrect heparin concentrations, or interruption of the infusion.

The most appropriate time to obtain the APTT during intermittent i.v. bolus heparin therapy has not been determined. Suggested sampling times have ranged from just before a dose to one hour before a dose. The APTT is commonly obtained 30 minutes before a dose during intermittent i.v. bolus therapy and in the middle of the dosing interval when subcutaneous injections are used. A reliable interpretation of the APTT with intermittent i.v. bolus therapy depends upon appropriate timing of the injection and of blood sampling by laboratory personnel. This timing may not be realistically achievable in many institutions without rigid control.[100]

When necessary, changes in heparin infusion rate can be made at four- to six-hour intervals if coagulation studies can be rapidly obtained. Dosage adjustments should be made cautiously. APTT response to changes in heparin infusion rate are not always linear and increases in dosage should be made in small increments; e.g., 100–200 units/hr (Figure 1). If the APTT is dangerously low, an additional bolus injection along with the increased infusion rate may be necessary. Generally, these changes must be made on a trial and error basis.

Hattersley and associates[108] reported that the effect of heparin on the ACT is log-linear and developed an equation to adjust heparin infusion rates based upon their retrospective data. One prerequisite for this type of model is that the response of the particular coagulation test to changes in heparin infusion rate must be linear throughout the test's therapeutic range for heparin.

Other things that should be monitored periodically during heparin therapy include platelet counts (to detect potential heparin-induced thrombocytopenia), hematocrit, urinalysis (for presence of red blood cells), stool for occult blood, actual amount of heparin administered per day, and subjective evidence of bleeding. There is no agreement on how often platelet counts should be performed, but we would suggest three times per week.

Long-Term Therapy

In most patients treated for DVT or PE it is desirable to continue anticoagulant therapy after acute treatment with heparin to prevent recurrent thromboembolism. This is accomplished with oral administration of warfarin or with subcutaneous administration of heparin.

Heparin-Warfarin Conversion. Initiation of warfarin must occur before discontinuation of heparin. The period of overlap with the two anticoagulants should be four to six days.[14,44,109,110] There are several reasons for this overlap, the most obvious being the desire to protect the patient fully from recurrent thromboembolism. The onset of warfarin's effect is delayed for several days after beginning therapy, and the effect of heparin diminishes in a matter of minutes to hours after it is discontinued. Therefore, to prevent a break in the level of anticoagulation, it is necessary to await the full effect of warfarin before discontinuing heparin.

Following initiation of warfarin, the PT may increase into the therapeutic range within 36–72 hours. However, it has been shown experimentally that the early increase in prothrombin time is secondary to a reduction in the level of clotting factor VII. It is thought that the antithrombotic effect of warfarin can be attributed to a reduction in the levels of factors IX and X.[14,109] The latter clotting factors have half-lives of 20–30 hours, and concentrations of these factors decline over several days following warfarin administration. Therefore, a therapeutic prothrombin time in the first few days of warfarin therapy may not be protective against thromboembolism. It has recently been suggested that a brief hypercoagulability state may also be produced immediately following heparin discontinuation or after the first dose of warfarin.[109]

Warfarin therapy can be initiated at any time during heparin treatment. Because of the need for the four- to six-day overlap, it is useful to initiate warfarin as early as is practical. Heparin is often initiated as soon as the diagnosis of DVT or PE is suspected. When the diagnosis is confirmed and it becomes evident that anticoagulant therapy will be continued, warfarin should be started. Self et al.[111] showed that early administration of warfarin (within 24 hours after initiating heparin therapy) decreased the number of days on heparin and reduced the length of hospitalization compared with that in patients given warfarin later in the heparin course.

In the conversion period it is important to consider the effects of heparin on the PT. Heparin has been shown to increase the PT modestly. Sawyer et al.[112] reported an average PT increase of 1.8 seconds in patients on heparin infusions. The average APTT in these patients was 79.2 seconds (mean control value of 38.1 sec). In a subgroup of patients with APTT values exceeding 150 seconds, the PT increase ranged from 0.6 to 8.0 seconds. These increases are minimal and it is not necessary to interrupt the heparin infusion to obtain blood for determination of the PT. If patients are receiving intermittent bolus heparin therapy, the PT should be drawn at the time of the minimum heparin effect, i.e., just before the next heparin dose. When the heparin is discontinued, the PT may decrease slightly and the warfarin dose may need a small adjustment.

The effect of warfarin on the APTT is not well documented, although it appears that the APTT is increased. Some increase in the APTT may be anticipated when warfarin is begun.[113]

In summary, warfarin should be initiated as soon as it becomes apparent that oral anticoagulation will be used. Heparin should be continued for the recommended 7–10 days at full doses and overlapped with the warfarin for four to six days. The dosage of warfarin should be adjusted to stabilize the prothrombin ratio in the therapeutic range before heparin is discontinued.

Laboratory Monitoring. Previous recommendations for oral anticoagulation in the United States suggested that a therapeutic PT ratio (patient:control) should range from 1.5 to 2.5.[4,114] These recommendations were based upon data from clinical use in the 1940s, but the optimal therapeutic range had never been determined by rigorous testing. The suggested therapeutic prothrombin ratio of 1.5–2.5 has been shown to be successful clinically but is associated with a high risk of bleeding. In addition, thromboplastin reagents in previous studies were not well standardized, and PT values are not comparable when determined by different methods.

Thromboplastins used to measure the PT are derived from a number of different sources, including rabbit brain or human brain, and these thromboplastins differ in sensitivity.[114-118] For example, in a given patient population with a PT of 18 seconds using rabbit-brain thromboplastin, the PT might range from 22 to 80 seconds with human-brain thromboplastin. The most common reagents used in the United States are derived from rabbit brain, while in Great Britain over 95% of hospitals use the British Comparative Thromboplastin (BCT) derived from human brain.[115] A prothrombin ratio of 1.3–1.7 with rabbit-brain thromboplastin corresponds to a ratio of 2.0–4.0 with BCT (Table 5). A PT ratio of 2.0–2.5 using rabbit-brain thromboplastin exceeds the limit considered safe with BCT.[114] Clinicians monitoring warfarin therapy must be familiar with the reagents used in their laboratory and the sensitivities of those reagents.

An additional difficulty in determining the

therapeutic range for warfarin relates to the standardization of reagents. In Great Britain, thromboplastin reagents have been standardized. In the United States, PT results from different laboratories using different reagents may not be comparable.

These major differences in sensitivity and lack of standardization have complicated the interpretation of the older literature and have led to the use of different intensities of oral anticoagulation. The PT ratio of 1.5–2.5 recommended in North America is greater than that used elsewhere. This intensity is now considered excessive for venous thromboembolism by many authors.[114–116,119,120] Recommendations now being made suggest maintaining the PT ratio between 1.3 and 2.0 (using rabbit-brain thromboplastin) when treating venous thromboembolism.[109,114–117] Controlled clinical trials have confirmed these suggestions.[121–127]

Early studies demonstrated that the risk of bleeding was much lower when the PT ratio was 1.2–1.6.[121,122] Moschos et al.[122] suggested in 1964 that a ratio of 1.2–1.5 might be the optimal range based upon the incidence of bleeding. However, other studies suggested that it was necessary to use more intense anticoagulation to prevent recurrent thromboembolism.[39,125,126]

Clinical Efficacy of Warfarin versus Subcutaneous Heparin. Recent studies by Hull et al.[123,124,127] have helped to clarify the optimal level of long-term anticoagulation with warfarin and have evaluated the efficacy of warfarin versus subcutaneous heparin. In each of three studies, patients received a continuous i.v. infusion of heparin for 10 to 14 days. In the first study,[123] 68 patients with deep-vein thrombosis of the calf or proximal leg veins were treated. Patients were randomly assigned to receive either warfarin adjusted to achieve a PT ratio of 1.5–2.0 (rabbit-brain thromboplastin) or minidose heparin (5000 units subcutaneously every 12 hours). Calf-vein thrombosis was treated for six weeks and proximal-vein thrombosis for 12 weeks. There were no recurrent thromboembolic episodes in any patients with calf-vein thrombosis. In patients with proximal-vein thrombosis, significantly more patients receiving minidose heparin had recurrences when compared with warfarin-treated patients (47% versus 0%). However, bleeding occurred in significantly more patients receiving warfarin than in those on heparin (21% versus 0%).

In another randomized study, Hull et al.[124] administered warfarin or subcutaneous heparin for 12 weeks to 106 patients with proximal-vein thrombosis. Warfarin dosage was adjusted to maintain a PT ratio of 1.5–2.0 (rabbit-form thromboplastin), which was monitored weekly by the patients' family physicians. The dosage of subcutaneous heparin was adjusted in the hospital to maintain a APTT ratio midway between the dosing interval of 1.5. Once the heparin dose was established, no further monitoring was performed. New thromboembolic episodes occurred in 2 of 53 patients receiving heparin and in 1 of 53 receiving warfarin; all recurrences occurred when therapy was interrupted. Significantly more patients in the warfarin group experienced bleeding episodes.

In the third study these investigators compared "less intense" warfarin therapy to "conventional" warfarin therapy in 96 patients with proximal-vein thrombosis. The group receiving conventional treatment ($n = 49$) was monitored using Simplastin (rabbit-brain thromboplastin); PTs were maintained at 1.5–2.0 times the control value. The group receiving less intense therapy ($n = 47$) had PTs maintained at 2.0 times the control using the more sensitive Manchester method (human-brain thromboplastin), which corresponded to 1.3 times the control value with Simplastin. There was one case of recurrent thromboembolism in each group. Significantly more patients receiving conventional treatment had hemorrhage (22% versus 4%).[127]

These studies demonstrate that adjusted-dose heparin and less intense warfarin therapy are as effective as conventional warfarin therapy for treating proximal-vein thrombosis, and the risk of hemorrhage is significantly greater with the latter regimen. Minidose heparin is not effective for treating proximal-vein thrombosis after 10–14 days of intravenous heparin. At this time it is not known whether less intense warfarin therapy will be effective for treating thromboembolic disorders other than proximal deep-vein thrombosis of the leg. Another question that must be answered is whether a low intensity of anticoagulation can be maintained when monitoring is performed with thromboplastins derived from animal sources.

An advantage of heparin is that once the dosage is established, no further monitoring is necessary. However, the cost of heparin and syringes is con-

Table 5.
Comparison of Thromboplastins[114–118]

Reagent	Source	Therapeutic Range[a]
Manchester (British Comparative Thromboplastin or BCT)	Human brain	2.0–4.0
Simplastin (General Diagnostics)	Rabbit brain	1.3–1.7
Brain Thromboplastin (Ortho)	Rabbit brain	1.3–1.8
Thromboplastin C (Dade)	Rabbit brain	1.4–1.8
Thrombotest	Bovine brain	2.0–3.5

[a] Therapeutic prothrombin ratio (patient/control) recommended in Europe for venous thromboembolism.

siderably greater than the cost of warfarin. Hull et al.[128] performed a cost-effectiveness analysis and determined that the less intense warfarin therapy was the most cost effective.

Subcutaneous heparin may be preferred for patients in remote areas who cannot have their PT adequately monitored. Heparin may also be preferred for the treatment of thromboembolism during pregnancy. Heparin does not cross the placenta and does not cause embryopathy such as that associated with warfarin. However, the risk of stillbirth and neonatal mortality is quite high with heparin.[129–131]

Dosage and Administration of Warfarin. Initiation of warfarin with a loading dose does not hasten the anticoagulant effect, which is predominantly determined by the degradation of preformed clotting factors II, VII, IX, and X.[132] Loading doses may increase the risk of bleeding and make future dosage adjustments difficult. A common method of initiating therapy is to give warfarin sodium 10 mg daily for three days followed by dosage adjustments based upon daily PT measurements. However, in our experience this initial regimen may be excessive for 10–15% of patients, and a dosage adjustment may be necessary after the second warfarin dose.

A number of linear-regression techniques that are intended to predict warfarin maintenance-dose requirements have been described.[133–137] These methods rely upon the patient's initial PT response and predict a maintenance dose based upon population averages. These statistical associations may not be clinically applicable because of interpatient variability and differences between laboratories.[138,139] In addition, many of these methods were developed using a therapeutic PT range of 1.5–2.5. Carter and associates demonstrated in retrospective[140] and prospective[141] studies that two of these methods are unreliable and may prolong the time required for stabilization of the PT. These authors recommended that neither method be used clinically.

Computer-assisted programs that predict warfarin dosage and refine these predictions daily may be more reliable than a single linear-regression prediction.[142] The analog computer[141,143,144] or Bayesian forecasting[145] may be useful in predicting warfarin dosages, but further evaluations are necessary. Until thorough evaluations have been performed, warfarin prediction techniques should be considered investigational.

During the initial inpatient stabilization period, only very small dosage adjustments should be made if possible. Dosages should be withheld only when absolutely necessary to avoid an excessive decline in the PT.

Because of the necessary overlap with heparin and the time required to stabilize the warfarin dose, five to seven days of warfarin therapy are usually necessary before the patient is ready to be discharged from the hospital. To be considered stabilized, we believe the patient should have at least two to three consecutive daily PT ratios that are similar (e.g., 1.7, 1.8, and 1.7) while receiving the same warfarin dose. However, it is not mandatory that rigid stabilization be completed in the hospital if appropriate monitoring can be performed soon after discharge.

There are a number of dosage regimens that can be employed after the patient is discharged. One method is to dispense only one tablet strength (e.g., 5 mg) and have the patient take multiples or fractions of the tablets (e.g., 1½ tablets Monday, Wednesday, Friday, and one tablet all other days). With this method dosage adjustments are always made with 5-mg tablets, which eliminates confusion between tablet strengths but may be difficult for some patients.

Once patients are discharged, warfarin dosage requirements frequently change. This may be related to diet, exercise, or noncompliance. Therefore, a PT should be determined shortly after discharge and then weekly (Figure 3). The frequency of PT determinations can be gradually reduced to every two weeks and finally to every four weeks in reliable patients with stable PTs. Unexpectedly high or low PTs require evaluation of compliance

Figure 3. Algorithm for management of long-term warfarin therapy following hospital discharge.

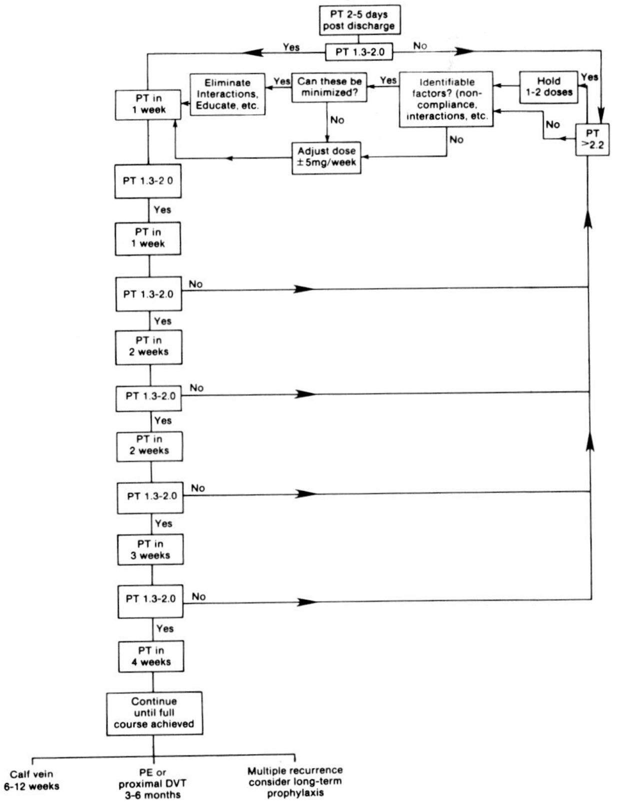

and potential drug interactions. If these have been ruled out, the warfarin dosage should be gradually adjusted (i.e., 5 mg per week or less) to achieve PTs in the therapeutic range. It may be necessary to hold one or two doses if the PT is dangerously elevated (i.e., PT ratio > 2.2).

Drug Interactions with Warfarin. The potential for harmful drug interactions is a constant concern during warfarin therapy. Concurrent drug therapy must be carefully supervised and appropriately monitored to maximize the safety and efficacy of anticoagulant treatment. Drug interactions have been shown to influence warfarin therapy in a number of ways. Drug interactions have increased the need for warfarin dosage adjustments,[146] have increased the percentage of prothrombin times outside the therapeutic range,[147] and have increased the number of bleeding episodes.[148] Drug interactions may potentially increase the risk of recurrent thromboembolism.

Several excellent resources are available for detailed information regarding warfarin drug–drug interactions[149–151]; these interactions will not be recounted here. Instead, a few general principles will be reviewed.

Drugs interact with warfarin by a number of different mechanisms (Table 6). If the mechanism of a potential interaction is understood, the clinician will understand how the interaction will be manifest (increased or decreased warfarin effect), the time course of the interaction (onset and duration of effect), and how best to manage the interaction.

Most discussions of drug interactions consider the effects of a drug added to a stable warfarin regimen. It must be remembered that interactions are also evident when warfarin is added to other drugs, when drugs are discontinued, or even when dosages are changed. In each of these cases, the clinical expression of the interaction may be different. For example, when phenobarbital is added to a stable warfarin regimen, the enzyme induction by the barbiturate will result in a gradual decrease in warfarin effect. Over a two-week period, the dosage of warfarin will need to be increased. If at a later time the dosage of phenobarbital was increased, additional changes in warfarin dosage might be needed. If the phenobarbital was discontinued, the enzyme induction would be gradually lost. The warfarin effect would increase and the dosage would need to be decreased. If warfarin was started in a patient already taking phenobarbital an interaction may go unnoticed, although an unusually high dosage of warfarin might be necessary to prolong the prothrombin time adequately.

The number of drugs used in patients receiving warfarin should be minimized to avoid interactions. Studies have shown that as the number of drugs used by a patient on warfarin increases, the stability of the warfarin effect decreases and the incidence of bleeding increases. If a drug is required, the drug that is least likely to interact, based on the best evidence available, should be used. It is prudent to suspect that any drug might potentially interact with warfarin; therefore, clinicians should be alert to changes in the prothrombin time when any drug is started, stopped, or when the dosage is changed.

Drug interactions have the potential to complicate the management of a patient on warfarin greatly. However, in most patients few problems occur. If concurrent drug use is minimized, carefully selected, and monitored appropriately, and if the patient takes his or her medication reliably, drug interactions are easily managed.

Table 6.
Mechanisms of Drug–Drug Interactions with Warfarin

Mechanism	Interacting Drug
Decrease bioavailability of warfarin	Cholestyramine, colestipol
Protein displacement	Phenylbutazone
Induction of warfarin-metabolizing enzymes	Barbiturates
Inhibition of warfarin-metabolizing enzymes	Cimetidine
Alter synthesis of clotting factors	Estrogens (increase synthesis); Androgens (decrease synthesis)
Alter hemostatic processes	Antiplatelet drugs, heparin

Adverse Effects of Thrombolytic and Anticoagulant Therapy

Thrombolytic Agents. *Hemorrhage.* Because the currently available thrombolytic agents produce an indiscriminate systemic effect on coagulation, bleeding is the major complication. Spontaneous bleeding occurs in approximately 20% of patients, an incidence similar to that seen in patients anticoagulated with heparin.[72,74] Bleeding occurs more frequently from cutdown and vessel-puncture sites and from other sites of trauma with thrombolytic agents than with heparin.[70–74,82] The reported incidence of serious bleeding (necessitating either blood transfusion or discontinuation of thrombolytic therapy) varies widely among studies and appears related to how frequently the investigators used invasive techniques.[77] Major bleeding has been reported to occur in 5–20% of patients treated with thrombolytic agents,[70–74,82] although with greater clinical experience the incidence in general practice may be as low as 5%.[77] With thrombolytic therapy, the incidence of central nervous system (CNS) bleeding is approximately 1%; with heparin it is 0.5%.[73,77]

Patient selection and careful patient management are crucial in trying to avoid bleeding complications. If serious bleeding should occur, the thrombolytic agent should be stopped. Fresh frozen plasma or cryoprecipitate can be given to reverse the hemostatic defect.[70,71,77] Normal hemostasis can usually be achieved in less than an hour. In emergencies, some authors[70,71] have advocated using aminocaproic acid to achieve immediate hemostasis, even though its clinical efficacy has not been proven.

Other Adverse Effects. Allergic reactions have been reported rarely with urokinase but occur in roughly 15% of patients treated with streptokinase.[71,82] Anaphylaxis has been rarely reported but does occur despite the previous administration of corticosteroids. One paper described a patient with IgE-mediated anaphylaxis to streptokinase who was subsequently shown to have a positive immediate-type hypersensitivity skin reaction to streptokinase.[152] These authors recommended that this skin test be used routinely before streptokinase therapy. Further clinical data are needed to support this recommendation. Other allergic symptoms, including urticaria, pruritus, flushing, nausea, vomiting, and musculoskeletal pain occur in approximately 15% of patients. Some of these symptoms might occur as a result of a delayed hypersensitivity reaction. Two cases of serum sickness associated with streptokinase therapy have been reported, raising the possibility of immune-complex formation.[153,154] For these reasons, corticosteroids are given before and during streptokinase therapy (e.g., hydrocortisone 100 mg every 12 hours). However, the efficacy of corticosteroids in preventing these reactions has not been proven.

Fever occurs in roughly 40% of patients treated with streptokinase and in 15% treated with urokinase. The fever is usually mild, but 3.5% of patients have temperatures greater than 104 °F.

Acute renal failure has also been associated with streptokinase therapy. Acute diffuse renal embolization from thrombi overlying ulcerative aortic atheromatous plaques was the presumed etiology in one case.[155] In two other cases, the clinical history was most consistent with an acute hypersensitivity-induced interstitial nephritis.[156,157] Both patients recovered, and the role of streptokinase in causing these reactions was not proven in either case.

Acute hepatitis attributed to streptokinase has been reported in one patient.[158] A 27-year-old woman developed fever and substantial alkaline phosphatase and SGOT elevations both on initial administration of streptokinase and with rechallenge. Guillain–Barré syndrome has occurred in association with streptokinase therapy in two patients.[159,160]

Adult respiratory distress syndrome (ARDS) has been described in association with streptokinase therapy for the treatment of PE.[161] ARDS has been observed in our institution in patients treated with streptokinase for acute coronary artery thrombosis, but the exact incidence has not been determined.

Heparin and Warfarin. *Hemorrhage.* Hemorrhage is the most obvious and the most worrisome side effect of anticoagulant therapy. The incidence of bleeding reported in the literature varies considerably. Coon and Willis[121] reported a 2% incidence of major bleeding (bleeding requiring blood replacement or discontinuation of the anticoagulant) in about 3800 courses of warfarin and heparin in both inpatients and outpatients. Minor bleeding (requiring only a dosage adjustment) was reported in an additional 4.8% of patients. The Boston Collaborative Drug Surveillance Program reported an incidence of hemorrhage from heparin and warfarin therapy of 17% and 9%, respectively, in 1600 inpatients on heparin and 1000 inpatients on warfarin.[162]

Although these figures are representative of the literature, there are many factors that can dramatically alter the incidence of bleeding in any particular patient population. The quality of monitoring and the intensity of anticoagulation are important variables influencing the expected frequency of bleeding. Patient selection is also very important.

The risk of bleeding increases as either the PT or the APTT increases. Fewer episodes of bleeding would be anticipated with a patient's PT (using rabbit-brain thromboplastin) maintained at 1.3–2.0 times the control value versus a range of 2.0–2.5 times the control value. This is the major finding in the recent studies examining the efficacy of less-intense anticoagulation. The majority of bleeding episodes occur as a result of excessively prolonged prothrombin or partial thromboplastin times, but bleeding may also occur when the PT or APTT are "therapeutic." [121] If the cause or source of bleeding is not obvious, an investigation may uncover a previously unknown lesion, such as a peptic ulcer or malignancy.

The risk of bleeding is high during the period in which both heparin and warfarin are being used. Initiation of warfarin therapy with a large loading dose can also produce an unnecessary bleeding risk. The concurrent use of antiplatelet agents with either warfarin or heparin increases the risk of hemorrhage.

Patient reliability is an important variable to consider when attempting to predict the incidence of hemorrhage during outpatient management of warfarin therapy. The patient willing to follow medication instructions and adhere to required follow-up visits will be an excellent candidate. Patients at the other end of the spectrum can be worrisome.

The most common signs of bleeding include melena, hematemasis, hematuria, hematoma, ecchymosis, and epistaxis. Table 4 lists a number of risk factors that have been identified or factors that may increase the probability of hemorrhage.[121,148,163,164]

Other Adverse Effects of Warfarin. Purple-toe syndrome is a rare adverse effect of warfarin therapy with only scattered case reports in the literature.[165,166] This adverse effect usually occurs three to eight weeks after warfarin is begun. The affected toes are painful, and toe color blanches with pressure and fades with elevation. The intensity of the pain and color can fluctuate from day to day. The mechanism of this effect is unknown but it is unrelated to PT prolongation. When this adverse reaction is observed it is recommended that the warfarin be discontinued. The discoloration may persist for weeks to months.

Skin infarction with gangrene and necrosis is another rare side effect of warfarin.[167] This side effect is also unrelated to the intensity of anticoagulation and may be the result of a direct toxic effect. It occurs within the first 10 days of warfarin use, and women are more likely to experience this effect than men. The most commonly involved sites include the thigh, breast, and buttocks.

Anticoagulation with warfarin during pregnancy poses several problems. Besides the obvious maternal risk of bleeding, warfarin can also cause fetal hemorrhage because it crosses the placenta. In addition, warfarin is teratogenic. A fetal warfarin syndrome (warfarin embryopathy) has been described. Typical features include nasal hypoplasia, small nares, and stippled epiphyses. These defects are associated with first-trimester exposure. Warfarin exposure in the second and third trimester has been associated with mental retardation, blindness, spasticity, and seizures. Hall et al.[129] described 418 pregnancies associated with exposure to warfarin; only 67% resulted in live births with no complications. Currently, it would seem undesirable to use warfarin during any part of pregnancy. This fact should be reviewed with any woman of child-bearing age receiving warfarin. Women who do not desire pregnancy should be counseled about adequate birth-control methods.

Other Adverse Effects of Heparin. Thrombocytopenia attributed to heparin has also been reported. The incidence of heparin-induced thrombocytopenia has varied considerably from study to study, ranging from less than 1% to 30%.[168-173] This adverse effect is more common in patients receiving beef-lung heparin than in those receiving porcine-intestine heparin. The onset of thrombocytopenia has been described as early as two days after the start of therapy but most commonly occurs after six days of therapy.[168,172,173] It has been suggested that there are different types of heparin-induced thrombocytopenias based on the time of onset. The early type of thrombocytopenia is described as mild, reversible, and not associated with major complications. The delayed type has been associated with bleeding or arterial thrombosis, or both. Whether or not it is useful to monitor for heparin-induced thrombocytopenia is controversial. Daily or every other day platelet counts have been advocated.[168,171,172] Others suggest that monitoring platelet counts will help detect the problem but will not allow prevention particularly of the delayed type of thrombocytopenia with its associated morbidity and mortality.[173] Until these issues are clarified, periodic platelet counts (every other day) seem to be appropriate. It is also prudent not to continue heparin administration longer than necessary.

Osteoporosis secondary to heparin is an adverse effect for which little information is available. It appears to be related to dose and duration of heparin therapy. Griffith[174] found evidence of osteoporosis in patients receiving greater than 15,000 units daily for six months or longer.

Heparin does not cross the placenta and holds some hope for treating DVT during pregnancy. Maternal hemorrhagic complications from heparin have been reported in about 10% of pregnancies.[129] There is no evidence that heparin is teratogenic; however, fetal and neonatal complications are observed frequently. Hall et al.[129] reported complications in 37 of 135 pregnancies during which heparin was administered. These complications included stillbirth and prematurity; fetal hemorrhage was not reported.

Information for the Patient

Warfarin. It is extremely important to enlist the cooperation of the patient being placed on warfarin. In fact, an unreliable patient can be considered a relative contraindication to anticoagulant therapy. Areas that need to be discussed with the patient include the following:

1. *Need for Strict Compliance.* The importance of taking warfarin and other medications as directed and of following instructions regarding prothrombin times and follow-up office visits must be stressed.
2. *Side Effects.* The sites and signs of bleeding as well as instructions on when and where to call if bleeding occurs should be reviewed.
3. *Dietary Instruction.* The patient should be told that no major dietary restrictions are necessary; however, no abrupt changes in dietary habits should be made. Rarely, diets with excessive quantities of vitamin K have interfered with warfarin therapy.[175]
4. *Frequent Prothrombin Times.* The patient needs to be aware of the required monitoring of prothrombin times and why this is necessary. Some patients question the need for continued monitoring of warfarin, and this issue is best addressed early in the course of treatment.
5. *Drug Interactions.* The patient should be informed that other drugs can greatly influence the effect of warfarin and should be told not to start or stop medication without first asking their physician. It may be useful to make specific recommendations regarding

the use of common nonprescription drugs; e.g., antacids, analgesics, and cold products.

The quantity of information to be learned requires both an oral presentation and written materials. Patients should not be expected to remember this much information without having some reference materials at home. There are a number of such materials available, including an excellent patient instruction brochure prepared by E.I. duPont de Nemours & Company.

It is also important for the patient to inform health-care personnel caring for them (e.g., pharmacist, physician, dentist) that they are taking warfarin. It may be useful to provide the patient with an identification card stating that the patient is receiving warfarin. Patients on long-term warfarin therapy may wish to wear a bracelet containing this information.

Subcutaneous Heparin. Subcutaneous heparin should be administered into the fatty tissue above the iliac crest or abdomen. The patient should be instructed to grasp a 1–2-inch area of fat, hold it away from deeper tissues, and inject into this tissue. The needle should not be moved while injecting. The patient should then apply pressure to the site for 1–2 minutes after injection but should not massage the area. Different sites should be used for each new injection. Severe bleeding or bruising should be reported to the patient's physician.

Conclusion

Although anticoagulants have been used clinically for almost 50 years, some of the most fundamental questions concerning anticoagulation have only recently been answered. Some of these answers have been aided by the development of more sophisticated diagnostic procedures.

Future clinical trials should further define the role of thrombolytics in acute DVT and PE. While they are being used with ever-increasing frequency, some authors suggest that thrombolytic agents should be used more liberally.

Still left unanswered is whether calf-vein thrombosis should be treated aggressively with anticoagulants or simply followed closely.

The use of less intense anticoagulation for proximal-vein DVT should certainly lower the hemorrhagic risk of long-term anticoagulation. However, it is yet to be determined if less intense anticoagulation can be used for pulmonary embolism or for arterial thromboembolic events.

References

1. McLean J. The thromboplastic action of cephalia. *Am J Physiol.* 1916; 41:250–7.
2. Best CH. Preparation of heparin and its use in the first clinical cases. *Circulation.* 1959; 19:79–86.
3. Barritt DW, Jordon SC. Anticoagulant drugs in the treatment of pulmonary embolism: a controlled trial. *Lancet.* 1960; 1:1309–12.
4. Carey LC, Williams RD. Comparative effects of dicoumarol, tromexan, and heparin on thrombus propagation. *Ann Surg.* 1960; 152:919–52.
5. Allen EV, Barker NW, Waugh JM. A preparation from spoiled sweet clover. *JAMA.* 1942; 120:1009–15.
6. Campbell HA, Link KP. Studies on the hemorrhagic sweet clover. IV. The isolation and crystallization of the hemorrhagic agent. *J Biol Chem.* 1941; 138:21–33.
7. Link KP. The discovery of dicumarol and its sequels. *Circulation.* 1959; 19:97–107.
8. Seidman M, Robertson DN, Link KP. Studies on 4-hydroxycoumarins: X. Acylation of 3-(α-phenyl-β-acetylethyl)-4-hydroxycoumarin. *J Am Chem Soc.* 1950; 72:5193–5.
9. Virchow RLK. Gesammelte Abhandlungen zur Wissenschaftlichen. In: Thrombose und Emboli. Vol IV. Berlin: Hamm-Grotesche Buchhandlung; 1862:219.
10. Shattil SJ, Bennett JS. Platelets and their membranes in hemostasis: physiology and pathophysiology. *Ann Intern Med.* 1981; 94:108–18.
11. Shattil SJ. Diagnosis and treatment of recurrent venous thromboembolism. *Med Clin North Am.* 1984; 68:577–600.
12. Hamer JD, Malone PC, Silver IA. The PO_2 in venous valve pockets: its possible bearing on thrombogenesis. *Br J Surg.* 1981; 68:166–70.
13. LeQuesne LP. Relation between deep vein thrombosis and pulmonary embolism in surgical patients. *N Engl J Med.* 1974; 291:1292–4.
14. Bell WR, Simon TL. Current status of pulmonary thromboembolic disease: pathophysiology, diagnosis, prevention, and treatment. *Am Heart J.* 1982; 103:239–62.
15. Gjöres JE. The incidence of venous thrombosis and its sequelae in certain districts of Sweden. *Acta Chir Scand.* 1956; 206(Suppl):1–88.
16. Bauer G. A roentgenological and clinical study of the sequels of thrombosis. *Acta Chir Scand.* 1942; 74(Suppl):5–115.
17. Bieger R, Boekhout-Mussert RJ, Hohmann F et al. Is streptokinase useful in the treatment of deep vein thrombosis? *Acta Med Scand.* 1976; 199:81–8.
18. Kakkar VV, Flanc C, Howe CT et al. Treatment of deep vein thrombosis. A trial of heparin, streptokinase and Arvin. *Br Med J.* 1969; 1:806–10.
19. Arnesen H, Hoiseth A, Ly B. Streptokinase or heparin in the treatment of deep vein thrombosis. *Acta Med Scand.* 1982; 211:65–8.
20. Johansson E, Ericson K, Zetterquist S. Streptokinase treatment of deep venous thrombosis of the lower extremity. *Acta Med Scand.* 1976; 199:89–94.
21. Arnesen H, Heilo A, Jakobsen E et al. A prospective study of streptokinase and heparin in the treatment of deep vein thrombosis. *Acta Med Scand.* 1978; 203:457–63.
22. Rösch J, Dotter CT, Seaman AJ et al. Healing of deep venous thrombosis: venographic findings in a randomized study comparing streptokinase and heparin. *Am J Roentgenol.* 1976; 127:553–8.
23. Olow B, Johanson C, Andersson J et al. Deep venous thrombosis treated with a standard dosage of streptokinase. *Acta Chir Scand.* 1970; 136:181–9.
24. Albrechtsson U, Anderson J, Einarsson E et al. Streptokinase treatment of deep venous thrombosis and the post thrombotic syndrome. *Arch Surg.* 1981; 116:33–7.
25. Thomas DP, Gurewich V, Ashford TP. Platelet adherence to thromboemboli in relation to the pathogenesis and treatment of pulmonary embolism. *N Engl J Med.* 1966; 274:953–6.
26. Sackner MA, Will DH, DuBois AB. The site of pulmonary vasomotor activity during hypoxia or serotonin administration. *J Clin Invest.* 1966; 45:112–21.
27. Rosoff CB, Salzman EW, Gurewich V et al. Reduction of platelet serotonin and the response to pulmonary emboli. *Surgery.* 1971; 70:12–9.
28. Thomas D, Stein M, Tanabe G et al. Mechanism of bron-

choconstriction produced by thromboemboli in dogs. *Am J Physiol.* 1964; 206:1207–12.
29. Gurewich V, Cohen ML, Thomas DP. Humoral factors in massive pulmonary embolism: an experimental study. *Am Heart J.* 1968; 76:784–94.
30. Stein M, Levy SE. Reflex and humoral responses to pulmonary embolism. *Prog Cardiovasc Dis.* 1974;17:167–74.
31. McIntyre KM, Sasahara AA. Hemodynamic and ventricular responses to pulmonary embolism. *Prog Cardiovasc Dis.* 1974; 17:175–90.
32. Dalen JE, Haynes FW, Hoppin FG et al. Cardiovascular responses to experimental pulmonary embolism. *Am J Cardiol.* 1967; 20:3–9.
33. Moser KM, Fedullo PF. Venous thromboembolism. Three simple decisions (Part I). *Chest.* 1983; 83:117–21.
34. Moser KM, Fedullo PF. Venous thromboembolism. Three simple decisions (Part 2). *Chest.* 1983; 83:256–60.
35. Moreno-Cabral R, Kistner RL, Nordyke RA. Importance of calf vein thrombophlebitis. *Surgery.* 1976; 80:735–42.
36. Havig O. Deep vein thrombosis and pulmonary embolism. *Acta Chir Scand.* 1977; 478(Suppl):1–92.
37. Menzoian JO, Sequeira JC, Doyle JE et al. Therapeutic and clinical course of deep vein thrombosis. *Am J Surg.* 1983; 146:581–5.
38. Barker NW, Nygaard KK, Walters W et al. A statistical study of postoperative venous thrombosis and pulmonary embolism. I. Incidence in various types of operations. *Mayo Clin Proc.* 1940; 15:769–73.
39. Coon WW, Willis PW. Thromboembolic complications during anticoagulant therapy. *Arch Surg.* 1972; 105:209–12.
40. Salzman EW, Deykin D, Shapiro RM et al. Management of heparin therapy: a controlled prospective trial. *N Engl J Med.* 1975; 292;1046–50.
41. Hattersley PG, Mitsuoka JC, King JH. Heparin therapy for thromboembolic disorders. A prospective evaluation of 134 cases monitored by the activated coagulation time. *JAMA.* 1983, 250:1413–6.
42. Nicolaides AN, DuPont PA, Desai S et al. Small doses of subcutaneous sodium heparin in preventing deep venous thrombosis after major surgery. *Lancet.* 1972; 2:890–3.
43. Sharma GVRK, Schoolman M, Cella G et al. Key references: pulmonary embolism. Part I. *Circulation.* 1983; 67:245–7, 474–7.
44. Ockelford PA, Hull R. Management of venous thrombosis and thrombophlebitis. *Drugs.* 1982; 24:152–62.
45. Greenfield LJ, Jay SJ. Immediate management of massive pulmonary embolism. *Chest.* 1982; 82:775–8.
46. Bomalaski JS, Martin GH, Hughes RL et al. Inferior vena cava interruption in the management of pulmonary embolism. *Chest.* 1982; 82:767–74.
47. Russell JC. Prophylaxis of postoperative deep vein thrombosis and pulmonary embolism. *Surg Gynecol Obstet.* 1983; 157:89–104.
48. Halkin H, Goldberg J, Modan M et al. Reduction of mortality in general medical inpatients by low-dose heparin prophylaxis. *Ann Intern Med.* 1982; 96:561–5.
49. Leyvraz PF, Richard J, Bachmann F et al. Adjusted versus fixed-dose subcutaneous heparin in the prevention of deep-vein thrombosis after total hip replacement. *N Engl J Med.* 1983; 309:954–8.
50. Multicenter Trial Committee. Dihydroergotamine–heparin prophylaxis of postoperative deep vein thrombosis. *JAMA.* 1984; 251:2960–6.
51. Tillet WS, Sherry, S. The effect in patients of streptococcal fibrinolysin (streptokinase) and streptococcal desoxyribonuclease on fibrinous, purulent and sanguinous pleural exudations. *J Clin Invest.* 1949; 28:173–90.
52. Tillett WS, Johnson AJ, McCarty WR. The intravenous infusion of the streptococcal fibrinolytic principle (streptokinase) into patients. *J Clin Invest.* 1955; 34:169–85.
53. Konttinen Y. Some observations on the effect of thrombin on the antifibrinolytic aspect of streptokinase. *Scand J Clin Lab Invest.* 1962; 14:568–9.
54. Kakkar VV, Howe CT, Laws JW et al. Late results of treatment of deep vein thrombosis. *Br Med J.* 1969; 1:810–11.
55. Tsapogas MJ, Peabody RA, Wu KT et al. Controlled study of thrombolytic therapy in deep vein thrombosis. *Surgery.* 1973; 74:973–84.
56. van de Loo JCW, Kriessmann A, Trübestein G et al. Controlled multicenter pilot study of urokinase–heparin and streptokinase in deep vein thrombosis. *Thromb Haemost.* 1983; 50:660–3.
57. Theiss W, Wirtzfeld A, Fink U et al. The success rate of fibrinolytic therapy in fresh and old thrombosis of the iliac and femoral veins. *Angiology.* 1983; 34:61–9.
58. Seaman AJ, Common HH, Rösch J et al. Deep vein thrombosis treated with streptokinase or heparin: a randomized study. *Angiology.* 1976; 27:549–56.
59. Robertson BR, Nilsson IM, Nylander G. Thrombolytic effect of streptokinase as evaluated by phlebography of deep venous thrombi of the leg. *Acta Chir Scand.* 1970; 136:173–80.
60. Gormsen J, Laursen B. Treatment of acute phlebothrombosis with Streptase. *Acta Med Scand.* 1967; 181:373–83.
61. Kiil J, Carvalho A, Sakso P et al. Urokinase or heparin in the management of patients with deep vein thrombosis. *Acta Chir Scand.* 1981; 147:529–32.
62. Watz R, Savidge GF. Rapid thrombolysis and preservation of valvular venous function in high deep vein thrombosis. *Acta Med Scand.* 1979; 205:293–8.
63. Robertson BR, Nilsson IM, Nylander G. Value of streptokinase and heparin in treatment of acute deep venous thrombosis. *Acta Chir Scand.* 1968; 134:203–8.
64. Robertson BR, Nilsson IM, Nylander G. Effect of streptokinase and heparin on patients with deep venous thrombosis: a coded examination. *Acta Chir Scand.* 1967; 133:205–15.
65. D'Angelo A, Mannucci PM. Outcome of treatment of deep-vein thrombosis with urokinase: relationship to dosage, duration of therapy, age of thrombus and laboratory changes. *Thromb Haemost.* 1984; 51:236–9.
66. Browse NL, Thomas ML, Pim HP. Streptokinase and deep vein thrombosis. *Br Med J.* 1968; 3:717–20.
67. Marbet GA, Eichlisberger R, Duckert F et al. Sequential treatment of deep leg vein thrombosis with porcine plasmin and low dose streptokinase. *Thromb Haemost.* 1982; 48:190–5.
68. Marbet GA, Eichlisberger R, Duckert F et al. Side effects of thrombolytic treatment with porcine plasmin and low dose streptokinase. *Thromb Haemost.* 1982; 48:196–200.
69. Duckert F, Müller G, Nyman D et al. Treatment of deep vein thrombosis with streptokinase. *Br Med J.* 1975; 1:479–81.
70. Sasahara AA, Sharma GVRK, Tow DE et al. Clinical use of thrombolytic agents in venous thromboembolism. *Arch Intern Med.* 1982; 142:684–8.
71. Bell WR, Meek AG. Guidelines for the use of thrombolytic agents. *N Engl J Med.* 1979; 301:1266–70.
72. Urokinase Pulmonary Embolism Trial Study Group. Urokinase pulmonary embolism trial—Phase 1 results. *JAMA.* 1970; 214:2163–72.
73. Urokinase Pulmonary Embolism Trial Study Group. Urokinase–streptokinase embolism trial—Phase 2 results. *JAMA.* 1974; 229:1606–13.
74. Ly B, Arnesen H, Eie H et al. A controlled clinical trial of streptokinase and heparin in the treatment of major pulmonary embolism. *Acta Med Scand.* 1978; 203:465–70.
75. Tibbutt DA, Davies JA, Anderson JA et al. Comparison by controlled clinical trial of streptokinase and heparin in treatment of life-threatening pulmonary embolism. *Br Med J.* 1974; 1:343–7.
76. Miller GAH, Sutton GC, Kerr IH et al. Comparison of streptokinase and heparin in treatment of isolated acute massive pulmonary embolism. *Br Med J.* 1971; 2:681–4.
77. National Institutes of Health. Thrombolytic therapy in treatment: summary of an NIH consensus conference. *Br*

Med J. 1980; 2:1585–8.

78. Sharma GVRK, Burleson VA, Sashara AA. Effect of thrombolytic therapy on pulmonary-capillary blood volume in patients with pulmonary embolism. *N Engl J Med.* 1980; 303:842–5.
79. Benotti JR, Ockene IS, Alpert JS et al. The clinical profile of unresolved pulmonary embolism. *Chest.* 1983; 84:669–78.
80. Cole RP. Thrombolytic therapy in thromboembolic disorders of the lung. *NY State J Med.* 1984; 84:1–2.
81. Hoechst-Roussel. Streptase package insert. Somerville, NJ; 1984 Jan.
82. Rutkowski DM, Burkle WS. Advances in thrombolytic therapy. *Drug Intell Clin Pharm.* 1982; 16:115–21.
83. Hassall E, Ulich TU, Ament ME. Pulmonary embolism and Malassezia pulmonary infection related to urokinase therapy. *J Pediatr.* 1983; 102:722–5.
84. Ludwig H. Results of streptokinase therapy in deep venous thrombosis during pregnancy. *Postgrad Med J.* 1973; 49(Suppl 5):65–7.
85. McTaggart DR, Ingram TG. Massive pulmonary embolism during pregnancy treated with streptokinase. *Med J Aust.* 1977; 1:18–20.
86. Simel DL, Moorman JR, Pryor SL et al. Is streptokinase safe during menses? *Arch Intern Med.* 1984; 144:841.
87. Deykin D. Current status of anticoagulant therapy. *Am J Med.* 1982; 72:659–64.
88. Bjork I, Lindahl U. Mechanism of the anticoagulant action of heparin. *Mol Cell Biochem.* 1982; 48:161–82.
89. Bjornsson TD, Levy G. Pharmacokinetics of heparin. I. Studies of dose dependence. *J Pharmacol Exp Ther.* 1979; 210:237–42.
90. Cipolle RJ, Seifert RD, Neilan BA et al. Heparin kinetics: variables related to disposition and dosage. *Clin Pharmacol Ther.* 1981; 29:387–93.
91. Hirsh J, van Aken WG, Gallus AS et al. Heparin kinetics in venous thrombosis and pulmonary embolism. *Circulation.* 1976; 53:691–5.
92. Simon TL, Hyers TM, Gaston JP et al. Heparin pharmacokinetics: increased requirements in pulmonary embolism. *Br J Haematol.* 1978; 39:111–20.
93. Elliott CG, Michocki RJ, Brown R et al. Heparin requirements in pulmonary embolism and venous thrombosis: a prospective study. *J Clin Pharmacol.* 1982; 22:102–9.
94. Glazier RL, Crowell EB. Randomized prospective trial of continuous vs intermittent heparin therapy. *JAMA.* 1976; 236:1365–7.
95. Mant MJ, O'Brien B, Thong KI et al. Hemorrhagic complications of heparin therapy. *Lancet.* 1977; 1:1133–5.
96. Wilson JR, Lampman J. Heparin therapy: a randomized prospective study. *Am Heart J.* 1979; 97:155–8.
97. Wilson JE, Bynum LJ, Parkey RW. Heparin therapy in venous thromboembolism. *Am J Med.* 1981; 70:808–16.
98. Self TH, Vanderbush RE. Cost of continuous infusion vs intermittent IV heparin. *Am Heart J.* 1980; 99:816–8.
99. Chenella FC, Gill MA, Kern JW et al. Improved method for estimating initial heparin infusion rates. *Am J Hosp Pharm.* 1979; 36:782–4.
100. Greenlaw CW, Henrietta GC, Stolley SN. Standardized heparin dosage schedule using pharmacokinetic principles. *Am J Hosp Pharm.* 1979; 36:920–3.
101. Hattersley PG. Progress report: the activated coagulation time of whole blood (ACT). *Am J Clin Path.* 1976; 66:899–904.
102. Kelton JG, Hirsh J. Bleeding associated with antithrombotic therapy. *Semin Hematol.* 1980; 17:259–91.
103. Wessler S, Morris LE. Studies in intravascular coagulation. IV. The effect of heparin and dicoumarol on serum-induced venous thrombosis. *Circulation.* 1955; 12:553–6.
104. Basu D, Gallus A, Hirsh J et al. A prospective study of the value of monitoring heparin treatment with the activated partial thromboplastin time. *N Engl J Med.* 1972; 287:324–7.
105. Poller L, Thomson JM, Palmer MK. Measuring partial thromboplastin-time: an international collaborative study. *Lancet.* 1976; 2:842–6.
106. Brandt JT, Triplett DA. Laboratory monitoring of heparin. Effect of reagents and instruments on the activated partial thromboplastin time. *Am J Clin Path.* 1981; 76:530–7.
107. Hattersley PG, Mitsuoka JC, King JH. Sources of error in heparin therapy of thromboembolic disease. *Arch Intern Med.* 1980; 140:1173–5.
108. Hattersley PG, Mitsuoka JC, Ignoffo RJ et al. Adjusting heparin infusion rates from the initial response to activated coagulation time. *Drug Intell Clin Pharm.* 1983; 17:632–4.
109. Wessler S, Gitel SN. Warfarin: from bedside to bench. *N Engl J Med.* 1984; 311:645–52.
110. Stein PD, Willis PW. Diagnosis, prophylaxis, and treatment of acute pulmonary embolism. *Arch Intern Med.* 1983; 143:991–4.
111. Self TH, Bauman JH, Brown JR et al. Concurrent initiation of heparin and warfarin therapy. *Am Heart J.* 1981; 102:470–1.
112. Sawyer WM, Raasch RH. Effect of heparin on prothrombin time. *Clin Pharm.* 1984; 3:192–4.
113. Kayser SR. Thrombosis. In: Katcher BS, Young LY, Koda-Kimble MA, eds. Applied therapeutics: The clinical use of drugs. San Francisco: Applied Therapeutics, Inc; 1983:338.
114. Loeliger EA. The optimal therapeutic range in oral anticoagulation: history and proposal. *Thromb Haemost.* 1979; 42:1141–52.
115. Poller L. Oral anticoagulants reassessed. *Br Med J.* 1982; 284:1425–6.
116. Bradlow BA. Oral anticoagulants in the 1980's: a reassessment of indication, dosage and laboratory control. *S Afr Med J.* 1983; 64:313–6.
117. Loeliger EA, Van den Basselaar AMHP, Broekmans AW. Intensity of oral anticoagulation in patients monitored with various thromboplastins. *N Engl J Med.* 1983; 308:1228–9.
118. Loeliger EA, Lewis SM. Progress in laboratory control of oral anticoagulants. *Lancet.* 1982; 2:318–20.
119. Poller L, Taberner DA. Dosage and control of oral anticoagulants: an international collaborative survey. *Br J Haematol.* 1982; 51:479–85.
120. Hull R, Hirsh J. Long-term anticoagulant therapy in patients with venous thrombosis. *Arch Intern Med.* 1983; 143:2061–3.
121. Coon WW, Willis PW. Hemorrhagic complications of anticoagulant therapy. *Arch Intern Med.* 1974; 133:386–92.
122. Moschos CB, Wong PCY, Sise HS. Controlled study of the effective level of long-term anticoagulation. *JAMA.* 1964; 190:799–805.
123. Hull R, Delmore T, Genton E. Warfarin sodium versus low-dose heparin in the long-term treatment of venous thrombosis. *N Engl J Med.* 1979; 301:855–8.
124. Hull R, Delmore T, Carter C. Adjusted subcutaneous heparin versus warfarin sodium in the long-term treatment of venous thromboembolism. *N Engl J Med.* 1982; 306:189–94.
125. Sevitt S, Innes D. Prothrombin-time and thrombotest in injured patients on prophylactic anticoagulant therapy. *Lancet.* 1964; 1:124–9.
126. Coon WW, Willis PW, Symons MS. Assessment of anticoagulant treatment of venous thromboembolism. *Ann Surg.* 1969; 170:559–68.
127. Hull R, Hirsh J, Jay R et al. Different intensities of oral anticoagulant therapy in the treatment of proximal-vein thrombosis. *N Engl J Med.* 1982; 307:1676–81.
128. Hull RD, Raskob GE, Hirsh J et al. A cost-effectiveness analysis of alternative approaches for long-term treatment of proximal venous thrombosis. *JAMA.* 1984; 252:235–9.
129. Hall JG, Pauli RM, Wilson KM. Maternal and fetal sequelae of anticoagulation during pregnancy. *Am J Med.* 1980;68:122–39.
130. Merril LK, VerBurg DJ. The choice of long-term anticoagulants for the pregnant patient. *Obstet Gynecol.* 1976; 47:711–4.

131. Tawes RL, Kennedy PA, Harris EJ et al. Management of deep venous thrombosis and pulmonary embolism during pregnancy. *Am J Surg.* 1982; 144:141–5.
132. O'Reilly RA, Aggeler PM. Studies on coumarin anticoagulant drugs: initiation of warfarin therapy without a loading dose. *Circulation.* 1968; 38:169–77.
133. Williams DB, Karl RC. A simple technique for predicting daily maintenance dose of warfarin. *Am J Surg.* 1979; 137:572–6.
134. Miller DR, Brown MA. Predicting warfarin maintenance dosage based on initial response. *Am J Hosp Pharm.* 1979; 36:1351–5.
135. Sawyer WT. Predictability of warfarin dose requirements: theoretical considerations. *J Pharm Sci.* 1979; 68:432–4.
136. Routledge PA, Davies DM, Bell SM et al. Predicting patients' warfarin requirements. *Lancet.* 1977; 2:854–5.
137. Dobrzanski S. Predicting warfarin dosage. *J Clin Hosp Pharm.* 1983; 8:247–50.
138. Chua LH, Dobrzanski S, Taylor P. Use of a warfarin dose prediction method. *J Clin Hosp Pharm.* 1984; 9:253–6.
139. Morrison GW. Predicting warfarin requirements. *Lancet.* 1979; 1:167–8.
140. Carter BL, Reinders TP, Hamilton RA. Prediction of maintenance warfarin dosage from initial patient response. *Drug Intell Clin Pharm.* 1983; 17:23–6.
141. Carter BL, Taylor JW, Reinders TP. Evaluation of two methods to predict maintenance warfarin dosage. *Drug Intell Clin Pharm.* 1984; 18:510.
142. Sheiner LB. Computer-aided long-term anticoagulation therapy. *Comput Biomed Res.* 1969; 2:507–18.
143. Howell JR. Um pequeno computador analogico aplicado na simulacao de dosagem de drogas em pacientes. *Ci and Cult.* 1976; 28(Suppl):878–80.
144. Rock WL, Reinders TP, Salter FJ et al. Evaluation of computer-assisted pharmacist consultation during initiation and stabilization of warfarin therapy. Paper presented to 14th Annual ASHP Midyear Clinical Meeting. Las Vegas, NV: 1979 Dec. 6.
145. Svec J, Coleman R, Mungall D et al. Bayesian pharmacokinetic/pharmacodynamic forecasting of prothrombin response to warfarin therapy. *Drug Intell Clin Pharm.* 1984; 18:513.
146. Williams JRB, Griffin JP, Parkins A. Effect of concomitantly administered drugs on the control of long term anticoagulant therapy. *Q J Med.* 1976; 45:63–73.
147. O'Malley K, Stevenson IH, Ward CA et al. Determinants of anticoagulant control in patients receiving warfarin. *Br J Clin Pharmacol.* 1977; 4:309–14.
148. May FE, Stewart RB, Cluff LE. Drug interactions and multiple drug administration. *Clin Pharmacol Ther.* 1977; 22:322–8.
149. Hansten PD. Drug interactions. 4th ed. Philadelphia, PA: Lea & Febiger; 1979.
150. Serlin MJ, Breckenridge AM. Drug interactions with warfarin. *Drugs.* 1983; 25:610–20.
151. Koch-Weser J, Sellers EM. Drug interactions with coumarin anticoagulants. *N Engl J Med.* 1971; 285:487–98, 547–58.
152. McGrath KG, Pattersen R. Anaphylactic reactivity to streptokinase. *JAMA.* 1984; 252:1314–17.
153. Toty WG, Romano T, Benian GM et al. Serum sickness following streptokinase therapy. *AJR* 1982; 138:143-4.
154. Straub PW, Boersma J, Rhymer K et al. Plasmocytosis following thrombolytic treatment with streptokinase. *Schweiz Med Wochenschr.* 1974; 104:1891–2.
155. Rieben FW, Waldeherr R, Oster P et al. Acute renal failure due to diffuse cholesterol embolization during streptokinase treatment. *Dtsch Med Wochenschr.* 1979; 104:1447–99.
156. Pick RA, Joswig BC, Cheung AK et al. Acute renal failure following repeated streptokinase therapy for pulmonary embolism. *West J Med.* 1983; 138:878–80.
157. Spargen L, Liljeqvist L, Ljungdahl I et al. Temporary changes in renal function following streptokinase therapy—a case report. *Acta Med Scand.* 1976; 199:335–6.
158. Sallen MK, Efrusy ME, Kniaz JL et al. Streptokinase induced hepatic dysfunction. *Am J Gastroenterol.* 1983; 78:523–4.
159. Eden KV. Possible association of Guillain-Barré Syndrome with thrombolytic therapy. *JAMA.* 1983; 249:2020–1.
160. Leaf DA, MacDonald I, Kliks B et al. Streptokinase and the Guillain-Barré syndrome. *Ann Intern Med.* 1984; 100:617.
161. Martin TR, Sandblom RL, Johnson RJ. Acute respiratory distress syndrome following thrombolytic therapy for pulmonary embolism. *Chest.* 1983; 83:151–3.
162. Lawson DH. Anticoagulants and hemostatics. In: Miller RR, Greenblatt DJ, eds. Drug effects in hospitalized patients. New York: John Wiley & Sons; 1976:101–8.
163. Moore FD, Osteen RT, Karp DD et al. Anticoagulants, venous thromboembolism, and the cancer patient. *Arch Surg.* 1981; 116:405–7.
164. Walker A, Jick H. Prediction of bleeding during heparin therapy. *JAMA.* 1980; 244:1209–12.
165. Feder W, Auerback R. "Purple Toes": an uncommon sequela of oral coumarin drug therapy. *Ann Intern Med.* 1961; 55:911–7.
166. Lebsack CS, Wiebert RT. "Purple Toes" syndrome. *Postgrad Med.* 1982; 71:81–4.
167. Horn JR, Danziger LH, David RJ. Warfarin-induced skin necrosis: report of four cases. *Am J Hosp Pharm.* 1981; 38:1763–8.
168. Cipolle RJ, Rodvold KA, Seifert R et al. Heparin-associated thrombocytopenia: a prospective evaluation of 211 patients. *Ther Drug Monit.* 1983; 5:205–11.
169. Bell WR, Royall RM. Heparin-associated thrombocytopenia: a comparison of three heparin preparations. *N Engl J Med.* 1980; 303:902–7.
170. Cines DB, Kaywin P, Bina M et al. Heparin-associated thrombocytopenia. *N Engl J Med.* 1980; 303:788–95.
171. Silver D, Kapsch DN, Tsoi EKM. Heparin-induced thrombocytopenia, thrombosis and hemorrhage. *Ann Surg.* 1983; 198:301–6.
172. Guay DRP, Richard A. Heparin-induced thrombocytopenia—association with a platelet aggregating factor and cross-sensitivity to bovine and porcine heparin. *Drug Intell Clin Pharm.* 1984; 18:398–401.
173. King DJ, Kelton JG. Heparin-associated thrombocytopenia. *Ann Intern Med.* 1984; 100:535–40.
174. Griffith GC, Nichols G, Asher JD et al. Heparin osteoporosis. *JAMA.* 1965; 193:91–4.
175. Quereshi GD, Reinders TP, Swint JJ et al. Acquired warfarin resistance and weight reducing diet. *Arch Intern Med.* 1981; 141:507–9.

Management of bronchiolitis

MILAP C. NAHATA, JULIE A. JOHNSON, AND DWIGHT A. POWELL

Abstract: The incidence, etiology, epidemiology, clinical presentation, treatment, prognosis, and prevention of bronchiolitis are discussed with a critical evaluation of the available studies on various therapeutic approaches.

Bronchiolitis is a lower respiratory-tract viral infection that affects 6–10% of all children below two years of age. Respiratory syncytial virus (RSV) is the usual pathogen. The symptoms range from mild wheezing to severe respiratory distress. An infected child usually has a fever, a rapid pulse, an increased breathing rate, and difficulty in breathing.

Because most of the infants hospitalized with bronchiolitis have hypoxemia, the administration of oxygen is the mainstay of therapy. Correct fluid therapy is essential to avoid dehydration and overhydration. Limited data are available on the use of drugs in the management of bronchiolitis. Although a variety of adrenergic drugs, theophylline, and corticosteroids are used, sound efficacy data are lacking, and most studies have documented a lack of therapeutic benefits. One study reported that the combined use of corticosteroids and albuterol may be beneficial in severely ill patients. Recent studies have shown that the continuous administration of ribavirin may decrease viral shedding. Antibiotics are not indicated unless a secondary bacterial infection is present.

Oxygen and fluid therapy have a clear role in the management of patients with bronchiolitis; however, no specific guidelines are available for the use of drugs in the treatment of these patients.

Index terms: Albuterol; Antivirals: Bronchiolitis; Fluids; Oxygen; Pediatrics; Ribavirin; Steroids, cortico-; Sympathomimetic agents
Clin Pharm. 1985; 4:297–303

Bronchiolitis is a lower respiratory-tract viral infection characterized by the acute onset of wheezing.[1] Annually, it affects 6–10% of all children less than two years of age.[2] Most patients with bronchiolitis are within the age range from two to nine months.[2]

It is surprising that bronchiolitis has been recognized in the medical literature for only a brief period. Bronchiolitis was first reported in a journal in 1941[3] and appeared in Textbook of Pediatrics in 1954.[4] The disease was generally considered to be pneumonia during the first half of this century.[5]

Although the majority of patients with bronchiolitis are never ill enough to be hospitalized, 1–2% of infants less than one year of age require careful observation and inpatient management.[1] At our hospital, about 150–200 infants with the diagnosis of bronchiolitis are admitted each year for an average stay of five days. Besides supplemental oxygen and general supportive care, a number of drugs including epinephrine, isoproterenol, theophylline, corticosteroids, and ribavirin have been reported to have possible therapeutic value in the management of this disease. However, because of conflicting reports, no clear guidelines are available for the use of drugs in the management of bronchiolitis. The objectives of this article are to summarize the important features of bronchiolitis and discuss the current concepts and controversies surrounding its management.

Etiology and Epidemiology

Respiratory syncytial virus (RSV) is the major cause of bronchiolitis. It is an etiologic agent in more than 80% of the cases during the yearly epidemic and about 50% of the total number of cases of bronchiolitis.[5] Parainfluenza viruses (types 1, 2, and 3) account for about 25% of all cases. Adenoviruses, *Mycoplasma pneumoniae*, rhinoviruses, and influenza viruses (types A and B) are each responsible for about 5% of the cases. Less than 5% of all cases are caused by enteroviruses, herpes viruses hominis, and mumps.[5]

Although some studies have reported bacterial etiologies including *Haemophilus influenzae*,[6,7] *Streptococcus pneumoniae*,[8] and mixed viral and bacterial infections,[9] bacteriologic and serologic studies have not provided a clear evidence for bacteria as important pathogens in this disease.[5,10,11]

Sporadic cases of bronchiolitis can occur at any time during the year, but the seasonal peak of yearly epidemics in the United States attributable to the primary pathogen, RSV, usually occurs between

MILAP C. NAHATA, PHARM.D., is Associate Professor of Pharmacy and Pediatrics, Colleges of Pharmacy and Medicine; JULIE A. JOHNSON is a senior pharmacy student; and DWIGHT A. POWELL, M.D., is Associate Professor and Chief, Section of Infectious Diseases, Department of Pediatrics, The Ohio State University and Children's Hospital, Columbus.

Address reprint requests to Dr. Nahata at the College of Pharmacy, The Ohio State University, 500 West 12th Avenue, Columbus, OH 43210.

This is **article 680-204-8509** in the **ASHP Continuing Education System.** See page 337 for learning objectives and test questions.

December and March.[2] Although most cases are reported in the winter, the time of the peak season for bronchiolitis may vary by geographic area.[12]

The virus is generally introduced to the infant by an older sibling or adult with a mild cold. Based on a study of nasal secretions from infants with acute bronchiolitis, RSV remains infectious for more than six hours on counter tops and for 30 minutes on cloth and paper tissue.[13] Thus, contact with clothing, furniture, or tissues contaminated by the secretions of infected children may be one way the disease spreads. This has been verified by the spread of RSV in volunteers who touched contaminated secretions and then their eyes and nasal mucosa.[14] Small-particle aerosols of RSV have not been documented to spread the disease.[12]

Clinical Presentation

Cough and coryza are the earliest symptoms of bronchiolitis. There is usually a gradual progression of the illness over a one- to seven-day period. A sudden progression to marked respiratory distress including tachypnea, lethargy, intercostal retractions, and wheezing can occur in many patients. About 50–80% of the children with bronchiolitis have fevers of 38.3–38.9 °C. The pulse is rapid, the respiratory rate is usually increased, and breathing is usually difficult and noisy. Other features include anorexia, restless sleep, vomiting, diarrhea, cyanosis, conjunctivitis, pharyngitis, and otitis media.[5,15,16]

The main pathophysiologic event that underlies these clinical characteristics is the partial obstruction of airflow in the bronchioles.[1] Airway lumen diameter is compromised by mucosal-cell swelling, intraluminal secretions, submucosal edema, and peribronchiolar infiltrates. Although the presence of bronchospasm has been questioned,[1] some infants appear to benefit from bronchodilator therapy. Decreased lumen size creates resistance to the movement of air during inspiration and expiration, resulting in increased work of breathing.

Air trapping in the alveoli and areas of microatelectasis results in a ventilation and perfusion imbalance, accounting for mild hypoxemia in most infants. Although the alveolar pressure of carbon dioxide ($P_{A_{CO_2}}$) is usually below normal, it is not as low as expected with the rapid respiratory rate. Hypoxemia and hypercarbia become worse as the severity of disease increases. Cyanosis, not present with mild hypoxemia, reflects severe oxygen desaturation and pending respiratory failure.[17–19] Infants with cyanotic congenital heart disease or underlying obstructive lung disease may develop severe and frequently fatal bronchiolitis following RSV infections.

The results of routine laboratory tests are of limited value. The findings from chest roentgenograms may vary,[5] but they usually show flattened diaphragms and hyperinflated lung parenchyma. Areas of atelectasis and infiltrates may be present. An examination of the comparative lung fields, pulmonary vascularity, and cardiac silhouette is helpful in differentiating bronchiolitis from foreign-body aspiration and congestive heart failure. Other diseases that must be considered in the differential diagnosis are cystic fibrosis, α-1-antitrypsin deficiency, pulmonary vascular anomalies, gastric esophageal reflux, and aspiration pneumonitis. The differentiation of bronchiolitis from reactive-airways disease may not be possible in the infant who has wheezing associated with a respiratory infection.[5]

Treatment

Although the importance of supportive treatment has been clearly established, limited data are available about the role of drugs in the management of bronchiolitis. The various therapeutic approaches that have been taken are described in this section.

Supportive Treatment. *Oxygen Therapy.* Because most infants with bronchiolitis have hypoxemia caused by ventilation and perfusion abnormalities, the administration of oxygen remains the mainstay of therapy.[1,20–22] The goal is to maintain the arterial oxygen tension between 70 and 90 torr. Generally, this can be achieved by administering 30–40% oxygen in a tent.[5] Although the oxygen should be humidified, the use of mist and aerosol is discouraged. The mist can act as an irritant causing reflex bronchoconstriction,[23] and the water does not reach the lower airways.[24] Temperatures within humidified tents should be monitored to maintain an isothermic environment. In addition, arterial blood gases should be monitored in patients with increasing respiratory rates, cyanosis, and agitation.[5] In infants with respiratory failure, intubation and mechanical ventilatory assistance are required.[25]

Fluid Therapy. Patients with bronchiolitis may be dehydrated because of a decrease in fluid intake and an increase in fluid loss by vomiting or rapid respiration. Although the fluid deficit should be corrected, overhydration must be avoided. Since pulmonary interstitial edema is present in patients with bronchiolitis, excess fluid can contribute to airway obstruction.[5] Furthermore, there is no evidence to suggest that overhydration promotes the clearance of mucous plugging in the respiratory tracts of these infants.[25]

Drug Treatment. A summary of available studies on drug therapy in bronchiolitis is presented in Tables 1–3. Bronchodilators (adrenergic agents and theophylline), corticosteroids, ribavirin, and ampicillin have been evaluated in patients with bronchiolitis. These studies are reviewed below.

Bronchodilators. Since it is difficult to differenti-

Table 1.
Studies of Bronchodilators in Children with Bronchiolitis

Reference No.	No. Patients (Age)	Drug and Dose[a,b]	Tests To Evaluate Therapy	Response to Therapy
26	10 (4–12 wk)	Isoproterenol, 2 mL of 0.2% solution (5 patients); metaproterenol, 2 mL of 0.2% solution (5 patients)	Pulmonary resistance by total-body plethysmogram	No consistent change in pulmonary resistance
27	7 (3–6 mo) 6 (6–12 mo) 3 (>12 mo)	Albuterol, 1 mL of 0.25% solution; three patients received isoproterenol, not albuterol	Pulmonary resistance by forced-oscillation technique	No appreciable change in pulmonary resistance
28	21 (2–17 mo)	Epinephrine, 2 mL of 0.4% solution (14 patients); phenylephrine 2 mL of 0.25% solution	Modified forced-oscillation technique	No improvement
29	32 (7–43 mo)	Albuterol, 1.5 mL of 0.5% solution	Forced-oscillation technique in all; total-body plethysmogram in 12 patients	No change in pulmonary resistance in patients <18 mo; the children >20 mo showed >15% fall in pulmonary resistance
30[c]	39 assessments in 25 patients (5–28 wk)	Water (12 assessments); albuterol, 5 mg (12 assessments); ipratropium bromide 250 mg (15 assessments)	Intrathoracic pressure swings and tidal volume to yield total work of breathing	Mean work of breathing decreased (18%) only with ipratropium; no change in clinical status for most; six patients receiving ipratropium improved
32[d]	64 (<18 mo)	Theophylline, 2–7 mg/kg every six hours (30 patients); of 30, 37% corticosteroids and 27% isoetharine; no theophylline or other drugs (34 patients)	Clinical response and length of hospitalization	No difference in treated versus untreated patients

[a] All drugs were evaluated after a single dose except for theophylline.
[b] The time the drug therapy was started (i.e., during or after acute illness) and the severity of disease were unclear.
[c] Double-blind randomized study.
[d] Retrospective study.

ate bronchiolitis from reactive-airways disease, bronchodilator therapy is usually considered. Few prospective studies, however, have supported the routine use of these drugs (Table 1).

Phelan and Williams[26] studied five infants who received nebulized isoproterenol and another five who received nebulized metaproterenol during an RSV epidemic. The clinical status of the infants and pulmonary function test results failed to show any therapeutic benefits from these single-dose regimens. Rutter and Milner[27] also reported a lack of effect with single-dose therapy using nebulized albuterol in 13 children and isoproterenol aerosol in 3 children. Lenney and Milner[28] found the single-dose treatment with nebulized phenylephrine in 7 children and nebulized epinephrine in 14 children to be ineffective. Another study by these investigators showed that nebulized albuterol resulted in a greater improvement in respiratory resistance in patients more than 18 months of age compared with younger patients. They suggested that the failure of albuterol therapy in children less than 18 months of age may have been attributable to the infants' poorly developed bronchial muscles.[29] However, these findings are of limited value because most patients with bronchiolitis are younger than 18 months. Stokes et al.[30] compared nebulized water, albuterol, and ipratropium bromide (an anticholinergic drug) in a double-blind study of 25 infants. They found a major improvement in 6 of 15 assessments with ipratropium bromide but no change in the nebulized water or albuterol groups.

Although the use of theophylline has been recommended by Welliver[25] and Ellis,[31] no studies are available to document the efficacy of theophylline in bronchiolitis. In a retrospective study,[32] the clinical response and length of hospitalization were not altered by theophylline therapy (Table 1).

Corticosteroids. Corticosteroids have been used with the hypothesis that their anti-inflammatory action may reduce bronchiolar inflammation and swelling.[33,34] The data on the efficacy of corticosteroids in bronchiolitis are shown in Table 2.

Table 2.
Studies of Corticosteroids in Children with Bronchiolitis

Reference No.	No. Patients (Age)	Drug and Dose[a]	Duration of Therapy	Tests To Evaluate Therapy	Reponse or Outcome
33[b,c]	44 (1.5–18 mo)	Methylprednisolone i.m. 5 mg/kg on day 1 and 2.5 mg/kg on day 2 (22 patients); placebo (22 patients); all received tetracycline and epinephrine	Every 12 hours until discharge	Severity score	No improvement in steroid or placebo group
34[b]	297 (<30 mo)	Betamethasone i.v./i.m. 1 mg/kg first dose then 0.5 mg/5 lb (148 patients); placebo (149 patients)	Every 12 hours for 72 hours	Clinical status, roentgenograms	Slight but insignificant change in clinical status in steroid group
35[b]	57 (1–25 mo)	Dexamethasone i.m. 0.1 mg/mL (31 patients); placebo (26 patients); 0.15 meg sodium chloride/mL; all received penicillin and streptomycin for five days	14 days; doses were 0.2 (day 1–9), 0.1 (day 10–11), 0.05 (day 12–13), 0.02 (day 14), mL/lb/day in four doses	Clinical status	No change in clinical status in either group
36[b,c]	32 (1–12 mo)	Dexamethasone i.m. 0.3 mg/kg followed by 0.1 mg/kg every eight hours (8 patients); albuterol 2.5 mg inhaled and 0.15 mg/kg every eight hours as syrup (8 patients); dexamethasone and albuterol (8 patients); and placebo (8 patients)	Seven days or until discharge, whichever occurred first	Clinical scores including respiratory rate, wheezing, cyanosis, accessory respiratory muscle use	Three groups similar and unresponsive but combination group had twice the rate of improvement

[a] The time the drug therapy was started (i.e., during or after acute illness) and the severity of disease were unclear.
[b] Double-blind study.
[c] Randomized study.

Three controlled studies with corticosteroids have failed to demonstrate any therapeutic benefit in children with bronchiolitis.[33-35] One recent study showed that a combination of dexamethasone and albuterol was more effective than placebo, dexamethasone alone, and albuterol alone.[36] The patients in the combined dexamethasone and albuterol group demonstrated a faster improvement in clinical scores and fewer complications when they were compared with the other groups. Because of the small number of patients in each group, these authors suggested that further studies be conducted before the use of such combined therapy is recommended. Despite a lack of clear evidence for the efficacy of corticosteroids in bronchiolitis, it has been suggested that these drugs should not be withheld in patients with life-threatening disease because of the fear of complications.[3] None of the available studies has reported adverse effects from corticosteroids in patients with bronchiolitis.

Anti-infective Therapy. A summary of the studies on the effect of antiviral and antibiotic drugs on bronchiolitis is presented in Table 3. Because RSV is the primary pathogen to cause bronchiolitis, the development of an antiviral agent may provide the most specific therapy for these patients. Ribavirin [1-β-D-ribofuranosyl-1*H*-1,2,4,-triazole-3-carboxamide; Virazole (ICN)] is an investigational synthetic nucleoside with antiviral properties in vitro against a variety of both RNA and DNA viruses. After the initial studies in a cotton-rat model and normal adult volunteers with an experimental RSV infection, ribavirin aerosol was studied by two groups in patients with bronchiolitis.[37,38] These controlled studies reported a significant improvement in the ribavirin group compared with the control group. Viral shedding, however, was not affected in one study, which may have been attributable to the short duration of the therapy.[37] No adverse effects were observed with the use of ribavirin aerosol in either study. It should be pointed

Table 3.
Studies of Anti-infective Agents in Children with Bronchiolitis

Reference No.	No. Patients (Age)	Drug and Dose[a]	Tests To Duration of Therapy	Response Evaluate Therapy	or Outcome
37[b]	26 (mean 3.8 mo)	Ribavirin aerosol, 10 mg/kg every 12 hours (12 patients); saline inhalation every 12 hours (14 patients)	Began after RSV[c] shedding noted and continued for five days	RSV titers and clinical status	No significant difference but earlier initiation and longer treatments may be beneficial
38[b]	33	Ribavirin aerosol, 0.82 mg/kg/hr (16 patients); water inhalation (17 patients)	Therapy began at about 1.5 days after admission and continued for 3–6 days	RSV titers, blood gases, and clinical score	Significant improvement and decreased RSV shedding with ribavirin
39[b,d]	44	Ampicillin, 125 mg every six hours (25 patients); placebo (19 patients); all received ephedrine, 16 mg every eight hours	Therapy continued until signs and symptoms disappeared	Clinical status	No improvement with ampicillin or placebo

[a] The time the drug therapy was started (i.e., during or after acute illness) and the severity of disease were unclear.
[b] Double-blind study.
[c] Respiratory syncytial virus.
[d] Randomized study.

out that ribavirin aerosol can be administered by the same equipment used to deliver oxygen or by endotracheal tube in infants requiring ventilatory assistance.[37,38] We are unaware of a convenient method for administering ribavirin aerosol at home to ambulatory patients.[38]

Since bronchiolitis is a viral illness, antibiotics are not indicated. Ampicillin offered no advantages when compared with placebo in one controlled study of patients with bronchiolitis.[39] Antibiotic therapy, however, should be considered during the course of therapy when a change in illness suggests the possibility of a secondary bacterial infection.[3] Bacterial culture samples (from the blood and tracheal aspirate) should be obtained before therapy.[3]

Limitations of Available Studies

In reviewing the available studies, several problems were identified:

1. Many investigations lacked well-controlled study designs;
2. The duration of therapy (e.g., single-dose versus several days) varied among the studies;
3. There was variation in the time the therapy was instituted (i.e., during or after acute illness)[30];
4. Uniform tests were not used to assess the pharmacologic and therapeutic effects;
5. A forced-oscillation method was used to measure lower-airway resistance in some studies, and its reliability in infants has been questioned[1];
6. There was missing information on the severity of illness in several studies;
7. Concomitant drugs were used in several studies;
8. Only a small number of patients were enrolled in some of the studies;
9. Blood gas concentrations were not consistently monitored to determine the efficacy of bronchodilators; and
10. Many investigators failed to perform virologic or serologic studies.

Therapeutic Approach

The limitations of the currently available studies on drug therapy may, in part, be responsible for the lack of a standard therapeutic approach for managing patients with bronchiolitis. There is no controversy about the importance of oxygen and fluid therapy. However, no uniform guidelines are available on the use of drugs beyond these supportive measures. Welliver[25] recommended the use of a test dose of epinephrine, since some patients appeared to benefit from such therapy. Theophylline therapy has been recommended for those patients responding to epinephrine; however, bronchodilators were not recommended for patients who failed to respond to test doses of epinephrine. Ellis[31] recommended the use of adrenergic aerosols as well as theophylline. Corticosteroids have been recommended for severely ill patients.[5,31] There is no clear evidence supporting the efficacy of any bronchodilator or corticosteroid in patients with bronchiolitis. The results of two studies with ribavirin appear promising and form the basis for the consideration of its use in severely ill patients.[38]

At our hospital, infants with bronchiolitis are generally managed with low concentrations of humidified oxygen. Arterial blood gases are monitored if the infant is cyanotic or has a respiratory rate >60 breaths/min. Ambient oxygen is adjusted to maintain the alveolar pressure of oxygen ($P_{A_{O_2}}$) > 60 mm Hg. Heart rates are routinely monitored, and infants less than two months of age are placed on apnea monitors. In all but the most mild cases, a trial of 1% isoetharine aerosol or subcutaneous epinephrine 1:1000, 0.01 mL/kg is given. If this treatment results in improved air movement and decreased wheezing, the child is given isoetharine aerosol every four hours or occasionally intravenous theophylline. Serum theophylline concentrations are carefully monitored with the realization that fivefold variations in theophylline clearance may be found in infants with bronchiolitis.[40] Patients who are unable to maintain $P_{A_{O_2}} > 50$ mm Hg with $F_{I_{O_2}} \geq 50\%$ or who maintain a $P_{A_{CO_2}} > 45$ mm Hg despite bronchodilator therapy are intubated and supported by mechanical ventilation because of the danger of respiratory failure.

Prognosis and Prevention

Because of the difficulty in distinguishing bronchiolitis from allergic respiratory disease, it is unclear if infants with bronchiolitis are at increased risk of developing reversible airways disease (asthma) as children or chronic obstructive pulmonary disease as adults. It has been found that about 50% of the patients with bronchiolitis have a subsequent episode of wheezing, and more than 75% of the patients have lung function abnormalities at their 12-month follow-up examinations after the acute illness.[41] In a study involving 23 infants with bronchiolitis who were re-evaluated at age 11 years, only 3 were found to have completely normal lung functions; 18 of the 23 children had oxygen tension values that were significantly lower than the control values.[42] The clinical importance of the continuing abnormal lung function is unknown. The mortality rate in patients with bronchiolitis has ranged from 2 to 5.5%.[43–45]

Because RSV is transmitted by direct contact from an adult or a sibling to an infant, handwashing is beneficial in preventing the spread of infection. The use of gowns and masks has been found unnecessary.[46] A 10-year study of acquired immunity to RSV showed that the induced immunity by the first infection had no demonstrable effect on illness associated with reinfection one year later; however, a considerable reduction in severity occurred with the third infection. These authors suggested that amelioration of illness rather than prevention of infection may be a realistic goal for immunoprophylaxis.[47] Various types of vaccines and immunoglobulins have been studied without success.[12]

Conclusion

Bronchiolitis is a common respiratory-tract illness in infants. Oxygen and fluid therapy have a clear role in the management of these patients. No evidence is available about the efficacy of bronchodilators and corticosteroids in bronchiolitis. Ribavirin can be considered in hospitalized patients with severe illness. Further studies are necessary to evaluate the role of ribavirin, combined use of corticosteroids and bronchodilators, vaccines, and immunoglobulins. Until specific guidelines are available, a variety of therapeutic approaches to managing patients with bronchiolitis will continue to be used.

References

1. Wohl ME, Chernick V. Bronchiolitis. *Am Rev Respir Dis.* 1978; 118:759–81.
2. Henderson FW, Clyde WA Jr, Collier AM et al. The etiologic and epidemiologic spectrum of bronchiolitis in pediatric practice. *J Pediatr.* 1979; 95:183–91.
3. Hubble D, Osborn GR. Acute bronchiolitis in children. *Br Med J.* 1941; 1:107–10.
4. Nelson WE. Viral or probable viral infections. In: Nelson WE, ed. Pediatrics. 6th ed. Philadelphia: W. B. Saunders Company; 1954:823–8, 1438–46.
5. Cherry JD. Bronchiolitis and asthmatic bronchitis. In: Feigin RD, Cherry JD, eds. Textbook of pediatric infectious diseases. Philadelphia: W. B. Saunders Company; 1981:178–86.
6. Wood SH, Buddingh GJ, Abberger BF Jr. An inquiry into the etiology of acute bronchiolitis of infants. *Pediatrics.* 1954; 13:363–72.
7. Sell SHW. Some observations on acute bronchiolitis in infants. *Am J Dis Child.* 1960; 100:31–9.
8. Macasaet FF, Kidd PA, Bolano CR et al. The etiology of acute respiratory infections. III. The role of viruses and bacteria. *J Pediatr.* 1968; 72:829–39.
9. Nichol KP, Cherry JD. Bacterial-viral interrelations in respiratory infections of children. *N Engl J Med.* 1967; 277:667–72.
10. Loda FA, Clyde WA Jr, Glezen WP et al. Studies on the role of viruses, bacteria, and *M. pneumoniae* as causes of lower respiratory tract infections in children. *J Pediatr.* 1978; 72:161–76.
11. Beem M, Wright FH, Fasan DM et al. Observations on the etiology of acute bronchiolitis in infants. *J Pediatr.* 1962; 61:864–9.
12. Hall CB. Respiratory syncytial virus. In: Feigin RD, Cherry JD, eds. Textbook of pediatric infectious diseases. Philadelphia: W. B. Saunders Company; 1981; 1247–67.
13. Hall CB, Geiman JM, Douglas RG Jr. Possible transmission by fomites of respiratory syncytial virus. *J Infect Dis.* 1980; 141:98–102.
14. Hall CB, Douglas RG Jr. Modes of transmission of respiratory syncytial virus. *J Pediatr.* 1981; 99:100–3.
15. Pratt EL. Acute bronchiolitis in infants. *Med Clin North Am.* 1944; 28:1098–107.
16. Gurwitz D, Mindorff C, Levison H. Increased incidence of bronchial reactivity in children with a history of bronchiolitis. *J Pediatr.* 1981; 98:551–5.
17. Downes JJ, Wood DW, Striker TW et al. Acute respiratory

failure in infants with bronchiolitis. *Anesthesiology.* 1968; 29:426–34.
18. Reynolds EOR. Bronchiolitis. In: Kendig EL Jr, ed. Disorders of the respiratory tract in children. Philadelphia: W. B. Saunders Company; 1967:272–82.
19. Wright FH, Beem MO. Diagnosis and treatment: management of acute viral bronchiolitis in infancy. *Pediatrics.* 1965; 35:334–7.
20. Ellis EF. Therapy of acute bronchiolitis. *Pediatr Res.* 1977; 11:263–4.
21. Mellins RB. Bronchiolitis—comments on pathogenesis and treatment. *Pediatr Res.* 1977; 11:268–9.
22. Simpson H, Matthew DJ, Inglis JM et al. Virological findings and blood gas tensions in acute lower respiratory tract infections in children. *Br Med J.* 1974; 2:629–32.
23. Taussig LM. Mists and aerosols: new studies, new thoughts. *J Pediatr.* 1974; 84:619–22.
24. Bau SK, Aspin N, Wood DE et al. The measurement of fluid deposition in humans following mist tent therapy. *Pediatrics.* 1971; 48:605–12.
25. Welliver RC. Bronchiolitis: update for managing patients this winter. *J Respir Dis.* 1982; 3:19–29.
26. Phelan PD, Williams HE. Sympathomimetic drugs in acute viral bronchiolitis. Their effect on pulmonary resistance. *Pediatrics.* 1969; 44:493–7.
27. Rutter C, Milner AD, Hillier EJ. Effect of bronchodilators on bronchiolitis and wheezy bronchitis. *Arch Dis Child.* 1975; 44:493–7.
28. Lenney W, Milner AD. Alpha and beta adrenergic stimulants in children under 18 months of age. *Arch Dis Child.* 1978; 53:107–9.
29. Lenney W, Milner AD. At what age do bronchodilator drugs work? *Arch Dis Child* 1978; 53:532–5.
30. Stokes GM, Milner AD, Hodges IGC et al. Nebulized therapy in acute severe bronchiolitis in infancy. *Arch Dis Child.* 1980; 58:279–83.
31. Ellis EF. Therapy of acute bronchiolitis. *Pediatr Res.* 1977; 11:263–4.
32. Brooks LJ, Cropp GJA. Theophylline therapy in bronchiolitis: a retrospective study. *Am J Dis Child.* 1981; 135:934–6.
33. Dabbousia IA, Tkachyk JS, Stamm SJ. A double-blind study of the effect of corticosteroids in the treatment of bronchiolitis. *Pediatrics.* 1966; 37:477–84.
34. Leer JA, Green JL, Heimlich EM et al. Corticosteroids treatment in bronchiolitis. *Am J Dis Child.* 1969; 117:495–503.
35. Sussman S, Grossman M, Magoffin R et al. Dexamethasone in obstructive respiratory tract infection in children: a controlled study. *Pediatrics.* 1964; 34:851–5.
36. Tal A, Bavilski C, Yohai D et al. Dexamethazone and salbutamol in the treatment of acute wheezing in infants. *Pediatrics.* 1983; 71:13–8.
37. Taber LH, Knight V, Gilbert BE et al. Ribavirin aerosol treatment of bronchiolitis associated with respiratory syncytial virus infection in infants. *Pediatrics.* 1983; 72:613–8.
38. Hall CB, McBride JT, Walsh EE et al. Aerosolized ribavirin treatment of infants with respiratory syncytial viral infection: a randomized double-blind study. *N Engl J Med.* 1981; 308:1443–7.
39. Field CMB, Connolly JH, Murtagh G et al. Antibiotic treatment of epidemic bronchiolitis—a double-blind trial. *Br Med J.* 1966; 1:83–5.
40. Franko TG, Powell DA, Nahata MC. Pharmacokinetics of theophylline in infants with bronchiolitis. *Eur J Clin Pharmacol.* 1983; 23:123–7.
41. Stokes GM, Milner GM, Hodges IGC et al. Lung function abnormalities after acute bronchrolites. *J Pediatr.* 1981; 93:871–4.
42. Kattan M, Keens TG, Lapierre JG et al. Pulmonary function abnormalities in symptom-free children after bronchiolitis. *Pediatrics.* 1977; 59:683-8.
43. Henderson AT, Rosenzweig S. Bronchiolitis in infancy. Clinical study with special emphasis on the cardiac complications. *U.S. Armed Forces Med. J.* 1951; 2:943–52.
44. Dennis JL, Palmer WM, Cleveland RW. Bronchiolitis in infants. Problem in practice. *JAMA.* 1960; 172:688–91.
45. Heycock JB, Noble TC. 1,230 cases of acute bronchiolitis in infancy. *Br Med J.* 1962; 2:879–81.
46. Hall CB, Douglas MD. Nosocomial respiratory syncytial viral infection: should gowns and masks be used? *Am J Dis Child.* 1981; 135:512–5.
47. Henderson FW, Collier AM, Clyde WA et al. Respiratory syncytial virus infections, reinfections and immunity: a prospective, longitudinal study in young children. *N Engl J Med.* 1979; 300:530–4.

“

Gaps in Our Knowledge about Hypertension

The long-term results of [antihypertensive] drug therapy over many decades remain unknown. Some studies raise questions about risks associated with drug therapy. The data from the Multiple Risk Factor Intervention Trial suggest that *mild* hypertensives with electrocardiographic abnormalities may have a higher mortality rate when treated with thiazide diuretics. Other recent work indicates that some antihypertensive drugs raise cholesterol levels or lower high-density lipoprotein levels so that the benefit of reduced blood pressure may be offset by an increased cardiovascular risk from lipid anomalies. Currently, we use different drugs empirically without often knowing the mechanisms by which blood pressure is reduced. It is hoped that future studies will explain the mechanism of action of the various antihypertensive drugs, will elucidate possible genetic and acquired differences in response to these drugs, and will clarify the etiologic heterogeneity of hypertension. Most importantly, it is hoped that we will learn how to predict the specific target organ risk of the various hypertensive complications more accurately. In the future, a "diagnosis" of "essential hypertension" in a given patient may be as archaic as would be a diagnosis of fever or anemia today without specifying the underlying causes. It is sobering to admit that although we have made extraordinary progress in biomedical research, large gaps remain in our understanding of the fundamental mechanisms of the biochemistry, genetics, physiology, pathology, and pharmacology of high blood pressure. More fundamental and epidemiologic research is badly needed.

—Burke W, Motulsky AG. Hypertension: some unanswered questions. *JAMA.* 1985; 253:2260–1. Editorial.

”

Management of antibiotic-associated pseudomembranous colitis

MARK H. GROSS

Abstract: The diagnosis, etiology, epidemiology, and drug therapy of antibiotic-associated pseudomembranous colitis (AAPMC) are reviewed.

AAPMC is an uncommon but potentially serious adverse reaction to therapy with almost any oral or injectable antibiotic and certain antineoplastic agents that alter intestinal flora. Proliferation of *Clostridium difficile* and subsequent release of clostridial cytotoxins cause pseudomembranous lesions and symptoms such as watery diarrhea, cramping abdominal pain, and low-grade fever. Symptoms can appear from four days after the start of antibiotic or antineoplastic therapy to 10 weeks after therapy has been discontinued.

Drug therapy of AAPMC is directed at reducing the amount of *Cl. difficile* in the colon and promoting normalization of intestinal flora. Mild cases of AAPMC may respond to discontinuation of the etiologic agent and replacement of fluid and electrolytes. Therapy with an anticlostridial antibiotic is indicated in severe cases; although a seven- to 10-day course of oral vancomycin hydrochloride is the most widely recognized therapy, the drug is expensive and unpalatable. Good results have been reported with oral metronidazole and with bacitracin, both of which are less expensive than vancomycin. For all of these therapies, relapse rates are 20–39%. Anion exchange resins may be useful in mild cases of AAPMC.

Successful management of AAPMC depends on a complex and ill-defined interrelationship between normal intestinal flora, patient immune response, antibiotic therapy, and the infecting clostridium strain. For moderate or severe cases of AAPMC, therapy should begin with metronidazole or bacitracin and vancomycin should be reserved for refractory cases, relapses, or patients with allergies to the other agents.

Index terms: Antibiotics; Anti-infective agents; Antineoplastic agents; Bacitracin; Costs; Enterocolitis; Metronidazole; Toxicity; Vancomycin
Clin Pharm. 1985; 4:304–10

Antibiotic-associated pseudomembranous colitis (AAPMC) is an uncommon but potentially serious adverse reaction to therapy with almost any oral or injectable antibiotic that alters colonic flora. A direct relationship between onset of disease, recent antibiotic therapy, and high concentrations of *Clostridium difficile* in the colon was established in the late 1970s; before that time, gastrointestinal surgery, intestinal obstruction, uremia, and *Staphylococcus aureus* overgrowth were all believed to be predisposing factors for AAPMC.[1] Although clindamycin therapy is implicated most frequently as the cause of this disease,[2] recent evidence indicates that clindamycin does not cause AAPMC any more frequently than do other commonly used antibiotics such as ampicillin or the cephalosporins.[3] AAPMC has also occurred after the administration of certain antineoplastic agents.[3] The antibiotics and antineoplastic agents that have been associated with pseudomembranous colitis are listed in Table 1.

Diagnosis and Etiology

The clinical features of AAPMC include watery diarrhea, cramping abdominal pain, low-grade fever, hypoalbuminemia, and leukocytosis.[11] Abdominal tenderness and bloody diarrhea occur in about 10% of cases, and fever occurs in up to 80%. Colonic perforation and toxic megacolon occur rarely.[12] Symptoms can appear from four days after the start of antibiotic therapy to 10 weeks after therapy with the offending drug is discontinued.[11,12]

Pathophysiologic changes can occur in any section of the colon, and the affected areas may not be detected if only a proctoscopic examination is performed. Pseudomembranous lesions resemble whitish-yellow raised plaques.[13] The colonic mucosa may be erythematous, edematous, friable, ulcerated, and necrotic.[11,13]

No single factor can substantiate the diagnosis of AAPMC. Diarrhea is a relatively common side effect of oral therapy with many antibiotics, and only 15–25% of such cases are caused by clostridial toxins.[14,15] Even if clostridial toxins are isolated, the diagnosis of AAPMC cannot be confirmed because some individuals are asymptomatic carriers of *Cl. difficile* and its cytotoxin.[16–18] Currently, the most useful diagnostic test is a cell-culture assay that produces a characteristic cytopathologic effect in the presence of *Cl. difficile* cytotoxin. If the cyto-

MARK H. GROSS, PHARM.D., is Clinical Pharmacist, Department of Pharmacy, Box 3089, Duke University Medical Center, Durham, NC 27710.

The secretarial assistance of Nita Ashby is acknowledged.
This is **article 680-204-8510** in the **ASHP Continuing Education System.** See page 338 for learning objectives and test questions.

Table 1.
Antibiotics and Antineoplastic Agents Associated with Pseudomembranous Colitis[2-10]

Antibiotics	
Amoxicillin	Neomycin
Amphotericin B	Penicillin G
Ampicillin[a]	Penicillin V
Carbenicillin	Rifampin
Cephalosporins[a,b]	Sulfamethoxazole–Trimethoprim
Chloramphenicol	Tetracycline
Clindamycin[a]	Ticarcillin
Cloxacillin	Tobramycin
Erythromycin	
Gentamicin	
Lincomycin	*Antineoplastics*
Methicillin	Cyclophosphamide
Metronidazole	Doxorubicin
Nafcillin	Fluorouracil
	Methotrexate

[a] Most frequently associated with pseudomembranous colitis.
[b] Includes cefazolin, cefotaxime, cefuroxime, cefoxitin, cefamandole, cephalexin, cephalothin, cephaloridine, cephradine, and moxalactam.

pathologic effect is prevented by pretreatment with clostridial antitoxin, *Cl. difficile* toxin is presumed to be present.[14]

Although visualization of pseudomembranous plaques is helpful, it is not always necessary for diagnosis, especially if the lesions are confined to the proximal colon or if colonoscopy would present a substantial risk to the patient. The diagnosis of AAPMC can be made if a positive cell-culture assay result accompanies clinical symptoms of AAPMC that are temporally associated with recent antibiotic use.

For AAPMC to occur, drug-induced alteration of colonic flora must be present. The disease can occur even if the infecting clostridial strain is sensitive to the causative antibiotic.[19] The theory that *Cl. difficile* can proliferate and cause disease only in an environment that lacks competing bacterial flora[20] has been confirmed by animal studies in which AAPMC could be produced only in antibiotic-treated animals or newborn animals with sterile intestines.[21,22]

In humans, increasing age is the only other important risk factor. AAPMC has been shown to occur more frequently in older adults than in children, and anticlostridial antibodies have been found more frequently in young adults than in elderly patients.[23]

Early observations that clindamycin was fatal to hamsters led investigators to search for a relationship between hemorrhagic cecitis and antibiotic therapy with clindamycin.[21,24] Bartlett et al.[25] isolated a cytopathologic substance from the feces of hamsters with clindamycin-induced hemorrhagic cecitis. This substance, which was purified from stool cultures of *Cl. difficile*, could induce enterocolitis in healthy animals if injected intracecally. In an analogous study using stool samples from patients with gastrointestinal complications of clindamycin or ampicillin therapy (diarrhea, pseudomembranous colitis), a substance purified from the stools of patients with pseudomembranous colitis was shown to be cytotoxic in cell cultures.[22] The substance also induced enterocolitis in hamsters if injected intracecally. Similar results were demonstrated when *Cl. difficile* cultured from the stool samples was injected into hamsters. Both cytotoxicity in cell culture and enterocolitis in hamsters were prevented by pretreatment with clostridial antitoxin; this antitoxin was later purified and found to be the antitoxin from *Clostridium sordellii*.[26]

The pathogenic cytotoxin of *Cl. difficile* has not yet been fully characterized, but at least two distinct components appear to be involved. Clostridial toxin A may be enterotoxic and toxin B may have cytotoxic properties.[27] A third factor, which alters motility, may also be present.[28]

Epidemiology

The incidence and distribution of AAPMC are poorly understood. Overall estimates of the incidence of AAPMC in the general population range from 0.001% to 10%, depending on geographic location.[12] Unlike other infectious diseases, AAPMC can result from proliferation of *Cl. difficile* acquired from both endogenous and exogenous sources.[29] Inconsistent isolation techniques and nonstandardized growth media have made epidemiologic studies difficult to interpret.

Clinical manifestation of AAPMC seems to depend on a number of interacting factors, including previous antibiotic therapy, competing intestinal flora, and the presence of *Cl. difficile*. *Cl. difficile* or clostridial antibodies are present in the intestinal flora of neonates but are rarely found in stool samples from adults.[16,17,30] Hafiz et al.[31] isolated *Cl. difficile* from the urinary tracts of 100% of adult men with nonspecific urethritis and 72% of adult women patients of a venereal disease clinic. However, variations in culture techniques have prevented these results from being replicated.[29] *Cl. difficile* has also been detected in stool samples from asymptomatic patients receiving antibiotics.[32]

Exogenous sources of *Cl. difficile* are also important in the epidemiology of AAPMC. Spores or viable organisms have been cultured from the hospital environment and from asymptomatic hospital personnel.[33-35] Fekety et al.[35] sampled multiple hospital sites with a clostridium-selective agar culture medium and obtained positive cultures from bedding, toilets, floors, and washbasins. Positive cultures were also obtained from fingers and stool specimens of asymptomatic hospital personnel who worked near patients with AAPMC. Viable spores have been obtained from inanimate objects up to five months after contamination.[35,36] For these reasons, several authors have recommended

Table 2.
Patient Response to Drug Therapy for Antibiotic-Associated Pseudomembranous Colitis

Reference No.	Daily Dose	Duration of Therapy (days)	No. Patients Treated	Patient Outcome Response	Failure	Relapse
Vancomycin Hydrochloride						
4	2 g	7–10	9	9	0	0
5	2 g	5–17	3	3[a]	0	3
39, 40	0.5–2 g	5–21	100	97[a]	3	26
41	500 mg	5	22	19	3	0
42	2 g	10	52	45	0	6
43	2 g	10	1	0	1	0
Metronidazole						
6	2 g	10	1	0	0	1
42	1 g	10	42	37	2	2
44	1.5–2 g	7–14	13	11	0	2
Bacitracin						
45	100,000 U	7–10	4	3	0	1
46	100,000 U	6–10	2	2	0	0

[a] Response to first course of therapy only.

that enteric isolation precautions be taken with patients with AAPMC.[18,29]

Drug Therapy

Drug therapy of AAPMC is directed at reducing the amount of *Cl. difficile* cytotoxin in the colon and promoting normalization of intestinal flora. Drug therapy should be initiated only after other forms of colitis have been ruled out and, optimally, after stool samples have been obtained, positive cell-culture assay results have been reported, and a colonoscopic examination has revealed the presence of pseudomembranous plaques.

The goal of drug therapy for mild attacks of AAPMC is to prevent progression of the disease by decreasing the amount of cytotoxin in the colon and promoting normalization of fecal flora. The etiologic agent should be discontinued and replacement therapy with appropriate fluids and electrolytes should be initiated.[11] Although the use of such antidiarrheal agents as diphenoxylate with atropine (Lomotil, Searle Laboratories) or loperamide (Imodium, Janssen Pharmaceutica) in mild cases of AAPMC has been reported, use of these drugs may worsen or prolong the clinical course.[37,38]

In severe cases of AAPMC, therapy with an anticlostridial antibiotic is indicated to eradicate the high concentrations of *Cl. difficile* and halt further production of cytotoxin. Vancomycin, metronidazole, and bacitracin have all been used in the treatment of AAPMC with varying degrees of success (Table 2). These antibiotics have sometimes been used in conjunction with anion exchange resins such as cholestyramine and colestipol. The costs associated with various therapeutic regimens for AAPMC are outlined in Table 3.

Table 3.
Costs of Drug Therapy for Antibiotic-Associated Pseudomembranous Colitis

Agent	Regimen	Cost[a] ($)
Vancomycin	500 mg q.i.d. × 7 days	530.60
	500 mg q.i.d. × 7 days	255.75[b]
	125 mg q.i.d. × 7 days	189.50
Metronidazole	250 mg q.i.d. × 10 days	21.70
Bacitracin	25,000 U q.i.d. × 7 days	110.50
Cholestyramine	4 g t.i.d. × 7 days	31.70

[a] 1984 Average wholesale price as listed in *Drug Topics Red Book Annual Pharmacists' Reference* (Oradell, NJ: Medical Economics Company Inc.; 1984).
[b] Cost of 10-g vial of powder for oral use.

Vancomycin. A 10-day course of therapy with vancomycin (as the hydrochloride salt) 500–2000 mg/day orally in four divided doses is the preferred therapy for AAPMC.[4,39] This regimen can produce fecal concentrations of vancomycin that are several hundred times the concentration needed to inhibit toxin-producing strains of *Cl. difficile*.[4,41] Diarrhea, cramping, and fever usually subside within two to four days after the initiation of therapy, and stool toxin titers usually decrease within one week.[11] Although vancomycin therapy is considered nonsystemic, measurable serum vancomycin concentrations have been found in patients with both normal and compromised renal function during oral vancomycin therapy.[47,48]

Relapses occur frequently despite the extreme sensitivity of *Cl. difficile* to vancomycin, the absence of vancomycin-resistant strains, and easily achievable bactericidal concentrations of vancomycin. Chang et al.[45] reported that 20 of 100 patients with AAPMC experienced one or more relapses following therapy with vancomycin. Bartlett et al.[40] reported a 14% relapse rate among 79 patients treated with vancomycin 500–2000 mg/day for 6 to 21 days; relapses occurred 4 to 21 days after vancomycin therapy was discontinued. Of 19 patients who received a second course of vancomycin therapy, 79% responded positively. Recent cumulative data from Bartlett et al.[39] demonstrated that of 100 patients treated with vancomycin, 91% had a good response to therapy (i.e., patients improved promptly and recovered without changes in treatment), 6% had a fair response (i.e., patients had definite improvement with some changes in therapy needed or some symptoms persisting), and 3% were treatment failures (i.e., no response was seen with or without changes in therapy). However, 26% of those patients suffered from one to six relapses, and AAPMC was a major or contributing cause of death in three of those patients.

Failure to obtain bactericidal concentrations of vancomycin does not seem to be the cause of relapses; relapses can occur even when fecal vancomycin concentrations are 3000 $\mu g/g$, no resistant strains have been isolated, and minimum inhibitory concentrations are 2 $\mu g/mL$ or less.[39,43] George et al.[5] described three patients with recurring AAPMC, one of whom died after receiving vancomycin therapy for a second relapse. An early case report by Marrie et al.[49] discussed a patient in whom a relapse of AAPMC did respond to a second course of vancomycin therapy. Eglinton et al.[43] described a patient with AAPMC who did not respond to two courses of therapy with vancomycin 500 mg orally every six hours even though stool cultures revealed *Cl. difficile* that was susceptible to vancomycin at 0.25 $\mu g/mL$.

The reports of relapses of AAPMC contradict the theory that, to cure clostridial pseudomembranous colitis, very high colonic concentrations of vancomycin should be used even if the strain is extremely sensitive. Although *Cl. difficile* is a spore-forming bacillus, resistant spores have not been isolated from the colon. Reinfections may therefore be caused by introduction of spores from exogenous sources before the host's normal gut flora are reestablished.

No clostridium strains that are resistant or tolerant to vancomycin have been isolated, although resistance to clindamycin and tetracycline has been shown.[18] Many oral antibiotics are associated with AAPMC, but it is unlikely that vancomycin causes AAPMC even though it can cause lethal enterocolitis in hamsters.[50]

Paradoxically, some patients improve clinically even when cytotoxin can be isolated from stool.[39] It is possible that competing intestinal flora reduce the number of pathogenic bacteria in the colon. The host may also develop an immune response. However, cure implies eradication of the infectious agent, a negative cytotoxin assay, and no clinical symptoms of disease.

Metronidazole. Metronidazole has also been used to treat AAPMC. Teasley et al.[42] found no significant differences in relapse rates or number of treatment failures among 94 patients who received 10-day courses of therapy with either vancomycin or metronidazole. Treatment failed in two of 51 patients who received metronidazole. Treatment failure was defined as persistence of four or more watery stools per day after six days of antibiotic treatment. Relapse was defined as recurrence within 21 days of diarrhea and *Cl. difficile* or cytotoxin in a patient whose bowel pattern had returned to normal after previous treatment with a 10-day course of vancomycin or metronidazole. Six of 52 patients receiving vancomycin and two of 42 patients receiving metronidazole suffered relapses. The findings of this study have been challenged because of the relatively small sample sizes of each group (which may mask differences between the two regimens).[51]

Patients with AAPMC whose symptoms do not improve after therapy with metronidazole may require therapy with vancomycin to eradicate *Cl. difficile* toxin; the converse of this statement may also be true. Cherry et al.[44] described 13 patients whose diarrhea resolved within five days of beginning therapy with metronidazole 1.5–2.0 g/day orally. Two patients who suffered relapses were later cured by vancomycin therapy. Portnoy et al.[6] described one patient who was cured by vancomycin therapy after one 10-day course of metronidazole therapy and a second course of therapy with metronidazole plus cholestyramine both were unsuccessful. In contrast, Eglinton et al.[43] described a patient who was cured by metronidazole therapy after two courses of vancomycin therapy were unsuccessful.

"Pulse" therapy with metronidazole may be used in conjunction with standard metronidazole therapy in patients whose clinical response to treatment is poor, or this therapy may be used alone after a 10-day course of metronidazole therapy to eradicate any remaining viable organisms or spores and prevent a relapse of AAPMC. Mitchell and Gaver[52] successfully treated one patient who had had no reponse to vancomycin therapy with three cycles of 10-day "pulses" of metronidazole 750 mg orally q.i.d. followed by five days without drug. This patient suffered no relapses during a six-month follow-up period.

Thus, relapses of AAPMC can respond to a second seven- to 10-day course of the same drug. The most important preventive measure against relapses may be limiting patient exposure to viable spores from the surrounding environment and from personnel who might be asymptomatic carriers of spores.

Despite its economic advantage and possible therapeutic equivalence to vancomycin, metronidazole is not an ideal drug for AAPMC. Unlike vancomycin, metronidazole is absorbed before it reaches the colon but may still be active in the large intestine because of biliary excretion.[53] Although systemic absorption of metronidazole exposes the patient to potential side effects, adverse reactions are usually minimal.[54]

A number of studies have implicated oral metronidazole as a cause of AAPMC.[7-9] Saginur et al.[7] reported a patient in whom clinical and cytopathological evidence of AAPMC followed therapy with metronidazole. Metronidazole given concurrently with other antimicrobials was associated with colitis in four patients described by Kappas et al.[8] However, these findings should not discourage use of metronidazole in the treatment of AAPMC, especially if the infecting clostridium strain is sensitive to metronidazole.

Indeed, metronidazole may be useful in any case of AAPMC that is not directly associated with the previous use of this drug. Although most data indicate that metronidazole is probably clinically equivalent to vancomycin in terms of rates of response and relapse, larger clinical studies are needed before metronidazole can be considered therapeutically superior, equivalent, or inferior to vancomycin. Evidence indicates that metronidazole can be used successfully as first-line therapy in a majority of patients, with vancomycin reserved for treatment of refractory cases or relapses. Intravenous metronidazole may also be preferred therapy for patients who cannot tolerate oral medications.[39]

Bacitracin. Bacitracin is another alternative therapy for AAPMC. Like vancomycin, bacitracin is active against anaerobes and is not absorbed after oral administration. Chang et al.[45] successfully treated four patients with 25,000 U (500 mg) of bacitracin powder for intravenous use dissolved in water and taken orally four times daily for 10 days. Two of these patients had previously received unsuccessful therapy with vancomycin. Tedesco[46] successfully treated two patients, one who had received two unsuccessful courses of vancomycin therapy and one who was allergic to vancomycin, with a similar bacitracin regimen. Young et al.[55] found bacitracin 80,000 U/day orally to be significantly less effective in eradicating *Cl. difficile* from stool than vancomycin 500 mg/day orally, but symptomatic improvement and eradication of cytotoxin were similar in patients receiving bacitracin or vancomycin. The authors suggested that therapy with bacitracin should be considered an alternative to vancomycin therapy for AAPMC.

A comparison of cost-effectiveness of vancomycin, metronidazole, and bacitracin indicates that empiric therapy with bacitracin or metronidazole may be more cost-effective than vancomycin therapy when there is a high probability of AAPMC. However, vancomycin therapy is probably more cost-effective in patients known to have toxin-positive stools but an otherwise low probability of disease.[56]

Exchange Resins. By binding clostridial enterotoxins in the colon, anion exchange resins such as cholestyramine or colestipol may be useful in patients with mild cases of AAPMC. Resins are thought to be ineffective in severe cases of AAPMC because they only bind toxins and do not eradicate *Cl. difficile*. Although Kreutzer and Milligan[10] reported that the good results they witnessed in 12 patients who received cholestyramine 4 g orally for 3–19 days were unrelated to severity of disease, Tedesco et al.[57] found that the resins were effective only in patients with milder symptoms. Keighley[58] treated 17 patients with either colestipol or a placebo and found that 36% responded to colestipol compared with 22% who responded to placebo.

Simultaneous use of cholestyramine resin and vancomycin has been advocated, but resins have been shown to bind vancomycin in vitro. Some authors have recommended that the two drugs be administered several hours apart to avoid this interaction.[11] However, King and Barriere[59] assessed the in vitro antibacterial activity of vancomycin-cholestyramine suspensions and found that binding of vancomycin to cholestyramine did not affect the antibiotic activity of vancomycin. Resins may best be used in conjunction with an antibiotic to suppress the effects of cytotoxins in patients who do not respond to other therapies. Tedesco[11] treated nine such patients with two courses of vancomycin 125 mg orally q.i.d. followed by vancomycin dosages gradually tapered over a two-week period plus colestipol hydrochloride 4 g b.i.d. Colestipol therapy was then maintained without vancomycin therapy until normal colonic flora could be re-established.

Other Approaches. Unorthodox approaches to treatment of AAPMC have included rectal administration of normal stool flora and injections of clostridial antitoxin. Based on the assumption that AAPMC results from altered colonic flora, Bowden et al.[60] administered enemas of stool from normal subjects to patients with AAPMC and noted favorable results in 13 of 16 patients. Anticipated poor patient acceptance of this therapy, as well as the danger of transmitting other enteric diseases, should limit its widespread use even if positive results are replicated.

The antitoxin produced by *Cl. sordellii* can neutralize in vitro the clostridial cytotoxins A and B, which are thought to be pathogenic.[22] Therefore, the antitoxin could theoretically serve as an antidote, but preliminary animal data do not prove this hypothesis. Bartlett[39] administered intraperitoneal or intracardiac injections of antitoxin to hamsters but failed to confer protection against cytotoxins and disease. However, this does not rule out the development of a human vaccine against cytotoxins once human antibodies are isolated and purified in large quantities.

Conclusion

Antibiotic-associated pseudomembranous colitis cannot always be cured simply by a two-week course of a potent anticlostridial agent. Relapses may occur in 20–39% of patients even if the clostridial strain is exquisitely sensitive to the antimicrobial. Eradication of *Cl. difficile* seems dependent on the complex and ill-defined interaction between normal stool flora, immune response, antibiotics, and the infecting strain.

Vancomycin has been considered the drug of choice for AAPMC, but it is very expensive, its bitter taste makes oral administration unpleasant, and rates of relapse up to 39% have been reported. Metronidazole is a less expensive agent that may be as effective as vancomycin, but its disadvantages include systemic absorption and a possible role as a cause of AAPMC. Bacitracin may also be an alternative to vancomycin. It has good activity against anaerobes, minimal oral absorption, and lower cost, but more comparative studies are needed to prove its effectiveness.

Mild cases of AAPMC may respond to therapy with binding resins such as cholestyramine or colestipol and supportive fluids and electrolytes. A rational and cost-effective approach to treating moderate or severe AAPMC may be to start therapy with metronidazole or bacitracin, and reserve vancomycin therapy for refractory cases, relapses, or patients with allergies to the other agents.

References

1. Bartlett JG, Gorbach SL. Pseudomembranous enterocolitis (antibiotic-related colitis). *Adv Intern Med.* 1977; 22:455–76.
2. Tedesco FJ, Barton RW, Alpers DH. Clindamycin-associated colitis: a prospective study. *Ann Intern Med.* 1974; 81:429–33.
3. Silva J, Fekety R, Werk C et al. Inciting and etiologic agents of colitis. *Rev Infect Dis.* 1984; Suppl 6:S214–21.
4. Tedesco F, Markham R, Gurwith M. Oral vancomycin for antibiotic-associated pseudomembranous colitis. *Lancet.* 1978; 2:226–8.
5. George WL, Volpicelli NA, Stiner DB et al. Relapse of pseudomembranous colitis after vancomycin therapy. *N Engl J Med.* 1979; 301:414–5.
6. Portnoy D, Soneji A, Murray A et al. Pseudomembranous colitis: multiple relapses after treatment with metronidazole. *Can Med Assoc J.* 1981; 124:1603–5.
7. Saginur R, Hawley CR, Bartlett JG. Colitis associated with metronidazole therapy. *J Infect Dis* 1980; 141:772–3.
8. Kappas HA, Shinagawa N, Arabi Y et al. Diagnosis of pseudomembranous colitis. *Br Med J.* 1978; 1:675–8.
9. Daly J, Chowdory KVJ. Pseudomembranous colitis secondary to metronidazole. *Dig Dis Sci.* 1983; 28:573–4.
10. Kreutzer EW, Milligan FD. Treatment of antibiotic-associated pseudomembranous colitis with cholestyramine resin. *Johns Hopkins Med J.* 1978; 143:67–72.
11. Tedesco FJ. Pseudomembranous colitis: pathogenesis and therapy. *Med Clin North Am.* 1982; 66:655–63.
12. Silva J, Fekety R. Clostridial and antimicrobial enterocolitis. *Annu Rev Med.* 1981; 32:327–33.
13. George WL. Antimicrobial agent-associated colitis and diarrhea: historical background and clinical aspects. *Rev Infect Dis.* 1984; 6 (Suppl):S208–13.
14. Bartlett JG, Dzink J. Clinical and laboratory observations in *Clostridium difficile. Am J Clin Nutr.* 1980; 33:2521–6.
15. Burdon DW, George RH, Mogg GAG et al. Faecal toxin and severity of antibiotic-associated pseudomembranous colitis. *J Clin Pathol.* 1981; 34:548–51.
16. George WL, Rolfe RD, Mulligan ME et al. Infectious diseases 1979—antimicrobial agent-induced colitis: an update. *J Infect Dis.* 1979; 140:266–8.
17. Viscidi R, Willey S, Bartlett JG. Isolation rates and toxigenic potential of *Clostridium difficile* isolates from various patient populations. *Gastroenterology.* 1981; 81:5–9.
18. Burdon DW. *Clostridium difficile*: the epidemiology and prevention of hospital-acquired infections. *Infection.* 1982; 10:203–4. Editorial.
19. Dzink J, Bartlett JG. In vitro sensitivities of *Clostridium difficile* isolates from patients with antibiotic-associated pseudomembranous colitis or diarrhea. *Antimicrob Agents Chemother.* 1980; 17:695–8.
20. Bartlett JG. Antibiotic-associated pseudomembranous colitis. *Hosp Pract.* 1981; 16:85–95.
21. Bartlett JG, Onderdonk AB, Cisneros RJ et al. Clindamycin-associated colitis due to a toxin-producing strain of *Clostridium* in hamsters. *J Infect Dis.* 1977; 136:701–5.
22. Bartlett JG, Chang TW, Gurwith M et al. Antibiotic-associated pseudomembranous colitis due to toxin-producing Clostridia. *N Engl J Med.* 1978; 298:531–4.
23. Nakamura S, Mikawa M, Nakashio S et al. Isolation of *Clostridium difficile* from the feces and antibodies in sera of young and elderly patients. *Microbiol Immunol.* 1981; 25:345–51.
24. Rifkin G, Silva J, Fekety R. Intestinal and systemic toxicity of fecal extracts from hamsters with clindamycin-induced colitis. Paper presented to 17th Interscience Conference on Antimicrobial Agents and Chemotherapy. New York, NY: 1977 Oct 12.
25. Bartlett JG, Chang TW, Moon N et al. Antibiotic-induced lethal enterocolitis in hamsters: studies with eleven agents and evidence to support the pathogenic role of toxin-producing Clostridia. *Am J Vet Res.* 1978; 39:1525–30.
26. Rifkin GD, Fekety FR, Silva J et al. Antibiotic-induced colitis: implication of a toxin neutralized by *Clostridium sordellii* antitoxin. *Lancet.* 1977; 2:1103–5.
27. Taylor NS, Thorne G, Bartlett JG. Comparison of two toxins produced by *Clostridium difficile. Infect Immun.* 1981; 1036–43.
28. Justus PG, Martin JL, Goldberg DA et al. Myoelectric effects of *Clostridium difficile:* motility-altering factors distinct from the cytotoxin and enterotoxin in rabbits. *Gastroenterology.* 1982; 83:836–43.
29. Mulligan M. Epidemiology of *Clostridium difficile*-induced intestinal disease. *Rev Infect Dis.* 1984; 6 (Suppl):S222–8.
30. George RH, Hartley S. Antibodies to *Clostridium difficile* cytotoxin in a pediatric population. *Am J Dis Child.* 1983; 137:1024–5.
31. Hafiz S, McEtegart MG, Mortan RS et al. *Clostridium difficile* in the urogenital tract of males and females. *Lancet.* 1974; 1:420–1.
32. Mulligan ME, Edelstein MAC, George WL. Effect of cefoxitin therapy on fecal flora. Paper presented to the 80th Annual Meeting of the American Society of Microbiology. Washington, DC: 1980 Sep 20.
33. Mulligan ME, Rolfe RD, Finegold SM et al. Contamination of a hospital environment by *Clostridum difficile. Curr Microbiol* 1979; 3:173–5.
34. Pierce PF Jr, Wilson R, Silva J et al. Antimicrobial-associated pseudomembranous colitis: an epidemic investigation of a cluster of cases. *J Infect Dis.* 1982; 145:269–71.
35. Fekety R, Kim KH, Brown D et al. Epidemiology of antibiotic-associated colitis: isolation of *Clostridium difficile* from the hospital environment. *Am J Med.* 1981; 70:906–8.

36. Kim K, Fekety R, Batts DH et al. Isolation of *Clostridium difficile* from the environment and contacts of patients with antimicrobial associated colitis. *J Infect Dis.* 1981; 143:42–50.
37. Pittman F. Lomotil and antibiotic colitis. *Ann Intern Med.* 1975; 83:124–5.
38. Novak E, Lee DG, Seckman CE et al. Unfavorable effect of atropine-diphenoxylate therapy in lincomycin-caused diarrhea. *JAMA.* 1976; 235:1451–4.
39. Bartlett JG. Treatment of antibiotic-associated pseudomembranous colitis. *Rev Infect Dis.* 1984; 6 (Suppl):S235–41.
40. Bartlett JG, Tedesco FJ, Shull S et al. Symptomatic relapse after oral vancomycin therapy of antibiotic-associated pseudomembranous colitis. *Gastroenterology.* 1980; 78:431–4.
41. Keighley MRB, Burdon DW, Arabi Y et al. Randomized controlled trial of vancomycin for pseudomembranous colitis and post-operative diarrhea. *Br Med J.* 1978; 2:1667–9.
42. Teasley DG, Olson MM, Gerding DN et al. Prospective, randomized study of metronidazole versus vancomycin for clostridium-associated diarrhea and colitis. *Lancet.* 1983; 2:1043–6.
43. Eglinton GS, Mayes GR, Potts DW. Pseudomembranous colitis unresponsive to oral vancomycin therapy. *South Med J.* 1982; 75:1279–80.
44. Cherry RD, Portnoy D, Jabbari M. Metronidazole: an alternative therapy for antibiotic-associated colitis. *Gastroenterology.* 1982; 82:849–51.
45. Chang TW, Gorbach SL, Bartlett JG et al. Bacitracin treatment of antibiotic-associated pseudomembranous colitis and diarrhea caused by *Clostridium difficile* toxin. *Gastroenterology.* 1980; 78:1584–6.
46. Tedesco FJ. Bacitracin therapy in antibiotic-associated pseudomembranous colitis. *Dig Dis Sci.* 1980; 25:783–4.
47. Dudley MN, Quintiliani R, Nightingale CH et al. Absorption of vancomycin. *Ann Intern Med.* 1984; 101:144.
48. Spizter PG, Eliopoulous GM. Systemic absorption of enteral vancomycin in a patient with pseudomembranous colitis. *Ann Intern Med.* 1984; 100:523–4.
49. Marrie TJ, Faulkner RS, Badley BW. Pseudomembranous colitis: isolation of 2 species of cytotoxic Clostridia and successful treatment with vancomycin. *Can Med Assoc J.* 1978; 119:1058–60.
50. Bartlett JG, Chang TW, Moon N et al. Antibiotic-induced lethal enterocolitis in hamsters: studies with eleven agents and evidence to support the pathogenic role of toxin-producing clostridia. *Am J Vet Res.* 1978; 39:1525–30.
51. Gordon RS. Prospective, randomized study of metronidazole versus vancomycin for clostridium-associated diarrhea and colitis. *Lancet.* 1983; 2:1417. Letter.
52. Mitchell SR, Gaver WR. Intermittent therapy with metronidazole for relapse of pseudomembranous colitis. *JAMA.* 1984; 251:3082. Letter.
53. Nielsen ML, Justsen T, Goldman P. Excretion of metronidazole in human bile. *Scand J Gastroenterol.* 1977; 12:1003–8.
54. Brogden RN, Heel RC, Speight TM et al. Metronidazole in anaerobic infections: a review of its activity, pharmacokinetics, and therapeutic use. *Drugs.* 1978; 16:387–417.
55. Young GP, Ward P, McDonald M et al. Comparison of oral bacitracin with vancomycin in the therapy of antibiotic-associated colitis. *Gastroenterology.* 1984; 86:1306. Abstract.
56. Cuchura GJ, Tally FP, Chang T et al. Cost effective strategies for the management of suspected *Clostridium difficile*-associated diarrhea. *Clin Res.* 1983; 31:691. Abstract.
57. Tedesco FJ, Napier J, Gamble W et al. Therapy of antibiotic-associated pseudomembranous colitis. *J Clin Gastroenterol.* 1979; 1:51–5.
58. Keighley MRB. Antibiotic-associated pseudomembranous colitis: pathogenesis and management. *Drugs.* 1980; 20:49–56.
59. King C, Barriere SL. Analysis of the in vitro interaction between vancomycin and cholestyramine. *Antimicrob Agents Chemother.* 1981; 19:326–9.
60. Bowden TA, Mansberger AR, Lykins LE. Pseudomembranous enterocolitis: mechanisms of restoring floral homeostasis. *Am Surg.* 1981; 47:178–83.

“

New Look at Vancomycin

Vancomycin was isolated in the mid-1950s from a strain of *Streptomyces orientalis* that had been found in a sample of soil from a jungle path in Borneo. It was highly active and bactericidal against staphylococci, including the penicillin-resistant strains that had emerged in the early 1950s as an important cause of hospital-acquired infection. The original formulations contained visible impurities and were referred to as Mississippi mud; probably these impurities caused many of the adverse reactions associated with vancomycin in the early days. Because of these reactions vancomycin was prescribed sparingly, and it was used hardly at all after the introduction in the early 1960s of the penicillinase-stable penicillins cloxacillin and methicillin for the treatment of penicillin-resistant staphylococcal infections. During the past decade new indications have emerged; and, to the gratification of clinicians, the drug seems to have lost some of its tendency to cause adverse reactions. . . .

Except in antibiotic-associated pseudomembranous colitis, for which it is probably the drug of first choice, vancomycin is still generally regarded as a second-line antibiotic. Important indications include the treatment of prophylaxis of endocarditis caused by gram-positive organisms in penicillin-allergic patients and the treatment of serious infections caused by gram-positive organisms resistant, or not responding, to standard antibiotics. These include infections in patients undergoing renal dialysis and those who are immunocompromised or have prosthetic heart valves or shunts for the relief of hydrocephalus. Vancomycin has also been used successfully to treat severe infections caused by coagulase-negative staphylococci in newborn babies. . . .

—Anon. Born-again vancomycin. *Lancet.* 1985; 1:677–8. Editorial

”

Research

Evaluation of the vancomycin-clearance:creatinine-clearance relationship for predicting vancomycin dosage

Gary R. Matzke, John M. Kovarik, Michael J. Rybak, and Steve C. Boike

Abstract: Four methods of predicting vancomycin maintenance doses on the basis of the relationship between total-body or renal clearance of the drug and creatinine clearance were evaluated retrospectively using data from 24 patients who received vancomycin hydrochloride.

Data for 18 men and 6 women with creatinine clearances of 10–130 mL/min were used; the mean (± S.D.) vancomycin maintenance dose was 22.0 ± 11.2 mg/kg/day. The actual vancomycin maintenance dose needed to sustain an average steady-state vancomycin concentration of 15 mg/L was determined based on individual pharmacokinetic values. Predicted vancomycin maintenance doses were generated using the vancomycin-clearance:creatinine-clearance relationships derived separately by Nielsen, Moellering, Rotschafer, and Matzke. Orthogonal regression analysis was used to determine relationships between actual and predicted maintenance doses. Predictive ability of each method was assessed for bias (mean error) and precision (root mean squared error).

Mean error and root mean squared error (± S.D.), respectively, for the four methods were as follows: Nielsen −262 ± 451, 522 ± 718; Moellering −91 ± 439, 448 ± 547; Rotschafer 192 ± 602, 632 ± 682; and Matzke −76 ± 101, 408 ± 517. Doses predicted by the Nielsen relationship were significantly lower than the actual vancomycin maintenance doses. Use of the Rotschafer relationship resulted in substantial overprediction, which increased as creatinine clearance declined. Doses predicted by the Moellering and Matzke relationships were slightly less than but not significantly different from the actual dose. The Matzke method demonstrated the least bias and was the most precise.

Of these methods for predicting vancomycin maintenance dose, the Moellering and Matzke methods probably yield clinically similar degrees of accuracy and are superior to the Nielsen and Rotschafer methods.

Index terms: Antibiotics; Blood levels; Dosage; Excretion; Methodology; Pharmacokinetics; Vancomycin; Vancomycin hydrochloride
Clin Pharm: 1985; 4:311–5

Vancomycin was first introduced in 1956 for the treatment of staphylococcal infections. Early reports of nephrotoxicity[1-3] and ototoxicity[4-6] and the development of penicillinase-resistant penicillins limited its utility. Isolation of methicillin-resistant strains of *Staphylococcus aureus* in the late 1960s led to a re-evaluation of vancomycin. Currently, vancomycin hydrochloride is the drug of choice for the treatment of methicillin-resistant staphylococcal infections and is an alternative to penicillin for staphylococcal and streptococcal infections. It is also widely used in combination with an aminoglycoside against enterococci.[7]

Vancomycin's resurgence has spawned an increase in investigations of its pharmacology and pharmacokinetics. Several evaluations have been reported in patients with various degrees of renal insufficiency.[8-11] Relationships between pharma-

Gary R. Matzke, Pharm.D., is Associate Professor, College of Pharmacy, University of Minnesota, and Co-Director, Drug Evaluation Unit, Hennepin County Medical Center, Minneapolis, MN. John M. Kovarik is a Pharm.D. candidate, College of Pharmacy, University of Minnesota, Minneapolis. Michael J. Rybak, Pharm.D., is Assistant Professor, and Steve C. Boike, Pharm.D., is Adjunct Assistant Professor, College of Pharmacy and Allied Health Professions, Wayne State University and Detroit Receiving Hospital and University Health Center, Detroit, MI.

Address reprint requests to Dr. Matzke at the Drug Evaluation Unit, Hennepin County Medical Center, 701 Park Avenue, Minneapolis, MN 55415.

The secretarial assistance of Kim Podany and the artistic assistance of Diane Erickson are acknowledged.

cokinetic values and physiological functions (such as between vancomycin total-body clearance and creatinine clearance) have been assessed. Dosing guidelines for the use of vancomycin in patients with decreased renal function have resulted from these investigations.

Our study was undertaken to evaluate the relationship between total-body or renal vancomycin clearance and creatinine clearance for the purpose of predicting vancomycin maintenance doses in patients with various degrees of renal function.

Methods

Pharmacokinetic data for 24 patients (18 men, 6 women) ranging in age from 27 to 71 years (mean ± S.D. = 37.5 ± 10.8 years) were retrospectively reviewed (Table 1). For all patients, vancomycin therapy had been ordered by their attending physicians at Detroit Receiving Hospital in Detroit, Michigan, for the treatment of methicillin-resistant staphylococcal infections. Prescribed maintenance doses ranged from 4.5 to 44.1 mg/kg/day (mean ± S.D. = 22.0 ± 11.2 mg/kg/day). Creatinine clearance (CL_{cr}) was determined by the method of Cockroft and Gault[12]:

$$CL_{cr} = BW\ (140 - \text{age})/\text{serum creatinine} \times 72$$

where BW = lean body weight.

Blood samples for serum vancomycin concentration determinations were drawn at steady state after an average of 18 days of therapy (range = 2 to 43 days). Samples were obtained from a forearm vein in the arm contralateral to that used for drug administration 30 minutes before and 60 minutes after a one-hour infusion. Vancomycin concentrations were determined by fluorescence-polarization immunoassay (TDx, Abbott Diagnostics, Irving, TX). The minimum quantifiable concentration was 0.6 mg/L. The interassay coefficient of variation for this procedure was less than 10% over the range of concentrations measured.

The log vancomycin concentration–time data were analyzed by one of the Detroit investigators to determine the elimination rate constant (k) and half-life ($t_{1/2}$) for each patient. Volume of distribution (V) was determined by the method of Sawchuk and Zaske.[13] Total-body clearance (CL) was calculated as the product of the volume of distribution and the elimination rate constant. Vancomycin clearance was assumed to be dose independent. Each patient's actual maintenance dose (D_m) needed to sustain an average steady-state concentration of 15 mg/L was determined from the total-body clearance using the following equation:

$$D_m\ (\text{mg/day}) = \text{CL (L/hr)} \times 24\ (\text{hr/day}) \times 15\ (\text{mg/L}) \quad (1)$$

Predicted maintenance doses were calculated for each patient using the nomogram of Moellering et al.[8] (Moellering) and the dosing equation of Nielsen et al.[9] (Nielsen). Predicted total-body clearances were calculated from the vancomycin–creatinine clearance relationships of Rotschafer et al.[10] (Rotschafer) and Matzke et al.[11] (Matzke). Clearance values for each patient were substituted into Equation 1 to yield the predicted daily maintenance doses needed to achieve an average steady-state serum concentration of 15 mg/L.

Scatter plots of the data were obtained by plotting predicted versus actual vancomycin clearance and predicted versus actual maintenance doses (Figure 1). Relationships were assessed by orthogonal regression analysis. Estimated and actual maintenance doses were also compared by analysis of variance. Differences were subsequently assessed with Student's t test for paired data.

Percentage error in dosage prediction was calculated as follows:

$$\text{Percentage error} = [(\text{predicted dose} - \text{actual dose}) \times 100]/\text{actual dose} \quad (2)$$

Predictive ability of each of the four methods was assessed for bias (mean error) and precision (root mean squared error), as follows:

$$\text{Mean error} = (1/n) \sum_{i=1}^{n} \text{pe} \quad (3)$$

$$\text{Root mean squared error} = \sqrt{(1/n) \sum_{i=1}^{n} (\text{pe})^2} \quad (4)$$

where prediction error (pe) is predicted dose mi-

Table 1.
Pharmacokinetic Data for 24 Study Patients

Patient Weight (kg)	V (L/kg)	$t_{1/2}$ (hr)	k (hr^{-1})	CL (mL/min)	CL_{cr} (mL/min)
71	1.51	9.15	0.076	136	130
68	0.72	4.98	0.139	114	103
74	0.33	4.88	0.142	58	101
51	0.53	5.43	0.128	57	100
84	0.58	5.14	0.135	110	100
71	0.44	4.70	0.147	77	98
60	0.78	8.20	0.085	66	88
54	0.43	4.92	0.141	54	83
66	0.47	7.40	0.094	48	80
80	0.68	9.75	0.071	64	80
69	0.21	3.66	0.189	45	79
70	0.50	6.94	0.100	58	75
99	0.35	15.90	0.044	25	73
72	0.52	5.27	0.132	80	69
81	0.23	10.45	0.066	21	66
63	0.46	8.15	0.085	41	45
75	0.36	5.87	0.118	53	43
58	0.25	4.07	0.170	40	40
80	0.38	20.00	0.035	18	30
79	0.65	39.80	0.017	15	27
47	0.74	22.67	0.031	18	21
56	0.68	26.00	0.027	17	18
71	0.61	48.20	0.014	11	18
73	0.99	83.20	0.008	10	10

Figure 1. Scatter plots of predicted versus actual vancomycin maintenance doses for the four dosage-prediction methods.

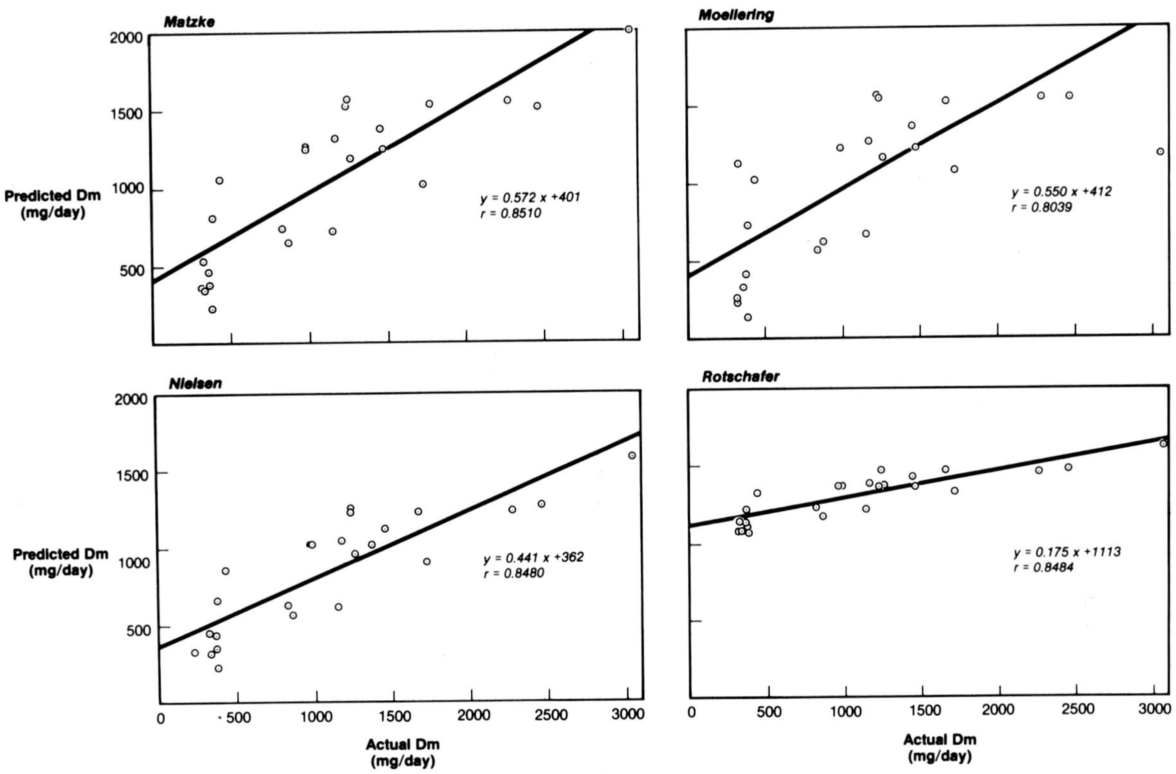

nus actual dose and n is the number of dosage pairs. Proportions were compared by chi-square analysis. The $p < 0.05$ level was chosen as significant for all statistical analyses.

Results

Pharmacokinetic data for the study population are listed in Table 1. The ability of each method to estimate total-body or renal vancomycin clearance from creatinine clearance is the basis for the method's predictive accuracy. Orthogonal regression analysis of predicted versus actual clearance showed nearly identical correlation among the methods that assessed total-body clearance (Moellering 0.804; Matzke 0.848; Rotschafer 0.848). Despite the similar degrees of correlation, there was marked dissimilarity in the slope and intercept of these relationships: Moellering (0.667; 12.076), Matzke (0.633; 15.567), and Rotschafer (0.177; 51.462).

Predicted maintenance doses for the Nielsen and Matzke methods were confined within a range of error that was much narrower than the range for the Moellering and Rotschafer doses (Figure 2). The Nielsen-predicted vancomycin-maintenance-dose frequency distribution is negatively skewed. This method significantly underpredicted vancomycin maintenance doses. No statistical differences between actual and estimated vancomycin maintenance doses were observed with the other three methods.

The Rotschafer relationship was the least precise; it substantially overpredicted maintenance doses (Table 2). Although the correlation of Moellering-predicted vancomycin maintenance dose with actual vancomycin maintenance dose was the poorest, this method demonstrated bias and precision second only to the method of Matzke et al. The method of Matzke et al. yielded the highest degree of correlation and precision and the least bias.

With the Rotschafer relationship, bias increased and precision decreased as creatinine clearance declined. This was particularly apparent among patients with creatinine clearances of 30 mL/min or less (mean error ± S.D. = 756 ± 47 and root mean squared error ± S.D. = 757 ± 263) and was not observed with the other three methods. The bias and precision, respectively, of the other three methods in this patient group were Nielsen, −3 ± 109 and 88 ± 100; Matzke, 35 ± 109 and 114 ± 121; and Moellering, 74 ± 338 and 346 ± 448.

Discussion

Dosing methods have been proposed for other agents with narrow therapeutic ranges, such as the aminoglycosides, theophylline, and digoxin. Some

Figure 2. Frequency distribution of observed percentage error with which vancomycin maintenance doses were predicted.

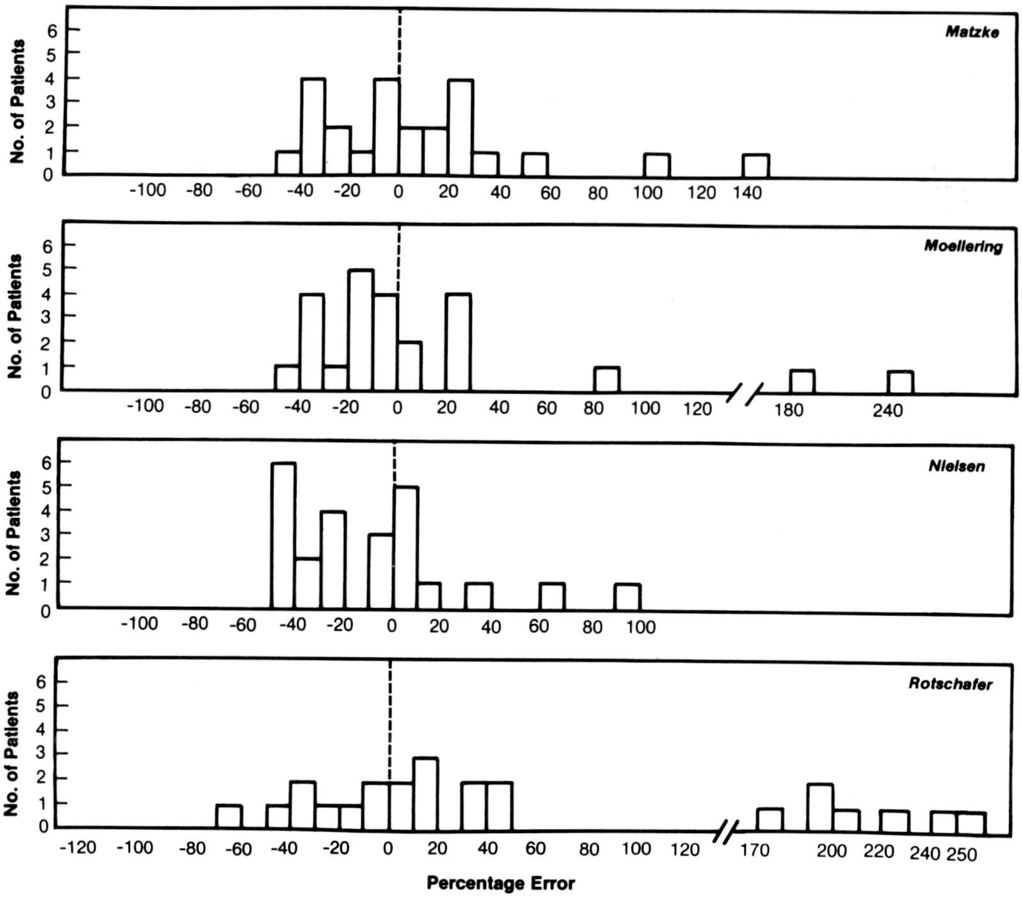

Table 2.
Correlation, Bias, and Precision of Vancomycin Maintenance Dose Predictions versus Actual Dosages

Prediction Method	Correlation Coefficient	Bias (mean error, mg/day)	Precision (root mean squared error, mg/day)
Nielsen	0.848	−262 ± 451	522 ± 718
Moellering	0.804	−91 ± 439	448 ± 547
Rotschafer	0.848	192 ± 602	632 ± 682
Matzke	0.851	−76 ± 401	408 ± 517

of these dosing methods have been evaluated (retrospectively, prospectively, or both) for accuracy.[14-18] An assessment of vancomycin-dosing guidelines for pediatric patients was recently reported by Alpert et al.[19] They found that when age-specific guidelines of Schaad et al.[20] were used, 30–70% of peak and 25–35% of trough serum vancomycin concentrations exceeded the desired maximum values. Although insufficient data were reported for full characterization of the predictive accuracy of the guidelines of Schaad et al.,[20] these data suggest that the proposed vancomycin dosing guidelines for adult patients should also be carefully evaluated.

Therapeutic average steady-state concentrations[8,9] (15–20 mg/L) and peak and trough concentrations[7,10,11] (20–40 mg/L and <10 mg/L, respectively) have been proposed. For purposes of comparison in this evaluation, the attainment of an average steady-state concentration was chosen since the Nielsen and Moellering methods are based on this goal and cannot be altered to predict the vancomycin maintenance dose necessary to attain desired peak and trough serum concentrations. The four vancomycin dosing methods assessed in this evaluation incorporate the relationship between renal or total-body vancomycin clearance and creatinine clearance as the means of predicting the maintenance dose for a given patient. A high degree of correlation between total-body vancomycin clearance and creatinine clearance was observed in the original reports of Moellering et al.[8] and Matzke et al.[11] These two dosing models demonstrated the greatest accuracy in this evaluation (i.e., smallest percentage error). Rotschafer et al.[10] reported a poor correlation between these two variables; using their method, substantial variability, decreasing accuracy as creatinine clearance declines, and extensive overprediction were observed. The method of Nielsen et al.[9] is based on the relationship between vancomycin renal clearance and creatinine clearance. Although a strong correlation between these variables was reported, the use of this relationship resulted in significant underprediction of the actual maintenance doses for this patient population.

Conclusion

This study suggests that the Matzke method should produce the most precise and least biased estimate of desired vancomycin dosages. The Moellering method would probably yield a clinically similar degree of accuracy. The marked imprecision and bias of the Rotschafer relationship suggest that this correlation should be used with caution, if at all. The Nielsen method was significantly biased but more precise than the Rotschafer correlation; its use would tend to provide the most conservative initial prediction, but its underprediction of maintenance doses could result in early clinical failures.

The toxicity profile of vancomycin and interpatient variability should be considered when selecting desired serum concentrations. Since all of these methods were associated with marked predictive variability for some patients, vancomycin dosages should be based on prospective, individualized pharmacokinetic monitoring.

References

1. Kirby WM, Perry DM, Bauer AW. Treatment of staphylococcal septicemia with vancomycin. *N Engl J Med.* 1960; 162:49–55.
2. Waisbren BA, Kleinerman L, Shemp J et al. The comparative toxicity and clinical effectiveness of vancomycin, ristocetin, and kanamycin. *Antibiot Ann.* 1959–60; 497–515.
3. Woodley DW, Hall WH. The treatment of severe staphylococcal infections with vancomycin. *Ann Intern Med.* 1961; 55:235–49.
4. Geraci JE, Heilman FR, Nichols DR et al. Antibiotic therapy of bacterial endocarditis: VI. Vancomycin for acute micrococcal endocarditis. *Proc Staff Meet Mayo Clin.* 1958; 33:172–81.
5. Louri DB, Kaminski T, Buchman J. Vancomycin in severe staphylococcal infections. *Arch Intern Med.* 1961; 107:125–40.
6. Dutton AAC, Elmer PC. Vancomycin: report on treatment of patients with severe staphylococcal infections. *Br Med J.* 1959; 1:114–9.
7. Cunha BA, Ristuccia AM. Clinical usefulness of vancomycin. *Clin Pharm.* 1983; 2:417–24.
8. Moellering RC, Krogstad DJ, Greenblatt DJ. Vancomycin therapy in patients with impaired renal function: a nomogram for dosage. *Ann Intern Med.* 1981; 94:343–6.
9. Nielsen HE, Hanson HE, Korsager B et al. Renal excretion of vancomycin in kidney disease. *Acta Med Scand.* 1975; 197:261–4.
10. Rotschafer JC, Crossley K, Zaske DE et al. Pharmacokinetics of vancomycin: observations in 28 patients and dosage recommendations. *Antimicrob Agents Chemother.* 1982; 22:391–4.
11. Matzke GR, McGory RW, Halstenson CE et al. Pharmacokinetics of vancomycin in patients with various degrees of renal function. *Antimicrob Agents Chemother.* 1984; 25:433–7.
12. Cockroft DW, Gault MH. Prediction of creatinine clearance from serum creatinine. *Nephron.* 1976; 16:31–41.
13. Sawchuk RJ, Zaske DE. Pharmacokinetics of dosing regimens which utilize multiple intravenous infusions: gentamicin in burn patients. *J Pharmacokinet Biopharm.* 1976; 4:183–95.
14. Russell WL, McNeeley DJ, Yost RL et al. Confirmation of a computer-derived nomogram to predict gentamicin serum concentrations. *Am J Hosp Pharm.* 1978; 35:570–3.
15. Abel SR, Aronoff GR. Accuracy of a micro-computer program for tobramycin consult services. *Clin Pharmacol Ther.* 1984; 35:224.
16. Johnson MH, Burkle WS. Evaluation of the Chiou method for determining theophylline dosages. *Clin Pharm.* 1984; 3:174–8.
17. Lopez LM, Russell WL, Hemmes RJ et al. Inadequacy of FDA dosing guidelines for intravenous theophylline. *Drug Intell Clin Pharm.* 1984; 18:987–91.
18. Lalonde RL, Pao D. Correlation coefficient versus prediction error in assessing the accuracy of digoxin dosing methods. *Clin Pharm.* 1984; 3:178–83.
19. Alpert G, Campos JM, Harris MC et al. Vancomycin dosage in pediatrics reconsidered. *Am J Dis Child.* 1984; 138:20–2.
20. Schaad UB, McCracken GH, Nelson JD. Clinical pharmacology and efficacy of vancomycin in pediatric patients. *J Pediatr.* 1980; 96:119–26.

Twice-daily moxalactam versus gentamicin and clindamycin in patients with penetrating abdominal trauma

LARRY D. CROTS, FAROUCK N. OBEID, H. MATHILDA HORST, AND BRACK A. BIVINS

Abstract: The effectiveness and total costs of moxalactam administered every 12 hours versus a combination of gentamicin and clindamycin for prophylactic use in patients with penetrating abdominal trauma were compared.

Fifty patients scheduled for laparotomy after penetrating abdominal wounds were randomly assigned to receive either clindamycin phosphate 600 mg every six hours with gentamicin (as the sulfate salt) 3–5 mg/kg/day in three divided doses or moxalactam disodium 2 g every 12 hours. Therapy was begun preoperatively and continued for a minimum of three days in patients without hollow-organ injury and five days in patients with hollow-organ injury; total duration of therapy could not exceed four weeks. Patients receiving moxalactam also received phytonadione 10 mg intramuscularly once a week.

Although wound cultures from several patients were positive for *Staphylococcus epidermidis, Pseudomonas aeruginosa,* and enterococci, no symptomatic infections developed. No direct toxic effects of moxalactam or gentamicin–clindamycin were seen; transient abnormalities in blood-coagulation tests or serum creatinine concentration occurred in several patients. Although mean drug costs per patient for moxalactam and gentamicin–clindamycin were similar, the mean cost of therapy per patient was $125.23 higher for the combination regimen than for moxalactam when laboratory, personnel-time, and supply costs were added to drug costs.

Moxalactam given every 12 hours was a safe and effective alternative to the combination of gentamicin and clindamycin for preventive use in the study patients with penetrating abdominal trauma.

Index terms: Antibiotics; Aminoglycosides; Clindamycin phosphate; Costs; Gentamicin sulfate; Moxalactam disodium; Phytonadione; Toxicity; Wounds

Clin Pharm. 1985; 4:316–20

Antimicrobial spectra of new cephalosporins compare favorably with spectra of combination therapy with aminoglycosides. The new cephalosporins may also be less toxic than the aminoglycosides.[1-4] However, the high cost per dose of the new cephalosporins has been a major drawback to their acceptance.[5,6] A recent study of total costs of antimicrobial therapy—antibiotic costs, administration costs, and monitoring costs—suggests that cost per dose may be a misleading indicator of the actual cost of antimicrobial therapy.[6] In selecting a prophylactic antibiotic from clinically equivalent agents, considerations should include available administration routes, dosing frequency, side effects, toxicity, and cost.[4]

We evaluated the effectiveness and the cost of twice-daily administration of the third-generation cephalosporin moxalactam versus combination therapy with gentamicin and clindamycin for prophylactic use in patients with penetrating abdominal injuries.

Methods

This study was conducted during the six-month period from July 1 to December 31, 1983. The study was approved by the institutional review board, and written consent was obtained from all participants.

Clinical Management. Fifty consecutive patients scheduled to undergo laparotomy for penetrating abdominal wounds were randomly assigned to receive therapy with one of two antibiotic regimens. Patients in group 1 received clindamycin phosphate (Cleocin, The Upjohn Company) 600 mg every six hours with gentamicin (as the sulfate salt; Garamycin, Schering Corporation) 3–5 mg/kg/day in three equal doses; gentamicin dosages were adjusted to achieve peak serum gentamicin concentrations of approximately 6 μg/mL and trough concentrations of approximately 1.5 μg/mL. Patients in group 2 received moxalactam disodium (Moxam, Eli Lilly and Company) 2 g

LARRY D. CROTS is Clinical Pharmacist; FAROUCK N. OBEID, M.D., and H. MATHILDA HORST, M.D., are staff surgeons; and BRACK A. BIVINS, M.D., is Division Head, Division of Trauma Surgery, Henry Ford Hospital, Detroit, MI.

Address reprint requests to Mr. Crots at the Department of Pharmacy, Henry Ford Hospital, 2799 West Grand Boulevard, Detroit, MI 48202.

Supported in part by a grant from Eli Lilly and Company, Indianapolis, IN.

 0278-2677/85/0501-0316$01.25.

every 12 hours; they also received phytonadione (Aquamephyton, Merck, Sharp & Dohme) 10 mg intramuscularly once a week as part of the protocol.

Group assignment was based on sequence of entry into the study, using a previously randomized list that was kept blind from the investigators by packaging. After a patient was entered into the study, the group assignment was revealed to the investigators. Patients who had received an antimicrobial agent during the three-day period immediately preceding pretherapy evaluation or who required concomitant therapy with an antibiotic other than those included in the study protocol were excluded.

Management of the penetrating abdominal injuries was uniform throughout the study period. Laparotomies for local wound exploration or diagnostic peritoneal lavage (or both) were performed on selected patients who had stab wounds without overt signs of visceral injury. In patients with gunshot wounds, exploratory laparotomies were performed routinely unless the missile tract was superficial to the peritoneum. Antibiotic therapy was initiated in the emergency room as soon as the decision for abdominal exploration was made and was continued according to the patient's injury pattern: three days minimum for patients without hollow-organ injury, five days minimum for patients with hollow-organ injury. Therapy could be continued beyond the minimum period at the discretion of the investigator but could not exceed four weeks.

Baseline laboratory testing included complete blood count with differential, serum electrolytes and enzymes (including calcium, phosphorus, magnesium, SGOT, SGPT, LDH, alkaline phosphatase, creatine phosphokinase, creatinine, total bilirubin, total protein, albumin, cholesterol, triglycerides, blood urea nitrogen, uric acid, and glucose), blood-coagulation tests (prothrombin time, partial thromboplastin time, and platelet count), urinalysis (including microscopic examination), erythrocyte-sedimentation rate, and Coombs' test. Laboratory tests were repeated as clinically indicated. Prothrombin time and partial thromboplastin time were also determined before and after moxalactam therapy for patients in group 2.

Aerobic and anaerobic cultures and sensitivities of organisms isolated from blood, wound, and intraperitoneal fluid were obtined within four hours of the first dose of antibiotic. In vitro susceptibility to moxalactam was tested using the minimum inhibitory concentration method, and susceptibility to gentamicin and clindamycin was tested using the Kirby-Bauer disk-diffusion method. The absence of a pathogen did not exclude patients from the study.

Clinical and demographic data were collected at the time of entry into the study. Patients were monitored with physical examination, laboratory tests, and vital-signs measurement daily during the study period and three times weekly thereafter until discharge; a follow-up physical examination was performed 14 to 30 days after discharge.

Cost Analysis. Total costs of therapy—including drugs, laboratory tests, personnel time, and supplies—were analyzed. Drug and supply costs were based on the actual contract cost of the drugs and supplies to the institution. Laboratory costs were based on actual costs to the institution ($8.10 per determination of serum aminoglycoside concentration and $7.92 per determination of both prothrombin time and partial thromboplastin time). Pharmacy and nursing labor costs were based on institutional time-study data, which indicated a labor cost of $1.22 per intermittent i.v. infusion.

Patients were evaluated for success or failure of the therapeutic regimen. Failure was defined as clinical evidence of continued or new infection accompanied by a temperature higher than 38 °C on two occasions six hours apart, a white blood cell count greater than 20,000/cu mm, abscess formation, wound infection, or a positive blood culture. Success was defined as recovery without evidence of infection.

Results

Clinical Management. Of the 50 study patients, 25 patients were assigned to group 1 (clindamycin-gentamicin therapy) and 25 patients were assigned to group 2 (moxalactam therapy). The groups were comparable in age, weight, and sex (Table 1). Pertinent clinical data are shown in Table 2.

Prolonged prothrombin times (longer than 14 seconds) and partial thromboplastin times (longer than 40 seconds) were seen in two patients in group 1 and one patient in group 2; the greatest elevation (56 seconds) occurred in group 1. These times returned to normal within eight hours with-

Table 1.
Demographic Characteristics of Patients Treated with Gentamicin-Clindamycin (Group 1) or Moxalactam (Group 2)

Characteristic	Group 1	Group 2
No. patients (no. men)	25 (23)	25 (23)
Age (years)		
Mean	27.0	27.1
Range	17–57	18–62
Weight (kg)		
Mean	71.8	74.7
Range	59–84	59–136
No. patients with hollow-organ injuries	12	11
Length of hospital stay (days)		
Mean	10.4	9.5
Range	3–28	3–21
Total hospital stay for all patients (days)	261	238

out administration of phytonadione. In one patient in group 2, serum creatinine concentration increased to more than 2.0 mg/dL but returned to normal within 48 hours. None of these abnormal laboratory values could be related clearly to either antibiotic regimen, and the study drugs were not discontinued.

Four patients in group 2 had positive peritoneal cultures, compared with three patients in group 1. Peritoneal cultures from one patient in group 2 were positive for enterococcus (minimum inhibitory concentration less than 16 μg/mL for moxalactam) shortly after initiation of antibiotic therapy. This patient had multiple gunshot wounds to the chest, abdomen, and extremities and an elevated temperature during the first eight days of hospitalization. The fever, which was attributed to impaired pulmonary function caused by the gunshot wounds and indwelling chest tubes, resolved after chest percussion and nasotracheal suctioning, and the patient did not develop a symptomatic enterococcal infection. Another patient in group 2 became infected with *Staphylococcus epidermidis* in a wound site that had previously been infected with a different bacterium; minimum inhibitory concentrations were not obtained, and no further antibiotics were administered. One patient in group 1 had a persistent fever attributed to atelectasis, which gradually resolved. Positive *Staph. epidermidis* cultures obtained from another group 1 patient were related to a contaminated i.v. catheter.

Cultures taken from two patients in group 2 after antibiotic therapy had been discontinued grew enterococci and *Staph. epidermidis;* minimum inhibitory concentrations were not determined, but the patients did not develop symptoms of infection. Similarly, cultures of the wound drainage from one patient in group 1 taken after antibiotic therapy had been discontinued grew *Pseudomonas aeruginosa* sensitive to gentamicin and *Staph. epidermidis* resistant to gentamicin, clindamycin, and moxalactam, but the patient did not develop symptoms of infection.

Cost Analysis. The total costs of therapy for patients receiving gentamicin and clindamycin (group 1) or moxalactam (group 2) are presented in Table 3. The total cost of therapy for the 25 patients in group 1 was $3130.75 more than therapy for patients in group 2. The cost of antibiotics alone represented 57% of total therapy costs for group 1 and 76% of total therapy costs for group 2.

The mean cost of therapy per patient was $125.23 more in group 1 than in group 2. This represents an approximate 38% greater cost for combination therapy than for single-agent therapy. Since the mean drug cost per patient was similar for both groups ($260.23 for group 1 and $254.95 for group 2), most of the difference in the total costs of therapy was because of differences in laboratory costs, personnel time, and supply costs.

Table 2.
Characteristics of Antibiotic Therapy and Number of Laboratory Tests in Patients Receiving Gentamicin–Clindamycin (Group 1) or Moxalactam (Group 2)

Variable	Group 1	Group 2
Antibiotic Therapy		
Duration (days)		
Total	135	149
Mean	5.4	6
Range	3–15	3–18
Total no. doses	405 (gentamicin) 540 (clindamycin)	298
Mean daily dose	372 mg (gentamicin) 2.4 g (clindamycin)	4 g
Laboratory Tests		
Cultures		
Total no. determinations	165	173
No. determinations per patient	6.6	6.9
Determinations of serum gentamicin concentration		
Total no. determinations	52	0
Mean no. determinations per patient	2	0
PT/PTT determinations[a]		
Total no. determinations	0	69
Mean no. determinations per patient	0	2.8

[a] PT = prothrombin time, PTT = partial thromboplastin time.

Table 3.
Total Costs of Therapy[a] in Patients Receiving Gentamicin–Clindamycin (Group 1) or Moxalactam (Group 2)

Variable	Group 1	Group 2
Number of doses	405 (gentamicin) 540 (clindamycin)	298
Drug costs ($)		
Antibiotics	6,505.65	6,329.52
Phytonadione	0	44.24
Total	6,505.65	6,373.76
Laboratory charges ($)		
Serum gentamicin concentration determinations[b]	421.20	0
PT/PTT determinations[c]	0	546.48
Pharmacy and nursing personnel time[d] ($)	1,152.90	363.56
Supply costs ($)		
I.V. solutions	567.00	178.80
Administration sets	2,362.50	745.00
Syringes	236.25	74.50
Needles	47.25	14.90
Filter straws (for clindamycin ampuls)	135.00	0
Total cost of therapy ($)	11,427.75	8,297.00
Mean cost of therapy per patient ($)	457.11	331.88
Mean cost of therapy per day ($)	84.65	55.68

[a] Based on total costs for 25 patients in each group.
[b] Using EMIT assay.
[c] PT = prothrombin time, PTT = partial thromboplastin time.
[d] Calculated as number of doses multiplied by mean cost of personnel time per dose (based on institutional data showing the mean cost of preparing and administering an intermittent drug dose to be $1.22).

Costs for serum creatinine determinations were not included in the calculation of laboratory costs because the number of serum creatinine determinations obtained in each group was similar. Personnel time required for aminoglycoside dosage adjustments by the clinical pharmacists also was not included in the analysis; there were seven such adjustments for patients in group 1 that, if included, would have increased the cost of combination therapy.

Discussion

Antimicrobial therapy for patients with traumatic injuries is preventive rather than truly prophylactic, because the antibiotic is administered after contamination has occurred. In the preantibiotic era, abdominal trauma with bowel injury was almost invariably fatal. Use of penicillin in the 1940s led to a 30–40% decrease in mortality rates, and subsequent broad-spectrum regimens have been associated with mortality rates of 4–15%.[7] In trauma patients who are potentially exposed to mixed-flora contamination as a consequence of their injuries, broad-spectrum coverage has been considered necessary and has usually been achieved with combination therapy.[7-9]

The newer cephalosporins, with their extended spectra and relatively low toxicities, have been considered attractive alternatives to combination therapy. Stone et al.[8] found three third-generation agents (moxalactam, cefotaxime, and cefoperazone) equivalent to the combination of gentamicin and clindamycin in the treatment of polymicrobial surgical sepsis. In that study, moxalactam was administered every eight hours. Schentag et al.[10] also found that moxalactam given every eight hours was equivalent to the combination of tobramycin and clindamycin in the treatment of abdominal sepsis, but they specifically excluded patients with abdominal trauma from their study.

Our results indicate that moxalactam given every 12 hours is as effective as the combination of gentamicin and clindamycin in the management of penetrating abdominal trauma. Although appropriate duration of antimicrobial therapy in trauma is currently under study, we used a 72-hour minimum period as a compromise between the short (24-hour) and long (5-day) regimens reported.[7-12] The 72-hour period corresponds to recommendations by Crenshaw et al.[13] for minimum duration of therapy.

No symptomatic infections developed in patients in either group. Although two patients in group 2 had positive cultures (*Staph. epidermidis* and enterococci) after moxalactam was discontinued, we did not find enterococcal overgrowth that has been associated with the newer cephalosporins.[11]

Direct toxic effects of moxalactam or gentamicin and clindamycin were not identified in our patients, and we did not find the prolonged prothrombin times and partial thromboplastin times reported by Schentag et al.[10] Phytonadione was administered prophylactically to patients receiving moxalactam; two patients in group 1 and one patient in group 2 had minimal elevations in prothrombin time and partial thromboplastin time without evidence of bleeding. Similarly, renal impairment seen in 29% of older septic patients studied by Schentag et al.[10] was not seen in our patients. An increase in serum creatinine concentration in one of our patients could not be related directly to his antibiotic therapy.

The mean drug costs per patient for moxalactam therapy and combination gentamicin and clindamycin therapy were almost identical ($254.95 and $260.23, respectively). However, when laboratory, personnel time, and supply costs were added to drug costs, the mean cost of therapy per patient was $125.23 higher for the combination regimen than for moxalactam. Administration and monitoring costs were responsible for 23% of group 2 costs and 51% of group 1 costs.

Our results are in agreement with those of Rapp et al.,[6] who demonstrated in a retrospective study that single-agent therapy with a first-generation cephalosporin was less expensive than combination therapy with an aminoglycoside. Schentag et al.[10] also found no difference in cost between moxalactam given every eight hours and combination therapy with tobramycin and clindamycin, but they did not consider personnel or monitoring costs in their analysis.

Conclusion

Moxalactam given every 12 hours was a safe and effective alternative to a combination of gentamicin and clindamycin for preventive use in the study patients with penetrating abdominal injuries.

References

1. Thompson RL, Wright AJ. Cephalosporin antibiotics. *Mayo Clin Proc.* 1983; 58:79–87.
2. Neu HC. The new beta-lactamase-stable cephalosporins. *Ann Intern Med.* 1982; 97:408–19.
3. DiPiro JT, Bivins BA, Record KE et al. The prophylactic use of antimicrobials in surgery. *Curr Probl Surg.* 1983; 20:69–132.
4. DiPiro JT, Record KE, Bivins BA. Evaluation of new cephalosporins for prophylaxis of surgical infection. *Clin Pharm.* 1982; 1:135–40.
5. Barza M. Three generations of cephalosporins. *Clin Pharm.* 1982; 1:165–7.
6. Rapp RP, Bannon CL, Bivins BA. The influence of dose frequency and agent toxicity on the cost of parenteral antibiotic therapy. *Drug Intell Clin Pharm.* 1982; 16:935–8.
7. Thadepalli H. Principles and practice of antibiotic therapy for post-traumatic abdominal injuries. *Surg Gynecol Obstet.* 1979; 148:937–46.
8. Stone HH, Strom PR, Fabian TC et al. Third-generation cephalosporins for polymicrobial surgical sepsis. *Arch Surg.*

1983; 118:193–200.
9. Moore FA, Moore EE, Mill MR. Preoperative antibiotics for abdominal gunshot wounds. *Am J Surg*. 1983; 146:762–5.
10. Schentag JJ, Wels PB, Reitberg DP et al. A randomized clinical trial of moxalactam alone versus tobramycin plus clindamycin in abdominal sepsis. *Ann Surg*. 1983; 198:35–41.
11. Dougherty SH, Flohr AB, Simmons RL. Breakthrough enterococcal septicemia in surgical patients. *Arch Surg*. 1983; 118:232–8.
12. Oreskovich MR, Dellinger EP, Lennard ES et al. Duration of preventative antibiotic administration for penetrating abdominal trauma. *Arch Surg*. 1982; 117:200.
13. Crenshaw C, Glanges E, Webber C et al. A prospective random study of a single agent versus combination antibiotics as therapy in penetrating injuries of the abdomen. *Surgery*. 1983; 156:289–94.

Research Notes

Acyclovir pharmacokinetics in a patient on continuous ambulatory peritoneal dialysis

SHIV K. SETH, JAMES A. VISCONTI, LEE A. HEBERT, AND HARVEY C. KRASNY

Clin Pharm. 1985; 4:320–2

Acyclovir is an antiviral agent shown to be a potent inhibitor of replication of the Herpesvirus group. It is an acyclic analogue of deoxyguanosine. In the cell infected with herpes simplex virus, acyclovir is selectively phosphorylated to the monophosphate by the virus-coded deoxypyrimidine kinase[1] and is subsequently converted to the diphosphate and triphosphate by host-cell enzymes.[2] Acyclovir triphosphate is a potent inhibitor (suicide inactivator) of the herpesvirus DNA polymerase.[3] Elimination of acyclovir in healthy subjects occurs primarily by glomerular filtration and tubular secretion. In patients with anuria and end-stage renal disease, the total body clearance decreases and half-life increases substantially. Krasny et al.[4] reported a plasma half-life of 5–6 hours for acyclovir during hemodialysis and a plasma dialysis clearance of 113 mL/min.

Continuous ambulatory peritoneal dialysis (CAPD) is a frequently used alternative to hemodialysis. Many antibiotics that are efficiently hemodialyzed have shown very low plasma clearance in patients on CAPD. Recently, we investigated the pharmacokinetics of acyclovir after intravenous administration of the drug for treatment of herpes zoster in a patient with end-stage renal disease who was receiving CAPD.

Case Report. Our patient was a 54-year-old, white man who was admitted to University Hospital with hepatosplenomegaly. His white blood cell count was 2100/cu mm; hemoglobin and hematocrit were 9.8 g/dL and 29%, respectively; platelet count was 102,000/cu mm; BUN was 101 mg/dL; and serum creatinine was 6.7 mg/dL. Analysis of bone marrow aspirate was consistent with myeloproliferative syndrome. A splenectomy was performed, and an open renal biopsy revealed membranoproliferative glomerulonephritis. The patient became anuric and was started on CAPD. Subsequently, he developed fever, chills, and rash that began with crops of vesicles associated with severe pain. The vesicles were distributed over the left shoulder and neck area.

A diagnosis of shingles (herpes zoster) was made, and the patient was started on acyclovir (as the sodium salt) 200 mg i.v. administered once daily over 60 minutes. Other medications the patient received during hospitalization included aspirin, calcium carbonate, allopurinol, dipyridamole, propranolol, hydralazine, docusate sodium, and meperidine. After beginning acyclovir therapy, the patient showed dramatic improvement, with a decrease in pain and crusting of the herpetic lesions. By the seventh day of acyclovir therapy, the lesions were not painful to touch and acyclovir therapy was discontinued. Throughout hospitalization the dialysate was clear and there was no evidence of peritonitis.

Methods. During acyclovir therapy, blood and peritoneal dialysate samples were obtained for determination of acyclovir concentration. All blood samples were collected in heparinized tubes and centrifuged; the supernatant plasma was then frozen at −20 °C. Plasma and peritoneal dialysate concentrations of acyclovir were determined using

SHIV K. SETH, PH.D., is Clinical Assistant Professor, and JAMES A. VISCONTI, PH.D., is Professor of Pharmacy Practice, College of Pharmacy, The Ohio State University, Columbus, OH. LEE A. HEBERT, M.D., is Professor of Medicine and Director of the Department of Nephrology, College of Medicine, The Ohio State University, Columbus. HARVEY C. KRASNY, PH.D., is Senior Research Scientist, Burroughs Wellcome Company, Research Triangle Park, NC.

Presented in the Clinical Research Forum at the 19th Annual ASHP Midyear Clinical Meeting, Dallas, TX, December 4, 1984.

a radioimmunoassay highly specific for acyclovir.[5] The assay sensitivity was 2.2 ng/mL, and the coefficient of variation was within 10%.

Peak and trough plasma concentrations of acyclovir were obtained on days 4–7 of acyclovir therapy. Blood samples for pharmacokinetic analyses were also drawn 1.5, 2, 4, 8, 12, 16, and 23.5 hours after the start of infusion on day 4.

Three dialysis-fluid exchanges were performed daily. The first two exchanges consisted of an 8-hour and a 6-hour dwell time with 1.5% Dianeal solution; the final exchange consisted of a 10-hour dwell time with 4.25% Dianeal solution. The total dialysate returned after each exchange was collected to determine total recovery of acyclovir. The patient was permitted to move around freely to allow proper mixing of the dialysate.

Pharmacokinetic values for acyclovir were calculated using a standard model-independent approach. Calculations were based on data from blood samples obtained after the fourth dose. The area under the plasma concentration–time curve during the 24-hour sampling period (AUC_{0-24}) at steady state was calculated by the trapezoidal method, using 1.6 μg/mL as the predose concentration. The elimination rate constant (γ_z) was calculated by regression analysis of the terminal phase of the plasma concentration–time curve.

Elimination half-life was calculated as $0.693/\gamma_z$. Total body clearance (CL) was calculated as dose in milligrams divided by AUC_{0-24} in mg·hr/L. Volume of distribution (V) during the elimination phase was calculated as follows:

$$V = CL/\gamma_z$$

The CAPD clearance was calculated as follows:

$$CL_{CAPD} = Ad/AUC_{0-24}$$

where *Ad* equals the amount of drug recovered in the dialysate fluid during the 24-hour sampling period. The fraction of the i.v. dose recovered in the CAPD fluid during the study period was also calculated.

Results. Table 1 shows peak and trough concentrations (C) of acyclovir in plasma, concentrations in the dialysate, and the total amount of acyclovir recovered from the dialysate used in each treatment. The peak and trough plasma concentrations on days 4–7 indicated that steady state was achieved. Decreases in the dialysate concentration of acyclovir during the 24-hour period after a dose corresponded to decreases in plasma concentrations (Figure 1). Acyclovir pharmacokinetic values in plasma are shown in Table 2.

Table 1.
Acyclovir Concentrations (μg/mL) in Plasma and Dialysate and Recovery of Acyclovir from Dialysate

Day	Time after Dose (hr)	*C*	Total Acyclovir (μg) in Dialysate
Plasma Samples			
3	12.0	2.2	
4	1.5	6.4	
4	2.0	5.3	
4	4.0	4.1	
4	8.0	3.2	
4	12.1	2.5	
4	16.0	2.3	
4	23.5	1.6	
5	1.6	5.6	
5	23.8	1.3	
6	1.7	5.2	
6	23.5	1.3	
7	1.5	4.9	
Dialysate Samples			
3	14–24	2.0	5886
4	0–8[a]	3.3	6412
4	8–14[b]	1.9	4832
4	13–23[c]	1.6	3429
5	0–7	3.2	7498
5	8–14	2.6	6612
5	14–24	1.6	2981
6	0–8	3.3	6090
6	8–14	1.0	3882
6	14–24	1.4	2468

[a] First exchange.
[b] Second exchange.
[c] Third exchange.

Figure 1. Concentrations of acyclovir in plasma and dialysate fluid.

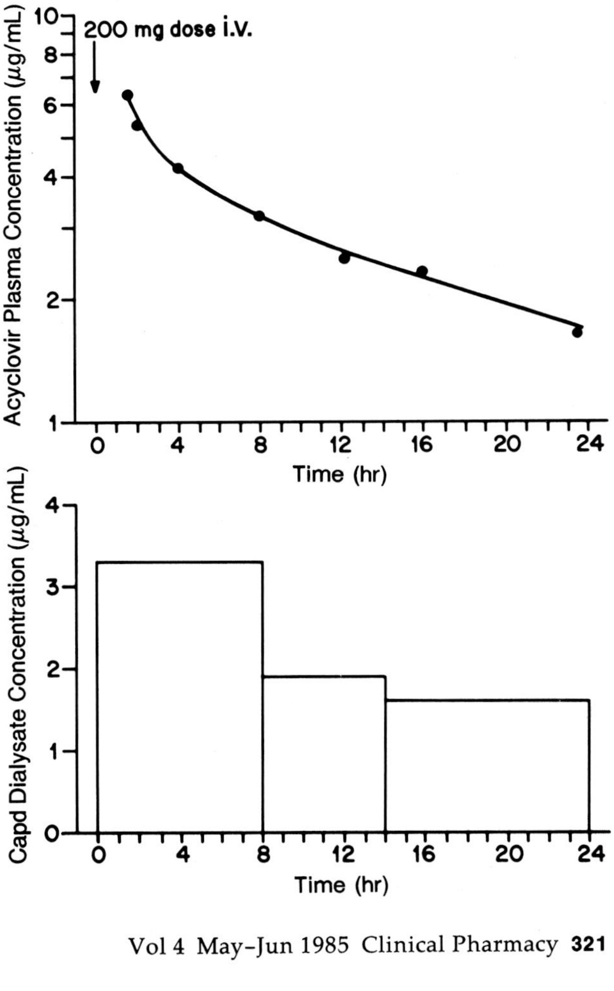

Table 2.
Acyclovir Pharmacokinetic Values

Variable	Value
AUC_{ss0-24} (mg·hr/L)	68.6
Volume of distribution (L)	62.0
Elimination rate constant (hr^{-1})	0.047
Elimination half-life (hr)	14.7
Total body clearance (mL/min)	48.6
CAPD clearance (mL/min)	3.6
Percentage of dose recovered in dialysate	7.3

Discussion. The total body clearance of acyclovir in our CAPD patient was 48.6 mL/min, and the elimination half-life was 14.7 hours, compared with 327 mL/min and 2.5 hours, respectively, in humans with normal renal function.[6] The contribution of peritoneal dialysate clearance to total body clearance was 7.3%, since the fraction of dose recovered in dialysate during the 24-hour collection period at steady state was only 7.3% of the acyclovir dose. In patients with end-stage renal disease undergoing intermittent hemodialysis, the acyclovir dialysis clearance (113 mL/min) and the plasma elimination half-life (5.4 hours during dialysis)[4] were closer to those values found in normal subjects.

Conclusion. These preliminary results in a single CAPD patient indicate that peritoneal dialysis may not be as efficient as hemodialysis in removing acyclovir from plasma.

References

1. Fyfe JA, Keller PM, Furman PA et al. Thymidine kinase from herpes simplex virus phosphorylates the new antiviral compound, 9-(2-hydroxyethoxymethyl) guanine. *J Biol Chem.* 1978; 253:8721–7.
2. Miller WH, Miller RL. Phosphorylation of acyclovir (acycloguanosine) monophosphate by GMP kinase. *J Biol Chem.* 1980; 255:7204–7.
3. Furman PA, St. Clair MH, Spector T. Acyclovir triphosphate is a suicide inactivator of herpes simplex virus DNA polymerase. *J Biol Chem.* 1984; 259:9575–9.
4. Krasny HC, Liao SH, deMiranda P et al. Influence of hemodialysis on acyclovir pharmacokinetics in patients with chronic renal failure. *Am J Med.* 1982; 73:202–4.
5. Quinn RP, deMiranda P, Gerald L et al. A sensitive radioimmunoassay for the antiviral agent BW 248U [9-(2-hydroxyethoxymethyl) guanine]. *Anal Biochem.* 1979; 98:319–28.
6. Blum MR, Liao S, deMiranda P. Overview of acyclovir pharmacokinetic disposition in adults and children. *Am J Med.* 1982; 73 (Suppl):186–92.

Appearance of ranitidine in breast milk following multiple dosing

Gregory L. Kearns, Richard F. McConnell, Jr., John M. Trang, and Ronald B. Kluza

Clin Pharm. 1985; 4:322–4

Ranitidine hydrochloride (Zantac, Glaxo, Inc., Research Triangle Park, NC 27709) is an H_2-receptor antagonist that, unlike cimetidine, does not contain an imidazole group.[1] The excretion of ranitidine into breast milk following a single oral dose has been described.[2] We studied the excretion of ranitidine into the breast milk of a lactating mother following the administration of multiple doses.

Methods. A 34-year-old, multigravida white woman who had taken four oral doses of ranitidine hydrochloride for reflux esophagitis inquired whether the drug had been transferred to her infant by nursing. To evaluate the presence of ranitidine in breast milk, informed consent was obtained to study serum and paired breast-milk samples collected during a dosing interval. At the time of the study, the mother had taken four 150-mg (2.44 mg/kg) doses of ranitidine (as the hydrochloride salt) at 0700 and 1900 daily. Her 54-day-old, 4.8-kg infant had been exclusively breast-fed since birth at four-hour intervals for 10 to 15 minutes on each breast. The infant weighed 3.4 kg at birth (39-weeks gestational age) and had a normal neonatal course. Both the infant and mother were healthy at the time of the evaluation, and the postnatal growth and development of the infant were within normal limits.

Immediately preceding the fifth scheduled ranitidine dose at 0700 on the day of the study, a 5-mL

Gregory L. Kearns, Pharm.D., is Assistant Professor of Pharmaceutics and Pediatrics, University of Arkansas for Medical Sciences, Little Rock. Richard F. McConnell, Jr., M.D., is Head, Asthma Allergy Clinic, Arlington, TX; at the time of this study, he was a postdoctoral fellow, Division of Allergy, Department of Pediatrics, The Louisiana State University School of Medicine, Shreveport. John M. Trang, Ph.D., is Assistant Professor of Pharmaceutics and Interdisciplinary Toxicology, University of Arkansas for Medical Sciences. Ronald B. Kluza, Ph.D., is Dean, College of Pharmacy, Drake University, Des Moines, IA; he was Professor and Chairman, Department of Pharmaceutics, University of Arkansas for Medical Sciences, at the time of this study.

Address reprint requests to Dr. Kearns at the Department of Pharmaceutics, Slot 522, University of Arkansas for Medical Sciences, 4301 W. Markham, Little Rock, AR 72205.

The assistance of Christopher Warner, Ph.D., Glaxo, Inc., for performing the serum and breast-milk ranitidine analyses; Janet K. McConnell, M.S.N., P.N.P., for collecting the samples and reviewing the manuscript; and Cindy Blot, for her technical and editorial help, is acknowledged.

venous blood sample was obtained and both breasts were emptied of milk by manual expression. The 0700 dose (150 mg) of ranitidine was administered orally with 100 mL of tap water. Breast-feeding was withheld during the subsequent 12-hour period, and the infant was given a commercial infant formula.

At 1.5, 5.5, and 12 hours following the 0700 ranitidine dose, 5 mL venous blood samples were collected in glass specimen tubes that did not contain anticoagulants. At each blood sampling time, a 10-minute manual expression of milk from each breast was completed. Milk samples (approximately 75 to 80 mL each) from both breasts were pooled (with the exception of the 5.5-hour postdose sample) and frozen at −70 °C. The pH of the breast-milk samples ranged from 7.0 to 7.15. Venous blood samples were permitted to clot at room temperature and were centrifuged at 5000 *g* for 10 minutes to obtain the serum, which was then frozen at −70 °C. Ranitidine therapy was discontinued following the 12-hour postdose sampling interval. The mother was given an antacid regimen, and breast-feeding was resumed the following morning.

Ranitidine concentrations were determined in 1-mL alkalinized samples of serum and homogenized breast milk using the reverse-phase high-pressure liquid chromatography (HPLC) method described by Mihaly et al.[3] The analyses of serum and milk samples were performed by the manufacturer of ranitidine (Glaxo Group Research Limited, Ware, Hertfordshire, UK).

Results. The observed ranitidine concentrations in breast milk and serum and the resultant milk-to-serum (M:S) ratios for each sampling point are shown in Table 1. The observed peak ranitidine concentration in both milk and serum occurred at the 5.5-hour postdose sampling interval. Disparate milk and serum concentration profiles were found, with the milk concentrations of ranitidine declining during the apparent absorption phase in serum. The ranitidine elimination half-life estimate, using the 5.5- and 12-hour postdose serum concentrations, was 2.91 hours.

Table 1.
Ranitidine Milk and Serum Concentrations and Milk-to-Serum Ratios during Multiple Dosing

Time after Dose (hr)	Ranitidine Concentration (ng/mL) Milk	Serum	Milk:Serum Ratio
predose[a]	993	53[a]	18.73
1.5	722[b]	106	6.81
5.5	2610	309	8.44
12.0	1569	66[a]	23.77

[a] Predose samples were obtained immediately before the fifth dose of ranitidine 150 mg (as the hydrochloride salt).

[b] The mean ranitidine concentration in pooled milk samples from the right (708 ng/mL) and left (736 ng/mL) breasts.

An examination of the M:S ratios following drug administration revealed an apparent accumulation of ranitidine in milk with the highest observed M:S ratio occurring 12 hours after drug administration. In serum, the difference between the predose and 12-hour postdose ranitidine concentrations (13 ng/mL) was minimal as expected for near steady-state conditions. The disparity in breast-milk concentrations at these times (576 ng/mL), however, suggested that steady-state conditions had not yet been achieved in milk.

Discussion. Ranitidine is a weak base (pKa 8.2) and is 15% bound to plasma protein.[1] It is freely soluble in water and alcohol, very slightly soluble in chloroform (data on file, Glaxo, Inc.), and slightly less lipid soluble than cimetidine (a structurally related H_2-receptor antagonist).[2] Using an average value of 7 for the pH of human breast milk,[4] the theoretical M:S ratio for ranitidine is 6.49, based on a rearrangement of the Henderson-Hasselbalch equation.[5] Applying these same calculations to breast milk with a pH of 7.15, the M:S ratio for ranitidine would be 2.36. While our observed value at 1.5 hours following drug administration (6.81) was in agreement with the estimated value for a milk pH of 7 (6.49), our observed predose (18.73) and 12-hour postdose (23.77) M:S ratios were markedly different. The data in Table 1 show that the time of the minimum ranitidine concentration in milk lagged behind that in serum by approximately two hours. This was consistent with other studies of nadolol,[5] atenolol,[6] and cimetidine[7] excretion into breast milk, where lag times have been demonstrated for the appearance of maximum drug concentrations in milk when compared with serum. Although the actual peak serum concentration of ranitidine in our patient could have been obscured by our choice of sampling times, the patient's estimated serum half-life for ranitidine (2.91 hours) based on the 5.5- and 12-hour postdose serum concentrations was in agreement with values reported (2.1 to 3.1 hours) following the oral administration of ranitidine hydrochloride in adults.[1,8] This finding indicated that the ranitidine serum concentrations approximated steady-state conditions in our patient.

The absolute values of the M:S ratios for ranitidine and their variability over the 12-hour dosing interval in our patient cannot be attributed solely to changes in the pH of the milk. Other physicochemical and physiologic factors, which we were unable to control in our clinical study, may have contributed to the variability in the observed ratios. The volume of the milk samples obtained by manual expression may not have accurately reflected the volume consumed by the infant during feeding. As the volume of milk removed from the breast can influence the concentration of many xenobiotics in breast milk,[4,9] the variability in the milk volume obtained for our samples could have altered the observed ranitidine M:S ratios. Accordingly, it would be difficult to extrapolate our ratio data directly to the calculation of the ranitidine dose transferred to an infant via breast milk.

The lipid solubility of ranitidine may also have contributed to the disparity in the serum and milk concentration–time curve. Compounds with poor lipid solubility would be expected to produce a milk concentration–time curve that, relative to plasma, reflects a delayed time to peak concentration and a decreased apparent terminal elimination rate constant of the drug from breast milk.[9] This was apparently the case in our subject (Table 1), where ranitidine, a less lipid-soluble compound, accumulated in the "deep" pharmacokinetic compartment represented by breast milk.[4,9] Finally, the diurnal variation in milk production and the constituents of breast milk[9] could have contributed to the variability in the ranitidine M:S ratios observed in our subject.

The discordant disposition of ranitidine in the milk and serum following multiple dosing in our patient may also provide a possible explanation for the variable M:S ratios observed within a dosing interval. Riley et al.[2] reported median milk to plasma ratios of 1.92:1, 2.78:1, and 6.70:1 for samples collected at 2, 4, and 8 hours, respectively, following the oral administration of a single 150-mg dose of ranitidine (as the hydrochloride salt) in six lactating women. This trend of increasing ranitidine M:S ratios following single-dose administration[2] was also apparent following the administration of multiple doses in our patient.

Cimetidine (pKa 6.8) has also been reported to achieve higher concentrations in breast milk following repeated dosing, with milk to plasma ratios ranging from 4:6 to 11:8.[7] Physicochemical or pharmacokinetic relationships common to both cimetidine and ranitidine may contribute to their breast-milk disposition profiles during multiple-dose administration. Furthermore, physiologic factors associated with lactation[4,9] may influence common physicochemical and pharmacokinetic factors, resulting in extreme variability in the M:S ratios reported for both ranitidine[2] and cimetidine.[7]

Because of the variable M:S ratios for ranitidine, it is not feasible to estimate the infant dose by equations that assume a constant M:S ratio during a dosing interval.[9] The lack of data on ranitidine disposition in infants also precludes assessing the potential pharmacokinetic or pharmacodynamic consequences of administering the drug to an infant via breast milk. The manufacturer of ranitidine states that "caution should be exercised when Zantac is administered to a nursing mother."[10] While our data cannot be used either to support or to refute this recommendation, it appears that attempts to schedule infant feeding between one and two hours following maternal drug administration would result in reduced exposure of the infant to ranitidine via breast milk. This would be in contrast to nursing toward the end of a 12-hour dosing interval (i.e., > eight hours after a dose), when the largest M:S ratio was observed in our patient.

Conclusion. A pharmacokinetic approach examining the rates of appearance and disappearance of ranitidine in breast milk, the cumulative areas under the serum concentration–time curves for both the mother and infant, and the area under the breast-milk concentration–time curves will be required before the disposition of ranitidine in breast milk can be properly evaluated. Prospective, controlled studies of steady-state breast-milk disposition of ranitidine in a larger population of lactating women are needed to address properly both the scientific and clinical aspects of breast-feeding during ranitidine therapy.

References

1. Brogden RN, Carmine AA, Heel RC et al. Ranitidine: a review of its pharmacology and therapeutic use in peptic ulcer disease and other allied disease. *Drugs.* 1982; 24:267–303.
2. Riley AJ, Crowley P, Harrison C. Transfer of ranitidine to biological fluids: milk and semen. In: Misiewicz JJ, Wormsley KG, eds. The clinical use of ranitidine. Oxford: Medicine Publishing Foundation Series, Medicine Publishing Foundation. 1981; 5:77–86.
3. Mihaly GW, Drummer OH, Marshall A et al. High pressure liquid chromatographic determination of ranitidine, a new H_2-receptor antagonist in plasma and urine. *J Pharm Sci.* 1980; 69:1155–7.
4. Wilson JT. Pharmacokinetics of drug excretion. In: Wilson JT, ed. Drugs in breast milk. New York: ADIS Press Australasia Pty Ltd.; 1981; 15–33.
5. Devlin R, Duchin K, Fleiss P. Nadolol in human serum and breast milk. *Br J Clin Pharmacol.* 1981; 12:393–6.
6. White WB, Andreoli JW, Wong SH et al. Atenolol in human plasma and breast milk. *Obstet Gynecol.* 1984; 63:42–5.
7. Somogyi A, Gugler R. Cimetidine excretion into breast milk. *Br J Clin Pharmacol.* 1979; 7:627–9.
8. Sewing KF. Pharmacodynamics and pharmacokinetics of ranitidine in man. In: Misiewica JJ, Wormsley KG, eds. The clinical use of ranitidine. Oxford: Medicine Publishing Foundation Series, Medicine Publishing Foundation. 1981; 5:32–40.
9. Wilson JT. Determinants and consequences of drug excretion in breast milk. *Drug Metab Rev.* 1983; 14:619–52.
10. Glaxo, Inc., Zantac product information. Research Triangle Park, NC; 1984 Sep.

Warfarin absorption in a patient with short-bowel syndrome

MARK E. LEHMAN, KENNETH W. KOLB, GLENN R. BARNHART, LAWRENCE D. WAGMAN, AND WILLIAM H. BARR

Clin Pharm. 1985; 4:325–6

Short-bowel syndrome is a clinical entity denoting the loss of an extensive portion of the small bowel. It is difficult to define the term more accurately because the normal adult gut may be anywhere from 350 to 650 cm in length. The loss of more than 80% of the bowel results in profound nutritional losses.[1] Not only is the nutritional state of the patient in question, but the absorptive surface available for oral drug therapy is also a major concern. Mitchell et al.[2] reported a case in which a patient with approximately 100 cm of residual gut was able to absorb adequate amounts of warfarin sodium to elicit an anticoagulant response. We recently had the opportunity to study the oral absorption, serum concentrations, and consequent anticoagulant effect of warfarin sodium in a patient with less than 15 cm of jejunum.

Methods. The patient was a 76-year-old black woman who had been admitted to Medical College of Virginia Hospital on January 18, 1984, with a diagnosis of possible perforated diverticular abscess. She was found to have extensive small-bowel necrosis, and approximately two thirds of the small bowel had to be surgically resected. Forty-eight hours postoperatively, the patient was found to have necrotic terminal ileum and proximal right colon; following a second resection of the necrotic bowel and formation of an end jejunostomy, only 12–15 cm of jejunum remained.

During the course of hospitalization, the patient received intravenous heparin therapy to treat documented deep-vein thrombosis with the dose adjusted to keep the activated partial thromboplastin time at 1.5–2 times control. On February 23 (day 1) the patient was given an initial 20-mg dose of warfarin sodium in an effort to switch to oral anticoagulant therapy. Following the administration of this 20-mg dose, serum samples were collected at 0.5, 1, 2, 4, 8, 12, and 24 hours to be assayed for warfarin concentration in an effort to determine the extent of drug absorption. The warfarin elimination half-life was determined by regression analysis.

The patient did well over the next several weeks and was eventually discharged on April 21 (day 59); at the time of discharge, the dose of warfarin necessary to maintain the prothrombin time at approximately 1.6 times control was 2.5 mg daily. Figures 1 and 2 summarize the patient's warfarin dosage and response to anticoagulant therapy during hospitalization. Serum warfarin concentrations were determined just before the evening dose on February 27 (day 5) and one hour before dosing on April 20 (day 58).

On two separate occasions, 24-hour jejunostomy drainage collections were obtained and assayed for warfarin content following doses of 10 and 2.5 mg to ascertain the extent of warfarin absorption. The percentage of warfarin absorbed was determined by the following formula:

Figures 1 and 2. The patient's warfarin sodium dosage (top figure) and prothrombin time ratio response (bottom figure) during hospitalization are shown.

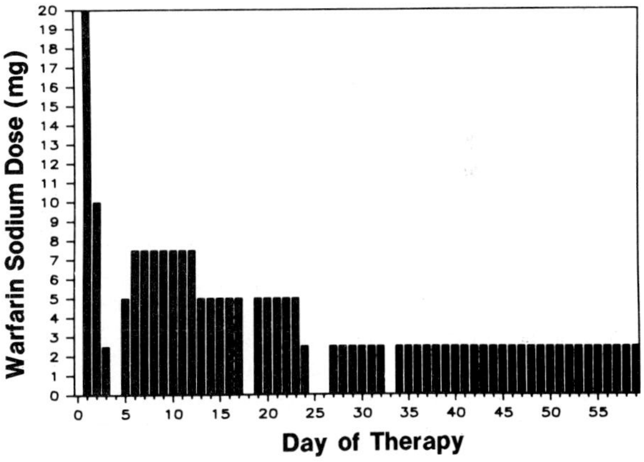

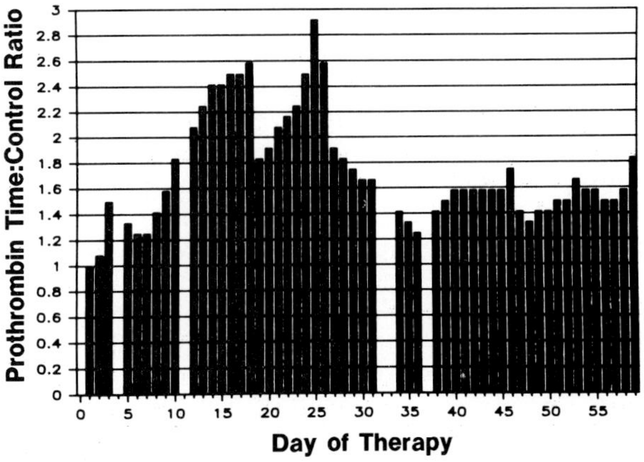

MARK E. LEHMAN, PHARM. D., is Assistant Professor, Department of Pharmacy and Pharmaceutics, School of Pharmacy, Medical College of Virginia (MCV). KENNETH W. KOLB, PHARM. D., is Assistant Clinical Professor, Department of Pharmacy, MCV Hospitals. GLENN R. BARNHART, M.D., is Fellow, and LAWRENCE D. WAGMAN, M.D., is Surgical Resident, Department of Surgery, MCV Hospitals. WILLIAM H. BARR, PH.D., is Professor and Chairman, Department of Pharmacy and Pharmaceutics, School of Pharmacy, MCV, Virginia Commonwealth University, Richmond.

Address reprint requests to Dr. Lehman at the School of Pharmacy, P.O. Box 581, MCV Station, Richmond, VA 23298-0001.

The support of the nursing staff of the General Surgery Service, MCV Hospital, is acknowledged.

Percent Absorbed = Dose − Amount Recovered/Dose × 100

where dose is the warfarin dose in milligrams, and amount recovered is the product of the concentration (mg/L) of warfarin sodium in the 24-hour jejunostomy collection and the volume (L) of jejunostomy collection.

All samples were assayed for warfarin content, using the high-performance liquid chromatography (HPLC) method developed by Vanhaelen-Fastre' and Vanboelen.[3]

Results. The elimination rate constant, as calculated from the serum warfarin concentrations taken on day 1, was 0.57 hr^{-1} ($r^2 = 0.98$). The half-life of racemic warfarin was 12.1 hours. The peak serum warfarin concentrations occurred at or before 0.5 hours following oral tablet administration.

The serum warfarin concentration just before the evening dose on day 5 was 0.65 mg/L. The steady-state serum concentration obtained one hour before dosing on day 58 before discharge was 1.2 mg/L. The amount of warfarin recovered in the 24-hour collection of jejunostomy drainage on day 2 was 0.72 mg. The calculated absorption of the 10-mg dose administered just before the start of the drainage collection was 92.8%. At steady state (day 57), only 0.1 mg of warfarin was recovered from the 24-hour jejunostomy drainage collection following the administration of 2.5 mg of warfarin sodium. The calculated absorption of this dose was 96.1%.

Discussion. Warfarin has been reported to be rapidly and completely absorbed following oral administration in patients with normal small-bowel conditions.[4,5] Mitchell et al.[2] reported a case of a 41-year-old man with 100 cm of small bowel intact who was successfully anticoagulated with warfarin doses of 5–7.5 mg daily. Warfarin concentrations determined from serum and gastrointestinal drainage samples were not reported. The authors concluded that successful anticoagulation might be possible in other patients with the same degree of small-bowel resection.

The patient we described exhibited complete and rapid absorption of oral warfarin therapy. The reported average absorption rate is greater than 90% in normal volunteers, while in this patient the calculated absorption was 92.8% and 96.1% on two separate occasions.[5] The time of peak warfarin absorption estimated in this patient (0.5 hr) was slightly faster than the usual reported time to peak of 60–90 minutes.[4] Although the relationship between the serum concentration of warfarin and its anticoagulant effect is indirect and complex, this patient had serum concentrations generally thought to be above the apparent minimum effective plasma warfarin concentration needed for anticoagulation.[6]

The halflife of 12.1 hours in this patient was shorter than the mean half-life reported in studies using HPLC assays, but was within the range reported for most studies.[4–6]

Conclusion. The pharmacologic response, absorption, and serum warfarin concentrations in this patient with approximately 15 cm of residual jejunum showed that warfarin was rapidly and almost completely absorbed. It appears that patients with short-bowel syndrome, regardless of the amount of small bowel remaining, can be effectively anticoagulated with oral warfarin sodium therapy.

References

1. Wright HK, Olson MD. Short bowel syndrome. *Curr Probl Surg*. 1971; 3:51.
2. Mitchell JF, Maas LC, Barger RC et al. Successful oral anticoagulant therapy in a patient with short bowel syndrome. *Am J Hosp Pharm*. 1977; 34:171–2.
3. Vanhaelen-Fastre' R,Vanboelen M. High performance liquid and thin layer chromatography of coumarin anticoagulants and their degradation products. *J Chromatogr*. 1976; 129:397–402.
4. O'Reilly RA, Aggeler PM, Leong LS. Studies on the coumarin anticoagulant drugs: the pharmacodynamics of warfarin in man. *J Clin Invest*. 42: 1542–51.
5. Breckenridge A, Orme M. Kinetics of warfarin absorption in man. *Clin Pharmacol Ther*. 1974; 14:955–61.
6. Nagashima R, O'Reilly RA, Levy G. Kinetics of pharmacologic effects in man: the anticoagulant action of warfarin. *Clin Pharmacol Ther*. 1969; 10:22–35.

Drug Experience

Straightforward reports of unusual drug experiences are included in this section. These may be confirmations of previously reported drug experiences or brief apparent first reports. While selected references may be cited, the purpose of a Drug Experience report is not to present an extensive review of the literature.

A related section, Grand Rounds, includes papers that are well-documented patient case reports with a thorough review of the important literature to help put the case in perspective.

Gentamicin elimination in a patient undergoing continuous ultrafiltration

MARK E. LEHMAN AND KENNETH W. KOLB

Clin Pharm. 1985; 4:327–30

Continuous arteriovenous ultrafiltration (CAVU) is a relatively new technique that is used to remove both water and solutes in patients with acute renal failure who are unable to tolerate conventional hemodialysis.[1] Hypotension, vascular instability, and electrolyte imbalances frequently occur during and after hemodialysis, and these conditions may preclude hemodialysis in medically unstable patients. When hemodialysis cannot be safely employed, CAVU can be used as an effective alternative. It offers the advantages of easy operation, greater hemodynamic stability, less fluctuation in serum electrolytes, and augmented fluid removal and input. The CAVU system facilitates the removal of fluid and electrolytes, as well as small- and medium-sized molecules (molecular weight < 5000 daltons).[1-9]

MARK E. LEHMAN, PHARM.D., is Assistant Professor, Department of Pharmacy and Pharmaceutics, School of Pharmacy, Medical College of Virginia (MCV), Virginia Commonwealth University, and KENNETH W. KOLB, PHARM.D., is Assistant Clinical Professor, Department of Pharmacy, MCV Hospitals, Richmond.

Address reprint requests to Dr. Lehman at the School of Pharmacy, P.O. Box 581, MCV Station, Richmond, VA 23298-0001.

The editorial assistance of William L. Rock, Pharm.D., and the support of the nursing staffs of the general medical and surgical intensive care units, MCV Hospitals, are acknowledged.

Presented at the 19th Annual ASHP Midyear Clinical Meeting, Dallas, TX, December 4, 1984.

In this report, we describe the case of a patient who underwent CAVU during gentamicin therapy and present a pharmacokinetic analysis of the effects of CAVU on gentamicin elimination. In a literature search, we found no information on the removal of aminoglycosides by CAVU. Since CAVU removes plasma water and the distribution of gentamicin in this compartment is extensive, it is likely that some drug would be removed. In patients who are critically ill from both sepsis and acute renal failure, and in whom changes in drug clearance could influence outcome of therapy, it is important to know whether a substantial amount of drug would be removed by CAVU.

Case Report. *Clinical Course.* A 73-year-old black woman came to our emergency room with a three-day history of a tender umbilical mass associated with nausea, vomiting, and constipation. The diagnosis upon admission included a presumed gangrenous small bowel secondary to an incarcerated umbilical hernia. She had a history of insulin-dependent diabetes mellitus, congestive heart failure, hypertension, and chronic renal failure. On admission, she was receiving NPH insulin, furosemide, digoxin, hydralazine, and nitroglycerin ointment. Admission laboratory tests and vital signs showed a BUN of 77 mg/dL, serum creatinine of 5.3 mg/dL, blood pressure of 126/77 mm Hg, and weight of 69.4 kg.

The patient was taken to surgery, and an incarcerated umbilical hernia and gangrenous small bowel were found. The gangrenous bowel was resected, and the hernia was repaired. She was transferred to the recovery room in guarded condition and was started on cefoxitin 1 g (as the sodium salt) i.v. every eight hours. Over the next several days, the patient's urine output decreased. On hospital day 5, her serum creatinine was 6.8 mg/dL and her blood urea nitrogen was 85 mg/dL. On day 11, an increased white blood cell count with a shift to the left (24,000 with 35% bands) was noted. A computed tomography scan performed on hospital day 12 showed fluid collection around the area of the anastomosis.

On day 13, surgical re-exploration revealed a perianastomotic leak and abscess formation. The abscess was drained, and an ileostomy was formed. Postoperative sputum, blood, and urine cultures were positive for enteric streptococci. *Enterobacter cloacae*, and *Pseudomonas aeruginosa* sensitive to piperacillin and gentamicin. On day 14 the patient began a regimen of these antibiotics with the dose of each adjusted for renal failure [piperacillin 4 g i.v. (as the sodium salt) every 12 hours and gentamicin 130 mg i.v. (as the sodium salt) every 24 hours].

The patient was essentially anuric at this point so it was decided that CAVU should be initiated in an effort to control her fluid volume. On hospital day 15 a Scribner shunt was inserted, and CAVU was begun. The patient's weight at this time was 89.6 kg. On day 17 the gentamicin regimen was discontinued and moxalactam 1 g i.v. (as the sodium salt) every 12 hours was added to the piperacillin regimen in an effort to minimize potentially nephrotoxic agents. The CAVU was extremely effective in removing excess fluid, with the patient losing an average of 4–5 kg per day. However, her condition continued to decline over the next several days, and hemodialysis was used to replace CAVU on day 22. On day 26, she experienced cardiopulmonary arrest and attempts to resuscitate her were unsuccessful.

Pharmacokinetic Analysis. CAVU was performed with the use of a Diafilter-30 ultrafiltration cartridge (Amicon Company, Danvers, MA) and conventional hemodialysis blood tubing (Gambro Inc., Barrington, IL). The entire circuit was flushed before use with two liters of heparinized saline. Circulatory access was obtained via a forearm Quinton-Scribner arteriovenous cannula. The filtrate port of the ultrafiltration cartridge was connected to a wall suction unit with a collection chamber attached.[10] Nurses in the intensive-care unit controlled the rate of ultrafiltration by adjusting the pressure gradient created by the wall suction unit. The ultrafiltration cartridge was changed daily by a dialysis technician. A continuous arterial infusion of heparin was administered at rates that would keep the clotting time between 175 and 219 seconds, or about two times the control value. Blood samples for gentamicin concentration were taken from the arterial line.

On hospital day 15, the patient received gentamicin 130 mg (as the sulfate salt) intravenously over 30 minutes beginning at 1400 hours. At approximately 1900 hours, CAVU was begun. Simultaneous ultrafiltrate and serum samples to be assayed for gentamicin content were collected at 5.5, 6.25, 11.25, 17.25, and 29.25 hours following gentamicin administration. In addition, each time the ultrafiltrate collection unit was emptied, an aliquot was collected, and the volume was recorded. All blood samples were immediately transferred to the toxicology lab, where the serum was extracted and frozen at −70 °C pending assay. The ultrafiltrate samples were refrigerated and transferred to the toxicology laboratory on the morning of day 17. The gentamicin concentration of each aliquot was determined using the TDX assay (fluorescent polarization, Abbott Laboratories).

The amount of gentamicin in each ultrafiltrate collection was calculated by multiplying the ultrafiltrate gentamicin concentration by the volume of the collection. The average rate of gentamicin removal by ultrafiltration was determined by dividing the amount of gentamicin removed in a collection period by the amount of time over which the collection took place. The average flow rate during each collection period was determined by dividing the volume of the ultrafiltrate collected by the duration of that collection period. The average flow rate during the entire period was calculated by dividing the total volume of ultrafiltrate collected by the total time of collection. The clearance of drug by ultrafiltration was determined by dividing the average rate of removal by the calculated serum gentamicin concentration at the midpoint of the collection period. The overall average clearance was calculated by taking a weighted average of all the individual clearance values, i.e., dividing the sum of the products of the individual clearance values and the duration of each collection period by the duration of the total procedure. The elimination rate constant (k) for gentamicin during ultrafiltration was determined using linear regression analysis of five serum gentamicin concentrations obtained during the collection period. This k was then used to estimate the serum gentamicin concentrations at the time of each ultrafiltrate collection.

The volume of ultrafiltrate collected and the gentamicin concentrations in the collected ultrafiltrate are presented in Tables 1 and 2. The total volume of ultrafiltrate removed in 23.75 hours was 7655 mL. Although the desired flow rate was 400 mL/hr, the actual flow rate ranged from 100 to 900 mL/hr, with an average flow rate of 322.3 mL/hr.

A total of 27.5 mg of gentamicin was removed by ultrafiltration during the 23.75-hour collection period. The average rate of gentamicin removal during each collection period ranged from 0.4 to 3.1 mg/hr with a mean of 1.6 ± 0.8 mg/hr. The ultrafiltration clearance of gentamicin ranged from 0.09 to 0.75 L/hr, with a weighted average for ultrafiltration clearance of 0.27 L/hr. The elimination rate constant (k) of gentamicin during ultrafiltration was 0.0106

Table 1.
Simultaneous Ultrafiltrate and Serum Gentamicin Concentrations

Hours After CAVU Initiation	Hours After End of Gentamicin Infusion	Gentamicin Concentration (mg/L)	
		Ultrafiltrate	Serum
0.25	5.5	4.5	5.2
1	6.25	4.5	5.1
6	11.25	4.2	4.8
12	17.25	4.1	4.6
24	29.25	3.5	4.0

hr^{-1} ($r = 0.997$), and the half-life ($t_{1/2}$) was calculated as 65.38 hours ($t_{1/2} = 0.693/k$).

Discussion. This case illustrates the removal of gentamicin by CAVU. The importance of the removal of 27.5 mg of gentamicin in a 24-hour period by CAVU could not be assessed in this patient because a prefiltration serum concentration was not obtained to calculate total body gentamicin stores. Also, an accurate determination of the patient's ability to eliminate gentamicin could not be made because of her rapidly deteriorating renal function and clinical state and the short duration of gentamicin therapy. However, it seems logical to postulate that the ultrafiltration clearance of gentamicin could be substantial in a septic patient with markedly impaired renal clearance, such as this patient.

The gentamicin elimination rate during hemodialysis is generally considered constant over the dialysis period because the blood flow rate is assumed to be constant. Of note in this case was the variability in ultrafiltration flow rates when wall suction was used to produce negative pressure and was manually adjusted by nursing personnel (Table 2). We thought that the flow rate of each interval would be similar; however, we did not find this to be the case. Both the average rate of gentamicin removal and the ultrafiltration clearance of gentamicin appear to be affected by the ultrafiltration flow rate (Figures 1 and 2). The following equation was derived from linear regression analysis to estimate clearance at various flow rates in this patient:

$$\text{Clearance (L/hr)} = 0.85\,[\text{flow (L/hr)}] - 0.0024 \quad (r = 0.998)$$

The importance of monitoring the flow rate can be illustrated by calculating the clearance of gentamicin at the extremes of flow rate. At a flow rate of 100 mL/hr, the gentamicin clearance would have been approximately 0.08 L/hr. By comparison, at the much faster flow rate of 900 mL/hr, the clearance would have been approximately 0.76 L/hr. In practice, with critically ill patients, these differences in gentamicin ultrafiltrate clearance could be clinically important.

Table 2.
Ultrafiltrate Data

Collection Period: Hours After CAVU Initiation	Collection Period: Hours After End of Gentamicin Infusion[a]	Volume of Ultrafiltrate Collected (mL)	Gentamicin Concentration of Ultrafiltrate (mg/L)	Ultrafiltrate Flow Rate (mL/hr)
0–1.75	5–7	700	4.1	400
1.75–2.75	7–8	450	3.9	450
2.75–3.75	8–9	350	4.3	350
3.75–5.75	9–11	500	3.7	250
5.75–8.75	11–14	700	3.6	233
8.75–15.75	14–21	700	3.7	100
15.75–16.75	21–22	900	3.4	900
16.75–17.75	22–23	750	3.6	750
17.75–19.75	23–25	800	3.3	400
19.75–21.75	25–27	950	3.4	475
21.75–23.75	27–29	855	3.3	428

[a] The CAVU was initiated 5.25 hours after the end of the gentamicin infusion.

Figure 1. Correlation of calculated average rate of gentamicin removal by ultrafiltration versus ultrafiltrate flow rate ($r = 0.986$).

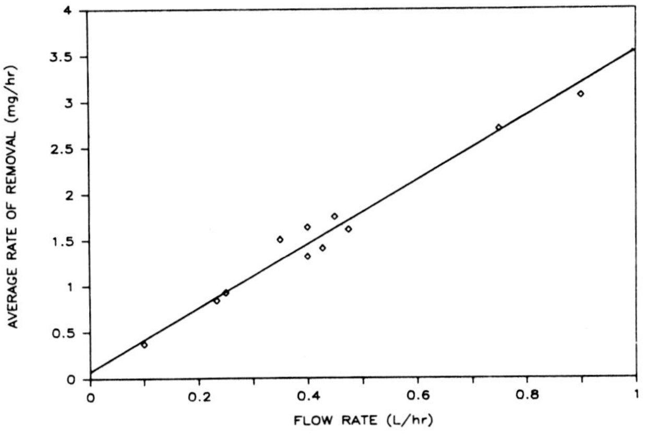

Figure 2. Correlation of ultrafiltrate clearance of gentamicin versus ultrafiltrate flow rate ($r = 0.998$).

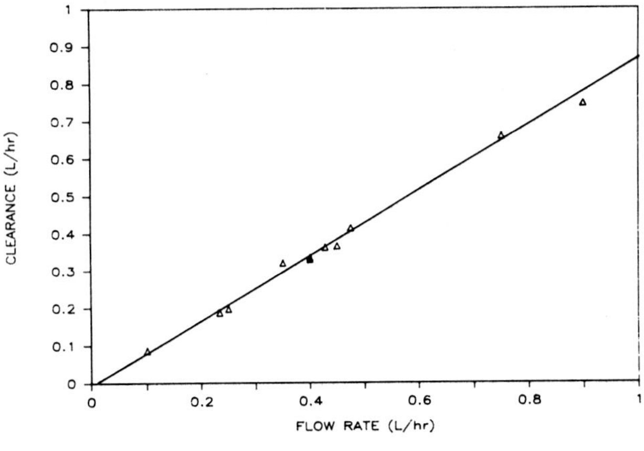

The potential in vitro inactivation of aminoglycoside antibiotics (in this case gentamicin) by piperacillin was minimized by preparing all blood samples for assay immediately after sampling.[11-13] Preparation consisted of centrifugation, decanting the serum portion, and freezing at −70 °C until assay. However, this could not be done for the ultrafiltrate samples, and so the amount of gentamicin reported in the ultrafiltrate may have been less than the actual amount present. If this was the case, then the amount of drug removed by CAVU was actually greater than what we are able to report, which may increase the importance of this route of gentamicin elimination.

Conclusion. CAVU is a therapeutic tool that is used to alleviate fluid overload in critically ill patients. It acts as an extracorporeal route of drug elimination for drugs such as gentamicin, and therefore, should be considered when making dosing adjustments in patients undergoing CAVU. For these patients, serum drug concentrations need to be monitored routinely to determine the extent of extracorporeal drug removal and ensure therapeutic antimicrobial serum concentrations. CAVU would be expected to have the greatest effect on elimination of drugs that are small- or medium-sized molecules, those that are distributed primarily into extracellular fluid, and drugs that exhibit little or no protein or tissue binding. As the use of CAVU increases, prospective pharmacokinetic studies will be needed to determine the effect of CAVU on pharmacokinetic variables.

References

1. Kramer P, Wigger W, Rieger J et al. Arteriovenous haemofiltration: a new and simple method for treatment of overhydrated patients resistant to diuretics. *Klin Wschr.* 1977; 55:1121–2.
2. Synhaivsky A, Kurtz S, Wochos D et al. Acute renal failure treated by slow continuous ultrafiltration. *Mayo Clin Proc.* 1983; 58:729–33.
3. Lauer A, Saccaggi A, Ronco C et al. Continuous arteriovenous hemofiltration in the critically ill patient. Clinical use and operational characteristics. *Ann Intern Med.* 1983; 99:455–60.
4. Kramer P, Seegers A, DeVivie R et al. Therapeutic potential of hemofiltration. *Clin Nephrol.* 1979; 11:145–9.
5. Paganini EP, Nakamoto S. Continuous slow ultrafiltration in oliguric acute renal failure. *Trans Am Soc Artif Intern Organs.* 1980; 26:201–4.
6. Silverstein ME, Ford CA, Lysaght MJ et al. Treatment of severe fluid overload by ultrafiltration. *N Engl J Med.* 1974; 291:747–51.
7. Kramer P, Bohler J, Kehr A et al. Intensive care potential of continuous arteriovenous hemofiltration. *Trans Am Soc Artif Intern Organs.* 1980; 26:28–32.
8. Henderson LW, Besarab A, Michaels A et al. Blood purification by ultrafiltration and fluid replacement (diafiltration). *Trans Am Soc Artif Intern Organs.* 1967; 13:216–26.
9. Kaplan AA, Longnecker RE, Folkert YW. Continuous arteriovenous hemofiltration: a report of six months' experience. *Ann Intern Med.* 1984; 100:358–67.
10. Kaplan AA, Longnecker RE, Folkert YW. Suction-assisted continuous arteriovenous hemofiltration. *Trans Am Soc Artif Intern Organs.* 1983; 29:408–13.
11. Chanbusarakum P, Murray PR. Analysis of the interaction between piperacillin, ticarcillin, or carbenicillin and aminoglycoside antibiotics. *Antimicrob Agents Chemother.* 1978; 14:505–6.
12. Pickering LK, Rutherford I. Effect of concentration and time upon inactivation of tobramycin, gentamicin, netilmicin and amikacin by azlocillin, carbenicillin, mecillinam, mezlocillin and piperacillin. *J Pharmacol Exp Ther.* 1981; 21:345–9.
13. Thompson MB, Russo ME, Saxon BJ et al. Gentamicin inactivation by piperacillin or carbenicillin in patients with end-stage renal disease. *Antimicrob Agents Chemother.* 1982; 21:268–73.

Pentobarbital coma for treating intractable seizures in a neonate

TIMOTHY E. WELTY AND ROBERT L. KRIEL

Clin Pharm. 1985; 4:330–2

Anesthetic barbiturates have been used successfully to treat intractable seizures and increased intracranial pressure (ICP) in patients as young as six months old.[1-3] Recently, our neonatal intensive-care unit cared for a newborn infant who was treated with pentobarbital coma to control seizures that were related to increased ICP and were refractory to phenobarbital. Since we are unaware of literature reports describing the use of pentobarbital coma in neonates, we describe the clinical outcome and pharmacokinetics of pentobarbital in this patient.

Case Report. A 41–42-week gestation, 4150-g infant girl was admitted to our neonatal intensive-care unit three hours after birth. She was the product of an uneventful first pregnancy for a 32-year-old woman. Labor lasted for nine hours and was complicated by late decelerations occurring approximately 7.5 hours after labor had started. Upon delivery the infant was intensely meconium stained, had one- and five-minute Apgar scores of 3 and 3, and was intubated within two minutes. The initial physical examination was unremarkable. The infant's head circumference was 35.5 cm.

TIMOTHY E. WELTY, PHARM.D., is Clinical Pharmacist, St. Elizabeth Hospital, Lafayette, and Assistant Professor of Clinical Pharmacy, Purdue University, West Lafayette, IN. At the time of this study, he was a research fellow in neuropharmacology and pharmacokinetics, Department of Pharmaceutical Services, St. Paul-Ramsey Medical Center, St. Paul, MN. ROBERT L. KRIEL, M.D., is Director, Department of Pediatric Neurology, St. Paul-Ramsey Medical Center, and Associate Professor of Pediatric Neurology, University of Minnesota, Minneapolis.

Address reprint requests to Dr. Welty at the Pharmacy Department, St. Elizabeth Hospital. P.O. Box 7501, Lafayette, IN 47903.

Supported in part by the Medical Education and Research Foundation of St. Paul-Ramsey Medical Center, St. Paul, MN.

Three hours after delivery, the infant began to have seizures along with the clinical signs of increased ICP. Over the next four hours the infant received 140 mg of phenobarbital sodium intravenously in three divided doses. Glycerol was sterilized for intravenous use as described by MacDonald and Uden,[4] and 4 g every six hours for eight doses was administered. Ampicillin 200 mg i.v. every 12 hours (as the sodium salt) and gentamicin 10 mg i.v. every 12 hours (as the sulfate salt) were also given for 36 hours. The respirator rate was increased to hyperventilate the infant. In spite of serum phenobarbital concentrations ranging from 33.5 to 35.5 mg/L, eight hours after starting the phenobarbital therapy the neurologist's examination and EEG interpretation indicated that the seizures were persisting. Pancuronium bromide 0.15–0.2 mg i.v. was given every hour as needed to provide better control of respirations and continued for 24 hours.

On the second day of life, the infant's head circumference increased to 36.5 cm. The anterior fontanelle was bulging, and the sutures were separated. Since the neurologic status of the infant continued to deteriorate, coma was induced with pentobarbital sodium in an effort to control seizures and prevent progressive neurologic damage. The pentobarbital dose was adjusted to control the seizures and ICP.[5]

The infant was maintained on a respirator, and continuous EEG monitoring was used to detect seizure activity. Phenobarbital was discontinued, and a loading dose of pentobarbital sodium 40 mg (9.6 mg/kg) was infused over one hour. A maintenance infusion of pentobarbital sodium 1 mg/kg/hr was then started with the goal of achieving a serum concentration of approximately 10 mg/L.[2,3,5] Serum concentrations were measured by a modified gas chromatography assay that separated the pentobarbital from phenobarbital and had a sensitivity of 1 mg/L.[6] Electroencephalographic monitoring and serum concentration determinations were used to guide the dosage adjustments.

Serum pentobarbital concentrations were measured at 1, 25, and 48 hours after discontinuation of the infusion. The terminal elimination rate and half-life were estimated on the basis of a linear-regression analysis of the three serum concentrations. The apparent volume of distribution was estimated from a serum concentration achieved one hour after the initial loading dose.

Pentobarbital sodium was administered intermittently over a period of three days. Three additional loading doses of pentobarbital were given after starting the infusion because a resident physician thought that the seizures had not been controlled. Later, the pentobarbital infusion was stopped for 24 hours because of concern about excessive electroencephalographic suppression. The infusion rate of pentobarbital ranged from 0.5 to 2.0 mg/kg/hr (Figure 1). Several serum pentobarbital concentrations were determined, and the measurements ranged from 10.0 to 20.5 mg/L (Figure 1). Retrospective analysis of clinical data showed that the seizures were originally controlled at pentobarbital concentrations above 15.0 mg/L, in spite of the resident physician's initial evaluation.

A neurologic examination of the infant one month later revealed a head circumference of 36.2 cm, normal spontaneous movements of the lower extremities, and spasticity with restricted activity in the upper extremities. A computed tomography scan showed moderately dilated lateral ventricles and extensive decreased density in both hemispheres, suggesting cerebral atrophy.

Discussion. Pentobarbital coma has gained increasing acceptance in the treatment of both increased intracranial pressure[2] and status epilepticus.[3,5] Previous reports of pentobarbital use and pharmacokinetics have been limited to adults and children.[2,7,8] This case represents the first literature report of clinical and pharmacokinetic data on pentobarbital use for this indication in a neonate.

The apparent volume of distribution, terminal elimination half-life, and elimination rate constant in our patient were 1.0 L/kg, 21 hours, and 0.33 hr^{-1}, respectively. Plotting on a logarithmic scale, the elimination portion of the serum concentration–time curve demonstrated a better fit with a one-compartment pharmacokinetic model. This differs from previous pentobarbital pharmacokinetic modeling[7,8] and is most likely related to the completion of the distribution phase during the loading infusion of pentobarbital. In addition, the

Figure 1. Pentobarbital serum concentrations (top) correlated with pentobarbital doses (bottom). Loading doses of pentobarbital were infused over one hour. The broken line represents the elimination portion of the curve.

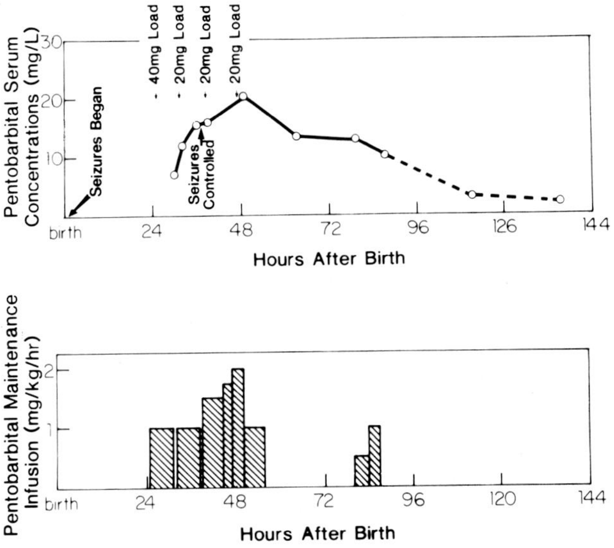

pharmacokinetic values in this infant were similar to those that have been reported in adults.[7,8]

As the serum pentobarbital concentrations approached 20 mg/L, the neurologist thought that the normal EEG patterns had been suppressed excessively. This led to the temporary discontinuation of the pentobarbital infusion. These EEG changes may have been attributable to the unusual sensitivity of the neonatal cerebral cortex to pentobarbital or to an interaction between phenobarbital and pentobarbital at phenobarbital concentrations of approximately 35 mg/L. The precise reason for these changes at reasonable pentobarbital serum concentrations is unclear from this case, but clinicians should be aware of this problem when using pentobarbital in neonates.

Conclusion. This case demonstrates the potential for using pentobarbital coma in neonates with refractory seizures and increased ICP. In spite of a poor neurologic outcome, which was probably inevitable, the pentobarbital did control seizures in this patient.

References

1. Brown AS, Horton JM. Status epilepticus treated by intravenous infusions of thiopentone sodium. *Br Med J.* 1967; Jan:27–8.
2. Schaible DH, Cupit GC, Swedlow DB et al. High-dose pentobarbital pharmacokinetics in hypothermic brain-injured children. *J Pediatr.* 1982; 100 (4):655–60.
3. Goldberg MA, McIntyre HB. Barbiturates in the treatment of status epilepticus. *Adv Neurol.* 1983; 34:499–503.
4. MacDonald JT, Uden DL. Intravenous glycerol and mannitol therapy in children with intracranial hypertension. *Neurology.* 1982; 32:437–40.
5. Young GB, Blume WE, Bolton CF et al. Anesthetic barbiturates in refractory status epilepticus. *Can J Neurol Sci.* 1980; 7 (4):291–2.
6. Stern EL, Caron GP. Measuring barbiturates, sedatives, and anticonvulsants in serum by gas-liquid chromatography. *Am J Med Technol.* 1977; 43(9):834–42.
7. Brodie BB, Burns JJ, Mark LC et al. The fate of pentobarbital in man and dog and a method for its estimation in biological material. *J Pharmacol Exp Ther.* 1953; 109:26–34.
8. Ehrnedo M. Pharmacokinetics and distribution properties of pentobarbital in humans following oral and intravenous administration. *J Pharm Sci.* 1974; 63:1114–8.

Potentiation of warfarin anticoagulation by topical testosterone ointment

SARAH MCQUADE LORENTZ AND ROBERT T. WEIBERT

Clin Pharm. 1985; 4:333–5

There is substantial evidence indicating that 17-alkylated androgens can increase the hypoprothrombinemic effect of oral anticoagulants. This interaction has resulted in hemorrhagic complications in anticoagulated patients. Anabolic steroids including methandrostenolone, norethandrolone, and oxymetholone have been shown to interact with oral anticoagulants.[1-10] An early report suggested that non-17-alkylated androgens, like testosterone esters, may not interact with warfarin.[8] In the patient described in this case report, the anticoagulant effect of warfarin increased markedly after the application of a vaginal ointment of testosterone propionate, a non-17-alkylated androgen.

Case Report. A 69-year-old white woman with chronic atrial fibrillation and left atrial enlargement received anticoagulation therapy with warfarin (Coumadin, Dupont, Wilmington, DE). She had been monitored by the University of California–San Diego Medical Center anticoagulation clinic during 16 months of warfarin therapy with doses ranging from 5 to 6.1 mg daily. Throughout this period, she had also taken a combination product of hydrochlorothiazide and triamterene (Dyazide, Smith Kline & French, Philadelphia, PA) one twice daily, digoxin (Burroughs Wellcome, Research Triangle Park, NC) 0.25 mg twice daily, and propanolol hydrochloride (Ayerst Laboratories, New York, NY) 20 mg four times daily.

The most recent warfarin dose had been 7.5 mg Sunday and 5 mg daily for the rest of the week (week 0). At this time, the prothrombin time (PT) by the quick one-stage method using Dade Thromboplastin-C[a] on a Lancer Coagulyzer[b] was 16.8 seconds (control 10.5 seconds) with a prothrombin

SARAH MCQUADE LORENTZ, PHARM.D., is Home Care Pharmacist, Department of Pharmacy, University of California–San Diego Medical Center, and ROBERT T. WEIBERT, PHARM.D., is Associate Clinical Professor, School of Pharmacy, University of California–San Francisco.

Address reprint requests to Dr. Lorentz at the Department of Pharmacy H-765, UCSD Medical Center, 225 Dickinson Street, San Diego, CA 92103-9981.

Presented at the 17th Annual ASHP Midyear Clinical Meeting, Los Angeles, CA, December 6, 1982.

time ratio (PTR) of 1.6 (Figure 1). At week 3, she was found to have lichen sclerosus et atrophicus, and treatment was started with a 2% testosterone propionate in a petrolatum ointment, which was applied twice daily to the vulvar and vaginal lesions. She returned for a routine anticoagulation follow-up examination after two weeks of testosterone treatment. At this time (week 5), the PT was 29.4 seconds (control 10.3 seconds) with a PTR of 2.9 (Figure 1). The increase in the PT could not be related to alcohol ingestion, medication changes, dietary changes, or other factors known to enhance anticoagulation.

The patient showed no signs of hemorrhage and the warfarin therapy was discontinued for two days and then restarted with 2.5-mg doses alternating with 5-mg doses every other day. One week later, the PTR was 1.7 and remained stable for the following two weeks. Over the next month, the patient decreased use of the testosterone ointment, and the PTR dropped to 1.2 (Figure 1, week 14). The warfarin dosage was then increased to 5 mg, but she also resumed twice-daily use of the testosterone ointment. The following week (week 15), the PTR was 1.6, and a serum testosterone concentration was 5667 pg/mL (normal 50–400 pg/mL) (Figure 1, week 15). Five weeks later, the PTR was 2.8. Again, the warfarin therapy was stopped for two days, and the regimen of alternating 5-mg with 2.5-mg doses was started. After one week, the PTR was 1.7 (Figure 1, week 21).

Over the next six weeks, the patient's use of the testosterone ointment was gradually tapered. The warfarin dose was increased to an average daily amount of 4.2 mg, and eventually it was increased to 5 mg daily. Her responses to the anticoagulant therapy remained stable. A serum testosterone concentration determined three months after she had discontinued using the ointment was 541 pg/mL (Figure 1, week 39).

Discussion. Substantial amounts of the 2% testosterone propionate ointment were absorbed via the vaginal and vulvar route. This topical absorption was shown by a 10-fold increase in the serum testosterone concentration, which was 5667 pg/mL during and 541 pg/mL after use of the ointment.

The twice-daily use of the testosterone ointment caused a 78% increase in PT. The second course produced a 65% increase in PT. A 25% reduction in the warfarin dosage was needed to get the PTR to return to the therapeutic range. Additionally, as the use of the testosterone ointment was reduced, the patient's PTR decreased, and the warfarin dose was increased.

The mechanism of action of androgenic steroid–warfarin interactions remains unclear. The interactions among warfarin and the 17-alkylated testosterone derivatives, including methandrostenolone, norethandrolone, methyltestosterone, danazol, and oxymetholone, have been explained by a variety of mechanisms. These include decreased formation of clotting factors, increased degradation of clotting factors, and increased anticoagulant receptor-site affinity. It has also been hypothesized that the fibrinolytic activity of anabolic steroids may contribute to hemorrhagic events.[1–13]

Conclusion. Alkylated androgens are known to potentiate the effects of oral anticoagulants, and our experience with this patient showed that a non-17-alkylated androgen testosterone propionate, could interact with warfarin. This case also demonstrated the substantial absorption of the testosterone ointment by the vulvar and vaginal routes. Although individual differences in topical absorption are likely, clinicians should be aware of possible systemic effects of applying testosterone via this route. The potentially harmful interaction of the testosterone ointment and anticoagulation therapy can be safely managed with careful monitoring and an appropriate reduction in the warfarin dose.

Figure 1. Clinical results from a course of warfarin and 2% testosterone propionate ointment showing changes in prothrombin time ratios, mean warfarin dose, and serum testosterone concentrations. At point A (during use of testosterone ointment) serum concentration was 5667 pg/mL; at point B (three months after ointment was discontinued) serum testosterone concentration was 541 pg/mL. The normal range of serum testosterone in postmenopausal women is 50–400 pg/mL.

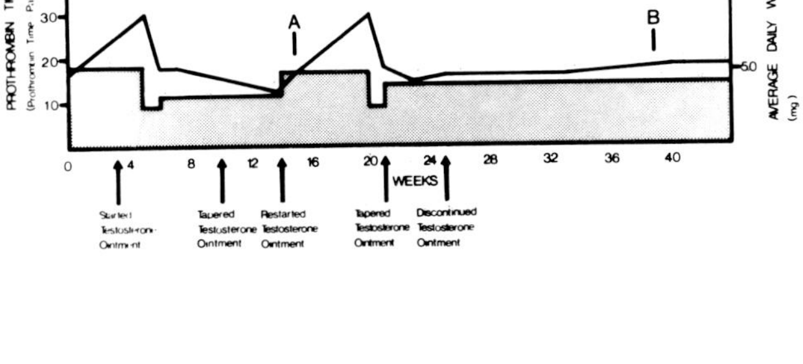

[a] B4216-50 Dade Diagnostics Inc., Aguada, Puerto Rico 00602.

[b] Lancer Coagulyzer II, Sherwood Medical Industries, Inc., 1831 Olive Street, St. Louis, MO 63013.

References

1. Pyorala K, Kekki M. Decreased anticoagulant tolerance during methandrostenolone therapy. *Scand J Clin Lab Invest.* 1963; 15:367–74.
2. Pyorala K, Kekki M. Anabolic steroids and anticoagulant requirements. *Lancet.* 1963; 2:360–1.
3. Murakami M, Odake K, Matsuda T. Effects of anabolic steroids on anticoagulant therapy. *Jpn Circ J.* 1965; 29:243–50.
4. McLaughlin GE, McCarty DJ Jr, Segal BL. Hemarthrosis complicating anticoagulant therapy. *JAMA.* 1966; 196:1020–1.
5. Schrogie JJ, Solomon HM. The anticoagulant response to bishydroxycoumarin II. The effect of D-thyroxine, clofibrate and norethandrolone. *Clin Pharmacol Ther.* 1967; 8:70–7.
6. Robinson BHB, Hawkins JB, Ellis JE. Decreased anticoagulant tolerance with oxymetholone. *Lancet.* 1971; 1:1356.

7. Longridge RGM, Gillam PMS, Barton GM. Decreased anticoagulant tolerance with oxymetholone. *Lancet*. 1971; 1:90.
8. Edwards MS, Curtis JR. Decreased anticoagulant tolerance with oxymetholone. *Lancet*. 1971; 1:491.
9. DeOya JC, Del Rio A, Noya M et al. Decreased anticoagulant tolerance with oxymetholone in paroxysmal nocturnal haemoglobulinemia. *Lancet*. 1971; 2:259.
10. Ekert H, Muntz RH, Colebatch JG. Decreased anticoagulant tolerance with oxymetholone. *Lancet*. 1971; 2:609.
11. Husted S, Andreason F, Foged L. Increased sensitivity to phenprocoumon during methyltestosterone therapy. *Eur J Clin Pharmacol*. 1976; 10:209–16.
12. Goulbourne IA, Macleod DA. An interaction between Danazol and warfarin. *Br J Obstet Gynaecol*. 1981; 88:950–1.
13. Small M, Lowe GDO, McCune G et al. Danazol and oral anticoagulants. *Scott Med J*. 1982; 27:331–2.

Dermatologic reaction to a sustained-release theophylline product

STEPHEN MENDEL, CHARLES A. BECK, JR., AND JEAN A. RUMSFIELD

Clin Pharm. 1985;4:334–335

The use of theophylline has increased greatly in the past 10–15 years. It is used as a prophylactic agent for controlling bronchospasm in patients with asthma.[1] Sustained-release theophylline preparations are now available that provide constant steady-state serum theophylline concentrations; Theo-Dur (Key Pharmaceuticals, Miami, FL) is widely used for this purpose.

Allergic reactions to aminophylline (theophylline ethylenediamine)[2,3] have been attributed to the ethylenediamine component rather than to the active drug.[4,5] Our literature search failed to document any allergic reactions to theophylline alone. We recently treated a patient who demonstrated an allergic reaction to Theo-Dur.

Case Report. A 25-year-old man, weight 160 lb (72.5 kg), height 71 in, with no history of allergies or asthma was admitted to the emergency room on the evening of July 25, 1983, with chief complaints of shortness of breath and coughing. His blood pressure was 112/70 mm Hg, his temperature was 98.3 °F (36.8 °C), and his respiratory rate was 38 per minute. Physical examination revealed expiratory wheezing; no other abnormalities were found. The patient was diagnosed as suffering from acute asthma and was treated with two doses of terbutaline sulfate 0.25 mg subcutaneously and one 300-mg tablet of Theo-Dur (lot 334202). Prescriptions for Theo-Dur and cephalexin were given to the patient, who was to have them filled at a community pharmacy.

At 6 a.m. the next morning, the patient again was admitted to the emergency room with a diffuse, erythematous, maculopapular, pruritic rash over his entire body (including the palms of his hands). The patient was admitted to the hospital, and therapy consisting of aminophylline (Aminophyllin, G. D. Searle) 42 mg intravenously each hour (0.58 mg/kg/hr), cephalexin (Keflex, Dista) 500 mg every six hours, and guaifenesin (Robitussin, A. H. Robins Company, Richmond, VA) 5 mL four times a day was begun. He was also given one dose of diphenhydramine (Benadryl, Parke Davis) 50 mg intramuscularly followed by 25 mg orally every six hours, and calamine lotion was applied as needed.

The laboratory data revealed an erythrocyte sedimentation rate of 63 mm/hr and a white blood cell count of 7600, with a differential count of 57 segmented neutrophils, 19 band neutrophils, 2 eosinophils, 14 lymphocytes, and 8 monocytes.

Over the next three days the rash subsided, therapy with Theo-Dur (lot 334202) 300 mg every 12 hours was begun, and the patient was given an albuterol inhaler (Proventil, Schering). Within 24 hours the rash reappeared. Theo-Dur therapy was stopped, and the patient was given aminophylline 42 mg per hour intravenously and a bolus dose of methylprednisolone sodium succinate (Solu-Medrol, Upjohn) 500 mg. The rash subsided and therapy with prednisone 30 mg orally each day was begun.

On August 1, 1983, cephalexin was discontinued and Theo-Dur was restarted at a dose of 450 mg every 12 hours. Within 12 hours, the rash again appeared.

The Theo-Dur was discontinued and therapy with another sustained-release theophylline product (Slo-Phyllin Gyrocaps, William H. Rorer, Inc., Fort Washington, PA) was begun at a dose of 375 mg every 12 hours. The rash disappeared and the patient was discharged three days later (August 4) on a regimen of Slo-Phyllin Gyrocaps 375 mg every 12 hours. The patient's medication course is in Figure 1.

Discussion. We initially suspected that the patient was allergic to one of the inert ingredients used in the manufacturing of Theo-Dur. We contacted the manufacturer of Theo-Dur to obtain a list of tablet ingredients. Two ingredients in particular, beeswax and cornstarch, caught our attention because many people are sensitive to bee stings and some people are sensitive to corn. Upon careful questioning, the

STEPHEN MENDEL, PHARM.D., is Clinical Pharmacist, Department of Pharmacy Services, University Hospitals of Cleveland, Cleveland, OH. CHARLES A. BECK, JR., M.D., is Medical Director, Respiratory Therapy Services, Ingalls Memorial Hospital, Harvey, IL. JEAN A. RUMSFIELD, PHARM.D., is Clinical Assistant Director, College of Pharmacy, University of Illinois, Chicago.

Address reprint requests to Dr. Mendel at the Department of Pharmacy Services, University Hospitals of Cleveland, Cleveland, OH 44106.

Figure 1. Medication course in relation to appearance of rash; + = rash present, ± = rash fading, − = no rash.

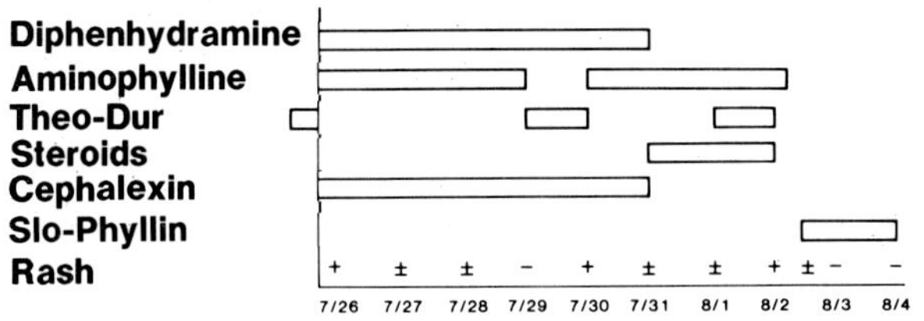

patient denied allergy to either of these.

Allergy to cephalexin was also considered because cephalosporins are frequently implicated in dermatologic reactions (up to 13% incidence).[6] A review of this patient's previous history revealed that he had received cephalexin four to five years before admission without adverse effect. Although sensitization could not be ruled out, this patient's rash subsided while he was receiving cephalexin. In addition, the cephalexin had been discontinued before the last positive rechallenge with Theo-Dur.

Once we determined that therapy with Slo-Phyllin Gyrocaps did not cause a rash in this patient, we contacted William H. Rorer, Inc. and asked for a list of excipients used in that product. The company indicated that no ingredients except sugars and dyes are added.

One disease state that could have been responsible for a dermatologic eruption of the type seen in this patient is syphilis; unfortunately, no test for syphilis was performed.

Adverse drug reactions are common, and the skin is more frequently affected than any other organ system.[7] The rate of all cutaneous reactions per course of drug therapy is estimated to be 3 per 1000.[8] Any drug can potentially produce a rash; unfortunately, no tests are currently available to confirm that a single medication is the cause of a particular eruption.[6] Methods that are available to help the clinician determine the cause of a dermatologic reaction include skin testing, radioallergosorbent test, hemagglutination (to detect drug-specific IgM and IgG), and rechallenge. In this case report, rechallenge was the only method used to determine the cause of the reaction.

Theophylline is generally considered unlikely to cause an allergic reaction.[5,6] Skin testing has been suggested as a method for predicting allergy to aminophylline, theophylline, or ethylenediamine, although the nonspecific irritant effect of ethylenediamine can cloud the interpretation.[5] Skin testing with components of Theo-Dur and Slo-Phyllin Gyrocaps might have been more precise for determining the cause of reaction in this patient. However, many authors think than an accurate history and rechallenge with the drug under careful observation can be more useful than provocative skin testing.[5]

Conclusion. We were unable to determine a definite cause for this patient's allergic skin rash. Our first hypothesis of a theophylline allergy proved incorrect. The most likely explanation is an unusual hypersensitivity reaction to the sustained-release theophylline product Theo-Dur.

References

1. Hendeles L, Weinberger M. Theophylline: a state of the art review. *Pharmacotherapy.* 1983; 3:2–44.
2. Tag J, Weissborg D. Allergies to aminophylline. *Acta Allergol.* 1958; 12:39.
3. Provost TT, Jillson GF. Ethylenediamine and contact dermatitis. *Arch Dermatol.* 1967; 96:231–4.
4. Davis L, Cupit G, Shimomura S. Ethylenediamine hypersensitivity. *Drug Intell Clin Pharm.* 1978; 42:482–3.
5. Kradjan WA, Lakshminarayn S. Allergy to aminophylline: lack of predictability by skin testing. *Am J Hosp Pharm.* 1981; 38: 1031–3.
6. Swinyer LJ. Determining the cause of drug eruptions. *Primary Care.* 1982; 10(3):369–87.
7. Cluff LE, Caranosos GH, Stewart RB, eds. Clinical problems with drugs. Philadelphia: W.B. Saunders Company; 1975:80.
8. Arndt KA, Jick H. Rates of cutaneous reactions to drugs. *JAMA.* 1976; 235:918–23.

CP Continuing Education

The ASHP Continuing Education system gives readers a self-assessment mechanism for selected articles in Clinical Pharmacy *and the* American Journal of Hospital Pharmacy. *It also allows readers to obtain continuing education credit for these articles.*

For the purpose of CE-credit enrollment, a blank answer sheet is published at the end of each installment of the column for the CE articles in that issue. An enrollee accumulates these answer sheets until the enrollment is submitted, using the form that is published in the May–June and November–December issues of Clinical Pharmacy *and in the June and December issues of the* American Journal of Hospital Pharmacy. *Any combination of tests within a 12-month period, from both* Clinical Pharmacy *and* American Journal of Hospital Pharmacy, *may be included in an enrollment. More complete details about enrollment in the system will appear in the semiannual enrollment form.*

All education aspects of the program are directed by Warren E. McConnell, Ph.D., Special Assistant in the ASHP Executive Office.

Article 680-204-8508 (see page 279)
Qualifies for 2.0 hours of CE credit

Pathophysiology and treatment of deep-vein thrombosis and pulmonary embolism

Learning Objectives

After studying this article, the reader should be able to

1. Identify the three mechanisms responsible for thromboembolism.
2. Compare and contrast the mechanisms of action of thrombolytic agents, heparin, and warfarin.
3. List recommended treatment regimens for streptokinase, urokinase, and intravenous heparin for the acute treatment of deep-vein thrombosis and pulmonary embolism.
4. List recommended durations of warfarin therapy for acute deep-vein thrombosis and pulmonary embolism.
5. Identify at least one blood coagulation test for monitoring therapy with thrombolytic agents, heparin, and warfarin and compare the usefulness of the respective tests in terms of predicting efficacy and toxicity of therapy with each drug.

Self-assessment Questions

For each question there is one best answer only.

1. The major danger of deep-vein thrombosis is

   a. Hypercoagulability.
   b. Destruction of venous valves.
   c. Embolization.
   d. All of the above alternatives are correct.
   e. Alternatives b and c only are correct.

2. Factors that may predispose to the development of deep-vein thrombosis include

   a. Pregnancy.
   b. Prothrombin deficiency.
   c. Carcinoma.
   d. All of the above alternatives are correct.
   e. Alternatives a and c only are correct.

3. Laboratory monitoring of thrombolytic therapy is used primarily to

   a. Minimize bleeding complications.
   b. Ensure that a lytic state is achieved.
   c. Monitor antibodies to the drug.
   d. Determine when to stop therapy.
   e. Determine dosage adjustments during therapy.

4. Large loading doses of heparin are given to patients with pulmonary embolism to prevent

   a. Thrombocytopenia.
   b. Pulmonary-arteriolar vasodilation.
   c. Prostaglandin release.
   d. Alternatives b and c are both correct.
   e. None of the above alternatives is correct.

5. The blood component that causes lysis of fibrin clots after activation by streptokinase or urokinase is

   a. Prothrombin.
   b. Plasmin.
   c. Thrombin.
   d. Protein C.
   e. Antithrombin III.

6. The recommended duration of streptokinase treatment in patients with massive pulmonary embolism is

a. 96 hours.
b. 72 hours.
c. 48 hours.
d. 24 hours.
e. 12 hours.

7. Thromboplastins used as reagents for prothrombin tests are derived from all of the following sources except

a. Cows.
b. Pigs.
c. Humans.
d. Rabbits.
e. All of the above alternatives are correct.

8. Risk factors for hemorrhage with anticoagulant therapy include

a. Severe hypertension.
b. Age over 60.
c. Cancer.
d. All of the above alternatives are correct.
e. Alternatives a and b only are correct.

9. Estrogens may interact with warfarin by which of the following mechanisms?

a. Induction of warfarin-metabolizing enzymes.
b. Increased synthesis of clotting factors.
c. Displacement of warfarin from plasma proteins.
d. Decreased bioavailability of warfarin.
e. Estrogens do not interact with warfarin.

10. Which of the following thrombolytic drug regimens is appropriate for a 100-kg patient with a massive pulmonary embolism?

a. Urokinase 250,000 IU i.v. over 10 min, then 100,000 IU/hr i.v. for 12 hours.
b. Streptokinase 250,000 IU i.v. over 30 min, then 100,000 IU/hr for 72 hours.
c. Streptokinase 4,400 IU i.v. over 10 min, then 4,400 IU/hr for 24 hours.
d. Urokinase 4,400 IU i.v. over 10 min, then 4,400 IU/hr for 12 hours.
e. None of the above regimens is appropriate.

Article 680-204-8509 (see page 297)
Qualifies for 1.0 hour of CE credit

Management of bronchiolitis

Learning Objectives

As a result of studying this article, the reader should be able to

1. State the incidence of bronchiolitis in the age groups usually affected.
2. Describe the pathogenesis of bronchiolitis.
3. Describe the clinical presentation and prognosis of bronchiolitis.
4. List three basic approaches to treatment of bronchiolitis.
5. Describe measures that may be beneficial in prevention of bronchiolitis.

Self-assessment Questions

For each question there is one best answer only.

1. Bronchiolitis results in hospitalization of what percentage of infants with the disease?

a. 1–2%.
b. 10–20%.
c. 40–50%.
d. 60–80%.

2. Bronchiolitis may be easily differentiated from reactive-airways disease in an infant with a respiratory infection by assessing

a. Chest X-ray films.
b. Respiratory rate.
c. White blood cell count and differential.
d. None of the above alternatives is correct.

3. The best preventive measure for bronchiolitis is

a. Vaccination.
b. Handwashing.
c. Prophylactic antibiotics.
d. Prophylactic ribavirin.

4. The major cause of bronchiolitis is

a. Bacterial infection, usually with *Haemophilus influenzae* type B.
b. *Mycoplasma pneumoniae* infection.
c. Respiratory syncytial virus infection.
d. Mixed bacterial–viral infection.

5. The preferred anti-infective agent in patients with bronchiolitis is

a. Ampicillin.
b. Ribavirin.
c. Cefaclor.
d. None of the above alternatives is correct.

6. An important element in bronchiolitis therapy is oxygen, which should be administered

a. After intubation of the infant.
b. Humidified in an oxygen tent.
c. At a concentration of 80–100%.
d. Until arterial oxygen tension reaches 100 torr.

7. Corticosteroids should generally be avoided in children with nonlife-threatening bronchiolitis because of

a. The danger of adrenal suppression.
b. The potential for interactions with theophylline.
c. Lack of proven efficacy.
d. None of the above alternatives is correct.

8. Drug therapy of bronchiolitis requiring hospitalization should include

a. Antibiotics.
b. Antiviral therapy.
c. Bronchodilators.
d. None of the above alternatives is correct.

9. The recommended approach to general therapy of bronchiolitis in hospitalized patients includes

a. Oxygen therapy.
b. Theophylline therapy.
c. Anti-infectives.
d. Alternatives a and b are both correct.

10. Bronchiolitis occurs most frequently

a. During the spring "hay fever" season.
b. During the winter "flu" season.
c. In day-care centers where infants are concentrated.
d. In hospital nurseries where proper handwashing is not adhered to.

Article 680-204-8510 (see page 304)
Qualifies for 1.0 hour of CE credit

Management of antibiotic-associated pseudomembranous colitis

Learning Objectives

As a result of studying this article the reader should be able to

1. List the most common etiologic agents of antibiotic-associated pseudomembranous colitis (AAPMC).
2. Name the causative organism of AAPMC and discuss the importance of endogenous and exogenous routes of transmission.
3. List the major criteria used to establish the diagnosis of AAPMC.
4. Recommend an appropriate regimen for the treatment of AAPMC.
5. State the usual dosages and adverse drug reactions for the drugs used most commonly to treat AAPMC.

Self-assessment Questions

For each question there is one best answer only.

1. AAPMC occurs most commonly after therapy with

a. Clindamycin.
b. Vancomycin.
c. Antineoplastic agents.
d. None of the above alternatives is correct.

2. Which of the following criteria establish the diagnosis of AAPMC?

a. Positive results for a cell-culture assay for clostridial cytotoxin accompanied by clinical symptoms of AAPMC.
b. Diarrhea temporally associated with recent antibiotic use.
c. Isolation of clostridial toxins from samples of stool.
d. Visualization of pseudomembranous plaques.

3. Which of the following statements regarding the incidence of AAPMC is not true?

a. AAPMC will not occur if the infecting clostridial strain is susceptible to the causative antibiotic.
b. Elderly patients are at greater risk for developing AAPMC than are young adults.
c. AAPMC occurs only in the presence of drugs that alter the colonic flora.
d. *Clostridium difficile* and clostridial spores present in the hospital environment can contribute to the development of AAPMC.

4. Which of the following statements regarding the drug therapy of AAPMC is true?

a. Drug therapy should be initiated as soon as clinical symptoms of AAPMC appear, even if the diagnosis has not been confirmed.
b. Mild cases of AAPMC may respond to discontinuation of the etiologic agent and replacement of fluids and electrolytes.
c. The use of antidiarrheal agents can hasten the clinical course of AAPMC by permitting intestinal healing.
d. A therapeutic regimen for AAPMC should always include an anticlostridial antibiotic.

5. The high relapse rate associated with vancomycin therapy for AAPMC can be attributed to

a. A growing number of vancomycin-resistant strains of *Clostridium difficile.*
b. Failure to achieve measurable serum concentrations in some patients.
c. Reinfection with clostridial spores before normal intestinal flora have been restored.
d. Vancomycin's induction of a second episode of AAPMC.

6. Which of the following factors has limited the widespread use of metronidazole in the treatment of AAPMC?

a. Prohibitively high costs associated with metronidazole therapy.
b. Frequent adverse reactions.
c. Lack of clinical equivalence to vancomycin therapy.
d. None of the above alternatives is correct.

7. Bacitracin can be considered a feasible alternative to vancomycin in which of the following situations?

a. Relapses of AAPMC following vancomycin therapy.
b. Moderate cases of AAPMC in vancomycin-allergic patients.
c. Alternatives a and b are both correct.
d. None of the above alternatives is correct.

8. Which of the following statements about the use of anion-exchange resins in treating AAPMC is true?

a. Exchange resins can successfully inactivate clostridial toxins by binding them in the colon.
b. Resins may be most useful when used as adjuncts to antibiotic therapy.
c. Exchange resins should not be used as adjuncts to antibiotic therapy because they bind antibiotics.
d. Alternatives a and b are both correct.

9. Unorthodox approaches to the treatment of AAPMC have included which of the following?

   a. Rectal administration of vancomycin.
   b. Rectal administration of normal stool flora.
   c. Injections of clostridial antitoxins.
   d. Alternatives b and c are both correct.

10. Which of the following regimens represents the most cost-effective approach to treating moderate or severe cases of AAPMC?

   a. Discontinuation of the etiologic agents and replacement of fluid and electrolytes.
   b. A 10-day course of oral metronidazole or bacitracin, with vancomycin reserved for relapses and refractory cases.
   c. A 10-day course of oral vancomycin alone.
   d. A 10-day course of oral vancomycin and exchange resins, with metronidazole and bacitracin reserved for relapses and refractory cases.

Answer sheet

May–June 1985 ***Clinical Pharmacy***

Note: An enrollment form for the ASHP Continuing-Education System appears in this issue. Please accumulate all the answer sheets you wish to use in one enrollment and submit them at one time with a completed enrollment form.

Place an X in the box(es) at the top of the column(s) corresponding to the test(s) you are taking. Darken the boxes corresponding to the correct answers.

☐ 680-204-8508 2.0 hours	☐ 680-204-8509 1.0 hour	☐ 680-204-8510 1.0 hour
a b c d e	a b c d	a b c d
1. ☐☐☐☐☐	1. ☐☐☐☐	1. ☐☐☐☐
2. ☐☐☐☐☐	2. ☐☐☐☐	2. ☐☐☐☐
3. ☐☐☐☐☐	3. ☐☐☐☐	3. ☐☐☐☐
4. ☐☐☐☐☐	4. ☐☐☐☐	4. ☐☐☐☐
5. ☐☐☐☐☐	5. ☐☐☐☐	5. ☐☐☐☐
6. ☐☐☐☐☐	6. ☐☐☐☐	6. ☐☐☐☐
7. ☐☐☐☐☐	7. ☐☐☐☐	7. ☐☐☐☐
8. ☐☐☐☐☐	8. ☐☐☐☐	8. ☐☐☐☐
9. ☐☐☐☐☐	9. ☐☐☐☐	9. ☐☐☐☐
10. ☐☐☐☐☐	10. ☐☐☐☐	10. ☐☐☐☐

ASHP Use Only
(2.0)8508______(3)
(1.0)8509______(3)
(1.0)8510______(3)

ASHP CE instructions and enrollment form

Instructions

1. The system is flexible. You may, within a 12-month period, select any combination of tests from the *American Journal of Hospital Pharmacy* and *Clinical Pharmacy* to give you the number of credits you need.
2. An Answer Sheet is published at the end of each installment of the CE column. An Enrollment Form is published in the May-June and November-December issues of *CP* and in the June and December issues of *AJHP*.
3. Complete only one Enrollment Form, but note on the form all the tests you are taking. Staple together all answer sheets for one enrollment.
4. Tests included in one enrollment must have been published within the past 24 months. Once a particular test is included in an enrollment, it may not be included in a subsequent enrollment.
5. The passing score on each test is 70%. Within four weeks of receiving your enrollment, ASHP will mail you a CE certificate or notify you that certain tests were failed. Failed tests may be retaken only one time, without additional cost. There are no refunds for failed tests.
6. ASHP is approved by the American Council on Pharmaceutical Education as a provider of continuing pharmaceutical education (Provider Number 680-204). (The following states recognize ACPE-approved providers: AK, AR, AZ, FL, IA, ID, IN, KS, KY, LA, MA, ME, MI, MS, MT, NE, NH, NM, NV, OH, OR, SD, WA, and WY [also Puerto Rico].) Most states that recognize ACPE-approved providers will accept credit earned through journal CE programs; however, since some states have restrictions on the number of credit hours or CE units they will accept toward the total requirement, it is advised that readers check with their respective state board of pharmacy if they are uncertain about the board's regulations.
7. Send your Enrollment Form, Answer Sheet(s), and check (made payable to ASHP) to:

ASHP CE
American Society of Hospital Pharmacists
4630 Montgomery Avenue
Bethesda, MD 20814

Enrollment Form

Name____

Address______________________________________

City____________________State____________Zip________

Tests included in this enrollment:

Test Number	*Hours of Credit*

(Write additional numbers and hours on a separate sheet and attach it to this form.)

Total hours __________

Total fee($) enclosed __________

Fee Schedule
$3.50/hour
$15.00 minimum/enrollment

Current Literature

Book Reviews

Antimicrobial Therapy

Edited by Angela M. Ristuccia and Burke A. Cunha.

Published by Raven Press, 1140 Avenue of the Americas, New York, NY 10036, 1984. xvi + 618 p. Price $98.50.

This text is divided into five major sections. "Clinical Aspects" contains chapters dealing with antibiotic selection, resistance, synergy, effect of antibiotics on the immune response, kinetics and antibiotic blood concentrations, and empiric therapy. "Microbiological Aspects" deals exclusively with susceptibility testing. "Antibiotics" has 13 chapters dealing with major classes of antibacterial agents and a chapter devoted to side effects. "Antibiotic Tissue Penetration" contains 17 chapters dealing with basic principles of tissue penetration, the effect of protein binding, and penetration into various tissues and fluids. Finally, "Analytical Methods" contains four chapters describing various techniques to measure antibiotic concentrations in biologic tissues and fluids. The book should have been called *Antibacterial Therapy* since there are no chapters on antitubercular, antifungal, antiviral, or antiparasitic drugs.

The editors intended for this book to serve a dual role: a resource for clinicians and a reference text for those involved in antibiotic research. My estimate is that the book is divided roughly into equal portions for these two roles; sections in the book clearly are of little use to the clinician (e.g., susceptibility testing of *Mycoplasmas* and *Chlamydia*, analytical methods, and much of the tissue penetration material).

There are sections of individual chapters that, on the surface, appear to be research related, but that may be of use to the clinician. Conversely, many chapters would seem to be of enormous utility to the clinician but contain large amounts of material that would be of primary interest only to an investigator. For these reasons, I had some difficulty in evaluating this book. Adding to the dilemma was the inconsistency in content, style, and organization in chapters intended to be similar (e.g., in the "Antibiotics" section). Some chapters appear to have been poorly edited, while others are sparkling examples of grammar, spelling, and organization.

There is a substantial amount of redundancy in material, since several antibiotic chapters contain information on assay procedures, side effects, or tissue penetration that may be repeated in the chapter on antibiotic side effects or in the sections on tissue penetration or analytical methods (e.g., the chapter on aminoglycosides).

Overall, the book is well referenced and comprehensive, and the individual chapter authors are well known and highly qualified to write on the subject matter.

Given all of the above reservations regarding this book, I would recommend it to the clinician for the amount of material on antibiotic pharmacology and the principles of antibiotic therapy. I would recommend the rest of the book to those involved in antibiotic research, particularly for the methodology in the tissue penetration and analytical methods sections.

The price of nearly $100 may dissuade many potential users. I could almost envision two texts from this one, each appealing to separate audiences and each at a more reasonable price.

Reviewed by Steven L. Barriere, Pharm.D., College of Pharmacy, The University of Michigan, Ann Arbor, MI 48109.

Critical Care: A Comprehensive Approach

By Roger C. Bone.

Published by the American College of Chest Physicians, 911 Busse Highway, Park Ridge, IL 60068, 1984. 532 p. Price $49.95.

This book is a welcome addition to the limited number of textbooks dealing with the management of critically ill patients. The text, supported by the Council on Critical Care of the American College of Chest Physicians, consists of 36 chapters mainly authored by experts in their fields.

Most chapters deal with cardiopulmonary topics applicable to intensive-care settings, including mechanical ventilation and weaning techniques; respiratory and hemodynamic monitoring; status asthmaticus; thoracic surgery and trauma; arrhythmia detection and management; acute myocardial infarction; congestive heart failure; and cardiogenic shock. A wide range of additional topics are also included: gastrointestinal hemorrhage; nutrition; cerebral resuscitation; burn patients; and drug overdose. The book may be divided into chapters dealing with groups of disorders, which are general reviews and limited in detail, and chapters addressing specific diseases.

Overall, the text is well written except for minor typographical errors and provides numerous tables and figures that supplement the discussion. Unfortunately most of the chapters have a rather limited reference list.

In order to adequately provide "a comprehensive approach," the authors review the pathophysiology of each disease state, highlighting the implications to the critically ill patient. In addition, the authors place in perspective the pertinent historical, physical, and laboratory findings as well as an overview of drug- and nondrug-related treatment modalities. State-of-the-art monitoring variables for treatment interventions are also discussed.

Continued on page 347

Current Literature *Continued from page 342*

Controversies in the management of the critically ill patient are raised, but the authors do not consistently provide detailed discussions or recommendations regarding the best approach to these controversies. This is especially true of the drug-related issues in seriously ill patients, such as the use of corticosteroids or naloxone in the treatment of septic shock; the role of labetalol or nifedipine in the treatment of hypertensive emergencies; the use of crystalloid or colloid solutions for fluid resuscitation; and the use of third-generation cephalosporins in the intensive-care unit.

Of the two chapters dealing specifically with drug use, the pulmonary-drug chapter is a more informative section than the cardiovascular-drug chapter. For example, the discussions on encainide, flecainide, lorcainide, and amiodarone are limited to two paragraphs. Certain chapters do provide complete drug-treatment recommendations (acute myocardial infarction, endocrine emergencies), whereas others do not (recognition and management of arrhythmias, gastrointestinal hemorrhage).

Therefore, the text is most useful in reviewing recent developments in critical care. This book provides a basic understanding of the management of the critically ill patient. The book would be of value to the clinical pharmacist involved in the intensive-care setting. However, a supplemental source would be needed to address adequately the pharmacologic issues in this patient population.

Reviewed by Erkan Hassan, Pharm.D., Department of Clinical Pharmacy, School of Pharmacy, University of Maryland, Baltimore, MD 21201.

The Psychopharmacology of Lithium

By F. Neil Johnson.

Published by Oxford University Press, 200 Madison Ave., New York, NY 10016, 1984. ix + 327 p. Price $69.00.

The stated purpose of this book is to attempt to pull together existing strands of evidence that provide clues to a psychological model of lithium action. After summarizing the existing evidence, the author proposes a psychological model of lithium action. The book is divided into three sections: a brief review of lithium therapy, an exhaustive review of lithium's behavioral actions, and the development of a psychological model that can be used to explain not only the action of lithium but also the affective disorders.

The first chapter provides a basic review of lithium's clinical uses, factors associated with therapeutic effectiveness, the procedural routine, adverse effects, and contraindications. This chapter is designed to outline briefly the principles of lithium therapy but is not comprehensive. Because the chapter is so brief, none of the clinical aspects of lithium therapy is discussed in any detail.

The second chapter lays the groundwork for the following 14 chapters. The need for a common conceptual language—involving a behaviorally based model—between the psychopharmacologist and the psychiatrist is emphasized. These 14 chapters attempt to "isolate and identify the information which is currently available

Continued on page 350

Please turn page for brief sum

1 One-dose protection that lasts longer than the surgery*

12-hour protection eliminates the need for intraoperative dosing

Precef should usually be administered 1 hour before the operation to achieve an effective concentration in the wound tissues

1 One-dose protection against the most common surgical pathogens

Excellent coverage of both gram-negative and gram-positive pathogens*

Well tolerated IM or IV

- Excellent safety record, less than 2% incidence of adverse reactions in 1,534 patients treated with Precef†
- No cases of drug-related pseudomembranous colitis have been reported; however, this condition has been reported with the use of other cephalosporins and other broad-spectrum antibiotics, and its occurrence should be borne in mind

1 One-dose economy

Lower drug acquisition costs than with multi-dose regimens

Lower costs for infusion sets and diluents

1 One-dose simplicity

Simplest possible dosage for most general surgical prophylactic procedures – one gram, one dose – which means fewer IVs

Gives you more control; eliminates potential problems with follow-up doses and helps prevent inappropriate use

Reduces chance of administration errors

*Against possible infections due to susceptible pathogens.
†Refer to Official Package Circular for complete information on side effects.

ull prescribing information.

Current Literature *Continued from page 347*

upon which a behavioral model of lithium action may ultimately be based." Chapters 3 through 15 provide a thorough review of lithium's actions on each of the following: sensory systems; motor systems; perceptual processes; intellectual functioning; response selection and initiation; acquisition and retention processes; feelings, moods, and emotional states; verbal behavior; sleep; social behavior; miscellaneous unlearned behavior patterns; circadian and other rhythms in behavior; and drug-induced behavior. Each chapter contains introductory comments, a presentation of the available data separated into human and animal studies, and concluding remarks. All studies discussed are clearly referenced.

The remainder of the book is, in my opinion, the most interesting from a theoretical point of view. Based on the preceding evidence, as well as evidence provided in the remaining chapters, Johnson develops a stimulus-processing model of lithium action and affective disorders. Two propositions underlie the model: (1) Lithium impairs the efficiency of stimulus analytic processes and (2) only the processing of stimuli of around threshold physical intensities is affected. Mania is proposed to result from an overprocessing of external stimulation (analyzer hypersensitivity). When this hypersensitivity reaches a critical level, emergency homeostatic mechanisms are called into play that suppress analyzer sensitivity to a level below normal. The resultant analyzer subsensitivity is proposed to then give rise to symptoms of depression. Thus, lithium's effectiveness in the prophylaxis and acute treatment of mania is proposed to result from its ability to suppress stimulus processing and thereby prevent the manic episode.

This book is a reference text. It should prove useful to clinicians and researchers who are looking for specific information regarding lithium's effects on specific behaviors or behavioral systems. It is thoroughly referenced and well indexed. It also offers a fascinating conceptualization of affective disorders and lithium action. However, it contains no practical or clinical information on how to use lithium in the treatment of affective disorders; I cannot recommend it for purchase by most pharmacists. For those with a particular interest in lithium, it provides an interesting theoretical model and a good reference for lithium's effects on behavior.

Reviewed by Janet L. Kinney, Pharm.D., College of Pharmacy, University of Arizona, Tucson, AZ 85721.

Books Received

Books are listed as received; selected books may be reviewed in Book reviews in subsequent issues.

The Aging Process: Therapeutic Implications, edited by Robert N. Butler and Alexander G. Bearn. Published by Raven Press, 1140 Avenue of the Americas, New York, NY 10036, 1985. xii + 337 p. Price $45.00.

Alfentanil: Pharmacology and Uses in Anaesthesia, by Carl C. Hug, Jr., and Michael Chaffman. Published by ADIS Press, 15 Rawene Road, Birkenhead, Auckland 10, New Zealand, 1984. x + 115 p. Price $32.00.

Continued on page 354

A Money-Saving Regimen That *Works*

The following is a brief summary of prescribing information. For complete prescribing information, please see SK&F literature or PDR.

INDICATIONS AND USAGE

Monocid (sterile cefonicid sodium, SK&F) is indicated in the treatment of infections due to susceptible strains of the microorganisms listed below:

LOWER RESPIRATORY TRACT INFECTIONS, due to *Streptococcus pneumoniae* (formerly *D. pneumoniae*); *Klebsiella pneumoniae*; *Escherichia coli*; and *Hemophilus influenzae* (ampicillin-resistant and ampicillin-sensitive).

URINARY TRACT INFECTIONS, due to *Escherichia coli*; *Proteus mirabilis* (indole-negative *Proteus*); and *Klebsiella pneumoniae*.

SKIN AND SKIN STRUCTURE INFECTIONS, due to *Staphylococcus aureus* and *S. epidermidis*; *Streptococcus pyogenes* (Group A *Streptococcus*) and *S. agalactiae* (Group B *Streptococcus*).

SEPTICEMIA, due to *Streptococcus pneumoniae* (formerly *D. pneumoniae*) and *Escherichia coli*.

BONE AND JOINT INFECTIONS, due to *Staphylococcus aureus*.

SURGICAL PROPHYLAXIS

Administration of a single 1 gram dose of 'Monocid' before surgery may reduce the incidence of postoperative infections in patients undergoing surgical procedures classified as contaminated or potentially contaminated (e.g., colorectal surgery, vaginal hysterectomy, or cholecystectomy in high-risk patients), or in patients in whom infection at the operative site would present a serious risk (e.g., prosthetic arthroplasty, open heart surgery). Although cefonicid has been shown to be as effective as cefazolin in prevention of infection following coronary artery bypass surgery, no placebo-controlled trials have been conducted to evaluate any cephalosporin antibiotic in the prevention of infection following coronary artery bypass surgery or prosthetic heart valve replacement.

In cesarean section, the use of 'Monocid' (after the umbilical cord has been clamped) may reduce the incidence of certain postoperative infections.

When administered one hour prior to surgical procedures for which it is indicated, a single 1 gram dose of 'Monocid' provides protection from most infections due to susceptible organisms throughout the course of the procedure and for approximately 24 hours after administration. Intraoperative and postoperative administration of 'Monocid' is not necessary. Daily doses of 'Monocid' may be administered for two additional days in patients undergoing prosthetic arthroplasty or open heart surgery.

Therapy with 'Monocid' may be initiated pending results of susceptibility studies. Treatment should be adjusted according to findings.

Before using 'Monocid' concomitantly with other antibiotics, the prescribing information for those agents should be reviewed for contraindications, warnings, precautions and adverse reactions. Renal function should be carefully monitored.

CONTRAINDICATIONS

'Monocid' is contraindicated in persons who have shown hypersensitivity to cephalosporin antibiotics.

WARNINGS

BEFORE THERAPY WITH 'MONOCID' IS INSTITUTED, CAREFUL INQUIRY SHOULD BE MADE TO DETERMINE WHETHER THE PATIENT HAS HAD PREVIOUS HYPERSENSITIVITY REACTIONS TO CEPHALOSPORINS, PENICILLINS, OR OTHER DRUGS. THIS PRODUCT SHOULD BE GIVEN CAUTIOUSLY TO PENICILLIN-SENSITIVE PATIENTS. ANTIBIOTICS SHOULD BE ADMINISTERED WITH CAUTION TO ANY PATIENT WHO HAS DEMONSTRATED SOME FORM OF ALLERGY, PARTICULARLY TO DRUGS. SERIOUS ACUTE HYPERSENSITIVITY REACTIONS MAY REQUIRE EPINEPHRINE AND OTHER EMERGENCY MEASURES.

Pseudomembranous colitis has been reported with the use of cephalosporins (and other broad-spectrum antibiotics); therefore, it is important to consider that diagnosis in patients who develop diarrhea in association with antibiotic use.

Treatment with broad-spectrum antibiotics alters normal flora of the colon and may permit overgrowth of Clostridia. Studies indicate a toxin produced by *Clostridium difficile* is one primary cause of antibiotic-associated colitis. Cholestyramine and colestipol resins have been shown to bind the toxin *in vitro*.

Mild cases of colitis may respond to drug discontinuance alone. Moderate to severe cases should be managed with fluid, electrolyte and protein supplementation as indicated. When the colitis is not relieved by drug discontinuance and when it is severe, oral vancomycin is the treatment of choice for antibiotic-associated pseudomembranous colitis produced by *C. difficile*. Other causes of colitis should also be considered.

PRECAUTIONS

General: With any antibiotic, prolonged use may result in overgrowth of nonsusceptible organisms. Careful observation is essential, and appropriate measures should be taken if superinfection occurs.

Drug Interactions: Nephrotoxicity has been reported following concomitant dministration of other cephalosporins and aminoglycosides.

ncy: (Category B.) Reproduction studies have been performed in mice, ts at doses up to an equivalent of 40 times the usual adult ve revealed no evidence of impaired fertility or harm to the There are, however, no adequate and well-controlled ien. Because animal reproduction studies are not an response, this drug should be used in pregnancy

Pe

arean section, 'Monocid' should be administered has been clamped.

is excreted in human milk in low concentrations. hen 'Monocid' is administered to a nursing woman.

tiveness in children have not been established.

ADVERSE REACTIONS

'Monocid' is generally well tolerated and adverse reactions have occurred infrequently. The most common adverse reaction has been pain on I.M. injection. On-therapy conditions occurring in greater than 1% of 'Monocid'-treated patients were:

Injection Site Phenomena (5.7%): Pain and/or discomfort on injection; less often, burning, phlebitis at I.V. site.

Increased Platelets (1.7%).

Increased Eosinophils (2.9%).

Liver Function Test Alterations (1.6%): Increased alkaline phosphatase, increased SGOT, increased SGPT, increased GGTP, increased LDH.

Less frequent on-therapy conditions occurring in less than 1% of 'Monocid'-treated patients were:

Hypersensitivity Reactions: Fever, rash, pruritus, erythema, myalgia and anaphylactoid-like type reactions have been reported.

Hematology: Decreased WBC, neutropenia, positive Coombs' test.

Diarrhea.

DOSAGE AND ADMINISTRATION

General

The usual adult dosage is 1 gram of 'Monocid' given once every 24 hours, intravenously or by deep intramuscular injection. Doses in excess of 1 gram daily are rarely necessary; however, in exceptional cases dosage of up to 2 grams given once daily have been well tolerated. When administering 2 gram I.M. doses once daily, one-half the dose should be administered in different large muscle masses.

Surgical Prophylaxis

When administered one hour prior to appropriate surgical procedures (see Indications and Usage), a 1 gram dose of 'Monocid' provides protection from most infections due to susceptible organisms throughout the course of the procedure and for approximately 24 hours after administration. Intraoperative and postoperative administration of 'Monocid' is not necessary. Daily doses of 'Monocid' may be administered for two additional days in patients undergoing prosthetic arthroplasty or open heart surgery.

In cesarean section 'Monocid' should be administered only after the umbilical cord has been clamped.

General Guidelines for Dosage of 'Monocid', I.V. or I.M.

Type of Infection	Daily Dose (grams)	Frequency
Uncomplicated Urinary Tract	0.5	once every 24 hours
Mild to Moderate	1	once every 24 hours
Severe or Life-Threatening	2*	once every 24 hours
Surgical Prophylaxis	1	1 hour preoperatively

*When administering 2 gram I.M. doses once daily, one-half the dose should be administered in different large muscle masses.

Impaired Renal Function

Modification of 'Monocid' dosage is necessary in patients with impaired renal function. Before prescribing, consult Dosage and Administration section of complete prescribing information.

HOW SUPPLIED

'Monocid' is supplied in vials equivalent to 500 mg. and 1 gram of cefonicid; in "Piggyback" Vials for I.V. admixture equivalent to 1 gram of cefonicid; and in Pharmacy Bulk Vials equivalent to 10 grams of cefonicid.

BRS-MC:L11

Smith Kline &French Laboratories **SK&F**

ONE DOSE
ONE GRAM
ONCE DAILY

MONOCID®
IV/IM
brand of sterile
cefonicid sodium
(lyophilized)

Continued from page 350

American Hospital Formulary Service – Drug Information 1985. Published by the American Society of Hospital Pharmacists, 4630 Montgomery Ave., Bethesda, MD 20814, 1985. xvii + 1793 p. Price $50/year; $80/year (outside U.S. and Canada); $35/year (students); includes initial bound volume plus three supplements.

Annual Drug Data Report, Vol. VI, 1984, J. R. Prous, editor. Published by J. R. Prous, S.A., Apartado de Correos 540, Barcelona, Spain, 1984. x + 485 p. Price $200.

Applied Virology, edited by Edouard Kurstak. Published by Academic Press, Inc., Orlando, FL 32887, 1984. xxv + 518 p. Price $59.00, £45.50.

Arzneimittel vor, während oder nach der Mahlzeit? Ein Leitfaden für Ärzte und Apotheker, by F. W. H. M. Merkus. Published by Wissenschaftliche Verlagsgesellschaft mbH, Birkenwaldstrasse 44, 7000 Stuttgart 1, West Germany, 1984. 112 p. Price DM 5.

Clinical Guide to Parenteral Micronutrition, edited by Thomas G. Baumgartner. Published by Educational Publications, Ltd., 2020 Ruby St., Melrose Park, IL 60160, 1984. xii + 388 p. Price $29.95.

Contemporary Writings on Long Term Care Pharmacy, Volume III. Published by the American Society of Consultant Pharmacists, 2300 Ninth St. South, Arlington, VA 22204, 1985. ii + 135 p. Price $10 (ASCP members), $15 (nonmembers).

Current Medical Diagnosis and Treatment 1985, edited by Marcus A. Krupp, Milton J. Chatton, and David Werdegar. Published by Lange Medical Publications, Drawer L, Los Altos, CA 94022, 1985. 1157 p. Price $27.50.

Detecting and Counting Medication Errors in Long Term Care Facilities, by Health Information Designs, Inc. Published by the American Society of Consultant Pharmacists, 2300 Ninth St. South, Arlington, VA 22204, 1984. iii + 141 p. Price $20 (ASCP members), $30 (nonmembers).

The Diuretic Manual, edited by Jules B. Puschett and Arthur Greenberg. Published by Elsevier Science Publishing Co., Inc., 52 Vanderbilt Avenue, New York, NY 10017, 1985. xiv + 175 p. Price $29.95 (dfl-110.00).

Drug Consultant, 1985-1986, edited by Rhoda M. Michaels and G. R. Brown. Published by M. J. Powers & Co. Publishers, Inc., One Wiley Drive, Somerset, NJ 08873, 1985. viii + 383 p. Price $18.95.

Evaluation and Treatment of Chronic Pain, edited by Gerald M. Aronoff. Published by Urban & Schwarzenberg, Inc., 7 East Redwood Street, Baltimore, MD 21202, 1985. xliv + 684 p. Price $65.00.

Pediatric Medications: An Emergency and Critical Care Reference, by Carolyn M. Stewart and Linda B. Stewart. Published by Aspen Systems Corporation, 1600 Research Blvd., Rockville, MD 20850, 1984. xxv + 453 p. Price $45.00.

Remington's Pharmaceutical Sciences, 17th Edition. Published by the Mack Printing Company, Easton, PA 18042, 1985. xvi + 1984 p. Price $85.00.

Review of the Public Health Service's Response to AIDS. Published by the Office of Technology Assessment, Congress of the United States, 1985. Available from the Superintendent of Documents, Government Printing Office, Dept. SSMC, Washington, DC 20402 (#052-003-00984-6). 168 p. Price $5.50.

New Periodical

Journal of Geriatric Drug Therapy, James Cooper, editor. Published quarterly, beginning Spring 1986, by The Haworth Press, Inc., 28 East 22nd St., New York, NY 10010. Price (U.S., Canada, Mexico) $24.00 for individuals, $32.00 for institutions, and $42.00 for libraries, plus postage and handling ($2 U.S., $7 Canada and Mexico); (foreign) $38.80, $48.40, and $60.80 for the same groups, respectively, postage and handling included. Introductory discount of $7.00 for individuals if payment accompanies subscription order.

This journal will focus specifically on drug therapy and related issues concerning the geriatric patient. Its goal will be to cover important findings and promote the exchange of controversial, innovative, and timely views related to geripharmacotherapy. It will publish original studies of drug efficacy and safety in geriatric patients; innovative drug therapy services for geriatric patients in ambulatory, long-term care, and hospital settings; updates on drug-related problems of misuse and adverse reactions in the elderly; and practical drug therapy information for physicians, nurses, pharmacists, and other health professionals in both the geriatric and the drug therapy fields. Articles will also cover therapeutic and pharmacokinetic as well as educational, social, psychological, and regulatory/economic considerations in geriatric drug therapy and pharmacy services.

Advertising Index

American Society of Hospital Pharmacists
- Clinical Pharmacy, 354A, 354B, inside back cover
- Clinical Research Forum, 267
- Guidelines for Administration of Intravenous Medications to Pediatric Patients, 339

Beecham Laboratories
- Timentin, 271–278

Biotrack, Inc.
- Warfcalc, 341

Bristol Laboratories, Division of Bristol-Myers Company
- Cefadyl, 251–252
- Mexate, 243–244
- Precef, 348–350

Ingham Medical Center
- Position Available, 347

International Pharmaceutical Federation
- 45th International Congress, 351

Lederle Laboratories, A Division of American Cyanamid Company
- Maxzide, 249–250

Roche Laboratories, Division of Hoffmann-La Roche Inc.
- Coactin, 253–254, 343–346
- Institutional, 268–270
- Rocephin, 259–264

Smith Kline & French Laboratories
- Ancef, 246–247
- Cefizox, inside front cover
- Monocid, 352–353
- Tagamet, 265–266

Stuart Pharmaceuticals, Division of ICI Americas, Inc.
- Institutional, outside back cover

The University of Michigan
- Positions Available, 347

The Upjohn Company
- Micronase, 256–258

July–August 1985 Volume 4, Number 4 Coden: CPHADV ISSN: 0278-2677

CLINICAL PHARMACY

Drug Reviews

393 **New β_2-adrenergic agonist aerosols**
H. William Kelly

404 **Current status of cardiac glycoside drug interactions**
Piet M. Hooymans and Frans W. H. M. Merkus

Therapy Reviews

414 **Whole-bowel irrigation for mechanical colon cleansing**
Katherine A. Michael, Joseph T. DiPiro, Talmadge A. Bowden, and Francis J. Tedesco

425 **Use of carbamazepine in psychiatric disorders**
Lois J. Birkhimer, Judy L. Curtis, and Michael W. Jann

434 **Aluminum-related osteomalacia in renal-failure patients**
Karen E. Vick and Curtis A. Johnson

Research

440 **Multicenter evaluation of six methods for predicting warfarin maintenance-dose requirements from initial response**
William T. Sawyer, Timothy E. Poe, Bruce R. Canaday, John S. Weiner, Dennis M. Williams, C. Edwin Webb, and Mark J. Ellison

Research Notes

446 **Gastrointestinal transit times of cathartics used with activated charcoal**
Edward P. Krenzelok

448 **Theophylline pharmacokinetics in paraplegic subjects**
Jack L. Segal, Christopher M. Smith, Stanley K. Gordon, and Ibrahim M. Eltorai

Editorials

452 **Reservoir aerosol delivery systems**
Karen J. Tietze

453 **Transdermal nitroglycerin patches**
Stephen H. Curry

Drug Experience

455 **Metallic taste associated with tetracycline therapy**
Louis D. Magnasco and Andrew J. Magnasco

357 **News**
Nonsedating antihistamine terfenadine approved by FDA . . . Auranofin approved for second-line therapy of rheumatoid arthritis . . . Panel reviews sedation and anesthesia in the dental office . . . Ticarcillin-clavulanic acid marketed by Beecham . . . *Haemophilus* vaccine approved . . . Health implications of obesity explored at consensus conference . . . Inosiplex available for AIDS patients . . . Allopurinol approved for management of recurrent calcium oxalate stones

370 **Letters**
Oral acyclovir pharmacokinetics, Courtney Fletcher, Barbara Chinnock, Henry H. Balfour, Jr.; Bev L. True, Barry L. Carter . . . Hypersensitivity vasculitis associated with streptokinase, Robert F. Thompson, Mark A. Stratton, Warren A. Heffron . . . Change in enzyme content and manufacturer of Viokase, Rosemary R. Berardi, Carol L. Colvin

463 **CP Continuing Education**

468 **Current Literature**
Book Review: *Practice of Critical Care Pharmacy (Majerus, Dasta),* Larry H. Danziger . . . Books Received

468 **Advertising Index**

Instructions to Authors

CLINICAL PHARMACY gives priority to (1) studies that objectively evaluate drug effects in human trials, (2) evaluative review articles on the clinical uses of new drugs, and (3) evaluations of the current status of drug therapy in selected diseases. Contributions to the following sections are invited:

Drug Reviews: Detailed, analytical reviews on the clinical use of specific drugs, with preference given to new drugs and to evaluative rather than descriptive literature reviews.

Therapy Reviews: Articles that focus primarily on a disease state (rather than on a drug or drug class) and its treatment. These reviews foster an understanding of the pathophysiology of a disease and the related treatment.

Research: Reports of well-conducted original research on drug effects in humans.

Research Notes: Short research reports, such as updates on previously published work, confirmations of previous findings, or original research of modest scope.

Grand Rounds: Patient case reports and literature reviews combined in a way that gives them high educational value.

Drug Experience: Straightforward reports, with selected literature references, of unusual drug experiences.

Therapy Consultation: Brief advice, in a question-and-answer format, on how to handle specific drug-therapy problems. Readers are invited to submit questions, which the editor will forward to appropriate consultants for answering.

Letters: Short comments on previously published work or about potential problems, apparent trends, or controversies in drug therapy or clinical research.

Commentaries: Well-reasoned expressions of opinion on drug-therapy or clinical-research issues.

The editors have the sole authority to decide in which section to publish an accepted manuscript.

Manuscripts are subject to review by qualified outside reviewers, as well as by the editors, and will be accepted for publication only if they are believed to represent an important contribution to the literature. All papers submitted for publication must be accompanied by a completed copy of a manuscript checklist. The checklist appears on page 105 of the January–February 1985 issue. Authors of especially important original work may request "fast-track" review of their papers. Authors may suggest appropriate reviewers for their papers.

Accepted materials become the permanent and sole property of ASHP and may not be published or reprinted elsewhere without written permission from both the author and the editor.

The editors reserve the right to revise all materials submitted, if necessary. The publisher assumes no responsibility for the statements and opinions advanced by contributors to CLINICAL PHARMACY.

CLINICAL PHARMACY accepts manuscripts prepared according to the specifications of the Uniform Requirements for Manuscripts Submitted to Biomedical Journals (*Am J Hosp Pharm.* 1982; 38:1538–43). CLINICAL PHARMACY's manuscript checklist (page 105, January-February 1985 issue) generally conforms to the Uniform Requirements.

Under the terms of the Copyright Revision Act of 1976 (Public Law 94-553) it is necessary to have the rights of the authors transferred to the publisher in order to provide for the widest possible dissemination of professional and scientific literature. Accordingly, all transmittal letters accompanying manuscripts submitted for publication, including contributions for the Letters column, must contain the following language: "In consideration of the American Society of Hospital Pharmacists (ASHP) taking action in reviewing and editing my (our) submission, the author(s) undersigned hereby transfer(s), assign(s), or otherwise convey(s) all ownership rights in the submission and all copyright ownership to ASHP. In the event that such work is not published by ASHP, all said rights shall be released." We regret that we cannot consider manuscripts for publication that are not accompanied with transmittal letters containing the above language signed by all authors.

Authors must certify in their letter of transmittal that none of the material in their manuscript has been published previously nor is under consideration or been accepted for publication elsewhere. If this certification cannot be made, suitable explanation must be offered.

Six copies of all manuscripts should be submitted. Manuscripts should be typewritten with double spacing (including tables) on one side of good quality, 21.6 × 27.9-cm white paper, and with margins of at least 2.5 cm. For guidance on style, authors should consult the manuscript checklist, recent issues of CLINICAL PHARMACY, and the *Council of Biology Editors Style Manual*, fifth edition. *The American Heritage Dictionary of the English Language* and the AMA's *Manual for Authors and Editors* contain helpful advice on correct usage.

Galley proofs are sent to authors for inspection against the original manuscript and for correction. Unnecessary alterations in galley proof must be avoided. Extensive alterations will be charged to the author. An order form for reprints is sent to the corresponding author after galley proofs have been cleared.

CLINICAL PHARMACY (ISSN 0278-2677) is published bimonthly by the American Society of Hospital Pharmacists, 4630 Montgomery Avenue, Bethesda, MD 20814. Joseph A. Oddis, Executive Vice President. Second class postage is paid at Bethesda, MD, and at additional mailing offices. **Postmaster: Send address changes to: ASHP, 4630 Montgomery Avenue, Bethesda, MD 20814.**

Annual Subscription Rate:	*USA*	*Non-USA*
ASHP Member	$35	$40
ASHP Student Member	$25	$30
Institutions and Nonmembers	$55	$60

The cost of single copies is $9. Airmail delivery outside of the continental United States is available for an additional charge of $36 per year. Requests to replace missing issues free of charge are honored only up to six months after date of issue.

Advertising for CLINICAL PHARMACY is accepted in accordance with the Statement of Advertising Policy of the American Society of Hospital Pharmacists (see *Am J Hosp Pharm.* 1981; 38:1045). For additional information, contact the Advertising Representative (William McCausland Associates, Inc., P.O. Box 189, Pitman, NJ 08071. Phone 609-589-5454).

All articles published, including editorials, letters, and book reviews, represent the opinions of the authors and do not reflect the official policy of the American Society of Hospital Pharmacists or the institution with which the author is affiliated, unless this is clearly specified.

Microfilm and microfiche editions are available for purchase. Contact University Microfilms, 300 N. Zeeb Road, Ann Arbor, MI 48106.

Articles in CLINICAL PHARMACY are abstracted and indexed in *Current Contents, Clinical Sciences, Excerpta Medica, Index Medicus, Inpharma, International Pharmaceutical Abstracts*, and *Reactions*.

News

Nonsedating antihistamine terfenadine approved by FDA

FDA approval of terfenadine (Seldane, Merrell Dow), the first of a new class of nonsedating antihistamines, could offer good news for the estimated 40 million Americans who suffer from allergies but fear the sedation caused by conventional antihistamines. The drug, which was approved May 5, was already available in more than 20 countries; it has become the largest-selling antihistamine in some of these markets. According to Sorkin and Heel,[1] terfenadine offers a worthwhile improvement in adverse-effect profile over traditional antihistamines and could become an agent of choice (along with other nonsedating antihistamines) in patients requiring an H_1 antagonist.

Terfenadine is a peripheral selective H_1-histamine-receptor antagonist. Unlike other antihistamines that act on central H_1-histamine receptors, terfenadine does not penetrate the cerebrospinal fluid, which may explain its lack of CNS effects. Also, terfenadine does not impair psychomotor performance, adversely affect subjective feelings, or enhance the depressant effects of concomitantly administered alcohol or benzodiazepines.

Terfenadine is well absorbed from the gastrointestinal tract and is rapidly and extensively biotransformed into two metabolites; a carboxylic acid metabolite has antihistaminic activity. Concentrations following a single dose peak at about two hours, the distribution half-life is 3.4 hours, and the elimination half-life is 20.25 hours. Terfenadine is extensively (97%) bound to human serum protein.

The drug is indicated for the relief of symptoms associated with seasonal allergic rhinitis such as sneezing, rhinorrhea, pruritus, and lacrimation. Clinical studies have shown that terfenadine is comparable to other antihistamines and superior to placebo in alleviating the symptoms of seasonal allergic rhinitis.

The most frequently reported adverse effect from the use of terfenadine is sedation (14%), which is comparable to the incidence with placebo. Other reported adverse effects in patients taking the drug for 7–14 days include drowsiness (9%), headache (6.3%), fatigue (2.9%), dizziness (1.4%), gastrointestinal distress (4.6%), and dry mouth (2.3%).

The recommended dose for terfenadine for adults and children 12 years and older is 60 mg twice daily. The prescription drug became available May 20; the wholesale price of 60-mg tablets in bottles of 100 is $43.86.

1. Sorkin EM, Heel RC. Terfenadine. A review of its pharmacodynamic properties and therapeutic efficacy. *Drugs.* 1985; 29:34–56.

Auranofin approved for second-line therapy of rheumatoid arthritis

Smith Kline & French's oral gold compound, auranofin (Ridaura), was marketed in early June for treatment of rheumatoid arthritis when first-line agents (nonsteroidal anti-inflammatory agents) fail. Auranofin, which was reviewed in the March–April 1984 *CP*, was under consideration at FDA for 3.5 years; its approval seemed to be delayed following the benoxaprofen incidents in August 1982.

Like other gold-containing compounds, auranofin can cause gold toxicity, which is characterized by a fall in hemoglobin, leukopenia below 4000 leukocytes/cu mm, granulocytes below 1500/cu mm, platelets below 150,000/cu mm, proteinuria, hematuria, pruritus, rash, stomatitis, or persistent diarrhea. SKF advises performing baseline blood tests and monthly monitoring with complete blood count with differential, platelet count, and urinalysis. In 18 comparative trials, 12.3% of auranofin patients discontinued therapy because of side effects (compared with 33.9% of injectable-gold patients).

Auranofin is approved for use in adults with rheumatoid arthritis who have had an inadequate response to (or are intolerant of) full doses of nonsteroidal anti-inflammatory agents. Its therapeutic benefits may not be apparent for three to four months or for up to six months in some patients. Auranofin is contraindicated in patients with histories of necrotizing enterocolitis, pulmonary fibrosis, exfoliative dermatitis, bone-marrow aplasia, or other severe hematologic disorders.

The drug is available as 3-mg capsules in bottles of 60. The usual daily dosage is 6 mg, given either as a single dose or as two 3-mg doses. The suggested wholesale price to pharmacists is $34.20 per 60 capsules.

Panel reviews sedation and anesthesia in the dental office

Selection of a particular drug for controlling apprehension, anxiety, fear, and pain in dental patients rests with the practitioner, but sedation and general anesthesia should be used only in offices with adequate facilities and appropriately trained personnel. An NIH Consensus Development Conference held April 22–24 in Bethesda, MD, reached this conclusion after considering factors related to anesthesia and sedation in the dental office. Included were the training necessary for safe and effective use, indications and contraindications for use

Continued on page 362

The Only First-Generation

ANCEF ANCEF ANCEF

brand of sterile

CEFAZOLIN SODIUM IV/IM

(LYOPHILIZED) Injection: 500 mg. and 1 gram vials

The following is a brief summary of prescribing information. For complete prescribing information, please see SK&F literature or *PDR*.

INDICATIONS

Bone and joint infections due to *Staphylococcus aureus* and other indicated infections due to susceptible organisms. See complete prescribing information for a complete list of indications.

CONTRAINDICATIONS

'ANCEF' IS CONTRAINDICATED IN PATIENTS WITH KNOWN ALLERGY TO THE CEPHALOSPORIN GROUP OF ANTIBIOTICS.

WARNINGS

BEFORE CEFAZOLIN THERAPY IS INSTITUTED, CAREFUL INQUIRY SHOULD BE MADE CONCERNING PREVIOUS HYPERSENSITIVITY REACTIONS TO CEPHALOSPORINS AND PENICILLIN. CEPHALOSPORIN C DERIVATIVES SHOULD BE GIVEN CAUTIOUSLY IN PENICILLIN-SENSITIVE PATIENTS.

SERIOUS ACUTE HYPERSENSITIVITY REACTIONS MAY REQUIRE EPINEPHRINE AND OTHER EMERGENCY MEASURES.

There is some clinical and laboratory evidence of partial cross-allergenicity of the penicillins and the cephalosporins. Patients have been reported to have had severe reactions (including anaphylaxis) to both drugs.

Any patient who has demonstrated some form of allergy, particularly to drugs, should receive antibiotics cautiously. No exception should be made with regard to 'Ancef'.

Pseudomembranous colitis has been reported with the use of cephalosporins (and other broad-spectrum antibiotics); therefore, it is important to consider its diagnosis in patients who develop diarrhea in association with antibiotic use.

Treatment with broad-spectrum antibiotics alters normal flora of the colon and may permit overgrowth of clostridia. Studies indicate a toxin produced by *Clostridium difficile* is one primary cause of antibiotic-associated colitis. Cholestyramine and colestipol resins have been shown to bind the toxin *in vitro*.

Mild cases of colitis may respond to drug discontinuance alone.

Moderate to severe cases should be managed with fluid, electrolyte and protein supplementation as indicated.

When the colitis is not relieved by drug discontinuance or when it is severe, oral vancomycin is the treatment of choice for antibiotic-associated pseudomembranous colitis produced by *C. difficile*. Other causes of colitis should also be considered.

PRECAUTIONS

General—Prolonged use of 'Ancef' may result in the overgrowth of non-susceptible organisms. Careful clinical observation of the patient is essential.

When 'Ancef' is administered to patients with low urinary output becaus of impaired renal function, lower daily dosage is required (see Dosage and Administration).

'Ancef', as with all cephalosporins, should be prescribed with caution in individuals with a history of gastrointestinal disease, particularly colitis.

Drug Interactions—Probenecid may decrease renal tubular secretion of cephalosporins when used concurrently, resulting in increased and more prolonged cephalosporin blood levels.

Drug/Laboratory Test Interactions—A false positive reaction for glucose in the urine may occur with Benedict's solution, Fehling's solution, or with Clinitest® tablets, but not with enzyme-based tests such as Clinistix and Tes-Tape®.

Positive direct and indirect antiglobulin (Coombs) tests have occurred; these may also occur in neonates whose mothers received cephalosporins before delivery.

Carcinogenesis/Mutagenesis—Mutagenicity studies and long-term studies in animals to determine the carcinogenic potential of 'Ancef' hav not been performed.

Continued from page 357

in different age groups, appropriate agents providing the greatest margin of safety, and proper management and monitoring of the patient.

Use of sedative and anesthetic techniques in the dental office is often necessary for controlling pain and anxiety in the patient. Dental patients are generally in good health, procedures are usually short, the depth of anesthesia and level of sedation are often minimal, and patient fear and apprehension rather than nature of the procedure frequently determine whether sedation is used at all; these patients differ markedly from most hospitalized patients requiring anesthesia. In healthy anxious adults, sedation and local anesthesia relieve pain and discomfort; use of sedative techniques in patients with medical conditions that increase risks is contraindicated. For complex procedures general anesthesia can be used, but it is contraindicated in unhealthy adults. Indications for use in the elderly are similar to those in younger adults, although the practitioner must consider (1) the effect of age on the pharmacokinetic properties of drugs and (2) the increased risk of drug interactions (since many elderly patients are on long-term drug regimens). Young children who require extensive treatment or who are disabled are candidates for sedation; however, the panel recommends that procedures on such patients be performed in the hospital.

Drug groups used for sedation and general anesthesia in dental patients are similar to those used in the hospital. These drug groups include benzodiazepines, barbiturates, alcohols, opioid analgesics, antihistamines, phenothiazines, and nitrous oxide/oxygen. Drugs that induce sedation at low doses but that are considered general anesthetics are halogenated inhalation agents, ultrashort-acting barbiturates, and the dissociative agent ketamine. Accessory agents include the antimuscarinics and glycopyrrolate (for sedation and general anesthesia) and the neuromuscular blocking agents (for general anesthesia).

The panel concluded that proper monitoring of patients and training of personnel are needed to manage patients. Dental facilities should be equipped with suction and monitoring equipment, emergency drugs, and equipment capable of delivering oxygen under positive pressure. Personnel should be trained using the American Dental Association's Guidelines for Teaching the Comprehensive Control of Pain and Anxiety, Parts I and III; at least one year of practical training in sedation and general-anesthesia administration was also recommended.

Ticarcillin–clavulanic acid marketed by Beecham

A second product containing the β-lactamase inhibitor clavulanic acid in a fixed-dose combination has been marketed by Beecham Laboratories. Timentin is a combination of clavulanate potassium with ticarcillin disodium; available only for injection, it joins the oral product Augmentin (amoxicillin–potassium clavulanate) in Beecham's U.S. antibiotic line.

Ticarcillin–clavulanate potassium is indicated for treating infections caused by susceptible organisms (including *Klebsiella, Escherichia coli, Pseudomonas aeruginosa,* and *Staphylococcus aureus)* in several serious infections, such as septicemia, lower respiratory infections, bone and joint infections, skin and skin-structure infections, and complicated and uncomplicated urinary-tract infections. Combination therapy with aminoglycosides has been synergistic against some *Ps. aeruginosa* strains.

Timentin is available in vials containing ticarcillin 3 g (as the disodium salt) and clavulanic acid 100 or 200 mg (as the potassium salt). The two strengths are referred to by the company as 3.1-g and 3.2-g (depending on the clavulanic acid content) vials or piggyback bottles. The 3.1-g vial will cost $9.35.

Beecham claims that sales of Augmentin make it "the most successful antibiotic ever launched in the U.S. marketplace." More than 200,000 new prescriptions are written for Augmentin each month, the company reports, and sales are now at $740,000 per week.

The next β-lactamase inhibitor likely to be marketed is sulbactam, a Pfizer product. It will be marketed as a single agent for injection rather than in fixed-dose combinations; clinical studies thus far have used sulbactam in combination with ampicillin in patients with peritonitis, perforated bowel or appendix, and gynecologic or urologic infections.

Haemophilus vaccine approved

A vaccine to protect children 18 months to 6 years of age against *Haemophilus influenzae* type b (Hib), the leading cause of bacterial meningitis in the U.S., was approved April 16 by FDA. The polysaccharide vaccine is relatively safe, but the vaccine's effectiveness in those who are at highest risk for contracting the disease (children less than 24 months old) is questionable.

The new vaccine, b-Capsa I, has been recommended for use in all children 24 months and older and in children 18 months or older in high-risk groups, such as those attending day-care centers, by the advisory committee on immunization practices of the Centers for Disease Control. The new vaccine is manufactured by Praxis Biologics and is distributed by Mead Johnson's Nutritional Division.

A recent study in *JAMA*[1] used a decision-tree analytic model to compare the outcomes of alternative strategies for immunizing children against Hib and related complications. The cost-effectiveness model compared different strategies for use of the vaccine, including universal immunization and use in high-risk groups.

The authors varied the efficacy rate for 18-month-old infants from 25 to 90% in their analysis. The break-even point was at about 50% in the cost-benefit model. They concluded that any protection provided by the Hib vaccine would result in a favorable cost-effectiveness ratio, even if protection were only for the minority of children that contract the disease after 18 months of age.

Ward,[2] in an accompanying editorial, criticized the study for failing to show more than a partial effectiveness in the critical age group. He said that any Hib vaccine that was less than 50% effective in 18-month-old children would have problems becoming widely accepted. Ward did recommend that children 24 months and older be vaccinated, especially those enrolled in day-care centers.

Continued on page 367

Continued from page 362

The marketed vaccine—and that used in the *JAMA* study—was a polysaccharide vaccine composed of polyribosyl-ribitol-phosphate (PRP). Another vaccine, called PRP-D, that covalently binds a protein carrier to PRP is now being tested in Alaskans (who are at high risk for Hib) in an NIH-sponsored trial. The protein carrier in PRP-D is being used to increase immunogenicity in infants younger than 18 months. The PRP-D vaccine is being investigated by Connaught Laboratories. The study will be completed in 1987.

1. Cochi SL, Broome CB, Hightower AW. Immunization of U.S. children with *Haemophilus influenzae* type b polysaccharide vaccine. *JAMA*. 1985; 253:521–9.
2. Ward JI. Is *Haemophilus influenzae* type b disease preventable? *JAMA*. 1985; 253:554–6. Editorial.

Health implications of obesity explored at consensus conference

Obesity as a risk factor in hypertension, hyperlipidemia, diabetes, heart disease, and cancer was the subject of a February 11–13 NIH Consensus Development Conference in Bethesda, MD. The consensus panel concluded that the "evidence is now overwhelming that obesity . . . is clearly associated" with these conditions and that obese patients have a higher mortality ratio and more excess deaths per 1000 per year than nonobese people.

Defining obesity as weight greater than 20% higher than desirable weight, the panel noted that obese people should be advised to reduce their weights for health reasons. "Weight reduction is also highly desirable," the panel reported, "even in patients with less degrees of obesity" in certain situations. These included

- Patients with a history of noninsulin-dependent diabetes mellitus or a family history of diabetes mellitus;
- Women with a history of gestational diabetes or history of giving birth to large-for-gestational-age infants;
- Patients with idiopathic hypertension; and
- Patients with hypertriglyceridemia or hypercholesterolemia.

Copies of the panel's complete statement are available at no cost from the National Institutes of Health, Office of Medical Applications of Research, Building 1, Room 216, Bethesda, MD 20205.

Inosiplex available for AIDS patients

FDA has approved the "compassionate" use of inosiplex (Isoprinosine, Newport Pharmaceuticals) in patients with acquired immunodeficiency syndrome (AIDS). AIDS patients have been reportedly traveling to Mexico to obtain the drug, where it is available without a prescription.

Inosiplex has not been approved by FDA as safe and effective for any indication. Physicians who wish to obtain the product must contact Newport Pharmaceuticals (in Newport Beach, CA), qualify as investigators, and agree to work within a research protocol.

Allopurinol approved for management of recurrent calcium oxalate stones

Allopurinol (Zyloprim, Burroughs Wellcome) has been approved by FDA for the management of recurrent calcium oxalate stones in patients with hyperuricemia. The drug was previously indicated only for the management of patients with signs and symptoms of primary or secondary gout and for patients receiving cancer therapy who are prone to increases in serum and urinary uric acid concentrations.

Allopurinol is indicated for the management of recurrent calcium oxalate stones in patients whose urinary uric acid excretion exceeds 800 mg/day (men) or 750 mg/day (women). The recommended dose for treating recurrent stones in hyperuricemic patients is 200–300 mg/day in divided doses or as a single daily dose.

News Briefs

• New labeling about the effect of food on absorption of Searle's **sustained-release theophylline product** Theo-24 has been approved by FDA; patients receiving 900 mg or more of the once-daily product should take doses at least one hour before eating a high-fat meal (such as a bacon-and-eggs breakfast).

• Sales of **oxyphenbutazone (Tandearil)** have been discontinued in the U.S. by its manufacturer, Ciba-Geigy. Additionally, the company has received FDA approval to amend the labeling for **phenylbutazone (Butazolidin)** to include indications for four severe arthritic conditions: active ankylosing spondylitis, acute gouty arthritis, active rheumatoid arthritis, and acute attacks of degenerative joint disease of the hip and knees.

• **One-dose therapy of vulvovaginal candidiasis** is the approved indication for Mycelex-G 500 mg (clotrimazole, Miles Laboratories); severe vulvovaginitis requires multiple-dose therapy, and possible pathogens other than *Candida* (e.g., *Trichomonas* and *Gardnerella vaginalis*) must be ruled out.

• Limiting the length of the therapy to 14 days with 0.05% **betamethasone dipropionate ointment** (Diprolone Ointment, Schering Laboratories) is no longer necessary, according to the revised product labeling. However, no more than 45 grams of the ointment should be applied weekly.

• A patient-information brochure about **Chlamydia,** a sexually transmitted disease affecting 3–10 million people annually, is available from the American Social Health Association, 260 Sheridan Avenue, Palo Alto, CA 94306. Enclose a stamped, self-addressed envelope to get a free copy of the brochure, which was funded through a grant from Lederle Laboratories.

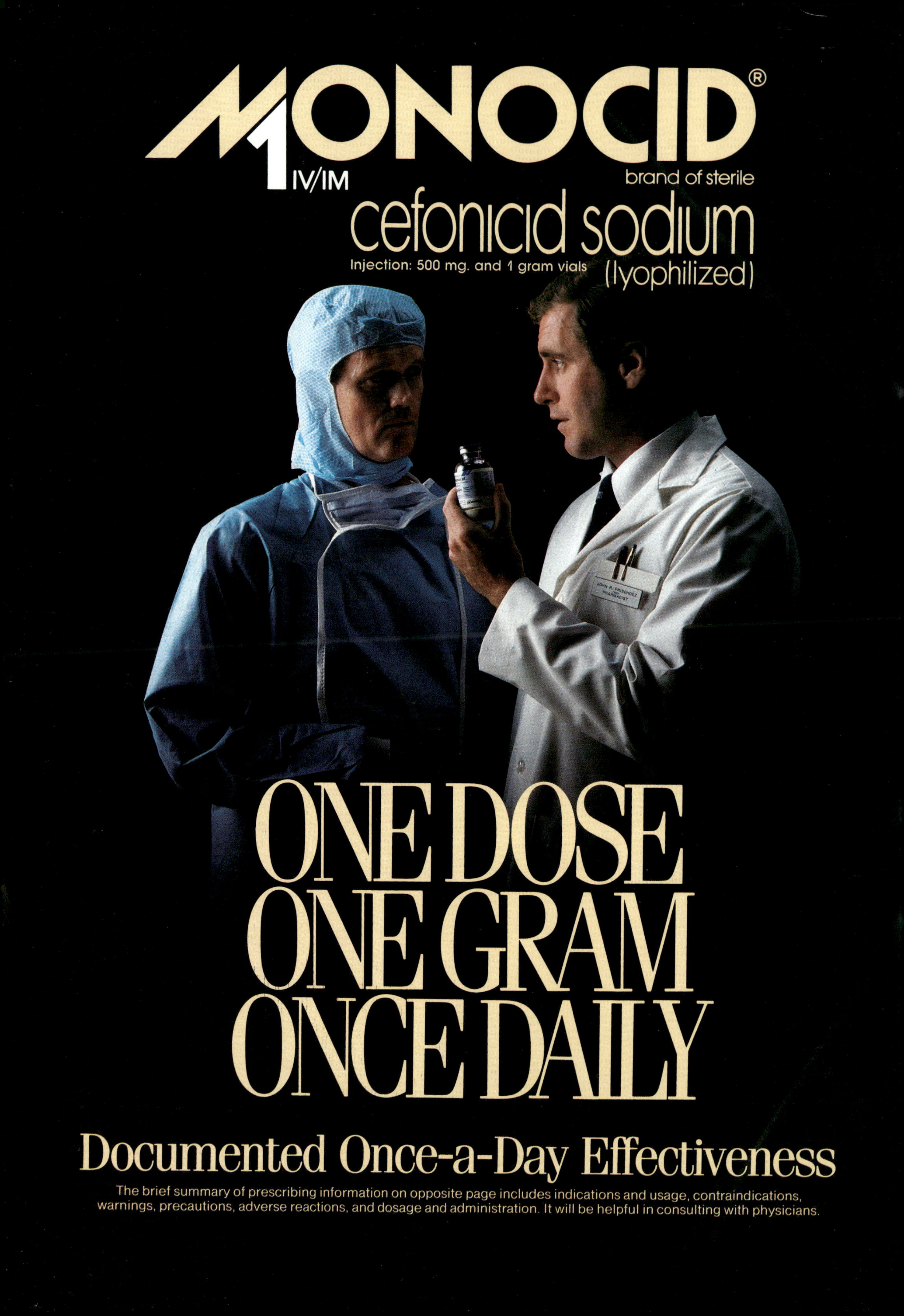
MONOCID®
IV/IM
brand of sterile
cefonicid sodium
Injection: 500 mg. and 1 gram vials (lyophilized)
ONE DOSE
ONE GRAM
ONCE DAILY
Documented Once-a-Day Effectiveness
The brief summary of prescribing information on opposite page includes indications and usage, contraindications, warnings, precautions, adverse reactions, and dosage and administration. It will be helpful in consulting with physicians.

A Money-Saving Regimen That *Works*

The following is a brief summary of prescribing information. For complete prescribing information, please see SK&F literature or PDR.

INDICATIONS AND USAGE

Monocid (sterile cefonicid sodium, SK&F) is indicated in the treatment of infections due to susceptible strains of the microorganisms listed below:

LOWER RESPIRATORY TRACT INFECTIONS, due to *Streptococcus pneumoniae* (formerly *D. pneumoniae*); *Klebsiella pneumoniae*; *Escherichia coli*; and *Hemophilus influenzae* (ampicillin-resistant and ampicillin-sensitive).

URINARY TRACT INFECTIONS, due to *Escherichia coli*; *Proteus mirabilis* (indole-negative *Proteus*); and *Klebsiella pneumoniae.*

SKIN AND SKIN STRUCTURE INFECTIONS, due to *Staphylococcus aureus* and *S. epidermidis*; *Streptococcus pyogenes* (Group A *Streptococcus*) and *S. agalactiae* (Group B *Streptococcus*).

SEPTICEMIA, due to *Streptococcus pneumoniae* (formerly *D. pneumoniae*) and *Escherichia coli.*

BONE AND JOINT INFECTIONS, due to *Staphylococcus aureus.*

SURGICAL PROPHYLAXIS
Administration of a single 1 gram dose of 'Monocid' before surgery may reduce the incidence of postoperative infections in patients undergoing surgical procedures classified as contaminated or potentially contaminated (e.g., colorectal surgery, vaginal hysterectomy, or cholecystectomy in high-risk patients), or in patients in whom infection at the operative site would present a serious risk (e.g., prosthetic arthroplasty, open heart surgery). Although cefonicid has been shown to be as effective as cefazolin in prevention of infection following coronary artery bypass surgery, no placebo-controlled trials have been conducted to evaluate any cephalosporin antibiotic in the prevention of infection following coronary artery bypass surgery or prosthetic heart valve replacement.

In cesarean section, the use of 'Monocid' (after the umbilical cord has been clamped) may reduce the incidence of certain postoperative infections.

When administered one hour prior to surgical procedures for which it is indicated, a single 1 gram dose of 'Monocid' provides protection from most infections due to susceptible organisms throughout the course of the procedure and for approximately 24 hours after administration. Intraoperative and postoperative administration of 'Monocid' is not necessary. Daily doses of 'Monocid' may be administered for two additional days in patients undergoing prosthetic arthroplasty or open heart surgery.

Therapy with 'Monocid' may be initiated pending results of susceptibility studies. Treatment should be adjusted according to findings.

Before using 'Monocid' concomitantly with other antibiotics, the prescribing information for those agents should be reviewed for contraindications, warnings, precautions and adverse reactions. Renal function should be carefully monitored.

CONTRAINDICATIONS
'Monocid' is contraindicated in persons who have shown hypersensitivity to cephalosporin antibiotics.

WARNINGS
BEFORE THERAPY WITH 'MONOCID' IS INSTITUTED, CAREFUL INQUIRY SHOULD BE MADE TO DETERMINE WHETHER THE PATIENT HAS HAD PREVIOUS HYPERSENSITIVITY REACTIONS TO CEPHALOSPORINS, PENICILLINS, OR OTHER DRUGS. THIS PRODUCT SHOULD BE GIVEN CAUTIOUSLY TO PENICILLIN-SENSITIVE PATIENTS. ANTIBIOTICS SHOULD BE ADMINISTERED WITH CAUTION TO ANY PATIENT WHO HAS DEMONSTRATED SOME FORM OF ALLERGY, PARTICULARLY TO DRUGS. SERIOUS ACUTE HYPERSENSITIVITY REACTIONS MAY REQUIRE EPINEPHRINE AND OTHER EMERGENCY MEASURES.

Pseudomembranous colitis has been reported with the use of cephalosporins (and other broad-spectrum antibiotics); therefore, it is important to consider that diagnosis in patients who develop diarrhea in association with antibiotic use.

Treatment with broad-spectrum antibiotics alters normal flora of the colon and may permit overgrowth of Clostridia. Studies indicate a toxin produced by *Clostridium difficile* is one primary cause of antibiotic-associated colitis. Cholestyramine and colestipol resins have been shown to bind the toxin *in vitro.*

Mild cases of colitis may respond to drug discontinuance alone. Moderate to severe cases should be managed with fluid, electrolyte and protein supplementation as indicated. When the colitis is not relieved by drug discontinuance and when it is severe, oral vancomycin is the treatment of choice for antibiotic-associated pseudomembranous colitis produced by *C. difficile.* Other causes of colitis should also be considered.

PRECAUTIONS
General: With any antibiotic, prolonged use may result in overgrowth of nonsusceptible organisms. Careful observation is essential, and appropriate measures should be taken if superinfection occurs.

Drug Interactions: Nephrotoxicity has been reported following concomitant administration of other cephalosporins and aminoglycosides.

Pregnancy: (Category B.) Reproduction studies have been performed in mice, rabbits and rats at doses up to an equivalent of 40 times the usual adult human dose and have revealed no evidence of impaired fertility or harm to the fetus due to 'Monocid'. There are, however, no adequate and well-controlled studies in pregnant women. Because animal reproduction studies are not always predictive of human response, this drug should be used in pregnancy only if clearly needed.

Labor and Delivery: In cesarean section, 'Monocid' should be administered only after the umbilical cord has been clamped.

Nursing Mothers: 'Monocid' is excreted in human milk in low concentrations. Caution should be exercised when 'Monocid' is administered to a nursing woman.

Pediatric Use: Safety and effectiveness in children have not been established.

ADVERSE REACTIONS
'Monocid' is generally well tolerated and adverse reactions have occurred infrequently. The most common adverse reaction has been pain on I.M. injection. On-therapy conditions occurring in greater than 1% of 'Monocid'-treated patients were:

Injection Site Phenomena (5.7%): Pain and/or discomfort on injection; less often, burning, phlebitis at I.V. site.

Increased Platelets (1.7%).

Increased Eosinophils (2.9%).

Liver Function Test Alterations (1.6%): Increased alkaline phosphatase, increased SGOT, increased SGPT, increased GGTP, increased LDH.

Less frequent on-therapy conditions occurring in less than 1% of 'Monocid'-treated patients were:

Hypersensitivity Reactions: Fever, rash, pruritus, erythema, myalgia and anaphylactoid-like type reactions have been reported.

Hematology: Decreased WBC, neutropenia, positive Coombs' test.

Diarrhea.

DOSAGE AND ADMINISTRATION
General
The usual adult dosage is 1 gram of 'Monocid' given once every 24 hours, intravenously or by deep intramuscular injection. Doses in excess of 1 gram daily are rarely necessary; however, in exceptional cases dosage of up to 2 grams given once daily have been well tolerated. When administering 2 gram I.M. doses once daily, one-half the dose should be administered in different large muscle masses.

Surgical Prophylaxis
When administered one hour prior to appropriate surgical procedures (see Indications and Usage), a 1 gram dose of 'Monocid' provides protection from most infections due to susceptible organisms throughout the course of the procedure and for approximately 24 hours after administration. Intraoperative and postoperative administration of 'Monocid' is not necessary. Daily doses of 'Monocid' may be administered for two additional days in patients undergoing prosthetic arthroplasty or open heart surgery.

In cesarean section 'Monocid' should be administered only after the umbilical cord has been clamped.

General Guidelines for Dosage of 'Monocid', I.V. or I.M.

Type of Infection	Daily Dose (grams)	Frequency
Uncomplicated Urinary Tract	0.5	once every 24 hours
Mild to Moderate	1	once every 24 hours
Severe or Life-Threatening	2*	once every 24 hours
Surgical Prophylaxis	1	1 hour preoperatively

*When administering 2 gram I.M. doses once daily, one-half the dose should be administered in different large muscle masses.

Impaired Renal Function
Modification of 'Monocid' dosage is necessary in patients with impaired renal function. Before prescribing, consult Dosage and Administration section of complete prescribing information.

HOW SUPPLIED
'Monocid' is supplied in vials equivalent to 500 mg. and 1 gram of cefonicid; in "Piggyback" Vials for I.V. admixture equivalent to 1 gram of cefonicid; and in Pharmacy Bulk Vials equivalent to 10 grams of cefonicid.

BRS-MC:L11

Smith Kline &French Laboratories SK&F

ONE DOSE
ONE GRAM
ONCE DAILY

MONOCID® IV/IM
brand of sterile
cefonicid sodium
(lyophilized)

Letters

The Letters *column is a forum for rapid exchange of ideas among readers of* CP. *Liberal criteria are applied in the review of submissions to encourage contributions to this column.*

The Letters *column includes the following types of contributions: (1) comments, addenda, and minor updates on previously published work, (2) alerts on potential problems related to drug therapy or clinical research, (3) observations or comments on trends in drug therapy or clinical research, and (4) brief expressions of opinion about controversies in drug therapy or clinical research.*

Letters need not be submitted with the journal's manuscript checklist. The following conditions, however, must be adhered to: (1) the body of the letter must be no longer than two typewritten pages, (2) the use of references, tables, and illustrations should be minimized, (3) the authors' names, affiliations, and mailing addresses must be typed at the end of the letter in the format used by CP, *and (4) the entire letter (including references, tables, and authors' names) must be typed double spaced on plain white paper (not letterhead). Following acceptance of a letter, the authors are required to sign an exclusive publication statement and a copyright-transferral form.*

Oral acyclovir pharmacokinetics

We would like to provide some additional discussion on the pharmacokinetics and dosing of oral acyclovir. In their recent article in *Clinical Pharmacy,* True and Carter[1] report that only a small amount of acyclovir is eliminated in the stool. While less than 2% of intravenously administered acyclovir is eliminated in the stool,[2] this does not seem to be the case for the orally administered drug. One patient in a study by Straus et al.[3] eliminated 15–25% of the administered dose in a 24-hour stool collection. It is reasonable to expect the poor gastrointestinal absorption of oral acyclovir to contribute to increased elimination of the drug in the stool.

True and Carter conclude that each dose of oral acyclovir should not exceed 400 mg. Their reference for this conclusion deserves further comment. Twenty immunocomprised patients with herpesvirus infections were enrolled in the study by deMiranda and Blum.[4] Eight patients received oral acyclovir 200 mg, six received 400 mg, and six received 600 mg every four hours for a total of 31 doses. The mean peak plasma concentrations obtained on day 6 failed to show a proportional increase from the 400-mg to the 600-mg dosing schedules. There was no crossover design, however, and interpatient variability in the pharmacokinetic values must be expected. True and Carter failed to examine the relative constant urinary recovery of unchanged drug, the area under the curve, and the estimated (from urinary excretion data) bioavailability of oral acyclovir of 20.6%, 22.5%, and 17.3%, respectively, for the 200-, 400-, and 600-mg dosages. The study authors concluded that "the net absorption of acyclovir is nearly proportional to the dose in the 200- to 600-mg dose range."[4] The pharmacokinetic data of a recent study by Selby et al.[5] compared with those of deMiranda and Blum suggest that within the 200- and 800-mg dose range, AUC increases proportionately and urinary excretion of acyclovir is relatively constant. Although saturable or dose-dependent absorption has been shown in dogs,[6] it has not been shown in human subjects taking 200–800 mg of oral acyclovir in absolute bioavailability studies. It is premature to conclude that oral acyclovir doses in excess of 400 mg should not be administered, especially in light of current investigations that are using 800-mg dosing schedules.

1. True BL, Carter BL. Update on acyclovir: oral therapy for herpesvirus infections. *Clin Pharm.* 1984; 3:607–13.
2. deMiranda P, Good SS, Laskin OL et al. Disposition of intravenous radioactive acyclovir. *Clin Pharmacol Ther.* 1981; 30:662–72.
3. Straus SE, Smith HA, Brickman C et al. Acyclovir for chronic mucocutaneous herpes simplex virus infections in immunocompromised patients. *Ann Intern Med.* 1982; 96:270–7.
4. deMiranda P, Blum MR. Pharmacokinetics of acyclovir after intravenous and oral administration. *J Antimicrob Chemother.* 1983; 12:29–37.
5. Selby P, Blake S, Mbidde EK et al. Amino (hydroxyethoxymethyl) purine: a new well-absorbed prodrug of acyclovir. *Lancet.* 1984; 2:1428–30.
6. Krasny HC, deMiranda P, Blum MR et al. Pharmacokinetics and bioavailability of acyclovir in the dog. *J Pharmacol Exp Ther.* 1981; 216:281–8.

COURTNEY FLETCHER, PHARM.D.
Department of Pharmaceutical Services

BARBARA CHINNOCK
Clinical Virology Research Laboratory

Continued on page 372

NEW from SK&F: Single-Dose Unit

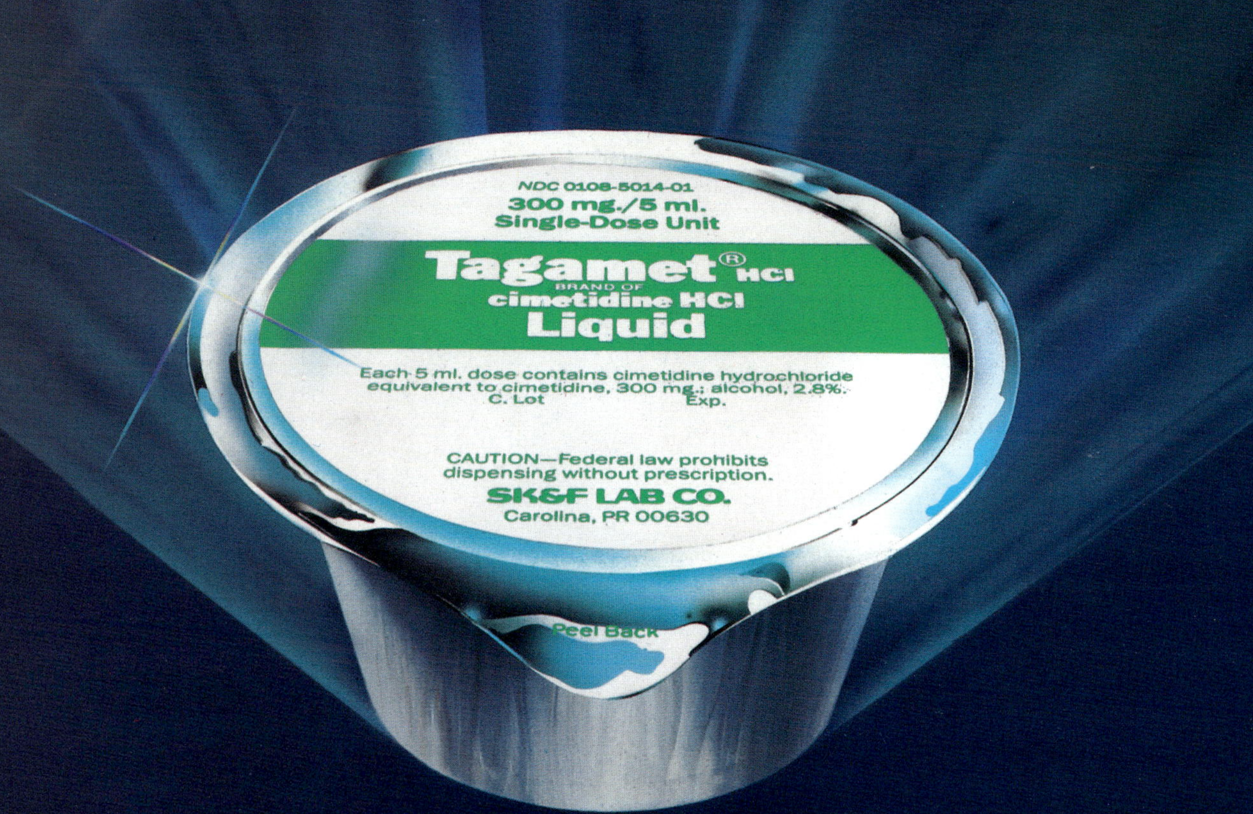

Tagamet® HCl Liquid

BRAND OF **cimetidine HCl** 300 mg./5 ml.*

- Appropriate for hospital and nursing home use
- Additional flexibility of administration
- The only H_2-antagonist in oral liquid form

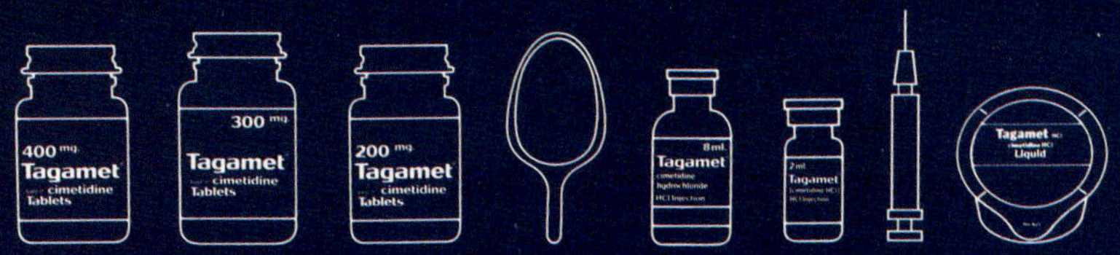

Continuing Innovation in Dosage Versatility

*Each 5 ml. (1 dose) contains cimetidine hydrochloride equivalent to cimetidine, 300 mg.; alcohol, 2.8%.
Please refer to brief summary of prescribing information on adjacent page.

SK&F LAB CO.
Carolina, P.R. 00630

Letters *Continued from page 370*

Henry H. Balfour, Jr., M.D.
Departments of Laboratory Medicine and Pathology and Pediatrics

University of Minnesota Health Sciences Center
Box 611, Mayo, 420 Delaware Street, SE
Minneapolis, MN 55455

We appreciate the comments of Fletcher, Chinnock, and Balfour; however, some of their statements deserve further discussion.

Our recommendation that single oral doses of acyclovir larger than 400 mg not be used was based on the limited amount of pharmacokinetic data available at the time of our review. As Fletcher et al. point out, the study by deMiranda[1] had a small sample size (eight patients) and lacked a crossover design. While acyclovir serum concentrations did not significantly increase with doses above 400 mg, this could be attributed to patient variability. However, Fletcher et al. fail to refer to the study by Brigden et al.[2] in which six male volunteers did receive oral acyclovir in a crossover design. As the dosage of acyclovir was increased from 100 to 600 mg, the percentage recovered in the urine decreased from 13.2 to 6%. Further, blood concentrations did not increase significantly when the dose was increased from 400 to 600 mg. The area under the plasma–time curve (AUC) was 3.2 times greater with three doses of 200 mg each, administered at four-hour intervals, than with one single dose of 600 mg.

The statement by Fletcher et al. that "the pharmacokinetic data of a recent study by Selby et al.[3] . . . suggest that within the 200- to 800-mg dose range, the AUC increases proportionately" is misleading. Selby et al. compared a single 800-mg oral dose of acyclovir with a single dose of an investigational prodrug of acyclovir. While this dosage resulted in excellent serum concentrations with chronic dosing, no comparison was made of this single large dose with smaller divided doses of equivalent total quantity. Therefore, it is not known if the subjects in this study would have achieved similar concentrations had the 800-mg dose been administered in a divided schedule. In addition, this study used acyclovir in tablet form, while the product used in the Brigden study[2] and the marketed drug are micronized formulations in capsules.

The pharmacokinetic data concerning oral acyclovir are limited. However, the data of Bridgen et al.,[2] who first proposed dose-limited absorption, and the data of the deMiranda group[1] suggest that single doses above 400 mg may not result in a proportional increase in serum concentrations. Until more extensive pharmacokinetic data are available, it seems reasonable, and possibly more cost-effective, to administer oral acyclovir in smaller divided doses rather than in doses greater than 400 mg.

1. deMiranda P, Blum MR. Pharmacokinetics of acyclovir after intravenous and oral administration. *J Antimicrob Chemother.* 1983; 12:29–37.
2. Brigden D, Fowle A, Rosling A. Acyclovir, a new antiherpetic drug: early experience in man with a systemically administered drug. In: Collier LH, Oxford J, eds. Developments in antiviral therapy. London: Academic Press; 1980:53–62.

Continued on page 383

Continued from page 372

3. Selby P, Blake S, Mbidde EK et al. Amino (hydroxyethoxymethyl) purine: a new well-absorbed prodrug of acyclovir. *Lancet*. 1984; 2:1428–30.

BEV L. TRUE, PHARM.D., Clinical Pharmacy Fellow in Family Practice
BARRY L. CARTER, PHARM.D., Assistant Professor

College of Pharmacy
University of Iowa
Iowa City, IA 52242

Hypersensitivity vasculitis associated with streptokinase

Currently, there is one case in the literature of a serum sickness-like reaction in a patient receiving streptokinase.[1] We recently encountered another patient with a similar illness following the use of streptokinase for acute pulmonary embolization. With the increasing use of this drug, it is likely that such allergic reactions will be encountered more frequently.

A 47-year-old physically active man was hospitalized after 12 hours of malaise, fatigue, dyspnea on exertion, and three hours of pleuritic right-chest pain. He denied cough, fever, chills, trauma, and periods of prolonged inactivity. He was taking no medication and had no known allergies.

Except for a right lateral chest-wall friction rub, physical examination was normal. Ventilation–perfusion scan demonstrated a perfusion defect in the right lung. Digital subtraction angiography, done with Conray-60 contrast material, confirmed the presence of pulmonary emboli. There were no clues, then or subsequently, to suggest a source of venous thrombi.

Following a 250,000-unit loading dose, streptokinase 100,000 units/hour was administered via peripheral vein continuously for the next 26 hours. Intravenous infusion of heparin was started three hours after discontinuation of streptokinase and was continued for seven days. Daily warfarin was also started at the same time.

Rapid improvement occurred during the first two or three hospital days and, by the fifth hospital day, the patient felt well (while receiving only heparin and warfarin). Six days following discontinuation of streptokinase, he awoke with abdominal pain, malaise, fatigue, and bilateral wrist pain. Abdominal examination was unremarkable, temperature was normal, and there was tenderness and reduced range of motion in both wrists, without swelling or increased warmth. The following morning, these joints were normal, but the patient still

Continued on page 386

When a type II diabetic patient needs more than diet, unique MICRONASE® Tablets (glyburide) are a logical first choice.

Choosing antidiabeti

1. Micronase—a rational choice in type II diabetes

Insulin levels are normal or elevated in most patients with type II diabetes, although insulin action is markedly impaired. MICRONASE helps normalize the tissue response to endogenous insulin.

Initially, MICRONASE helps lower serum glucose in responsive patients by stimulating the release of additional insulin. As therapy continues, MICRONASE is believed to promote peripheral glucose metabolism by helping to correct defects at the cellular receptor and postreceptor levels.

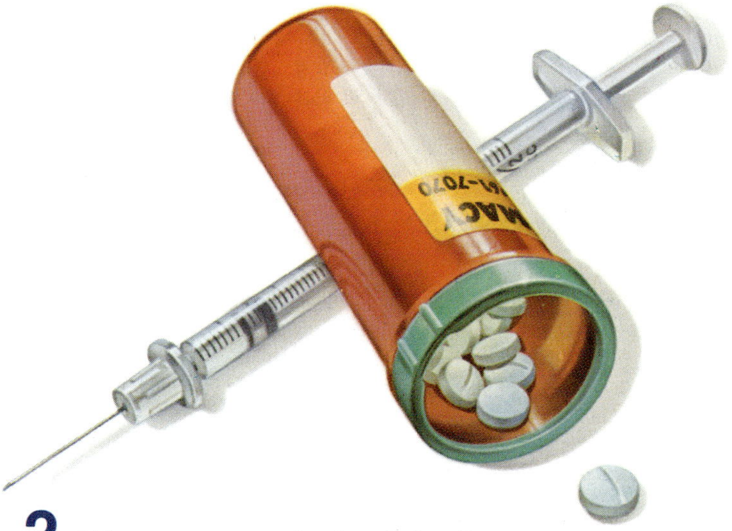

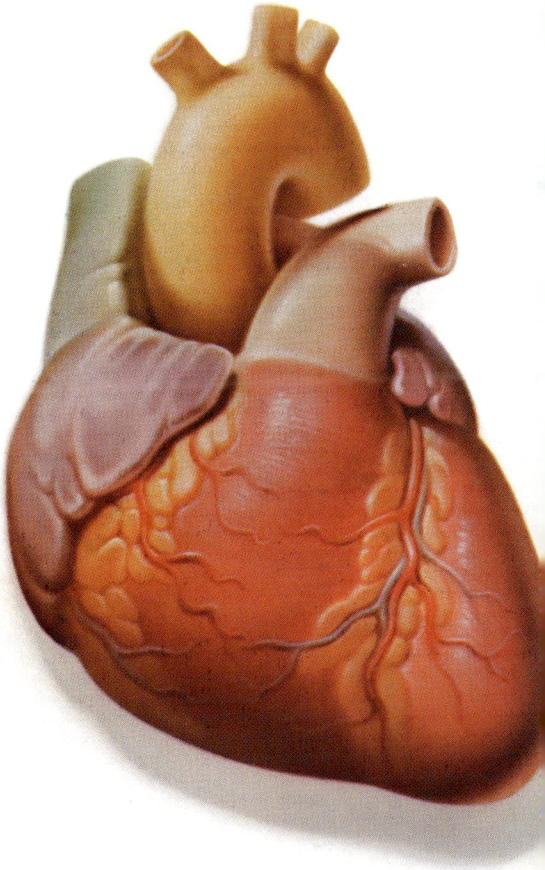

2. Micronase—a single, daily dose provides 24-hour glycemic control

MICRONASE provides 24-hour control of blood glucose with a single, daily, low-milligram dose. MICRONASE may be taken with food, since food intake does not appear to affect its bioavailability.

3. Micronase—for the type II diabetic patient who is also hypertensive: Control without risk of water retention

This may also be significant for the type II diabetic pat with congestive heart failure. MICRONASE actually cau mild diuresis.

herapy today

Micronase—an important consideration in type II diabetic patient with renal impair-nt: Control plus unique dual excretion... % urine, 50% bile

nination of MICRONASE equally in bile and urine reduces the of drug accumulation, which may result in hypoglycemia. RONASE should be used with caution in patients with renal airment; however, in a single-dose study, plasma clearance of RONASE was prolonged only in patients with severe renal airment.

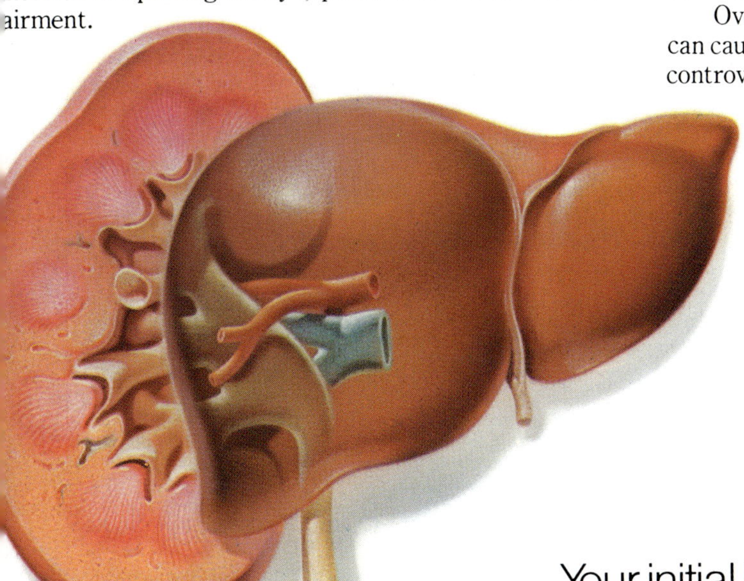

5. Micronase—for the patient who fails on other diabetic therapy: Potency and dosage flexibility

MICRONASE may prove effective when other drugs fail. Five mg of MICRONASE is approximately equivalent to 250 mg of chlorpropamide or 500 mg of acetohexamide in its ability to lower blood glucose. The dosage range of MICRONASE allows for greater dosage flexibility than other agents.

Overdosage of sulfonylureas, including MICRONASE, can cause hypoglycemia. Although the interpretations are controversial, the UGDP study reported in 1970 that the use of tolbutamide, an oral hypoglycemic drug, was associated with increased cardiovascular mortality.

Upjohn The Upjohn Company
Kalamazoo, MI 49001

Your initial Rx in type II diabetes

Micronase®

glyburide, **5 mg** Tablets

For brief summary of prescribing information, please turn page.

Letters *Continued from page 383*

noted malaise, fatigability, and abdominal pain. Later that day, a rash on the buttocks was noted; by the end of the day, this rash covered most of the buttocks and lower extremities. The rash was nonpruritic, palpable, and purpuric. Platelet count at the time was 360,000 with prothrombin time 1½ times control. That evening, urine microscopic examination showed 30 red blood cells per high-power field, without casts or proteinuria.

A presumptive diagnosis of hypersensitivity vasculitis, probably secondary to streptokinase, was made. Heparin had been stopped three hours before the rash was noted, while warfarin was continued. Additional laboratory studies done the day after the appearance of the rash revealed normal values for the third component of complement (C_3), platelet count, and serum creatinine, and negative circulating immune complexes. Total hemolytic complement was reduced to 26 units (normal, 50–200 units). Microscopic hematuria persisted for only 12 hours. While the rash improved rapidly over four days, fatigability and generalized weakness resolved slowly over the next six weeks.

Our patient's clinical picture best fits that of Henoch-Schönlein purpura, a subtype of the hypersensitivity vasculitides. The evidence that streptokinase was the provocative antigen is circumstantial. We found a single case report of a similar reaction, which was labeled "serum sickness" and attributed to streptokinase.[1] That patient developed fever, edema, arthralgia, palpable purpura, transient proteinuria, and low total hemolytic complement six days after cessation of intra-arterial streptokinase infusion. Although leukocytoclastic vasculitis with localized skin necrosis has been reported following subcutaneous heparin,[2] systemic hypersensitivity vasculitis has not been reported with this drug. Warfarin therapy is occasionally associated with dermatological reactions, such as dermal gangrene; with histological features of leukocytoclastic vasculitis; and an instance of fever, chills, and purpura associated with warfarin therapy has been reported.[3] Our patient, however, subsequently tolerated long-term warfarin therapy. Given the above information, we believe that the agent most likely to have caused this syndrome was streptokinase.

1. Totty WG, Romano T, Benian GM et al. Serum sickness following streptokinase therapy. *AJR.* 1982; 138:143–4.
2. Kearsley JH, Jeremy RW, Coates AS. Leukocytoclastic vasculitis and skin necrosis following subcutaneous heparin calcium. *Aust NZ J Med.* 1982; 12(3):288–9.
3. Tanay A, Yust I, Brenner S et al. Dermal vasculitis due to coumadin hypersensitivity. *Dermatologia.* 1982; 165:178–85.

ROBERT F. THOMPSON, M.D., Assistant Professor
Department of Family, Community and Emergency Medicine

MARK A. STRATTON, PHARM.D., Assistant Professor
College of Pharmacy
Department of Family, Community and Emergency Medicine

WARREN A. HEFFRON, M.D., Professor and Chairman
Department of Family, Community and Emergency Medicine

School of Medicine
University of New Mexico
Albuquerque, NM 87131

Continued on page 388

WHY VIBRAMYCIN® IV'S (DOXYCYCLINE HYCLATE) 48-HOUR STABILITY SAVES YOU MORE MONEY THAN ANY OTHER DOXYCYCLINE

Twice the stability at room temperature reduces product waste

When reconstituted, Vibramycin IV is the only injectable doxycycline hyclate with 48-hour stability at room temperature as documented in its package insert. This allows you to store it for twice as long as any other injectable doxycycline. This superior reconstituted shelf life applies to the most common diluents–Sodium Chloride Injection 0.9%, USP, or 5% Dextrose Injection, USP.

Longer stability means less waste. Because of Vibramycin IV's extended reconstituted life, unused preparations need not be discarded. And standardized dosages (100 mg or 200 mg) enhance the probability that these preparations will be used, thus making them even more economical.

Extended stability brings greater convenience and efficiency to your pharmacy. Now, you can prepare "piggybacks" less frequently for greater savings of time and labor.

Of course, 48-hour reconstituted stability isn't the only way we keep your costs down. Vibramycin IV is bid at competitive prices. And guaranteed availability helps ensure that you'll never run out of Vibramycin IV.

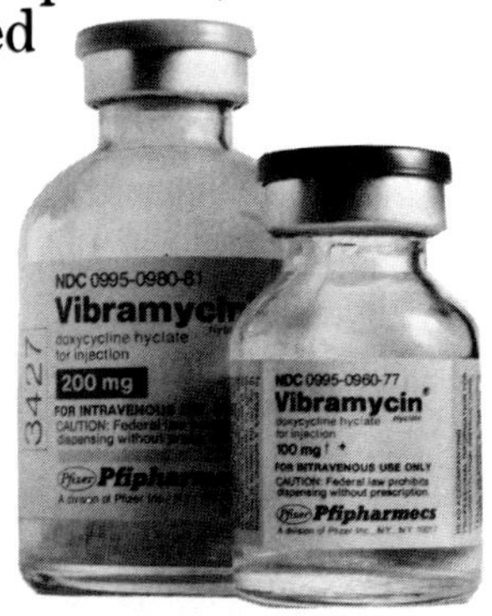

When you add up all these cost-saving features, you'll see why Vibramycin IV is the most economical choice in doxycycline.

VIBRAMYCIN® IV
(DOXYCYCLINE HYCLATE)
The original, and now the most cost effective

Pfizer
Pfipharmecs Division
New York, NY 10017

Please see following page for brief summary of prescribing information.

Letters *Continued from page 386*

Change in enzyme content and manufacturer of Viokase

The recent review article, "Management of Maldigestion Associated with Pancreatic Insufficiency,"[1] incorrectly reports the current enzyme content and manufacturer of Viokase tablets.

Viokase tablets and powder are currently manufactured by A. H. Robins Co. and were reformulated under the Viobin label in March 1984 to contain pancrelipase instead of pancreatin. The correct labeled enzyme potencies of available Viokase dosage forms are as follows[2]:

	Each tablet	Each 0.7 g powder (¼ tsp)
Lipase USP units	8,000	16,800
Protease, USP units	30,000	70,000
Amylase, USP units	30,000	70,000

The fact that the authors incorrectly reported the enzyme content is not surprising to us, since most current references, including the *American Hospital Formulary Service—Drug Information 85*,[3] are in error. In response to our telephone request, A. H. Robins confirmed the product formulation change, the date of reformulation, and the fact that pharmacists and physicians were not notified in advance of the change (Schneiweiss F, A. H. Robins Co. Written communication. 1985 Jan 31).

Although the actual change in labeled enzyme content per dosage unit may not be important therapeutically for most patients with pancreatic insufficiency, the new Viokase formulation is now very similar to at least two other pancreatic enzyme preparations, Cotazym capsules (Organon) and Ku-Zyme HP capsules (Kremers-Urban). We believe this similarity to be important, since hospitals with formularies may wish to purchase only one pancrelipase preparation. Moreover, hospital pharmacies could request the manufacturers to bid for this purchase, resulting in a possible price reduction.

In our opinion, the fact that health professionals were not informed prospectively concerning this formulation change is unfortunate, since considerable confusion already exists regarding the pancreatic enzyme content of commercial products.

1. Perry RS, Gallagher J. Management of maldigestion associated with pancreatic insufficiency. *Clin Pharm.* 1985; 4:161–9.
2. Robins AH. Viokase package insert. Richmond, VA; 1984 Jul.
3. McEvoy GK, ed. American Hospital Formulary Service—Drug Information 85. Bethesda, MD: American Society of Hospital Pharmacists, Inc.; 1985:1290.

Rosemary R. Berardi, Pharm.D., Associate Professor of Pharmacy
Carol L. Colvin, Pharm.D., Clinical Assistant Professor of Pharmacy

College of Pharmacy
University of Michigan
Ann Arbor, MI 48109-1065

Drug Reviews

New β_2-adrenergic agonist aerosols

H. WILLIAM KELLY

Abstract: The β_2-adrenergic agonists are reviewed in terms of their dose–response characteristics, and two newer agents, fenoterol hydrobromide and bitolterol mesylate aerosols, are reviewed in relation to older agents.

The fenoterol aerosol contains a more potent β_2-adrenergic agonist dose per puff than the other aerosols but, when given in equipotent doses, offers no advantage over available agents. Bitolterol mesylate is a prodrug that is hydrolyzed to the active β_2-adrenergic agonist colterol by lung esterases. Bitolterol demonstrates an improved bronchoselectivity in animals, but there are insufficient comparative data in humans. Tachycardia is the dose-limiting toxicity for all β_2-adrenergic agonists. Currently available data do not suggest an important improvement in duration of action for the newer agents over terbutaline or albuterol.

Aerosol administration improves bronchoselectivity of all the agents. Optimal use of β_2-adrenergic agonist aerosols requires understanding of the variable dose–response characteristics. The type of delivery system and patient technique are important variables in determining the dose delivered. Tube-spacer devices attached to aerosol canisters can significantly improve delivery of the β_2-adrenergic agonists to the lungs in patients unable to synchronize actuation and inspiration. They provide minimal to no improvement in patients who can perform the appropriate technique.

Aerosol administration is the route of choice for β_2-adrenergic agonists for prophylaxis of exercise-induced bronchospasm; albuterol and terbutaline provide a prolonged duration of action with excellent β_2-adrenergic selectivity. Patients should be carefully instructed in the optimal use of metered-dose inhalers, and some patients may benefit from use of tube-spacers.

Index terms: Aerosols; Bitolterol mesylate; Bronchial spasm; Fenoterol hydrobromide; Sympathomimetic agents; Toxicity
Clin Pharm. 1985; 4:393–403

Selective β_2-adrenergic agonists are playing an increasingly greater role in clinicians' treatment of asthma and other obstructive airways diseases. Last year, a metered-dose aerosol form of terbutaline sulfate became available in the United States. Bitolterol mesylate, as a metered-dose aerosol, was released in April of this year, and the metered-dose inhaler of fenoterol hydrobromide is expected to receive Food and Drug Administration approval soon. There are numerous other investigational β_2-adrenergic agonists undergoing premarketing clinical trials. These newer agents are being marketed first as aerosol preparations, which reflects changing attitudes of clinicians toward use of aerosols. This attitudinal change is the result of a large volume of research investigating optimal use of β_2-adrenergic agonists.

In this review, I will compare the newer β_2-adrenergic agonists bitolterol mesylate (Tornalate, Breon–Winthrop) and fenoterol hydrobromide (Berotec, Boehringer–Ingelheim) with the β_2-adrenergic aerosols already available. To accomplish this, I will evaluate the pharmacologic principles of the dose–response characteristics of the β_2-adrenergic agonists. The optimal use of β_2-adrenergic aerosols, including the use of spacer devices, will be discussed.

Pharmacology

A complete review of the pharmacology of adrenergic bronchodilators is beyond the scope of this article; for more detailed discussions the reader should refer to several excellent reviews.[1-4] Fig-

H. WILLIAM KELLY, PHARM.D., is Associate Professor of Pharmacy and Pediatrics, College of Pharmacy and School of Medicine, University of New Mexico, Albuquerque, NM. This manuscript was prepared while Dr. Kelly was on sabbatical at the University of North Carolina at Chapel Hill.

Address reprint requests to Dr. Kelly at the College of Pharmacy, University of New Mexico, Albuquerque, NM 87131.

This is **article 680-204-8511** in the **ASHP Continuing Education System.** See page 463 for learning objectives and test questions.

ure 1 compares the chemical structures of the β-adrenergic agonists. The reader should note that bitolterol mesylate is a prodrug that requires hydrolysis by esterase to colterol, a catecholamine similar to terbutaline and albuterol, for pharmacologic activity.

Alterations in the chemical structures of these compounds determine molar potency, relative selectivity, oral activity, and duration of action. This section will focus on potency and β_2 selectivity, while oral activity and duration of action will be discussed in the next section on clinical pharmacology.

Potency. Figure 2 depicts classical dose–response curves. The curves are plotted in Figure 2a on a linear concentration axis and in Figure 2b on a logarithmic concentration axis. The ordinate is defined as the percentage of the maximal response.

An understanding of the characteristics of the dose–response curves explains some of the apparently conflicting data in the literature. Assuming that the ordinate represented bronchial smooth muscle relaxation, curves A and B would represent β_2-adrenergic agonists with differing affinities for the β_2 receptor.[5] In this case the log dose–response curve B is shifted to the right of A, but the slope and maximal attainable response are equal, so that drugs A and B are full agonists that differ only in potency (dose required to produce the response). On the other hand curve C represents a partial agonist that differs in efficacy or "intrinsic activity."[5] In this case both the slope of the log dose–response curve and the maximal response are altered. As stated previously, alterations in the chemical structure of the adrenergic agents may alter potency or efficacy at the receptor.[3,6]

On a molar basis, isoproterenol is the most potent of the β_2 agonists currently available. Altering the catechol ring structure to a resorcinol (metaproterenol, terbutaline) or a saligenin (albuterol) decreases the affinity for the β_2 receptor, while enlarging the group on the terminal amine increases the affinity. In vitro preparations of cholinergic-contracted bronchial smooth muscle[1] and anesthetized animal models[7] of bronchospasm clearly demonstrate the relative potency of the various agents. In most studies to date, all the agents are full β_2-adrenergic agonists with the following relative potencies: colterol > isoproterenol > fenoterol ≥ albuterol > terbutaline ≥ isoetharine > metaproterenol > bitolterol.[1,7,8] Therefore, if administered in equipotent doses, all these agents will produce the same degree of smooth muscle relaxation or bronchodilation.

The potency differences between preparations are largely reflected in their recommended dosages in Table 1. With the exception of fenoterol, the dose per actuation of metered-dose aerosol of each drug gives an approximately equipotent dose. This has been confirmed in clinical trials; the fenoterol dose per actuation, which is approximately twice that of albuterol, produces greater bronchodilation

Figure 1. Chemical structures of the β_2-adrenergic agonists.

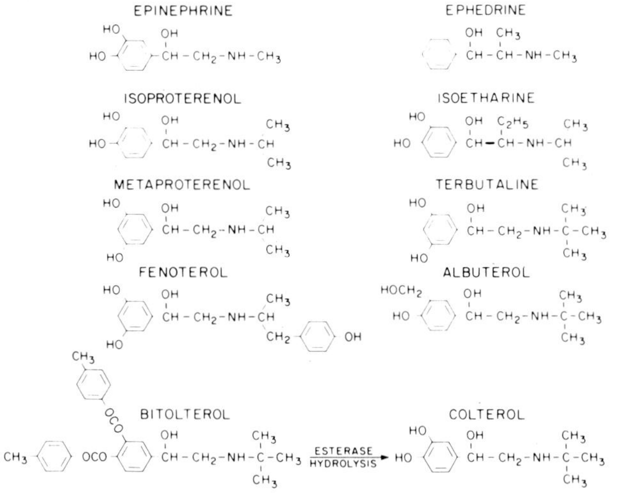

Figure 2. Pharmacologic dose–response curves. In figure A, the dose is plotted on a linear scale; in figure B, the dose is plotted on a logarithmic scale. Curves A and B represent compounds with different potencies (receptor affinity). Curve C represents a compound that is a partial agonist with a different potency and efficacy (intrinsic activity) at the receptor. ED_{50} represents the dose that produced 50% of maximal response.

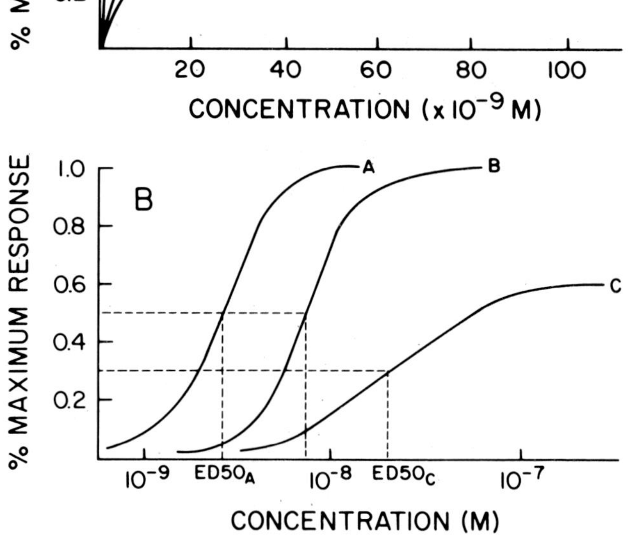

Table 1.
β_2-Adrenergic Aerosol Preparations and Dosages

Drug	Preparations[a]	Dosages: Pediatric	Dosages: Adult
Isoproterenol Hydrochloride and Sulfate			
Various manufacturers	0.25% (1:400) 2.5 mg/mL 0.50% (1:200) 5 mg/mL 1.0% (1:100) 10 mg/mL	0.05–0.1 mg/kg every two to four hours.	One to two inhalations of 0.25% solution by hand-bulb nebulizer; 2.5 mL of 0.05% solution via nebulizer every two to four hours.
Isuprel Mistometer (Breon) Norisodrine Aerotrol (Abbott) Medihaler-Iso (Riker) Norisodrine sulfate (Aerohaler, Abbott)	131 μg/spray 120 μg/spray 80 μg/spray 45 μg/spray 110 μg/spray	One to two inhalations every four to six hours.	One to two sprays every two to four hours as needed.
Isoetharine			
Isoetharine hydrochloride inhalation (Roxane)	0.1%, 0.125%, 0.2%	0.1–0.2 mg/kg every two to four hours.	3–5 mg undiluted via nebulizer with oxygen at 4–6 L/min over 15–20 minutes every two to four hours.
Bronkosol unit dose (Breon) Various manufacturers	0.25% 0.5%, 1%		0.5 and 1% solutions diluted 1:3 with 0.9% sodium chloride every two to four hours.
Bronkometer (Breon)	340 μg/spray	One to two sprays every four to six hours; may increase to every two hours for acute attacks.	One to two sprays every four to six hours; may increase to every two hours for acute attacks.
Metaproterenol			
Alupent (Boehringer Ingelheim) Metaprel (Dorsey)	5% (50 mg/mL) solution for nebulization 0.6% unit dose vial of 2.5 mL (15 mg)	0.25–0.5 mg/kg every two to four hours; maximum 15 mg as single dose.	5–15 inhalations of 5% undiluted from hand-bulb nebulizer every two to six hours as needed or 0.3 ml (15 mg) diluted with 2.5 mL of 0.9% sodium chloride in nebulizer every two to four hours.
Metered dose inhalers (MDI): Alupent (Boehringer Ingelheim) Metaprel (Dorsey)	0.65 mg/puff[b] (300 puffs) powder suspension	One to two puffs every four to six hours and before exercise.	Two to three puffs every four to six hours and before exercise.
Albuterol			
Ventolin (Glaxo) Proventil (Schering)	90 μg/puff[b] (200 puffs) powder suspension	One to two puffs every four to six hours and before exercise.	One to two puffs every four to six hours and before exercise.
	0.5% (5 mg/mL) solution for nebulization (not available in U.S.)	0.05–0.15 mg/kg every two to six hours as needed.	2.5–5 mg every two to six hours as needed.
Terbutaline			
Brethaire (Geigy) inhaler	0.2 mg/puff[b] (300 puffs) powder suspension	One to two puffs every four to six hours and before exercise.	One to two puffs every four to six hours and before exercise.
Brethine (Geigy) Bricanyl (Merrell Dow)	0.1% (1 mg/mL) solution in 0.9% sodium chloride for injection (not approved for this use)	0.1–0.3 mg/kg every two to six hours as needed.	5–7 mg (5–7 mL) undiluted every four to six hours as needed.
Bitolterol Mesylate			
Tornalate (Breon)	0.37 mg/spray[b] (300 sprays) solution	One to three sprays every four to six hours.	One to three sprays every four to six hours.
Fenoterol Hydrobromide			
Berotec MDI (Boehringer Ingelheim)	0.16 mg/puff[b] (300 puffs) powder suspension	One to two puffs every four to six hours.	One to two puffs every four to six hours.

[a] All products are solutions unless otherwise noted.
[b] FDA requires that the amount of the drug that reaches the patient be on the label as opposed to the amount released from the canister with each actuation. Thus, products released in the U.S. have an apparent lower dose per actuation.

as well as side effects when compared puff for puff.[9] When fenoterol and albuterol are administered in equipotent doses, there is no apparent advantage for either agent.[10,11] Although colterol, the active metabolite of bitolterol, is more potent than isoproterenol, bitolterol appears much less potent, probably as a result of incomplete hydrolysis.[8,12]

The β_2-adrenergic agonists all produce the typical dose–response curves in asthmatic patients whether given orally,[13] by injection,[14] or by inhalation.[15] The apparent difference in potency from various modes of administration is a function of the percentage of dose administered that reaches the receptor sites. By observing the characteristics of the dose–response curves in Figure 2, two key principles for evaluating comparative studies in the literature become obvious. First, the linear portion of the curve falls within the range of 20 to 80% of maximal response, and thereafter even very large dose increases will fail to produce significantly greater bronchodilation. This occurs frequently in clinical dose-range studies where the lowest dose used produces near maximal bronchodilation; even exponential increases in dose fail to produce further clinically important bronchodilation.[16,17] Second, the log-dose characteristic requires that exponential increases in dose are necessary for each incremental improvement within the linear portion of the curve. In other words, an increase from four to eight inhalations is required to give the same percentage of improvement as an increase from two to four inhalations of the same dose. Therefore, if linearly incremental doses are administered or if the improvement in pulmonary function is plotted against a linear increment in dose (Figure 2a), the data may be misinterpreted as showing a lack of further significant bronchodilation with increased dose.[18]

Physiologic Determinants of the Dose-Response Curve. A major determinant of the clinical dose–response curve is the physiologic condition of the patient's airways.[19] Karlsson and Persson[20] demonstrated a shift to the right of the isoproterenol dose–response curve between in vitro spontaneously contracted tracheal rings and those contracted with carbachol. Increasing the carbachol concentration (thus maximizing the degree of contraction) further shifted and flattened the curve, apparently decreasing both the potency and efficacy of isoproterenol. In vitro studies on isolated human bronchial smooth muscle[1] and in vivo studies in normal subjects and mild asthmatics[21] have not shown significant differences in the β_2-adrenergic agonist dose–response curves. However, there is evidence that the degree of bronchial constriction significantly alters the dose–response curve. Barnes and Pride[22] demonstrated a greater variability in dose–response curves to inhaled albuterol in asthmatics than in normal subjects. The dose that produced 50% of maximal response (ED_{50}) was significantly correlated with the baseline pulmonary function in the asthmatics. However, even the baseline pulmonary functions are a poor predictor of response in acutely ill asthmatics and in asthmatics recovering from acute attacks.[23–25] Patients often demonstrate a greater response during recovery than during onset and progression of an acute asthma attack at the same baseline pulmonary functions. Patients with severe obstruction who do not respond to the usual dose often respond to higher doses.[15,25]

Further evidence for the shift in dose–response curves comes from the apparent difference between the bronchodilator dose–response curve and the dose–response curve for the prevention of exercise- or chemical-induced bronchospasm in asthmatics.[26,27] The challenge agent acts like a functional antagonist in the in vitro model, shifting the dose–response curve to the right; greater concentrations of β_2-adrenergic agonist are required to prevent bronchoconstriction from the challenge than are needed to produce maximal dilation of spontaneously constricted bronchioles.[5] In reverse, the β_2-adrenergic agonists can be considered as partial functional antagonists of the constricting event that can be overcome by increasing the dose of the challenge.[28] This is consistent with the experimental dose–response curves produced in vitro.[5,20] In other words, as the degree of constriction increases, the bronchodilation dose–response curve progressively shifts to the right as pictured in Figure 2b.

Because bronchoprovocation tests present a uniform stimulus that results in a relatively reproducible degree of bronchoconstriction,[29,30] they may provide a better means of demonstrating differences between β_2-adrenergic agonists than the ability to reverse spontaneous bronchoconstriction in stable asthmatics.[26,27,31] In this regard, it is interesting to note that some in vitro studies using maximal contraction with carbachol have demonstrated a difference in the efficacies (intrinsic activity) among the β_2-adrenergic agonists.[32] Patients with the greatest degree of reactivity to the provocation require larger doses of β_2-adrenergic agents for protection,[33] so care should be taken in extrapolating results from comparative studies using bronchoprovocation to clinical practice.

Selectivity. Increasing the size of the terminal amino group on β-adrenergic agonists (Figure 1) improves their selectivity for the β_2 receptor.[3,4,7] The tertiary butyl group (terbutaline, albuterol, bitolterol) appears to provide optimal β_2-receptor selectivity; the three agents are only partial agonists (Figure 2, curve C) in isolated cardiac preparations.[7,8,34] Increasing the size of the moiety further (as in fenoterol) produces a full agonist in cardiac tissue.[7] The separation of the dose–response curves for tracheal relaxation and cardiac stimulation appears great enough to provide excellent bronchoselectivity for fenoterol in the usual therapeutic doses,[11] but differences may become more apparent when higher dosages are given.[35] Isoproterenol and metaproterenol—two nonselective agents—typically fail to demonstrate a significant separation of the bronchial and cardiac dose–response curves in the anesthetized dog model[7] or in humans[36] when given intravenously.

Despite the demonstration of β_2 selectivity, cardiac stimulation with tachycardia is still the major dose-limiting toxicity of all these agents.[1-4] The chronotropic response is thought to be a reflexive baroreceptor-mediated response to the β_2-adrenergic vasodilation.[2,3,7] The recent findings that the ratio of β_1:β_2-adrenergic receptors is approximately 65:35 in the left atrium and ventricle[37] and 50:50 in the right atrium and ventricle[38] raise new questions regarding the mechanism of the chronotropic effect.[38] Some clinical evidence suggests that β_2-adrenergic stimulation produces as great or greater chronotropic response as β_1-adrenergic stimulation.[39,40] Improving β_2 selectivity even further would not appear to improve bronchoselectivity further. Bronchoselectivity is significantly enhanced by administering these agents directly into the lung by aerosol.

Bitolterol mesylate represents another approach to improving bronchoselectivity. In the rat and dog, intravenously administered tritium-labeled bitolterol is preferentially retained in the lung (compared with plasma or heart).[12,41] Esterase activity also appears to be greater in the lung than the heart in dogs and other animal species.[8] This results in a greater separation of bronchodilation and cardiac stimulation dose–response curves in the anesthetized dog than in the albuterol or colterol curves. Because of their similar structures, colterol and albuterol have similar separation of bronchodilation and cardiac stimulation.[8] Clinical trials in man have demonstrated that bitolterol produces less cardiovascular stimulation than isoproterenol[42-44] but not less than metaproterenol[45] or albuterol[46] when each product is administered as a metered-dose aerosol in the manufacturers' recommended doses.

Clinical Pharmacology

Duration of Action. The duration of effect for drugs that reversibly bind at the receptor is determined by the rate of removal of the drug from the receptor site and the minimum effective concentration of drug required to produce a clinical response. Thus, if the dose–response curve is shifted to the right (Figure 2b, curve A to curve B) as a result of a bronchoprovocation, the duration will appear shortened when compared with bronchodilation.[26,27] At the other end of the curve, if the concentration required to produce maximal response is exceeded, the duration depends on the time required for the fall to the maximum effective concentration in addition to the time required to fall from maximum to minimum effective concentration. For a drug that undergoes first-order elimination with rapid equilibrium (one compartment), the duration of response can be estimated by:

$$\text{Duration} = (2.303/k)\log(X_0/X_{min})$$

where X_0 is the beginning concentration, X_{min} is the minimum effective concentration, and k is the first-order elimination rate of the drug.[47] Increasing the dose at near maximal effective concentrations will increase the duration of action without affecting intensity of response. This has been illustrated by Ruffin et al.[48] in a dose–response study with aerosolized albuterol (Figure 3) in which increasing doses increased the duration without a significant change in peak response.

Comparative studies between bronchodilators with similar elimination characteristics, such as fenoterol and albuterol, will demonstrate significant differences in duration, but *not* intensity, when given in nonequipotent doses that approach maximum intensity.[9] The apparent advantage disappears when the drugs are given in equipotent doses.[10]

The rate of removal from the receptor site and elimination rate from the body of the β_2-adrenergic agonists are determined by their chemical structure. Catecholamines are removed from the recep-

Figure 3. Mean increases in forced expiratory volume at one second (FEV_1) for nine asthmatics administered 5, 2.5, 1.0, 0.5, 0.25, and 0 mg of albuterol by nebulizer. With the two highest doses, the peak effect is the same but the duration differs. If these had been two different agents, an apparent advantage for the agent administered at the higher dose could have been claimed. Reprinted with permission of the author and the publisher.[48]

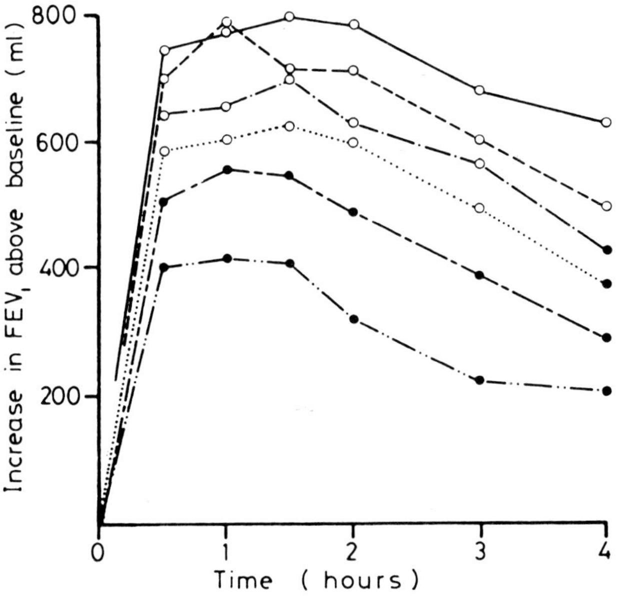

tor sites by catechol-specific tissue uptake and metabolized by catechol-O-methyltransferase, and conjugated with sulfate in the intestinal wall and liver.[3] The resorcinols are conjugated with sulfate and glucuronide and excreted unchanged in the urine.[3,49,50] Albuterol is conjugated with sulfate and excreted unchanged.

When the β_2-adrenergic agonists are administered systemically, changes in serum concentrations and pulmonary functions correlate closely.[51–53] Because of difficulties with analysis, few pharmacokinetic studies have been performed; the available pharmacokinetic data are summarized in Table 2. The large interpatient variability in elimination rates for each product would be expected to result in a significant variability in duration of action and this has been confirmed by numerous clinical trials.[1–4]

Colterol and isoproterenol, both catecholamines, have the same duration of action when administered systemically in equipotent doses.[8] The prolonged duration of action of bitolterol mesylate is thought to result from its slow hydrolysis in the lung.[8,12] Bitolterol mesylate gave a more prolonged duration of action than albuterol when administered in a dose that gave a greater peak effect than albuterol.[46] When administered in doses that gave similar peak effects, bitolterol and metaproterenol did not differ significantly in duration of bronchodilation.[45]

The other major determinant of duration of response is the physiologic status of the patient. Patients with severe bronchoconstriction have shortened durations of response.[3,6] Bronchodilation following a single dose of β_2-adrenergic agent is a limited test of duration because of the variability in bronchomotor tone in stable asthmatics, the relative ease in reversing mild to moderate spontaneous bronchoconstriction, and the inability to predict responsiveness from baseline pulmonary functions.[19] This is most striking in studies comparing duration for bronchodilation to duration for protection against exercise-induced bronchospasm in which the duration for protection is much shorter.[26,29] Studies using various means of bronchoprovocation may reflect a more clinically important duration of response by reflecting a more accurate concentration–response curve.

Clinically, it is more important to know the dose required to prevent or reverse bronchoconstriction from a triggering stimulus than to produce bronchodilation in a stable, symptom-free asthmatic patient. This is particularly true in patients with severe chronic asthma who require chronic maintenance bronchodilators for control of their symptoms. At least one study demonstrated that a group of chronic asthmatic patients were able to discern the difference between the short-acting catecholamine rimiterol and terbutaline; they preferred the longer-acting terbutaline for control of their symptoms.[55]

Metaproterenol by aerosol will provide adequate protection from exercise-induced bronchospasm for one hour but generally offers no protection at two hours.[29,56] The protective effect from isoproterenol is lost within an hour.[26,29,56] Albuterol provides significant protection for two hours in most patients and has been reported to provide varying degrees of protection for up to four to six hours in some patients.[56,57] Fenoterol protects against exercise-induced bronchospasm for two hours but not for four hours.[58] The duration of the protective effect from terbutaline and bitolterol has not been studied.

Systemic versus Aerosol Administration. The advantages and disadvantages of aerosolized versus systemic administration of β_2-adrenergic agonists have been adequately reviewed elsewhere.[3,6] The major advantage of aerosol administration is equivalent or greater bronchodilation and protection from exercise-induced bronchospasm with significantly fewer systemic side effects.[1–4,14] The theoretical advantage for systemic administration is improved delivery to peripheral airways and greater bronchodilation in small airways for a given degree of bronchodilation in the larger central

Table 2.
Pharmacokinetic Variables for the β_2-Adrenergic Agonists

Drug	Oral Bioavailability (%)	Time to Peak Plasma Concentration (hr)	Elimination Half-life (hr)	Reference No.
Albuterol[a]	5–11	3–4	5.6 ± 2.3	51
Bitolterol[b]	N.A.[c]	0.5–2	3.0	12
Fenoterol[b]	6–10	2	6–7.5	11
Metaproterenol[b]	10	2–4	6.0[d]	54
Terbutaline[a]	11–33	2–4	3.5 ± 0.6	50, 52, 62

[a] Drug concentrations analyzed by high-performance liquid chromatography.
[b] Drug concentrations analyzed by radiolabeling techniques, which measure metabolites as well as parent drug.
[c] Not applicable.
[d] Beta elimination half-life; the α half-life is 6.0 minutes.

airways.[13,59] Recent evidence suggests that the site of bronchodilation is primarily determined by the site of the limitation in prebronchodilator airflow and not by the route of administration of the bronchodilator.[60,61] Studies in patients with acute asthma attacks in which bronchial deposition of aerosols might be expected to be compromised have also failed to demonstrate any benefit of systemic therapy over aerosols.[3,6] This has been confirmed in patients hospitalized with status asthmaticus.[6]

Another theoretical advantage of oral therapy over aerosol therapy is less interpatient and intrapatient variability in dose–response curves resulting from a less variable method of administration. Unfortunately, there is a significant interpatient variability in elimination of β_2-adrenergic agonists. Also, all the β_2-adrenergic agonists undergo significant and variable first-pass metabolism following oral administration,[3,11,49–52] and there is considerable interpatient variability in absorption rate and extent.[62] Thus, in recent years, the focus has turned to improving aerosol administration.

Inhalation Technique and Devices

Numerous studies investigating the optimal delivery of β_2-adrenergic aerosols have been performed and recently reviewed.[3,63,64] A number of the studies have shown conflicting results; the basic dose–response relationship explains how this might occur. In a patient with significant bronchoconstriction and low response (Figure 2, curve C), a 50% improvement in deposition of a bronchodilator may not result in a significant increase in pulmonary functions as it would in a more responsive (curves A and B) patient. Also, if the patients were highly responsive and the standard method produced a near 80% of maximal improvement, the alternate method may significantly improve aerosol deposition without significantly altering pathophysiology. The ultimate dose–response characteristics for aerosol administration are dependent on the dose delivered to the airway and the physiologic characteristics of the airway. For aerosol administration, the dose delivered is dependent on the mechanical characteristics of the device that generates the aerosol and on patient variables.

Delivery-System Characteristics. Device-dependent variables for aerosol delivery such as particle size, density, and hygroscopicity have been extensively reviewed elsewhere.[63,65] The most commonly used delivery systems for the β_2-adrenergic agonists are the fluorocarbon-propelled metered-dose canisters and the jet nebulizers with or without intermittent positive-pressure breathing (IPPB). Numerous trials comparing the metered-dose canisters with nebulization and IPPB have failed to demonstrate a significant advantage for any method.[3,64,66] The dose–response curves from two studies by Nelson and coworkers for albuterol[15] and terbutaline[67] clearly illustrate this lack of significant difference from the methods. The slopes of the dose–response curves from each method are the same. The right shift of the dose–response curve for the nebulization is a result of loss of medication in the nebulizer, air, and tubing.[3]

A recent study by Shim and Williams[68] demonstrated that three inhalations (1.95 mg) of metaproterenol from a metered-dose canister gave similar bronchodilation as 15 mg of metaproterenol by jet nebulizer. By weighing the nebulizer before and after the treatment and taking into consideration that inspiration only accounts for one third of the respiratory cycle, they estimated that only 10–15% (2–2.25 mg) of the instilled solution was inhaled by the patient.

The differences in dosage recommendations in Table 1 are a result of the difference in delivery to the patient. It should be pointed out that the doses in Table 1 are recommended starting doses. Various nebulizers differ in their efficiency of delivery so that dosages may have to be tailored to the nebulizer system as well as to the patient's response.[64,65] Radioisotope techniques have shown that IPPB leads to greater loss of aerosol in the tubing and patient's mouth and throat and decreased delivery to the patient's lungs compared with nebulization with quiet breathing.[3] Nebulization is equally effective by face mask or mouthpiece[3] (when just using a mouthpiece, a patient should use a noseclip).

The metered-dose canisters are the most convenient form for administering aerosol β_2-adrenergic agonists as well as the most cost-effective. Using radiolabeled Teflon particles, Newman et al.[69] demonstrated that, following actuation of a Freon-propelled canister, 8.8% (4.7–14.8%) of a dose was deposited in the lungs, 80% (70–89%) was initially deposited in the mouth then swallowed, and the remaining 9.8% was recovered from the canister and expired air (1.0%). These figures have been confirmed with pharmacokinetic studies showing that 0.8–10% of an inhaled dose is absorbed from the lungs.[50,70] Although 80–90% of an inhaled dose is swallowed, the extensive first-pass metabolism in the gastrointestinal wall and liver prevents the drug from reaching therapeutically effective serum concentrations.[50,70] A recent study demonstrated a physiologically small but statistically significant bronchodilation from mouth spraying with fenoterol without inhalation, presumably from buccal absorption, which would avert a first pass through the liver.[71]

Since Muir and Davies[72] reported that a slow deep inhalation increased the deposition of aerosols in the lungs, it has become increasingly recognized that inhalational technique is a major determinant of the dose delivered. A number of investigators have advocated various techniques to increase delivery, such as holding the canister away from the open mouth and timing the actuation late (80% of vital capacity) in inspiration. Often the recommendations resulted from studies of radiolabeled aerosols.[72] Recently, studies have shown that patients who have been prescribed metered-dose canisters use inappropriate techniques.[73-75] However, what is considered appropriate may differ between investigators. It is important to establish first what technique provides optimal physiologic results and then what variations produce a clinically important variability from that result.

In a series of elegant studies using physiologic response[76] as well as radiolabeled aerosols,[77] Newman and coworkers have shown that the two most important variables are speed of inhalation and duration of breath holding. With a slow, deep inhalation (approximately 30 L/min) and 10-second breath holding, the time of actuation during inspiration (20, 50, or 80% of vital capacity) was not a factor. They also demonstrated that the "open mouth" method was not superior to the standard "closed mouth" method. In contrast to Heimer et al.,[78] they found that four inhalations of terbutaline in rapid succession produced a further significant bronchodilation (approximately two times) over two inhalations.[76] Their study also showed a significant degree of bronchodilation when actuation preceded inspiration although not as great as during inspiration. This has recently been confirmed in children who generally have difficulty in coordinating actuation with inspiration.[79] Table 3 gives simple instructions for optimal use of a metered-dose inhaler.

Causes of Inappropriate Technique. The causes of inappropriate technique are many. Lack of patient instruction by physician and pharmacist is an important factor.[74,75] Kelling et al.[80] reported that only 40% of nonpulmonary physicians knew the appropriate inhalation technique. Patients are often not able to understand the written directions supplied by the manufacturer without a demonstration.[74] Patients who are initially instructed in appropriate technique slowly develop poor technique if not periodically checked.[73,74] Some patients are never able to develop adequate coordination; the most common error is actuation after inspiration is completed. These patients can often obtain adequate results by learning to actuate the canister before inhalation[76,79] or by using various tube-spacer devices.

Tube-spacers: Advantages and Disadvantages. Tube-spacers are devices that come in all sizes and shapes (Table 4 and Figure 4) and attach to the mouthpiece of an aerosol canister. The primary purpose of all tube-spacer devices is to act as a holding chamber in which the medication is sprayed before inhalation by the patient. The advantages of tube-spacers is that they decrease loss of drug in the oropharynx, decrease the need for accurate synchronization, and improve the deposition of the aerosol into the conducting airways.[81,82]

Clinically, the addition of a spacer device has been shown to decrease oropharyngeal side effects from inhaled corticosteroids[83] and significantly improve the bronchodilation from β_2-adrenergic agonists in patients unable to coordinate a pressurized canister alone.[84] Studies in which technique was not a variable have shown minimal to no significant improvement with addition of a tube-spacer.[85-88] This is not surprising considering the small and variable increase in dose that reaches the lung as a result of the tube-spacer. Newman et al.[81] demonstrated that the addition of a tube-spacer increased whole lung aerosol deposition to 11.5–13.0% from 7.8% with the actuator alone. However, a greater percentage of the amount reaching the lung was deposited in the conducting airways. In some clinical situations this may be important.

The disadvantages of tube-spacers are the increased cost and inconvenience. However, their cost is less than that of a home compressed-air nebulizer or an emergency-room visit for an acute attack of asthma. Metered-dose canisters with tube-spacers are as effective as nebulizers for treating acute asthma attacks.[3]

Conclusion

Aerosol administration is the route of choice for β_2-adrenergic agonists for prophylaxis of exercise-induced bronchospasm and reversal of acute bron-

Table 3.
Technique for Inhalation of Metered-Dose Aerosols

1. Shake the canister thoroughly.
2. Place the mouthpiece between the lips, making sure that the teeth and tongue are out of the way.
3. Breathe out steadily.
4. Actuate the canister while taking a *slow*, deep breath.
5. Hold the breath at full inspiration for 10 seconds.
6. Wait at least one minute before the next inhalation from the canister.

Table 4.
Types of Tube-spacers

Inspirease (Key Pharmaceuticals, Inc.)	A collapsible bag with a flow indicator whistle.[89]
Inhal-Aid (Key Pharmaceuticals, Inc.)	Plastic spherical chamber with a flow meter and one-way valves for directed airflow.[90]
Aerochamber (Monaghan Medical Co.)	Cylinder with one-way valve that traps aerosol until inhaled by subject.[87]
Nebuhaler (A.B. Dracho, Lund, Sweden)	750-mL conical spacer with a one-way valve at the mouthpiece.[82]
Brethancer (Geigy Pharmaceuticals)	10-cm open-ended telescopic tube.[81,84]

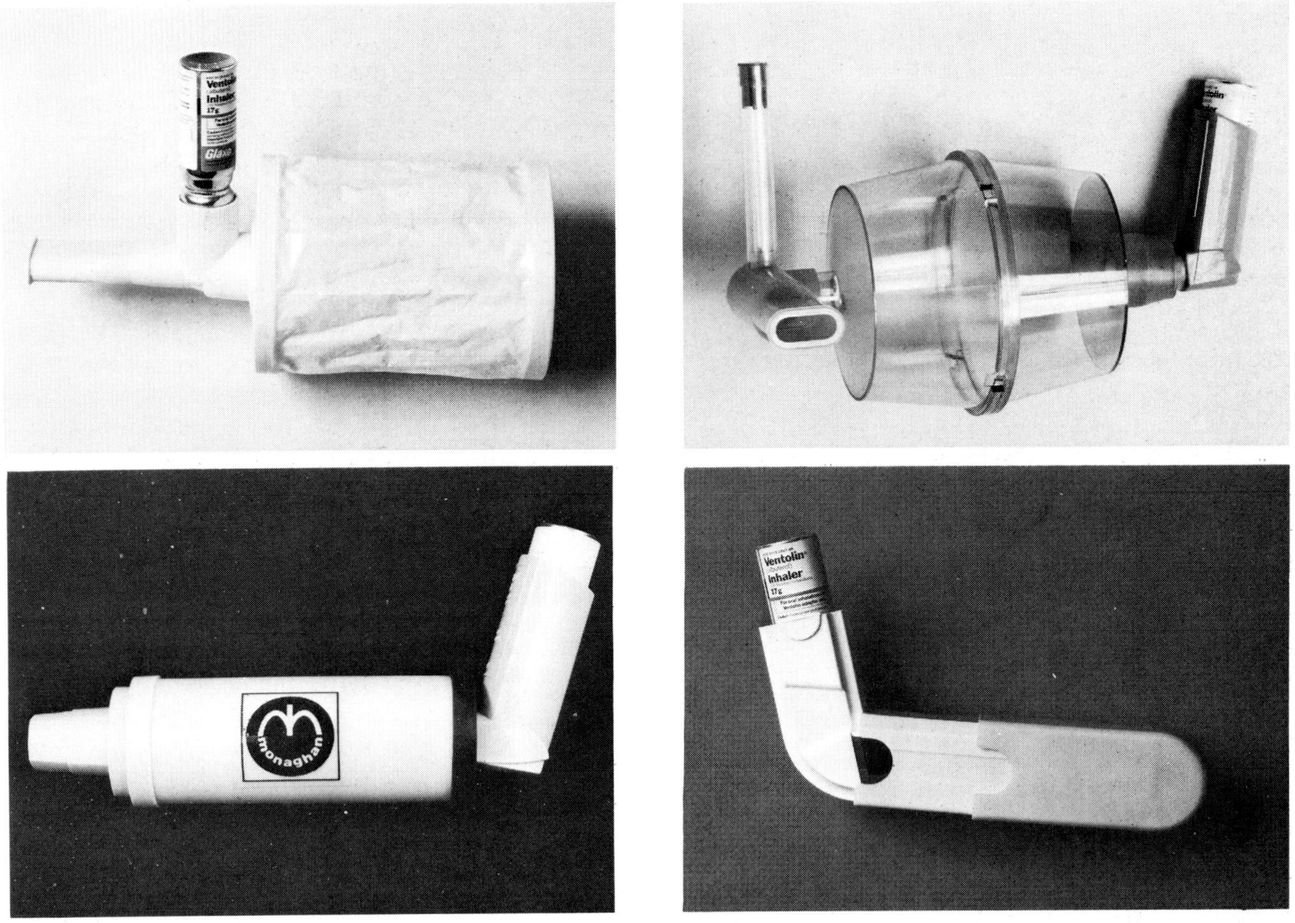

Figure 4. Four types of tube-spacers are shown here. On the upper left is the Inspirease device, which is marketed by Key Pharmaceuticals; also produced by Key is Inhal-Aid, shown on the upper right. Monaghan Medical's Aerochamber is pictured in the lower left, and Geigy's Brethancer is shown on the lower right. See Table 4 for descriptions of these tube-spacers.

chospasm. Albuterol and terbutaline provide a prolonged duration of action with excellent β_2-adrenergic selectivity. Fenoterol offers no advantage when used in equipotent dosages. Bitolterol mesylate, a prodrug, is an attempt to improve bronchoselectivity and duration of action; current data do not indicate that it is an important improvement over the other agents.

Patients should be carefully instructed in the optimal use of metered-dose inhalers. The technique should be kept simple and periodically checked. Tube-spacers provide an excellent alternative for those patients unable to synchronize their inhaler actuation with inspiration. They offer little to no advantage to patients able to perform the appropriate technique.

References

1. Svedmyr N, Simonsson BG. Drugs in the treatment of asthma. *Pharmacol Ther* [B]. 1978; 3:397–440.
2. Paterson JW, Woolcock AJ, Shenfield GM. State of the art: bronchodilator drugs. *Am Rev Respir Dis.* 1979; 120:1149–88.
3. Nelson HS. Beta-adrenergic therapy. In: Middleton E, Reed CE, Ellis EF, ed. Allergy: principles and practice. 2nd ed. St. Louis: C.V. Mosby Company; 1983:511–27.
4. Galant SP. Current status of beta-adrenergic agonists in bronchial asthma. *Pediatr Clin North Am.* 1983; 30:931–42.
5. van den Brink FG. General theory of drug-receptor interactions: drug-receptor interaction models. Calculation of drug parameters. In: van Rossum JM, ed. Kinetics of drug action. New York: Springer-Verlag; 1977:170–254.
6. Kelly HW. Controversies in asthma therapy with theophylline and the β_2-adrenergic agonists. *Clin Pharm.* 1984; 3:386–95.
7. Brittain RT, Jack D. Recent work on selective beta-adrenoceptor stimulants. In: Weiss EB, Segal MS, ed. Bronchial asthma: mechanisms and therapeutics. Boston: Little, Brown and Company; 1976:739–48.
8. Minatoya H. Studies on bitolterol, di-*p*-toluate ester of *n*-tert-butylarterenol: a new long-acting bronchodilator with reduced cardiovascular effects. *J Pharmacol Exp Ther.* 1978; 206:515–27.
9. Huhti E, Poukkula A. Clinical comparison of fenoterol and albuterol administered by inhalation: a double-blind study. *Chest.* 1978; 73:348–51.
10. Lawford P, Dowd DE, Palmer KNV. A comparison of the duration of action of fenoterol and salbutamol in asthma. *Curr Med Res Opin.* 1981; 7:349–51.
11. Heel RC, Brogden RN, Speight TM et al. Fenoterol: a review of its pharmacological properties and therapeutic efficacy in asthma. *Drugs.* 1978; 15:3–32.
12. Shargel L, Dorrbecker SA. Physiological disposition and metabolism of [3-H] bitolterol in man and dog. *Drug Metab Dispos.* 1976; 4:72–8.

13. Larsson S, Svedmyr N. Bronchodilating effect and side effects of beta-2-adrenoceptor stimulants by different modes of administration (tablets, metered aerosol and combinations thereof). A study with salbutamol in asthmatics. *Am Rev Respir Dis.* 1977; 116:861–9.
14. Thiringer G, Svedmyr N. Comparison of infused and inhaled terbutaline in patients with asthma. *Scand J Respir Dis.* 1976; 57:17–24.
15. Nelson HS, Spector SL, Whitsett TL et al. The bronchodilator response to inhalation of increasing doses of aerosolized albuterol. *J Allergy Clin Immunol.* 1983; 72:371–5.
16. Ruffin RE, Montgomery JM, Newhouse MT. Aerosol fenoterol by intermittent positive pressure breathing in asthmatic patients. *Clin Pharmacol Ther.* 1979; 25:821–5.
17. Tattersfield AE. Autonomic bronchodilators. In: Clark TJH, Godfrey S, eds. *Asthma.* 2nd ed. London: Chapman and Hall; 1983:301–35.
18. Williams MH, Kane C. Dose response of patients with asthma to inhaled isoproterenol. *Am Rev Respir Des.* 1975; 111:321–4.
19. Menendez R, Kelly HW. Pulmonary-function testing in the evaluation of bronchodilator agents. *Clin Pharm.* 1983; 2:120–8.
20. Karlsson J-A, Persson CGA. Influence of tracheal contraction on relaxant effects in vitro of theophylline and isoprenaline. *Br J Pharmacol.* 1981; 74:73–9.
21. Conolly ME, Tashkin DP, Hui KKP et al. Selective subsensitization of beta-adrenergic receptors in central airways of asthmatics and normal subjects during long-term therapy with inhaled salbutamol. *J Allergy Clin Immunol.* 1982; 70:423–31.
22. Barnes PJ, Pride NB. Dose-response curves to inhaled beta-adrenoceptor agonists in normal and asthmatic subjects. *Br J Clin Pharmacol.* 1983; 15:677–82.
23. Rebuck AS, Read J. Assessment and management of severe asthma. *Am J Med.* 1971; 51:788–98.
24. Shenfield GM, Hodson ME, Clarke SW et al. Patterns of response to isoprenaline in asthmatic patients. *Br J Dis Chest.* 1975; 69:273–8.
25. Mitchell CA, Armstrong JG, Bartholomew MA et al. Nebulized fenoterol in severe asthma: determinants of the dose response. *Eur J Respir Dis.* 1983; 64:340–6.
26. Eggleston PA, Beasley PP. Bronchodilation and inhibition of induced asthma by adrenergic agonists. *Clin Pharmacol Ther.* 1981;29:505–10.
27. Ahrens RC, Bonham AC, Maxwell GA et al. A method for comparing the peak intensity and duration of action of aerosolized bronchodilators using bronchoprovocation with methacholine. *Am Rev Respir Dis.* 1984; 129:903–6.
28. Rossing TH, Weiss JW, Breslin FJ et al. Effects of inhaled sympathomimetics on obstructive response to respiratory heat loss. *J Appl Physiol.* 1982; 52:1119–23.
29. Anderson S, Seale JP, Ferris L et al. An evaluation of pharmacotherapy for exercise-induced asthma. *J Allergy Clin Immunol.* 1979; 64:612–24.
30. Juniper EF, Frith PA, Dunnett C et al. Reproducibility and comparison of responses to inhaled histamine and methacholine. *Thorax.* 1978; 33:705–10.
31. Choo-Kang YFJ, Simpson WT, Grant IWB. Controlled comparison of the bronchodilator effects of three beta-adrenergic stimulant drugs administered by inhalation to patients with asthma. *Br Med J.* 1969; 2:287–9.
32. O'Donnell SR, Wanstall JC. Evidence that the efficacy (intrinsic activity) of fenoterol is higher than that of salbutamol on beta-adrenoceptors in guinea-pig trachea. *Eur J Pharmacol.* 1978; 47:333–40.
33. O'Byrne PM, Morris M, Roberts R et al. Inhibition of the bronchial response to respiratory heat exchange by increasing doses of terbutaline sulphate. *Thorax.* 1982; 37:913–7.
34. Tandon MK. Cardiopulmonary effects of fenoterol and salbutamol aerosols. *Chest.* 1980; 77:429–31.
35. Raper C, Malta E. Salbutamol: agonistic and antagonistic activity at beta-adrenoceptor sites. *J Pharm Pharmacol.* 1973; 26:661–3.
36. MacEwoy JDS, Vall-Spinosa A, Paterson JW. Assessment of orciprenaline and isoproterenol infusions in asthmatic patients. *Am Rev Respir Dis.* 1973; 108:490–500.
37. Heitz A, Schwartz J, Velly J. β-adrenoceptors of the human myocardium: determination of β_1 and β_2 subtypes by radioligand binding. *Br J Pharmacol.* 1983; 80:711–7.
38. Robberecht P, Delhaye M, Taton G et al. The human heart beta-adrenergic receptors. 1. Heterogeneity of the binding sites: presence of 50% beta-1- and 50% beta-2-adrenergic receptors. *Mol Pharmacol.* 1983; 24:169–73.
39. Lofdahl C-G, Svedmyr N. Selectivity of beta-adrenergic stimulating and blocking agents. *Eur J Respir Dis* (Suppl 136). 1984; 65:101–12.
40. Greefhorst APM, Herwaarden CLA. Ventilatory and haemodynamic effects of prenalterol and terbutaline in asthmatic patients. *Eur J Clin Pharmacol.* 1983; 24:173–8.
41. Shargel L, Dorrbecker SA, Levitt M. Physiological disposition and metabolism of *n*-t-butylarterenol and its di-*p*-toluate ester (bitolterol) in the rat. *Drug Metab Dispos.* 1976; 4:65.
42. Petty TL, Scoggin CH, Rollins DR et al. Bitolterol compared to isoproterenol in advanced chronic obstructive pulmonary disease. *Chest.* 1984; 86:404–8.
43. Kass I, Mingo TS. Bitolterol mesylate (WIN 32784) aerosol. A new long-acting bronchodilator with reduced chronotropic effects. *Chest.* 1980; 78:283–7.
44. Pinnas JL, Bernstein IL, Bronsky EE et al. Safety and efficacy study of bitolterol and isoproterenol nebulizer solutions. *J Allergy Clin Immunol.* 1985; 75(2):163. Abstract.
45. Cockcroft DW, Berscheid BA, Dosman JA et al. Comparison of bitolterol mesylate and metaproterenol sulphate. *Curr Ther Res.* 1981; 30:817–24.
46. Orgel HA, Kemp JP, Tinkelman DG et al. Bitolterol and albuterol metered-dose aerosols: comparison of two long-acting beta-2-adrenergic bronchodilators for treatment of asthma. *J Allergy Clin Immunol.* 1985; 75:55–62.
47. Kinetics of pharmacologic response. In: Gibaldi M, Perrier D, eds. Pharmacokinetics. 2nd ed. New York: Marcel Dekker, Inc. 1982: 221–69.
48. Ruffin RE, Obminski G, Newhouse MT. Aerosol salbutamol administration by IPPB: lowest effective dose. *Thorax.* 1978; 33:689–93.
49. Davies DS. Pharmacokinetic studies with inhaled drugs. *Eur J Respir Dis.* 1982; 63(Suppl 119):67–72.
50. Ripe E, Hornblad Y, Tegner K. Oral administration of terbutaline in asthmatic patients. *Eur J Respir Dis.* 1984; 65(Suppl 134):171–9.
51. Oosterhuis B, Braat MCP, van Boxtel CJ. Analysis of beta-sympathicomimetics in man with high performance liquid chromatography using mode sequencing and electrochemical detection. *Eur J Respir Dis.* 1984; 65(Suppl 135):153–6.
52. van den Berg W, Leferink JG, Maes RAA et al. The effects of oral and subcutaneous administration of terbutaline in asthmatic patients. *Eur J Respir Dis.* 1984; 65(Suppl 134):181–93.
53. Lonnerholm G, Foucard T, Lindstrom B. Oral terbutaline in chronic childhood asthma; effects related to plasma concentrations. *Eur J Respir Dis.* 1984; 65(Suppl 134):205–10.
54. Dengler HJ, Hengstmann JH. Metabolism and pharmacokinetics of orciprenaline in various animal species and man. *Arch Intl Pharmacodyn.* 1976; 223:71–87.
55. Paterson IC, Willey RF, Shotter MV et al. Objective and subjective comparisons of terbutaline and rimiterol bronchodilator aerosols. *Br J Dis Chest.* 1975; 69:267–72.
56. Sly RM. Beta-adrenergic drugs in the management of asthma in athletes. *J Allergy Clin Immunol.* 1984; 73:680–5.
57. Higgs CMB, Laszlo G. The duration of protection from exercise-induced asthma by inhaled salbutamol, and a comparison with inhaled reproterol. *Br J Dis Chest.* 1983; 77:262–9.
58. Konig P, Hordvik NL, Serby CW. Fenoterol in exercise-induced asthma: effect of dose on efficacy and duration of action. *Chest.* 1984; 85:462–4.

59. Tashkin DP, Trevor E, Chopra SK et al. Sites of airway dilatation in asthma following inhaled versus subcutaneous terbutaline. Comparison of physiologic tests with radionuclide lung images. *Am J Med.* 1980; 68:14–26.
60. Fairshter RD, Wilson AF. Relationship between the site of airflow limitation and localization of the bronchodilator response in asthma. *Am Rev Respir Dis.* 1980; 122:27–32.
61. Shaw RJS, Waller JF, Hetzel MR et al. Do oral and inhaled terbutaline have different effects on the lung? *Br J Dis Chest.* 1982; 76:171–6.
62. Davies DS. Pharmacokinetics of terbutaline after oral administration. *Eur J Respir Dis.* 1984; 65(Suppl 134):111–7.
63. Crompton GK, Moren F, Simonsson BG. Inhalation therapy in the management of airway obstruction. *Eur J Respir Dis.* 1983; 63(Suppl 119):1–125.
64. Shim C. Adrenergic agonists and bronchodilator aerosol therapy in asthma. *Clin Chest Med.* 1984; 5:659–68.
65. Swift DL. Aerosols and humidity therapy. Generation and respiratory deposition of therapeutic aerosols. *Am Rev Respir Dis.* 1980; 122(Suppl):71–7.
66. Stiksa G. Indications for continuous aerosol therapy. *Eur J Respir Dis* 1982; 63(Suppl 119):89–96.
67. Weber RW, Petty WE, Nelson HS. Aerosolized terbutaline in asthmatics. Comparison of dosage strength, schedule, and method of administration. *J Allergy Clin Immunol.* 1979; 63:116–21.
68. Shim CS, Williams MH. Effect of bronchodilator therapy administered by canister versus jet nebulizer. *J Allergy Clin Immunol.* 1984; 73:387–90.
69. Newman SP, Pavia D, Moren F et al. Deposition of pressurized aerosols in the human respiratory tract. *Thorax.* 1981; 36:52–5.
70. Davies DS. The fate of inhaled terbutaline. *Eur J Respir Dis.* 1984; 65(Suppl 134):141–7.
71. Rodenstein D, Stanescu DC. Mouth spraying versus inhalation of fenoterol aerosol in healthy subjects and asthmatic patients. *Br J Dis Chest.* 1982; 76:365–73.
72. Dolovich M, Ruffin RE, Roberts R et al. Optimal delivery of aerosols from metered dose inhalers. *Chest.* 1981; 80(Suppl):911–5.
73. Shim C, Williams MH. The adequacy of inhalation of aerosol from canister nebulizers. *Am J Med.* 1980; 69:891–3.
74. Crompton GK. Problems patients have using pressurized aerosol inhalers. *Eur J Respir Dis.* 1982; 63(Suppl 119):101–4.
75. Epstein SW, Manning CPR, Ashley MJ et al. Survey of the clinical use of pressurized aerosol inhalers. *Can Med Assoc J.* 1979; 120:813–6.
76. Newman SP, Pavia D, Clarke SW. How should a pressurized beta-adrenergic bronchodilator be inhaled? *Eur J Respir Dis.* 1981; 62:3–21.
77. Newman SP, Pavia D, Garland N et al. Effects of various inhalation modes on the deposition of radioactive pressurized aerosols. *Eur J Respir Dis.* 1982; 63(Suppl 119):57–65.
78. Heimer D, Shim C, Williams MH. The effect of sequential inhalations of metaproterenol aerosol in asthma. *J Allergy Clin Immunol.* 1980; 66:75–7.
79. Rivlin J, Mindorff C, Levison H et al. Effect of administration technique on bronchodilator response to fenoterol in a metered-dose inhaler. *J Pediatr.* 1983; 102:470–2.
80. Kelling JS, Strohl KP, Smith RL et al. Physician knowledge in the use of canister nebulizers. *Chest.* 1983; 83:612–4.
81. Newman SP, Moren F, Pavia D et al. Deposition of pressurized suspension aerosols inhaled through extension devices. *Am Rev Respir Dis.* 1981; 124:317–20.
82. Newman SP, Millar AB, Lennard-Jones TR et al. Improvement of pressurized aerosol deposition with Nebuhaler spacer device. *Thorax.* 1984; 39:935–41.
83. Toogood JH, Baskerville J, Jennings B et al. Use of spacers to facilitate inhaled corticosteroid treatment of asthma. *Am Rev Respir Dis.* 1984; 129:723–9.
84. Pedersen S. Aerosol treatment of bronchoconstriction in children with or without a tube spacer. *N Engl J Med.* 1983; 308:1328–30.
85. Weeke ER. Reported clinical experiences with inhaled terbutaline aerosol via spacer devices. *Eur J Respir Dis.* 1982; 63(Suppl 119):105–9.
86. Morris J, Milledge JS, Moszoro H et al. The efficacy of drug delivery by a pear-shaped spacer and metered dose inhaler. *Br J Dis Chest.* 1984; 78:383–7.
87. Dirksen H. Addition of a spacer device as an alternative in treatment with a metered dose inhaler. *Eur J Respir Dis.* 1983; 64(Suppl 130):42–7.
88. Swinburn PD, Sexton M. Inhaled bronchodilators: a comparison of different methods of inhaling. *NZ Med J.* 1981; 94:340.
89. Tobin MJ, Jenouri G, Danta I et al. Response to bronchodilator drug administration by a new reservoir aerosol delivery system and a review of other auxiliary delivery systems. *Am Rev Respir Dis.* 1982; 126:670–5.
90. Chang B, Sly RM, Eby D et al. Delivery of albuterol aerosol by Inhal-Aid to young children. *J Allergy Clin Immunol.* 1985; 75(2):159. Abstract.

Current status of cardiac glycoside drug interactions

PIET M. HOOYMANS AND FRANS W.H.M. MERKUS

Abstract: The effects of concomitant drug therapy on the absorption, distribution, and elimination of digoxin and digitoxin are reviewed.

A number of agents can increase or decrease the absorption of digoxin and digitoxin from the gastrointestinal tract by altering GI motility, binding the drugs through physical adsorption, altering the properties of the intestinal wall, or altering the bacterial flora of the intestine. The steady-state serum concentrations of digoxin and digitoxin can be affected if the changes in absorption are of sufficient magnitude, and adjustments in digoxin or digitoxin dosage may be required. A reduction in digoxin and digitoxin protein binding has occurred during concomitant administration of heparin and cardiac glycosides. Since digitoxin is more highly protein bound than digoxin, interactions that involve changes in protein binding are of much greater clinical importance with digitoxin.

A number of drugs increase or decrease the elimination of digoxin and digitoxin, and subtherapeutic or toxic concentrations of the cardiac glycosides often result. Drugs that induce hepatic microsomal enzymes can increase the elimination of digitoxin, which is eliminated mainly by hepatic biotransformation. Digoxin is eliminated mainly by renal excretion; renal clearance of digoxin may be increased by vasodilators and thyroid hormones and decreased by quinidine, verapamil, amiodarone, and potassium-sparing diuretics. The clinical importance of changes in serum concentrations of the cardiac glycosides that result from alterations in glycoside elimination requires further study, as does the importance of preliminary reports of interactions between cardiac glycosides and diazepam, captopril, and combination therapy with quinidine–pentobarbital or quinidine–rifampin.

Because the cardiac glycosides have a narrow therapeutic range, patients receiving concomitant therapy with agents that might affect the absorption, distribution, or elimination of the cardiac glycosides should be monitored carefully for symptoms of digitalis toxicity or undertreatment.

Index terms: Absorption; Amiodarone; Anticoagulants; Anti-inflammatory agents; Antithyroid drugs; Calcium antagonists; Cardiac drugs; Cimetidine; Digitoxin; Digoxin; Diuretics; Drugs, body distribution; Excretion; Gastrointestinal drugs; Heparin; Metabolism; Quinidine; Thyroid drugs; Vasodilating agents
Clin Pharm. 1985; 4:404–13

Cardiac glycosides are often administered concomitantly with other drugs for the prophylactic management or treatment of congestive heart failure and arrhythmias. Because the cardiac glycosides have a narrow therapeutic range, any alterations in their absorption, distribution, protein binding, or elimination that result from concomitant drug therapy can be important clinically. This review will discuss the effects of other drugs on the pharmacokinetics of digoxin and digitoxin; these cardiac glycosides were chosen for discussion because of their widespread use and the differences in their pharmacokinetic variables.

Interactions Caused by Altered Absorption

Several drugs can affect the absorption of cardiac glycosides in the GI tract[1–5] (Table 1). These interactions can be categorized according to mechanism, including altered GI motility, physical adsorption, changes in intestinal wall properties, and altered bacterial flora.

Alteration of GI Motility. Drugs such as metoclopramide, which accelerates gastric emptying and intestinal motility, and propantheline, which decreases intestinal motility, can affect the bioavailability of digoxin tablets with a poor dissolution profile.

In patients receiving maintenance therapy with slowly dissolving digoxin tablets, concurrent administration of propantheline bromide 15 mg three times daily increased serum digoxin concentrations by 30%, and concurrent administration of metoclopramide hydrochloride 10 mg three times daily lowered serum digoxin concentrations by 35%.[6] However, the absorption of digoxin from oral preparations that provide high bioavailability does not appear to be affected by simultaneous administration of drugs that alter gastrointestinal motility. Propantheline did not increase digoxin absorption when digoxin was administered as a liquid,[6] and neither propantheline nor metoclopramide significantly affected the extent of digoxin absorption from rapidly dissolving tablets.[7,8]

PIET M. HOOYMANS, PH.D., is Associate Director of the Pharmacy Department and the Clinical Pharmacokinetics and Toxicology Laboratory, Hospital Sittard, the Netherlands. FRANS W.H.M. MERKUS, PH.D., is Professor of Biopharmaceutics at the University of Amsterdam, the Netherlands, and Director of the Pharmacy Department and the Clinical Pharmacokinetics and Toxicology Laboratory, Hospital Sittard.

Address reprint requests to Dr. Hooymans at the Hospital Sittard, Walramstraat 23, 6131 BK Sittard, the Netherlands.

This is **article 680-204-8512** in the **ASHP Continuing Education System.** See page 464 for learning objectives and test questions.

Table 1.
Substances That Affect Absorption of Digoxin from Tablets

Substance (amount)	% Decrease in Absorption	Reference No.
Liquid antacids—aluminum hydroxide, magnesium hydroxide, magnesium trisilicate (60 mL)[a]	30	1
Kaolin–pectin suspension (60 mL)[a]	40	1
Cholestyramine resin (4–8 g)[a]	20–30	2
Dietary fiber (5–15 g)[a]	15–20	2,3
Activated charcoal (10 g)[a]	80	3
Aminosalicylic acid (8 g daily)	20	2
Neomycin (2–4 g daily)	40	4
Sulfasalazine (2–6 g daily)	20	5

[a] When administered simultaneously with digoxin dose.

Physical Adsorption. The interaction between cardiac glycosides and antacids may not be important in most clinical situations. Concurrent administration of antacids has been reported to reduce the bioavailability of digoxin; in healthy volunteers, simultaneous administration of digoxin tablets and single high doses of liquid antacids (60 mL of 4% aluminum hydroxide gel suspension, 60 mL of 8% magnesium hydroxide gel, or 60 mL of magnesium trisilicate) resulted in a significant reduction (approximately 30%) in digoxin absorption.[1] However, digoxin absorption was not reduced when a 10-mL dose of either aluminum hydroxide mixture, BPC, or magnesium trisilicate mixture, BPC, was administered three times daily to patients.[9]

Administration of antacids in tablet form did not lower steady-state digoxin concentrations.[10] A single high dose of liquid antacid had less effect on digoxin absorption when digoxin was administered orally in soft gelatin capsules than when currently available tablet preparations of digoxin were administered.[11] In patients receiving maintenance therapy with digitoxin, a 20-mL dose of magnesium-aluminum hydroxide suspension administered three or four times daily did not significantly affect steady-state plasma digitoxin concentrations when the antacid was given one or two hours after the digitoxin dose.[12]

Physical adsorption of digoxin to kaolin–pectin preparations, hypocholesterolemic agents (such as cholestyramine resin and colestipol), dietary fiber, or activated charcoal can result in a pronounced decrease in digoxin absorption. In healthy volunteers, administration of digoxin tablets simultaneously with either 60 mL of a kaolin–pectin suspension of usual strength or 90 mL of a concentrated kaolin–pectin suspension resulted in decreases in mean digoxin absorption of approximately 40% and 60%, respectively.[1,13] The extent of digoxin absorption was not altered when kaolin–pectin suspension was administered two hours after a dose of digoxin, but a 20% decrease in digoxin absorption was evident when kaolin–pectin suspension was administered two hours before a dose of digoxin.[13] Kaolin–pectin suspension impaired digoxin absorption from soft gelatin capsules less than from currently available tablets.[11]

Administraton of cholestyramine resin 4–8 g[2] or dietary fiber 5–15 g[2,3] simultaneously with digoxin reduced digoxin absorption by 20–30% and 15–20%, respectively. The decrease in digoxin bioavailability appeared to be related to both the dose of cholestyramine and the proximity of time of administration of the two drugs. Simultaneous administration of cholestyramine resin 4 g eight times daily shortened the half-life of digitoxin from six to four days in normal volunteers.[14,15] However, simultaneous administration of colestipol 5 g four times daily did not significantly decrease digitoxin half-life.[16]

The absorption of digoxin was almost completely prevented when activated charcoal 50 g was ingested immediately after a dose of digoxin.[17] An 80% reduction in digoxin absorption after simultaneous intake of activated charcoal 10 g has been reported.[3] After therapy with activated charcoal 2 g three times daily for 12 days, the plasma concentrations of digoxin and digitoxin in cardiac patients were decreased by approximately 30% and 18%, respectively.[3]

The decrease in plasma digoxin and digitoxin concentrations following administration of activated charcoal might have been caused by either decreased absorption or interference with the enterohepatic circulation of digoxin and digitoxin. Decreased absorption is not the likely mechanism because activated charcoal was administered 4 hours after and 12 hours before the doses of digoxin and digitoxin. Enterohepatic circulation of drug appeared to be greater for digitoxin than for digoxin; however, activated charcoal 3 g three times daily did not significantly shorten the half-life of digitoxin in healthy volunteers (8.8 days with and 8.0 days without charcoal).[3]

In fasting patients, decreased cardiac glycoside absorption can usually be avoided by administering digoxin or digitoxin 60–90 minutes before administering an agent to which digoxin or digitoxin might adsorb. Interference with the enterohepatic circulation of digoxin and digitoxin is of minor clinical importance in most situations. Treatment of digoxin and digitoxin intoxications by interfering with the enterohepatic circulation of the cardiac glycosides has been reported, but discussion of these studies is outside the scope of this article.

Alteration of Intestinal Wall Properties. Neomycin, sulfasalazine, and aminosalicylic acid decrease the absorption of digoxin,[2,4,5] possibly by altering the properties of the intestinal wall. Separating administration of digoxin from administration of these drugs does not prevent the interaction. After two weeks of concurrent administration of aminosalicylic acid 2 g four times daily, the absorption of a single dose of digoxin was reduced by 20%.[2] A 40% reduction in digoxin absorption has been reported in subjects who received digoxin in addition to neomycin 2–4 g daily.[4] After six days of treatment with sulfasalazine 2–6 g daily, the absorption of a single dose of digoxin was decreased by approximately 20%.[5]

An increasing number of patients are receiving cytotoxic drug therapy, and it is well known that cytotoxic drugs can damage the intestinal mucosa and decrease the absorption of other drugs. No studies of this potential interference with digoxin absorption have been published.

Interference with the absorption of β-acetyldigoxin by cytotoxic agents has been reported. This cardiac glycoside has the general properties of digoxin; it is deacetylated to digoxin as it passes through the intestinal wall. The rate and extent of absorption of β-acetyldigoxin have been reduced by concurrent treatment with the following combinations of drugs: cyclophosphamide, vincristine, procarbazine, and prednisone; cyclophosphamide, vincristine, cytarabine, and prednisone; or doxorubicin, bleomycin, and prednisone. The mean steady-state serum digoxin concentration during cytotoxic drug therapy is about 50% lower than before chemotherapy. The absorption of β-acetyldigoxin returns to initial levels approximately one week after the last dose of cytotoxic drug is administered.[18]

In contrast, concurrent cytotoxic drug therapy does not lead to a reduction in steady-state plasma digitoxin concentrations. This difference is probably caused by digoxin's absorption in an area of the intestine that is more sensitive to chemotherapeutic effects than the area located more distally where digitoxin is absorbed.[19] Although attainment of peak digitoxin concentrations may be delayed during cytotoxic chemotherapy, this delay is not relevant clinically in patients receiving chronic digitoxin therapy.

Alterations of Intestinal Bacterial Flora. An interesting interaction has been reported between digoxin and erythromycin (this interaction may also occur with tetracycline).[20] Approximately 10% of patients receiving digoxin tablets metabolize about 40% of a digoxin dose to cardioinactive compounds such as dihydrodigoxin and dihydrodigoxigenin. The bacterial flora of the intestine contribute greatly to this metabolic process; *Eubacterium lentum*, a common anaerobe in human gut flora, is the organism believed to be responsible for converting digoxin to cardioinactive metabolites in the intestine.[21] Concurrent administration of erythromycin arrests this metabolic process, presumably by altering the intestinal flora. As a result, the serum digoxin concentration approximately doubles. A patient has been described in whom erythromycin-induced digoxin toxicity occurred.[22]

The largest increases in serum digoxin concentration during concurrent antibiotic therapy are seen when digoxin tablets of limited bioavailability are used. When encapsulated liquid concentrates of digoxin (which have a high bioavailability) are used, production of dihydrodigoxin is much lower than when digoxin tablets of standard dissolution rate are used.[23]

Interactions Caused by Altered Protein Binding

An interaction between heparin and cardiac glycosides that results in alteration of glycoside protein binding has been reported in patients on hemodialysis.[24] In these patients, the free fractions of digitoxin and digoxin rose from 2.6 to 6.9% and from 78.3 to 87.1%, respectively, during dialysis. The reduction in protein binding was believed to be caused by heparin-induced release of free fatty acids that displaced digitoxin and digoxin from their albumin-binding sites. However, recent evidence suggests that the increase in free fatty acid concentrations results from in vitro hydrolysis of plasma triglycerides by lipases that are released after heparin administration.[25] When this hydrolysis was blocked, heparin administration did not alter the binding of digitoxin to albumin in patients on hemodialysis.[26]

Since digitoxin is more highly protein bound than digoxin (98% versus 25%), drug interactions that involve changes in protein binding are of much greater clinical importance with digitoxin.

Interactions Caused by Altered Elimination

Other clinically important interactions result from changes in the rate of removal of cardiac glycosides from the body. Some drugs alter the hepatic transformation of digitoxin; others affect digoxin's renal clearance.

Enzyme Inducers. Digitoxin is eliminated mainly by hepatic biotransformation, and drugs that induce hepatic microsomal enzymes may increase the elimination of digitoxin. Phenobarbital accelerates the formation of highly polar metabolites of digitoxin (such as digoxin).[27,28] In patients who received phenobarbital 60 mg three times daily during digitoxin therapy, the steady-state concentration of digitoxin decreased by approximately 50%.[28] Concurrent therapy with phenytoin 900 mg daily in one patient and phenylbutazone 300 mg daily in another patient on digitoxin maintenance therapy resulted in approximately 50% reductions in plasma digitoxin concentrations.[29]

A decrease in serum digitoxin concentrations of approximately 50% has also been observed during concurrent treatment with rifampin; in one report, the serum digitoxin half-life decreased from 8.2 to

4.5 days.[30] A significant reduction in digitoxin half-life was seen in volunteers who received rifampin 1.2 g for eight days.[31] Two patients in whom concurrent therapy with rifampin 600 mg daily caused a decrease in serum digitoxin concentrations have been described.[32,33]

Because digoxin elimination is dependent on renal function, rifampin's effects on digoxin metabolism are most notable in patients with poor renal function. One patient on dialysis developed symptoms of congestive heart failure when plasma digoxin concentrations decreased after initiation of rifampin therapy.[34] The digoxin dosage requirements of two other patients on dialysis increased substantially when rifampin therapy was started and decreased by approximately 50% when rifampin was discontinued.[35] A substantial increase in digoxin elimination has also been reported in a patient with only moderately impaired renal function.[36]

Vasodilators. Intravenous administration of sodium nitroprusside and hydralazine caused a 50% increase in renal clearance of digoxin in patients with chronic congestive heart failure.[37] The increase in digoxin clearance was probably caused by an increase in tubular secretion of digoxin, but the results of the study might have been influenced by the short periods of urine collection. Further studies are needed to determine the effects of vasodilator therapy on digoxin elimination.

Antiarrhythmic Agents. *Quinidine.* Since the first reports of an interaction between digoxin and quinidine appeared,[38-42] more than 100 articles on this subject have been published, including several review articles.[43-48] An increase in serum digoxin concentration occurs in more than 90% of patients who receive concomitant therapy with digoxin and quinidine. The serum digoxin concentration begins to increase upon initiation of quinidine therapy and doubles in most patients, although as much as a threefold increase in concentration can occur; attaining a new steady-state digoxin concentration usually requires less than a week but may take longer.[49,50]

The mechanism of the digoxin–quinidine interaction is complex. A reduction in renal clearance of digoxin after quinidine administration has been reported during maintenance therapy with digoxin[51-53] and following a single dose of digoxin.[54,55] The decrease in renal clearance of digoxin is about 40% in cardiac patients on digoxin maintenance therapy. The observed decrease in renal clearance may be caused by an effect of quinidine on the renal tubular handling of digoxin.

The extrarenal clearance of digoxin also decreases in the presence of quinidine.[56] This decrease is especially important in patients with poor renal function; in patients on hemodialysis, serum digoxin concentrations tend to double.[57] The cause of decreased extrarenal clearance of digoxin is unknown.

In studies of quinidine's influence on the volume of distribution of digoxin, both no change and a decrease have been reported.[49,50,54,55,58] Studies of cardiac patients on digoxin maintenance therapy indicate that a 20–40% decrease in digoxin distribution volume during concomitant quinidine administration is likely.[50,58] A 23% decrease in the ratio of digoxin concentration in skeletal muscle to that in serum during concomitant quinidine therapy has been reported in patients with atrial fibrillation[59]; approximately 50% of a dose of digoxin distributes into skeletal muscle. The decrease in the volume of distribution of digoxin is probably responsible for the acute rise in serum digoxin concentrations that occurs upon initiation of quinidine therapy, while the decrease in renal clearance of digoxin is probably responsible for the increase in steady-state serum digoxin concentrations.

The systemic availability of digoxin decreases 15% during concomitant quinidine administration,[60] but this finding is not in agreement with the results of another study.[61] Any effect of quinidine on the extent of digoxin absorption probably does not contribute to the digoxin–quinidine interaction.

Reports of the magnitude of quinidine-induced increases in the serum digoxin concentration are conflicting. Most data suggest a twofold to threefold increase if serum quinidine concentrations are in the therapeutic range. Serum digoxin concentration may double as a result of doubling the dose of quinidine in an individual patient,[51,62] but in general, there is no correlation or only a weak correlation between serum quinidine concentrations and the magnitude of changes in the serum digoxin concentration in a group of patients.[49,53,63] Therefore, the serum quinidine concentration cannot be used to predict change in serum digoxin concentration.

Of interest is the observation that the decrease in digoxin distribution volume is positively correlated with plasma quinidine concentrations and occurs only at therapeutic plasma quinidine concentrations. Changes in renal clearance of digoxin occur even at subtherapeutic concentrations of quinidine.[58,64] Conflicting results have been reported concerning the relation between plasma quinidine concentrations and decreases in the renal and extrarenal clearance of digoxin.[58,64]

Evidence from several studies indicates that the elevated digoxin concentrations during concomitant administration of quinidine and digoxin may result in a correspondingly increased therapeutic effect. In two studies of healthy volunteers, the positive inotropic effects of digoxin were reduced during concomitant treatment with quinidine despite an increase in serum digoxin concentration.[55,65] However, the results of these studies were complicated by the negative inotropic effects of quinidine. Quinidine-induced increases in the steady-state serum digoxin concentration were accompanied by proportional increases in the inotropic effects of digoxin in two studies of healthy volunteers who received maintenance doses of digoxin and quinidine,[66,67] while the inotropic effects of digoxin were decreased during concomitant quinidine therapy in another study.[68] These three studies appear to be most relevant to the clinical setting. Leahey et al.[69] reported that three patients on digoxin maintenance therapy had ECG findings that suggested enhanced digitalis effect; one patient had clinical evidence of an increased hemodynamic effect after concomitant quinidine administration. These effects paralleled the increase in serum digoxin concentration.

Several case reports mentioned adverse effects of digoxin during concomitant administration with quinidine.[39,40] Data provided by the Boston Collaborative Drug Surveillance Program obtained before the first reports of a digoxin–quinidine interaction were published indicated that cardiac and gastrointestinal symptoms of digitalis toxicity occurred more commonly in patients treated with both digoxin and quinidine than in comparable patients treated with digoxin alone.[70] However, most of this difference could be accounted for by the frequency with which clinically similar adverse reactions occur in patients receiving quinidine alone. Elderly patients appear to have been an exception; the incidence of adverse effects among elderly patients receiving both digoxin and quinidine was substantially higher than among elderly patients receiving either digoxin or quinidine alone.

Adverse effects that result from the digoxin-quinidine interaction can be prevented to some extent if the digoxin maintenance dose is decreased by one half at the start of quinidine therapy. Such an adjustment should keep the serum digoxin concentration within the normal range. Quinidine-induced increases in the serum digoxin concentration are highly variable; it is therefore desirable to monitor serum digoxin concentration and patient symptoms when quinidine is administered with digoxin.

Interactions have also been observed between digoxin and quinine,[71,72] a stereoisomer of quinidine, and between digoxin and hydroxychloroquine,[73] a semisynthetic quinine derivative.

Compared with digoxin, relatively few studies have reported an interaction between digitoxin and quinidine, and the results of these studies are conflicting. No difference in the steady-state digitoxin concentration was observed between a group of patients who were treated with digitoxin and quinidine and another group of patients treated only with digitoxin.[74] The effect of quinidine on the steady-state serum digitoxin concentration is difficult to measure because of the long half-life of digitoxin (about seven days). Although one report described a 32% mean increase in the serum digitoxin concentration after 10 days of concomitant administration of digitoxin and quinidine,[75] this is too short a period to establish a new steady-state serum digitoxin concentration.

The same authors reported that the steady-state serum digitoxin concentrations in two patients increased from 26 to 34 ng/mL and from 16 to 22 ng/mL, respectively, after approximately two months of concomitant administration of quinidine and digitoxin.[75] In three healthy volunteers, the mean steady-state serum digitoxin concentration increased from 11.4 to 18.5 ng/mL after 45 days of simultaneous administration of quinidine 180 mg three times daily (trough quinidine concentration 0.8 μg/mL), and a further increase to 24.1 ng/mL occurred after the dose of quinidine was doubled (trough quinidine concentration 2.1 μg/mL).[76] Kuhlmann et al.[77] also reported an interaction between digitoxin and quinidine in healthy volunteers.

One study of the effects of concomitant quinidine therapy on digitoxin pharmacokinetics following a single dose of digitoxin found no change in total body clearance of digitoxin,[78] while two other studies reported decreases in total body digitoxin clearance of 29%[79] and 63%.[80] The conflicting results of these studies may be explained by differences in blood quinidine concentrations; the steady-state serum quinidine concentrations of patients in these studies were 1.4–1.6 μg/mL,[78] 1.3–2.9 μg/mL,[79] and 2.0–3.5 μg/mL.[80]

Since no change in digitoxin volume of distribution during quinidine therapy has been shown,[78-80] concomitant administration of quinidine and digitoxin seems to carry no risk of an acute rise in serum digitoxin concentration. However, close monitoring of the serum digitoxin concentration and careful observation of patients for symptoms of digitalis toxicity are recommended when digitoxin and quinidine are given concomitantly.

Calcium-Channel Blockers. Verapamil hydrochloride (240–360 mg daily) increased the steady-state serum digoxin concentration by about 70% in patients[81,82] and healthy subjects.[83] Symptoms suggestive of digoxin toxicity were observed in approximately 15% of patients who were treated with both drugs.[81] Since verapamil-induced increases in the serum digoxin concentration have been accompanied by intensified glycoside effects in healthy volunteers,[83,84] digoxin dosage adjustment may be necessary in patients who are receiving verapamil.

Changes in the pharmacokinetics of digoxin during concomitant administration of digoxin and of verapamil include reductions in renal clearance (20%), extrarenal clearance (60%), and volume of distribution (23%).[85] However, verapamil-induced changes in digoxin pharmacokinetics may be transient. In a longitudinal study of healthy volunteers, the serum digoxin concentration increased from 0.21 to 0.34 ng/mL after one week of concomitant verapamil administration, and renal clearance of digoxin fell from 198 to 128 mL/min.[86] These changes resolved gradually, and after six weeks renal clearance of digoxin returned to the initial rate and plasma digoxin concentration decreased to 0.27 ng/mL. Because the observed serum digoxin concentrations in this study were very low and close to the limits of detection of the digoxin assay, further study is needed to investigate the effect of long-term verapamil therapy on digoxin pharmacokinetics.

Steady-state serum digoxin concentration may increase by 53% during coadministration of verapamil 240 mg daily and digoxin, and by 155% during coadministration of verapamil hydrochloride 240 mg daily, quinidine sulfate 480 mg daily, and digoxin.[87] Although the effect of quinidine alone on serum digoxin concentration was not evaluated in this study, these findings suggest that verapamil and quinidine have additive effects on the serum digoxin concentration. Only a small increase (approximately 30%) in the steady-state serum digoxin concentration was found in patients taking tiapamil.[88]

Diltiazem hydrochloride 90 mg daily did not cause a significant change in digoxin half-life or volume of distribution after a single dose of digoxin in healthy volunteers.[89] Of the three studies that evaluated the effect of concurrent diltiazem therapy (120–240 mg daily) on steady-state digoxin concentration, one reported no significant change,[90] while increases of 36%[91] and 22%[92] were reported in the other two studies. A small increase (20–30%) in serum digoxin concentration during concomitant diltiazem therapy is most likely.

There probably is no clinically relevant pharmacokinetic interaction between nifedipine and either digoxin or digitoxin. A 45% increase in the steady-state serum digoxin concentration was observed in healthy volunteers who received digoxin plus nifedipine 10 mg three times daily.[83] However, another study in healthy subjects reported no alteration of digoxin concentration during concomitant therapy with nifedipine 20 mg three times daily.[93] No significant change in the total body clearance of digoxin was apparent during concomitant administration of nifedipine 30–40 mg daily,[94,95] and nifedipine 30–60 mg daily did not significantly affect steady-state digoxin concentrations in cardiac patients who received both drugs.[96] Nifedipine did not alter the pharmacokinetics of digitoxin in patients.[97]

Amiodarone. Amiodarone, an antiarrhythmic agent, elevates the steady-state serum digoxin concentration by approximately 80% in patients. The increase in serum digoxin concentration contributes to the gastrointestinal, cardiac, and neurologic effects observed in some patients during combination therapy with digoxin and amiodarone.[98–102] The interaction between digoxin and amiodarone has also been described in a patient on hemodialysis.[103] The amiodarone–digoxin interaction appears to be of greater magnitude in children than in adults.[104]

Other Antiarrhythmic Drugs. Relatively high serum concentrations of disopyramide (mean 5.05 μg/mL) caused an increase of only 15% in the steady-state serum digoxin concentration.[105] Disopyramide is a suitable alternative to quinidine in patients receiving maintenance therapy with digoxin, especially since other studies have found that any interaction between these two drugs is not clinicaly important.[106–108] The antiarrhythmic agents ajmaline, aprindine, lidoflazine, lidocaine, propafenone,[51] mexiletine,[109] procainamide,[106] lorcainide,[110] sparteine,[110] and tocainide[111] do not elevate the steady-state serum digoxin concentration, while flecainide causes an increase of about 15%.[112,113]

The effects of antiarrhythmic agents on the steady-state serum digoxin concentration are summarized in Table 2.

Thyroid Hormones and Antithyroid Agents. Hyperthyroid patients appear to require larger doses of digitalis, while hypothyroid patients need smaller doses. Altered sensitivity to digitalis in patients with thyroid disease and changes in digitalis pharmacokinetics, especially in hyperthyroid patients, may explain the interaction. Increased clearance of cardiac glycosides is the most likely explanation for the decrease in serum digoxin and digitoxin concentrations in hyperthyroid patients.[114,115] Concurrent treatment of thyroid disease with thyroid hormones or antithyroid agents may require digitalis dosage adjustment.

Potentially Important but Unproven Interactions

Potassium-Sparing Diuretics. Spironolactone reduces digoxin clearance by 35%, apparently as a

Table 2.
Effects of Antiarrhythmic Agents on Serum Steady-State Digoxin Concentrations

Antiarrhythmic Agent	% Increase in Digoxin Concentration	Reference No.
Ajmaline	0	51
Amiodarone	80	98–102
Aprindine	0	51
Diltiazem	25	91–92
	0	90
Disopyramide	15	105
	0	106–108
Flecainide	15	112, 113
Lidocaine	0	51
Lidoflazine	0	51
Lorcainide	0	110
Mexiletine	0	109
Nifedipine	45	83
	0	93, 96
Procainamide	0	106
Propafenone	0	51
Quinidine	100	38–42
Sparteine	0	110
Tiapamil	30	88
Tocainide	0	111
Verapamil	70	81–83

result of inhibition of renal tubular secretion of digoxin by spironolactone or its metabolites.[116] In healthy volunteers, administration of both spironolactone and quinidine simultaneously with digoxin caused significantly greater decreases in digoxin clearance than the decreases caused by either drug alone.[117] Patients on digoxin maintenance therapy who received spironolactone 100 mg daily had increased steady-state serum digoxin concentrations; mean serum digoxin concentration increased from 0.8 to 1.0 ng/mL, but one patient's serum digoxin concentration increased from 1.0 to 3.5 ng/mL.[118] No changes in steady-state serum digoxin concentration were observed in elderly patients who received successive doses of hydrochlorothiazide, spironolactone–hydrochlorothiazide combination, and triamterene–hydrochlorothiazide combination.[119]

Spironolactone and its metabolites can interfere with commonly used radioimmunoassays for digoxin. The false elevation of serum digoxin concentration is usually small and depends on the digoxin-binding antibody that is used. Interference is more likely in patients with hepatic dysfunction.[120,121] In normal subjects, the total and extrarenal digoxin clearance decreased by approximately 20% and 70%, respectively, during daily administration of triamterene 150 mg.[116] Amiloride 10 mg daily doubled renal clearance of digoxin and blocked extrarenal digoxin clearance; as a result, total body clearance of digoxin tended to decrease.[122] The clinical significance of the interaction between digoxin and triamterene or amiloride, especially in patients with poor renal function, remains to be established.

Amiloride and spironolactone may alter the pharmacologic effects of digoxin. In healthy volunteers, amiloride suppressed digoxin's inotropic effect, spironolactone caused minor decreases of the inotropic effect, and triamterene did not alter this effect.[116,122] Studies in patients with heart disease are needed to clarify the clinical importance of differences between the potassium-sparing diuretics with respect to digoxin pharmacodynamics.

Reports of the effects of spironolactone on the pharmacokinetics of digitoxin are conflicting. Both a 20% decrease[123] and a 30% increase[15] in digitoxin half-life have been attributed to concomitant administration of spironolactone. Further studies are needed to confirm these interactions with potassium-sparing diuretics and determine their clinical relevance.

Cimetidine. Concomitant administration of cimetidine resulted in a 25% decrease in steady-state serum digoxin concentrations in patients.[124] These results contrast with those of other studies in which cimetidine was found to have no effect on the area under the plasma digoxin concentration versus time curve.[125,126]

Nonsteroidal Anti-inflammatory Agents. There are conflicting data from several studies of interactions between digoxin and nonsteroidal anti-inflammatory agents. In preterm infants with reduced renal function, addition of indomethacin to a digoxin regimen resulted in a 55% increase in serum digoxin concentrations.[127] Significant increases in serum digoxin concentration have been observed in healthy volunteers during concomitant therapy with ibuprofen (15% increase), indomethacin (25%), diclofenac (29%), and aspirin (31%).[128] However, other studies in healthy volunteers do not indicate that important interactions occur between digoxin and indomethacin[129,130] or digoxin and aspirin.[131]

In a study performed in ambulatory patients, a significant increase in mean serum digoxin concentration (60%) was reported after seven days of concurrent administration of ibuprofen and digoxin; however, no significant increase was observed after 28 days of concomitant therapy.[132] Patient noncompliance might have been a complicating factor.

Based on the available data, no conclusive statement can be made concerning interactions between digoxin and nonsteroidal anti-inflammatory agents.

Preliminary Studies and Case Reports

The clinical importance of several preliminary reports of pharmacokinetic interactions with the cardiac glycosides has not been confirmed. These interactions include the following:

- Diazepam administered simultaneously with digoxin in healthy volunteers reduced urinary excretion of digoxin with a resulting increase in digoxin half-life.[133]
- During concomitant therapy with captopril, the serum digoxin concentrations in patients with congestive heart failure were 25% higher than during therapy with digoxin alone.[134]
- Accelerated quinidine metabolism was observed in a patient who also received daily doses of digoxin and pentobarbital; discontinuation of pentobarbital produced a sharp increase in serum digoxin concentration.[135]
- In a patient receiving concurrent therapy with digoxin, quinidine, and rifampin, discontinuation of rifampin therapy caused an increase in serum digoxin concentration.[36]
- Cimetidine caused an increase in the serum concentrations of both digitoxin and quinidine in a patient receiving all three drugs; it is unclear whether the increase in digitoxin concentration was related to a direct effect of cimetidine or a cimetidine-induced increase in serum quinidine concentration.[136]

Conclusion

Clinically important pharmacokinetic interactions can occur when digoxin or digitoxin is administered concomitantly with other drugs. Digoxin dosage should be reduced during concomitant therapy with quinidine, verapamil, or amiodarone. Drugs that induce hepatic microsomal enzymes increase the elimination of digitoxin. In some patients, the serum digoxin concentration increases during erythromycin therapy. Doses of kaolin–pectin suspension, cholestyramine, and activated charcoal should be spaced as far as possible from doses of cardiac glycosides to avoid interference with cardiac glycoside absorption. Absorption of digoxin is reduced during concomitant therapy with sulfasalazine, aminosalicylic acid, or neomycin. To date, the clinical importance of other interactions has not been confirmed.

References

1. Brown DD, Juhl RP. Decreased bioavailability of digoxin due to antacids and kaolin-pectin. *N Engl J Med.* 1976; 295: 1034–7.
2. Brown DD, Juhl RP, Warner SL. Decreased bioavailability of digoxin due to hypocholesterolemic interventions. *Circulation.* 1978; 58:164–72.
3. Reissell P, Manninen V. Effect of administration of activated charcoal and fibre on absorption, excretion and steady state blood levels of digoxin and digitoxin. Evidence for intestinal secretion of the glycosides. *Acta Med Scand.* 1982; Suppl 668:88–90.
4. Lindenbaum J, Maulitz RM, Butler VP. Inhibition of digoxin absorption by neomycin. *Gastroenterology.* 1976; 71:399–404.
5. Juhl RP, Summers RW, Guillory JK et al. Effect of sulfasalazine on digoxin bioavailability. *Clin Pharmacol Ther.* 1976; 20:387–94.
6. Manninen V, Apajalahti A, Melin J et al. Altered absorption of digoxin in patients given propantheline and metoclopramide. *Lancet.* 1973; 1:398–400.
7. Manninen V, Apajalahti A, Simonen H et al. Effect of propantheline and metoclopramide on absorption of digoxin. *Lancet.* 1973; 1:1118–9. Letter.
8. Johnson BF, O'Grady J, Bye C. The influence of digoxin particle size on absorption of digoxin and the effect of propantheline and metoclopramide. *Br J Clin Pharmacol.* 1978; 5:465–7.
9. Cooke J, Smith JA. Absence of interaction of digoxin with antacids under clinical conditions. *Br Med J.* 1978; 2:1166–7. Letter.
10. Vöhringer HF, Kuhlmann J, Rietbrock N. Der Einfluss von Antacida auf die Plasmakonzentration von Digoxin beim Menschen. *Dtsch Med Wochenschr.* 1976; 101:106–8.
11. Allen MD, Greenblatt DJ, Harmatz JS et al. Effect of magnesium-aluminum hydroxide and kaolin-pectin on absorption of digoxin from tablets and capsules. *J Clin Pharmacol.* 1981; 21:26–30.
12. Kuhlmann J. Plasmaspiegel und renale Elimination von Digitoxin bei Langzeittherapie mit Aluminium-Magnesium-Hydroxid-Gel. *Dtsch Med Wochenschr.* 1984; 109:59–61.
13. Albert KS, Ayres JW, Di Santo AR et al. Influence of kaolin-pectin suspension on digoxin bioavailability. *J Pharm Sci.* 1978; 67:1582–6.
14. Caldwell JH, Greenberger NJ. Interruption of the enterohepatic circulation of digitoxin by cholestyramine. *J Clin Invest.* 1971; 50:2626–37.
15. Carruthers SG, Dujovne CA. Cholestyramine and spironolactone and their combination in digitoxin elimination. *Clin Pharmacol Ther.* 1980; 27:184–7.
16. van Bever RJ, Duchateau AM, Pluym BF et al. The effect of colestipol on digitoxin plasma levels. *Arzneimittelforsch.* 1976; 26:1891–3.
17. Neuvonen PJ, Elfving SM, Elonen E. Reduction of absorption of digoxin, phenytoin and aspirin by activated charcoal in man. *Eur J Clin Pharmacol.* 1978; 13:213–8.
18. Kuhlmann J, Zilly W, Wilke J. Effects of cytostatic drugs on plasma level and renal excretion of beta-acetyldigoxin. *Clin Pharmacol Ther.* 1981; 30:518–27.
19. Kuhlmann J, Wilke J, Rietbrock N. Cystostatic drugs are without significant effect on digitoxin plasma level and renal excretion. *Clin Pharmacol Ther.* 1982; 32:646–51.
20. Lindenbaum J, Rund DG, Butler VP et al. Inactivation of digoxin by the gut flora: reversal by antibiotic therapy. *N Engl J Med.* 1981; 305:789–94.
21. Dobkin JF, Saha JR, Butler VP et al. Digoxin-inactivating bacteria: identification in human gut flora. *Science.* 1983; 220:325–7.
22. Friedman HS. Erythromycin-induced digoxin toxicity. *Chest.* 1982; 82:202. Letter.
23. Rund DG, Lindenbaum J, Dobkin JF et al. Decreased digoxin cardioinactive-reduced metabolites after administration as an encapsulated liquid concentrate. *Clin Pharmacol Ther.* 1983; 34:738–43.
24. Storstein L, Janssen H. Studies on digitalis. VI. The effect of heparin on serum protein binding of digitoxin and digoxin. *Clin Pharmacol Ther.* 1976; 20:15–23.
25. Giacomini KM, Giacomini JC, Blaschke TF. Absence of effect of heparin on the binding of prazosin and phenytoin to plasma proteins. *Biochem Pharmacol.* 1980; 29:3337–40.
26. Lohman JJ, Hooymans PM, Koten ML et al. Effect of heparin on digitoxin protein binding. *Clin Pharmacol Ther.* 1985; 37:55–60.
27. Jelliffe RW, Blankenhorn DH. Effect of phenobarbital on digitoxin metabolism. *Clin Res.* 1966; 14:160. Abstract.
28. Solomon HM. Interactions between digitoxin and other drugs in man. *Am Heart J.* 1972; 83:277–80.
29. Solomon HM, Reich S, Spirt N et al. Interactions between digitoxin and other drugs in vitro and in vivo. *Ann NY Acad Sci.* 1971; 179:362–9.
30. Peters U, Hausamen TU, Grosse-Brockhoff F. Einfluss von Tuberkulostastika auf die Pharmakokinetiek des Digitoxins. *Dtsch Med Wochenschr.* 1974; 99:2381–6.
31. Zilly W, Breimer DD, Richter E. Pharmacokinetic interactions with rifampicin. *Clin Pharmacokinet.* 1977; 2:61–70.
32. Boman G, Eliasson K, Odar-Cederöf I. Acute cardiac failure during treatment with digitoxin—an interaction with rifampicin. *Br J Clin Pharmacol.* 1980; 10:89–90. Letter.
33. Poor DM, Self TH, Davis HL. Interaction of rifampin and digitoxin. *Arch Intern Med.* 1983; 143:599.
34. Novi C, Bissoli F, Simonati V et al. Rifampin and digoxin: possible drug interaction in a dialysis patient. *JAMA.* 1980; 244:2521–2. Letter.
35. Gault H, Longerich L, Dawe M et al. Digoxin–rifampin interaction. *Clin Pharmacol Ther.* 1984; 35:750–4.
36. Bussey HI, Merritt GJ, Hill EG. The influence of rifampin on quinidine and digoxin. *Arch Intern Med.* 1984; 144: 1021–3.
37. Cogan J, Humphreys MH, Carlson CJ et al. Acute vasodilator therapy increases renal clearance of digoxin in patients with congestive heart failure. *Circulation.* 1981; 64:973–6.
38. Kaufmann G. Is there a need for new cardiac glycosides? For more blood level determinations? In: Bodem G, Dengler HJ, eds. Cardiac glycosides. New York: Springer; 1977:410–21.
39. Ejvinsson G. Effect of quinidine on plasma concentrations of digoxin. *Br Med J.* 1978; 1:279–80.
40. Leahey EB, Reiffel JA, Drusin RE et al. Interaction between quinidine and digoxin. *JAMA.* 1978; 240:533–4.
41. Doering W, König E. Anstieg der Digoxinkonzentration im Serum unter Chinidinmedikation. *Med Klin.* 1978; 73: 1085–8.
42. Hooymans PM, Merkus FW. Effects of quinidine on plasma concentration of digoxin. *Br Med J.* 1978; 2:1022. Letter.

43. Hooymans PM, Merkus FW. Mechanism of the digoxin-quinidine interaction. *Pharm Int.* 1980; 1:158–61.
44. Wood BG, Rietbrock N. Digitalis–quinidine interactions. *Trends Pharmacol Sci.* 1982; 3:118–22.
45. Bigger JT, Leahey EB. Quinidine and digoxin: an important interaction. *Drugs.* 1982; 24:229–39.
46. Bussey HI. The influence of quinidine and other agents on digitalis glycosides. *Am Heart J.* 1982; 104:289–302.
47. Fichtl B, Doering W. The quinidine–digoxin interaction in perspective. *Clin Pharmacokinet.* 1983; 8:137–54.
48. Bussey HI. Update on the influence of quinidine and other agents on digitalis glycosides. *Am Heart J.* 1984; 107: 143–6.
49. Schenck-Gustafsson K, Dahlquist R. Pharmacokinetics of digoxin in patients subjected to the quinidine–digoxin interaction. *Br J Clin Pharmacol.* 1981; 11:181–6.
50. Ochs HR, Bodem G, Greenblatt DJ. Impairment of digoxin clearance by coadministration of quinidine. *J Clin Pharmacol.* 1981; 21:396–400.
51. Doering W. Quinidine–digoxin interaction: pharmacokinetics, underlying mechanism and clinical implications. *N Engl J Med.* 1979; 301:400–4.
52. Dahlquist R, Ejvinsson G, Schenck-Gustafsson K. Effect of quinidine on plasma concentration and renal clearance of digoxin. A clinically important drug interaction. *Br J Clin Pharmacol.* 1980; 9:413–8.
53. Mungall DR, Robichaux RP, Perry W et al. Effects of quinidine on serum digoxin concentration. *Ann Intern Med.* 1980; 93:689–93.
54. Hager WD, Fenster P, Mayersohn M et al. Digoxin–quinidine interaction: pharmacokinetic evaluation. *N Engl J Med.* 1979; 300:1238–41.
55. Steiness E, Waldorff S, Hansen PB. Reduction of digoxin-induced inotropism during quinidine administration. *Clin Pharmacol Ther.* 1980; 27:791–5.
56. Hooymans PM, Holford NH, Massie BM et al. Quinidine decreases both renal and metabolic clearance of digoxin. *Am J Cardiol.* 1980; 45:453. Abstract.
57. Doering W, Fichtl B, Herrmann M et al. Quinidine–digoxin interaction: evidence for involvement of an extrarenal mechanism. *Eur J Clin Pharmacol.* 1982; 21:281–5.
58. Pedersen KE, Christiansen BD, Klitgaard NA et al. Changes in steady state digoxin pharmacokinetics during quinidine therapy in cardiac patients: influence of plasma quinidine concentration. *Acta Pharmacol Toxicol.* 1983; 52:357–63.
59. Schenck-Gustafsson K, Jogestrand T, Nordlander R et al. Effect of quinidine on digoxin concentration in skeletal muscle and serum in patients with atrial fibrillation. *N Engl J Med.* 1981. 305:209–11.
60. Pedersen KE, Christiansen BD, Klitgaard NA et al. Effect of quinidine on digoxin bioavailability. *Eur J Clin Pharmacol.* 1983; 24:41–7.
61. Hager WD, Mayersohn M, Graves PE. Digoxin bioavailability during quinidine administration. *Clin Pharmacol Ther.* 1981; 30:594–9.
62. Risler T, Peters U, Grabensee B et al. Untersuchungen zur Interaktion von Chinidin und Digoxin beim Menschen. *Dtsch Med Wochenschr.* 1979; 104:1523–6.
63. Friedman HS, Chen TS. Use of control steady state serum digoxin levels for predicting serum digoxin concentration after quinidine administration. *Am Heart J.* 1982; 104:72–6.
64. Leahey EB, Bigger JT, Butler VP et al. Quinidine–digoxin interaction: time course and pharmacokinetics. *Am J Cardiol* 1981; 48:1141–6.
65. Hirsh PD, Weiner HJ, North RL. Further insights into digoxin–quinidine interaction: lack of correlation between serum digoxin concentration and inotropic state of the heart. *Am J Cardiol.* 1980; 46:863–7.
66. Belz GG, Doering W, Aust PE et al. Quinidine–digoxin interaction: cardiac efficacy of elevated serum digoxin concentration. *Clin Pharmacol Ther.* 1982; 31:548–54.
67. Schenck-Gustafsson K, Jogestrand T, Brodin L et al. Cardiac effects of treatment with quinidine and digoxin, alone and in combination. *Am J Cardiol.* 1983; 51:777–82.
68. Das G, Barr CE, Carlson J. Reduction of digoxin effect during the digoxin–quinidine interaction. *Clin Pharmacol Ther.* 1984; 35:317–21.
69. Leahey EB, Reiffel JA, Heissenbuttel RH et al. Enhanced cardiac effect of digoxin during quinidine treatment. *Arch Intern Med.* 1979; 139:519–21.
70. Walker AM, Cody RJ, Greenblatt DJ et al. Drug toxicity in patients receiving digoxin and quinidine. *Am Heart J.* 1983; 105:1025–8.
71. Wandell M, Powell JR, Hager D et al. Effect of quinine on digoxin kinetics. *Clin Pharmacol Ther.* 1980; 28:425–30.
72. Aronson JK, Carver JG. Interaction of digoxin with quinine. *Lancet.* 1981; 1:1418. Letter.
73. Leden I. Digoxin–hydroxychloroquine interaction? *Acta Med Scand.* 1982; 211:411–2.
74. Storstein L, von der Lippe A, Amlie J et al. Is there an interaction between digitoxin and quinidine? *Circulation.* 1979; 60(Suppl II):230. Abstract.
75. Peters U, Risler T, Grabensee B et al. Interaktion von Chinidin und Digitoxin beim Menschen. *Dtsch Med Wochenschr.* 1980; 105:438–42.
76. Kreutz G, Keller F, Gast D et al. Digitoxin–quinidine interaction achieving steady-state conditions for both drugs. *Naunyn Schmiedebergs Arch Pharmacol.* 1982; 319:R 82.
77. Kuhlmann J, Nohrmann M, Marcin S. Effects of quinidine on plasma level and renal excretion of digitoxin achieving steady state conditions. *Arch Pharm.* 1984; 325:R 85. Abstract.
78. Ochs HR, Pabst J, Greenblatt DJ et al. Noninteraction of digitoxin and quinidine. *N Engl J Med.* 1980; 303:672–4.
79. Fenster PE, Powell JR, Graves PE et al. Digitoxin–quinidine interaction: pharmacokinetic evaluation. *Ann Intern Med.* 1980; 93:698–701.
80. Garty M, Sood P, Rollins DE. Digitoxin elimination reduced during quinidine therapy. *Ann Intern Med.* 1981; 94:35–7.
81. Klein HO, Lang R, Weiss E et al. The influence of verapamil on serum digoxin concentration. *Circulation.* 1982; 65: 998–1003.
82. Schwartz JB, Keefe D, Kates RE et al. Acute and chronic pharmacodynamic interaction of verapamil and digoxin in atrial fibrillation. *Circulation.* 1982; 65:1163–70.
83. Belz GG, Doering W, Munkes R et al. Interaction between digoxin and calcium antagonists and antiarrhythmic drugs. *Clin Pharmacol Ther.* 1983; 33:410–7.
84. Pedersen KE, Thayssen P, Klitgaard NA et al. Influence of verapamil on the inotropism and pharmacokinetics of digoxin. *Eur J Clin Pharmacol.* 1983; 25:199–206.
85. Pedersen KE, Dorph-Pedersen A, Hvidt S et al. Digoxin–verapamil interaction. *Clin Pharmacol Ther.* 1981; 30:311–6.
86. Pedersen KE, Dorph-Pedersen A, Hvidt S et al. The long-term effect of verapamil in plasma digoxin concentration and renal digoxin clearance in healthy subjects. *Eur J Clin Pharmacol.* 1982; 22:123–7.
87. Doering W. Effect of coadministration of verapamil and quinidine on serum digoxin concentration. *Eur J Clin Pharmacol.* 1983; 25:517–21.
88. Lessem J, Bellinetto A. Interaction between digoxin and calcium antagonist. *Am J Cardiol.* 1982; 49:1025. Abstract.
89. Yoshida A, Fujita M, Kurosawa N et al. Effects of diltiazem on plasma level and urinary excretion of digoxin in healthy subjects. *Clin Pharmacol Ther.* 1984; 35:681–5.
90. Schrager BR, Pina I, Frangi M et al. Diltiazem, digoxin interaction? *Circulation.* 1983; 68(Suppl III):368. Abstract.
91. Oyama Y, Fujii S, Kunda K. Digoxin–diltiazem interaction. *Am J Cardiol.* 1984; 53:1480–1.
92. Rameis H, Magometschnigg D, Ganzinger U. The diltiazem–digoxin interaction. *Clin Pharmacol Ther.* 1984; 36: 183–9.
93. Schwartz JB, Migliore PJ. Effect of nifedipine on serum digoxin concentration and renal digoxin clearance. *Clin Pharmacol Ther.* 1984; 36:19–24.

94. Pedersen KE, Dorph-Pedersen A, Hvidt S et al. Effect of nifedipine on digoxin kinetics in healthy subjects. *Clin Pharmacol Ther.* 1982; 32:562–5.
95. Zylber-Katz E, Koren G, Levy M. Pharmacokinetic study of digoxin and nifedipine coadministration. *Clin Pharmacol Ther.* 1984; 35:286. Abstract.
96. Schwartz JB, Raizner A, Akers S. The effect of nifedipine on serum digoxin concentrations in patients. *Am Heart J.* 1984; 107:669–73.
97. Kuhlmann J, Marcin S, Franck KH. Effects of nifedipine on pharmacokinetics and pharmacodynamics of beta-acetyl-digoxin and digitoxin in patients. *Klin Wochenschr.* 1984; 62:451–7.
98. Moysey JO, Jaggarao NS, Grundy EN et al. Amiodarone increases plasma digoxin concentrations. *Br Med J.* 1981; 282:272.
99. Berdeaux A, Valette H, Auzepy P et al. Influence de l'amiodarone sur la digoxinemie. *Nouv Presse Med.* 1981; 10: 3650.
100. Nademanee K, Kannan R, Hendrickson J et al. Amiodarone–digoxin interaction during treatment of resistant cardiac arrhythmias. *Am J Cardiol.* 1982; 49:1026. Abstract.
101. Nager G, Nager F. Interaction between amiodarone and digoxin. *Schweiz Med Wochenschr.* 1983; 113:1727–30.
102. Douste-Blazy P, Montastruc JL, Bonnet B et al. Influence of amiodarone on plasma and urine digoxin concentrations. *Lancet.* 1984; 1:905. Letter.
103. Mingardi G. Amiodarone and plasma digoxin levels. *Lancet.* 1984; 1:1238. Letter.
104. Koren G, Hesslein P, McLeod SM. Kinetics of amiodarone-associated digoxin toxicity in children. *Clin Pharmacol Ther.* 1984; 35:252. Abstract.
105. Manolas EG, Hunt D, Sloman G. Effects of quinidine and disopyramide on serum digoxin concentrations. *Aust NZ J Med.* 1980; 10:426–9.
106. Leahey EB, Reiffel JA, Giardina EV et al. The effect of quinidine and other oral antiarrhythmic drugs on serum digoxin. *Ann Intern Med.* 1980; 92:605–8.
107. Wellens HJ, Gorgels AP, Braat SJ et al. Effect of oral disopyramide on serum digoxin levels. A prospective study. *Am Heart J.* 1980; 100:934–5.
108. Risler T, Burk M, Peters U et al. On the interaction between digoxin and disopyramide. *Clin Pharmacol Ther.* 1983; 34: 176–80.
109. Day T, Hunt D. Interaction between mexiletine and digoxin. *Med J Aust.* 1983; 2:630.
110. Doering W, König E. Chinidin erhöht den Digoxin-Spiegel. *Med Klin.* 1981; 76:395–8.
111. Lohman JJ, Hooymans PM, Verhey MT et al. The effect of tocainide on digoxin serum level and renal clearance. *Pharm Weekbl [Sci].* 1983; 5:346.
112. Tjandramaga TB, Verbesselt A, Hecken A et al. Oral digoxin pharmacokinetics during multiple-dose flecainide treatment. *Arch Int Pharmacodyn Ther.* 1982; 260:302–3.
113. Lewis GP, Holtzman JL. Interaction of flecainide with digoxin and propranolol. *Am J Cardiol.* 1984; 53:52–7B.
114. Aronson JK. Clinical pharmacokinetics of digoxin 1980. *Clin Pharmacokinet.* 1980; 5:137–49.
115. Ochs HR, Greenblatt DJ, Bodem G et al. Disease-related alterations in cardiac glycoside disposition. *Clin Pharmacokinet.* 1982; 7:434–51.
116. Waldorff S, Hansen PB, Egeblad H et al. Interactions between digoxin and potassium-sparing diuretics. *Clin Pharamacol Ther.* 1983; 33:418–23.
117. Fenster PE, Hager WD, Goodman MM. Digoxin–quinidine–spironolactone interaction. *Clin Pharmacol Ther.* 1984; 36:70–3.
118. Steiness E. Renal tubular secretion of digoxin. *Circulation.* 1974; 50:103–7.
119. Finnegan TP, Spence JD, Cape RD. Potassium-sparing diuretics: interaction with digoxin in elderly men. *Geriatrics.* 1984; 32:129–31.
120. DiPiro JT, Cote JR, DiPiro CR et al. Spironolactone interference with digoxin radioimmunoassay in cirrhotic patients. *Am J Hosp Pharm.* 1980; 37:1518–21.
121. Paladino JA, Davidson KH, McCall BB. Influence of spironolactone on serum digoxin concentration. *JAMA.* 1984; 251:470–1. Letter.
122. Waldorff S, Hansen PB, Kjaergard H et al. Amiloride-induced changes in digoxin dynamics and kinetics: abolition of digoxin-induced inotropism with amiloride. *Clin Pharmacol Ther.* 1981; 30:172–6.
123. Wirth KE, Frolich JC, Hollifield JW et al. Metabolism of digitoxin in man and its modification by spironolactone. *Eur J Clin Pharmacol.* 1976; 9:345–54.
124. Fraley DS, Britton HL, Schwinghammer TL et al. Effect of cimetidine on steady-state serum digoxin concentrations. *Clin Pharm.* 1983; 2: 163–5.
125. Jordaens L, Hoegaerts J, Belpaire E. Noninteraction of cimetidine with digoxin absorption. *Acta Clin Belg.* 1981; 36: 109–10.
126. Ochs HR, Gugler R, Guthoff T et al. Effect of cimetidine on digoxin kinetics and creatinine clearance. *Am Heart J.* 1984; 107:170–2.
127. Koren G, Soldin S, McLeod SM. Interaction of digoxin with commonly coadministered drugs—two different renal mechanisms. *Clin Res.* 1983; 31:249A. Abstract.
128. Isbary J, Doering W, König E. Der Einfluss von Tiaprofensäure auf die Digoxinkonzentration im Serum im Vergleich zu anderen Antirheumatika. *Z Rheumatol.* 1982; 41:164. Abstract.
129. Rau R, Konstantinidou D, Diembeck W. Zur Frage einer Interaktion zwischen Digoxin und Indomethacin. *Z Rheumatol.* 1982; 41:164. Abstract.
130. Finch MB, Johnston GD, Kelly JG et al. Pharmacokinetics of digoxin alone and in the presence of indomethacin therapy. *Br J Clin Pharmacol.* 1984; 17:353–5.
131. Fenster PE, Comess KA, Hanson CD et al. Kinetics of the digoxin–aspirin combination. *Clin Pharmacol Ther.* 1982; 32:428–30.
132. Quattrocchi FP, Robinson JD, Curry RW et al. The effect of ibuprofen on serum digoxin concentrations. *Drug Intell Clin Pharm.* 1983; 17:286–8.
133. Castillo-Ferrando JR, Garcia M, Carmona J. Digoxin levels and diazepam. *Lancet.* 1980; 2:368. Abstract.
134. Cleland JG, Dargie HJ, Hodsman GP et al. Interaction of digoxin and captopril. *Br J Clin Pharmacol.* 1984; 17:214. Abstract.
135. Chapron DJ, Mumford D, Pitegoff GI. Apparent quinidine-induced digoxin toxicity after withdrawal of pentobarbital. *Arch Intern Med.* 1979; 139:363–5.
136. Polish LB, Branch RA, Fitzgerald GA. Digitoxin–quinidine interaction: potentiation during administration of cimetidine. *South Med J.* 1981; 74:633–4.

Therapy Reviews

Whole-bowel irrigation for mechanical colon cleansing

KATHERINE A. MICHAEL, JOSEPH T. DIPIRO, TALMADGE A. BOWDEN, AND FRANCIS J. TEDESCO

Abstract: The physiology, solution composition, indications, efficacy, and safety of whole-bowel irrigation (WBI) for mechanical bowel cleansing are reviewed.

WBI with isotonic electrolyte solutions produces diarrhea when the infusion rate exceeds the capacity of the intestine to distend and absorb the solution. A number of solutions are used for WBI, including 0.9% sodium chloride, balanced electrolyte solutions, lactated Ringer's, mannitol, and electrolyte solutions containing polyethylene glycol 3350 (PEG). WBI solution administration rates vary from 15–90 mL/min, by oral ingestion or nasogastric tube, with total volumes ranging from 1 to 20 L. The onset of diarrhea occurs as soon as 20 minutes with clearing of the effluent as early as 90 minutes. Faster administration rates appear to shorten overall cleansing time.

Two PEG-electrolyte lavage solutions (ELSs) have recently gained FDA approval. The recommended dosage rate is 1.2–1.8 L/hr orally or by nasogastric tube until rectal effluent is clear. In most patients, this requires a maximum of 4–6 L. Initial data indicate that PEG-ELSs are safe for elderly patients and for patients who have an increased risk of fluid overload, but these solutions have not been evaluated in children, pregnant women, or patients with inflammatory bowel disease.

WBI is an effective alternative to other regimens for removing fecal material and reducing bowel lumen bacterial counts before colonoscopy and colorectal surgery. Retention of excess WBI solution may interfere with the quality of barium enema radiographs; this can be minimized by completing the irrigation the evening before the examination. Gastrointestinal side effects occur in about one third of the patients following WBI, but do not generally require discontinuing the irrigation. Solutions containing PEG with sodium sulfate as the primary electrolyte result in the least net water and electrolyte movement and are preferred over other solutions.

Index terms: Drug administration rate; Electrolytes; Flow; Gastric lavage; Irrigating solutions; Toxicity
Clin Pharm. 1985; 4:414–24

Mechanical bowel cleansing regimens are customarily used before gastrointestinal surgical, endoscopic, or radiographic procedures. The ideal colon evacuant should act rapidly and require minimal preoperative hospital stay. It should leave no residual fecal material, gas, fluid, or oil droplets, be readily acceptable to the patient, be easily administered (preferably by the oral route), and should not increase patient morbidity.[1-3] No universally accepted method for bowel cleansing currently exists. Often, a regimen that is considered effective by the physician causes the patient discomfort, while mild regimens may not result in prompt and complete bowel evacuation and, therefore, may be unacceptable to the physician.

Whole-bowel irrigation (WBI), which produces volumogenic diarrhea by ingestion of relatively large volumes of electrolyte solutions, is a technique for preparation of the bowel before surgery or diagnostic procedures. WBI has become popular because colon cleansing can often be achieved in a much shorter period of time compared with other techniques. A number of solutions have been used for WBI; those containing an isotonic electrolyte profile in combination with polyethylene glycol have gained recent popularity. This article reviews

KATHERINE A. MICHAEL, PHARM.D., is Research Associate, Department of Pharmacy Practice, College of Pharmacy, University of Georgia (UGA), Athens. JOSEPH T. DIPIRO, PHARM.D., is Assistant Professor of Pharmacy, College of Pharmacy, UGA, and Assistant Adjunct Professor of Surgery, Medical College of Georgia (MCG). TALMADGE A. BOWDEN, M.D., is Professor of Surgery, Department of Surgery, and FRANCIS J. TEDESCO, M.D., is Professor of Medicine and Chief, Section of Gastroenterology, MCG, Augusta.

Address reprint requests to Dr. DiPiro at the Medical College of Georgia, Room CJ-112, Augusta, GA 30912.

The assistance of Susan E. Baldwin in preparing this manuscript is acknowledged.

This is **article 680-204-8513** in the **ASHP Continuing Education System.** See page 465 for learning objectives and test questions.

the literature on WBI regimens including discussions on the physiology of volumogenic diarrhea, the composition of WBI solutions, and the indications for the use of these solutions, and their efficacy and safety.

Physiology of Volumogenic Diarrhea

Diarrhea produced by the ingestion of large amounts of fluid (volumogenic diarrhea) results from the relationships among the fluid flow rate through the gut, the total fluid volume entering the intestine, and the gut's absorptive capacity. In 1965, Dillard and colleagues[4] performed dye dilution studies on small-bowel segments to describe these relationships. These investigators found that infusion of 0.9% sodium chloride solution above a certain critical flow rate resulted in faster fluid transit time and produced diarrhea rather than increasing (distending) intestinal volume. Love et al.[5] found similar results with total intestinal perfusion. When an isotonic electrolyte solution containing sodium chloride, potassium chloride, and sodium bicarbonate was ingested at rates less than 70 mL/min, the ingestion rate was directly proportional to the intestinal volume. However, at flow rates greater than 70 mL/min, the intestinal volume remained relatively constant and increasing flow rates resulted in faster fluid transport through the gut. Apparently, a limit is reached beyond which the gut is resistant to dilatation and increasing flow rates are handled by proportionally decreasing transit times. The absorptive capacity of the bowel appears to reach a maximum at similar flow rates. At these flow rates where intestinal volume and absorptive capacity reach a maximum, the fluid volume (mL/kg of body weight) required to produce diarrhea remains relatively constant and is not influenced by the solution osmolarity or temperature.[6] Therefore, WBI with isotonic electrolyte solutions produces diarrhea when the infusion rate exceeds the capacity of the intestine to distend and absorb the solution.

Solutions and Administration Techniques for Whole-Bowel Irrigation

The various solutions used for WBI are outlined in Table 1. The electrolyte concentrations in the majority of solutions are isotonic to reduce the possibility of serum electrolyte disturbances during irrigation, and all but the hypertonic mannitol solutions have an osmolarity similar to plasma.

Mannitol solutions have been studied as an adjunct and an alternative to electrolyte solutions.[7–13] When taken orally in quantities of greater than 40 g, mannitol, a poorly absorbed carbohydrate, produces osmotic diarrhea[11] with little or no fluid absorption.[7,9]

In 1980, Davis et al.[14,15] introduced a new solution for WBI designed to prevent net fluid and electrolyte changes. This solution contains polyethylene glycol (average molecular weight of 3350) and sodium sulfate in addition to the sodium chloride, potassium chloride, and sodium bicarbonate that are in previously used solutions.

Polyethylene glycol 3350 (PEG) is a mixture of ethylene glycol polymers commonly used in ointment and suppository bases. PEG has also been used as a nonabsorbable volume marker in intestinal perfusion and flow studies with the assumption that it does not influence water and electrolyte

Table 1.
Solutions Used for Whole-Bowel Irrigation

	Concentrations of Ingredients (meq/L)								
Solutions	Sodium	Potassium	Chloride	Bicarbonate	Sulfate	Mannitol	Polyethylene Glycol	Osmolarity (mOsm/L)	Reference No.
0.9% sodium chloride	154	...	154	...	...	...	...	308	4, 7, 9, 27, 28 32, 34
Sodium chloride with potassium chloride	140–154	4–13	144–167	...	...	...	...	288–334	8, 27, 33, 57
"Balanced" electrolyte solutions	132–140	10	112–121	30–35	...	...	...	254–306	23, 24, 26, 28, 30, 31, 36 61, 62, 64, 65
	35	2.4	28.4	8.8	...	...	...	75	67
Lactated Ringer's[a]	130	4	109	...	...	...	...	273	29, 58
Mannitol 5%	...	...	...	...	...	50 g/L	...	274	7, 8
10%	...	...	...	...	...	100 g/L	...	549	7, 9, 10–12
20%	...	...	...	...	...	200 g/L	...	1098	12
Balanced electrolyte solution with mannitol and polyethylene glycol	125	10	35	20	80	80	5 g/L	273	14
Balanced electrolyte solution with polyethylene glycol	125	10	35	20	80	...	59.0–60.0 g/L	263–280	1, 14, 36–39, 51 55, 56, 63 64, 66

[a] Also contains calcium 3 meq/L and lactate 28 meq/L.

movement.[16-19] To test this assumption, Davis et al.[15] studied water and electrolyte absorption rates in 30-cm segments of jejunum and ileum in 22 normal subjects. The solutions tested contained sodium 135 meq/L, potassium 5 meq/L, chloride 110 meq/L, bicarbonate 30 meq/L, xylose 10 meq/L, and PEG 1, 2, 5, 10, or 20 g/L. Multilumen nasogastric tubes placed under fluoroscopic guidance were used to administer the solution and to withdraw samples of fluid from different intestinal segments for measurement of electrolytes and osmolarity. PEG was shown to inhibit jejunal and ileal absorption of water, sodium, and chloride, with higher concentrations of PEG resulting in a greater degree of inhibition. The inhibition of water, sodium, and chloride absorption by PEG was thought to be caused by the osmotic pressure across intestinal mucosal cell membranes and possibly because of the inhibition of active sodium or chloride secretion in the bowel lumen.[15] Although the authors of this study questioned the validity of previous intestinal flow-rate calculations where PEG was used as a marker, they introduced the idea of using PEG to prevent fluid absorption with WBI fluids.

In an effort to develop a WBI solution with minimal effects on water and electrolyte absorption and secretion, these same investigators studied several electrolyte solutions containing varying concentrations of sodium chloride, potassium chloride, sodium bicarbonate, and sodium sulfate with mannitol or PEG or both.[14] Sodium sulfate was added because active sodium absorption is markedly reduced when sulfate is substituted for chloride,[20] and sulfate itself is a poorly absorbed anion.[21] The solutions were administered to normal volunteers by nasogastric tube at a rate of 20–30 mL/min. Rectal effluent was analyzed for osmolality and PEG and electrolyte concentrations. Net water and electrolyte movement was also calculated. The concentrations of electrolytes and PEG in the solution were adjusted until negligible movement of water and electrolytes occurred. The final solution, containing sodium chloride 1.47 g/L, sodium sulfate 5.68 g/L, potassium chloride 0.75 g/L, sodium bicarbonate 1.68 g/L, and PEG 59.0 g/L (sodium 125 meq/L, chloride 35 meq/L, potassium 10 meq/L, bicarbonate 20 meq/L, sulfate 80 meq/L), was associated with mild water secretion (60 mL/hr) and near zero net movement of electrolytes. Two WBI products using this PEG-electrolyte solution formulation recently gained FDA approval.[a,b]

Techniques for administering WBI solutions vary considerably. Solution administration rates vary from 15 to 90 mL/min, by oral ingestion or by nasogastric tube,[22,23] with total volumes ranging from 1 to 20 liters.[24,25] Some investigators have used warmed solutions,[7,9,22,25-34] while others have chilled or flavored the irrigant to improve palatability.[1,9-13,23,35-39] The onset of diarrhea occurs as soon as 20 minutes[29] after beginning irrigation with clearing of the effluent occurring as early as 90 minutes[26] or as late as 12 hours.[33] Faster rates of administration appear to shorten overall cleansing time,[23,40] but the relationship of irrigation administration rate and time to colon cleansing has not been specifically evaluated.

Evaluation of Mechanical Bowel Cleansing

Criteria for the effectiveness of bowel cleansing by WBI vary with the procedure for which the bowel is being prepared. Although no definite standards exist, some general statements can be made concerning what constitutes adequate bowel cleansing.

The primary goal of mechanical bowel preparation before colorectal surgery is to rid the bowel of feces. Removal of fecal material from the bowel with resultant collapse of the intestine facilitates handling of the bowel at operation and reduces patient morbidity and mortality.[41,42] Although mechanical bowel preparation alone does not reduce the concentration of residual microorganisms in the colon at the time of operation,[43,44] it does reduce the total number of bacteria and possibly the rate of wound infections and potentially fatal anastomatic leaks.[31,45-48] Therefore, mechanical bowel cleansing regimens for colorectal surgery should be evaluated by their ability to remove fecal contents, reduce bacterial counts, and prevent postoperative infectious complications.

Thorough cleansing of the colon is also essential for satisfactory diagnostic examinations. Inadequate bowel preparation for colonoscopy and barium enema may lead to incorrect or misleading diagnosis and is frequently the cause of repeat examination.[3,49,50] For colonoscopic examination, excess fluid residue, easily aspirated through the colonoscope, does not present a major problem.[10,37,51] However, solid fecal residue interferes with visualization of the bowel mucosa and must be removed.[52,53]

The diagnostic quality of a barium enema radiograph is proportional to the degree of colon cleansing. Residual solid, liquid, and gaseous colonic contents are difficult to distinguish from pathologic lesions.[49,54] While excess fluid does not necessarily interfere with a single-contrast barium enema, it may prevent the adequate barium coating of the mucosa necessary for a diagnostic double-air-contrast barium enema.[55,56]

Clinical Studies

It is difficult to compare the results of the different studies of WBI as a colon cleansing technique for several reasons. One problem is that the patient characteristics, solutions, and administration techniques vary considerably. Second, efficacy is not always evaluated objectively. Furthermore, although several blinded and randomized comparative studies are available, the control groups did not receive consistent mechanical bowel preparations. Our review includes all English-language clinical studies of WBI preparation for colorectal surgery, colonoscopy, and barium enema with a special emphasis on the comparative studies with well-defined, objective efficacy criteria.

Colorectal Surgery. WBI with 0.9% sodium chloride, lactated Ringer's, and other "balanced" electrolyte solutions before colorectal surgery has been judged successful in 80–94% of cases.[26–28,33,48,57] The studies evaluated fecal matter and free fluid in the gut and collapse of the gut mucosa at operation, although not all assessments were objective. Only two controlled trials have been conducted that compared electrolyte WBI to other methods for preoperative preparation of the colon. Chung et al.[58] compared the efficacy of WBI with lactated Ringer's solution to a regimen consisting of a clear liquid diet, magnesium citrate, and 0.9% sodium chloride solution enemas in 41 patients scheduled for colon surgery. Patients in the WBI group were given a regular diet until noon the day before surgery, after which they were allowed nothing by mouth. On the afternoon before surgery, six liters of warmed lactated Ringer's solution was infused by nasogastric tube over three hours. The WBI method more frequently resulted in collapse of the small and large intestine, as judged at the time of surgery, while the clear liquid/magnesium citrate/enema regimen resulted in more fluid retained in the small intestine, although the difference was not significant. In 30 of the 41 patients requiring colon resection, solid and liquid colonic content was measured in the resected segments. Only four patients had visible feces in the lumen, and no significant differences between the groups in the amount of retained feces was found. Subjective assessment of the quality of the bowel preparation noted unsatisfactory results only rarely with either regimen. Christensen and colleagues[30] compared the effectiveness of WBI with a solution containing sodium chloride 6 g/L, sodium bicarbonate 2.5 g/L, and potassium chloride 0.75 g/L with a regimen consisting of a fluid diet, oral cascara sagrada, and 0.9% sodium chloride solution enemas in 100 patients scheduled for colorectal surgery. Patients in the WBI group received the solution by nasogastric tube at a rate of 3–4 L/hr until the rectal effluent was clear. The mean volume administered was 8.8 L over a period of 2.75 hours. Collapse of the small and large intestine, as evaluated at surgery by a blinded investigator, was more frequent after WBI than after the fluid diet/cascara/enema preparation.

Two additional studies have compared WBI using electrolyte solutions with mannitol for colorectal surgery. In a prospective study of 42 patients requiring bowel preparation for surgery, Donovan et al.[9] compared a regimen using 0.9% sodium chloride solution at 3–6 L/hr (control) with an identical regimen preceded by 500 mL of 20% mannitol. The study was not randomized, as patients with constipation or suspected stenosis were placed in the mannitol group. In the WBI/mannitol group, 86% of patients had successful preparations, defined as little or no fecal residue in the colon at operation, compared with 52% in the control (WBI only) group. Mannitol significantly reduced the time and amount of irrigant required to produce clear fecal effluent. These results were confirmed by Minevini et al.[7] who found WBI with 0.9% sodium chloride solution plus 50 g of 10% mannitol superior to either agent alone, as judged by fecal residue present at the time of surgery.

PEG-electrolyte lavage solutions (PEG-ELSs) have been evaluated as a preoperative bowel preparation in one published study, and information from two recent abstracts of studies is also available. Ambrose et al.[1] compared WBI with a PEG-ELS containing sodium sulfate, sodium chloride, potassium chloride, sodium bicarbonate, and PEG 59.1 g/L (Table 1) with a regimen consisting of oral liquid sennoside plus retrograde rectal washout. Seventy-seven patients were randomly allocated to receive either liquid sennoside/rectal washout or WBI with PEG-ELS orally or by nasogastric tube. Patients in the WBI groups ingested the solution at a rate of 1–2 L/hr until the rectal effluent became clear. The average volume of PEG-ELS consumed was 4.5 L over a period of four hours. Preparation effectiveness was assessed at the time of surgery according to the amount of fecal residue present in the colon. Eight-two percent of patients in the WBI groups had adequate preparation (no residue or only fluid residue) compared with 77% in the liquid sennoside/rectal washout group. Poor preparation (solid fecal residue) was noted in 23% of the liquid sennoside/rectal washout group compared with 17% in the WBI groups; none of these differences were significant. Comparing these results with previous studies,[7] the authors concluded that the PEG-ELS was an effective alternative to mannitol and 0.9% sodium chloride solution for preoperative WBI. Fleites et al.[59] compared the efficacy of WBI with PEG-ELS (sodium sulfate, sodium chloride, potassium chloride, sodium bicarbonate, PEG 59.1 g/L) to a three-day regimen of restricted diet, bisacodyl, magnesium citrate, and enemas in patients undergoing elective colonic resection. The PEG-ELS was as effective as the diet/cathartic/enema preparation as judged by residual fecal material in the bowel. Because the WBI was rapid and well tolerated, the authors considered it the preparation of choice for elective colonic resection. DiPalma et al.[60] found the PEG-ELS plus bisacodyl tablets superior to a regimen of clear liquids, magnesium citrate, liquid sennosides, and enemas for preparation before colon surgery in 31 patients, but specific rating criteria were not given.

WBI, like other mechanical bowel-cleansing regimens, reduces the total number of colonic bacteria but not the concentration of residual microorganisms in the bowel lumen.[26,42] WBI alone has not proven acceptable in preventing postoperative wound infection and sepsis.[31,48] Gottrup et al.[48] studied infection rates following WBI with 0.9% sodium chloride solution in 135 patients undergoing elective colorectal surgery. The patients were randomly assigned to receive WBI alone, WBI plus intravenous metronidazole, or WBI plus ampicillin and metronidazole. Abdominal wound infection rates were greatest in the group that received WBI alone (32%) and least in the group that received WBI plus ampicillin and metronidazole (2%). Intra-abdominal abscesses also occurred more frequently in the group that received no antimicrobial agents than in either of the other two groups, but the difference was not statistically significant. The incidence of postoperative infection was related to the preparation effectiveness when antimicrobial agents were not given, but this relationship was not significant when antimicrobial agents were administered. Both Chung[58] and Christensen[30] observed similar postoperative infection rates in patients who received WBI and in those who received liquid diet, enemas, and magnesium citrate or cascara when both groups were given identical preoperative antibiotic regimens of intramuscular gentamicin/clindamycin or intravenous ampicillin/metronidazole. However, better intestinal evacuation with WBI decreased the incidence of anastomotic leaks, which can lead to lethal septic complications.[30,33] In contrast, Guttrup et al.[48] found no correlation between bowel content and clinical signs of anastomotic leakage following preparation with WBI with or without antibiotics. The authors postulated that surgical technique was more important in determining the incidence of anastomotic leak than the degree of bowel cleansing.

Colonoscopy. WBI has been extensively evaluated as a cleansing regimen before colonoscopy. Rhodes and colleagues[61] compared the effectiveness of WBI with a preparation consisting of a clear liquid diet for three days plus magnesium sulfate, bisacodyl tablets, and suppositories given the day before examination in 60 patients undergoing colonoscopy. On the morning of the examination, patients in the WBI group ingested 2.5–3.5 L of an isotonic electrolyte solution containing sodium chloride 6.14 g/L, potassium chloride 0.75 g/L, and sodium bicarbonate 2.95 g/L over one hour. The adequacy of the preparation was evaluated at the time of examination using a predefined rating scale. Small accumulations of feces not interfering with a thorough examination were considered good results while no more than small bits of adherent feces were judged excellent. Good or excellent results were obtained in 93% of patients in the WBI group compared with 77% in the diet/magnesium sulfate/bisacodyl group. In another study using an identical solution and rating scale, the same investigators found an 85% success rate with WBI that improved to 95% when 10 mg of oral metoclopramide was given 30 minutes before the irrigation to promote gastric emptying.[62] Other studies have confirmed successful colon preparation in greater than 90% of patients prepared for colonoscopy with isotonic electrolyte or 0.9% sodium chloride WBI, although no objective assessment criteria were specified.[27,28] One investigator found that a 2000-mL 0.9% sodium chloride solution enema on the morning of colonoscopy was necessary for a consistently clean bowel in patients prepared the evening before colonoscopy with 0.9% sodium chloride irrigation.[32]

Gilmore et al.[8] compared WBI using 0.9% sodium chloride solution plus potassium chloride 1 g/L with irrigation using 5% mannitol in 38 patients being prepared for colonoscopy. The adequacy of preparation was judged by blinded colonoscopists according to fecal residue, volume of fluid, and overall acceptability, although no specific assessment criteria were mentioned. One hundred percent of patients in the group receiving 0.9% sodium chloride solution had excellent or satisfactory preparations compared with 88% in the mannitol group. The volume of residual fluid in both groups was more than that experienced after other mechanical bowel preparations but was easily aspirated during the examination. Newstead et al.[10] confirmed these results, reporting an excellent preparation (no fecal or fluid residue) in 88% of 50 patients receiving 500 mL of 10% mannitol orally the evening before colonoscopy.

PEG-ELS has been evaluated as a colon-cleansing method before colonoscopy in several studies.[36,37,51,63] The solution, consisting of sodium chloride, sodium sulfate, potassium chloride, sodium bicarbonate, and PEG 59.1 g/L (Table 1), was ingested orally at rates of 12.5–30 mL/min in volumes ranging from 1.2 to 8 liters. Fecal evacuant was usually clear within three hours. Good to excellent colon cleansing, with little or no fecal residue, and adequate bowel-wall visualization were achieved in 95% of patients. When compared with a three-day regimen of clear liquid diet, magnesium citrate, oral bisacodyl, and tap-water enemas in a randomized, blinded study, the PEG-ELS resulted in significantly better bowel-wall visualization and significantly less fecal residue.[37] In a similar randomized, blinded study, the PEG-ELS resulted in a cleaner colon than a regimen of a three-day minimal residue diet, magnesium citrate, bisacodyl tablets, and tap-water enemas, but the difference was not significant.[63] Although both preparations were considered adequate, the investigators in each of these studies considered the PEG-ELS the preparation of choice for colonoscopy. Preparation with this solution resulted in up to a liter of residual fluid in the bowel, but this was easily aspirated through the colonoscope and was less of a problem if WBI was performed the evening before rather than the morning of the examination.[36,51] Adler et al.[64] demonstrated significantly better colonoscopy preparation with a PEG-ELS compared with a balanced electrolyte solution containing sodium 133 meq/L, potassium 9.4 meq/L, chloride 112 meq/L, and bicarbonate 30 meq/L, although the criteria for effectiveness were not objective.

Barium Enema. Two blinded, controlled studies have compared WBI using isotonic electrolyte solutions with regimens consisting of castor oil plus tap water or 0.9% sodium chloride solution enemas for bowel cleansing before single-contrast barium enema examination.[24,65] In both studies, a solution containing sodium chloride 6.5 g/L, sodium bicarbonate 2.5 g/L, and potassium chloride 0.75 g/L was ingested at a rate of 1 liter every 40 minutes until the rectal effluent was clear. The volume of solution required ranged from 1 to 6 liters. Preparation adequacy was evaluated according to amount of gas and feces on abdominal scout films, gas and feces interference on barium enema, and clarity of mucosal pattern on radiographs. No significant difference was noted between the two groups in each study except for the presence of gas on scout films and barium enema radiographs that was more pronounced in the WBI group. Success rates in patients who completed the preparation were 85% and 86%, respectively, in the WBI group for each study compared with 95% and 90%, respectively, in the castor oil/enema groups in the two studies. Twelve percent of patients in the WBI groups were unable to complete the preparation; the cause of this was not mentioned. When results from patients not able to complete the regimen were included in the statistical analysis, the success rates for WBI dropped to 76.6% and 83.3%, respectively, in the two studies.[24,65] In another study of 60 patients requiring single-contrast barium enema, a three-day regimen consisting of a clear liquid diet, magnesium citrate, and bisacodyl produced good (small amount of feces not interfering with examination) to excellent (no visible feces) results in 63% of patients compared with 86% success in the group prepared with WBI. Poor preparation, requiring further cleansing and repeat examination, occurred in one patient in each group.[61]

When compared with a regimen consisting of a low residue diet, magnesium sulfate, castor oil, and bisacodyl suppositories as preparation for single-contrast barium enema, WBI with 1 L of 10% mannitol produced significantly better quality examinations with less fecal residue.[13]

PEG-ELS has not been evaluated as a preparation for single-contrast barium enema, but one subjective report indicated that this solution was acceptable.[39]

WBI has also been evaluated as a preparation for double-contrast barium enema with mixed results. In a study of healthy men prepared with an isotonic solution of sodium chloride, potassium chloride, and sodium bicarbonate, Skucas et al.[23] subjectively rated 10 of 12 examinations excellent, particularly with regard to coating of the mucosa. Fluid retention was not detectable in eight examinations, and only a minimal amount was detected in two. Retained stool could be detected in only two subjects. Similar results were noted by King et al.[29] in a controlled study comparing WBI using lactated Ringer's solution with a preparation consisting of castor oil and retrograde colonic lavage. Diagnostic quality was judged according to fecal matter present in the bowel. Success rates were 85% in the WBI group compared with 62% in the alternative group. The only observed undesirable effect of WBI on the quality of the examination was a significant degree of contrast-media dilution produced by retained lavage solution in the terminal small bowel and proximal colon. This occurred in only a few patients and in no case was sufficient to make the examination nondiagnostic. The authors postulated that dilution with irrigation fluid could be avoided if the time between completion of the preparation and start of the examination was longer than the minimum of one hour used in this study. However, Skucas[23] found minimal problem with fluid retention when examinations were begun as soon as 40 minutes after completion of WBI.

In contrast to these results, Bakran et al.[22] found WBI with 0.9% sodium chloride solution inadequate as preparation for double-contrast barium enema. This regimen was compared with a group that received liquid senna extract (X-prep, Gray Pharmaceutical Co., Norwalk, CT) the evening before examination followed by retrograde colonic lavage immediately before the barium enema. In both groups, one to three hours elapsed between the completion of the preparation and the beginning of the examination. No significant difference in residual feces between the groups was noted; however, the degree of solution retention in the saline lavage group with resultant poor mucosal coating presented a major problem in diagnostic quality of the examinations.

Lee et al.[12] evaluated WBI using 200 g of mannitol with and without retrograde colonic washout for double-contrast barium enema preparation and found this to be inferior to a regimen of liquid senna extract plus colonic washout. The radiographs were assessed under blinded conditions for amount and particle size of fecal residue. Although the mannitol produced a more severe purgation, it did not result in better fecal clearance. Foord et al.[11] evaluated several methods of administering mannitol as a preparation for double-contrast barium enema. The preparations were again assessed according to amount and particle size of fecal residue. As a result of this work, the authors recommended a regimen consisting of three days of a low residue diet with liquids only on the day before examination plus 1 L of 10% mannitol in four divided doses on the evening before the barium enema. Delaying the examination until the afternoon allowed for better clearance of fecal and fluid residue. This regimen, although acceptable, appears to negate the advantage of rapid preparation with WBI. The quality of mucosal coating after air insufflation was not specifically addressed in either study.[11,12] In a subjective evaluation, Palmer et al.[13] found significantly better mucosal coating after WBI after 1 L of 10% mannitol compared with a regimen of a low residue diet, castor oil, magnesium, and bisacodyl suppositories. Twenty-one of 23 patients in the mannitol group had adequate (7 of 21) to good (14 of 21) barium mucosal coating after air insufflation.

Davis and Smith[66] evaluated WBI using a solution consisting of sodium sulfate, sodium chloride, potassium chloride, sodium bicarbonate, and 80 m*M* per liter of mannitol as a preparation for double-contrast barium enema. This solution was similar to the PEG-ELS developed by these investigators except mannitol was substituted for the PEG (Table 1). Twenty patients were prospectively randomized to receive either WBI with the mannitol/electrolyte solution or a two-day regimen consisting of a low residue diet, bisacodyl tablets, magnesium sulfate, and tap-water enemas with bisacodyl tannex. Patients in the WBI group ingested the solution at a rate of 1.8–2.0 L/hr until the rectal effluent was clear. The mean (± S.D.) volume ingested was 3.5 ± 0.5 L over an average of 2.7 ± 0.5 hr. Examination was delayed until at least six hours after completing the irrigation. The radiographs were graded under blinded conditions on five points: amount of gas on scout film, amount of feces on scout film, amount of feces on barium study, residual fluid on barium enema, and quality of mucosal coating. WBI appeared better at removing feces; however, no statistical evaluation was performed. Both preparations produced adequate mucosal coating, but those in the diet/bisacodyl/magnesium sulfate/enema group had better scores in this category. There was more residual fluid following WBI, but this was minimal and did not interfere with the adequacy of the examinations. Patients in the WBI group also did not score as well with respect to gas on the scout films. The authors concluded that WBI with the mannitol/electrolyte solution was at least as effective as the alternative preparation.

WBI with PEG-ELSs has been evaluated as a preparation for double-contrast barium enema in several comparative studies. In a randomized, blinded study of 36 patients scheduled for double-contrast barium enema, WBI with a solution composed of sodium sulfate, sodium chloride, potassium chloride, sodium bicarbonate, and PEG 59.1 g/L was compared with a two-day mechanical bowel preparation consisting of a clear liquid diet, magnesium citrate, bisacodyl tablets, and enemas.[37] The PEG-ELS was ingested the evening before the examination at a rate of 1–1.25 L/hr until the rectal effluent cleared, with a mean ± S.D. volume of 3.5 ± 0.2 L consumed. The radiographs were scored according to the amount and particle size of residual fecal material. No significant difference in the quality of examination between the two groups was found; however, successful preparations were obtained in only 70% of both groups. Residual fluid did not appear to be a problem although the quality of the mucosal coating was not specifically addressed. In a similar study, Girard et al.[55] compared WBI using PEG-ELS with a regimen of a low residue/liquid diet, magnesium sulfate, and bisacodyl tablets (control) as preparation for double-contrast barium enema. The PEG-ELS was ingested at a rate of 1.5 L/hr on the evening before the examination. An average of 2.8 L was required to produce a clear rectal effluent. Both methods were adequate at removing fecal material but the diet/magnesium sulfate/bisacodyl control group had significantly more radiographs with no residual feces (excellent preparation) or only small, nonadherent particles (good preparation). Diagnostic quality mucosal coating was seen in only 33% of the WBI group compared with 71% of the control group. However, when 20 mg of bisacodyl tablets was taken immediately following WBI, fecal clearance was greatly improved, and the number of radiographs with diagnostic quality mucosal coating increased to 74%. The authors concluded that WBI with PEG-ELS plus oral bisacodyl was a reasonable alternative for double-contrast barium enema preparation. Finally, in a brief report, Thoeni[56] noted his results in 10 patients prepared for double-contrast barium enema with PEG-ELS WBI. The colon was free of feces in all patients, but none of the examinations was diagnostic because excess fluid in the colon prevented adequate mucosal coating.

The reasons for these conflicting reports concerning the effectiveness of WBI preparation for double-contrast barium enema are not readily apparent. Wide variations exist in solutions used, technique of administration, rates of ingestion, quantity of fluid ingested, employment of ancillary drugs to promote gastric emptying, and the interval between completion of the irrigation and performance of the examination. Additionally, the type of barium used, the method of its preparation, or barium density may all influence the quality of the barium radiograph.[66]

Adverse Reactions

Gastrointestinal complaints including nausea, vomiting, cramping, bloating, and abdominal distention are the most frequently reported side effects of WBI.[9,11,22–24,29,31,33,36,37,40,51,55,61,65] The incidence of these side effects ranged from 0 to 100% in the various trials.[29,32,58] It is difficult to compare these studies because different fluid administration rates and volumes were used, solutions were given orally or by nasogastric tube, and patient characteristics were not consistent. Overall, the prevalence of mild gastrointestinal discomfort appears to be about 33%, with even fewer patients requiring discontinuation or alteration of the fluid. Although these reactions are generally not serious, Sogge and Butler[67] have reported a case of Mallory-Weiss syndrome secondary to severe vomiting in a 65-year-old patient prepared for colonoscopy by WBI with an isotonic solution of sodium chloride, potassium chloride, and sodium bicarbonate. The vomiting was thought to be caused by delayed gastric emptying and an extremely rapid solution administration rate of 3.5 liters over 40 minutes. The addition of metoclopramide (given orally or parenterally) at the start of WBI or during WBI has been advocated by some to reduce gastrointestinal distress,[8,22,25,30–32,34,55] while other authors believe its routine use is not justified.[37,58] In a placebo-controlled trial by Rhodes et al.,[62] metoclopramide 10 mg administered orally 30 minutes before beginning the irrigation significantly decreased the incidence of bloating and nausea. Vomiting and cramping were also decreased but the difference was not significant. In contrast, Brady et al.[68] found no significant difference in the overall incidence of gastrointestinal complaints or preparation effectiveness between patients receiving premedication with 10 or 20 mg of oral metoclopramide and placebo. Rhodes et al.[62] used much faster solution administration rates in their patients (3 L/hr) than were used in the Brady study (1.5 L/hr).[68] This could account for a high incidence of symptoms associated with volume overload that may be relieved by metoclopramide. Slower and carefully controlled fluid administration rates may also decrease gastrointestinal discomfort.[22,29,34,58]

Water and sodium absorption with potential circulatory overload is a major concern with WBI. Several investigators have measured weight gain and electrolyte changes during WBI. Weight gained from ingestion of 1–15 L of electrolyte irrigation solutions ranged from a mean of 1.1 to 2.3 kg.[22–24,27,28,30,58,65] Weight gain during WBI may be partially attributable to retained fluid in the bowel;[23] however, actual fluid and electrolyte absorption has been documented by changes in fecal water and electrolytes and packed red-cell volume.[22,61,64] One study reweighed patients the day following the procedure and found that an initial average weight gain of 1.6 kg decreased to 0.5 kg 24 hours later.[58] Although changes have been noted in blood urea nitrogen, hematocrit, hemoglobin and serum, fecal and urine electrolytes following electrolyte WBI, they have not been found to be clinically important.[22–24,27,31,58,61,65] It is important to note that nearly all studies of electrolyte WBI excluded elderly patients and patients with congestive heart failure, renal disease, and inflammatory bowel disease. Some investigators administered furosemide prophylactically to prevent fluid overload.[30,68] Smith et al.[25] used WBI with 0.9% sodium chloride solution to treat constipation in 70 elderly patients (mean age 80 yr), some of whom had a history of cardiac failure. All patients received 40 mg of furosemide before the lavage. Weight changes ranged from −3.0 to +5.9 kg (mean weight gain of 1.0 kg), and no significant changes in hemoglobin, blood urea nitrogen, serum electrolytes, or osmolality occurred. Most investigators agree, however, that WBI with electrolyte solutions is contraindicated in patients with congestive heart failure, renal failure, and possibly inflammatory bowel disease because greater fluid absorption is likely with abnormal bowel mucosa.

WBI with mannitol solutions appears to cause less fluid absorption than 0.9% sodium chloride and other electrolyte solutions. In a study comparing WBI using 0.9% sodium chloride solution with an identical regimen preceded by 500 mL of 20% mannitol, no significant changes in serum electrolytes occurred in either group, but mannitol significantly decreased fluid absorption from 2.7 to 1.2 L.[9] These results were confirmed by Minervini et al.[7] who found that sodium and water retention was reduced when mannitol was added to 0.9% sodium chloride irrigation while mannitol alone resulted in an insignificant fluid gain and a slight decrease in serum sodium concentration. No changes in serum potassium concentrations occurred in any of the groups. In a study by Newstead et al.,[10] patients irrigated with 500 mL of 10% mannitol experienced an average net fluid loss of 478 mL and an average weight loss of 1.89 kg, although no serious complications were noted. WBI with 5% mannitol has also resulted in decreased body weight, blood pressure, and plasma volume.[8] In the same study, 12 patients prepared with a combination of 10% mannitol and 0.9% sodium chloride had a less significant decrease in plasma volume.[8]

Although mannitol may be an effective addition or alternative to electrolyte WBI in patients at risk for fluid overload, its safety has been questioned. In 1979, Bigard et al.[69] reported a case of fatal colonic explosion during colonoscopic electrosurgical polypectomy after bowel preparation with a mannitol-containing oral lavage solution. Two gases produced by colonic bacteria, hydrogen, and methane, are combustible and potentially explosive if the oxygen concentration of the gas mixture is greater than 5%. Although the production of methane has no clear-cut relation to diet, colonic bacteria require a constant supply of exogenous substrate, primarily unabsorbed carbohydrate, to produce hydrogen. Rigorous bowel-cleaning preparation for colonoscopy reduces intestinal gases to below dangerous levels; however, mannitol preparation has been shown to increase the number of gas-producing bacteria (primarily *E. coli*) and concentrations of hydrogen and methane to potentially explosive levels.[70-74] Mannitol has also been associated with an increase in postoperative sepsis caused by *E. coli*.[75] Routine use of carbon dioxide insufflation during colonic polypectomy has been recommended to prevent the possibility of explosion,[71,76] but most authors agree that an alternative osmotic cathartic, which will not provide a nutrient for gas-producing bacteria, is more practical.[70,72,77]

PEG–WBI solutions were specifically developed to prevent the fluid and electrolyte disturbances seen with isotonic electrolyte solutions and mannitol.[14] Initially tested in normal volunteers, the solution containing PEG 59.1–60.0 g/L and sodium sulfate, as the major electrolyte (Table 1), has resulted in minimal water and electrolyte absorption or secretion.[1,14,15,36,37,51,55,63,64] Use in small numbers of elderly patients and patients with congestive heart failure, renal failure, chronic obstructive pulmonary disease, and cirrhosis indicates that PEG-ELSs may be safe in patients who have an increased risk of circulatory overload.[1,14,36,37,64] Combustible levels of hydrogen and methane have not been found after WBI with PEG-ELSs.[1,14,63]

Recently, concern has been expressed regarding the safety of orally administered polyethylene glycol in man.[78-83] Fecal recovery following the oral ingestion of PEG has been reported to range from 96.3 to 100.1%.[16,18,19] Oral ingestion of 4 L of commercially available PEG-ELSs (containing PEG 60.0 g/L) could result in a potential systemic dose of 9.6 g of PEG assuming 4% absorption.[78] A recent abstract indicated absorption of only 0.3% following a 240-g oral dose of PEG,[84] but plasma concentrations of PEG have not yet been determined. Absorption of lower-molecular-weight polyethylene glycols from topical preparations has resulted in increased serum osmolality and toxicity similar to ethylene glycol ingestion, but these results cannot be extrapolated to higher-molecular-weight compounds.[85-87] More extensive pharmacologic studies are needed to confirm the safety of PEG in man.

In a recent study, no abnormalities in colonic mucosal histology were found following the ingestion of 3–4 L of PEG-ELS, whereas magnesium citrate plus liquid sennosides resulted in flattened surface epithelial cells, an increase in lamina propria edema, and depletion of goblet cells, which could interfere with pathologic diagnoses.[88]

Patient acceptance of WBI, particularly with PEG-ELSs, has been good, with a large number of patients who had previously received other bowel preparations preferring the lavage method.[24,26-28,32,36,51,58,61,63,68] In a survey of patient opinion, the most common complaints with WBI were gastrointestinal distress, discomfort of nasogastric tubes used to administer the solutions, and prolonged sitting on the commode during the preparation. Only 5% stated that they would refuse a repeated preparation if necessary.[34]

FDA-Approved PEG-Electrolyte Lavage Solutions

Two PEG-ELSs[a,b] have recently gained FDA approval for mechanical bowel cleansing before gastrointestinal examination. The recommended administration rate is 1.2–1.8 L/hr orally or by nasogastric tube until rectal effluent is clear.[89,90] In most patients this will require a maximum of 4–6 L. The rapid ingestion of 200–300 mL every 10 minutes rather than slow continuous drinking is preferred. One company recommends a continuous rate of 20–30 mL/min for nasogastric tube administration.[90] The patient should fast for three to four hours before ingesting the solution.[89,90] Routine use of metoclopramide premedication is probably not justified but may be helpful in patients with delayed gastric emptying.

The use of flavoring agents in the solutions is not recommended because of the possible fermentation of added ingredients to potentially explosive gases.[73,89,90] The addition of any sugar to the solution may also stimulate the absorption of sodium in the small bowel.[23]

Conclusion

WBI is an effective alternative for rapid mechanical bowel cleansing before colorectal surgery or colonoscopy. Excessive fluid retention may interfere with the quality of barium enema radiographs; however, this problem may be minimized by completing the irrigation the evening before the examination.

Solutions containing PEG with sodium sulfate as the primary electrolyte result in less net water and electrolyte movement than other balanced electrolyte solutions and do not present the risks of dehydration and production of potentially explosive colonic gas seen with mannitol. Therefore, these PEG-ELSs are preferred over other solutions for WBI. The primary patient complaints with PEG-ELSs are salty taste and abdominal fullness.

Initial data indicate that PEG-ELSs are safe for use in stable patients at increased risk for fluid overload, such as those with chronic renal failure and congestive heart disease. WBI is contraindicated in patients with actual or suspected ileus, gastric-outlet obstruction, or bowel perforation. Its safety has not been determined in children, pregnant women, or patients with inflammatory bowel disease.

---

[a] Golytely, Braintree Laboratories, Inc., Braintree, MA 02184.
[b] Colyte, Edlaw Preparations, Inc., Farmingdale, NY 11735.

References

1. Ambrose NS, Johnson M, Burdon DW et al. A physiological appraisal of polyethylene glycol and a balanced electrolyte solution as a bowel preparation. *Br J Surg*. 1983; 70:428–30.
2. Hughes K, Mann S, Cooke MBD et al. A new oral bowel evacuant (Picolax) for colon cleansing. *Clin Radiol*. 1983; 34:75–7.
3. Brouwers JRBJ, van Ouwerkerk WPL, deBoer SM et al. A controlled trial of senna preparations and other laxatives used for bowel cleansing prior to radiological examination. *Pharmacology*. 1980; 20(Suppl 1):58–64.
4. Dillard RL, Eastman H, Fordtran JS. Volume-flow relationship during the transport of fluid through the human small intestine. *Gastroenterology*. 1965; 49:58–66.
5. Love AHG, Mitchell TG, Phillips RA. Water and sodium absorption in the human intestine. *J Physiol*. 1968; 195:133–40.
6. Shehadeh Z, Grantham RN, Brecher GA, et al. Effects of infusion rate and osmolarity on volumogenic diarrhea. *Gastroenterology*. 1969; 57:24–9.
7. Minervini S, Alexander-Williams J, Donovan IA et al. Comparison of three methods of whole bowel irrigation. *Am J Surg*. 1980; 140:400–2.
8. Gilmore IT, Ellis WR, Barrett GS et al. A comparison of two methods of whole gut lavage for colonoscopy. *Br J Surg*. 1981; 68:388–9.
9. Donovan IA, Arabi Y, Keighley MRB et al. Modification of the physiological disturbances produced by whole gut irrigation by preliminary mannitol administration. *Br J Surg*. 1980; 67:138–9.
10. Newstead GL, Morgan BP. Bowel preparation with mannitol. *Med J Aust*. 1979; 2:582–3.
11. Foord KD. Oral mannitol as a preparation for double-contrast barium enema. *Clin Radiol*. 1982; 33:467–9.
12. Lee JR, Hares MM, Keighley MRB. A randomised trial to investigate X-prep, oral mannitol and colonic washout for double-contrast barium enema. *Clin Radiol*. 1981; 32:591–4.
13. Palmer KR, Khan AN. Oral mannitol: a simple and effective bowel preparation for barium enema. *Br Med J*. 1979; 2:1038.
14. Davis GR, Santa Ana CA, Morawski SG et al. Development of a lavage solution associated with minimal water and electrolyte absorption of secretion. *Gastroenterology*. 1980; 78:991–5.
15. Davis GR, Santa Ana CA, Morawski SG et al. Inhibition of water and electrolyte absorption by polyethylene glycol (PEG). *Gastroenterology*. 1980; 79:35–9.
16. Wilkinson R. Polyethylene glycol 4000 as a continuously administered non-absorbable faecal marker for metabolic balance studies in human subjects. *Gut*. 1971; 12:654–60.
17. Allen LH, Raynolds WL, Margen S. Polyethylene glycol as a quantitative fecal marker in human nutrition experiments. *Am J Clin Nutr*. 1979; 32:427–40.
18. Shields R, Harris J, Davies MW. Suitability of polyethylene glycol as a dilution indicator in the human colon. *Gastroenterology*. 1968; 54:331–3.
19. Soergel KH, Hogan WJ. On the suitability of poorly absorbed markers as dilution indicators in the gastrointestinal tract. *Gastroenterology*. 1967; 52:1056–7.
20. Turnberg LA, Bieberdorf FA, Morkawski SG et al. Interrelationships of chloride, bicarbonate, sodium and hydrogen transport in the human ileum. *J Clin Invest*. 1970; 49:557–67.
21. Wilson TH. Fluid and electrolytes. In: Intestinal absorption. Philadelphia: WB Saunders Company; 1962:152.
22. Bakran A, Bradley JA, Bresnihan E et al. Whole gut irrigation: an inadequate preparation for double contrast barium enema examination. *Gastroenterology*. 1977; 73:28–30.
23. Skucas J, Cutcliff W, Fischer HW. Whole-gut irrigation as a means of cleaning the colon. *Radiology*. 1976; 121:303–5.
24. Levy AG, Benson JW, Hewlett EL et al. Saline lavage: a rapid, effective, and acceptable method for cleansing the gastrointestinal tract. *Gastroenterology*. 1976; 70:157–61.
25. Smith RG, Currie JEJ, Walls ADF. Whole gut irrigation: a new treatment for constipation. *Br Med J*. 1978; 1:396–7.
26. Hewitt J, Reeve J, Rigby J et al. Whole-gut irrigation in preparation for large-bowel surgery. *Lancet*. 1973; 2:337–40.
27. Crapp AR, Tillotson P, Powis SJA et al. Preparation of the bowel by whole-gut irrigation. *Lancet*. 1975; 2:1239–40.
28. Chambers CE, Carter HG. Saline lavage: a rapid, safe, effective method of whole-gut irrigation for bowel preparation. *S Med J*. 1978; 71:1065–6.
29. King DM, Downes MO, Heddle RM. An alternative method of bowel preparation for barium enemas. *Br J Radiol*. 1979; 52:388–9.
30. Christensen PB, Kronborg O. Whole-gut irrigation versus enema in elective colorectal surgery: a prospective, randomized study. *Dis Colon Rectum*. 1981; 24:592–5.
31. Raahave D, Hansen OH, Carstensen HE et al. Septic wound complications after whole bowel irrigation before colorectal operations. *Acta Chir Scand*. 1981; 147:215–8.
32. Glass RL, Winship DH, Rogers WA. Comparison of intragastric infusion with conventional mechanical bowel preparation. *Dis Colon Rectum*. 1981; 24:589–91.
33. Hartzenberg HB, McQuaide JR. Whole-gut irrigation as a preparation for colorectal surgery. *S Afr Med J*. 1982; 62:91–3.
34. Downing R, Dorricott NJ, Keighley MRB et al. Whole gut irrigation: a survey of patient opinion. *Br J Surg*. 1979; 66:201–2.
35. Hares MM, Nevah E, Minervini S et al. An attempt to reduce the side effects of mannitol bowel preparation by intravenous infusion. *Dis Colon Rectum*. 1982; 25:289–91.
36. Goldman J, Reichelderfer M. Evaluation of rapid colonoscopy preparation using a new gut lavage solution. *Gastrointest Endosc*. 1982; 28:9–11.
37. Ernstoff JJ, Howard DA, Marshall JB et al. A randomized blinded clinical trial of a rapid colonic lavage solution (golytely) compared with standard preparation for colonoscopy and barium enema. *Gastroenterology*. 1983; 84:1512–6.
38. Soergel KH, Wood CW, Brook J et al. More on "golytely." *Gastroenterology*. 1982; 83:729. Letter.
39. Meadows JO, Conyers CT. Golytely: preparation of choice for colonoscopy. *Gastrointest Endosc*. 1983; 29:256. Letter.
40. Inman VL, Jankowski NL. An ideal prep. *Soc Gastrointest Assist News*. 1979; 1:22–3.
41. Nichols RL, Gorbach SL, Condon RE. Alteration of intestinal microflora following preoperative mechanical preparation of the colon. *Dis Colon Rectum*. 1971; 14:123–7.
42. Nichols RL, Condon RE. Preoperative preparation of the colon. *Surg Gynecol Obstet*. 1971; 132:323–37.
43. Nichols RL, Condon RE, Gorbach SL et al. Efficacy of preoperative antimicrobial preparation of the bowel. *Ann Surg*. 1972; 176:227–32.
44. Arabi Y, Dimock F, Burdon DW et al. Influence of bowel preparation and antimicrobials on colonic microflora. *Br J Surg*. 1978; 65:555–9.
45. Hawley PR. Etiology of colonic anastomotic leaks. *Proc R Soc Med*. 1970; 63:752.
46. Barker K, Graham NG, Mason MC et al. The relative significance of preoperative oral antibiotics, mechanical bowel preparation and preoperative peritoneal contamination in the avoidance of sepsis after radical surgery for ulcerative colitis and Crohn's disease of the large bowel. *Br J Surg*. 1971; 58:270:3.
47. Irvin TT, Goligher JC. Etiology of disruption of intestinal anastomosis. *Br J Surg*. 1973; 60:461–4.
48. Gottrup F, Diederich P, Sorensen K et al. Prophylaxis with whole gut irrigation and antimicrobials in colorectal surgery. *Am J Surg*. 1985; 149:317–22.
49. Miller RE. The clean colon. *Gastroenterology*. 1976; 70:289–90.
50. Kendrick RGM, MacKenzie S, Beckly DE. A comparison of four methods of bowel preparation for barium enema. *Clin Radiol*. 1981; 32:95–7.
51. Thomas G, Brozinsky S, Isenberg JI. Patient acceptance and effectiveness of a balanced lavage solution (golytely) versus

the standard preparation for colonoscopy. *Gastroenterology.* 1982; 82:435–7.
52. Williams W, Teague R. Colonoscopy: a progress report. *Gut.* 1973; 14:990–1003.
53. Overholt BF. Colonoscopy: a review. *Gastroenterology.* 1975; 68:1308–20.
54. Dodds WJ, Scanlon T, Shaw DK et al. An evaluation of colon cleansing regimens. *Am J Roentgenol.* 1977; 128:57–9.
55. Girard CM, Rugh KS, DiPalma JA et al. Comparison of golytely lavage with standard diet/cathartic preparation for double-contrast barium enema. *Am J Roentgenol.* 1984; 142:1147–9.
56. Thoeni RF. More on "golytely." *Gastroenterology.* 1982; 83:729–30. Letter.
57. Grace RH. Whole gut irrigation. *Coloproctology.* 1980; 5:297–300.
58. Chung RS, Gurll NJ, Berglund EM. A controlled clinical trial of whole gut lavage as a method of bowel preparation for colonic operations. *Am J Surg.* 1979; 137:75–81.
59. Fleites RL, Marshall JB, Eckhauser ML et al. The efficacy and safety of golytely as a single day surgical bowel preparation for colonic resection. *Gastroenterology.* 1984; 86:1174. Abstract.
60. DiPalma JA, Brady CE, Girard CM et al. Comparison of golytely versus standard colon cleansing methods for diagnostic radiology and colon surgery. *Gastroenterology.* 1984; 86:1063. Abstract.
61. Rhodes JB, Zvargulis JE, Williams CH et al. Oral electrolyte overload to cleanse the colon for colonoscopy. *Gastrointest Endosc.* 1977; 24:24–6.
62. Rhodes JB, Engstrom J, Stone KF. Metoclopramide reduces the distress associated with colon cleansing by an oral electrolyte overload. *Gastrointest Endosc.* 1978; 24:162–3.
63. DiPalma JA, Brady CE, Stewart DL et al. Comparison of colon cleansing methods in preparation for colonoscopy. *Gastroenterology.* 1984; 86:856–60.
64. Adler M, Quenon M, Even-Adin D et al. Whole gut lavage for colonoscopy—a comparison between two solutions. *Gastrointest Endosc.* 1984; 30:65–7.
65. Mathur MS, Maheshwari RK, Chadda VS et al. Evaluation of oral saline lavage for gastrointestinal tract radiology. *Am J Proctocol Gastroenterol Colon Rectal Surg.* 1979; 30:11–5.
66. Davis GR, Smith HJ. Double-contrast examination of the colon after preparation with Golytely (a balanced lavage solution). *Gastrointest Radiol.* 1983; 8:173–6.
67. Sogge MR, Butler ML. Mallory-Weiss syndrome induced by the oral electrolyte overload technique for colonoscopy preparation. *Gastrointest Endosc.* 1980; 26:51–2.
68. Brady CE, DiPalma JA, Pierson WP. Golytely lavage—is metoclopramide necessary? *Am J Gastroenterol.* 1985; 80:180–4.
69. Bigard MA, Gaucher P, Lassalle C. Fatal colonic explosion during colonoscopic polypectomy. *Gastroenterology.* 1979; 77:1307–10.
70. Keighley MRB, Taylor EW, Hares MM et al. Influence of oral mannitol bowel preparation on colonic microflora and the risk of explosion during endoscopic diathermy. *Br J Surg.* 1981; 68:554–6.
71. Taylor EW, Bentley S, Youngs D et al. Bowel preparation and the safety of colonoscopic polypectomy. *Gastroenterology.* 1981; 81:1–4.
72. La Brooy SJ, Fendick CL, Avgerinos A et al. Potentially explosive colonic concentrations of hydrogen after bowel preparation with mannitol. *Lancet.* 1981; 1:634–6.
73. Bond JH, Levitt MD. Factors affecting the concentration of combustible gases in the colon during colonoscopy. *Gastroenterology.* 1975; 68:1445–8.
74. Avgerinos A, Kalantzis N, Rekoumis G et al. Bowel preparation and the risk of explosion during colonoscopic polypectomy. *Gut.* 1984; 25:361–4.
75. Hares MM, Greca F, Youngs D et al. Failure of antimicrobial prophylaxis with cefoxitin or metronidazole and gentamicin: is mannitol to blame? *J Hosp Infec.* 1981; 2:127–33.
76. Rogers BHG. The safety of carbon dioxide insufflation during colonoscopic electrosurgical polypectomy. *Gastrointest Endosc.* 1974; 20:115–7.
77. Bond JH, Levitt MD. Colonic gas explosion—is a fire extinguisher necessary? *Gastroenterology.* 1979; 77:1349–50.
78. DiPiro J, Bowden TA, Sisley JF et al. Golytely solution for colonoscopy preparation. *Gastrointest Endosc.* 1984; 30:116–7. Letter.
79. Lifton LJ. On the safety of "golytely." *Gastroenterology.* 1984; 86:214. Letter.
80. Davis GR. On the safety of "golytely." *Gastroenterology.* 1984; 86:214–5. Letter.
81. Marshall JB, McCullough AJ. On the safety of "golytely." *Gastroenterology.* 1984; 86:215. Letter.
82. DiPalma JA, Brady CE. On the safety of "golytely." *Gastroenterology.* 1984; 86:215–6.
83. Meadows JO. On the safety of Golytely. *Gastrointest Endosc.* 1985; 31:108. Letter.
84. Brady CE, DiPalma JA, Morawski SG et al. Urinary excretion of polyethylene glycol (PEG-3350) and sulfate (SO_4) after Golytely lavage. *Gastroenterology.* 1985; 88:1334.
85. Bruns DE, Herold DA, Rodeheaver GT et al. Polyethylene glycol intoxication in burn patients. *Burns.* 1982; 9:49–52.
86. Anon. Topical PEG in burn ointments. *FDA Drug Bull.* 1982; 12:25–6.
87. Kulick MI, Lewis NS, Bansal V, Warpeha R. Hyperosmolality in the burn patient: analysis of an osmolal discrepancy. *J Trauma.* 1980; 20:223–8.
88. Pockros PJ, Foroozan P. Golytely lavage versus a standard colonoscopy preparation: effect on normal colonic mucosal histology. *Gastroenterology.* 1985; 88:545–8.
89. Braintree Laboratories. Golytely package insert. Braintree, MA; 1984 Jun.
90. Edlaw Preparations. Colyte package insert. Farmingdale, NY; 1984 Oct.

Use of carbamazepine in psychiatric disorders

LOIS J. BIRKHIMER, JUDY L. CURTIS, AND MICHAEL W. JANN

Abstract: Use of carbamazepine for the treatment of psychiatric disorders is reviewed.

Carbamazepine's mechanism of action may be related to inhibition of kindling (repeated subtherapeutic electrical stimulation) in the temporal lobe and limbic system. In most published studies, carbamazepine was useful in affective disorders, especially in patients with bipolar manic disorders. In controlled, double-blind studies in patients with primary affective or schizoaffective disorders, carbamazepine significantly decreased manic symptoms and showed some antidepressant effect. Synergistic effects have been observed when carbamazepine is used with lithium. Carbamazepine has been reported to decrease symptoms in patients with aggression, dyscontrol syndromes, schizophrenia, and alcohol withdrawal syndrome, but few of these studies have been controlled, comparative trials; carbamazepine may be useful in patients with these disorders who do not respond to conventional therapies.

Beneficial effects of carbamazepine in psychiatric disorders are usually observed with doses of 400–1600 mg/day and serum concentrations of 8–12 μg/mL. Carbamazepine is useful alone or in combination with other agents for bipolar affective disorders, especially in patients who are intolerant of or unresponsive to lithium. Serum carbamazepine concentration, hematological profile, and serum electrolytes should be monitored carefully to minimize the risk of toxicity.

Index terms: Antidepressants; Antimanic agents; Blood levels; Carbamazepine; Drug interactions; Lithium; Mental disorders; Psychotherapeutic agents; Toxicity
Clin. Pharm. 1985; 4:425–34

Carbamazepine (5-carbamyl-5*H*-dibenzo[*b,f*]azepine) is an anticonvulsant drug used for the treatment of psychomotor and grand mal seizures.[1] It is the drug of choice for trigeminal neuralgia and other paroxysmal pain syndromes.[2] In addition to its extensive use in neurology, carbamazepine is emerging as one of the most intriguing agents used in psychiatry. The drug has been accepted by many clinicians as an effective alternative to lithium in the treatment of affective disorders.[3] Additional indications for carbamazepine therapy include aggressive behavior, schizophrenia, and other psychiatric illnesses. This article will review the pharmacokinetics, adverse effects, and drug interactions of carbamazepine; examine its various applications in psychiatry; and make recommendations regarding therapeutic drug monitoring.

Pharmacokinetics

Single-dose studies have shown that absorption of carbamazepine occurs within 6–24 hours after oral administration. However, during long-term therapy, carbamazepine concentrations peak 3–6 hours after administration.[4] In animal studies, comparison between intravenous and oral administration of carbamazepine has indicated a bioavailability range of 58–87%.[4] In six normal human volunteers, the bioavailability of carbamazepine from a propylene glycol solution was 79%.[5] Four patients showed a marked increase in absorption when carbamazepine was taken with meals; absorption was increased because the solubility of carbamazepine is augmented by bile secreted after meals.

The plasma protein binding of carbamazepine using in vitro methods has been reported at 70–80%.[6,7] The effects of hepatic and renal diseases on carbamazepine protein-binding capacity have been investigated[7]; there were no significant differences in protein binding between patients with renal disease and normal volunteers. Patients with hepatic disease had a slightly lower percentage of bound carbamazepine. Carbamazepine is a neutral and lipophilic compound. In animal models, it penetrates into all tissues and organs.[4] In single-dose studies with normal volunteers receiving carbamazepine orally, the volume of distribution ranges between 0.79 and 1.86 L/kg.[6]

The metabolism of carbamazepine occurs via hepatic mechanisms and proceeds in a variety of pathways, forming different compounds. Two of the three metabolic pathways involve the formation of conjugates. The most important pathway is the formation of carbamazepine-10,11 epoxide (CBZ-E), an active metabolite with anticonvulsant

LOIS J. BIRKHIMER, PHARM.D., is Clinical Assistant Professor of Pharmacy and JUDY L. CURTIS is a Pharm.D. candidate and Psychiatric Pharmacy Resident, The University of Texas at Austin. MICHAEL W. JANN, PHARM.D., is Senior Research Scientist, College of Pharmacy, The University of Texas at Austin, and Clinical Assistant Professor of Pharmacology, The University of Texas Health Science Center at San Antonio.

Address reprint requests to Dr. Jann at The University of Texas Health Science Center at San Antonio, Department of Pharmacology, Clinical Pharmacy Programs, 7703 Floyd Curl Drive, San Antonio, TX 78284.

The assistance of Diana Lovelace and Debbie Robison with manuscript preparation is acknowledged.

properties.[4] Whether CBZ-E has psychotropic effects remains to be determined. Carbamazepine can induce its own metabolism. Bertilsson et al.[8] found that clearance of carbamazepine in children doubled from autoinduction and that this effect was complete within a month. Similar effects have been reported in adults.[9] The mean half-life of carbamazepine has been reported as 35.6 hours in adults and 16.9 hours in children in single-dose studies. During multiple-dose studies, the effect from autoinduction reduces the half-life to 15–28 hours.[4] More extensive information on carbamazepine pharmacokinetics has been published previously.[1,2,4,6]

Mechanism of Action

The precise mechanism of action for the therapeutic effects of carbamazepine in affective and other psychiatric disorders remains to be elucidated. Structurally, carbamazepine resembles chlorpromazine and imipramine (Figure 1). Like imipramine, carbamazepine causes blockade of the neurotransmitter norepinephrine at the presynaptic neuron.[10] Carbamazepine has also been shown to block the release of norepinephrine in vitro.[10] These properties may partially explain carbamazepine's efficacy in modulating both mania and depression.[10,11] Carbamazepine's pharmacological effects on dopaminergic mechanisms are uncertain. The drug does not displace H^3 spiroperidol binding or affect the dopamine metabolite homovanillic acid. Therefore, the antimanic effects are probably not mediated by direct blockage of postsynaptic dopamine receptors.[10,12] An extensive review of the proposed biochemical (Table 1) and pharmacological mechanisms of carbamazepine efficacy in psychiatric illnesses is beyond the scope of this article; these mechanisms have been previously described.[12]

The mechanism of action for carbamazepine's psychotropic activity may be related to the anticonvulsant properties of the drug. In animal models, carbamazepine is the most effective agent for inhibiting the kindling phenomenon in the limbic system and temporal lobe region.[11] Kindling is described as repeated subthreshold electrical stimulation that culminates in the development of major motor seizures or psychopathology. Behavioral changes associated with kindling of the amygdala and other related limbic structures have shown a wide variety of symptoms. Stimulation in different animal models has produced increased aggression, rage reactions, and bizarre behavior.[11] Intense fear, mood changes, and pressured speech have been observed in humans.[13,14] Carbamazepine's stabilizing effect on the kindling phenomenon is a com-

Figure 1. Chemical structure of carbamazepine (left) compared with structures of chlorpromazine (top) and imipramine.

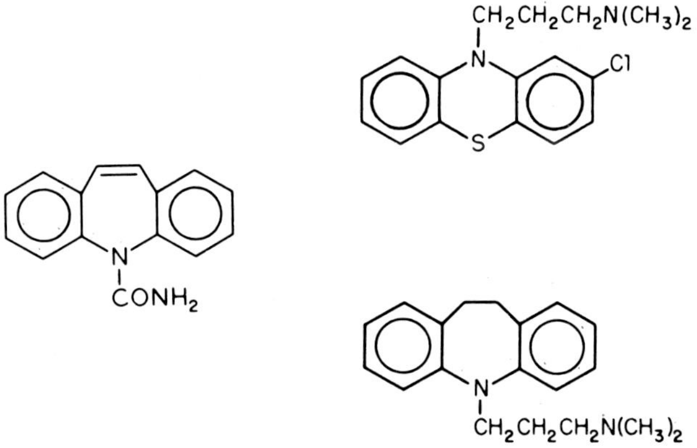

Table 1.
Biochemical Effects of Carbamazepine

Neurotransmitter System	Biochemical Effects	Comments
Norepinephrine	Blocks both reuptake and stimulus-induced release	May explain efficacy in both mania and depression
Dopamine	Apparently none	Does not displace H^3 spiroperidol binding
Serotonin	Reported to increase tryptophan levels	Serotoninergic mechanism underlies affective disorder
γ-aminobutyric acid (GABA)	High dose, chronic treatment decreases turnover rate	Lithium also can decrease turnover
Acetylcholine	Reported to increase and decrease release	Apparently not significant
Cyclic nucleotides	Inhibits accumulation of cyclic AMP	Lithium also decreases cyclic AMP
Thyroid hormones	Significant decrease in T_3 and T_4; slight decrease in TSH	Hormone levels decrease more in carbamazepine responders
Cortisol	Increases urinary free cortisol	Produces false-positive dexamethasone test
Opioid peptides	No significant effect	High baseline CSF levels may predict carbamazepine response
Somatostatin	Decreases CSF levels	No correlation with carbamazepine response
Vasopressin	Increases plasma levels	Opposite effect of lithium

mon link that may explain its efficacy in treating seizures, paroxysmal syndromes, and psychiatric disorders. The kindling model may be useful in understanding the development of psychopathology as a result of an ictal process or following an ictal event that manifests as psychiatric symptoms.[11]

Affective Disorders

Usefulness of carbamazepine in treating affective disorders was first suggested by Japanese investigators in the early 1970s.[15–17] In preliminary trials of 150 patients, beneficial antimanic and prophylactic response was seen in 103 (83%) of 124 patients with manic symptoms. Because these were uncontrolled open trials, conclusions are limited. Other psychotropic agents, including lithium, various antipsychotics, imipramine, desipramine, and diazepam, were allowed. Carbamazepine doses ranged from 200 to 1200 mg/day, and none of the studies reported serum concentrations. The Japanese experience, however, prompted several investigators in the United States to study carbamazepine use in psychiatric disorders.

Ballenger and Post[18,19] were the first to report results in two double-blind, placebo-controlled trials of carbamazepine in affective disorders. They assessed antimanic, antidepressant, and prophylactic effects in psychiatric patients. Both studies used identical methods. Subjects were diagnosed as having primary affective or schizoaffective disorder, according to the Research Diagnostic Criteria.[20] Following a two-week placebo washout period, carbamazepine treatment was initiated at 200 mg twice daily and titrated upward to maintain serum concentrations of 8–12 μg/mL. Maximum doses generally ranged from 600 to 1600 mg/day, although one subject received 2000 mg/day.[19] A second placebo period of several days to weeks followed the trial. In subjects who relapsed on placebo, carbamazepine therapy was resumed. Raters who were blind to the drug trial assessed the subjects twice daily using the Bunney–Hamburg scale, which is a global rating of depression, mania, psychosis, anxiety, and anger. Subjects reported their moods and side effects daily. The patients were also assessed using the Brief Psychiatric Rating Scale (BPRS) three times a week. Response in mania was quantified as follows: marked response = decrease of 4 or more points on the rating scales; moderate response = decrease of 2 to 4 points; partial response = decrease of 1 to 2 points; and poor response = decrease of less than 1 point. Antidepressant response was assessed by decreased scores as follows: good response = decrease of more than 2 points, moderate response = decrease of more than 1.5; partial response = 1.0–1.5; and poor response = decrease of less than 1 point.

The preliminary trial included 10 patients: six bipolar manic, two unipolar depressed, and two schizoaffective.[18] Seven of the 10 subjects responded favorably to carbamazepine with either antimanic, antidepressant, or prophylactic effects. Four of the responding subjects had failed to respond to lithium therapy, two carbamazepine responders later required the addition of antipsychotics to fully resolve their symptoms, and one carbamazepine nonresponder later responded to lithium. No statistical analysis was reported.

Ballenger and Post's second report[19] discussed 24 subjects who completed the clinical trial. However, results were analyzed for only 22 subjects (plus some patients from the preliminary trial). Nine bipolar manic and 13 depressed subjects (seven bipolar depressed, four unipolar depressed, two bipolar–schizoaffective) were evaluated. Of the nine manic subjects, improvement was marked in four, moderate in one, partial in two, and poor in two. Total sleep time was significantly increased ($p < 0.01$, paired t test). Improvement in mania was significant ($p < 0.05$, paired t test). Antimanic effects were observed within the first week of treatment and continued throughout the trial. Seven of the nine patients had previously received lithium therapy with poor or equivocal response. Prophylactic effects were noted in five patients (two had complete resolution of symptoms, three showed a decrease in severity or incidence of episodes) for periods of up to 22 months of therapy. Major relapses were seen in four of the nine patients when placebo was substituted for carbamazepine.

Antidepressant response to carbamazepine was considered good in four, moderate in one, partial in two, and poor in six of the 13 depressed patients but was not statistically significant ($p < 0.10$, paired t test). Antidepressant effects were observed after two weeks of carbamazepine therapy; this response time is similar to response times observed with other antidepressant agents. Significant improvement in total sleep time was noted ($p < 0.05$, paired t test). Four carbamazepine responders and two nonresponders had previous incomplete or poor response to lithium. In three subjects, carbamazepine prevented recurrence of depressive episodes for up to 22 months. In contrast to manic patients, only one depressed subject had a major clinical relapse when placebo was substituted for carbamazepine; six others had limited or probable relapses.

Prophylactic effects were also reported by Post et al.,[21] who followed seven patients (six bipolar, one recurrent depressive confusional psychosis) for an average of 1.7 years. These patients exhibited rapid, cycling mood swings and had been resistant to lithium therapy. The average dose of carbamazepine was 1285 mg/day, with an average serum concentration of 11.3 μg/mL. Three patients received carbamazepine only, and two were maintained on concomitant neuroleptics (one on a tricyclic antidepressant and one on lithium). The group experienced a 65% yearly reduction in manic and depressive episodes while receiving carbamazepine therapy ($p < 0.02$, paired t test). Recurrent episodes were shorter and less severe than before carbamazepine treatment. Six of the seven patients relapsed when carbamazepine was discontinued.

These findings are consistent with those of other investigators. Okuma and associates[22] performed a double-blind study of carbamazepine versus chlorpromazine in patients with endogenous manic psychosis. Of 60 patients, 41 were bipolar, 11 monopolar manic, 7 in their first manic episode, and 1 bipolar mixed. Carbamazepine doses ranged from 300 to 900 mg/day (serum concentration 2.7–11.7 μg/mL), while doses of chlorpromazine ranged from 150 to 450 mg/day. Patients were assessed by the Clinical Psychopharmacology Research Group (CPRG) rating scale for mania.[23] Moderate to marked improvement was noted in 70% of the carbamazepine group compared with 60% of the chlorpromazine patients, not a significant difference ($Z = 1.611$, Mann–Whitney U test). Antimanic effects were observed within 10 days in 65.7% of the carbamazepine patients and in 50% of the chlorpromazine group. The incidence of side effects was significantly lower in the carbamazepine group.

More recent evidence confirms the role of carbamazepine in prophylaxis of affective disorders. Jann et al.[24] performed a retrospective, longitudinal review of 11 patients (seven bipolar manic, one bipolar depressed, two schizoaffective, and one mentally retarded with hyperactivity) treated with carbamazepine. Seven patients (64%) responded to carbamazepine with serum concentrations in the range of 5.3–10.8 μg/mL. Of the seven bipolar patients who had manic symptoms previously refractory to lithium, five responded to carbamazepine.

In another long-term study, Kishimoto et al.[25] observed 32 patients receiving carbamazepine over an average 6.25-year period. Subjects conformed to DSM III criteria for bipolar affective disorder, had frequent mood changes, and had failed numerous previous therapies with antipsychotics and antidepressants. Carbamazepine doses ranged from 200 to 1200 mg/day; serum concentrations were 6–10 μg/mL. Patients were allowed to continue stable doses of lithium and other unspecified psychotropic agents; in four cases, however, these agents were withdrawn during carbamazepine therapy. Overall, a prophylactic effect was observed in 75% of the patients; 12% had complete inhibition and 63% had partial inhibition of symptoms. The most frequently observed effect of carbamazepine was the absence or reduced intensity of episodes; a greater effect was observed in manic compared with depressed episodes. Patients whose illnesses began before the age of 20 had complete inhibition of symptoms ($p < 0.01$, Fisher's exact test).

Nolen[26] studied carbamazepine as an adjunctive therapy for 12 bipolar patients without history of seizure disorder. In most cases antipsychotics and antidepressants were also continued. Patients were maintained on lithium with serum concentrations of 0.8–1.2 meq/L; carbamazepine was added and the dosage was titrated to achieve serum concentrations of 6–12 μg/mL. Rating scale information was not reported, but combined therapy was considered very effective in two, markedly effective in two, slightly effective in two, and ineffective in two patients during the six-month trial.

Overall response and antidepressant response may correlate better with serum and cerebrospinal fluid (CSF) concentrations of CBZ-E than with concentrations or dose of carbamazepine itself.[27] Eighteen bipolar patients were treated with carbamazepine alone at an average dose of 1055 mg/day. Mean serum and CSF concentrations of carbamazepine were 6.55 ± 0.06 μg/mL and 2.06 ± 0.10 μg/mL, respectively. These values compared with mean CBZ-E serum concentrations of 1.44 ± 0.2 μg/mL and CBZ-E CSF concentrations of 0.91 ± 0.09 μg/mL. These preliminary data indicate that CBZ-E may possess active psychotropic properties.[27]

Synergistic effects of combination therapy with carbamazepine and other psychotic agents have been suggested. Folks and associates[28] noted antimanic and antidepressant effects from carbamazepine in eight of 10 patients who were nonresponsive to or unable to take lithium. Four patients had bipolar disorders, three were schizoaffective, and three had affective syndromes associated with CNS disturbances (two had epilepsy; one had cerebral palsy). The authors suggested synergism between carbamazepine and lithium and between carbamazepine and tricyclic antidepressants. Lipinski and Pope,[29] Keisling,[30] and Warren and Crismon[31] have reported good response to combined carbamazepine treatment in manic patients not controlled by previous therapy with standard agents. Results of trials with carbamazepine in affective disorders are summarized in Table 2; study design, number of patients, carbamazepine dosage range and serum concentrations, and percentage of clinical responses are presented.

These reports suggest that carbamazepine, alone or in combination with other psychoactive agents, is potentially useful in treating patients with affective disorders. Patients with bipolar manic disorders showed the greatest improvement; less efficacy was demonstrated in depressed, schizoaffective and organic–affective patients. The majority of studies lacked accurate monitoring of target symptoms. The rating scales used (e.g., the Brief Psychiatric Rating Scale) assess psychotic symptoms rather than specific manic or depressive symptoms. Use of the Biegel–Murphy Mania Rating Scale or Hamilton Depression Scale would have provided more accurate assessment of affective target symptoms.[3]

Table 2.
Carbamazepine Use in Affective Disorders

Reference No.	Diagnosis	*n*	Design	Duration	Carbamazepine dose (mg/day)	Serum Carbamazepine Concentration (μg/mL)	Concurrent Drug Therapy	Overall Response (%)
15	Bipolar	10	Open	1–11 mo	200–600	NR[a]	Yes	90
16	Bipolar	50	Open, controlled trial	175 days	400–1200	NR	Yes	76
17	Bipolar	90	Open	NR	200–1200	NR	Yes	71
18	Bipolar manic Unipolar depressed Schizo-affective	6 2 2	Double blind, placebo controlled	56 days	600–1600	8–12	No	70
19	Bipolar manic Bipolar depressed Unipolar depressed Schizo-affective	9 7 4 2	Double blind, placebo controlled	60 days	600–1600	8–12	No	55
21	Bipolar manic Recurrent depression	6 1	Blind or open	Average 1.7 yr	Average 1285	Average 11.3	Yes	65
22	Bipolar manic Unipolar First manic episode Bipolar mixed	41 11 7 1	Double blind, chlorpromazine	42 days	380–540	2–11	No	70 carbamazepine 60 chlorpromazine
24	Bipolar manic Bipolar depressed Schizo-affective Mentally retarded with hyperactivity	7 1 2 1	Retrospective, longitudinal drug-use review	2 yr	NR	5.3–10.8	Yes	64
25	Bipolar	32	Open, controlled	Average 6.25 yr	200–1200	6–10	Yes	75
26	Bipolar	12	Open	3 yr	Titrated to plasma concentration	6–12	Yes	50
28	Bipolar Schizo-affective Organic-affective	4 3 3	Case study	NR	600–1600	8–12	Yes	80
29	Bipolar	3	Case study	NR	NR	8.5–9.5	Yes	100
30	Bipolar Schizo-affective	2 1	Case study	NR	NR	8–9	Yes	100
31	Bipolar	1	Case study	NR	600	7–8	Yes	100

[a] NR = not reported.

Lack of statistical power was a problem, since patient populations were small in most of the studies. Placebo-controlled studies can be difficult to implement in manic and depressed patients, especially in patients who do not respond to conventional pharmacologic intervention. Further trials are necessary to define the precise role of carbamazepine in affective disorders.

Aggressive Behavior, Schizophrenia, and Other Psychiatric Disorders

Carbamazepine has been used in a variety of nonaffective psychiatric disorders. Numerous case studies report its efficacy in patients with aggression, dyscontrol syndromes, schizophrenia, and alcoholism. Unfortunately, there are few controlled comparative trials using carbamazepine in these disorders.

Hakola and Laulaumaa[32] first reported the use of carbamazepine in eight violent schizophrenic women who had had nonspecific EEG findings. Episodes of violent behavior decreased in all patients. In four patients, schizophrenic symptoms also improved. Specific information regarding violent behavior and schizophrenic symptoms was not reported. Post and Luchins[33] reported the use of carbamazepine in two studies of violent nonepileptic schizophrenic patients. The first study was conducted with seven violent patients with normal EEGs who were hospitalized on chronic-care wards. Patient records were reviewed for three separate six-week periods—before carbamazepine was initiated, before it was discontinued, and after it was discontinued. During these periods, episodes of physical aggression, verbal hostility, and use of "p.r.n." medication were documented. A significant ($p = 0.01$, two-way analysis of variance) decrease in aggressive episodes was observed during carbamazepine treatment. The second study compared 11 violent patients who had normal EEGs with eight patients who had abnormal EEGs for six-week periods before and during carbamazepine therapy. Aggressive episodes were reduced by 54% in the normal-EEG patients and 38% in the patients with abnormal EEGs.

Klein et al.[34] studied 43 patients with "excited psychoses" (manic, schizophrenic, and schizoaffective disorders). Patients were assigned to two treatment groups; 20 patients received placebo plus haloperidol and 23 received carbamazepine plus haloperidol. Haloperidol doses were individually titrated. Carbamazepine doses were as high as 1200 mg/day with serum concentrations of 8–12 μg/mL. More improvement was noted in the group receiving combined therapy than in the placebo-haloperidol group.

Neppe[35] used carbamazepine in 13 nonresponsive psychiatric patients who had EEG abnormalities but no evidence of seizure disorder. Patients received carbamazepine 200 mg or placebo three times a day in a double-blind crossover design. Eight of the 11 patients who completed the study showed overall improvement, based on the various clinical rating scales (BPRS, Global Assessment, and Overall Clinical Rating).

Curtis and associates[36] retrospectively reviewed five adolescents and children receiving carbamazepine for conduct disorder, socialized-aggressive disorder, and explosive disorder. Three patients had abnormal EEGs with seizures; the other two had normal EEGs. All patients demonstrated fewer episodes of aggressive behavior. The number of p.r.n. medication doses and "time-outs" decreased significantly ($p < 0.05$). Serum carbamazepine concentrations were maintained between 6.4 and 8.4 μg/mL. One patient showed a greater improvement with combined lithium and carbamazepine therapy.

Carbamazepine may be useful in treating alcohol withdrawal syndromes.[37] In Scandinavian studies, carbamazepine was effective in reducing the length and severity of withdrawal symptoms such as anxiety, irritability, tremor, hallucinations, and sleep disturbance. Seizure incidence during withdrawal also decreased in patients receiving carbamazepine. Ballenger and Post[38] suggest that repeated episodes of alcohol withdrawal may result in a lower seizure threshold, similar to the kindling model.

Kaplan et al.[39] used carbamazepine in six bulimic patients. Five patients did not respond. The one patient who responded dramatically had a history suggestive of bipolar disorder. The authors suggested a possible link between bulimia and affective illness.

Reid et al.[40] studied 12 severely or profoundly retarded overactive patients in a double-blind crossover trial. Five patients were epileptic; seizure types were not reported. Carbamazepine doses ranged from 400 to 600 mg/day; no serum concentrations were reported. Patients in Group A were predominantly overactive and showed mood elevation. Group B exhibited severe and multiple behavior problems, including irritability, self-injury, stripping, and noisiness. The tendency was for Group A to improve and Group B to deteriorate; however, the difference was not statistically significant.

Other studies and case reports of carbamazepine use in treating schizophrenia, aggression, and other psychiatric disorders[41–44] are summarized in Table 3.

The majority of trials and case reports using carbamazepine in nonaffective disorders were not designed using placebo control periods or standardized rating scales. The lack of statistical power and significance is more prominent in these reports than in trials in affective disorders. Despite these study limitations, carbamazepine therapy can be

Table 3.
Reports of Carbamazepine Use in Nonaffective Disorders

Reference No.	Diagnosis	*n*	EEG Abnormal ?	Carbamazepine Dose (mg/day)	Serum Carbamazepine Concentration (μg/mL)	Concurrent Drug Therapy	Results
38	Schizophrenia Psychotic episodes	4 2	Yes (3 patients)	400–800	8 (1 patient)	Phenytoin 300 mg/day, diazepam 20 mg/day (1 patient)	Improvement in psychotic episodes and emotional lability
41	Prenatal rubella, aggressive	1	Yes	600	8.7	Primidone 750 mg/day, chlorpromazine 450 mg/day	Patient was able to leave institution and marry
42	Mental retardation, aggressive behavior, generalized seizures	1	Yes	1200	NR[a]	Valproic acid 700 mg/day	Aggressive behavior decreased from a mean of 15 outbursts/day to a mean of 3/day
43	Interictal fear, temporal lobe epilepsy	1	Yes	1000	8.9	None	Shorter and decreased episodes of fear in both patients
44	Paroxysmal behavior disorder	2	Yes (1 patient)	NR	6–8	Phenobarbital (1 patient)	Disappearance of paroxysmal behavior

[a] NR = not reported.

useful in patients who do not respond to conventional drug therapy.

Adverse Effects

The adverse effects of carbamazepine involve various physiological functions and organ systems. The hematological toxicity of carbamazepine has been extensively reviewed.[45] Between 1964 and 1981, only 20 cases of carbamazepine-associated aplastic anemia were reported. Thrombocytopenia and persistent leukopenia occur in approximately 2% of patients.[46] To date, three case reports have been published in the psychiatric literature describing hematological toxicities.[47–49] In two of these[47,48] the patients recovered promptly when carbamazepine was discontinued. In the remaining case report, fatal agranulocytosis in a chronic schizophrenic patient was treated with combined carbamazepine (400 mg/day) and haloperidol (15 mg/day).[49]

Neurological toxicity is reported in up to 60% of patients receiving carbamazepine. The most common symptoms of carbamazepine neurotoxicity are diplopia (16%), drowsiness (11%), blurred vision (6%), and equilibrium disturbance (3%).[50] These effects usually occur within the first two to three weeks of therapy and subside spontaneously or with a decrease in dosage. Neurotoxic symptoms are observed at therapeutic serum concentrations; therefore, careful patient supervision is required.[50] Therapeutic doses of carbamazepine caused dystonic reactions in four patients.[51] Orofacial dyskinesia has been described during carbamazepine intoxication in a patient who ingested 24 g.[52] The movements disappeared as the patient recovered. The patient's seizure control remained poor, and carbamazepine was restarted at 600 mg/day. The dyskinetic movements returned and carbamazepine was discontinued, with resolution of dyskinesia within three days.

Gastrointestinal side effects occur in 15% of patients treated with carbamazepine.[53] The most frequent symptoms are nausea, vomiting, and diarrhea. Granulomatous hepatitis and jaundice have been reported.[54,55] There are a few cases of carbamazepine-induced atrioventricular heart block.[56,57] Induction of the syndrome of inappropriate antidiuretic hormone and water intoxication by carbamazepine have been reported.[58–60] Several patients had hyponatremia, with serum sodium levels as low as 124 meq/L.[58–60] Based on these findings, baseline serum electrolyte assessment and routine monitoring are recommended for patients receiving carbamazepine.

Drug Interactions

As previously discussed, carbamazepine is almost entirely metabolized by the hepatic microsomal enzyme system and can induce its own metabolism. Other drugs that are extensively metabolized by the liver can cause changes in carbamazepine metabolism; conversely, carbamazepine can interfere with metabolism of the other drugs. Phenytoin, phenobarbital, primidone, and erythromycin have been reported to reduce carbamazepine serum concentrations.[61,62] In contrast, valproic acid, propoxyphene, and isoniazid have been reported to elevate carbamazepine concentrations.[61,63] Carbamazepine can increase the metabolism of theophylline and warfarin.[64,65] Neurotoxicity has been reported when lithium is used with carbamazepine[66,67]; plasma lithium and carbamazepine concentrations were within accepted therapeutic ranges. The symptoms reported were ataxia, horizontal nystagmus, hyperreflexia, and coarse tremors. Delirium was reported in one patient receiving carbamazepine and haloperidol 15 mg/day.[68] The patient had a low serum carbamazepine concentration (3.7 μg/mL). The delirium cleared within 12 hours after carbamazepine was discontinued. The interaction of carbamazepine and haloperidol was reported in three schizophrenic patients.[69] Plasma haloperidol concentrations decreased approximately 60% when carbamazepine was introduced. However, when carbamazepine was discontinued in one patient, plasma haloperidol levels increased from 17 to 107 ng/mL. These patients did not experience any adverse effects.

Therapeutic Drug Monitoring

Carbamazepine therapy can be associated with serious side effects and drug interactions. The drug has been used extensively for seizure disorders and trigeminal neuralgia, and the same monitoring procedures and cautions must be observed when carbamazepine is used for psychiatric disorders.

Therapy should be initiated at low doses, 100–200 mg daily for adults and 10 mg/kg/day for children. Doses should be individualized to the patient's response, side effects, and serum concentrations. The psychiatric literature suggests that serum concentrations be maintained between 8 and 12 μg/mL for maximum benefit.[19]

The following tests should be performed before carbamazepine therapy is begun:

1. Complete blood cell count with differential and platelet count,
2. Liver enzyme studies,
3. Serum electrolyte concentrations,
4. BUN, urine specific gravity, and serum creatinine concentration,
5. Neurological assessment with EEG (optional), and
6. ECG if the patient is over 40 years old or has preexisting cardiac disease.

Routine Monitoring

Serum carbamazepine concentrations should be obtained weekly during the dosage titration phase, one week after any dosage adjustment, and monthly once steady state is reached. Serum concentrations will decrease as a result of carbamazepine's autoinductive properties; up to six weeks may be required for maximal enzyme induction to occur. Therefore, serum carbamazepine concentrations should be obtained twice monthly to demonstrate that steady state has been achieved before beginning monitoring on a less frequent schedule. Hematologic studies and electrolyte monitoring should be performed every two weeks for two months and every three months thereafter.[46] A complete blood cell count and liver enzyme concentrations should be obtained immediately if rash or fever occurs.[46]

Conclusion

A growing body of literature supports the use of carbamazepine in psychiatric disorders. Serum concentrations of 8–12 μg/mL are optimal. Alone or in combination with other psychoactive agents, carbamazepine is useful for treating bipolar affective disorder. Carbamazepine may be especially useful in patients who are intolerant of or do not respond to lithium therapy. Use of carbamazepine in aggression, schizophrenia, and other disorders requires further study. As the use of carbamazepine in psychiatry increases, more reports of toxicity can be expected. Baseline hematological studies and monitoring of serum electrolytes and hepatic function, and appropriate monitoring of serum carbamazepine concentrations throughout therapy, will minimize the risks and maximize therapeutic effects.

References

1. Gamstrop I. Treatment with carbamazepine: children. In: Penry JK, Dalby DD, eds. Advances in neurology. New York: Raven Press; 1975:237–46.
2. Parsonage M. Treatment with carbamazepine: adults. In: Penry JK, Dalby DD, eds. Advances in neurology. New York: Raven Press; 1975:221–34.
3. Jann MW, Garrelts J, Ereshefsky L et al. Alternative drug therapies for mania: a literature review. *Drug Intell Clin Pharm.* 1984; 18:577–89.
4. Pynnonen S. Pharmacokinetics of carbamazepine in man: a review. *Ther Drug Monit.* 1979; 1:409–31.
5. Levy RH, Pitlick WH, Troupin AS et al. Pharmacokinetics of carbamazepine in normal man. *Clin Pharmacol Ther.* 1975; 17:657–68.
6. Bertilsson L. Clinical pharmacokinetics of carbamazepine. *Clin Pharmacokinet.* 1978; 3:128–43.
7. Hooper WD, Dubetz DK, Bochner et al. Plasma protein binding of carbamazepine. *Clin Pharmacol Ther.* 1975; 17:433–40.
8. Bertilsson L, Hojer B, Tybring G et al. Autoinduction of carbamazepine metabolism in children examined by a stable isotope technique. *Clin Pharmacol Ther.* 1979; 27:83–8.
9. Pynnonen S, Frey H, Sillanpaa M. The auto-induction of carbamazepine during long-term therapy. *Int J Clin Pharmacol.* 1980; 18:247–52.
10. Post RM, Rubinow DR, Uhde TW. Biochemical mechanisms of action of carbamazepine in affective illness and epilepsy. *Psychopharmacol Bull.* 1984; 20:585–94.
11. Post RM, Uhde TW, Putnam FW et al. Kindling and carbamazepine in affective illness. *J Nerv Ment Dis.* 1982; 170:717–31.
12. Post RM, Ballenger JC, Uhde TW et al. Efficacy of carbamazepine in manic-depressive illness: implications for underlying mechanisms. In: Post RM, Ballenger JC, eds. Neuro-

biology of mood disorders. Baltimore: Williams & Wilkins; 1984:777–817.

13. Heath RG, Monroe RR, Mickle W. Stimulation of the amygdaloid nucleus in a schizophrenic patient. *Am J Psychiatry*. 1955; 111:862–3.
14. Stevens JR, Mark VH, Erwin F et al. Deep temporal stimulation in man: long latency, long lasting psychological changes. *Arch Neurol*. 1969; 21:159–67.
15. Takezaki H, Hanoalea M. The use of carbamazepine in the control of manic-depressive psychosis and other manic-depressive states. *Clin Psych*. 1971; 13:173–83.
16. Okuma T, Kishimoto A, Inove K et al. Antimanic and prophylactic effects of carbamazepine (Tegretol) on manic-depressive psychosis. A preliminary report. *Folia Psychiatr Neurol Jpn*. 1973; 27:283–97.
17. Okuma T, Kishimoto A, Inove K et al. Antimanic and prophylactic effects of carbamazepine on manic-depressive psychosis. *Seishin-Ingaku Kenkyusho Gyosekishu*. 1975; 17:617–30.
18. Ballenger JC, Post RM. Therapeutic effects of carbamazepine in affective illness: a preliminary report. *Commun Psychopharmacol*. 1978; 2:159–75.
19. Ballenger JC, Post RM. Carbamazepine in manic-depressive illness: a new treatment. *Am J Psychiatry* 1980; 137:782–90.
20. Okuma T, Inanaga K, Otsuki S et al. A preliminary double-blind study of the efficacy of carbamazepine in prophylaxis of manic-depressive illness. *Psychopharmacology*. 1981; 73:95–6.
21. Post RM, Uhde TW, Ballenger JC et al. Prophylactic efficacy of carbamazepine in manic-depressive illness. *Am J Psychiatry* 1983; 140:1602–4.
22. Okuma T, Inanaga K, Otsuki S et al. Comparison of the antimanic efficacy of carbamazepine and chlorpromazine: a double-blind controlled study. *Psychopharmacology*. 1979; 66:211–7.
23. Takahashi R, Ito K, Ito H, et al. Comparison of efficacy of lithium carbonate and chlorpromazine in mania by double-blind controlled study. *Rinsho-Hyoka*. 1974; 2:23–45.
24. Jann MW, Saklad S, Ereshefsky L. Carbamazepine for patients with affective target symptoms. *Drug Intell Clin Pharm*. 1984; 18:81. Letter.
25. Kishimoto A, Ogura C, Hazama H et al. Long-term prophylactic effects of carbamazepine in affective disorder. *Br J Psychiatry*. 1983; 143:327–31.
26. Nolen WA. Carbamazepine, a possible adjunct or alternative to lithium in bipolar disorders. *Acta Psychiatr Scand*. 1983; 67:218–25.
27. Post RM, Uhde TW, Ballenger JC et al. Carbamazepine and its −10,11 epoxide metabolite in plasma and CSF. *Arch Gen Psychiatry*. 1983; 40:673–6.
28. Folks DG, King LD, Dowdy SB et al. Carbamazepine treatment of selected affectively disordered inpatients. *Am J Psychiatry*. 1982; 139:115–7.
29. Lipinski JF, Pope HA. Possible synergistic action between carbamazepine and lithium carbonate in the treatment of three acutely manic patients. *Am J Psychiatry* 1982; 139:948–9.
30. Keisling R. Carbamazepine and lithium carbonate in the treatment of refractory affective disorders. *Arch Gen Psychiatry*. 1983; 40:223. Letter.
31. Warren JA, Crismon ML. Carbamazepine in bipolar disorder—mixed. *Clin Pharm*. 1982; 1:266–8.
32. Hakola H, Laulaumaa V. Carbamazepine in treatment of violent schizophrenics. *Lancet*. 1982; 1:1358.
33. Post RM, Luchins D. Carbamazepine in psychiatric syndromes: clinical and neuropharmacological properties. *Psychopharmacol Bull*. 1984; 20:569–71.
34. Klein E, Bental E, Lever B et al. Carbamazepine and haloperidol vs placebo and haloperidol in excited psychoses. *Arch Gen Psychiatry*. 1984; 41:165–70.
35. Neppe VM. Carbamazepine as adjunctive treatment in nonepileptic chronic inpatients with EEG temporal lobe abnormalities. *J Clin Psychiatry*. 1983; 44:326–31.
36. Curtis JL, Jann MW, Saklad S et al. Use of carbamazepine in children and adolescents. *Pharmacotherapy*. 1985; in press.
37. Bjorkqvist SE, Isohanni M, Makela R et al. Ambulant treatment of alcohol withdrawal symptoms with carbamazepine: a formal multicenter double-blind comparison with placebo. *Acta Psychiatr Scand*. 1976; 53:333–42.
38. Ballenger JC, Post RM. Carbamazepine in alcohol withdrawal syndrome and schizophrenic psychoses. *Psychopharmacol Bull*. 1984; 20:572–84.
39. Kaplan AS, Garfinkel PE, Darby PL et al. Carbamazepine in the treatment of bulimia. *Am J Psychiatry*. 1983; 104:1225–6.
40. Reid A, Naylor G, Kay D. A double-blind, placebo controlled, crossover trial of carbamazepine in overactive severely mentally handicapped patients. *Psychol Med*. 1981; 11:109–13.
41. Tunks E, Dermer S. Carbamazepine in the dyscontrol syndrome associated with limbic system dysfunction. *J Nerv Ment Dis*. 1977; 164:56–63.
42. Rapport M, Soni W, Fialkov M et al. Carbamazepine in behavior therapy for aggressive behavior. *Behav Modif*. 1983; 20:255–65.
43. Hermann B, Melyn M. Effects of carbamazepine on interictal psychopathology in TLE with ictal fear. *J Clin Psychiatry*. 1984; 45:169–71.
44. Garbutt JC, Loosen PT. Is carbamazepine helpful in paroxysmol behavior disorders? *Am J Psychiatry*. 1983; 140:1363–4.
45. Pisiotta A. Hematologic toxicity of carbamazepine. In: Penry JK, Dalby DD, eds. Advances in neurology. New York: Raven Press; 1975:355–68.
46. Hart RG, Easton J. Carbamazepine and hematological monitoring. *Ann Neurol*. 1982; 11:309–12.
47. Baciewicz G, Yerevanian BI. Thrombocytopenia associated with carbamazepine: a case report and review. *J Clin Psychiatry*. 1984; 45:315–6.
48. Warren JA, Steinbook RM. Case report of carbamazepine-induced reticulocytosis. *Am J Psychiatry*. 1983; 140:247–9.
49. Luchins DL. Fatal agranulocytosis in a chronic schizophrenic patient treated with carbamazepine. *Am J Psychiatry*. 1984; 141:687–8.
50. Reynolds EH. Neurotoxicity of carbamazepine. In: Penry JK, Dalby DD, eds. Advances in neurology. New York: Raven Press; 1975:345–53.
51. Jacombe D. Carbamazepine-induced dystonia. *JAMA*. 1979; 241:2263.
52. Joyce RP, Gunderson CH. Carbamazepine-induced orofacial dyskinesia. *Neurology*. 1980; 30:1333–4.
53. Suria A, Killam ER. Antiepileptic drugs: mechanism of action. *Adv Neurol*. 1980; 563–75.
54. Levy M, Goodman MW, Bruce J. Granulomatous hepatitis secondary to carbamazepine. *Ann Intern Med*. 1981; 95:64–5.
55. Ramsay ID. Carbamazepine-induced jaundice. *Br Med J*. 1967; 4:155.
56. Ladefoged SD, Mogelvang JC. Total atrioventricular block and syncopes complicating carbamazepine therapy. *Acta Med Scand*. 1982; 212:185–6.
57. Beermann B, Edhag O, Vallin H. Advanced heart block aggravated by carbamazepine. *Br Heart J*. 1975; 37:668–71.
58. Sordillo P, Sagransky DM, Mercado R et al. Carbamazepine-induced syndrome of inappropriate antidiuretic hormone secretion. *Arch Intern Med*. 1978; 138:299–301.
59. Perucca E, Garratt A, Hebdige S et al. Water intoxication in epileptic patients receiving carbamazepine. *J Neurol Neurosurg Psychiatry*. 1978; 41:713–8.
60. Henry DA, Lawson DH, Reavey P et al. Hyponatremia during carbamazepine treatment. *Br Med J*. 1977; 7:83–4.
61. Finn AL. Anticonvulsants. In: Mungall D. Applied clinical pharmacokinetics. New York: Raven Press; 1983:103–26.
62. Wong YY, Ludden TM, Bell RB. Effect of erythromycin on carbamazepine kinetics. *Clin Pharmacol Ther*. 1982; 33:460–4.
63. Wright JM, Stokes EF, Sweeney VP. Isoniazid-induced carbamazepine toxicity and vice versa. *N Engl J Med*. 1982; 307:1325–7.

64. Rosenberry KR, Defusco CJ, Mansmann HC et al. Reduced theophylline half-life induced by carbamazepine therapy. *J Pediatr*. 1983; 102:472–4.
65. Hansen JM, Stersback-Nielsn K, Skovsted L. Carbamazepine induces accelerated diphenylhydantoin and warfarin metabolism in man. *Clin Pharmacol Ther*. 1971; 12:539–42.
66. Shukla S, Godwin CD, Long LEB et al. Lithium-carbamazepine neurotoxicity and risk factors. *Am J Psychiatry*. 1984; 141:1604–7.
67. Chaudry RP, Waters BGH. Lithium and carbamazepine interaction: possible neurotoxicity. *J Clin Psychiatry*. 1983; 44:30–1.
68. Kanter GL, Yerevanian BI, Ciccone JR. Case report of a possible interaction between neuroleptics and carbamazepine. *Am J Psychiatry*. 1984; 141:1101–2.
69. Jann MW, Ereshefsky L, Saklad SR et al. Effects of carbamazepine on plasma haloperidol levels. *J Clin Psychopharmacol*. 1985; 5:106–9.

Aluminum-related osteomalacia in renal-failure patients

Karen E. Vick and Curtis A. Johnson

Abstract: The pathophysiology, clinical presentation, prevention, and treatment of aluminum-related osteomalacia in renal-failure patients are reviewed.

Aluminum-related osteomalacia can develop in patients exposed to high concentrations of aluminum either in dialysis solutions or through gastrointestinal aluminum absorption from aluminum-containing antacids used to treat hyperphosphatemia. Although the exact etiology of aluminum-related osteomalacia is unknown, aluminum is believed to inhibit bone mineralization by forming an inhibitory complex with citric acid at physiologic concentrations. The complex is deposited along bone mineralization fronts and in bone marrow. The major symptoms of aluminum-related osteomalacia include skeletal pain, fractures, and vertebral collapse. The disease is difficult to diagnose because patients may have normal or slightly elevated serum concentrations of calcium, phosphate, alkaline phosphatase, and parathyroid hormone. Direct measurement of bone aluminum content (using biopsy) is often needed to confirm diagnosis. The aluminum-chelating agent deferoxamine mesylate can be used to measure bone aluminum content indirectly.

Aluminum intoxication can be managed either by preventing exposure to aluminum or by removing deposited aluminum from bone. New standards restrict aluminum content in dialysis solutions, and prevention now focuses on the use of aluminum-free phosphate binders for treatment of hyperphosphatemia. Calcium carbonate may be as effective as aluminum-containing antacids in controlling serum phosphate concentrations, but it should be used cautiously in patients who are hypercalcemic or at risk of developing metastatic calcification. Chelation therapy with deferoxamine has improved the symptoms and bone histology in a small number of patients. Clinical improvements have been seen in patients receiving intravenous deferoxamine 2–6 g per week for 20 weeks. The few reported adverse reactions to deferoxamine include pain at the injection site, skin flushing, erythema, urticaria, hypotension, and shock. Treatment with vitamin D analogues has been unsuccessful.

Although few patients have been studied, the use of deferoxamine in treating aluminum-related osteomalacia in renal-failure patients has improved clinical symptoms and bone histology. The exact etiologies of the condition and valid preventive approaches remain elusive.

Index terms: Aluminum; Antacids; Deferoxamine; Heavy metal antagonists; Osteomalacia; Solutions; Toxicity
Clin Pharm. 1985; 4:434–9

Aluminum accumulation in the bones of patients with renal failure was first reported in 1971 by Parsons et al.[1] The importance of this observation was not recognized until Alfrey et al.[2] suggested that aluminum was a contributing factor in the development of dialysis encephalopathy syndrome (dialysis dementia). Shortly thereafter, patients who were diagnosed as having dialysis encephalopathy syndrome were observed to have frequent osteomalacic fractures.[3] Initial reports of aluminum accumulation in patients receiving hemodialysis led investigators to suspect that dialysate was the source of aluminum. Recently, aluminum intoxication also has been observed in nondialyzed patients receiving aluminum-containing antacids to control hyperphosphatemia.[4] In addition to the skeletal and neurologic damage caused by exposure to aluminum, accumulation of alumi-

Karen E. Vick is Pharmacy Resident, University of Wisconsin Hospital and Clinics, Madison. Curtis A. Johnson, Pharm.D., is Clinical Associate Professor, Schools of Pharmacy and Medicine, University of Wisconsin, Madison.

Address reprint requests to Dr. Johnson at 425 North Charter Street, Madison, WI 53706.

num in a patient with chronic renal disease may cause microcytic anemia.[5]

Renal osteodystrophy is a bone disease resembling osteomalacia or osteitis fibrosa cystica that is commonly seen in patients with progressive renal failure.[6,7] Osteitis fibrosa cystica, a condition in which calcified bone is resorbed and replaced with fibrous tissue, occurs most frequently. It results usually from secondary hyperparathyroidism that is accompanied by low serum calcium concentrations and vitamin D deficiency.[8] Osteomalacia—a gradual softening and bending of the bone because of failure of osteoid tissue to calcify—usually occurs in the presence of normal or elevated serum calcium concentrations. In osteomalacia the parathyroid hormone (PTH) concentration is lower than that usually found in patients with end-stage renal disease.

Hsu et al.[6] investigated the incidence, age at onset, and progression of the radiographic, histologic, and biochemical characteristics of renal osteodystrophy in 50 children with chronic renal failure. During a 10-year observation period, 79% of the patients developed radiographic symptoms of osteodystrophy. All children whose renal failure was diagnosed before three years of age developed renal osteodystrophy. In those who had a later onset of renal failure, 60% developed bone disease. In a second evaluation Palma et al.[7] studied the records of 327 late-stage or terminally ill renal-failure patients who underwent bone-marrow biopsies. Of those patients given biopsies, 54% showed pure osteitis fibrosa cystica, 34% showed osteomalacia with osteitis fibrosa cystica, and 12% showed neither abnormality. The histologic features of both types of osteodystrophy have been associated with the accumulation of aluminum in bone.[9,10]

This article describes the pathophysiology and clinical presentation of aluminum-related osteomalacia, discusses ways to prevent its development, and examines the use of chelation therapy and vitamin D analogues for treatment of the disease.

Pathophysiology

Aluminum-related osteomalacia appears to develop because of exposure to aluminum in two ways. High concentrations of aluminum have been present in some hemodialysis fluids.[11,12]; current recommendations are that dialysate solutions contain no more than 10 μg of aluminum per liter.[13] Another route of aluminum exposure is through oral absorption of aluminum from aluminum-containing antacids.[14] Most patients with advanced renal disease require aluminum-containing antacids to control elevated serum phosphorus concentrations. Chronic use of aluminum-containing antacids increases the risk of developing osteomalacia particularly in children.[4,15] Other possible means of aluminum exposure include total parenteral nutrient[16] and albumin solutions.[17]

Animal studies have been conducted to explore the interaction between aluminum and bone.[18,19] Evidence to date indicates that aluminum interacts with citrate—at physiologic concentrations of citrate—to form a potent growth inhibitor of calcium phosphate crystals and bone mineralization.[20] Other polyvalent cations such as iron (+3), beryllium, and chromium may also interact with citric acid to form metal–citrate complexes. Growth inhibition results from adsorption of the complexes to calcium phosphate crystals, which stunts further growth of the crystals and thereby inhibits bone mineralization. In its complexed form, aluminum is deposited along mineralization fronts in bone where crystal growth normally occurs.[20]

Other mechanisms of aluminum-induced bone disease have been proposed, but no in vivo human data are available. Bachra and van Harskamp[21] demonstrated that the addition of small amounts of aluminum to a highly supersaturated solution of calcium and phosphorus caused precipitation of phosphate. The precipitated phosphate then served as a nucleus around which calcium apatite crystals deposited. Whether this mechanism occurs during in vivo dystrophic calcification remains unclear.

Another mechanism involves aluminum interference with phosphatase activity,[10] which alters the normal mineralization of bone.[22] The role of this mechanism in human osteomalacia is unclear since all available data are from animal studies.

Aluminum deposition may occur throughout the entire reticuloendothelial system, not just in mineralized bone, based on Kaye's observations of positive aluminum stains in the marrow of patients with aluminum in mineralized bones.[23] Pierides et al.[24] observed heavy iron deposition in both mineralized bone and marrow of patients with advanced osteomalacia, which suggests yet another etiology for the development of osteomalacia since iron (+3) can form complexes with citric acid.

The relationship between PTH, calcium, and aluminum has not been defined. Patients with aluminum-related osteomalacia often have normal serum concentrations of PTH and a decreased responsiveness of the parathyroid glands to low serum calcium concentrations.[25] Aluminum deposits in the parathyroid glands may be responsible for this effect.[26] Low concentrations of PTH alone may contribute to suppressed bone growth.

As proposed by Boyce et al.,[27] a combination of factors may lead to the development of hypercalcemia. Often serum calcium concentrations are normal to mildly elevated in patients with this aluminum-related disease. Initially, many patients with progressive renal disease develop hypocalcemia and are treated with vitamin D. This treatment increases calcium absorption and raises serum calcium concentrations; however, aluminum deposition blocks the uptake of calcium into the bone, and the resultant hypercalcemia leads to diminished PTH release.

Clinical Presentation

The major symptoms of aluminum-related osteomalacia include skeletal pain, fractures, and vertebral collapse.[28] Diagnosis can be difficult because specific laboratory findings are often confusing; a patient may have a normal to elevated serum calcium concentration, a moderately elevated serum phosphate concentration, a normal to moderately elevated serum alkaline phosphatase concentration, and a normal to moderately elevated serum PTH concentration.[28]

To diagnose the disease, a bone biopsy with either specific staining for aluminum or a direct measurement of aluminum content is required.[29] Most investigators administer a tetracycline to label bone before performing a biopsy. Aluminum content can be measured by spectrophotometry, energy-dispersive roentgenographic analysis, or specific histochemical stains. Because most laboratories are not equipped to perform these diagnostic procedures, many must be performed in referral centers.[29]

Because it is difficult to obtain a direct measurement of aluminum in bone, the use of the aluminum-chelating agent deferoxamine mesylate to measure aluminum content indirectly has been proposed.[29,30] Deferoxamine, a heavy-metal antagonist, is a sideochrome produced as the ferric complex by *Streptomyces pilosus*.[31] After the ferric component is removed, the metal-free ligand is used as the mesylate salt. Deferoxamine chelates a metal ion to the three hydroxamic groups of the molecule. The complex formed in plasma by this chelation is water soluble and is readily excreted by the kidneys or cleared by hemodialysis[32] or peritoneal dialysis.[33] The rate of complex formation appears to be pH dependent and occurs rapidly in an acidic environment.[31]

To evaluate the use of deferoxamine as a diagnostic agent, Milliner et al.[29] administered 40 mg/kg of intravenous deferoxamine infused over two hours to 54 patients on hemodialysis. Serum aluminum concentrations increased within two hours after drug administration. Peak serum aluminum concentrations, which ranged from 164 to 1566% of baseline, occurred 24–40 hours after the infusion. In patients with biopsy-documented aluminum-related osteodystrophy, peak concentrations of aluminum were 733 ± 326 μg/L, significantly higher than the 307 ± 122 μg/L in patients without aluminum-related bone disease. The change in serum aluminum concentration after the intravenous infusion correlated with bone aluminum content. An improvement in parathyroid function (increased PTH secretion) also was noted after the infusion. Based on an incremental change in serum aluminum concentrations of more than 200 μg/L, the diagnostic specificity of the test was only 50% (i.e., only 50% of patients who did not have the disease had an increase of 200 μg/L or less). Use of an increment of 300 μg/L improved the specificity to 71%.

Prevention

Aluminum intoxication can be treated by removing deposited aluminum from bone or prevented by eliminating exposure to aluminum. As previously stated, standards now restrict the aluminum content in hemodialysis solutions.[13] Since commercial preparations of peritoneal dialysate now available in this country contain nontoxic amounts of aluminum,[34] efforts to reduce aluminum exposure are directed at improving current methods of treating hyperphosphatemia (Table 1).

Aluminum-containing antacids, which have contained primarily aluminum hydroxide, have been used extensively for their phosphate-binding capability. At one time it was believed that aluminum taken orally was not absorbed by the gastrointestinal tract. Subsequent study has demonstrated that aluminum absorption by this route may be substantial, which may present a risk to patients.[14] Interest is growing in the search for alternative aluminum-free phosphate binders.

Slatopolsky et al.[35] studied the effects of calcium carbonate for treating hyperphosphatemia. In a study of 10 patients, serum phosphate concentrations were maintained equally with either calcium carbonate or aluminum-containing antacids. It should be noted that, during the control period when neither drug was administered, the mean serum phosphate concentration in these patients was only modestly elevated.

Despite the widespread interest in using calcium carbonate, only limited data comparing the therapeutic effects of calcium and aluminum are available. Calcium should be used cautiously in patients with hypercalcemia or in whom there is substantial risk of developing metastatic calcification. Likewise, calcium should be administered carefully to patients receiving vitamin D preparations because of the potential risk of hypercalcemia. One prudent approach would be to control initial hyperphosphatemia using the smallest possible dose of an aluminum-containing antacid, and, when serum phosphate concentrations have been reduced, convert the patient to calcium carbonate.

Polyuronic acid, another nonaluminum-containing phosphate binder, has been under investigation.[36] In a study involving dogs, this agent was as effective as aluminum hydroxide and calcium carbonate for treating hyperphosphatemia. Additional experience with this compound will be necessary before it can be recommended for use in humans.

Aluminum-related osteomalacia has been recently recognized as a major clinical problem in renal patients, and little is known about whether the prevention of aluminum exposure will stop development of the disease. Since it will be some time before preventive measures can be evaluated, patients who already have the disease or who develop it despite preventive efforts must be treated.

Treatment

Deferoxamine mesylate and vitamin D analogues have been used to treat aluminum-related osteomalacia. The only successes have been with deferoxamine (Table 1).

Chelation Therapy. The use of deferoxamine mesylate to treat osteomalacia was first reported by Brown et al.[37] Weekly administration of the drug to two patients during dialysis led to increased joint flexibility, diminished skeletal pain, improved ambulation, and improved posture. In spite of the clinical improvement, the bone structure of these patients remained abnormal, and little change was noted in the bone aluminum content. To date chelation therapy with deferoxamine appears to be the only successful treatment for aluminum-related osteomalacia because it is able to facilitate the removal of aluminum from bone. Use of deferoxamine has led to improvements in patients' symptoms and bone histology.

Malluche et al.[38] described the use of long-term intermittent infusions of deferoxamine in seven patients on hemodialysis or continuous ambulatory peritoneal dialysis (CAPD). Patients receiving hemodialysis were given 14.25 mg/kg/hr of deferoxamine intravenously three times per week during the first two hours of dialysis. Patients on CAPD received 85 mg/kg of deferoxamine intravenously once a week. Increased serum aluminum concentrations were noted in all patients following treatment, as were improved bone histology, decreased bone aluminum content, increased mineralization, decreased lamellar osteoid. The amount of aluminum removed from bone and the total amount of aluminum removed by the hemodialyzer were calculated for two patients. Aluminum removal from bone was estimated by multiplying the observed decrease in bone aluminum content by the dry weight of the skeleton. In both patients, total body aluminum removal exceeded the amount of aluminum removed from bone, which suggests that aluminum was removed from other sites of accumulation. The authors also noted that PTH secretion increased, perhaps as a result of aluminum removal from the parathyroid glands.

In another study, clinical improvement was seen in 14 of 16 patients receiving 2–6 g of intravenous deferoxamine per week for 20 weeks.[39] Follow-up bone biopsies were not reported.

The results from the above studies are limited because of the small number of patients studied. In all cases patients reported symptomatic clinical improvement. Malluche et al.[38] reported no serious side effects or cases of iron-deficiency anemia after 2.5–8 months of therapy involving more than 400 deferoxamine infusions. Brown[37] and Nebeker[39] also found no serious adverse drug effects. The reported changes in bone histology varied from histological improvement[38] to no improvement.[37] Nebeker[39] did not perform follow-up biopsies. The clinical improvement seen with deferoxamine therapy may benefit the patient even though a direct cost-benefit analysis has not been performed.

The risk of aluminum intoxication to patients receiving CAPD remains unknown. Since peritoneal dialysate contains negligible amounts of aluminum, the primary source of aluminum for these patients is aluminum-containing antacids.

Rottembourg et al.[34] demonstrated that the transfer of aluminum across the peritoneal membrane depends on serum aluminum concentrations. Other factors such as dialysate pH may also be important. Because peritoneal dialyzability of aluminum is improved in the presence of high serum aluminum concentrations, there has been interest in using deferoxamine in patients on CAPD to decrease the serum aluminum content.

Hercz et al.[40] recently reported on the use of intravenous and intraperitoneally administered deferoxamine in patients on peritoneal dialysis. A 40-mg/kg intraperitoneal dose of deferoxamine was administered in the overnight dialysate exchange, which led to increased aluminum removal compared with baseline and no observed adverse effects. The authors also found that equal doses of intraperitoneal and intravenous deferoxamine had similar effects on the removal of aluminum from peritoneal-dialysis patients. The effect of one dose persisted for several days with both methods. Should intraperitoneal dosing prove successful, self-administration of deferoxamine may become possible.

At present, deferoxamine has not been approved by FDA for use as a chelating agent for aluminum.

Table 1.
Approaches to Preventing and Treating Aluminum-Related Osteomalacia

Prevention
Reduce aluminum content in dialysis solutions
Reduce doses of aluminum hydroxide in antacids
Use nonaluminum-containing phosphate binders (calcium carbonate)
Treatment
Chelate aluminum with deferoxamine
Increase bone mineralization using vitamin D analogues

The drug's popularity is increasing among nephrologists because of its clinical effectiveness and apparent lack of adverse effects. Although the frequency of adverse reactions has not been determined, the most commonly reported toxicity has been pain at the injection site. Other reported side effects are skin flushing, erythema, urticaria, hypotension, and shock following rapid i.v. infusion. A possible histamine-liberating property of the drug may cause these effects. To avoid such responses, the manufacturer recommends that the drug be given intramuscularly or by slow i.v. infusion. Long-term therapy with deferoxamine has been associated with allergic-type reactions, blurred vision, leg cramps, tachycardia, and fever. Cataracts have developed in patients following long-term use of the drug; periodic slit-lamp examinations are recommended.

The dose of deferoxamine required for aluminum chelation is not well established. The dose needed to treat aluminum intoxication is presumably higher than that required for iron intoxication because of the decreased affinity of deferoxamine for aluminum compared with iron. For the treatment of iron intoxication, doses greater than 6 g/day are not approved. Intravenous infusion rates should not exceed 15 mg/kg/hr.

Vitamin D Therapy. Vitamin D analogues have also been used to treat aluminum-related osteomalacia. Neither calcitriol (1α,25-dihydroxyvitamin D_3) nor calcifediol (25-hydroxyvitamin D_3) has improved symptoms of the disease or bone histology. In early trials, approximately two thirds of the patients treated with 24,25-dihydroxyvitamin D_3 showed improved symptoms and histology.[41] Further investigation has revealed no benefit from 24,25-dihydroxyvitamin D_3 alone; however, combined therapy with calcitriol may be of value.[42]

To investigate the value of treatment with vitamin D preparations, it will be necessary to differentiate between osteitis fibrosa cystica (usually vitamin D responsive) and osteomalacia. Patients with mixed disease may show a variable response, complicating the interpretation of results.

Conclusion

Aluminum appears to be the etiologic agent for a vitamin D-resistant osteomalacia common in long-term dialysis patients or in renal-failure patients consuming aluminum-containing antacids. Aluminum has been localized histochemically in the osteomalacic bone of patients with chronic renal failure. The exact pathogenesis of this disorder is only now becoming understood; no one mechanism is responsible for the condition in all patients. Efforts at prevention have consequently not been uniformly successful. The chelating agent deferoxamine is proving efficacious in reducing pain, increasing ambulation, and improving the histologic effects of aluminum on bone. At present clinical experience is limited to a small number of patients. Although dosage recommendations and treatment plans remain empiric, further study of this drug is warranted.

References

1. Parsons V, Davies C, Goode C et al. Aluminum in bone from patients with renal failure. *Br Med J.* 1971; 4:273–5.
2. Alfrey AC, LeGendre GR, Kaehny WD. The dialysis encephalopathy syndrome. Possible aluminum intoxication. *N Engl J Med.* 1976; 294:184–8.
3. Pierides AM, Edwards WG, Cullum UX et al. Hemodialysis encephalopathy with osteomalacic fractures and muscle weakness. *Kidney Int.* 1980; 18:115–24.
4. Andreoli SP, Bergstein JM, Sherrard DJ. Aluminum intoxication from aluminum-containing phosphate binders in children with azotemia not undergoing dialysis. *N Engl J Med.* 1984; 310:1079–84.
5. Wills MR, Savory J. Aluminum poisoning: dialysis encephalopathy, osteomalacia, and anaemia. *Lancet.* 1983; 2:29–34.
6. Hsu AC, Kooh SW, Fraser D et al. Renal osteodystrophy in children with chronic renal failure: an unexpectedly common and incapacitating complication. *Pediatrics.* 1982; 20:742–50.
7. Palma FJ, Ellis HA, Cook DB et al. Osteomalacia in patients with chronic renal failure before dialysis or transplantation. *Q J Med.* 1983; 207:332–48.
8. Alfrey AC. Chronic renal failure: manifestations and pathogenesis. In: Schrier RW, ed. Renal and electrolyte disorders. Boston: Little, Brown & Co.; 1980:409–41.
9. Ott SM, Maloney NA, Coburn JW et al. The prevalence of bone aluminum deposition in renal osteodystrophy and its relation to the response to calcitriol therapy. *N Engl J Med.* 1982; 307:709–13.
10. Ihle B, Buchanan M, Stevens B et al. Aluminum associated bone disease: clinico-pathologic correlation. *Am J Kidney Dis.* 1982; 2:255–63.
11. Ward MK, Feest TG, Ellis HA et al. Osteomalacic dialysis osteodystrophy: evidence for a water-borne aetiologic agent, probably aluminum. *Lancet.* 1978; 1:841–5.
12. Walker GS, Aaron JE, Peacock M et al. Dialysate aluminum concentration and renal bone disease. *Kidney Int.* 1982; 21:411–5.
13. Association for the Advancement of Medical Instrumentation. Standard for hemodialysis system. Arlington, VA: Association for the Advancement of Medical Instrumentation; 1982.
14. Kaehny WD, Hegg AP, Alfrey AC. Gastrointestinal absorption of aluminum from aluminum-containing antacids. *N Engl J Med.* 1977; 296:1389–90.
15. Alfrey AC. Aluminum intoxication. *N Engl J Med.* 1984; 310:1113–5.
16. Klein GL, Ott SM, Alfrey AC et al. Aluminum as a factor in the bone disease of long-term parenteral nutrition. *Trans Assoc Am Physicians.* 1982; 95:155–64.
17. Milliner DS, Shinaberger JH, Shuman P et al. Inadvertent aluminum administration during plasma exchange due to aluminum contamination of albumin-replacement solutions. *N Engl J Med.* 1984; 312:165–7.
18. Robertson JA, Felsenfeld AJ, Haygood CC et al. Animal model of aluminum-induced osteomalacia: role of chronic renal failure. *Kidney Int.* 1983; 23:327–35.
19. Goodman WG, Henry DA, Horst R et al. Parenteral aluminum administration in the dog: II. Induction of osteomalacia and effect on vitamin D metabolism. *Kidney Int.* 1984; 25:370–5.
20. Thomas WC, Meyer JL. Aluminum-induced osteomalacia: an explanation. *Am J Nephrol.* 1984; 4:201–3.
21. Bachra BN, van Harskamp GA. The effect of polyvalent metal ions on the stability of a buffer system for calcifica-

tion in vitro. *Calcif Tissue Res.* 1970; 4:359–65.
22. Lieberherr M, Grosse B, Cournot-Witmer G et al. In vitro effects of aluminum on bone phosphatases: a possible interaction with bPTH and vitamin D_3 metabolites. *Calcif Tissue Int.* 1982; 34:280–4.
23. Kaye M. Bone marrow aluminum storage in endstage renal disease. *Kidney Int.* 1984; 25:145. Abstract.
24. Pierides AM, Pierce-Myli M. Iron and aluminum osteomalacia in hemodialysis patients. *N Engl J Med.* 1984; 310:1113. Letter.
25. Ott SM. Aluminum-related osteomalacia. *Int J Artif Organs.* 1983; 6:173–5.
26. Morrissey J, Rothstein M, Mayor G et al. Suppression of parathyroid hormone release by aluminum. *Kidney Int.* 1982; 21:138. Abstract.
27. Boyce BF, Fell GS, Elder HY et al. Hypercalcaemic osteomalacia due to aluminum toxicity. *Lancet.* 1982; 2:1009–13.
28. Felsenfeld AJ, Gutman R, Llach F et al. Osteomalacia in chronic renal failure: a syndrome previously reported only with maintenance dialysis. *Am J Nephrol.* 1982; 2:147–54.
29. Milliner DS, Nebeker HG, Ott SM et al. Use of the deferoxamine infusion test in the diagnosis of aluminum-related osteodystrophy. *Ann Intern Med.* 1984; 101:775–80.
30. Smith AJ, Faugere MC, Abreo K et al. The value of single desferrioxamine (DFO) infusion for diagnosis of bone aluminum accumulation. *Kidney Int.* 1984; 25:154. Abstract.
31. Klaasen CD. Heavy metals and heavy-metal antagonists. In: Gilman AG, Goodman LS, Gilman A, eds. The pharmacological basis of therapeutics. New York: Macmillan Publishing Co., Inc. 1980:1615–37.
32. Milliner DS, Shinaberger JH, Miller JH et al. Removal of aluminum during hemodialysis: effect of desferrioxamine. Paper presented to National Kidney Foundation Meeting. Washington, DC: 1983 Dec 4.
33. Hercz G, Milliner DS, Shinaberger JH et al. Aluminum metabolism and removal during CAPD. *Kidney Int.* 1984; 25:257. Abstract.
34. Rottembourg J, Gallego JL, Jaudon MC et al. Serum concentration and peritoneal transfer of aluminum during treatment by continuous ambulatory peritoneal dialysis. *Kidney Int.* 1984; 25:919–24.
35. Slatopolsky E, Weerts C, Lopez S et al. Calcium carbonate is an effective phosphorous-binder in dialysis patients. Paper presented to American Society of Nephrology Meeting. Washington, DC: 1984 Dec 9.
36. Nebeker HG, Schneider HW, Coburn JW. A non-aluminum containing phosphate binder: polyuronic acid. Paper presented to American Society of Nephrology Meeting. Washington, DC: 1984 Dec 9.
37. Brown DJ, Dawborn JK, Ham KN et al. Treatment of dialysis osteomalacia with desferrioxamine. *Lancet.* 1982; 2:343–5.
38. Malluche HH, Smith AJ, Abreo K et al. The use of deferoxamine in the management of aluminum accumulation in bone in patients with renal failure. *N Engl J Med.* 1984; 311:140–4.
39. Nebeker HG, Milliner DS, Ott SM et al. Aluminum-related osteomalacia: clinical response to desferrioxamine. *Kidney Int.* 1984; 25:173. Abstract.
40. Hercz G, Salusky IB, Milliner DS et al. Effects of intraperitoneal and intravenous desferrioxamine on aluminum removal during CAPD. Paper presented to American Society of Nephrology Meeting. Washington, DC: 1984 Dec 9.
41. Ott SM, Recker RR, Coburn JW et al. Vitamin D therapy in aluminum-related osteomalacia. *Kidney Int.* 1983; 23:107. Abstract.
42. Hodsman AB, Wong EGC, Sherrard DJ et al. Preliminary trials with 24,25-dihydroxyvitamin D_3 in dialysis osteomalacia. *Am J Med.* 1983; 74:407–14.

"

Alternatives to Digitalis Glycosides

This limited value of digitalis as an inotropic agent is combined with a high incidence of adverse effects. Not surprisingly, therefore, investigators have been looking for a potent orally active inotropic agent suitable for use in patients with congestive heart failure. This search has concentrated on two classes of drugs: the β adrenergic agonists and the nonsympathomimetic, nonglycoside agents, the bipyridine derivatives. Orally active phosphodiesterase inhibitors have attracted less interest. . . .

If we assume that stimulation of the depressed myocardium is beneficial in the long term then the bipyridine group of drugs seem most likely to supersede the digitalis glycosides, either alone or in combination with treatment with vasodilators. Amrinone has many advantages, but the incidence of adverse side effects is unacceptably high. Milrinone, an equally effective compound, seems to be better tolerated and may prove to be the drug of choice in the future. Large clinical trials will be needed to show an overall favorable or unfavorable effect on mortality. The challenge remains that of developing a drug which not only produces symptomatic improvement in heart failure but also prolongs life expectancy.

—Johnston GD. Alternatives to the digitalis glycosides for heart failure. *Br Med J.* 1985; 290:803–4. Editorial.

"

Research

Multicenter evaluation of six methods for predicting warfarin maintenance-dose requirements from initial response

WILLIAM T. SAWYER, TIMOTHY E. POE, BRUCE R. CANADAY, JOHN S. WEINER, DENNIS M. WILLIAMS, C. EDWIN WEBB, AND MARK J. ELLISON

Abstract: Warfarin maintenance-dose requirements predicted by six mathematical methods based on initial response to therapy were compared with patients' actual dose requirements in a multicenter trial.

Data were collected for patients who had received an initial regimen of warfarin sodium 10 mg orally every 24 hours for three days and for whom a prothrombin time (PT) had been determined 16–20 hours after the third dose. Patients' individual dose requirements and PT values were recorded during one to three follow-up visits after discharge from one of seven medical centers. Prothrombin ratios (patient PT divided by control PT) calculated on day 4 were used for maintenance-dose prediction by five methods; a sixth method was based on the cumulative warfarin dose–PT response curve up to a PT value of 20 seconds.

For 54 men and 30 women who qualified for the study, 197 maintenance-dose–PT response measurements were recorded; 95 in the first four weeks of therapy, 76 during weeks 5–12, and 26 at 6–12 months after initial treatment. Prothrombin ratios were within the therapeutic range (PT 1.5–2.5 times the control value) in 154 observations, and the mean actual warfarin sodium maintenance dose associated with therapeutic response was 7.6 mg/day. For patients with therapeutic prothrombin ratios, dose predictions by the five methods using prothrombin ratios (PRs) correlated significantly with actual dose requirements. The formula that predicted doses numerically closest to the actual dose is as follows: Dose = 11.17 − 21.08 (log PR). Only 45 observations were obtained for the sixth prediction method, and the correlation between actual and predicted doses was not significant.

Initial warfarin maintenance-dose requirements can be predicted effectively based on one PT determination after administration of three daily 10-mg doses. Using these predictions, patient-specific maintenance-dose regimens may be determined earlier in therapy, resulting in potential cost savings from shorter hospital stays.

Index terms: Anticoagulants; Costs; Dosage; Hospitals; Methodology; Warfarin sodium
Clin Pharm. 1985; 4:440–6

WILLIAM T. SAWYER, M.S., is Assistant Director for Clinical Services, Department of Pharmacy, North Carolina Memorial Hospital, Chapel Hill, and Associate Professor of Clinical Pharmacy, School of Pharmacy, and Clinical Assistant Professor of Family Medicine, School of Medicine, University of North Carolina at Chapel Hill (UNCCH). TIMOTHY E. POE, PHARM.D., is Director of Pharmacy Education, Northwest Area Health Education Center (AHEC), Winston–Salem, NC, and Clinical Assistant Professor of Pharmacy, School of Pharmacy, UNCCH, and Assistant Professor of Family Medicine, Bowman–Gray School of Medicine, Winston–Salem. BRUCE R. CANADAY, PHARM.D., is Director of Pharmacy Education, Wilmington AHEC, Wilmington, NC, and Clinical Associate Professor of Pharmacy, School of Pharmacy, and Clinical Assistant Professor of Medicine, School of Medicine, UNCCH. JOHN S. WEINER, PHARM.D., is Director of Pharmacy Education, Fayetteville AHEC, Fayetteville, NC; Clinical Instructor, School of Pharmacy, UNCCH; and Clinical Associate, Duke University Medical Center, Durham, NC. DENNIS M. WILLIAMS, PHARM.D., is Director of Pharmacy, Orange–Chatham Comprehensive Health Services, Carrboro, NC, and Clinical Assistant Professor, School of Pharmacy, UNCCH. C. EDWIN WEBB, PHARM.D., is Director of Pharmacy Services, St. Joseph's Hospital, Asheville, NC. MARK J. ELLISON, PHARM.D., is Clinical Assistant Professor of Pharmacy, School of Pharmacy, UNCCH, and Instructor of Family Medicine, East Carolina University School of Medicine, Greenville. At the time of this study, Sawyer was Director of Pharmacy Education, Charlotte AHEC, Charlotte, NC; Williams was Associate Director of Pharmacy Activities, Area L Health Education Center, Tarboro, NC; and Webb was Director of Pharmacy Education, Mountain AHEC, Asheville, and Clinical Associate Professor of Pharmacy, School of Pharmacy, and Clinical Assistant Professor of Family Medicine, School of Medicine, UNCCH.

Address reprint requests to Mr. Sawyer at the Department of Pharmacy, North Carolina Memorial Hospital, Manning Drive, Chapel Hill, NC 27514.

The assistance of Claude U. Paoloni, Director of the UNC School of Pharmacy AHEC Program, and Eugene Mayer, M.D., Director of the North Carolina AHEC Program, and the technical assistance of Aileen MacMillan and Marie Mullis are acknowledged.

Supported in part by a grant from E. I. DuPont de Nemours and Company, Wilmington, DE.

Traditional methods for initiating oral anticoagulant therapy have been inefficient and potentially hazardous.[1-3] Initial administration of a large loading dose, although it produces rapid anticoagulation, does not hasten the onset of antithrombotic action and may predispose the patient to adverse effects, including bleeding and dermatologic reactions.[4-7] Determination of a satisfactory warfarin maintenance dose frequently involves a time-consuming empiric process of daily prothrombin time (PT) measurement and frequent dosage adjustments, necessitating extended hospitalizations.[8]

Recently, techniques for estimating warfarin maintenance dose as a function of initial response have been described.[9-14] In most of these methods, three daily 10-mg oral warfarin doses are administered initially and PT is measured 16–18 hours after the third dose.[9,10-13] Retrospective application of these methods in small patient populations in individual centers has produced encouraging results.[10-12,15,16] However, the methods have not been compared in a large, multicenter trial, and their current clinical application remains limited.

If the value of warfarin maintenance-dose estimation techniques could be demonstrated, these techniques could be used to enhance the efficiency of oral anticoagulant therapy. For this reason, we conducted a prospective, multicenter study to compare warfarin maintenance doses calculated using six previously published dose-prediction methods with maintenance doses actually required by patients after titration of anticoagulant therapy to therapeutic values.

Methods

Study Population. The study was conducted in seven medical facilities that are affiliated with the North Carolina Area Health Education Center (AHEC) program. The appropriate committee(s) in each facility reviewed and approved the study protocol. All patients requiring oral warfarin sodium for prevention or treatment of thromboembolic disease were prospectively considered for participation. So that we could evaluate warfarin-dose predictability under routine clinical conditions, we did not exclude patients who had other disease states (e.g., congestive heart failure, hepatic disease, or thyroid disease). However, we excluded patients who were concurrently receiving drugs known to affect warfarin pharmacodynamics or clinical response substantially.[16,17] Because of the minimal effect of heparin on warfarin response[18] and the intent to simulate standard clinical conditions, we did not exclude patients concurrently receiving heparin as long as the patient's partial thromboplastin time (PTT) when warfarin was initiated was equal to or less than two times the control value.

Patients were entered in the study if they met the following two criteria: (1) they had received a fixed initial warfarin dosage regimen consisting of 10-mg oral doses administered at 24-hour intervals for three days and (2) patient and control PT values had been obtained approximately 16–20 hours after the third 10-mg dose.

Prediction of Maintenance Dose. After the initial three days of warfarin administration, dosages were individually titrated to achieve and maintain therapeutic PT values of 1.5–2.5 times the control value. After discharge, each patient was seen at least once but not more than three times for study follow-up during maintenance therapy. At each visit, the patient's dose requirement and the measured patient and control PT values were recorded to evaluate response to maintenance therapy. To allow for stabilization of plasma warfarin concentration and PT response,[19,20] we included in our analysis only dose-response observations that were obtained after a daily dosage regimen had been administered continuously for at least 10 days. During maintenance therapy, blood samples for PT determinations were obtained in outpatient facilities associated with the medical centers involved in the study or in private physicians' offices.

Coagulation Studies. PT values were determined in all facilities by the standard one-stage Quick method,[21] although the thromboplastin reagent used varied among individual facilities. For each patient, PT measurements were reported as the prothrombin ratio (PR), calculated by dividing the patient PT by the control PT value.

Calculations. Prothrombin ratios (PRs) for day 4 of warfarin therapy were used to predict patient-specific warfarin maintenance doses by five methods, all involving initial administration of three 10-mg daily doses.[9-13] Although equations for two of these methods were originally derived as a function of a coagulation measurement other than the prothrombin ratio,[12,13] for purposes of this study we used techniques previously described[22,23] to standardize all formulas to a prothrombin-ratio response index. Equations for these five methods are as follows:

Method 1[12]: $$\text{Dose} = 7.6 \cdot \log\{[68.9/(3.636 \cdot \text{PR} - 2.636)] - 7.13\} - 3.33 \quad (1)$$

Method 2[11]: $$\text{Dose} = 11.17 - 21.08 (\log \text{PR}) \quad (2)$$

Method 3[10]: $$\text{Dose} = -10 (\text{PR} - 2.4) \quad (3)$$

Method 4[13]: $$\text{Dose} = 0.332 [100/(3.636 \cdot \text{PR} - 2.636) - 11.6] \quad (4)$$

Method 5[9]: $$\text{Dose} = 14.87 - (34.08 \cdot \log \text{PR}) \quad (5)$$

Maintenance dose for each patient was also estimated as a function of the area under the cumulative warfarin dose–PT response curve (AUC) up to a PT value of 20 seconds,[14] as follows:

Method 6: $$\text{Dose} = 0.0465 \cdot \text{AUC} + 1.5 \quad (6)$$

Maintenance-dose estimates were initially computed with a handheld programmable calculator

(TI-59, Texas Instruments, Inc., Lubbock, TX 79408), using a previously described program.[22] Before data analysis, dosage calculations were verified using a commercial pharmacokinetics software system (Data Med, Inc., Minneapolis, MN 55414) with a microcomputer (Apple IIe, Apple Computer, Inc., Cupertino, CA 95014).

Data Analysis. We used three statistical techniques to compare predicted and actual warfarin maintenance doses:

1. The correlation between predicted and actual doses was evaluated by linear regression analysis.
2. Paired predicted and actual dose requirements were directly compared using nonparametric statistical methods for matched data pairs (Wilcoxon signed ranks test).
3. Numerical differences between the predicted dose and actual dose were determined for each method, and the absolute values of these numerical differences were calculated. The absolute fractional differences (aFD) between paired values were then calculated with the following equation:
   aFD = |(predicted dose − actual dose)/actual dose| (7)

In therapeutically anticoagulated patients, the relationship between actual and predicted maintenance dose was evaluated for all observations and at each follow-up PT measurement. Actual and predicted dose values were also compared in patients with recorded prothrombin-ratio responses outside the therapeutic range. In addition, the influence of selected patient variables (age, sex, weight, initial prothrombin-ratio response, indication for therapy, study facility) on actual maintenance-dose requirements and dose predictability was evaluated using linear regression and analysis of variance. Where multiple classes (>2) of a variable were compared by analysis of variance, Duncan's multiple-range test was used. For all statistical analyses, an a priori $p < 0.05$ was considered significant. Computerized statistical support for data analysis included the Statistical Analysis System (SAS), version 82.4.[24]

Results

Data were analyzed for 84 patients (54 men and 30 women) who qualified for inclusion in the study (Table 1). The most frequent indications of warfarin administration included pulmonary embolism (27 patients) and deep-vein thrombosis (25 patients). Prothrombin ratio on day 4 ranged from 1.1 to 2.7 (mean 1.5). A total of 197 maintenance-dose–PT response measurements were recorded (the first measurement in all 84 patients, a second measurement in 74 patients, and a third in 39 patients). Follow-up observations were divided into three categories according to the time elapsed after initiation of therapy: 1–4 weeks, 5–12 weeks, and more than 12 weeks. Of the 197 follow-up measurements, 95 were recorded during the first four weeks of therapy (mean 18.2 days after initiation), 76 during weeks 5–12 (mean 47.2 days), and 26 between 6 and 12 months after initial treatment (mean 169.6 days).

To assess whether patients exhibited a "stable" PT response to a given maintenance dose of warfarin, we evaluated the range of PT values in patients having two or more follow-up observations during administration of the same warfarin dose. In 13 patients, three dose-response measurements were recorded during administration of the same maintenance dose; the mean difference between the highest and lowest PT value in each patient was 2.2 seconds. In each of the 13 patients, all three PT values were within the therapeutic range. In 39 additional patients, two dose-response measurements were made during administration of the same maintenance dose; both responses were within the therapeutic range in 27 patients and both were outside the therapeutic range in six patients. For the six remaining patients, one of two measurements was above the therapeutic range in three cases, while one was below the therapeutic range in the other three. However, for these six pairs of PT measurements, the mean difference between the two values was only 4.3 seconds.

Prothrombin ratios were within the therapeutic range (1.5–2.5) in 154 of the 197 observations (Table 2). Considering all observations, the mean actual maintenance warfarin dose associated with therapeutic response was 7.6 mg, and the most frequently administered actual dose was 7.5 mg.

Comparison of Prediction Methods. A significant correlation was observed between doses predicted with each of the fixed initial regimen methods (methods 1–5) and actual warfarin mainte-

Table 1.
Characteristics of 54 Men and 30 Women Included in Study

Variable	Value
Age (yr)	
Mean ± S.D.	53.1 ± 18.7
Range	19–91
Weight (kg)	
Mean ± S.D.	80.5 ± 20.6
Range	50–179.5
Height (cm)	
Mean ± S.D.	171.7 ± 9.6
Range	149.9–193.0
Initial prothrombin ratio	
Mean ± S.D.	1.5 ± 0.3
Range	1.1–2.7
Indication for anticoagulation	
Deep-vein thrombosis	25
Pulmonary embolus	27
Transient ischemic attack or embolic stroke	13
Atrial fibrillation	7
Recent myocardial infarction	5
Other	7

Table 2.
Warfarin Maintenance Doses Administered and Corresponding Prothrombin Ratios

Weeks after Initiation of Warfarin[a]	Administered Dose in mg[b]	Prothrombin Ratio[b]
All Patients		
1–4 (*n* = 84)	8.3 ± 3.0 (2.5–15.0)	2.1 ± 0.7 (1.1–5.4)
5–12 (*n* = 74)	7.5 ± 2.6 (2.5–12.5)	1.8 ± 0.4 (1.1–3.5)
>12 (*n* = 39)	7.3 ± 2.5 (3.8–12.5)	1.7 ± 0.2 (1.2–2.3)
Cumulative (*n* = 197)	7.8 ± 3.1 (2.5–15.0)	2.0 ± 0.7 (1.0–5.4)
Patients with Therapeutic Response (Prothrombin Ratio 1.5–2.5)		
1–4 (*n* = 69)	7.8 ± 2.9 (2.5–15.0)	1.9 ± 0.3 (1.5–2.5)
5–12 (*n* = 60)	7.5 ± 2.5 (2.5–12.5)	1.8 ± 0.2 (1.5–2.5)
>12 (*n* = 25)	7.5 ± 2.5 (3.8–12.5)	1.8 ± 0.2 (1.5–2.3)
Cumulative (*n* = 154)	7.6 ± 2.9 (2.5–15.0)	1.8 ± 0.3 (1.5–2.5)

[a] *n* = Number of observations.
[b] Mean ± S.D. (range).

nance-dose requirements in therapeutically anticoagulated patients (Table 3). Method 2 predicted maintenance-doses (mean 7.6 mg) that were numerically closest to actual dose (mean difference 0.0 mg) and were not significantly different from actual maintenance-therapy dose requirements among all observations and within each group. Doses predicted by method 1 (mean 6.2 mg) were significantly less than actual requirements (mean 7.6 mg) overall. Within each group, doses predicted by method 1 were significantly less than actual values at 1-4 and 5-12 weeks and equivalent to actual doses at determinations after more than 12 weeks. Doses predicted with methods 3-5 were significantly higher than actual maintenance dose values among all observations and within each time period. The mean numerical difference between actual dose and dose predicted by method 2 (0.0 mg) was significantly different from mean numerical differences for methods 1, 3, 4, and 5, which ranged from −1.2 to 2.6 mg. The results of evaluating absolute values of the numerical differences were consistent with these observations. Overall, absolute differences for method 2 (mean 1.8 mg) were significantly less than absolute differences for method 1 and methods 3-5. In addition, the mean absolute fractional difference for method 2 (29.0%) was not significantly different from the value for method 1 (mean 29.2%) and was significantly less than the values for methods 3-5 (45.5%, 43.2%, and 39.4%, respectively).

The relationship between maintenance doses predicted with method 6 (AUC) and patients' actual dose requirements was evaluated in a limited number of cases. Because method 6 requires daily PT measurements until a value of 20 seconds or greater is achieved, the method could be studied in only 45 observations in 23 patients. Although the mean dose predicted with method 6 (6.6 mg) was not significantly different from actual maintenance dose requirements (mean 6.7 mg) among these observations, the correlation between the two values (r = 0.19) was not significant. Direct evaluation of the relationship between the calculated area under the cumulative warfarin dose–PT response curve and actual dose requirements yielded similar results, with no significant correlation identified.

Table 3.
Predicted Warfarin Maintenance Dose Requirements in Patients with Therapeutic Response

Weeks after Initiation of Warfarin[a]	Predicted Dose in mg (Mean ± S.D.)	*r*	aD[b] (Mean ± S.D.)
Method 1			
1–4 (*n* = 69)	6.1 ± 1.9	0.50	2.3 ± 2.0
5–12 (*n* = 60)	6.4 ± 1.9	0.57	1.8 ± 1.5
>12 (*n* = 25)	6.1 ± 2.2	0.41	2.6 ± 1.6
Cumulative (*n* = 154)	6.2 ± 2.0	0.48	2.2 ± 1.8
Method 2			
1–4 (*n* = 69)	7.5 ± 1.8	0.50	1.9 ± 1.6
5–12 (*n* = 60)	7.7 ± 1.8	0.58	1.7 ± 1.2
>12 (*n* = 25)	7.6 ± 2.0	0.40	2.1 ± 1.7
Cumulative (*n* = 154)	7.6 ± 1.9	0.49	1.9 ± 1.5
Method 3			
1–4 (*n* = 69)	8.7 ± 3.2	0.47	2.6 ± 2.0
5–12 (*n* = 60)	9.2 ± 3.1	0.59	2.6 ± 1.7
>12 (*n* = 25)	9.1 ± 3.4	0.38	3.2 ± 2.3
Cumulative (*n* = 154)	9.0 ± 3.2	0.48	2.7 ± 2.0
Method 4			
1–4 (*n* = 69)	8.4 ± 3.9	0.48	2.7 ± 2.4
5–12 (*n* = 60)	8.4 ± 3.7	0.66	2.4 ± 1.8
>12 (*n* = 25)	9.3 ± 3.5	0.47	3.3 ± 2.4
Cumulative (*n* = 154)	8.5 ± 3.7	0.50	2.7 ± 2.2
Method 5			
1–4 (*n* = 69)	8.5 ± 3.0	0.49	2.3 ± 1.9
5–12 (*n* = 60)	8.8 ± 3.0	0.57	2.3 ± 1.7
>12 (*n* = 25)	8.5 ± 3.1	0.35	2.8 ± 2.3
Cumulative (*n* = 154)	8.6 ± 3.0	0.48	2.4 ± 1.9

[a] *n* = Number of observations.
[b] Absolute difference, in milligrams, between administered dose and predicted dose.

Influence of Patient Characteristics. Patients' indications for warfarin therapy influenced neither actual dose requirements nor maintenance-dose predictability as reflected by absolute differences between method 2 predictions and actual dose. However, patient sex, weight, and age influenced actual maintenance dose requirements. Women required significantly lower doses (mean 6.5 mg) than men (mean 8.2 mg). Dose requirements also correlated positively with patient weight and negatively with patient age. Method 2 absolute differences were not significantly related to patient sex and weight or age.

Influence of Study Facility. There were no significant differences in mean actual maintenance-dose values for five of the six study facilities. The mean administered maintenance dose (11.5 mg) for five observations at facility 4 was significantly higher than that observed in other facilities (Table 4). However, dose predictability with Method 2 was not significantly different among all facilities, and no significant differences in absolute-difference values were noted.

Discussion

Our results demonstrate a clinically important correlation between actual warfarin maintenance dose and doses predicted by simple numerical techniques. Heretofore, these dose-prediction methods have been in limited use because they were developed retrospectively in small patient populations in single facilities.[9–11] Our current results in a larger number of patients indicate that the evaluated methods of predicting maintenance dose on the basis of response to a fixed initial dosing regimen (10 mg/day) can be applied to data pooled from several facilities. The correlations between actual dose and maintenance-dose predictions were similar for each of the fixed-dose methods, even though the equations were derived by different investigators using different laboratory indices of anticoagulation in different facilities.

Clearly, these techniques do not capture all sources of variability in the prediction of patient warfarin dose requirements. Factors such as changes in individual patient sensitivity and compliance may influence dose predictability. However, much of the observed variability, which is reflected in the value of the correlation coefficient, may have been related to the methods. Both in the development of the prediction methods and in this study, a range of prothrombin-ratio responses (1.5–2.5), rather than an individual value, was used as a therapeutic endpoint. In addition, most actual maintenance doses (more than 70%) were prescribed in 2.5-mg increments, whereas predicted doses were estimated to the nearest 0.1 mg. Nonetheless, a strong statistical association was observed between the actual dose and predictions by the fixed-dose methods. In 18 patients whose maintenance doses were predicted using the calculated area under the cumulative warfarin dose–PT curve, correlations with actual dose were weaker.

In our current study, method 2 predictions were the most representative of actual dose requirements when mean doses, absolute differences, and correlation coefficients were considered. Overall, method 2 predicted maintenance doses within 2.5 mg of actual recorded maintenance doses in 133 observations; therapeutic response was obtained with predicted doses in 83% of these cases. These results suggest that method 2 maintenance-dose predictions represent acceptable initial maintenance-dose therapy in patients receiving warfarin.

Although method 1-predicted doses were significantly lower than actual doses, therapeutic response was noted in 82% of observations in which the actual dose was within 2.5 mg of the method 1 prediction, and method 1 absolute fractional differences were comparable to method 2 values. In contrast, methods 3–5 overpredicted actual dose requirements at each observation. These dose-prediction methods were originally developed in patients whose steady-state prothrombin ratios ranged from 1.5 to 2.5; however, the actual maintenance doses administered in our current study resulted in mean prothrombin ratios that were less than two times the control (1.84)—a partial explanation for the overpredictions with methods 3–5. More recent data suggest that optimal anticoagulation in proximal deep-vein thrombosis is achieved with a prothrombin ratio of 1.5–2.0 rather than with a greater level of anticoagulation.[25,26] These observations are also consistent with the greater potential clinical utility of method 2.

Appropriate clinical application of these techniques requires not only documentation of their potential value but also identification of their potential limitations. In our current study, 23 nontherapeutic prothrombin ratios in 18 patients were observed in association with actual doses that were within 2.5 mg of method 2-predicted doses. In nine of these measurements in nine patients, actual maintenance doses greater than method 2 predictions produced prothrombin-ratios above the

Table 4.
Method 2 Warfarin Maintenance-Dose Prediction by Study Facility

Facility	No. Patients	No. Observations	Actual Warfarin Dose (mg)	Warfarin Dose Predicted by Method 2 (mg)	aD[a]
1	13	19	7.9	7.8	2.2
2	4	11	6.7	7.7	1.3
3	4	9	7.8	7.4	2.2
4	5	5	11.5[b]	8.7	3.0
5	19	32	7.1	6.9	1.8
6	31	69	7.5	7.9	1.8
7	8	9	8.0	8.4	1.5

[a] Absolute difference in milligrams between dose administered and dose predicted by method 2.

[b] Significantly higher than actual doses in other six facilities.

therapeutic range. Prothrombin-ratio responses below 1.5 were observed in three additional measurements in three patients whose maintenance doses were less than the method 2-predicted values. Therefore, in 66% of patients (52% of measurements) having a prothrombin ratio outside the therapeutic range and a maintenance dose within 2.5 mg of the method 2-predicted value, actual dose deviated from predicted dose in a fashion consistent with the response. These results suggest that the common practice of administering warfarin in 2.5-mg dose increments may be too imprecise for certain patients. Although therapy with alternating daily doses (e.g., 7.5 one day and 5.0 mg the next) is occasionally used and 2-mg tablets are available, warfarin doses are most frequently prescribed in multiples of 2.5 mg.[5,10–11] More careful titration of maintenance dose is probably desirable in selected patients. For example, for one patient in our study the predicted maintenance dose was 6.9 mg. Administration of a 7.5-mg daily dose to that patient produced a prothrombin ratio of 3.1, while 5-mg daily doses resulted in a prothrombin ratio of 1.4.

For 44 therapeutic prothrombin-ratio responses in 24 patients receiving actual doses that varied from method 2 predictions by more than 2.5 mg, we compared actual and predicted maintenance doses. For 27 of these observations (in 16 patients) an actual maintenance dose greater than that predicted by method 2 (mean difference 3.5 mg) was required. Based on these observations, we believe that precise initial dose estimation may not be possible in certain cases and that subsequent titration to higher doses may be necessary. The data also suggest that the potential for adverse effects from excessive initial anticoagulation is limited. Of these 44 therapeutic prothrombin-ratios, 10 were greater than 2.0 after an actual dose greater than the method 2-predicted value, and 13 were less than 2.0 after an actual dose lower than the method 2 estimate.

Use of a small initial warfarin dosage (10 mg/day) minimizes potential toxicity yet produces an acceptable onset of antithrombotic and anticoagulant effects.[3,6,7] This approach allows for early estimation of maintenance dose based on initial response; therefore, the time-consuming empiric process of daily dosage adjustments in the inpatient setting should be unnecessary for most patients. Adjustments of actual maintenance dose may be necessary because of interpatient variability and factors such as compliance or diet,[27,28] but these subsequent dosage adjustments do not require an inpatient hospital stay. If dose estimation is difficult or impractical because of unusual initial response, microcomputer-based algorithms can be used with previously described techniques for characterizing patient response to anticoagulants.[8,29,30]

Conclusion

An approximate initial warfarin maintenance dose can be predicted using simple calculation techniques that require only one PT determination after the administration of three 10-mg doses. If these techniques are used, patient-specific maintenance-dose regimens may be determined earlier in therapy, resulting in potential cost savings from shorter hospital stays.

References

1. Bays RP. Unusual sensitivity to warfarin sodium. *J La State Med Soc.* 1965; 117:55–9.
2. Coon WW, Willis PW. Hemorrhagic complications of anticoagulant therapy. *Arch Intern Med.* 1974; 133:386–92.
3. Deykin D. Warfarin therapy. *N Engl J Med.* 1970; 282:691–4, 801–3.
4. Deykin D, Wessler S, Reimer S. Evidence for an anthrombotic effect of dicumarol. *Am J Physiol.* 1960; 199:1161–4.
5. Jones RR, Cunningham J. Warfarin skin necrosis. *Br J Dermatol.* 1979; 100:561–5.
6. O'Reilly RA, Aggeler PM. Studies on coumarin anticoagulant drugs: initiation of warfarin therapy without a loading dose. *Circulation.* 1968; 38:169–77.
7. Udall JA. "No-load" warfarin therapy. *N Engl J Med.* 1970; 283:1345–6.
8. Sawyer WT, Finn AL. Digital computer-assisted warfarin therapy. Comparison of two models. *Comput Biomed Res.* 1979; 12:221–31.
9. Carter B, Reinders TR. Prediction of maintenance warfarin dosage from initial patient response. *Drug Intell Clin Pharm.* 1983; 17:23–6.
10. McGhee JR, Evans R, Wolfson PM et al. Predictability of warfarin maintenance dosage based upon initial response. *JAOA.* 1981; 80:335–8.
11. Miller DR, Brown MA. Predicting warfarin and maintenance dosage based on initial response. *Am J Hosp Pharm.* 1979; 36:1351–5.
12. Routledge PM, Bell SM, Davies DM et al. Predicting patient's warfarin requirements. *Lancet.* 1977; 2:854–5.
13. Sawyer WT. Predictability of warfarin dose requirements: theoretical considerations. *J Pharm Sci.* 1979; 68:432–4.
14. Williams DB, Karl RC. A simple technique for predicting daily maintenance dose of warfarin. *Am J Surg.* 1979; 137:572–6.
15. Sharma NK, Routledge PA, Rawlins MD et al. Predicting the dose of warfarin for therapeutic anticoagulation. *Thromb Haemost.* 1982; 47:230–1.
16. Gordon BM, Wiser WH, Davis RJ. Warfarin maintenance dose prediction based on initial anticoagulant response. *Clin Pharm.* 1984; 3:297–9.
17. Hansten PD. Drug interactions. 4th ed. Philadelphia: Lea & Febiger; 1979.
18. Sawyer WT, Raasch RH. Effect of heparin administration on prothrombin time determination. *Clin Pharm.* 1984; 3:192–4.
19. Quick AJ, Hussey CV. Comparison of the Thrombotest with the one-stage prothrombin time. *N Engl J Med.* 1961; 265:1286–9.
20. Kazmier FJ, Spittell JA, Thompson JJ et al. Effect of oral anticoagulants on factors VII, IX, X and II. *Arch Intern Med.* 1965; 115:667–73.
21. O'Reilly RA. The pharmacodynamics of oral anticoagulant drugs. In: Spaet TH, ed. Progress in hemostasis and thrombosis. Vol. 2. New York: Grune & Stratton; 1974:175.
22. Canaday BR, Sawyer WT. A pocket calculator program for prediction of warfarin maintenance dose. *Comp Biol Med.* 1982; 12:179–87.

23. Sawyer WT. Warfarin. In: Mungall D, ed. Applied pharmacokinetics. New York: Raven Press, Pubs.; 1983.
24. Anon. SAS user's guide. Raleigh, NC: SAS Institute, Inc.; 1982.
25. Hull RH, Hirsh J, Jay R et al. Different intensities of oral anticoagulant therapy in the treatment of proximal-vein thrombosis. *N Engl J Med.* 1982; 307:1676–81.
26. Hull RD, Raskob GE, Hirsh J et al. A cost-effectiveness analysis of alternative approaches for long-term treatment of proximal venous thrombosis. *JAMA.* 1984; 252:235–9.
27. Hull JH, Murray WJ, Brown HS et al. Potential anticoagulant drug interactions in ambulatory patients. *Clin Pharmacol Ther.* 1978; 24:644–9.
28. O'Reilly RA, Rytand DA. "Resistance" to warfarin due to unrecognized vitamin K supplementation. *N Engl J Med.* 1980; 303:160–1.
29. Abbrecht PH, O'Leary TJ, Behrendt DM. Evaluation of a computer-assisted method for individualized anticoagulant therapy: retrospective studies using a pharmacodynamic model. *Clin Pharmacol Ther.* 1982; 32:129–36.
30. Sheiner LB. Computer-aided long-term anticoagulation therapy. *Comp Biomed Res.* 1969; 2:507–18.

Research Notes

Gastrointestinal transit times of cathartics used with activated charcoal

EDWARD P. KRENZELOK

Clin Pharm. 1985; 4:446–8

Orally administered activated charcoal is an effective adsorbent used in the management of many poisoning emergencies.[1–18] Because its network of internal and external pores creates a large surface area, activated charcoal can adsorb both organic and inorganic toxins in the molecular weight range of 100–1000.

Activated charcoal has been used in the management of poisonings for more than 150 years; however, in the last 20 years it has emerged from a subordinate role.[1–4] New applications include using activated charcoal instead of inducing emesis with syrup of ipecac or performing gastric lavage.[4,10,11] Additionally, multiple-dose activated charcoal is effective in enhancing nonrenal elimination of drugs already absorbed.[1,5–8,17]

The goal of using activated charcoal is to decrease systemic absorption of toxins, thereby reducing toxicity. Although activated charcoal avidly adsorbs toxins, this process has not been demonstrated to be irreversible.[1,2] Therefore, it is important to use a cathartic to hasten the elimination of the activated charcoal–toxin complex from the bowel.

This study was designed to compare times required for elimination of activated charcoal from the bowel when charcoal is administered alone and with commonly used cathartics.

Methods. Five healthy volunteers (four women and one man) participated in the study, which was approved by the human research committee. The study used a crossover design in which subjects served as their own controls. Intestinal transit time was determined after administration of each of four preparations:

1. Activated charcoal 50 g in an aqueous slurry (240 mL), with ginger ale 300 mL (control);
2. Activated charcoal 50 g in 70% sorbitol solution (240 mL), with ginger ale 300 mL;
3. Activated charcoal in an aqueous slurry (240 mL), with magnesium citrate 300 mL; and
4. Activated charcoal 50 g in an aqueous slurry (210 mL) with magnesium sulfate 15 g (30 mL of a 50% solution), with ginger ale 300 mL.

The subjects were instructed to fast from solid foods for 12 hours before ingestion of the activated charcoal–cathartic mixtures. Water, not to exceed 480 mL, could be consumed during the fasting period. The charcoal–cathartic mixture was to be consumed over no longer than 15 minutes. No solid food or liquid could be consumed for two hours after ingestion of the activated charcoal–cathartic mixtures. The subjects recorded the time that ingestion of the test dose was completed and the time that they noted the first macroscopic evidence of activated charcoal in their stools. The minimum time between test doses was one week.

In phases 1, 2, and 4, ginger ale (of the same brand and from the same case) was used to control for the effect of the carbonation of magnesium citrate and the influence it may produce on gastric transit of the activated charcoal. The aqueous activated charcoal was prepared as a single batch for this study by Paddock Laboratories, Minneapolis,

EDWARD P. KRENZELOK, Pharm.D., is Director, Pittsburgh Poison Center, and Associate Professor of Pediatrics and Pharmacy, University of Pittsburgh.

Address reprint requests to Dr. Krenzelok at the Pittsburgh Poison Center, Children's Hospital of Pittsburgh, 125 DeSoto Street, Pittsburgh, PA 15213.

Presented at the 1984 American Association of Poison Control Centers/American Academy of Clinical Toxicology Annual Scientific Meeting, San Diego, CA, October 10, 1984.

MN 55427 (lot E418678). In phase 2, Paddock Laboratories' brand of activated charcoal in 70% sorbitol solution (Actidose, lot CH18611) was used. A commercial preparation of magnesium citrate (Citroma, National Magnesia Company, Glendale, NY 11227) was used in phase 3. The magnesium sulfate for phase 4 was freshly prepared using magnesium sulfate, USP, and sterile water for injection.

The subjects were instructed to drink the ginger ale or the magnesium citrate in alternating sips with the activated-charcoal study solution and to document discomfort that accompanied ingestion of any of the study solutions.

Results. Four of the five subjects completed all four phases of the study. One woman dropped out after completing phase 2 because she became pregnant.

Bowel transit times for the three cathartic regimens and the activated charcoal alone are shown in Table 1. The average transit time from ingestion of the activated charcoal alone to excretion of a charcoal-colored stool was 24.9 hours (1491.25 minutes). None of the subjects experienced any discomfort or excessive numbers of stools. In all cases, stools were formed and not watery.

After administration of activated charcoal in a vehicle of 70% sorbitol, the mean time for activated charcoal to appear in the stool was 1.3 hours (77.25 minutes). All subjects experienced abdominal discomfort before evacuation of the first charcoal stool. All stools were liquid and occurred intermittently for six to eight hours. Substantial amounts of charcoal were present in each stool.

The combination of magnesium citrate and activated charcoal 50 g produced a charcoal-containing stool in an average of 4.1 hours (244.25 minutes). None of the subjects experienced abdominal discomfort. The stool was formed, and no further catharsis occurred for at least six to eight hours after the initial episode.

When magnesium sulfate 15 g was administered with activated charcoal 50 g, the average time for the appearance of a charcoal-colored stool was 16.7 hours (1003 minutes). No cramping or other abdominal discomfort was noted. The stools were formed, and no further catharsis occurred for at least six to eight hours.

Table 1.
Bowel Transit Times (min) for Activated Charcoal Administered Alone (Control) and with Cathartics

Treatment	Mean ± S.D. (n = 4)	Range
Activated charcoal	1491 ± 92.77	1380–1590
Activated charcoal with sorbitol	77 ± 27.04	57–117
Activated charcoal with magnesium citrate	244 ± 65.97	200–342
Activated charcoal with magnesium sulfate	1003 ± 436.74	500–1563

Discussion. Sorbitol produced the most rapid gastrointestinal transit; a charcoal-colored stool was evacuated in approximately one hour and catharsis continued for several hours. Magnesium citrate also produced a relatively rapid catharsis, compared with the control and magnesium sulfate. Magnesium citrate did not produce the frequency of catharsis associated with sorbitol. Magnesium sulfate, the standard cathartic used in conjunction with activated charcoal in the management of the poisoned patient, produced the slowest gastrointestinal transit and resulted in only one charcoal-containing stool in the first 24 hours.

Standard references vary regarding the recommended dose of magnesium sulfate. Current recommendations include using 250 mg/kg and using 15–30 g.[13,14] Three of our subjects received doses in excess of 250 mg/kg, while one received an insufficient cathartic dose if 250 mg/kg is optimal. Magnesium sulfate in doses of 30 g may produce cathartic effects more expeditiously.

Sorbitol is an effective cathartic that does not appear to compromise the adsorptive capacity of activated charcoal.[16] The rapid gastrointestinal transit time associated with sorbitol may be of concern because the activated charcoal may not have sufficient time to adsorb the toxin. However, Pond and colleagues demonstrated that the activated charcoal–sorbitol combination dramatically reduced phenobarbital levels and enhanced clearance in overdose patients.[17]

In the clinical setting, the use and elimination of activated charcoal can be affected by factors not considered in our study. For example, anticholinergic, narcotic, or sedative–hypnotic properties of the ingested substance (the toxin) may cause decreased bowel motility. Prolonged transit times may result in desorption of toxins from activated charcoal. Therefore, it is important to use a cathartic that promotes rapid evacuation of the activated charcoal–toxin complexes. Although the solutions administered in this study (except magnesium citrate) were blinded to eliminate bias, other factors that influence gastric motility, such as stress and physical activity, could not be controlled.

Conclusion. Addition of sorbitol to activated charcoal decreased the charcoal's gastrointestinal transit time in these four volunteers. Gastrointestinal transit time was shorter for sorbitol than for magnesium citrate or magnesium sulfate.

References

1. Neuvonen PJ. Clinical pharmacokinetics of oral activated charcoal in acute intoxications. *Clin Pharmacokinet.* 1982; 7:465–89.
2. Holt LE, Holz PH. The black bottle. *J Pediatr.* 1963; 63:306–14.
3. Hayden JW, Comstock EJ. Use of activated charcoal in acute poisoning. *Clin Toxicol.* 1975; 8:515–33.
4. Neuvonen PJ, Vartianen M, Tokola O. Comparison of activated charcoal and ipecac syrup in prevention of drug ab-

sorption. *Eur J Clin Pharmacol.* 1983; 24:557–62.
5. Goldberg MJ, Berlinger WG. Treatment of phenobarbital overdose with activated charcoal. *JAMA.* 1982; 247:2400–1.
6. Berg MJ, Berlinger WG, Goldberg MJ et al. Acceleration of the body clearance of phenobarbital by oral activated charcoal. *N Engl J Med.* 1982; 307:642–4.
7. Levy G. Gastrointestinal clearance of drugs with activated charcoal. *N Engl J Med.* 1982; 307:676–8.
8. Linden CH, Lewis PK, Rumack BH. Phenobarbital overdosage: treatment with multiple doses of activated charcoal. Paper presented to American Academy of Clinical Toxicology Annual Meeting. Boston, MA: 1983 Aug 8.
9. Kulig K, Bar-Or D, Rumack BH et al. Intravenous aminophylline overdose: enhanced elimination by gastrointestinal activated charcoal in experimental animals. Paper presented to American Academy of Clinical Toxicology Annual Meeting. Boston, MA: 1983 Aug 8.
10. Burton BT, Barron L, Bayer MJ et al. Comparison of activated charcoal and gastric lavage in the initial management of drug overdose. Paper presented to International Congress of Clinical Toxicology. Snowmass, CO: 1982 Aug 8–13.
11. Kulig K, Bar-Or D, Cantrill SV et al. Management of acutely poisoned patients without gastric emptying. *Ann Emerg Med.* 1985; 14:562–7.
12. Corby DG, Decker WJ. Management of acute poisoning with activated charcoal. *Pediatrics.* 1974; 54:324–8.
13. Wanke LA. Prevention of absorption: dilution, emesis, gastric lavage, adsorption, catharsis. In: Bayer MJ, Rumack BH, Wanke LA, eds. Toxicologic emergencies. Bowie, MD: Robert J. Brady; 1984:37–51.
14. Haddad LA. A general approach to the emergency management of poisoning. In: Haddad LA, Winchester JF, eds. Clinical management of poisoning and drug overdose. Philadelphia: W.B. Saunders Co.; 1983:4–18.
15. Sketris IS, Mowry JB, Czajka PA et al. Saline catharsis: effect on aspirin bioavailability in combination with activated charcoal. *J Clin Pharmacol.* 1982; 22:59–64.
16. Mayersohn M, Perrier D, Picchioni AL. Evaluation of a charcoal-sorbitol mixture as an antidote for oral aspirin overdose. *Clin Toxicol.* 1977; 11:561–7.
17. Pond SM, Olson KR, Osterloh JD et al. Randomized study of the treatment of phenobarbital overdose with repeated doses of activated charcoal. *JAMA.* 1984; 251:3104–8.
18. Cooney DO. Activated charcoal. New York: Marcel Dekker, Inc.; 1980.

Theophylline pharmacokinetics in paraplegic subjects

JACK L. SEGAL, CHRISTOPHER M. SMITH, STANLEY K. GORDON, AND IBRAHIM M. ELTORAI

Clin Pharm. 1985; 4:448–51

Pneumonia and bronchitis are the primary causes of death in patients with spinal cord injuries,[1] and bronchospasm is a major component in the pathophysiology of these diseases. Diminished vital capacity and varying degrees of respiratory muscle and diaphragmatic paralysis, particularly in tetraplegic patients,[2] directly influence the clinical course and outcome in these individuals.

Theophylline has been shown to cause bronchodilation and to function as a respiratory stimulant in humans. It acts directly in improving diaphragmatic contractility and renders the diaphragm less susceptible to fatigue.[3] The pharmacokinetics of theophylline has been extensively studied,[4] and general pharmacokinetic guidelines for rational theophylline dose adjustment have been defined.[5] However, these guidelines are dependent on principles derived from studies involving populations with intact neuraxes.

This study was undertaken to examine the influence of spinal cord injury[6] on the pharmacokinetics of theophylline following a single intravenous infusion of aminophylline and to provide criteria for a rational approach to drug therapy in this population.

Methods. Nineteen men between 20 and 60 years of age volunteered for the study. Twelve of the subjects were paraplegic with post-traumatic myelopathy of not less than one year duration. These subjects were considered to have "complete" spinal cord injuries as defined by the total loss of sweating, sensation, and voluntary muscle control below the cord level of injury. Seven of the study subjects were age- and gender-matched nonsmoking normal controls. Laboratory tests performed on all study participants included a complete blood count, electrocardiogram, chest roentgenogram,

JACK L. SEGAL, M.D., is Staff Physician, Department of Medicine; CHRISTOPHER M. SMITH is Research Technician; STANLEY K. GORDON, M.D., is Chief, Spinal Cord Injury Service; and IBRAHIM M. ELTORAI, M.D., is Assistant Chief, Spinal Cord Injury Service, Veterans Administration Medical Center, Long Beach, CA.

Address reprint requests to Dr. Segal at the Veterans Administration Medical Center (111GM), 5901 East Seventh Street, Long Beach, CA 90822.

Supported in part by the Spinal Cord Injury–Hemodialysis Foundation, Gustavus and Louise Pfeiffer Foundation, and Veterans Assistance League.

blood glucose, serum electrolytes, liver-function studies, and creatinine clearance measurement. Volunteers with febrile illness, hematocrit <35 volume %, creatinine clearance ≤75 mL/min, hepatic or cardiac disease, decubitus ulcers, or those >15% above ideal body weight were excluded from the study. None of the study subjects were receiving theophylline therapeutically, and all participants were asked to abstain from methylxanthine-containing substances or other substances that could interfere with the assay method during and for 48 hours before the study period.

The aminophylline infusion was administered at 0830 ± 1 hr of each study day to minimize the influence of circadian variations in metabolism on theophylline disposition. The subjects were segregated into smoking (>10 cigarettes/day) and non-smoking categories. Following a 30-minute intravenous infusion of aminophylline 6 mg/kg,[a] 5-mL blood samples were withdrawn from an indwelling heparinized catheter placed in a contralateral extremity; the initial 1.5 mL of each sample was discarded. Samples were withdrawn at the end of the infusion (0 time) and at 0.5, 1.0, 1.5, 2.0, 2.5, 3.0, 4.0, 5.0, 6.0, 9.0, 12.0, and 24.0 hours. Sera were separated immediately and frozen until assayed. Meals (exclusive of methylxanthines), smoking, and routine hospital activities were allowed during the study period.

Serum theophylline concentration was measured at ambient temperature by reverse-phase high-performance liquid chromatography.[7] A mobile phase of 6.5% acetonitrile in 0.01 *M* sodium acetate buffer with a pH of 4.0 was used at a flow rate of 1.5 mL/min. Peak-height ratios of each compound relative to the internal standard (β-hydroxyethyl theophylline) were measured at 254 nm. Neither the within-day or between-day coefficients of variation of the assay exceeded 5%.

Model-dependent pharmacokinetic analysis of the time course of serum theophylline concentrations was performed using a one-compartment open model.[8] Theophylline concentrations during the period of rapid equilibrium (before 1.5 hours) were excluded from evaluation since data from the early distribution phase were difficult to interpret accurately. Estimation of pharmacokinetic values and calculation of the area under the theophylline concentration–time curve from zero to infinity ($AUC_{0\to\infty}$) were made with ESTRIP.[9] Values obtained were used in calculating the volume of distribution (V) and total body clearance (CL).

Analysis of variance with post hoc analysis (method of Scheffé) was used to test for statistical significance between variances and means. A two-variable linear correlation analysis was used to examine the relationship between pharmacokinetic variables and patient age, cord level of injury, and time since injury.

Results and Discussion. Table 1 summarizes the pharmacokinetic data on theophylline in this study. None of the subjects experienced side effects or failed to complete the study. The elimination rate constant (k) for theophylline was largest in the

Table 1.
Pharmacokinetic Data on Theophylline[a]

Subjects	k (hr^{-1})	$t_{1/2}$ (hr)	CL (mL/min/kg)[b]	V (L)	V (L/kg body weight)
Control group (nonsmokers) (n = 7)	0.068	10.2	0.90	52.8	0.54
	0.084	8.3	0.75	37.9	0.54
	0.086	8.1	0.84	38.5	0.59
	0.107	6.5	0.82	33.4	0.46
	0.093	7.5	0.75	35.5	0.49
	0.061	11.4	0.38	30.9	0.38
	0.050	14.0	0.30	30.4	0.36
	0.078 ± 0.020	9.4 ± 2.6	0.68 ± 0.24	37.1 ± 7.6	0.48 ± 0.08
Paraplegic nonsmokers (n = 6)	0.109	6.4	0.64	31.7	0.35
	0.092	7.5	0.82	43.3	0.54
	0.128	5.4	1.02	28.3	0.48
	0.101	6.9	0.69	34.6	0.41
	0.079	8.8	0.51	36.2	0.39
	0.051	13.7	0.40	31.3	0.48
	0.093 ± 0.027	8.1 ± 3.0	0.68 ± 0.22	34.2 ± 5.2	0.44 ± 0.07
Paraplegic smokers (n = 6)	0.195	3.6	1.57	26.5	0.48
	0.054	12.7	0.30	30.2	0.33
	0.213	3.3	1.82	31.7	0.51
	0.277	2.5	2.80	36.8	0.61
	0.151	4.6	1.40	39.4	0.54
	0.151	4.6	1.00	40.9	0.39
	0.174 ± 0.074	5.2 ± 3.8	1.48 ± 0.84	34.3 ± 5.7	0.48 ± 0.10

[a] Means ± S.D. are given for each of the pharmacokinetic variables for all three groups. Literature values for $t_{1/2}$, CL, and V derived from Goodman and Gilman's *Pharmacologic Basis of Therapeutics*, 6th ed., 1980, p. 1732, are 9.0 ± 2.1 hours, 0.69 ± 0.30 mL/min/kg, and 0.50 ± 0.05 L/kg, respectively.

[b] A significant difference was demonstrated by analysis of variance between the means and variances of theophylline CL in the smoking paraplegic subjects versus the nonsmoking subjects and controls.

group of paraplegic smokers. Although the k value in the nonsmoking control group was less than the k value for the paraplegic nonsmokers, the difference between means was not significant and probably reflected the influence of recreational drug use in nonsmoking paraplegics.

A significant decrease in theophylline half-life ($t_{1/2}$) in the smoking paraplegic group was observed that was similar to that described in individuals with an intact neuraxis who smoke.[4] A difference of 11.5 hours was noted between the extreme values of the range of theophylline half-life values in all study subjects.

There was no significant difference in mean theophylline V demonstrated between any of the study groups, although an excellent correlation with literature values was found. The mean CL was greatest in smoking paraplegic subjects and reflected the induction of theophylline metabolism caused by cigarette smoking.[4]

In an earlier study of gentamicin pharmacokinetics in patients with spinal cord injuries, we observed wide interindividual variation (dispersion) in patient pharmacokinetic variables.[10] This study was characterized by similar findings. Wide interindividual variation in the clearance of theophylline was found in the smoking paraplegic subjects (Figure 1).

Two-variable linear correlation analysis of theophylline $t_{1/2}$ and CL in all paraplegic patients showed a significant negative association ($r = -0.79$). This tended to support our contention that a change in the magnitude of theophylline V is unlikely and that biotransformation rather than V is the main determinant of variations in theophylline CL in paraplegic subjects as it is in patients with intact neuraxes.[11] No statistically significant associations were noted between the values of pharmacokinetic variables and patient age, time elapsed since injury, or cord level of injury.

Figure 1. A comparison of the clearance of theophylline in controls (nonsmoking) and in the smoking (Δ) and nonsmoking (O) paraplegic subjects.

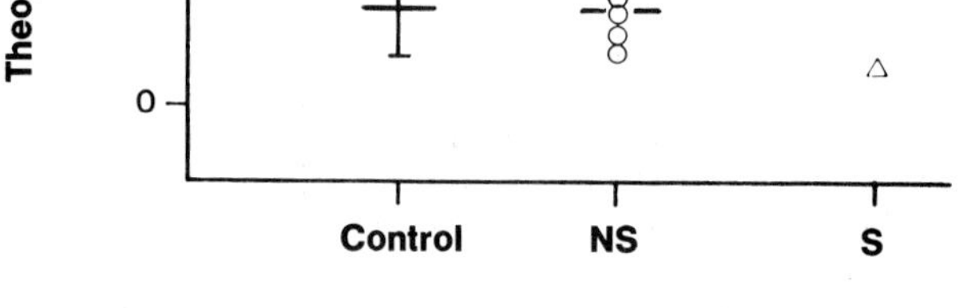

The increase in rate of elimination and clearance of theophylline in smoking paraplegic subjects is readily attributable to increased biotransformation caused by an induction of hepatic enzymes and is quantitatively similar to the increase seen in a population with intact neuraxes.[4]

The use of recreational drugs (marijuana) was suspected but could not be confirmed in several study subjects, and the influence of this unconfirmed activity on theophylline disposition could not be quantified. Pharmacokinetic variables for these individuals were reflective of a history of marijuana use; however, analysis of the nonsmoking paraplegic data following deletion of the values contributed by the marijuana-using subjects demonstrated no significant change in the mean values for the pharmacokinetic variables.

The practical implications of our observations concern unwary clinicians who can properly choose loading doses of theophylline but may fail to administer safe and effective maintenance doses. For example, consider the smoking paraplegic subject in our study who had a serum theophylline $t_{1/2}$ of 3.25 hours and an initial serum theophylline concentration of 15 μg/mL (median therapeutic concentration). If he had received the medication at an arbitrarily assigned dosing interval of eight hours, he would have reached a subtherapeutic serum theophylline concentration of less than 10 μg/mL in just over two hours. It can then be readily observed that this subject would maintain a subtherapeutic serum theophylline concentration for approximately 75% of the dosing interval. If the mean value for theophylline $t_{1/2}$ in this population (5.20 hours) was applied in a similar fashion, a subtherapeutic level would be present in approximately three hours and no improvement or advantage would be achieved. Mean values of pharmacokinetic variables obtained from the literature or calculated from data obtained in different populations will not ensure a safe or effective dosing regimen. A simple and effective method for predicting steady-state serum theophylline concentrations using individual patient variables should be applied.[12]

Conclusion. Based on our observations in a small number of subjects, the pharmacokinetics of theophylline in paraplegic subjects appear to be similar to those observed in subjects with intact neuraxes.

[a] Aminophylline Injection, USP, 500 mg/20 mL, Invenex Laboratories, Orlando, FL 32819, lot 058405S-F.

References

1. Frisbie JH, Kache A. Increasing survival and changing causes of death in myelopathy. *J Am Para Soc.* 1983; 6(3):51–9.
2. Ohry A, Molho M, Rozin R. Alterations of pulmonary function in spinal cord injured patients. *Paraplegia.* 1975; 13:101–8.

3. Aubier M, De Trover A, Sampson M et al. Aminophylline improves diaphragmatic contractility. *N Engl J Med.* 1981; 305(5):249–52.
4. Jusko WJ, Mark JG, Mangione A et al. Factors affecting theophylline clearances: age, tobacco, marijuana, cirrhosis, congestive heart failure, obesity, oral contraceptives, benzodiazepines, barbiturates, and ethanol. *J Pharm Sci.* 1979; 68(11):1358–66.
5. Jenne JW, Wyze E, Rood FS et al. Pharmacokinetics of theophylline: application to adjustment of the clinical dose of aminophylline. *Clin Pharmacol Ther.* 1972; 13:349–60.
6. Claus-Walker J, Halstead LS. Metabolic and endocrine changes in spinal cord injury. A four-part series. *Arch Phys Med Rehabil.* 1981–1982; 62(12):595–601; 63(11):569–80; 63(12):628–38.
7. Orcutt JJ, Kozak PP, Gilman SA et al. Micro-scale method for theophylline in body fluids by reverse-phase high-performance liquid chromatography. *Clin Chem.* 1977; 23(3):599–601.
8. Dvorchik BH, Vesell ES. Significance of error associated with use of the one-compartment formula to calculate clearance of thirty-eight drugs. *Clin Pharmacol Ther.* 1978; 23(6):617–21.
9. Don Brown R, Manno JE. ESTRIP, a BASIC computer program for obtaining initial polyexponential parameter estimates. *J Pharm Sci.* 1978; 67(12):1681–7.
10. Segal JL, Gray DR, Gordon SK et al. Pharmacokinetics of gentamicin in humans with spinal cord injury. *Clin Pharm.* 1984; 3:418–20.
11. Hendeles L, Weinberger M, Bighley L et al. Disposition of theophylline after a single intravenous infusion of aminophylline. *Am Rev Respir Dis.* 1978; 118:97–103.
12. Vozeh S, Kewitz G, Wenk M et al. Rapid prediction of steady-state serum theophylline levels in patients treated with intravenous aminophylline. *Eur J Clin Pharmacol.* 1980; 18:473–7.

Editorials

Reservoir aerosol delivery systems

Metered-dose inhaler (MDI) drug-delivery systems are convenient to use, portable, and deliver a small dose of drug directly to the site of action in the lungs, producing a more rapid onset of action and fewer side effects than with other routes of administration that produce systemic effects. In spite of these advantages, many patients are unable to use an MDI properly. Over the last decade reservoir aerosol delivery systems (RADSs) have been developed in an effort to overcome administration problems associated with MDIs. However, it is not well documented that RADSs are the answer to the problem. Many issues need to be addressed concerning the long-term benefits and potential risks associated with the use of RADSs.

Clinical response to an aerosolized drug depends on the amount of drug reaching the lungs. Particle deposition depends on particle size and airway-related factors such as flow rate, tidal volume, respiratory rate, and the amount of airway constriction.[1,2] Large particles do not flow well and tend to adhere to the back of the throat or to the bifurcations of the large airways. Metered-dose inhalers produce a variety of particle sizes. Approximately 8.8% of an MDI dose will reach the lungs.[3]

Moren and Anderson,[4] evaluating various tube-spacer devices (precursors of RADS), hypothesized that improved delivery of aerosolized drug to the lungs was secondary to droplet evaporation and decreased initial droplet velocity. Other investigators confirmed that similar types of tube spacers resulted in improved bronchodilation.[5–8] Some investigators[9–11] found no significant difference between the tube spacer and the MDI. It is difficult to compare the results of these studies since a variety of drugs, doses, measurements of pulmonary function, baseline patient status, and MDI educational techniques were used.

Early in 1984, Key Pharmaceuticals began marketing two RADSs, which are the only such devices commercially available currently. One device, the InspirEase, consists of a 700-mL, collapsible, 11.5-cm × 9-cm bag with a detachable mouthpiece. The mouthpiece contains a reed that produces a sound at inspiratory flow rates greater than 0.3 L/sec. To use the InspirEase, patients are advised to do the following: inflate the bag, actuate the cannister, inhale slowly through the mouthpiece until the bag is empty (without making a sound through the reed), hold the breath for five seconds, exhale back into the bag, and repeat the inhalation and exhalation procedure once. The second device, the Inhal-Aid, consists of a clear, rigid plastic chamber with a port for the MDI on one side and a mouthpiece on the other side. Attached to the mouthpiece is a clear plastic straw with an orange float that rises to the top of the straw at the proper inspiratory flow rate. Patients are instructed to activate the cannister, inhale slowly keeping the orange float at the top of the straw, hold the breath for five seconds, exhale, and repeat the inhalation and exhalation steps four times. The Inhal-Aid is approved for use in children; effectiveness of the InspirEase in children less than 12 years old has not been established.

There are no published studies of the Inhal-Aid RADS, and only one published study of the InspirEase RADS. In that study, Tobin et al.[12] compared the bronchodilating effects of one puff of metaproterenol delivered by MDI or InspirEase. Drug administration with InspirEase produced a mean percentage increase in specific airway conductance that was significant at all measurements. The forced expiratory volume at one second was not significantly different with either drug-delivery device, and the forced vital capacity was significantly different only at the 30-minute measurement. Improvement in pulmonary function may have resulted from the lower inspiratory flow rate, a more even distribution of aerosol throughout inspiration, a greater availability of medication through rebreathing, a longer contact time, or a decrease in patient errors.

Several questions about the use of RADSs still need to be addressed:

1. How much drug is lost in the reservoir? Tobin et al.[12] reported that 41% of a dose was lost in the InspirEase device after five inhalations from the bag. There are no studies determining the amount of drug lost in the InspirEase system after two inhalations (recommended procedure) or after any number of inhalations from the Inhal-Aid system.
2. Will sympathomimetic and corticosteroid drugs interact within the chambers? Both devices are prescribed for single-drug use, but many patients may not comply with this recommendation either for financial reasons or because of the inconvenience of transporting more than one device.
3. How frequently should the Inhal-Aid chamber be cleaned, and how often should a new reservoir bag be purchased for the InspirEase? The manufacturer recommends frequent cleaning of the Inhal-Aid device and replacement of the InspirEase reservoir every two weeks, but there are no published data available that address this point for either product.
4. What is the risk of fungal overgrowth and subsequent inhalation of fungi with the InspirEase RADS? The reservoir is an opaque, closed bag that might be expected to retain moisture.
5. Is there an interaction between the drug, the propellants, or both and the plastic surfaces?
6. Will patients continue to use the proper administration technique with the RADS over prolonged periods?
7. How safe are these devices? The Inhal-Aid has small parts that a child may inhale or swallow if left unsupervised.

Although patient acceptance of reservoir aerosol delivery systems appears to be high, the added cost, inconvenience, and exposure to potential problems does not justify the routine use of these devices by the majority of MDI users.

1. Newhouse MT, Ruffin RE. Deposition and fate of aerosolized drugs. *Chest.* 1978; 73(Suppl):936–43.
2. Miller WF. Aerosol therapy in acute and chronic respiratory disease. *Arch Intern Med.* 1973; 131:148–55.
3. Newman SP, Pavia D, Moren F et al. Deposition of pressurized aerosols in the human respiratory tract. *Thorax.* 1981; 36:52–5.
4. Moren F, Anderson J. Fraction of dose exhaled after administration of pressurized inhalation aerosols. *Int J Pharm.* 1980; 6:295–300.
5. Godden DJ, Crompton GK. An objective assessment of the tube spacer in patients unable to use a conventional pressurized aerosol efficiently. *Br J Dis Chest.* 1981; 75:165–8.
6. Pederson S. Aerosol treatment of bronchoconstriction in children with or without a tube spacer. *N Engl J Med.* 1983; 308:1328–30.
7. Spicer JE, Cayton RM, Frame MH et al. Influence of tube spacer on aerosol efficiency. *Lancet.* 1980; 2:1248.
8. Newman SP, Moren F, Pavia D et al. Deposition of pressurized suspension aerosols inhaled through extension devices. *Am Rev Respir Dis.* 1981; 124:317–20.
9. Bloomfield P, Crompton GK, Winsey NJP. A tube spacer to improve inhalation of drugs from pressurized aerosols. *Br Med J.* 1979; 2:1479.
10. Gomm SA, Keaney NP, Winsey NJP et al. Effect of an extension tube on the bronchodilator efficacy of terbutaline derived from a metered dose inhaler. *Thorax.* 1980; 35:552–6.
11. Prior JG, Nowell RV, Cochrane GM. High-dose inhaled terbutaline in the management of chronic severe asthma: comparison of wet nebulisation and tube spacer delivery. *Thorax.* 1982; 37:300–3.
12. Tobin MJ, Jenouri G, Danta I et al. Response to bronchodilator drug administration by a new reservoir aerosol delivery system and a review of other auxillary delivery systems. *Am Rev Respir Dis.* 1982; 126:670–5.

Karen J. Tietze, Pharm.D.
Philadelphia College of Pharmacy and Science
Philadelphia, PA 19104

Transdermal nitroglycerin patches

Transdermal nitroglycerin patches have now been on the U.S. market for about five years, and, despite widespread practitioner and consumer acceptance of these "high-tech" drug-delivery devices, questions are mounting about their efficacy in treating angina pectoris. Among the questions are:

1. Is the nitroglycerin delivery rate sufficient to relieve anginal pain, and are the patches clinically effective?
2. Is the patch delivery rate comparable with those of alternative dosage forms?
3. Does tolerance develop to transdermally administered nitroglycerin?
4. Is 24-hour therapy needed for angina pectoris?
5. Why have prescribers and patients accepted the patches so well?

Let's look at the available answers to these questions.

Delivery and efficacy are assessed through actual measurement of delivery rate and of serum drug concentrations. Data obtained are compared with studies of efficacy in humans. In recent studies of the delivery rate, the claim of 10-mg/day delivery from 10-mg/day patches was adequately confirmed.[1] Thus the products concerned appear to work as claimed; they are definitely a technological achievement. Mean plasma concentrations of nitroglycerin were relatively constant over a 24-hour period during the use of a single dose, again confirming manufacturers' claims. However, individual plasma concentrations fluctuated wildly. The reason for this is unknown, but it probably resulted from diurnal variations in disposition kinetics, not from erratic nitroglycerin delivery from the patches. Fluctuation probably has little clinical relevance.

Nitroglycerin ointment delivers two to four times the amount of nitroglycerin delivered by a 10-mg/day patch (when used according to package insert instructions) and, therefore, provides mean plasma nitroglycerin concentrations two to four times those obtained with a 10-mg/day patch. Thus, to match the ointment delivery rate, two to four 10-mg/day patches would be needed. Without doubt, the clinical efficacy of ointment and patches would then be equivalent, but only at a relative patch-to-ointment cost ratio of about 10:1.

The clinical efficacy of nitroglycerin ointment was established some 10 years ago[2]; in contrast, the efficacy of patches is in doubt.[3] During the last two years, some 15 papers have been published on this topic. Few studies have supported the efficacy claim.[3-5] There is a trend supporting the idea that efficacy is more likely to be shown in studies using relatively high doses (> 15 mg/day); this complements research on rate of delivery. However, another important trend is failure to show a 24-hour duration of effect, even though the drug remains detectable in blood for 24 hours. This raises the issue of tolerance.

Tolerance can be viewed as reduction in or disappearance of effect with continued drug administration. There are two major types of tolerance—pharmacokinetic and physiological. Pharmacokinetic tolerance is a reduction in drug concentrations with continued drug input; it results from increases in the rate of drug elimination with time. There is no evidence that this occurs with nitroglycerin. Physiological tolerance is an adaptive process, with tissue responsivity lost even though drug concentrations are maintained.

There is considerable evidence that physiological tolerance occurs with nitroglycerin. The 10-point drop in systolic blood pressure typically obtained initially with nitroglycerin is lost during the 24-hour period of administration of nitroglycerin with the skin patch. Whether this reflects the pharmacological mechanisms leading to relief of angina remains to be seen. However, it is proof that tolerance can occur. The real issue to be resolved is Does tolerance develop more prominently with continuous transdermal patch delivery, as opposed to intermittent sublingual or transdermal dosing? Evidence is accumulating that the answer to this question is Yes.

If tolerance is proved to be a problem, there will be major implications for transdermal nitroglycerin patches. There will be less of or no problem with the ointment, as this product gives three broad spikes associated with intermittent treatment every 24 hours. Continuous 24-hour patch therapy may prove to be inappropriate because of tolerance problems alone.

In fact, 24-hour therapy may be less needed than is commonly supposed. Angina pectoris can be a response to exercise, or it can occur at night during rest. Both types can occur in any one patient. But if a patient experiences only exercise-induced angina, then treatment may not be needed at night. If a patient experiences only nocturnal angina, then treatment may not be needed during the day. Thus a substantial proportion of patients may require only 8–16 hours of treatment in each 24-hour period. In these patients, any tolerance problem might go away if the patch were removed after the 8–16 hours needed for treatment. This interesting possibility deserves evaluation.

The final issue is the paradox of widespread physician and patient acceptance of patches despite academic skepticism. The roots of this appear to lie in the nature of the drug and the problem being treated. Some practitioners have said that, unless nitroglycerin-treated patients preferred nitroglycerin-induced headache over their perceived pain of angina, then they did not have angina in the first place. This statement recognizes the placebo effect. Presumably, placebo responders will respond to patches; they may even show an especially prominent response to the elegance and cosmetic acceptability of the patches, and the relatively high cost of patches may contribute to this. Also, there are undoubtedly some patients with angina who respond to low doses of nitroglycerin.

However, this leaves the most important group of patients, those who appear to need more than 15 mg/day, who cannot meet their nitroglycerin requirements without the use of multiple patches. For these patients there is a clear need for a low-cost patch with a larger surface area and a faster rate of delivery.

Currently available data raise some serious questions about the effectiveness of transdermal nitroglycerin patches for treating angina pectoris. Practitioners, researchers, product manufacturers, and the Food and Drug Administration should all be seeking answers to these questions, as well as questioning inappropriate use of these elegant but expensive devices.

1. Curry SH, Kwon H-R, Perrin JH et al. Plasma nitroglycerin and hemodynamic effects after sublingual, ointment and controlled-release doses. *Clin Pharmacol Ther.* 1984; 36:765–73.
2. Reichek N, Goldstein RE, Redwood DR et al. Sustained effects of nitroglycerin ointment in patients with angina pectoris. *Circulation.* 1984; 50:348–52.
3. Abrams J. The brief saga of transdermal nitroglycerin discs: paradise lost? *Am J Cardiol.* 1984; 54:220–4.
4. Crean PA, Ribeiro P, Crea F et al. Failure of transdermal nitroglycerin to improve chronic stable angina: a randomized, placebo-controlled, double-blind, double crossover trial. *Am Heart J.* 1984; 108:1494–500.
5. Reichek N, Priest C, Zimrin D et al. Antianginal effects of nitroglycerin patches. *Am J Cardiol.* 1984: 54:1–7.

Stephen H. Curry, Ph.D.
Division of Clinical Pharmacokinetics
College of Pharmacy
University of Florida
J. Hillis Miller Health Center
Gainesville, FL 32610

"

When To Use Third-Generation Cephalosporins

The conclusion must, therefore, be that we need much more evaluation—particularly clinical—of these new [third-generation cephalosporins]. Ideally, large multicenter trials should be set up to compare them alone and in various combinations, but this is perhaps asking too much. In the meantime their cost and the need to limit spread of resistance should limit their routine use. They should not be used for infections that can be treated with cheaper, well tried penicillins and cephalosporins. We suggest that they might be considered in the following groups of patients: (a) nonneutropenic patients with serious undefined sepsis, where they can probably be combined safely with most other antibiotics as necessary—for example, metronidazole if abdominal sepsis is suspected; (b) nonneutropenic patients with serious proved Gram-negative sepsis, when they can usually be used as sole antibiotics; (c) Gram-negative bacillary meningitis; (d) neutropenic patients with Gram-negative sepsis, when they should be combined with an aminoglycoside; and (e) patients with chronic relapsing infections such as those caused by *Ps. aeruginosa* in cystic fibrosis, where repeated courses of broad spectrum antibiotics may be necessary and toxic compounds, such as the aminoglycosides, may be better avoided.

The cephalosporins have been described as agents in search of diseases; indeed, the whole development of such powerful agents as the third-generation cephalosporins has been questioned. They have, nevertheless, arrived as genuine contenders for first line antibiotic treatment. Just which agent to use in which setting should become more apparent in the future. In the meantime the choice will have to depend on consideration of the spectrum of activity, pharmacokinetics, toxicity, and cost.

Further research is likely to be concerned with developing compounds capable of providing monotherapy for all infections—the holy grail of the pharmaceutical companies. Such an agent will require more predictable activity against a wider range of pathogens than offered by currently available drugs. In particular, better activity against staphylococci and *Bacteroides* spp is important.

—Gould IM, Wise R. Third generation cephalosporins. *Br Med J.* 1985; 290:878–9. Editorial.

"

Drug Experience

Straightforward reports of unusual drug experiences are included in this section. These may be confirmations of previously reported drug experiences or brief apparent first reports. While selected references may be cited, the purpose of a Drug Experience report is not to present an extensive review of the literature.

A related section, Grand Rounds, includes papers that are well-documented patient case reports with a thorough review of the important literature to help put the case in perspective.

Metallic taste associated with tetracycline therapy

LOUIS D. MAGNASCO
AND ANDREW J. MAGNASCO

Clin Pharm. 1985; 4:455–6

The tetracyclines are broad-spectrum antibiotics effective against a wide variety of organisms, including gram-positive and gram-negative bacteria, *Rickettsia* species, *Chlamydia* species, *Mycoplasma* species and others. They are considered the drugs of first choice (following immediate administration of amoxicillin and probenecid) in the treatment of gonococcal urethritis.[1]

Adverse reactions to tetracyclines are relatively common and consist mainly of gastrointestinal intolerance. The patient usually complains of anorexia, nausea, and vomiting.[1,2] This report describes a patient who experienced an alteration in sense of taste associated with the use of a tetracycline. Although such a side effect could theoretically result from the ability of the tetracyclines to cause fungal overgrowth in the mouth or increase circulating levels of blood urea nitrogen,[2–4] the alteration of taste in this patient was not accompanied by evidence of oral mycosis or abnormal laboratory test results.

Case Report. A 32-year-old, well-developed, well-nourished white man was admitted to the Stockton Medical Clinic (an after-hours, urgent-care clinic) on December 21, 1984, with a chief complaint of slight urethral discharge accompanied by burning during urination. He had no known allergies to medication, and a medication history yielded no pertinent results. The patient drank 2–3 cups of coffee per day and had smoked cigarettes for 15 years.

Physical examination revealed a very slight urethral discharge. Well-demarcated alopecia areata was also noted, but a dermatologist previously had attributed this condition to a reaction to aftershave lotion.

A tentative diagnosis of gonococcal urethritis was made and empiric antibiotic therapy was begun. The pharmacist was consulted and suggested immediate single doses of amoxicillin 3 g orally and probenecid 1 g orally, followed by tetracycline hydrochloride 500 mg orally four times daily for seven days. However, the patient refused the amoxicillin and probenecid, stating that the combination caused nausea and vomiting. Therapy was initiated instead with tetracycline hydrochloride 500 mg (Cyclopar 500, Parke-Davis, lot 386D3D) four times daily for 10 days. The patient was instructed to avoid all dairy products, antacids, and iron products and to take the medication on an empty stomach unless it upset his stomach, in which case he was to take it with food.

A gram stain and culture of the urethral exudate were ordered. Because the laboratory technician was ill, the results of both tests were not available for two days. The gram stain revealed a few gram-positive cocci but no gram-negative diplococci. The causative organism was identified as *Strepto-*

LOUIS D. MAGNASCO, PHARM.D., and ANDREW J. MAGNASCO, PHARM.D., are Vice Presidents, Magnasco Enterprises, Inc., Stockton, CA 95203.

Reprints of this article are not available.

coccus viridans resistant to penicillin, cloxacillin, ampicillin, and methicillin. The organism was sensitive to sulfamethoxazole–trimethoprim and cephalexin, with intermediate sensitivity to erythromycin and tetracycline.

The patient was asked to return to the clinic on December 24 but did not return until December 27. At that time, he complained of an intense, offensive metallic taste and a slight burning during urination. He reported to the pharmacist that the sensation was most intense 30–60 minutes after a dose and declined gradually until it ceased approximately 30 minutes before the next dose. The pattern was so regular that the patient used it to estimate the time for his next dose. He complained that the sensation was so powerful that it completely blocked out all other taste sensations. He reported no changes in his normal living or eating habits and said that he had never before experienced a similar taste sensation. He could not recall any previous therapy with tetracycline. All laboratory test results were within normal limits, and no oral overgrowth was noted.

Because of this adverse reaction, tetracycline was discontinued and therapy was begun with sulfamethoxazole 800 mg–trimethoprim 160 mg (H.R. Cenci Laboratories, Fresno, CA 93701, lot B41948) twice daily for 10 days. A follow-up call revealed that the patient had experienced no further episodes of taste alteration.

Discussion. The taste sensation described by this patient has been reported in patients taking metronidazole[5]; however, we know of no previous reports of this side effect in patients receiving tetracycline products. Although there are two tetracycline-associated conditions that could have caused this reaction, neither was present in this patient. Oral mycosis can result when tetracycline destroys normal protective flora and permits overgrowth of fungi such as *Candida* species.[3,6] Our patient showed no sign of oral mycosis. A second condition that could have caused the metallic taste is an increase in BUN associated with the catabolic effects of the tetracycline. This increased BUN can result in a metallic or ammonia-like taste,[2–4,7] but BUN was normal in our patient.

We suspected that the alteration in taste was a direct effect of the drug. This conclusion was supported by the temporal pattern of the metallic taste, which corresponded to times that have been reported for peak and trough tetracycline concentrations.[3,8,9]

Conclusion. A metallic taste experienced by patients receiving oral tetracycline hydrochloride may be considered a drug effect if BUN is normal and there is no evidence of oral mycosis.

References

1. Abramowicz M, ed. The Medical Letter handbook of antimicrobial therapy. Revised edition. New Rochelle, NY: The Medical Letter, Inc.; 1984.
2. Parke-Davis Division, Warner-Lambert Co. Tetracycline package insert. Morris Plains, NJ; 1983 Apr.
3. Sande M, Mandell G. Antimicrobial agents: tetracyclines and chloramphenicol. In: Goodman and Gilman's the pharmacological basis of therapeutics. 6th ed. Gilman AG, Goodman LS, Gilman A, eds. New York: Macmillan Publishing Co., Inc.; 1980; 1181–99.
4. Gambertoglio J. Renal disease. In: Herfindal E, Hirschman J, eds. Clinical pharmacy and therapeutics. Baltimore: Williams & Wilkins Co.; 1979:466–78.
5. Goldman P. Metronidazole. *N Engl J Med.* 1980; 303:1212–8.
6. Sohn C. Opportunistic fungal and viral infections. In: Katcher B, Young L, Koda-Kimble MA, eds. Applied therapeutics. San Francisco: Applied Therapeutics, Inc.; 1983:835–55.
7. Gambertoglio J, Mangini R, Robinson D. Kidney diseases. In: Katcher B, Young L, Koda-Kimble MA, eds. Applied therapeutics. San Francisco: Applied Therapeutics, Inc.; 1983:539–85.
8. Ludden T. Clinical pharmacokinetic consultation services. In: Evans W, Schentag J, Jusko W, eds. Applied pharmacokinetics. San Francisco: Applied Therapeutics, Inc.; 1980:4–25.
9. Winter M. Basic clinical pharmacokinetics. Spokane, WA: Applied Therapeutics, Inc.; 1980.

CP Continuing Education

The ASHP Continuing Education system gives readers a self-assessment mechanism for selected articles in Clinical Pharmacy *and the* American Journal of Hospital Pharmacy. *It also allows readers to obtain continuing education credit for these articles.*

For the purpose of CE-credit enrollment, a blank answer sheet is published at the end of each installment of the column for the CE articles in that issue. An enrollee accumulates these answer sheets until the enrollment is submitted, using the form that is published in the May–June and November–December issues of Clinical Pharmacy *and in the June and December issues of the* American Journal of Hospital Pharmacy. *Any combination of tests within a 12-month period, from both* Clinical Pharmacy *and* American Journal of Hospital Pharmacy, *may be included in an enrollment. More complete details about enrollment in the system will appear in the semiannual enrollment form.*

All education aspects of the program are directed by Warren E. McConnell, Ph.D., Special Assistant in the ASHP Executive Office.

Article 680-204-8511 (see page 393)
Qualifies for 1.0 hour of credit

New β_2-adrenergic agonist aerosols

Learning Objectives

As a result of studying this article the reader should be able to

1. Compare and contrast the new agents bitolterol and fenoterol with older β_2-adrenergic agonists.
2. Describe the relationship between chemical structures of these compounds and their molar potencies, relative selectivities, oral activities, and durations of action.
3. List the advantages and disadvantages of the systemic and aerosol routes of administration of β_2-adrenergic agonists.
4. Compare and contrast metered-dose inhalers, nebulizers, intermittent positive-pressure breathing, and tube-spacers in terms of delivery of β_2-adrenergic-agonist aerosols to β_2 receptors in the airways.
5. Name four common reasons for inappropriate patient technique in using a metered-dose inhaler.

Self-assessment Questions

For each question there is one best answer only.

1. The major dose-limiting toxicity of β_2-adrenergic agonists is
   a. Cardiac stimulation for all agents except those with a tertiary butyl group (terbutaline, albuterol, bitolterol).
   b. Cardiac stimulation for all agents except the nonselective ones (isoproterenol and metaproterenol).
   c. Cardiac stimulation for all agents because of a direct chronotropic effect on β receptors in the heart.
   d. Cardiac stimulation for all agents because of baroreceptor-mediated response to β_2-adrenergic vasodilation.

2. If administered in equipotent doses, isoproterenol and metaproterenol will
   a. Have different quantitative effects on bronchial smooth muscle.
   b. Have the same quantitative effects on bronchial smooth muscle.
   c. Provide different durations of protection from exercise-induced bronchospasm.
   d. Alternatives b and c are both correct.

3. In evaluating the response of a chronic asthmatic patient to inhaled β_2-adrenergic agonists, which of the following tests is most useful?
   a. Measurement of bronchodilation after a single dose in a stable patient.
   b. Determination of the dose required to prevent or reverse bronchoconstriction following a stimulant in a stable patient.
   c. Measurement of bronchodilation after multiple doses in a stable patient.
   d. Determination of the dose required to maintain bronchodilation for the longest period of time in a stable patient.

4. What percentage of an inhaled dose of β_2-adrenergic agonist aerosols reaches the β receptors in the bronchi?
   a. About 10%.
   b. About 30%.
   c. About 50%.
   d. About 70%.

5. A major determinant of a patient's response to a given dose of a β_2 agonist is
   a. Baseline pulmonary-function status.

b. Time since bronchospasm began.
c. Degree of bronchoconstriction present.
d. Type of stimulus causing bronchoconstriction.

6. When evaluating clinical results from studies of β_2-adrenergic agonists, it is important to remember that

a. Often the lowest dose used produces near maximal bronchodilation.
b. The linear portion of the dose–response curve is in the range of 20 to 80% of maximal bronchodilation.
c. Exponential increases in dose are required for each incremental improvement in the linear portion of the dose–response curve.
d. All of the above alternatives are correct.

7. Tube-spacers improve drug delivery in

a. Patients who use inhaled products more than three times a day.
b. Children who have difficulty holding inspired air for 10 seconds.
c. Patients unable to coordinate inspiration with activation of metered-dose inhalers.
d. Patients unresponsive to systemic β_2-adrenergic agonists.

8. Which of the following statements about the advantages of aerosol versus systemic therapy with β_2-adrenergic agonists is false?

a. Systemic therapy produces significantly greater bronchodilation in the small airways.
b. Aerosol therapy avoids the problem of liver metabolism that occurs with oral administration.
c. Aerosol administration provides bronchodilation similar to that resulting from systemic therapy.
d. Systemic therapy causes more side effects than aerosol-administered drug.

9. A dose–response graph for two drugs that are full agonists but have different potencies would have which of the following types of curves?

a. Two identical curves with the same slope and maximum values.
b. Two curves with the same slope but differing maximum values.
c. Two curves with differing slopes but the same maximum values.
d. Two parallel curves with identical slopes and maximum values.

10. For β_2-adrenergic agonist aerosols, the durations of action can be extended by

a. Increasing the dose of near maximal effective concentrations.
b. Delaying the removal of drug from the receptor site by altering the chemical structure.
c. Administering prodrugs that require metabolism in the body to pharmacologically active compounds.
d. All of the above alternatives are correct.

Article 680-204-8511 (see page 404)
Qualifies for 1.0 hour of CE credit

Current status of cardiac glycoside drug interactions

Learning Objectives

As a result of studying this article, the reader should be able to

1. Differentiate between digitoxin and digoxin in terms of potential drug interactions.
2. Describe four mechanisms for drug-induced alterations in digoxin and digitoxin absorption.
3. Describe the effects of altered protein binding on digoxin and digitoxin.
4. Name at least four drugs that alter the elimination of cardiac glycosides.
5. Differentiate between proven drug interactions with cardiac glycosides and potential interactions not yet fully substantiated.

Self-assessment Questions

For each question there is one best answer only.

1. All the following are known to interfere with the gastrointestinal absorption of digoxin and digitoxin except

a. Antacids.
b. Sucralfate.
c. Activated charcoal.
d. Kaolin–pectin.

2. Both digoxin and digitoxin are primarily metabolized by the

a. Hepatic microsomal system.
b. Proximal renal tubules.
c. Kupffer cells of the liver.
d. None of the above alternatives is correct.

3. Altered protein binding of which cardiac glycoside is clinically relevant?

a. Digitoxin.
b. Digoxin.
c. Alternatives a and b are both correct.
d. None of the above alternatives is correct.

4. Decreases in gastrointestinal motility will significantly

a. Increase absorption from rapidly dissolving oral digoxin tablets.
b. Increase absorption from rapidly dissolving oral digitoxin tablets.
c. Increase absorption from slowly dissolving digoxin tablets.
d. Increase absorption from slowly dissolving digitoxin tablets.

5. All of the following agents are known to interact with digoxin except

a. Heparin.
b. Erythromycin.

c. Aminosalicylic acid.
d. Quinidine.

6. Drug interactions with cardiac glycosides are important clinically because

a. Digoxin and digitoxin both have narrow therapeutic ranges.
b. Other drugs can alter absorption and elimination of both digoxin and digitoxin.
c. The drugs are used widely and monitoring of serum drug concentrations is common.
d. Alternatives a and b are both correct.

7. The cardiac glycoside–quinidine interaction results in

a. An increase in both the serum digoxin and digitoxin concentrations.
b. A decrease in serum digoxin concentration but an increase in the serum digitoxin concentration.
c. An increase in the serum digoxin concentration with no consistent effect on the serum digitoxin concentration.
d. No change in the serum digoxin concentration and an increase in the serum digitoxin concentration.

8. The cause of the neomycin–digoxin interaction is

a. Altered intestinal-wall properties.
b. Altered bacterial flora.
c. Altered protein binding.
d. Alternatives a and b are both correct.

9. The cause of the erythromycin–digoxin interaction is

a. Altered intestinal-wall properties.
b. Altered bacterial flora.
c. Altered protein binding.
d. Alternatives a and b are both correct.

10. The interaction between digoxin and calcium-channel blockers is clinically relevant for all but which of the following blockers?

a. Diltiazem.
b. Verapamil.
c. Nifedipine.
d. Alternatives a and c are both correct.

Article 680-204-8513 (see page 414)
Qualifies for 1.0 hour of CE credit

Whole-bowel irrigation for mechanical colon cleansing

Learning Objectives

After studying this article, the reader should be able to

1. Describe the physiology of volumogenic diarrhea produced by whole-bowel irrigation.
2. Identify three procedures for which whole-bowel irrigation has been evaluated.
3. Compare the efficacy of isotonic electrolyte solutions, mannitol solutions, and polyethylene glycol–electrolyte lavage solutions in whole-bowel irrigation.
4. Compare the safety of isotonic electrolyte solutions, mannitol solutions, and polyethylene glycol–electrolyte lavage solutions in whole-bowel irrigation.
5. List the ingredients in the preferred solution for whole-bowel irrigation and identify the recommended dosage and administration schedule for this solution.

Self-assessment Questions

For each question there is one best answer only.

1. The production of volumogenic diarrhea is a function of

a. Fluid flow rate in intestine.
b. Absorptive capacity of the intestine.
c. Fluid volume entering the intestine.
d. All of the above alternatives are correct.
e. Alternatives a and c only are correct.

2. Polyethylene glycol is added to whole-bowel irrigation solutions to

a. Inhibit intestinal absorption of water.
b. Inhibit bacterial growth in the irrigation solution.
c. Increase intestinal transit of the solution.
d. Alternatives a and b are both correct.
e. None of the above alternatives is correct.

3. Whole-bowel irrigation solutions successfully meet which of the following criteria for evaluating mechanical bowel-cleansing regimens for colorectal surgery?

a. Removal of fecal content.
b. Reduction of total colonic bacterial counts.
c. Prevention of postoperative infection.
d. All of the above alternatives are correct.
e. Alternatives a and b only are correct.

4. Gastrointestinal side effects such as nausea and vomiting during whole-bowel irrigation may be minimized by

a. Premedication with metoclopramide.
b. Decreasing fluid administration rates.
c. Sweetening the irrigation solution.
d. All of the above alternatives are correct.
e. Alternatives a and b only are correct.

5. The addition of mannitol to electolyte solutions for whole-bowel irrigation

a. Inhibits net electrolyte absorption from the intestinal lumen.
b. Favors the production of potentially explosive colonic gases.
c. May increase the incidence of postoperative sepsis from *Escherichia coli* organisms.
d. All of the above alternatives are correct.
e. Alternatives a and b only are correct.

6. The *major* problem with whole-bowel irrigation solutions that is avoided with polyethylene gly-

col-electrolyte lavage solutions is

a. Colonic gas production.
b. Fluid and electrolyte disturbance.
c. Colonic mucosal abnormalities.
d. Nausea and vomiting.
e. Mallory–Weiss syndrome.

7. Which of the following is *not* a contraindication to the use of whole-bowel irrigation?

a. Ileus.
b. Gastric-outlet obstruction.
c. Hemorrhoids.
d. Bowel perforation.
e. All of the above alternatives are contraindications.

8. The primary patient complaint(s) with polyethylene glycol–electrolyte lavage solutions is (are)

a. Vomiting.
b. Rectal pain.
c. Bitter taste.
d. Alternatives b and c are both correct.
e. None of the above alternatives is correct.

9. The addition of any sugar to whole-bowel irrigation solutions may

a. Stimulate the absorption of potassium in the small bowel.
b. Lead to the production of methane and hydrogen gas in the colon.
c. Produce excessive losses of sodium in the small bowel.
d. All of the above alternatives are correct.
e. Alternatives a and b only are correct.

10. The maximum volume of polyethylene glycol–electrolyte lavage solution usually required to produce a clear rectal effluent is approximately

a. 400 to 600 mL.
b. 20 to 30 mL/kg.
c. 1.2 to 1.8 L.
d. 4 to 6 L.
e. 6 to 12 L.

Answer sheet

July–August 1985 ***Clinical Pharmacy***

Note: An enrollment form for the ASHP Continuing-Education System appears in the May–June and November–December issues. Please accumulate all the answer sheets you wish to use in one enrollment and submit them at one time with a completed enrollment form.

Place an X in the box(es) at the top of the column(s) corresponding to the test(s) you are taking. Darken the boxes corresponding to the correct answers.

☐ 680-204-8511 1.0 hour a b c d	☐ 680-204-8512 1.0 hour a b c d	☐ 680-204-8513 1.0 hour a b c d e
1. ☐☐☐☐	1. ☐☐☐☐	1. ☐☐☐☐☐
2. ☐☐☐☐	2. ☐☐☐☐	2. ☐☐☐☐☐
3. ☐☐☐☐	3. ☐☐☐☐	3. ☐☐☐☐☐
4. ☐☐☐☐	4. ☐☐☐☐	4. ☐☐☐☐☐
5. ☐☐☐☐	5. ☐☐☐☐	5. ☐☐☐☐☐
6. ☐☐☐☐	6. ☐☐☐☐	6. ☐☐☐☐☐
7. ☐☐☐☐	7. ☐☐☐☐	7. ☐☐☐☐☐
8. ☐☐☐☐	8. ☐☐☐☐	8. ☐☐☐☐☐
9. ☐☐☐☐	9. ☐☐☐☐	9. ☐☐☐☐☐
10. ☐☐☐☐	10. ☐☐☐☐	10. ☐☐☐☐☐

ASHP Use Only
(1.0)8511______(3)
(1.0)8512______(3)
(1.0)8513______(3)

The Challenge:
Increase Pharmacy Productivity

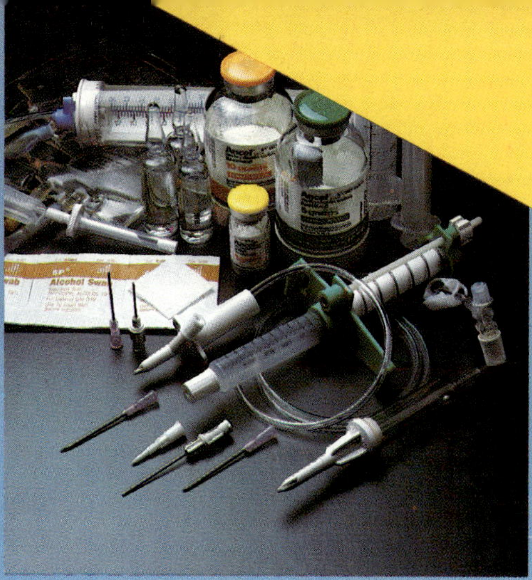

Now Available in 500 mg. Strength

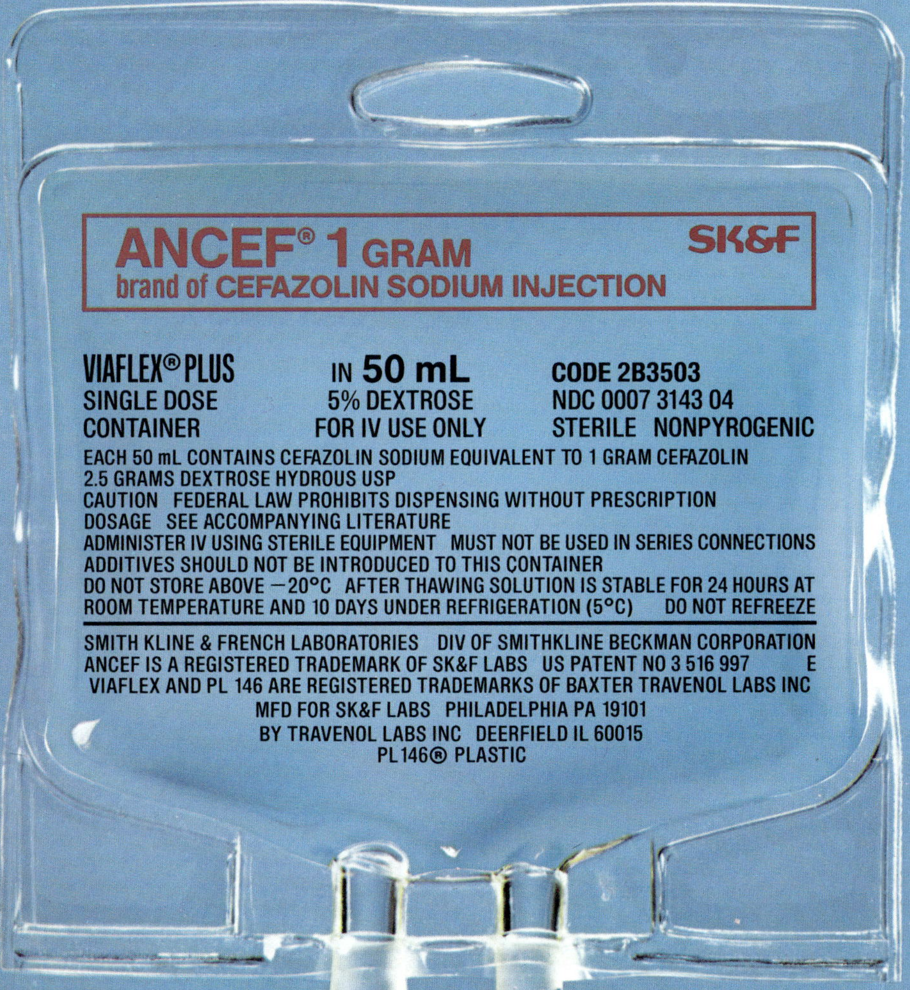

Our Response: ANCEF® 1 gram

brand of
CEFAZOLIN SODIUM INJECTION

The First Pre-Mixed, Injectable Cephalosporin

Ask Your Smith Kline &French Sales Representative About Availability in Your Area.

SK&F

MINI-BAG™ plastic containers are manufactured by Travenol Laboratories, Inc.

Smith Kline &French Laboratories
Philadelphia, PA

Current Literature

Book Review

Practice of Critical Care Pharmacy

Edited by Thomas C. Majerus and Joseph F. Dasta.

Published by Aspen Systems Corporation, 1600 Research Boulevard, Rockville, MD 20850, 1985. xvi + 315 p. Price $36.00.

Any clinician involved in the practice of critical care pharmacy will appreciate this text. The book is a compilation of the experiences of many of the leading clinical pharmacy experts practicing in critical care. It is divided into two sections. The first section deals with the emerging roles of the pharmacist in the area of critical care. It covers primarily what the practice of critical care pharmacy is and should be, how to begin implementation of critical care pharmacy programs, and how to justify such programs. It also briefly touches on the important relationship between nursing and pharmacy personnel in critical care areas.

The second section describes current and possible future avenues for pharmacy practitioners in critical care environments. It covers practices that have been established in specific critical care areas, such as in medical, surgical, pediatric, and neonatal units and the emergency room. This section is ideal as an aid for those pharmacists who wish to set up programs in the critical care setting. Important ideas are discussed on how to evaluate specific critical care needs, how to initiate new services, how to evaluate those services, and also, importantly, how to justify the newly created services. Many chapters also stress the value of pharmacy involvement in critical care areas in terms of better medical management of the patient, the potential for cost containment, and the potential for substantial research.

Throughout the text, the reader will find many important forms for documentation, evaluation of services, and educational programs. This type of material can be of benefit to those establishing programs in areas of critical care medicine.

This text is a perfect starting point for those clinical pharmacists or administrators wishing to initiate clinical pharmacy services in critical care medicine. Its value lies in the guidelines it presents for providing clinical pharmacy services and justifying such services in the critical care environment.

Reviewed by Larry H. Danziger, Pharm.D., Departments of Pharmacy and Surgery, Case Western Reserve University, University Circle, Cleveland, OH 44106.

Books Received

Books are listed as received; selected books may be reviewed in Book Reviews in subsequent issues.

Blue Book of Pharmacologic Therapeutics, by Gordon E. Johnson. Published by W. B. Saunders Company, West Washington Square, Philadelphia, PA 19105, 1985. xxi + 713 p. Price $24.95.

Guide for Adult Immunization, by Committee on Immunization, Council of Medical Societies, American College of Physicians. Published by American College of Physicians, 4200 Pine St., Philadelphia, PA 19104. xii + 132 p. Price $10 (1–5 copies), $8 (6–20 copies), $6.50 (21 or more copies).

Advertising Index

American Society of Hospital Pharmacists
Clinical Pharmacy, 468A, 468B, inside back cover
Beecham Laboratories
Timentin, 375–382
Biotrack, Inc.
Warfcalc, 389
Bristol Laboratories, Division of Bristol-Myers Company
Mexate, 373–374
Cal Lab East
Analysis Programs, 383
Lederle Laboratories, A Division of American Cyanamid Company
Maxzide, 391–392
Nash General Hospital
Position Available, 390
National Council on Patient Information and Education
Institutional, 451
Ochsner Foundation Hospital
Position Available, 390
Pfipharmecs, Division of Pfizer Corporation
Vibramycin, 387–388
Roche Laboratories, Division of Hoffmann-LaRoche Inc.
Coactin, 363–366
Institutional, 360–361
Rocephin, 457–462
Samford University
Positions Available, 390
Smith Kline & French Laboratories
Ancef, 358–359, 467
Cefizox, inside front cover
Monocid, 368–369
Tagamet, 371–372
Stuart Pharmaceuticals, Division of ICI Americas, Inc.
Institutional, outside back cover
The Upjohn Company
Micronase, 384–386
Veterans Administration
Positions Available, 390

News

Researchers discuss promising drugs for AIDS at Atlanta conference

The most extensive reports to date on drug therapy for patients with acquired immunodeficiency syndrome (AIDS) were presented at an international conference on AIDS held in Atlanta on April 14–17. This was the first meeting in the four-year history of AIDS at which scientists spoke seriously and with substantial data about attacking the disease in a fundamental way, rather than simply struggling against its many infectious and oncologic manifestations.

At least six agents have been shown to be potentially useful against the AIDS virus, and a few drugs are showing promise for enhancing the immune systems of AIDS patients. Clinical trials with these drugs are still in the early stages, and some have not been used yet in humans. Nonetheless, the fact that early studies with so many drugs have shown positive results is a milestone in AIDS research. Martin Hirsch, M.D., of Massachusetts General Hospital, commented, "I think it's truly amazing that in the less than one year that these searches have been going on, already six drugs have been shown to have some effect against the AIDS virus."

Epidemiology of AIDS. The continuing spread of AIDS, its lethal character, and the remote prospect of a vaccine (in light of the poor production of virus-neutralizing antibody in AIDS patients thus far) make the positive results of early clinical trials with the six antiviral agents welcome news. As of the beginning of August 1985, 11,300 cases of AIDS had been reported to the Centers for Disease Control (CDC). Of those patients who have had the disease for two years or more, more than 80% have died. The number of AIDS cases doubles every nine months or so.

There is every indication that the seeds for further spread of AIDS have already been sown. In his opening address, James Curran, M.D., head of the AIDS task force at CDC, told conference attendees that approximately 800 homosexual men were infected with the virus for every person diagnosed as having AIDS in 1980, based on retrospective serologic surveys. Applying that figure to today's situation, Curran speculated that as many as 0.5–1 million persons in the United States currently might be infected with the AIDS virus and that 10 to 15% of these persons will develop full-fledged AIDS during the next three years.

Since it seems likely that the current epidemic growth in the incidence of AIDS will continue for at least one more year, 20,000 cases will have been diagnosed by April 1986, Curran said. One factor that might change this rate of spread, he suggested, is a change in the sexual habits of homosexual men, the group that still makes up more than 70% of all AIDS cases. In San Francisco there has been a 75% decrease in rectal gonorrhea, a sign of a "drastic sexual revolution," according to Curran.

There is also the question of whether the disease will involve the heterosexual population. Although no more than 5% of AIDS cases to date have been attributed to heterosexual spread, some people fear that this figure will increase drastically. However, Curran predicted that "neither the rapidity of transmission nor the prevalence of AIDS will be as high among heterosexuals as among homosexuals or intravenous drug users."

The AIDS Virus. That drug treatments for AIDS are even a possibility is a result of the discovery of the AIDS virus. Three viruses linked to the disease have been identified by different researchers: lymphadenopathy-associated virus (LAV) was discovered by Luc Montagnier, M.D., and colleagues at the Institut Pasteur in Paris; human T-cell lymphotropic virus type III (HTLV-III, not closely related genetically to either HTLV-I or HTLV-II) was isolated by Robert Gallo, M.D., and coworkers at the National Cancer Institute; and AIDS-associated retrovirus (ARV) was found by Jay Levy, M.D., and his group at Stanford University. All three of these viruses are retroviruses, which are small, RNA-containing viruses in the same family as such animal tumor viruses as Rous sarcoma virus and feline leukemia virus; nucleic acid analyses indicate that they are probably variants of the same virus.

Since confirmation in early 1984 that the HTLV-III/LAV/ARV agent is the most likely cause of AIDS, screening for antiviral agents has been possible. The search has focused on agents that inhibit a key viral enzyme, reverse transcriptase, an RNA-dependent DNA polymerase that is essential for replication of the RNA genome. The enzyme uses the virus' RNA genetic material as a template and makes a corresponding DNA copy. This DNA copy is used to make further RNA copies for the replicated viruses and for the direction of protein synthesis.

Antiviral Agents. Six antiviral agents that inhibit viral replication in cell cultures and that are or shortly will be in clinical trials were discussed at the Atlanta conference; they are suramin sodium, HPA-23, trisodium phosphonoformate, ribavirin, α-interferon, and ansamycin.

Suramin Sodium. Suramin sodium is a derivative of naphthalene trisulfonic acid that has been used to treat onchocerciasis and trypanosomiasis for more than 50 years in African countries. After the discovery that suramin inhibits the viral reverse transcriptase in vitro,[1] suramin was tested in Phase I trials in seven AIDS patients with early Kaposi's sarcoma.

When used in trypanosomiasis, suramin has considerable toxicity, including fever, acute neurological deficits, hypersensitivity reactions, and abnormalities in liver function tests. However, even though the dose used investigationally in the seven AIDS patients (2 g/week for six weeks) was the same as the antiparasitic dose, little toxicity was observed, said Anthony Fauci, M.D., director of the National Institute of Allergy and Infectious Diseases. Fauci noted that in these AIDS patients, suramin attained blood concentrations that have been shown to inhibit virus replication in vitro. Also, there has been an inhibition in the ability to isolate the HTLV-III virus over time in these patients, a sign that the drug is having a beneficial effect.

HPA-23. HPA-23 is the code name for an investigational compound that is now being tested at the Institut Pasteur. It had been known for several years that HPA-23 inhibits retrovirus replication. The chemical composition of HPA-23 is very unusual; its molecular formula is $NaSb_9W_{21}O_{86}$. Jean-Claude Chermann, M.D., of the Institut Pasteur, calls it a three-dimensional cage; technically, it is a mineral ion condensate.

After initial toxicity tests in animals proved negative, HPA-23 was tested in a young hemophiliac with AIDS with encouraging results. Beginning in July 1983, French researchers treated this young man with 50–200 mg/day of HPA-23 given intravenously in three divided doses for 15 days. (The dose used now is 200 mg/day in all patients who tolerate it.) The AIDS virus could not be isolated during treatment even though it had been isolated before treatment, but the drug had to be stopped because of thrombocytopenia. Therapy with the drug was continued intermittently over the next several months, and the virus remained absent. The patient, who initially had brain toxoplasmosis, is now well and back at school.

In Paris, HPA-23 has been given to a total of 50 patients, some with end-stage AIDS, some with early AIDS, and some with AIDS-related complex (ARC). Many of these patients have been treated for only a short time. However, 2 of the first 4 patients treated had no virus after therapy,[2] and the virus can no longer be isolated in 13 of 15 patients who were treated with one course of HPA-23. About two thirds of all patients treated had a decrease in platelets requiring a reduction in drug dose or cessation of the drug. Said Chermann, "In our opinion, we have done successful Phase I and Phase II evaluations. We now need to do a randomized, controlled, multicenter trial."

Trisodium Phosphonoformate. At Massachusetts General Hospital, Hirsch and colleagues have been studying a pyrophosphate analog called trisodium phosphonoformate. This agent was developed and used in Sweden as an antiherpes drug. "It is a very potent inhibitor of HTLV-III reverse transcriptase in vitro at low doses," said Hirsch. "It is also a potent inhibitor of virus replication in vitro at concentrations easily achievable in vivo."

Phosphonoformate has a moderately convincing record of safety. More than 100 patients with viral diseases other than AIDS have been treated in Scandinavia "with apparently no toxicity," according to Hirsch.

Ribavirin. This antiviral with broad-spectrum in vitro activity has been in clinical testing for more than a decade. Ribavirin is approved in the United States for treatment of respiratory syncytial virus infection in infants via aerosol delivery. Recent trials have also demonstrated that ribavirin has some activity against the influenza virus. Some reduction in hemoglobin synthesis has been observed, but so far this does not appear to be a serious toxicity.

Although the exact mechanism of action of ribavirin is not known, the drug probably exerts its antiviral effect at the level of DNA synthesis. Joseph B. McCormick, M.D., and coworkers at CDC reported that ribavirin inhibits replication of LAV in lymphocytes in vitro at 50–100 μg/mL.[3] Similar data were presented at the Atlanta meeting by Clyde Crumpacker, M.D., of Harvard Medical School. Plans are under way to test ribavirin in patients with AIDS-related complex.

α-Interferon. This member of the interferon family "is an active inhibitor of HTLV-III replication," according to Hirsch.[4] The drug acts at very low doses that do not inhibit normal lymphocyte function and growth. Two randomized, controlled clinical trials using recombinant α-interferon in patients with AIDS and AIDS-related complex are under way. The trials will compare placebo with α-interferon 3 million units or 36 million units three times per week for 12 weeks.

According to Hirsch, "interferons have gotten very bad press, largely because patients treated in the terminal phases of illness did not respond." By working with patients who have AIDS-related complex or early AIDS, he and his colleagues hope to obtain better results.

Ansamycin. The most recent addition to the test battery for AIDS is ansamycin, an antibiotic used against disseminated mycobacterial infections (*Mycobacterium avium* and *M. tuberculosis*). In work from CDC presented at the Atlanta meeting, ansamycin was shown to inhibit replication of LAV in vitro, probably through its action on reverse transcriptase.

Immunoenhancer Therapy. Even if one of the previously mentioned compounds turns out to be an effective antiviral drug, it will need to be combined with immunoenhancers for a true cure of AIDS. "Inhibiting the virus is not enough," said Chermann. "It will also be necessary to reconstruct the immune system using immunomodulators and possibly by giving grafted immune cells." The reverse is also true: Grafting immune cells without killing the virus will be futile. Fauci and his colleagues at NIH performed bone marrow grafting in an AIDS patient who had a twin brother. "We believe that the reason the transplant failed was because the virus was still present and was killing the cells as we were infusing them," he said.

The most promising immunoenhancer currently is interleukin-2. Ample supplies to allow trials have become available through recombinant DNA technology. Some transient enhancement of immune function has been seen in patients treated with high doses of interleukin-2. At NIH, this compound was given by continuous infusion to 10 patients. Therapy was continued for two weeks, increasing doses from 250–2.5 million units/day. During four weeks of therapy there was a marked increase in the number of T-cells, according to Clifford H. Lane, M.D., of NIH. Also, in three of four patients treated with the highest doses of interleukin-2, Kaposi's sarcoma lesions regressed; however, no patient had a complete regression.

One substance that will most likely not be useful as an immunoenhancer in patients with AIDS is γ-interferon.

Continued on page 479

Continued from page 476

According to Fauci, "γ-interferon is prohibitively toxic at the doses required to affect the immune system."

Another material for which there is not good evidence of efficacy is isoprinosine (inosiplex), a complex of inosine, *p*-acetamidobenzoate, and 1-dimethylamino-2-propanol-1:3. A mystique surrounds isoprinosine, and in a scenario reminiscent of Laetrile, AIDS patients are reportedly traveling to Mexico to obtain it. Researchers say it produces no benefit, even in pre-AIDS. One report at the Atlanta conference concluded that isoprinosine, used as a single agent, is not an effective means of reversing immune abnormalities in patients with AIDS-related complex.

Vaccine Research. Although a vaccine to prevent infections with the HTLV-III/LAV family in viruses is probably the ultimate goal of AIDS research, it is not clear that such a vaccine is even possible. Neither Robin Weiss, M.D., director of the Chester Beatty Institute in London, nor Chermann and Montagnier of the Institut Pasteur have found substantial virus-neutralizing antibody in AIDS patients. This raises the possibility that the human immune system cannot mount an effective response to these viruses. No effective vaccines have yet been made against animal retroviruses. (A vaccine against feline leukemia virus was recently marketed in the United States, but its efficacy has been questioned. In addition, it is a crude preparation and would not be suitable for use in humans.)

At the Atlanta conference, Hirsch reported finding neutralizing antibody in a number of patients. However, the antibody was present only at a titer of 1:2 or 1:10; as Chermann commented, "antibody at 1:10 is nothing."

The use of passive antibody is also a theoretical possibility. AIDS virus expresses new antigens on the surface of the lymphocytes that it infects. Monoclonal antibodies directed against these viral surface antigens might destroy the infected lymphocytes and remove the infection. Such a tactic would have to be used early in the infection, when only a fraction of the patient's T-4 lymphocytes are infected. The search for appropriate monoclonal antibodies is now under way.

1. Misuya H, Popovic M, Yarchoan R et al. Suramin protection of T-cells in vitro against infectivity and cytopathic effect of HTLV-III. *Science*. 1984; 226:172–4.
2. Rozenbaum W, Dormont D, Spire B et al. Antimonialtungstate (HPA-23) treatment of three patients with AIDS and one with prodrome. *Lancet*. 1985; 1:450–1.
3. McCormick JB, Getchell JP, Mitchell SW et al. Ribavirin suppresses replication of lymphadenopathy virus in cultures of human adult T-lymphocytes. *Lancet*. 1984; 2:1367–9.
4. Ho DD, Rota TR, Kaplan JC et al. Recombinant human interferon ALFA-A suppresses HTLV-III replication in vitro. *Lancet*. 1985; 1:602–4.

William A. Check, Ph.D.
Clinical Pharmacy Correspondent

Data on dose-dumping of sustained-release theophylline published

The dose-dumping data on Theo-24, Searle's brand of once-daily theophylline, which were reported in the News column of the May–June 1984 *CP*,[1] have now been published in full.[2]

One of the authors of the article, Iowa physician Miles Weinberger, had been criticized in the lay press shortly after the problems with Theo-24 became known for failing to disclose industry consulting activity before advising FDA, but a select committee from the University of Iowa has cleared him of any improprieties.[3] Searle may now face problems—the *Washington Drug Letter*[4] reported June 17 that FDA staff has recommended prosecution of the company and five of its employees for withholding data suggesting "hazards, contraindications, and precautions" related to Theo-24.

The study data showed incomplete and variable absorption of Theo-24 (6 mg/kg) administered after an overnight fast (57–100% absorption, mean ± S.D. = 70.8 ± 16.7%). When the drug was administered after the eight healthy men volunteers ate a bacon-and-eggs breakfast, it was completely absorbed (86–135% absorption, mean ± S.D. = 111.4 ± 18.9%). Dose-normalized peak serum concentrations (expressed as the peak concentration/milligram per kilogram dose) averaged 0.65 ± 0.13 after fasting and 1.42 ± 0.22 after breakfast. Four subjects experienced toxicities when Theo-24 was taken postprandially.[2]

The *Washington Drug Letter* article[4] states that FDA officials have recommended prosecution of Searle because "the firm waited until several months after approval of Theo-24" to submit data on the dose-dumping effect of postprandially administered product. The Justice Department, and presumably other officials in HHS, must approve the recommendation before prosecution will occur.

1. Posey LM. Sustained-release theophylline bioavailability controversy mixes therapeutics, politics, money. *Clin Pharm*. 1984; 3:220, 222. News.
2. Hendeles L, Weinberger M, Milaretz G et al. Food-induced "dose-dumping" from a once-a-day theophylline product as a cause of theophylline toxicity. *Chest*. 1985; 87:758–65.
3. Weinberger M. My role as a clinical investigator and consultant to industry and the Food and Drug Administration (FDA). *J Allergy Clin Immunol*. 1985; 75:100.
4. Anon. Searle may face U.S. charges of withholding hazard data. *Washington Drug Lett*. 1985; 17(24):1.

Synthetic THC approved by FDA

Dronabinol (Marinol, Unimed, Inc., Somerville, NJ 08876-3587), a synthetic form of Δ-9-tetrahydrocannabinol (the principal psychoactive substance in marijuana) was approved by the Food and Drug Administration on June 6 for use in alleviating severe nausea and vomiting associated with cancer chemotherapy. The commercial availability of dronabinol is expected to have a major impact on the treatment of the estimated 50,000 patients each year who fail to respond adequately to conventional antiemetic therapy.

Approval of dronabinol follows more than a decade of extensive clinical trials and three years of consideration of the drug by FDA. More than 20,000 patients have been treated with the drug under a free federal distribution system managed by the National Cancer Institute; that program is expected to end with the commercial availability of dronabinol. However, the drug must be reclassified by DEA from Schedule I to Schedule II, and most states must also reschedule it before it can be prescribed

Continued on page 482

When a type II diabetic patient needs more than diet, unique MICRONASE® Tablets (glyburide) are a logical first choice.

Choosing antidiabeti

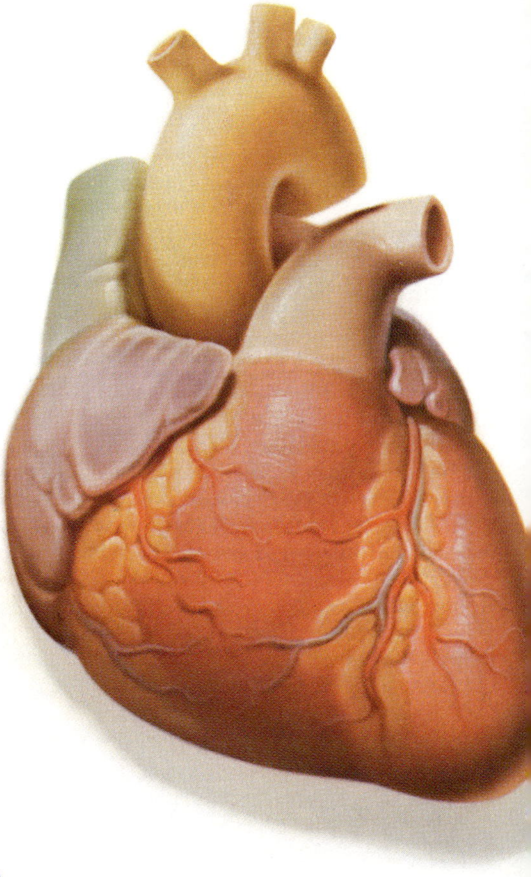

1. Micronase—a rational choice in type II diabetes

Insulin levels are normal or elevated in most patients with type II diabetes, although insulin action is markedly impaired. MICRONASE helps normalize the tissue response to endogenous insulin.

Initially, MICRONASE helps lower serum glucose in responsive patients by stimulating the release of additional insulin. As therapy continues, MICRONASE is believed to promote peripheral glucose metabolism by helping to correct defects at the cellular receptor and postreceptor levels.

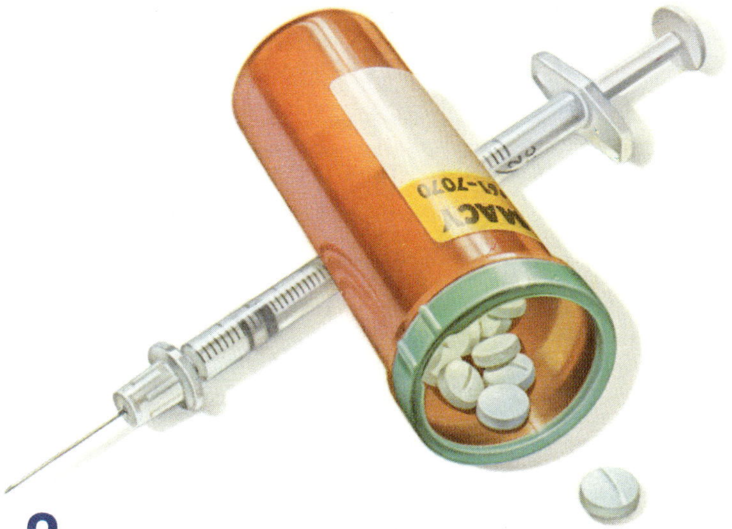

2. Micronase—a single, daily dose provides 24-hour glycemic control

MICRONASE provides 24-hour control of blood glucose with a single, daily, low-milligram dose. MICRONASE may be taken with food, since food intake does not appear to affect its bioavailability.

3. Micronase—for the type II diabetic patient who is also hypertensive: Control without risk of water retention

This may also be significant for the type II diabetic pa with congestive heart failure. MICRONASE actually ca mild diuresis.

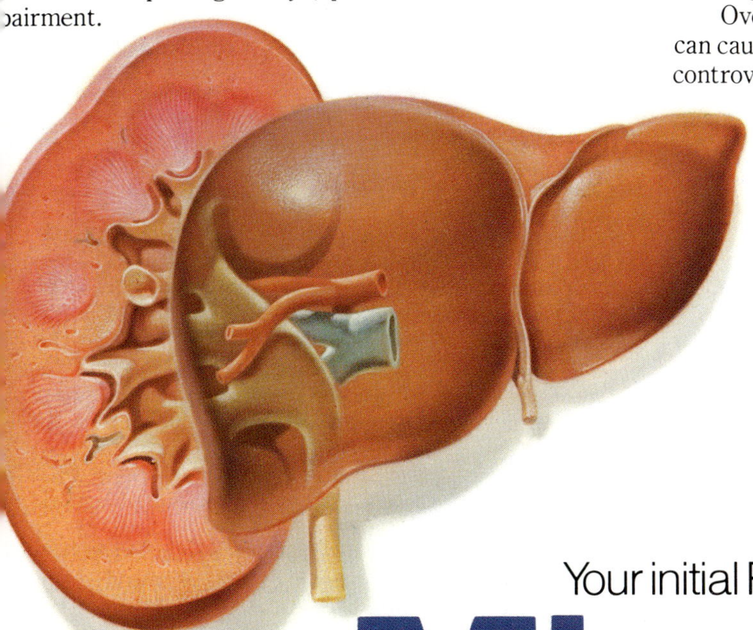

News *Continued from page 479*

and dispensed as a legal controlled substance.

Dronabinol is chemically synthesized and formulated in sesame oil. Following oral administration, peak plasma dronabinol concentrations occur in 2–3 hours; the elimination phase exhibits biphasic kinetics, with an α half-life of about four hours and a terminal half-life of 25–36 hours. The systemic availability of dronabinol is 10–20% relative to an i.v. dose; the principal active metabolite, 11-hydroxytetrahydrocannabinol, appears in the plasma in roughly the same milligram quantities as the parent drug.

Dronabinol is indicated for the treatment of the nausea and vomiting associated with cancer chemotherapy in patients who have failed to respond adequately to conventional antiemetic treatments. A substantial proportion of patients treated with dronabinol can be expected to experience disturbing psychotomimetic reactions not observed with other antiemetic agents.

The side effects of dronabinol include drowsiness, dizziness, muddled thinking, and brief impairment of coordination, sensory, and perceptual functions. Approximately 24% of patients treated with dronabinol reported experiencing a "high" (characterized by easy laughing, elation, and heightened awareness). In long-term controlled trials, only 7% of patients stopped using dronabinol because of intolerance to side effects.

The usual adult dose of dronabinol is 5 mg/sq m given 1–3 hours before the administration of chemotherapy and every 2–4 hours after chemotherapy for a total of four to six doses each day. The drug is supplied as round soft gelatin capsules containing 2.5, 5, or 10 mg of dronabinol in bottles of 50.

Study shows benefit in treating elderly hypertensive patients

Antihypertensive therapy can reduce cardiovascular mortality among elderly patients with high blood pressure by nearly 30%, according to a recently published study of 840 elderly hypertensive patients from the European Working Party on High Blood Pressure in the Elderly (EWPHE).[1]

The double-blind, placebo-controlled, multicenter EWPHE trial was the first large study to look specifically at morbidity and mortality of elderly hypertensive patients. The study was ended for ethical reasons in 1984 after 12 years because predetermined criteria of benefit for treated patients had been met.

During the trial, patients over the age of 60 with a sustained systolic blood pressure of 160–239 mm Hg and a sustained diastolic blood pressure of 90–110 mm Hg were randomly allocated to a placebo treatment group (n = 424) or an active treatment group (n = 416). Actively treated patients were given a combination of hydrochlorothiazide 25 mg and triamterene 50 mg (Dyazide, SKF), plus methyldopa (up to 2 g daily) if needed.

Analyses on randomized treatment in the double-blind part of the trial showed 29 fewer cardiovascular events and 14 fewer cardiovascular deaths per 1000 patient-years among patients on active therapy. The main

Continued on page 485

News *Continued from page 482*

benefits of treatment were a reduction in fatal myocardial infarction, severe congestive heart failure, and stroke; noncardiovascular mortality was not affected by active treatment. Overall intention-to-treat analysis, which included data on patients who dropped out of the double-blind part of the study, showed no significant reduction in mortality from all causes (9% reduction) but significant reductions in cardiac mortality (38%) and cardiovascular mortality (27%).

The results of this study raise the question, Should all elderly hypertensive patients now be treated? As the authors point out, caution must be exercised when extrapolating the results to the generality of elderly people with raised blood pressures. A *Lancet* editorial suggested that one of the major uncertainties in applying these results concerns the nature of the treatment used in the trial; since the EWPHE approach to stepped care was "rather unusual," the applicability of the results to other classes of antihypertensives appears questionable.[2]

The EWPHE study will not end the controversy over treatment of mild hypertension in elderly patients. As stated in the *Lancet* editorial, it seems likely that treating hypertension in the elderly according to the criteria now applied to younger patients will help at least some patients. At the same time, it seems likely that such treatment will lead to a greater likelihood of adverse effects and difficulties in compliance, which demand even greater vigilance and caution.

1. Amery A, Birkenhager W, Brixko P et al. Mortality and morbidity results from the European Working Party on High Blood Pressure in the Elderly trial. *Lancet*. 1985; 2:1349–54.
2. Anon. Treatment of hypertension in the over-60s. *Lancet*. 1985; 2:1369–70. Editorial.

Adjuvant chemotherapy useful in osteosarcoma, says NIH panel

Patients with osteosarcoma of the extremities who undergo limb-sparing surgery can benefit from adjuvant chemotherapy and radiation therapy, according to an NIH Consensus Development Conference panel. The December 3–5, 1984, deliberations of the panel addressed the effectiveness of limb-sparing treatment of adult soft-tissue sarcomas and osteosarcoma; the panel met in Bethesda, MD.

In general, the panel supported adjuvant therapy for patients with osteosarcoma but suggested that more study of patients with soft-tissue sarcomas is needed. Some centers have used regional (intra-arterial) chemotherapy and surgery, but results have not been superior to those of other approaches to treatment of soft-tissue sarcomas. Clinical trials in patients with osteosarcoma have shown comparable survival rates in patients receiving limb-sparing therapy plus chemotherapy in trials using amputation plus chemotherapy. Intra-arterial therapy has not been superior to intravenous chemotherapy; both are acceptable.

Single free copies of the panel's complete statement are available from the National Institutes of Health, Office of Medical Applications of Research, Building 1, Room 216, Bethesda, MD 20205.

Ceftazidime reaches U.S. market

Ceftazidime (Fortaz), the first injectable antibiotic in more than a decade to receive FDA's 1-A classification (indicating a new chemical entity with an important therapeutic gain over other available drugs), was marketed in early August by Glaxo. The semisynthetic third-generation cephalosporin has broad-spectrum activity and marked antipseudomonal activity.

Ceftazidime may be used alone or concomitantly with other antibiotics, such as aminoglycosides, vancomycin, and clindamycin. The drug has accumulated more than 500,000 patient days of use in 11 countries since 1983, and more than 440 U.S. patients were treated with ceftazidime under a compassionate-use protocol before the drug was approved by FDA.

Ceftazidime can be administered intravenously or intramuscularly. The drug is indicated for treating infections caused by susceptible organisms (including *Pseudomonas* species, *Klebsiella* species, *Escherichia coli*, *Haemophilus influenzae*, and methicillin-susceptible strains of *Staphylococcus aureus*) in several serious infections, such as lower respiratory tract infections, skin and skin structure infections, complicated and uncomplicated urinary tract infections, septicemia, and bone and joint infections.

Fortaz is available as 500-mg and 1- and 2-g vials, 1- and 2-g infusion packs, and 6-g pharmacy bulk packs. Glaxo has priced Fortaz at $11.08 per gram.

Lilly and SmithKline Beckman have both claimed marketing rights to ceftazidime under cross-licensing agreements entered into in 1969, and both are likely to market the drug next year.

Captopril approved for all degrees of hypertension

Captopril (Capoten, Squibb), the first angiotensin-converting-enzyme inhibitor, has been approved by FDA for use in mild and moderate hypertension. Because of concern that the drug impaired renal and immune function in some patients, FDA-approved labeling for captopril previously covered only hypertensive patients who had either failed to respond satisfactorily or developed unacceptable side effects on multidrug regimens. The recommended initial dose of captopril will remain 25 mg b.i.d. or t.i.d.; the drug is not recommended for use in patients with renal insufficiency.

News Briefs

• New labeling for **triazolam** (Halcion, Upjohn) that warns of a possible pharmacokinetic interaction between cimetidine and triazolam has been approved by FDA; in normal patients, coadministration with cimetidine resulted in a reduction in triazolam clearance, an increase in elimination half-life from 2.2 to 3.7 hours, and an approximate doubling of plasma concentration.

• Glaxo has received approval for labeling **ranitidine** (Zantac) for short-term treatment of active gastric ulcers; the drug was previously indicated only for short-term treatment of active duodenal ulcers.

• Searle has received FDA approval to amend the labeling for **intravenous metronidazole hydrochloride** (Flagyl I.V.) to include an indication for prophylactic use in elective colon and rectal surgery.

• **"Introduction to Pharmacokinetics,"** a self-paced, interactive, computer-assisted instruction program, is available from Pharmat, a publisher of continuing education materials for schools of pharmacy. The software package is intended for an IBM or similar computer; contact Pharmat, Inc., P.O. Box 3007, Lawrence, KS 66046, to obtain the name of the nearest school of pharmacy using Pharmat-developed materials.

• Limiting the length of the therapy to 14 days with 0.05% **betamethasone dipropionate ointment** (Diprolone Ointment, Schering Laboratories) is no longer necessary, according to the revised product labeling. However, no more than 45 grams of the ointment should be applied weekly.

• A patient-information brochure about **Chlamydia,** a sexually transmitted disease affecting 3 to 10 million people annually, is available from the American Social Health Association, 260 Sheridan Avenue, Palo Alto, CA 94306. Enclose a stamped, self-addressed envelope to get a free copy of the brochure, which was funded through a grant from Lederle Laboratories.

The Challenge:
Increase Pharmacy Productivity

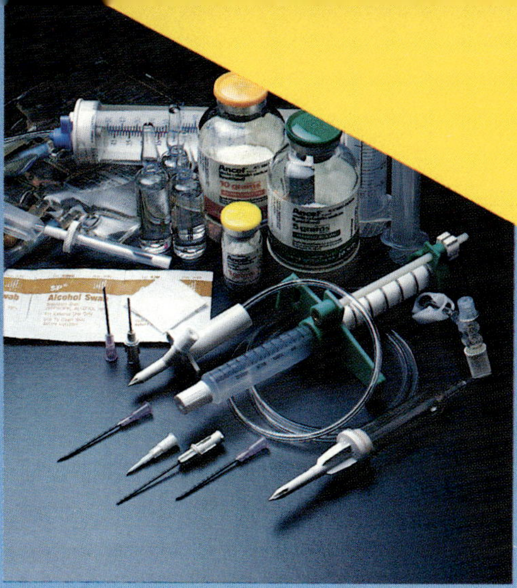

Now Available in 500 mg. Strength

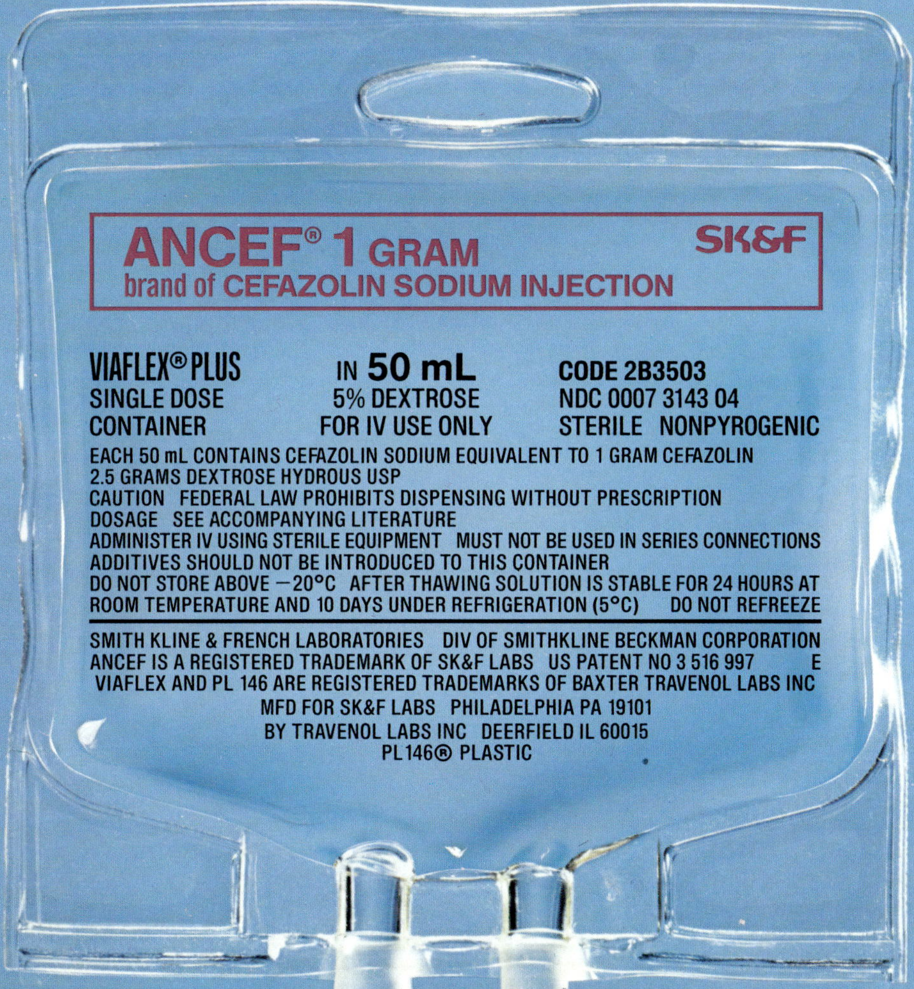

Our Response:

ANCEF®

1 gram

brand of

CEFAZOLIN SODIUM INJECTION

The First Pre-Mixed, Injectable Cephalosporin

Ask Your Smith Kline &French Sales Representative About Availability in Your Area.

SK&F

MINI-BAG™ plastic containers are manufactured by Travenol Laboratories, Inc.

Smith Kline &French Laboratories
Philadelphia, PA

Letters

The Letters *column is a forum for rapid exchange of ideas among readers of* CP. *Liberal criteria are applied in the review of submissions to encourage contributions to this column.*

The Letters *column includes the following types of contributions: (1) comments, addenda, and minor updates on previously published work, (2) alerts on potential problems related to drug therapy or clinical research, (3) observations or comments on trends in drug therapy or clinical research, and (4) brief expressions of opinion about controversies in drug therapy or clinical research.*

Letters need not be submitted with the journal's manuscript checklist. The following conditions, however, must be adhered to: (1) the body of the letter must be no longer than two typewritten pages, (2) the use of references, tables, and illustrations should be minimized, (3) the authors' names, affiliations, and mailing addresses must be typed at the end of the letter in the format used by CP, *and (4) the entire letter (including references, tables, and authors' names) must be typed double spaced on plain white paper (not letterhead). Following acceptance of a letter, the authors are required to sign an exclusive publication statement and a copyright-transferral form.*

Use of 0.9 % sodium chloride injection without heparin for maintaining indwelling intermittent injection sites

Two reports have recently appeared in the literature about the lack of clotting problems associated with the use of 0.9% sodium chloride injection without heparin to flush indwelling intermittent injection sites.[1,2] We have completed one study on our coronary-care unit using 0.9% sodium chloride injection alone to flush "heparin locks," and we are now conducting a second study on a surgical floor.

Our first study involved 100 patients and was to be discontinued immediately if the failure rate was greater than 10% in the first 20 patients. Each lock was flushed with 2 mL of 0.9% sodium chloride injection every 12 hours. If medications were given through the lock, it was flushed after each dose. The lock was considered a failure if it became blocked, and locks that became infiltrated were eliminated from the study. In most cases, the intravenous catheters that we used were 20-gauge, 1.25- or 1.5-inch in size (Deseret Medical Incorporated).

Upon completion of this study, the failure rate was 3%. The average length of time the catheters remained in place was 2.2 days. One patient's catheter remained patent for seven days; this patient received no i.v. medications. In fact, only 36 patients received any medications through the locks, and those medications were primarily boluses of morphine, furosemide, lidocaine, and atropine.

A larger study, now under way, involves two similar groups of general surgical patients and uses the same flushing procedures as above. One group of patients is receiving 0.9% sodium chloride injection, while the other group is receiving our normal flush solution containing heparin 10 units/mL. Thus far, there have been no failures in the group receiving 0.9% sodium chloride injection; evaluation of the heparin group has just begun and no meaningful results are available yet.

The savings our department has achieved by using flush solutions of 0.9% sodium chloride injection alone instead of with heparin is small, but the material savings to the hospital for the 29,000 heparin-lock doses administered yearly is about $20,000. Favorable results from our second study should allow us to adopt this new method. It also appears that a 12-hour flushing procedure is as adequate as the 8-hour one described previously.[1]

1. Epperson EL. Efficacy of 0.9% sodium chloride injection with and without heparin for maintaining indwelling intermittent injection sites. *Clin Pharm.* 1984; 3:626–9.
2. Schustek M. A cost effective approach to P.R.N. device maintenance. *NITA.* 1984; 7:527.

TERRY DEAN, Assistant Director of Pharmacy
PAM RIDLEY, Head Nurse–I.V. Team

Kitchener-Waterloo Hospital
835 King St., W.
Kitchener, Ontario N2G 1G3, Canada

In light of the economic pressures that hospitals face today, it was not at all surprising to see Epperson's paper, "Efficacy of 0.9% sodium chloride injection with and without heparin for maintaining indwelling intermittent injection sites" in a recent issue of *Clinical Pharmacy*.[1] Epperson is to be commended for exploring ways in which everyday costs in the practice of hospital pharmacy might be contained. However, his paper seems to have been focused more on cost containment than on what constitutes patency.

Since Heparin-Lock Flush Solution, USP, has been used successfully for more than a decade as the agent of choice in maintaining patency, we should exercise caution before adopting the findings of Epperson's report. In effect, the study's methods use subjective observation as a measure of patency. No attempt was made to determine whether any fibrin material had indeed formed within the catheter. Clot formation is a much more accurate measurement of a holding solution's ability to maintain patency. One of Epperson's references had reported earlier that sodium chloride alone was found not to be an adequate holding solution when the catheters themselves were examined for clot formation.[2]

We certainly agree with Epperson's conclusion that "Further controlled studies . . . are needed to confirm these results." It should be our intent to add to this body of knowledge before omitting heparin flush from heparin locks.

1. Epperson EL. Efficacy of 0.9% sodium chloride injection with and without heparin for maintaining indwelling intermittent injection sites. *Clin Pharm.* 1984; 3:626–9.
2. Hanson RS, Grant AM, Majors KR. Heparin lock maintenance with two units of sodium heparin in one milliliter of normal saline solution. *Surg Gynecol Obstet.* 1976; 142:373–6.

JOSEPH M. FERRARO, Assistant Director of I.V. Services
ROBERT F. GUANCI, Assistant Director of Pharmacy Services
ROBERT J. STONEBURNER, Director of Pharmaceutical Services

Department of Pharmacy and I.V. Services
Hampton General Hospital
3120 Victoria Boulevard
Hampton, VA 23669

My research on heparin-lock flushing solutions was performed for clinical as well as practical concerns —how to effectively eliminate heparin incompatibilities with many drugs that are given via heparin lock while avoiding the necessity of double-flushing the lock. It was conducted after a review of the literature revealed that a number of researchers had suggested or implied that heparin is not a necessary component of heparin-lock flushing solutions.

The study focused on the presence of phlebitis and the patency of the heparin lock. These are substantiated, practical considerations for the patient. The authors of the preceding letter propose to study the effect of heparinized saline versus nonheparinized saline on minute amounts of fibrin that may be found within a catheter. However, it needs to be established that fibrin particles have an important role in causing phlebitis in patients whose locks are routinely flushed with a solution. Unless fibrin particles can be demonstrated to affect rates of phlebitis or loss of patency directly, the question is merely academic and offers little to improving patient care.

To my knowledge, at least one manufacturer of prefilled syringes intends to underwrite just such a study as the one the authors propose. The motivations for, as well as the practical applications of, such a study remain unclear.

EDWARD L. EPPERSON, PHARM.D., Director of Pharmacy and I.V. Therapy
Rideout Memorial Hospital
726 Fourth Street
Marysville, CA 95901

Continued on page 494

MONOCID®

IV/IM

brand of sterile

cefonicid sodium

Injection: 500 mg. and 1 gram vials (lyophilized)

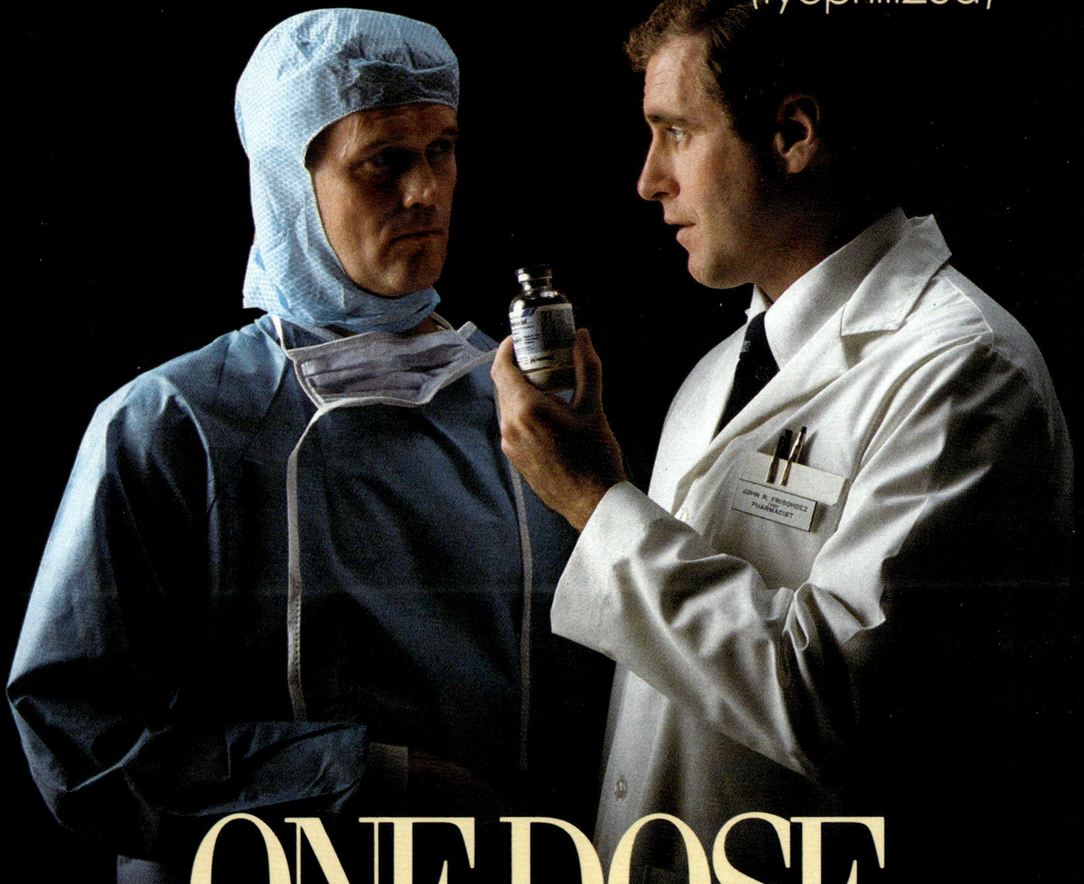

ONE DOSE ONE GRAM ONCE DAILY

Documented Once-a-Day Effectiveness

The brief summary of prescribing information on opposite page includes indications and usage, contraindications, warnings, precautions, adverse reactions, and dosage and administration. It will be helpful in consulting with physicians.

As safe as albumin or PPF

In comparative clinical studies, platelet counts, hematocrits, serum fibrinogen levels, prothrombin times (PT), and partial thromboplastin times (PTT) seen with Hespan were comparable to those seen with albumin or plasma protein fraction (PPF).[1,2]

Other studies demonstrate that when any reduction in platelet count or prolongation of PT or PTT does occur with Hespan, no increased bleeding results, even in patients with multiple trauma.[3-5] As with any volume expander, patients should be monitored for excessive hemodilution of coagulant factors or circulatory overload when large volumes are administered.

When Hespan-treated patients were monitored to detect localized or systemic sepsis, there was no evidence of a decrease in their ability to ward off infection or combat an established infection.[5]

Hespan is nonantigenic and, as with blood-derived colloids, any risk of allergic reaction is minimal. Hespan also has a negligible effect on subsequent blood typing or cross-matching.[6]

As effective as albumin or PPF

Comparative clinical studies have repeatedly demonstrated that Hespan is as effective as albumin or PPF in postoperative myocardial revascularization,[1-3] and hemorrhagic, traumatic, or septic shock.[4,5,7]

No significant differences between Hespan and albumin or PPF were noted in any efficacy parameter.[1-5,7] Hespan effectively maintained colloid osmotic pressure, restored plasma volume, and improved cardiac output and renal function in hypovolemic patients.[1-5,7] And, the volume-expanding effect of a single infusion of Hespan can persist for 24 hours or longer.

Half the price of albumin or PPF

Hespan offers a potential savings to your hospital of tens of thousands of dollars a year.

double the price.

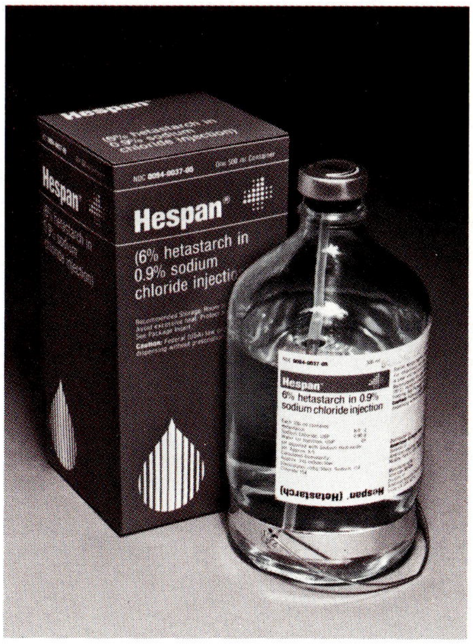

For additional information, contact the Medical Services Department, American Critical Care, 1600 Waukegan Road, McGaw Park, IL 60085. Phone 1-800-323-4980.

Lifesaving, moneysaving

HESPAN®
(hetastarch)

American Critical Care

American Hospital Supply Corporation

Please see references and brief summary of prescribing information on following page.

Letters *Continued from page 489*

The opioid–noradrenergic link in Gilles de la Tourette's syndrome

A substantial body of evidence has recently accumulated to suggest that central noradrenergic hyperactivity plays a role in the pathophysiology of a variety of withdrawal syndromes, including opiate withdrawal.[1] Clonidine, an α_2-adrenoreceptor agonist, has been shown to be effective in the management of acute opiate withdrawal.[1] It has also been shown to be beneficial in the management of Gilles de la Tourette's syndrome (TS), a condition in which excessive noradrenergic activity has been suggested to be of pathophysiologic importance.[2] It appears, thus, that the mechanisms underlying TS resemble those occurring during opiate withdrawal.

I recently suggested a role for the endogenous opioid system in the pathophysiology of TS and indicated that overactivity of the opioid system was critical in the pathogenesis of this condition.[3] Whatever the cause of the excessive endorphinergic tone found in TS, chronically increased opioid tone could lead to the development of subsensitivity and "down-regulation" of striatal and extrastriatal opiate receptors with a resultant decrease in the activity of this system ("autowithdrawal"). The latter mechanism could precipitate a compensatory increase in the activity of the noradrenergic system. Moreover, it is possible that in time this autotolerance process decreases itself, allowing the condition to reassert itself. Indeed, both normoactivity and hyperactivity of the noradrenergic system have been reported in TS.[2] Moreover, clonidine has been shown to benefit only a subgroup (50–60%) of patients, while others may experience exacerbation of symptoms with clonidine.[2]

It appears that in TS, alterations in the activity of the noradrenergic system do not reflect a basic underlying deficit intrinsic to central noradrenergic systems. Rather, central noradrenergic mechanisms are likely to become involved at some later stage in the pathophysiology of TS.[2] It is possible that noradrenergic mechanisms may be mobilized as part of a compensatory effort that follows alterations in the activity of the opioid system. In this case, a more rational approach to the therapy of TS should include the development of pharmacologic strategies aimed towards direct modulation of endogenous opioids. The use of an agent like pentazocine is likely to be beneficial. Such an agent (a partial agonist), while limiting the danger of opiate addiction, would antagonize overactivity of the opioid system and supplement such activity when the opioid system is hypoactive.

1. Glassman AH, Jackson WK, Walsh BT et al. Cigarette craving, smoking withdrawal, and clonidine. *Science*. 1984; 226:864–6.
2. Leckman JF, Cohen DJ. Recent advances in Gilles de la Tourette syndrome: implications for clinical practice and future research. *Psychiatr Dev*. 1983; 3:301–16.
3. Sandyk R. The effects of naloxone in Tourette syndrome. *Ann Neurol*. In press.

R. Sandyk, M.D., M.S., Research Assistant Professor of Neurology and Pharmacology
University of Arizona
Tucson, AZ 85724

Continued on page 502

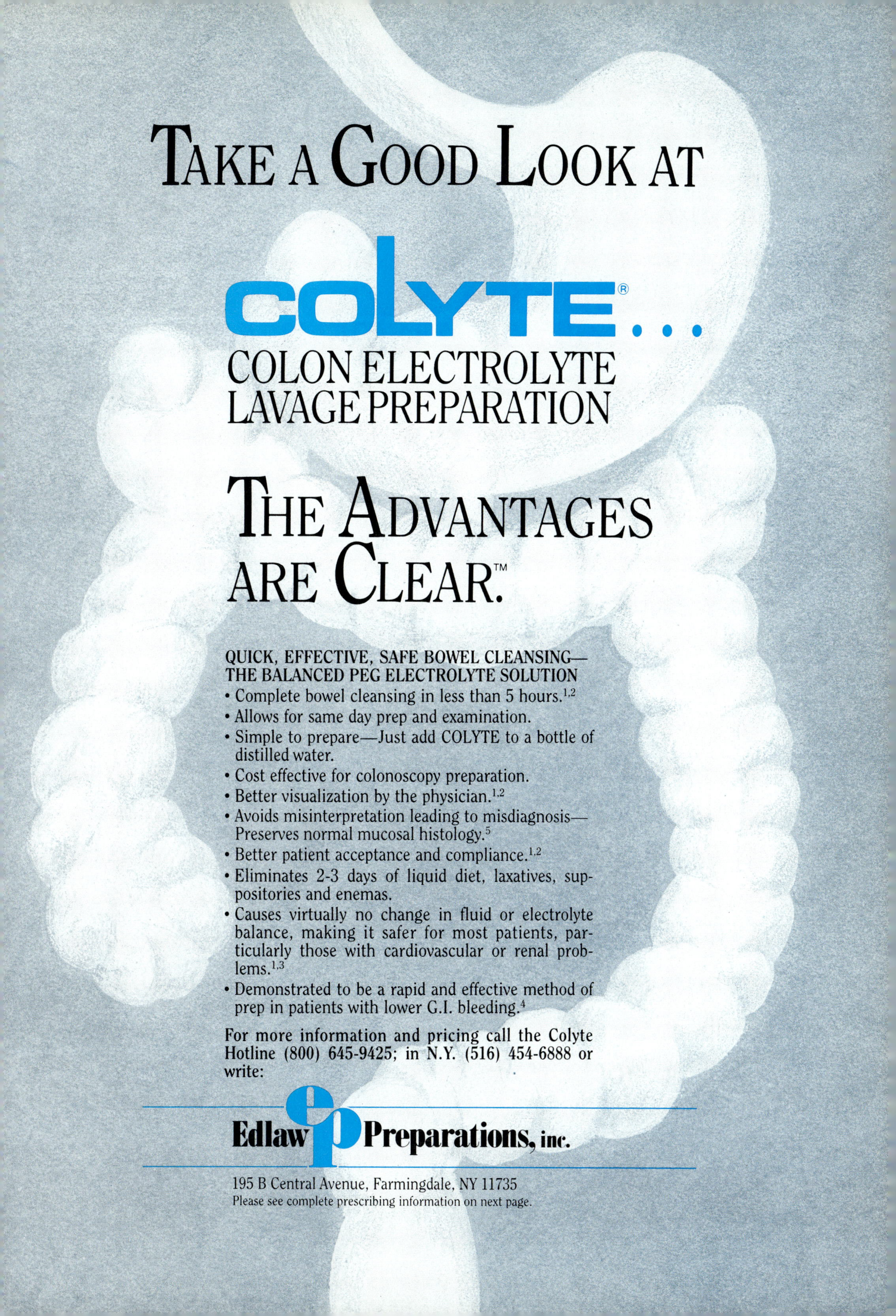
TAKE A GOOD LOOK AT
COLYTE®...
COLON ELECTROLYTE
LAVAGE PREPARATION
THE ADVANTAGES ARE CLEAR.™
QUICK, EFFECTIVE, SAFE BOWEL CLEANSING—
THE BALANCED PEG ELECTROLYTE SOLUTION
• Complete bowel cleansing in less than 5 hours.[1,2]
• Allows for same day prep and examination.
• Simple to prepare—Just add COLYTE to a bottle of distilled water.
• Cost effective for colonoscopy preparation.
• Better visualization by the physician.[1,2]
• Avoids misinterpretation leading to misdiagnosis—Preserves normal mucosal histology.[5]
• Better patient acceptance and compliance.[1,2]
• Eliminates 2-3 days of liquid diet, laxatives, suppositories and enemas.
• Causes virtually no change in fluid or electrolyte balance, making it safer for most patients, particularly those with cardiovascular or renal problems.[1,3]
• Demonstrated to be a rapid and effective method of prep in patients with lower G.I. bleeding.[4]
For more information and pricing call the Colyte Hotline (800) 645-9425; in N.Y. (516) 454-6888 or write:
Edlaw ep Preparations, inc.
195 B Central Avenue, Farmingdale, NY 11735
Please see complete prescribing information on next page.

Letters *Continued from page 494*

Beneficial hemodynamic effects of oral levodopa in a patient with cardiomyopathy

The use of the traditional positive inotropic agents in the treatment of heart failure has been successful for many years. Currently, the only oral inotropic agents used successfully are the digitalis glycosides. However, we recently used oral levodopa successfully to increase and maintain cardiac output in a patient with cardiomyopathy.

A 52-year-old woman who had stage IV ovarian carcinoma was recently admitted to the intensive-care unit of our hospital with severe cardiomyopathy believed to be secondary to doxorubicin therapy. An echocardiogram showed a dilated, hypokinetic left ventricle and no evidence of pericardial effusion. A Swan-Ganz pulmonary-artery catheter was inserted. The patient's initial hemodynamic status was as follows: pulse 80; blood pressure 86/64 mm Hg; pulmonary-capillary wedge pressure 19 mm Hg; pulmonary-artery pressure 42/19 mm Hg; central venous pressure 14 mm Hg; cardiac output 2.33 L/min; and cardiac index 1.30 L/min/sq m. Drug therapy was initiated with dopamine 5 μg/kg/min, digoxin 0.25 mg i.v., and transdermal nitroglycerin 2.5 mg every 24 hours. The dopamine infusion was increased to 15.8 μg/kg/min; however, the patient remained unresponsive and the cardiac output dropped to 1.63 L/min. Dopamine therapy was continued unchanged. On the second day of hospitalization, intravenous amrinone therapy was started at a dosage of 5 μg/kg/min. Cardiac output then increased to 3.36 L/min, cardiac index increased to 1.88 L/min/sq m, pulmonary-capillary wedge pressure decreased to 15 mm Hg, and pulmonary-artery pressure decreased to 30/21 mm Hg. However, by hospital day 5 the patient's platelet count had dropped from 161,000/cu mm on initiation of amrinone to 98,000/cu mm; at this time, amrinone therapy was discontinued. On the sixth hospital day, cardiac output was 2.4 L/min and cardiac index was 1.34 L/min/sq m. That morning, levodopa 100 mg orally every eight hours was started. Since the patient tolerated the levodopa well, the dose that evening was increased to 250 mg every six hours. The cardiac output at that time was 3.4 L/min and cardiac index was 1.90 L/min/sq m. The dopamine infusion had been decreased to 3.98 μg/kg/min and subsequently discontinued. Levodopa therapy was increased to 500 mg every six hours, and transdermal nitroglycerin was increased to 5 mg every 24 hours. Cardiac output continued to increase to 3.55 L/min and cardiac index increased to 1.98 L/min/sq m. At that time, the Swan-Ganz catheter was removed and the patient was transferred out of the intensive-care unit. Throughout her hospitalization, the patient's blood pressure remained between 120/68 and 88/60 mm Hg. The patient continued to improve and was discharged on hospital day 14 on the following medications: levodopa 500 mg orally every six hours, digoxin 0.25 mg orally every day, furosemide 40

Continued on page 504

Letters *Continued from page 502*

mg orally twice daily, spironolactone 50 mg orally twice daily, and transdermal nitroglycerin 5 mg daily.

The benefit of using oral levodopa in combination with digoxin to improve the inotropic action of the heart is evident in this patient. Our findings support those of Rajfer et al.[1] who also demonstrated that oral levodopa could be used to potentiate digoxin's hemodynamic effects in patients with heart failure.

1. Rajfer SI, Anton AH, Rossen JD et al. Beneficial hemodynamic effects of oral levodopa in heart failure: relation to the generation of dopamine. *N Engl J Med.* 1984; 310:1357–62.

Ronald W. Maddox, Pharm.D.
W. Stanley Arnold, M.D.
Van Odell Sliger, Pharm.D.

Mercer University
School of Pharmacy
345 Boulevard, N.E.
Atlanta, GA 30312

Procainamide-induced hypotension during CPR

Clinicians exercise great caution in administering cardioactive drugs to a conscious patient by intravenous bolus injection. Although the danger of rapid i.v. procainamide infusion is known in patients with intact circulation, there is no documentation of its potential consequences in patients receiving cardiopulmonary resuscitation (CPR).[1,2] It has been shown that near-normal systemic vascular resistance is usually present in human patients during cardiac resuscitation and that, in the animal model, the vasculature responds to pharmacologic agents.[3,4] We recorded femoral arterial pressure during cardiac resuscitation in an adult human patient to assess changes in systolic pressure following rapid i.v. administration of procainamide.

The patient, a 60-year-old insulin-dependent diabetic woman with a history of myocardial infarction, suffered cardiac arrest in her home. CPR was not performed by anyone present. When the paramedics arrived, they found the patient in ventricular fibrillation (VF) and began CPR, using a Michigan Instruments Thumper. This device was used until termination of the resuscitative efforts. Standard advanced life-support protocols of the American Heart Association were followed.[5] The patient received a 350-mg i.v. bolus injection of bretylium tosylate and was defibrillated 16 times. Despite therapy, she remained in VF. Twenty-four minutes after the patient arrived in the emergency department, a 20-gauge femoral arterial catheter was inserted to provide access for blood-gas sampling and continuous clinical monitoring of blood pressure. A Model 414 Tektronix pressure monitor with a Model 400 recorder was used to record arterial pressure at one-minute intervals. Arterial blood gases obtained at this time revealed a Po_2 of 110 torr, pH 7.41, and Pco_2 41 torr on 80% inspired oxygen.

Procainamide hydrochloride 500-mg i.v. (100 mg every three to five minutes) was ordered. However, the entire 500-mg dose was administered via a peripheral i.v. line over six minutes (see figure). Immediately after the infusion, systolic blood pressure fell rapidly and remained low despite i.v. administration of epinephrine and calcium chloride. After four additional defibrillations, the patient converted to an agonal idioventricular rhythm with electromechanical dissociation and was pronounced dead.

The marked drop in arterial pressure following i.v. procainamide administration in our patient is consistent with the known action of the drug and indicates that the vasculature in human beings is responsive to vasodilators during CPR.[1,2] Procainamide-induced hypotension is most pronounced at the end of the infusion period and persists for minutes to hours.[1] This was evident in our patient (see figure).

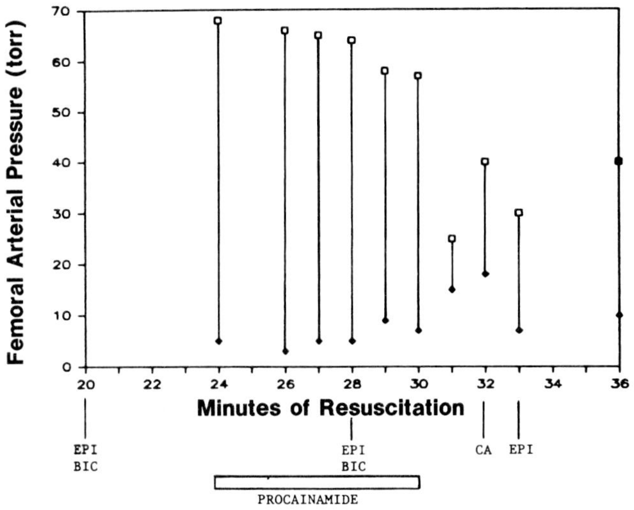

Systemic arterial pressure (□ = systolic, ◆ = diastolic) readings and times of epinephrine (EPI), sodium bicarbonate (BIC), and calcium chloride (CA) administration during cardiopulmonary resuscitation.

Our findings indicate the need to (1) administer drugs with vasodilating properties slowly during CPR, just as during more normal cardiovascular hemodynamic states; (2) continuously monitor arterial blood pressure during CPR to detect, and immediately attempt to treat, any adverse effects of therapy on systemic blood pressure; and (3) exercise caution about potential vasoactive drug interactions during CPR.

1. McClendon RL, Hansen WR, Kinsman JM. Hemodynamic changes following procainamide administered intravenously. *Am J Med Sci.* 1951; 222:375–81.
2. Stearns NS, Callahan EJ, Ellis LB. Value and hazards of intravenous procainamide ("Pronestyl") therapy. *JAMA.* 1952; 48:360–4.
3. Dohi S, Ujike Y, Nishikawa T et al. Pulmonary hemodynamics during external cardiac massage in humans. *Crit Care Med.* 1980; 8:123–6.
4. Pearson JW, Redding JS. Influence of peripheral vascular tone on cardiac resuscitation. *Anesth Analg.* 1965; 44:746–52.
5. Standards and guidelines for cardiopulmonary resuscitation (CPR) and emergency cardiac care (ECC). *JAMA.* 1980; 244:453–509.

Edgar R. Gonzalez, Pharm.D., Assistant Professor of Pharmacy Practice
University of Nebraska Medical Center
42nd and Dewey Avenue
Omaha, NE 68105

Joseph P. Ornato, M.D., Associate Professor of Internal Medicine
Medical College of Virginia
Virginia Commonwealth University
Richmond, VA 23298

Potentiation of opiate analgesia with ibuprofen

I was interested in the study by Weingart et al.[1] in which the nonsteroidal anti-inflammatory agent, ibuprofen, appeared to potentiate the analgesic effects of oral narcotics in cancer patients. This report adds further support to the possible role of the prostaglandins in mediating opioid analgesia.[2] In 1974, Collier and Roy[3] demonstrated that morphine blocks the ability of prostaglandins (PGE_1) to raise cyclic AMP levels in the rat's brain. Goldstein et al.[4] later showed that endorphins inhibited PGE_1-stimulated adenylate cyclase in neuroblastoma cells. Moreover, the analgesic effects of morphine have been shown to be reversed by intraventricular injection of PGE_1.[5] Interestingly, the analgesic effects of morphine have also been shown to be potentiated with lithium, a known inhibitor of PGE_1 biosynthesis.[6] Thus, it appears that the analgesic properties of the opiates could be enhanced by blockade of PGE_1 activity, an assumption supported by the Weingart study. Further, increased prostaglandin release in cancer patients having osteolytic metastasis[7] may possibly inhibit the analgesic effect of the opiates and thus be responsible for increased pain perception in these patients.[1]

1. Weingart WA, Sorkness CA, Earhart RH. Analgesia with oral narcotics and added ibuprofen in cancer patients. *Clin Pharm.* 1985; 4:53–8.
2. Horrobin DF. Possible roles of prostaglandins in mediating opioid actions. In: Endorphins and opiate antagonists in psychiatric research. New York: Plenum Medical Book Company; 1982:75–87.
3. Collier HOJ, Roy AC. Morphine-like drugs inhibit the stimulation by E prostaglandins of cyclic AMP formation by rat brain homogenates. *Nature.* 1974; 248:24–7.
4. Goldstein A, Cox BM, Kell WA et al. Endorphin from pituitary inhibits cyclic AMP formation in homogenates of neuroblastoma X glioma hybrid cells. *Nature.* 1977; 265:362–6.
5. Ferri S, Santagostino A, Braga PC et al. Decreased antinociceptive effect of morphine in rats treated intraventricularly with prostaglandin E_1. *Psychopharmacologica.* 1974; 39:231–6.
6. Jensen J. The effect of prolonged lithium ingestion on morphine actions in the rat. *Acta Pharmacol Toxicol.* 1974; 35:395–402.
7. Anon. Osteolytic metastases. *Lancet.* 1976; 2:1063–4.

R. Sandyk, M.D., M. Sc., Research Assistant Professor of Neurology and Pharmacology
University of Arizona
Tucson, AZ 85724

Drug Reviews

Pentamidine isethionate in the treatment of *Pneumocystis carinii* pneumonia

SUSAN DRAKE, VICTOR LAMPASONA, HAROLD L. NICKS, AND STEPHEN W. SCHWARZMANN

Abstract: The chemistry, antiprotozoal activity, pharmacology, clinical efficacy, adverse effects, dosage, administration, and hospital formulary considerations of pentamidine isethionate are reviewed.

Pentamidine, an aromatic diamidine, has been used since the 1940s to treat a variety of protozoal infections. It is now most commonly administered in the treatment of *Pneumocystis carinii* pneumonia (PCP). It is generally not metabolized, and it is stored or bound to tissue and excreted slowly as the parent compound.

Pentamidine is clearly effective in the treatment of PCP; however, the high incidence of adverse reactions associated with the drug led to the use of trimethoprim–sulfamethoxazole (TMP–SMX) as the first-line agent for PCP. Recent studies have reported a high incidence of adverse reactions, including leukopenia and hepatotoxicity, associated with the use of TMP–SMX therapy for PCP in patients with the acquired immunodeficiency syndrome (AIDS). The severity and frequency of these reactions suggest a possible new role for pentamidine in patients with AIDS who have PCP.

The recommended intramuscular and intravenous dosage of pentamidine isethionate for adults and children is 4 mg/kg/day for 14 days. Intramuscular administration is recommended; however, intravenous administration is a safe alternative if the dose is infused over a 60-minute period.

Pentamidine isethionate has specific application in the treatment of PCP as a second-line agent reserved for patients who cannot tolerate TMP–SMX.

Index terms: Antiprotozoals; Dosage; Formularies; Pentamidine isethionate; Pneumonia; Toxicity
Clin Pharm. 1985; 4:507–16

The antiprotozoal effect of pentamidine was discovered in the 1930s.[1] The drug was first used in the tropics during the 1940s to treat African trypanosomiasis and leishmaniasis.[2–5] A decade later, pentamidine was prescribed in Europe for *Pneumocystis carinii* pneumonia (PCP), and it substantially reduced the fatality rate from this disease in premature infants.[6]

Identified as an opportunistic protozoal infection, PCP has been diagnosed with increasing frequency since it was first described in the 1950s.[7,8] By 1967, 107 cases had been reported in the United States.[9] Unlike cases reported in Europe and the Orient where PCP was endemic and occasionally epidemic, its occurrence in the United States was at first sporadic. No specific age group was affected, and a variety of underlying diseases and infections were associated with the pneumonia in these early reports.[9]

In November 1967, the Parasitic Disease Drug Service of the Centers for Disease Control (CDC) began supplying investigational pentamidine to licensed physicians for the treatment of PCP and African sleeping sickness of the Gambian variety.[10,11] At that time, and until 1974, pentamidine was the most effective drug available for the treatment of PCP.[12] In 1974, however, Hughes et al.[12] documented the activity of trimethoprim–sulfamethoxazole (TMP–SMX) against *Pneumocystis carinii* in laboratory animals. This combination prod-

SUSAN DRAKE is Drug Information Specialist; VICTOR LAMPASONA, PHARM.D., is Associate Director for Clinical Services and Educational Programs and Clinical Pharmacokinetics Specialist; HAROLD L. NICKS, PHARM.D., was Clinical Resident, Department of Pharmaceutical Services; and STEPHEN W. SCHWARZMANN, M.D., is Chief of Infectious Diseases, Department of Medicine, Emory University Hospital, Atlanta.

Address reprint requests to Ms Drake at the Drug Information Center, Emory University Hospital, 1364 Clifton Road, NE, Atlanta, GA 30322.

The assistance of Mary Belknap, M.P.H., in the preparation of this manuscript is acknowledged.

This is **article 680-204-8515** in the **ASHP Continuing Education System.** See page 576 for learning objectives and test questions.

Figure 1. The chemical structure of pentamidine.

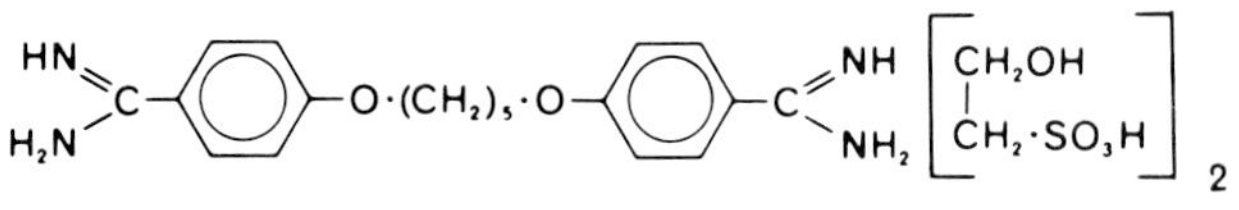

uct soon replaced pentamidine as the drug of choice because of similar efficacy and a reduced incidence of adverse reactions.[13] However, CDC continued supplying pentamidine to clinicians as alternative therapy in patients who were allergic to sulfa drugs or who failed to respond to TMP–SMX.

LyphoMed, Inc., received FDA approval to market pentamidine isethionate under the Orphan Drug Act and released Pentam 300 in October 1984.[14] This paper summarizes the current role of pentamidine isethionate in the treatment of PCP.

Chemistry

The chemical structure of pentamidine or 4,4-diamidinophenoxypentane di-(β-hydroxyethanesulfonate) is shown in Figure 1. This compound is structurally related to guanidine and its analog, synthalin, which was once used in the treatment of diabetes mellitus. Laboratory observations that synthalin also possessed activity against trypanosomes led to the structural modification and synthesis of the trypanocidal aromatic diamidines, 2-hydroxystilbamide, stilbamidine, propamidine, and pentamidine.[15,16]

The use of both the methanesulfonate and isethionate salt forms has been reported in the European and American literature. The dosage of pentamidine methanesulfonate is expressed in terms of the amount of pentamidine only; the dosage of pentamidine isethionate reflects the amount of pentamidine plus isethionate available.[17] Although it is important to be aware of both forms of the drug and the dosage adjustments required when converting from one to the other, this review deals with pentamidine isethionate, the only salt of pentamidine currently marketed.

Spectrum of Activity

Early investigations of aromatic diamidines, both in vitro and in laboratory animals, identified them as toxic to a number of protozoa with some degree of selectivity in their activity.[18-20] Both protozoans known to cause African sleeping sickness, *Trypanosoma rhodesiense* and *Trypanosoma gambiense*, were found sensitive to the diamidines; however, *Trypanosoma cruzi*, the causative organism of Chagas' disease, was resistant.[1,18] Pentamidine also exhibited some activity against *Trypanosoma congolense*, but only at toxic doses.[21]

In vitro studies demonstrated the activity of pentamidine against *Leishmania donovani*[22,23]; however, stilbamidine is the most potent leishmanocidal agent of the aromatic diamidines.[16] Pentamidine has been useful as second-line therapy for leishmaniasis resistant to antimony compounds.[24] Pentamidine also demonstrated activity against *Babesia canis* in puppies,[25] but its activity against *Babesia microti*, found in humans, has not been well established.[26]

Although certain aromatic diamidines possess antimalarial and antifungal properties, pentamidine has not exhibited any clinically important activity as an antimalarial or an antifungal agent.[24]

Most recently, pentamidine was found to be active against the protozoan parasite *Pneumocystis carinii*,[6] and it has been used extensively for that indication since the 1950s.[27]

Pharmacology

Mechanism of Action. The following mechanisms for the antiprotozoal activity of pentamidine have been proposed as a result of clinical and laboratory observations[25,28-30]:

1. Inhibition of dihydrofolate reductase,
2. Interference with aerobic glycolysis, and
3. Inhibition of oxidative phosphorylation and nucleic acid synthesis.

After Robbins[28] observed bone-marrow megaloblastosis and lowered serum folate concentrations in a patient treated with pentamidine, he speculated that folate antagonism may play a role in the drug's antiprotozoal activity. In vitro studies have confirmed that pentamidine inhibits dihydrofolate reductase, but to a lesser extent than methotrexate.[29] One problem with this proposed mechanism is the lack of therapeutic success against PCP with other folate antagonists such as methotrexate.[24]

Lourie and Yorke[25] proposed the second mechanism after they observed the greatest trypanocidal activity in species with a high degree of aerobic glycolysis and only minimal activity against species capable of anaerobic glycolysis. Finally, an in vitro study in mice tumor tissue showed inhibition of many cellular functions, especially in the energy-generating system of the cell. This suggested that the activity of pentamidine may involve impairment of oxidative phosphorylation and, to some extent, impairment of nucleic acid and protein synthesis.[31]

Pharmacokinetics. Studies of the pharmocokinetics of pentamidine have been hampered by poor assay technology. Quantitative data are sparse even today because of the lack of sensitive methods to analyze the presence of pentamidine in tissue and body fluids.[29]

Waalkes et al.[32] studied the pharmacokinetics of pentamidine in mice following a single intraperitoneal injection. After deposition in the tissue, pentamidine was excreted over a prolonged interval. The highest tissue concentrations were found in the kidneys, followed by the liver, and then other tissues. Essentially, no pentamidine was found in the brain tissue samples. Excretion occurred primarily through the kidneys, to a lesser extent in the feces, and in both cases as unchanged drug. The results and conclusions of Waalkes' study were similar to those reported by Waldman et al.[33]

Waalkes et al.[32] also determined the plasma and urinary concentrations of pentamidine isethionate in seven patients with malignant diseases who received pentamidine for PCP. The dosage was 4 mg/kg/day given intramuscularly for a maximum of 12 days. Plasma samples were obtained at intervals from 0.5 to 24 hours following each dose during the treatment period, and the determinations were generally found to be low. The mean peak concentration was 0.5 μg/mL one hour after injection, and the concentration remained essentially the same throughout the 24-hour period of evaluation. The highest plasma concentrations were found in patients with elevated blood-urea-nitrogen concentrations. The recovery of pentamidine in the urine was measured, and a mean of 17% (in a range from 11 to 29%) of the 4-mg/kg dose was excreted unchanged in the 24-hour period following administration. Decreasing amounts of the drug could be detected in urine up to eight weeks after the treatment period had ended. These data are consistent with findings in animals that pentamidine is not metabolized, but is stored or bound to tissues and excreted slowly as the unchanged drug.

Clinical Efficacy

Two types of host response to the *Pneumocystis carinii* organism have been identified. The first, infantile pneumonia, has appeared in premature infants and is responsible for the reported epidemics.[34] If untreated, the disease is associated with a 50% mortality rate.[6] The second type of host response is that observed in patients with PCP at all ages who have an underlying inherited or acquired immunodeficiency.[34] If untreated, the disease is almost always fatal.[9,10,35] In one survey of 107 adults and children in the United States with PCP during the period from 1955 to 1967, 102 (or 95%) of the patients died.[9]

When pentamidine became available, its use was first reported in the German literature in 1958 by Ivady and Paldy.[36] Pentamidine and two other aromatic diamidine compounds were prescribed for 19 infants with the epidemic form of PCP. By 1962, Ivady[6] treated an additional 212 cases of infantile PCP with pentamidine. The result was a reduction in the mortality rate from 50% (before 1958) to 3.5%. The greatest successes were seen with early diagnosis and therapy. Later, when pentamidine was used for adults and children, there was a 25–50% reduction in the mortality rate.[37]

In 1964 in London, Marshall et al.[38] successfully treated a child with PCP secondary to congenital hypogammaglobulinemia. In 1965, the first report of success with pentamidine in the United States again involved a child with congenital hypogammaglobulinemia.[39] Following these early experiences, a number of case reports[40–52] subsequently appeared in the English literature that further demonstrated the efficacy of pentamidine against PCP. Most of these cases involved children or adults with immune deficiencies, malignancies, or renal transplants. In several of these reports, the authors noted that the clinical response to pentamidine therapy was not apparent until after seven days of treatment or longer.[39,40,45] Most of the successfully treated patients received at least 10 days of therapy with pentamidine.

A number of reports of unsuccessful treatment with pentamidine have also appeared in the literature.[53–61] In most cases, the patients died before they could receive 10 days of pentamidine therapy, and many patients had received a previous unsuccessful course of therapy with TMP–SMX. Consequently, many of these patients did not receive pentamidine until the disease process had progressed substantially.

Evaluations involving large numbers of case reports have also appeared in the literature. The results of English-language studies are summarized in Table 1, and a description of each study is presented below.

Western et al.[10] of CDC were first to summarize clinical experiences with pentamidine in a large number of patients. During an 18-month period, 164 patients with proven or suspected PCP received pentamidine from the CDC. In 75 patients, the diagnosis was confirmed histologically. The patients ranged in age from less than 1 year to more than 60 years, with the largest group in the 20 years or older category. In most cases, the underlying disease process was cancer, although some patients had congenital immunologic disorders or had undergone organ transplantation. Seven patients also received pyrimethamine, a sulfa drug, or hydroxystilbamide, alone or in combination. In this study, 77% of the patients who received pentamidine for nine days or longer recovered.

In 1974, Walzer et al.[62] presented further data from CDC. Over a three-year period, 194 cases of confirmed PCP were analyzed. A total of 163 patients received pentamidine. The patient population was similar in age range and underlying disease process to that described by Western et al.,[10] although the largest number of patients fell in the $<$1-year-old category, followed by the groups aged 50–59, 5–9, and 10–19 years. The efficacy rates were similar to those found by Western et al.[10] Walzer et al. concluded that pentamidine was an effective agent if it was administered early in the course of the disease.

Goodell et al.[63] described their experience with 18 patients with neoplastic disease and proven or suspected PCP who were treated with pentamidine. Seven of 18 patients died during the acute phase of the pneumonia, and 6 of those who died received pentamidine for five days or less. Eleven patients survived, and four of those had their PCP diagnoses confirmed by needle biopsy. All of the surviving patients were treated for 6–14 days. Another 4 of the 11 survivors, who did not have biopsy-proven PCP, subsequently died of the underlying disease process. No evidence of *Pneumocystis carinii* was found on autopsy.

Rosen et al.[64] presented a report of 18 patients, mostly adults with neoplasms who had PCP documented by lung biopsy. One patient died before therapy was instituted, and 17 patients were treated with pentamidine for 14 days. Twelve patients had only PCP, five patients had mixed pulmonary lesions. Forty-one percent of the patients treated with pentamidine recovered. None of the patients with mixed pulmonary lesions survived.

Dutz et al.[65] described 33 infants with proven focal or massive diffuse PCP (i.e., infantile pneumonia). Eight patients with severe immunodeficiency had massive diffuse PCP, which progressed to respiratory crisis. Twenty-five patients with less severe immune deficiencies had focal PCP, which was characterized by small clumps of *Pneumocystis carinii* organisms localized in poorly aerated alveoli. A total of 12 patients received pentamidine, and 21 were untreated. All of the patients with focal PCP experienced an abatement of their symptoms with or without pentamidine treatment. Fifty percent of the patients with massive diffuse PCP treated with pentamidine survived, while only 33% of the patients who were not treated survived. These authors concluded that pentamidine is of little benefit once the diffuse PCP has reached the respiratory-crisis stage.

Eighty cancer patients with suspected or documented PCP were reviewed by the National Cancer Institute from 1967 to 1973.[66] Thirty of these patients had PCP documented by biopsy or autopsy, and 56 received pentamidine therapy. However, the authors did not indicate which of the treated patients had documented PCP infections. Of the 56 patients who received pentamidine, 31 received an adequate course of therapy (i.e., greater than seven days), and of those, 81% (25 of 31) survived. The remaining 25 patients, who received pentamidine, died before they could receive an optimal course of therapy.

Gentry et al.[67] reviewed the cases of 23 patients with PCP treated at the Stanford University Medical Center or Palo Alto Veterans Administration Hospital between the years 1962 and 1970. All patients except one were immunosuppressed secondary to drug therapy for malignancy, organ transplant, or collagen vascular disease. The remaining patient had congenital dysgammaglobulinemia. The patients ranged in age from 9 months to 68 years. In the cases in which an antemortem diagnosis of PCP was made, treatment with pentamidine was begun immediately. A total of 12 patients received pentamidine, 2 received pyrimethamine and sulfadiazine, and 10 received no therapy. The results of the pentamidine therapy are shown in Table 1.

Burke and Good[68] described the occurrence of PCP at the University of Minnesota Hospitals. Of 46 children and adults who contracted the disease, 22 were treated with pentamidine. Patients ranged in age from less than 1 year to 66 years of age. In most cases, the underlying disease was a malignant process. Ten of 22 patients survived, and 12 died. Four of the 10 survivors later died of the underlying disease process, but at autopsy no *Pneumocystis carinii* organisms were found. Eight of the 12 patients who died received pentamidine for 8 days or less, and the authors concluded that they could not be considered therapeutic failures.

Hughes et al.[69] reported their experience in treating PCP in children with malignancies. Pentamine was used for 41 of 51 patients who developed the disease. Twenty-eight (68%) of the treated patients recovered from the initial episode as determined by clinical observations and roentgenograms. Four patients had relapses within one year, and each received a second course of pentamidine therapy. One patient recovered, two died of com-

Table 1.
Clinical Use of Pentamidine Isethionate for *Pneumocystis carinii* Pneumonia (PCP)

Reference	Number of Patients	Drug Regimen[a] (mg/kg)	Duration of Treatment (days)	Percent Patients Recovered
Western et al.[10]	43	4	≥ 9	77
	32	4	1–8	9
Walzer et al.[62]	93	4	≥ 9	63
	70	4	<9	14
Goodell et al.[63]	12	4	6–10	92
	6	4	≤ 5	0
Rosen et al.[64]	17	4	14	41
Dutz et al.[65]				
Focal PCP	10	4	10	100
Massive diffuse PCP	2	4	10	50
Geelhoed et al.[66]	31	4	10–14	81
	25	4	<7	0
Gentry et al.[67]	8	4	10–14	63
	4	4	≤ 6	0
Burke and Good[68]	14	4	10–14	71
	8	4	<8	0
Hughes et al.[69]	41	150[b]	5	68
		100[b]	. . .	

[a] Administered intramuscularly.
[b] In this study, the dosage was 150 mg/sq m followed by 100 mg/sq m for the duration of the treatment.

plications unrelated to pentamidine,[70] and one died with extensive bilateral PCP found on autopsy.

Although a substantial amount of case-report data are available that compare the efficacy and toxicity of pentamidine in treating PCP with other therapeutic choices, there are few prospective, randomized clinical studies reported in the literature.[71-73]

Young and DeVita[71] reported the preliminary results of a study involving 21 patients at the National Institutes of Health who were randomly treated with pyrimethamine-sulfadiazine or pentamidine for suspected or documented PCP. Seven patients had PCP proven by open or percutaneous lung biopsy or percutaneous needle aspiration. Three patients were treated with pentamidine and four with pyrimethamine-sulfadiazine. Two of the three patients who were treated with pentamidine recovered, and the third patient died after 20 days of therapy. No *Pneumocystis carinii* or other infectious organisms were identified on autopsy.

Of four patients treated with pyrimethamine-sulfadiazine, two died within the first four days of therapy. One patient was cured, and the other received 14 days of pyrimethamine-sulfadiazine alone and an additional 10 days of combination therapy with pentamidine. Despite the combined therapy, this patient died, and no residual *Pneumocystis carinii* organisms were found on autopsy.

Toxicity was evaluated in all 21 patients involved in the study. Of the nine patients who received pentamidine therapy, 44% developed azotemia, and 33% developed local pain, abscess at injection, and abnormal liver-function test results. Twenty-two percent experienced hypotension, and in one patient, hypoglycemia and skin rash developed.

Forty-two percent of the patients treated with pyrimethamine-sulfadiazine developed azotemia, 58% hypotension, 25% abnormal liver function, and 17% anemia and skin rash. There were no increases in the incidence of adverse effects in patients who were treated with combination therapy. The authors suggested that both regimens were equally efficacious, but pentamidine may be more toxic (because of pain and abscess formation at the injection site). The comparative merits of both drugs may be better defined when more patients are evaluated on both regimens.

Siegel et al.[72] randomly assigned 25 pediatric cancer patients with documented PCP to treatment with either pentamidine or TMP-SMX. Fifteen patients received TMP-SMX 20 mg/kg/day (trimethoprim component) orally, and 10 received pentamidine isethionate 4 mg/kg/day intramuscularly. Patients who failed to respond to the initial therapy or who experienced life-threatening adverse reactions were switched to the alternate therapy. Results showed no significant difference in clinical or roentgenographic response. One patient who failed to respond to TMP-SMX therapy was given pentamidine, and two patients were switched from pentamidine to TMP-SMX therapy. Of those, one died after 14 days of therapy with extensive pulmonary involvement, and the rest recovered from their pneumonia.

The incidence of adverse effects was similar in both groups. Hematologic abnormalities and skin rash were the most common reactions in the TMP-SMX group. Hypoglycemia, abnormal renal function, and local reactions at the injection site were the most common findings in the pentamidine group.

Hughes et al.[73] reported data from 50 children randomly chosen to receive either pentamidine or TMP-SMX for documented PCP. For 14 days, 24 patients received pentamidine and 26 received TMP-SMX therapy. The patients who did not respond by at least three days of initial treatment were changed to the alternative regimen. Of the patients initially treated with TMP-SMX, 77% were cured (including three of nine patients who were changed to pentamidine therapy). Of the patients initially treated with pentamidine, 75% recovered (including four of nine patients who were changed to TMP-SMX therapy). Of 15 patients who were treated with pentamidine alone, 14 experienced an increase in blood-urea-nitrogen and creatinine values, hypoglycemia, inflammation at the injection site, or a combination of these adverse reactions. Only one patient treated with TMP-SMX alone developed a serious adverse effect involving an urticarial rash. The authors concluded that TMP-SMX was as effective as pentamidine against PCP and was associated with fewer adverse effects than pentamidine in the population studied.

In light of these findings, TMP-SMX became the drug of choice for PCP. Pentamidine became an alternative for patients who are allergic to sulfa drugs or show little or no clinical response to TMP-SMX, as measured by improving pulmonary status and reduction in fever within four days. In cases involving PCP in patients with acquired immunodeficiency syndrome (AIDS), however, there are a number of reports suggesting an incidence of adverse reactions to TMP-SMX therapy as high as 65%. These reactions have included leukopenia, hepatotoxicity, fever, rash, and immediate hypersensitivity reactions, and they have occurred most commonly during the second week of therapy.[74-76]

Gordin et al.[77] found a significantly increased incidence of adverse reactions in 38 AIDS patients treated with TMP-SMX. Of the 37 patients given TMP-SMX initially, 2 died within seven days. Of the remaining 35 patients, only 5 completed the course of therapy. Thirty patients were switched to pentamidine therapy. The incidence of rash with TMP-SMX was almost 10 times that seen in patients without AIDS treated with the drug. Hepatic toxicity occurred in 20% of patients and fever in 40%. Severe leukopenia (leukocyte count ≤ 2200/μL with a ≥1500/μL decrease) occurred in 29% of the patients and thrombocytopenia in 14%. In contrast, the overall incidence of toxicity associated with the pentamidine therapy was 43%, similar to that found by other authors in patients without AIDS.[62] Only 6 of 30 patients who received pentamidine experienced toxicity severe enough to require the discontinuation of the therapy.

Haverkos[78] retrospectively studied 282 cases of PCP confirmed by biopsy. Of these, 101 patients (group A) had AIDS, 31 were adults with known immunodeficiency (group B), and 150 were children with known immunodeficiency (group C). All patients received standard therapy, with most receiving TMP-SMX as initial treatment. More than half of the patients with AIDS were switched to pentamidine because of toxicity or lack of efficacy with TMP-SMX therapy. This rate of change was higher than that seen with groups B and C. Also in the group A patients, the duration of the therapy was longer and the rate of relapse was greater.

These observations suggest that pentamidine may be the drug of choice for patients with AIDS; however, further study is needed to determine the exact role of the drug in this patient population.

The combination of pentamidine with TMP-SMX therapy has not been evaluated in clinical trials. A preliminary study in rats compared pentamidine, TMP-SMX, a combination of the two, and trimethoprim alone.[79] The highest mortality rates were noted in the rats that received only pentamidine (48%) and pentamidine with TMP-SMX (45%). Another group of rats received TMP-SMX with half doses of pentamidine, and the mortality rate was 36%. In contrast, the mortality rate with TMP-SMX therapy alone was 21%. The authors suggested that the combination of pentamidine and TMP-SMX is no more effective than TMP-SMX alone, and it could even be harmful.

Adverse Reactions

Early reports in the English literature of experience with pentamidine contained little information on adverse reactions,[80] but as the drug gained widespread use, adverse effects began to be reported frequently. In a review of PCP in the United States, Walzer et al.[62] described the adverse reaction profile of pentamidine. Over a three-year period, 404 patients received the drug from CDC. Of those patients, 189 or 46.8% experienced a total of 347 adverse reactions. The most commonly reported, and often the most serious, adverse reaction was nephrotoxicity in 95 patients (23.5%). Azotemia occurred in patients who had not received other nephrotoxic agents and who had no history of renal impairment. It was usually mild and reversible. Of the 15 patients who experienced severe renal impairment, 14 died. In 12 of the 14 fatalities, pentamidine could not be considered the sole cause because other nephrotoxic antibiotics were administered, and conditions such as preexisting renal impairment and clinical complications such as bacterial sepsis were present.

Other adverse reactions included local reactions, such as pain and abscess at the injection site in 18.3%, abnormal liver function in 9.6%, hypotension in 9.6%, hypoglycemia in 6.2%, hematologic disturbances in 4.2%, skin rash in 1.5%, and hypocalcemia in 1.2%.

Similar adverse reactions have been reported with pentamidine in other reviews involving large numbers of patients.[10,66,68] In addition to the reactions described above, Western et al.[10] reported two deaths that were attributed to pentamidine. One patient, a three-year-old girl with acute lymphocytic leukemia, received pentamidine for 14 days and experienced a clearing of her pneumonitis. However, on day 14 of therapy, urticaria developed at the site of injection. The patient was discharged but returned three days later because of lethargy and irritability. At that time, an abscess was noted at the site of injection, and within a week, bullous lesions appeared and soon involved the total body surface. The patient died two weeks after completing a 14-day course of pentamidine therapy. Wang et al.,[81] who treated this patient stated that the skin lesions were characteristic of toxic epidermal necrolysis. In another case, an eight-year-old boy died after one dose of pentamidine from which he experienced gallop rhythm, tachycardia, pulmonary edema, and generalized convulsions.

Nephrotoxicity, as described by Walzer et al.,[62] has been reported by others[45,80] and is the major limiting toxicity of pentamidine therapy. In an attempt to elucidate the mechanism involved in pentamidine-induced renal toxicity, Makulu and Waalkes[82] demonstrated that pentamidine interacts with nucleic acids to form insoluble precipitates. They speculated that this process could occur within the kidney cells and deplete the nucleotide pool that is essential for energy-dependent functions of the kidney such as the regulation of the sodium and potassium balance.

These authors[82] also suggested that the interaction between pentamidine and nucleic acids may be responsible for the inflammatory reactions, such as sterile abscess, that have been observed after repeated injections of the drug.

The abnormal liver function that has been associated with pentamidine is usually in the form of elevations in transaminase concentrations of less than 175 units.[13]

In the past, the intravenous administration of pentamidine was associated with a high risk of hypotension, and for that reason, the CDC recommended intramuscular administration. Recently, the CDC examined the incidence of adverse reactions following intramuscular and intravenous administration in 108 patients with AIDS and found a higher incidence of hypotension following intramuscular administration.[83] These findings suggest that intravenous administration is acceptable if the medication is infused over at least one hour.

The incidence of hypoglycemia following pentamidine therapy may range from 6% to 40%,[62,71,84] and in some cases it has been sufficiently severe to require glucose therapy.[43,85–87] Symptoms can occur as early as two hours after an injection, but the greatest depression in blood glucose usually occurs during the first week of therapy, typically between the fifth and seventh days.[13]

Bryceson, as cited by Raia et al.,[88] suggested that the hypoglycemia results from a depletion of liver glycogen stores or, more likely, from a direct effect on the pancreas. The latter hypothesis is supported by reports of the development of diabetes mellitus[85,89,90] and pancreatitis[91] following pentamidine administration. Bouchard et al.[85] summarized reports of hypoglycemia that appeared in the American and foreign literature between 1943 and 1982. Of 90 reports of hypoglycemia, 28 patients subsequently developed diabetes mellitus 6–150 days after the first injection. These authors suggested that there may be an early cytolytic effect on the β-cells, resulting in insulin release and transient hypoglycemia, that is followed by β-cell destruction and insulin deficiency and eventually can lead to diabetes mellitus. The blood-glucose response to pentamidine resembles that noted with streptozotocin. It appears to be a cumulative and dose-dependent effect.[85]

Two cases of acute pancreatitis have been reported in patients receiving pentamidine.[91] In one patient, the pancreatitis recurred when rechallenged with pentamidine. The other patient also received prednisone but had received this drug for several years with no evidence of pancreatitis.

Hematologic effects have occurred infrequently with pentamidine. They include mild anemia and leukopenia, and with prolonged therapy, megaloblastic bone-marrow changes and thrombocytopenia.[92] In one case of thrombocytopenia, the patient's platelet count fell from 300,000/cu mm to 350/cu mm after two doses of pentamidine. Since there was a considerable increase in megakaryocytes in the bone marrow and transfused platelets did not survive in the circulation, the thrombocytopenia was attributed to the rapid destruction of the platelets.

More recently, CDC reported that of 179 AIDS patients with PCP who were treated with pentamidine, 26 (14.5%) developed leukopenia.[93] Leukocyte counts decreased by 50% or more during or after therapy. In 12 cases, pentamidine therapy was discontinued.

Finally, a rare complication of pentamidine therapy appears to be Herxheimer's reaction. In one case,[94] a 14-year-old boy suddenly developed fever, tachycardia, hypotension, and profound acidosis 11 hours after one dose of pentamidine. These symptoms persisted, and the patient died 10 hours later. Other reports of this reaction indicate that it most frequently occurs in severely ill patients with multiple parasitic infections.[11]

Dosage and Administration

The recommended intramuscular or intravenous dosage of pentamidine isethionate for adults and children is 4 mg/kg daily for 14 days,[14] although prolonged therapy of 14–21 days or more may be required for patients with AIDS.[78] Pentamidine is most commonly administered by intramuscular injection, but intravenous administration is a safe alternative if the dose is infused over a 60-minute period.[14]

Since pentamidine is eliminated primarily via the kidneys, a dosage adjustment is necessary in patients who have renal impairment. Bennett et al.[95] recommended that the dosing interval be extended in patients with compromised renal function. If the glomerular-filtration rate is less than 10 mL/min, a dose of 4 mg/kg should be administered every 48 hours, and if the rate is 10–50 mL/min, the dose should be administered every 24–36 hours.

The manufacturer of pentamidine has found that pentamidine is stable in infusion solution for up to 24 hours at room temperature. This is true of pentamidine in 5% dextrose injection at concentrations of 1 and 2.5 mg/mL and pentamidine in 0.9% sodium chloride injection at a concentration of 1 mg/mL. Further studies in disposable plastic syringes have shown that a concentration of 100 mg/mL is stable for up to 24 hours at room temperature.[a]

Toxicity monitoring should include the determination of serum creatinine daily or every other day, serum glucose daily or as required by clinical condition of the patient, and complete blood cell and platelet counts twice weekly. Since blood pressure has been reported to drop rapidly during infusion, it should be monitored appropriately. Although the occurrence of acute hypotension during infusion is uncommon, it can usually be adequately controlled by rapid volume replacement. If the intramuscular route is employed, daily observation of the injection site is mandatory, and if evidence of inflammation or pain develops, intravenous administration should be used.

Formulary Considerations

Pentamidine isethionate has specific application in the treatment of PCP as a second-line agent reserved for patients who cannot tolerate TMP-SMX. Although pentamidine was initially the drug of choice against PCP, TMP-SMX later assumed that role because it was found equally effective and less toxic. TMP-SMX is currently the first-line agent that should be on the formulary for treating PCP. Because of the problems associated with administering TMP-SMX to patients with AIDS, however, it may be appropriate for pentamidine to be available in institutions that treat a large number of patients with AIDS.

Cost and Availability

Pentam 300 (LyphoMed, Inc.) is available as a white, odorless powder in a single-dose vial containing 300 mg of pentamidine isethionate. Vials should be stored between 2 and 8 °C.[14] The current cost of the product is $39.49 per vial.[b]

Conclusion

Pentamidine isethionate has clearly been established as effective in the treatment of PCP, and at one time was the first-line agent for treatment of the disease. Considerable toxicity associated with the drug led to the use of TMP-SMX, which soon became the drug of choice for PCP. There is currently no evidence that a combination of these drugs is any more effective than either one alone. Recent reports of a high incidence of adverse effects in patients with AIDS treated with TMP-SMX suggest a possible new role for pentamidine in that patient population.

---

[a] Fruin DM. LyphoMed, Inc. Written communication. 1985 May 14.

[b] Fossey L. LyphoMed, Inc. Personal communication. 1985 Jul 19.

References

1. Rollo IM. Miscellaneous drugs used in the treatment of protozoal infections. In: Gilman AG, Goodman LS, Gilman A, eds. The pharmacologic basis of therapeutics. New York: MacMillan Publishing Co.; 1980:1071–2.
2. Saunders GFT. Preliminary report on the treatment of sleeping sickness by 4:4′-diamidino diphenoxy pentane. *Ann Trop Med Parasitol.* 1941; 35:169–74.
3. Lourie EM. Treatment of sleeping sickness in Sierra Leone. *Ann Trop Med Parasitol.* 1942; 36:113–31.
4. Saunders GFT, Holden JR, Hughes MH. Second report on the treatment of trypanosomiasis by pentamidine. *Ann Trop Med Parasitol.* 1944; 38:159–68.
5. Kirk R, Sati MH. The use of certain aromatic diamidines in the treatment of kala-azar. *Ann Trop Med Parasitol.* 1940; 34:181–97.
6. Ivady G, Paldy L. Treatment of *Pneumocystis carinii* pneumonia in infancy. *Natl Cancer Inst Monogr.* 1976; 43:201–5.
7. Hughes WT. *Pneumocystis carinii* pneumonitis. *Chest.* 1984; 85:810–3.
8. Lunseth JH, Kirmse TW, Prezyna AP et al. Interstitial plasma cell pneumonia. *J Pediatr.* 1955; 46:137–45.
9. Le Clair RA. Descriptive epidemiology of interstitial pneumocystic pneumonia. *Am Rev Respir Dis.*, 1969; 99:542–7.
10. Western KA, Perera DR, Schultz MG. Pentamidine isethionate in the treatment of *Pneumocystis carinii* pneumonia. *Ann Intern Med.* 1970; 73:695–702.
11. Anon. Informational material for physicians. Pentamidine isethionate (Lomidine). U.S. Department of Health and Human Services, Public Health Service. Atlanta, GA: Centers for Disease Control.
12. Hughes WT, McNabb PC, Makres TD et al. Efficacy of trimethoprim and sulfamethoxazole in the prevention and treatment of *Pneumocystis carinii* pneumonitis. *Antimicrob Agents Chemother.* 1974; 5:289–93.
13. Milder JE, Walzer PD, Powell RD. Treatment of *Pneumocystis carinii* pneumonia with trimethoprim–sulfamethoxazole and pentamidine: efficacy and toxicity. *South Med J.* 1979; 72:1626–8.
14. LyphoMed, Inc. Pentam 300 product literature. Melrose Park, IL; 1984.
15. Heathcote R. The diamidines: their pharmacological actions and their therapeutic uses in some tropical diseases. *J Trop Med Hyg.* 1946; 49:1–8.
16. Schoenbach EB, Greenspan EM. The pharmacology, mode of action and therapeutic potentialities of stilbamidine, pentamidine, propamidine and other aromatic diamidines—a review. *Medicine.* 1948; 27:327–77.
17. Anon. Pentamidine methanesulfonate to be distributed by CDC. *MMWR.* 1984; 33(17):225–6.
18. Briggaman RA. The aromatic diamidines. *Int J Dermatol.* 1977; 16:155–62.
19. Yorke W. Recent work on the chemotherapy of protozoal infections. *Trans R Soc Trop Med Hyg.* 1940; 33:463–82.
20. Lourie EM, Yorke W. The trypanocidal action of certain aromatic diamidines. *Ann Trop Med Hyg.* 1939; 33:289–304.
21. Daubney R, Hudson JR. The action of two aromatic diamidines on *Trypanosoma congolense* infections in cattle. *Ann Trop Med Hyg.* 1941; 35:175–86.
22. Adler S, Tchernomoretz I. The action of some aromatic diamidines on cultures of *Leishmania donovani. Ann Trop Med Parasitol.* 1945; 39:14–9.
23. Collier HOJ, Lourie EM. The action *in vitro* of diamidines and other compounds on *Leishmania donovani. Ann Trop Med Parasitol.* 1946; 40:88–100.
24. Young LS. *Pneumocystis carinii* pneumonia. New York: Marcel Dekker Inc; 1984.
25. Lourie EM, Yorke W. The action of certain aromatic diamidines on *Babesia canis* infections in puppies. *Ann Trop Med Parasitol.* 1939; 33:305–12.
26. Ruebush TK. *Babesia.* In: Mandell GL, Douglas RG, Bennett JE, eds. Principles and practice of infectious diseases. Canada: Wiley Medical Publications; 1979:2150–3.
27. Hughes WT. *Pneumocystis carinii* pneumonitis. *Antibiot Chemother.* 1981; 30:257–71.
28. Robbins JB. *Pneumocystis carinii* pneumonitis—a review. *Pediatr Res.* 1967; 1:131–8.
29. Waalkes TP, Makulu DR. Pharmacologic aspects of pentamidine. *Natl Cancer Inst Mongr.* 1976; 43:171–6.
30. Frenkel JK, Good JT, Shultz JA. Latent pneumocystis infection of rats, relapse and chemotherapy. *Clin Lab Invest.* 1966; 15:1559–65.
31. Bornstein RS, Yarbro JW. An evaluation of the mechanism of action of pentamidine isethionate. *J Surg Oncol.* 1970; 2:393–8.
32. Waalkes TP, Denham C, De Vita VT. Pentamidine: clinical pharmacological correlations in man and mice. *Clin Pharmacol Ther.* 1970; 11:505–12.
33. Waldman RH, Pearce DE, Martin RA. Pentamidine isethionate levels in lungs, livers and kidneys of rats after aerosol or intramuscular administration. *Am Rev Respir Dis.* 1973; 108:1004–6.
34. Hughes WT. *Pneumocystic carinii.* In: Mandell GL, Douglas RG, Bennett JE, eds. Principles and practice of infectious diseases. Canada: Wiley Medical Publication; 1979:2137–42.
35. Geelhoed GW, Levin BJ, Adkins PC et al. The diagnosis and management of *Pneumocystis carinii* pneumonia. *Ann Thorac*

Surg. 1972; 14:335–46.
36. Ivady G, Paldy L. Ein neues behandlungsverfahren der interstitiellen plasmazelligen pneumonie fruhgeborener mit funfuertigen stibium und aromatischen diamidinen. *Mschr Kinderheilk*. 1958; 106:10–5.
37. Anon. Pentamidine for *Pneumocystis carinii* pneumonia. *Med Lett Drug Ther*. 1985; 27(679):6–7.
38. Marshall WC, Weston HJ, Bodian M. *Pneumocystis carinii* pneumonia and congenital hypogammaglobulinemia. *Arch Dis Child*. 1964; 39:18–25.
39. Robbins JB, Miller RH, Arean VM et al. Successful treatment of *Pneumocystis carinii* pneumonitis in a patient with congenital hypogammaglobulinemia. *N Engl J Med*. 1965; 272:708–13.
40. Rodgers TS, Haggie MHK. *Pneumocystis carinii* pneumonia associated with hypogammaglobulinemia responding to pentamidine. *Lancet*. 1964; 1:1042. Letter.
41. Patterson JH, Lindsey IL, Edwards ES et al. *Pneumocystis carinii* pneumonia and altered host resistance: treatment of one patient with pentamidine isethionate. *Pediatrics*. 1966; 38:388–97.
42. Smith E, Gaspar IA. Pentamidine treatment of *Pneumocystis carinii* pneumonitis in an adult with lymphatic leukemia. *Am J Med*. 1968; 44:626–31.
43. Lillehei JP, Funke JL, Drage CW et al. *Pneumocystis carinii* pneumonia. *JAMA*. 1968; 206:596–600.
44. Einzig S, Hong R, Sharp HL. Successful treatment of *Pneumocystis carinii* in an immunologically deficient acute lymphatic leukemia patient. *Cancer*. 1969; 23:658–62.
45. DeVita VT, Emmer M, Levine A et al. *Pneumocystis carinii* pneumonia. *N Engl J Med*. 1969; 280:287–91.
46. Fortuny IE, Tempero KF, Amsden TW. *Pneumocystis carinii* pneumonia diagnosed from sputum and successfully treated with pentamidine isethionate. *Cancer*. 1970; 26:911–3.
47. Gentry LO, Remington JS. *Pneumocystis carinii* pneumonia in siblings. *J Pediatr*. 1970; 76:769–73.
48. Cohen ML, Weiss EB, Monaco AP. Successful treatment of *Pneumocystis carinii* and *Nocardia asteroides* in a renal transplant patient. *Am J Med*. 1971; 50:269–76.
49. Cohen ML, Weiss EB. *Pneumocystis carinii* pneumonia: percutaneous lung biopsy and review of literature. *Chest*. 1971; 60:195–9.
50. Friedman BA, Wenglin BD, Hyland RN et al. Roentgenographically atypical *Pneumocystis carinii* pneumonia. *Am Rev Respir Dis*. 1975; 111:89–96.
51. Mitsuyasu RT, Corwin HL, Harris AA et al. Failure of trimethoprim–sulfamethoxazole in the therapy of recurrent *Pneumocystis carinii* pneumonia. *Am Rev Respir Dis*. 1982; 125:762–5.
52. Trigg ME, Kohn DB, Sondel PM et al. Tracheal aspirate examination for *Pneumocystis carinii* cysts as a guide to therapy in *Pneumocystis* pneumonia. *J Pediatr*. 1983; 102:881–3.
53. Roberts FB, Nielsen HS. *Pneumocystis carinii* pneumonia: an unsuccessfully treated case. *Can Med Assoc J*. 1966; 94:1235–7.
54. Humphries KR, Ngan H, James K. *Pneumocystis carinii* pneumonia and reticuloses. *Thorax*. 1968; 23:100–4.
55. Lombardi DL, Mason JO, Hughes RK. *Pneumocystis* and *Mucormycosis* pneumonitis. *Chest*. 1970; 57:318–21.
56. Pappas G, Schroter G, Brettschneider L et al. Pulmonary surgery in immunosuppressed patients. *J Thorac Cardiovasc Surg*. 1970; 59:882–7.
57. Wang N, Huang S, Thurlbeck WM. Combined *Pneumocystis carinii* and cytomegalovirus infection. *Arch Pathol*. 1970; 90:529–35.
58. Pederson FK, Johansen S, Rosenkvist J et al. Refractory *Pneumocystis carinii* infection in chronic granulomatous disease: successful treatment with granulocytes. *Pediatrics*. 1979; 64:935–8.
59. Johnson JF, Rehder TL, Moore GF. *Pneumocystis carinii* pneumonia: review with a case study. *Drug Intell Clin Pharm*. 1981; 15:732–7.
60. Spangenthal S, Beer DJ, Snydman DR et al. *Pneumocystis carinii* and cytomegalovirus pneumonia in a previously healthy adult. *Am Rev Respir Dis*. 1982; 125:601–3.
61. Waldhorn RE, Tsou E, Kerwin DM. *Pneumocystis carinii* pneumonia in a previously healthy adult. *JAMA*. 1982; 247:1860–1.
62. Walzer PD, Perl DP, Krogstad DJ et al. *Pneumocystis carinii* pneumonia in the United States. *Ann Intern Med*. 1974; 80:83–93.
63. Goodell B, Jacobs JB, Powell RD et al. *Pneumocystis carinii*: the spectrum of diffuse interstitial pneumonia in patients with neoplastic disease. *Ann Intern Med*. 1970; 72:337–40.
64. Rosen PP, Martini N, Armstrong D. *Pneumocystis carinii* pneumonia. *Am J Med*. 1975; 58:794–802.
65. Dutz W, Post C, Jennings-Khodadad E et al. Therapy and prophylaxis of *Pneumocystis carinii* pneumonia. *Natl Cancer Inst Monogr*. 1976; 43:179–85.
66. Geelhoed GW, Hubbard SB, Powell RD et al. Clinical characteristics of *Pneumocystis carinii* pneumonia. *Am Surg*. 1979; 45:293–304.
67. Gentry LO, Ruskin J, Remington JS. *Pneumocystis carinii* pneumonia. *Calif Med*. 1972; 116:6–14.
68. Burke BA, Good RA. *Pneumocystis carinii* infection. *Medicine*. 1973; 52:23–51.
69. Hughes WT, Price RA, Kim H et al. *Pneumocystis carinii* pneumonitis in children with malignancies. *J Pediatr*. 1973; 82:404–15.
70. Hughes WT, Johnson WW. Recurrent *Pneumocystis carinii* pneumonia following apparent recovery. *J Pediatr*. 1971; 79:755–9.
71. Young RC, DeVita VT. Treatment of *Pneumocystis carinii* pneumonia: current status of the regimens of pentamidine isethionate and pyrimethamine–sulfadiazine. *Natl Cancer Inst Monog*. 1976; 43:193–200.
72. Siegel SE, Wolff LJ, Baehner RL et al. Treatment of *Pneumocystis carinii* pneumonitis. *Am J Dis Child*. 1984; 138:1051–4.
73. Hughes WT, Feldman S et al. Comparison of pentamidine isethionate and trimethoprim–sulfamethoxazole in the treatment of *Pneumocystis carinii* pneumonia. *J Pediatr*. 1978; 92:285–91.
74. Kovacs JA, Hiemenz JW, Macher AM et al. *Pneumocystis carinii* pneumonia: a comparison between patients with the acquired immunodeficiency syndrome and patients with other immunodeficiencies. *Ann Intern Med*. 1984; 100:663–71.
75. Engelberg LA, Lerner CW, Tapper ML. Clinical features of *Pneumocystis* pneumonia in the acquired immune deficiency syndrome. *Am Rev Respir Dis*. 1984; 130:689–94.
76. Small CB, Harris CA, Friedland GH et al. The treatment of *Pneumocystis carinii* pneumonia in the acquired immunodeficiency syndrome. *Arch Intern Med*. 1985; 145:837–40.
77. Gordin FM, Simon GL, Wofsy CB et al. Adverse reactions to trimethoprim–sulfamethoxazole in patients with acquired immunodeficiency syndrome. *Ann Intern Med*. 1984; 100:495–9.
78. Haverkos HW. Assessment of therapy for *Pneumocystis carinii* pneumonia. *Am J Med*. 1984; 76:501–8.
79. Kluge RM, Spaulding DM, Spain AJ. Combination of pentamidine and trimethoprim–sulfamethoxazole in the therapy of *Pneumocystis carinii* pneumonia in rats. *Antimicrob Agents Chemother*. 1978; 13:975–8.
80. Emmer M, DeVita VT. *Pneumocystis carinii* pneumonia and pentamidine isethionate toxicity. *Ann Intern Med*. 1968; 69:637–8. Letter.
81. Wang JJ, Freeman AI, Gaeta JF et al. Unusual complications of pentamidine in the treatment of *Pneumocystis carinii* pneumonia. *J Pediatr*. 1970; 77:311–4.
82. Makulu DR, Waalkes TP. Interaction between aromatic diamidines and nucleic acids: possible implications for chemotherapy. *J Natl Cancer Instit*. 1975; 54:305–9.
83. Navin TR, Fontaine RE. Intravenous versus intramuscular administration of pentamidine. *N Engl J Med*. 1984; 311:1701–2. Letter.
84. Murdoch JK, Keystone JS. Pentamidine and hypoglycemia.

Ann Intern Med. 1983; 99:879. Letter.
85. Bouchard P, Sai P, Reach I et al. Diabetes mellitus following pentamidine-induced hypoglycemia in humans. *Diabetes*. 1982; 31:40–5.
86. Grant AM, Sandler RM, Carrell RW. Hypoglycemic effect of pentamidine detected by glucose screen. *Lancet*. 1977; 2:510. Letter.
87. Sharpe SM. Pentamidine and hypoglycemia. *Ann Intern Med*. 1983; 99:128. Letter.
88. Raia JJ, Patton LR, Klein RA et al. Prolonged hypoglycemia during pentamidine therapy. *Clin Pharm*. 1983; 2:505–6. Letter.
89. Jha TK, Sharma VK. Pentamidine-induced diabetes mellitus. *Trans R Soc Trop Med Hyg*. 1984; 78:252–3.
90. Belehu A, Naafs B. Diabetes mellitus associated with pentamidine mesylate. *Lancet*. 1982; 1:1463–4. Letter.
91. Murphey SA, Josephs AS. Acute pancreatitis associated with pentamidine therapy. *Arch Intern Med*. 1981; 141:56–8.
92. Levy MA, Senior RM, Sneider RF. Severe thrombocytopenic purpura complicating pentamidine therapy for *Pneumocystis carinii* pneumonia. *Cancer*. 1974; 34:441–3.
93. Anon. Severe neutropenia during pentamidine treatment of *Pneumocystis carinii* pneumonia in patients with acquired immunodeficiency syndrome. *MMWR*. 1984; 33(6):65–7.
94. Stark FR, Crast F, Clemmer T et al. Fatal Herxheimer reaction after pentamidine in *Pneumocystis pneumonia*. *Lancet*. 1976; 1:1193. Letter.
95. Bennett WM, Muther RS, Parker RA et al. Drug therapy in renal failure: dosing guidelines for adults. *Ann Intern Med*. 1980; 93:62–89.

Aztreonam, a new monobactam antimicrobial

David R. P. Guay and Christopher Koskoletos

Abstract: The chemistry, in vitro activity, pharmacokinetics, adverse reactions, and clinical use of the monobactam antimicrobial aztreonam are reviewed.

Aztreonam, an investigational agent nearing approval in the United States and Canada, is the first in a class of monobactam antimicrobials to be evaluated extensively in vitro and in vivo. It has a narrow spectrum of activity, encompassing only aerobic gram-negative microorganisms including *Pseudomonas aeruginosa* and most multiply resistant Enterobacteriaceae. Aztreonam has no useful activity against gram-positive or anaerobic microorganisms. In preliminary studies, aztreonam achieved high tissue concentrations and was usually well tolerated. Approximately 65–75% of an administered dose is excreted unchanged into the urine, and the elimination half-life is 1.6–2.2 hours in subjects with normal renal function. Dosage should be adjusted in patients with renal impairment. Aztreonam was shown equivalent to gentamicin and cefamandole for treating serious urinary-tract infections and produced cure rates greater than 85% in gonococcal, lower respiratory tract, orthopedic, serious urinary tract, acute uncomplicated lower urinary-tract, gynecologic, and intra-abdominal infections. Development of resistance during therapy may be less likely with aztreonam than with other new cephalosporins.

Aztreonam will probably have an important role in antimicrobial therapy, but much further study is necessary to assess clinical efficacy and toxicity. The clinical importance of aztreonam's superior activity under anaerobic conditions compared with aminoglycosides and the theoretical reduced alteration in GI colonization resistance must be assessed in controlled trials. Evaluation of aztreonam versus ceftazidime, the carbapenems, and the carboxyquinolones is needed, and the likelihood of gram-positive superinfection, especially with enterococci, must be further assessed.

Index terms: Antibiotics; Aztreonam; Excretion; Half-life; Pharmacokinetics; Toxicity
Clin Pharm. 1985; 4:516–26

Aztreonam (Azactam, SQ 26,776, formerly known as azthreonam) is an antimicrobial of the monobactam class that is being developed by E. R. Squibb & Sons, Incorporated. Its chemical name is [2S-[2α,3β(Z)]]-2-[[[1-(2-amino-4-thiazolyl)-2-[(2-methyl-4-oxo-1-sulfo-3-azetidinyl)amino]-2-oxoethylidene]amino]oxy]-2-methylpropionic acid. The structures of the drug and its 3-aminomonobactamic acid nucleus are illustrated in Figure 1. The manufacturer is seeking approval for use of the drug in the treatment of infections caused by susceptible gram-negative microorganisms, including *Pseudomonas aeruginosa*. This article reviews the development, chemistry, pharmacoki-

David R. P. Guay, Pharm.D., is Clinical Research Fellow, Drug Evaluation Unit, Division of Nephrology, Department of Medicine, Hennepin County Medical Center, and Assistant Professor, College of Pharmacy, University of Minnesota, Minneapolis, MN; at the time this article was written, he was Clinical Coordinator and Scientific Staff Member, Departments of Pharmacy and Medicine, St. Boniface General Hospital, and Lecturer, Faculty of Pharmacy, University of Manitoba, Winnipeg, Manitoba, Canada. Christopher Koskoletos was an undergraduate pharmacy student at the University of Manitoba at the time this article was written.

Address reprint requests to Dr. Guay at the Drug Evaluation Unit, Division of Nephrology, Department of Medicine, Hennepin County Medical Center, 701 Park Avenue South, Minneapolis, MN 55415.

The secretarial assistance of Janine Unrau and Kim Podany is acknowledged.

This is **article 680-204-8516** in the **ASHP Continuing Education System.** See page 577 for learning objectives and test questions.

netics, adverse reactions, and clinical use of aztreonam in the treatment of infections caused by gram-negative microorganisms.

Chemistry and Structure–Activity Relationships

The screening of bacteria for the ability to produce β-lactam antibiotics resulted in the discovery of a new class of antibiotics known as the monobactams.[1-6] Unlike the penicillins and cephalosporins, these compounds are isolated from bacteria instead of from fungi. The most common producers of monocyclic β-lactams (monobactams) are from the genera *Gluconobacter* and *Acetobacter*, but *Chromobacterium*, *Agrobacterium*, and *Pseudomonas* species also synthesize monobactams.

All monobactams have the same basic nucleus (3-aminomonobactamic acid or 3-AMA) and exhibit certain structural similarities to other β-lactams (Figure 2). Starting with this basic nucleus, which is prepared synthetically, a broad variety of derivatives have been formed.[1,2,6,7] Aztreonam is one of these derivatives; in addition, the monobactams SQ 26,917 (Squibb) and RO172301 (Roche) are under investigation.

Figure 1. Graphic formulas of (left) aztreonam (SQ 26,776) and (right) 3-aminomonobactamic acid (3-AMA).

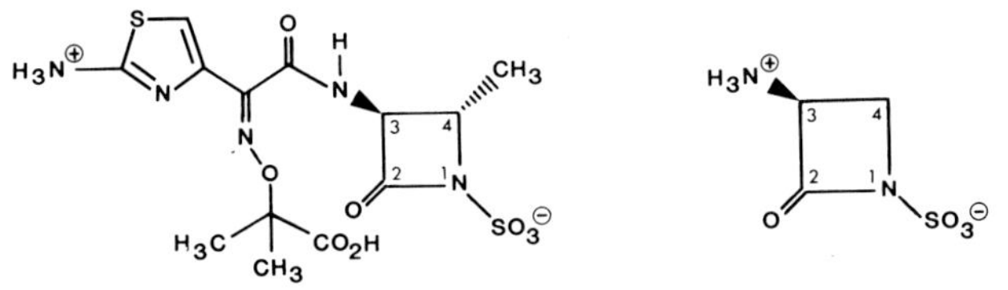

Figure 2. Graphic formulas of selected classes of β-lactam antimicrobials.

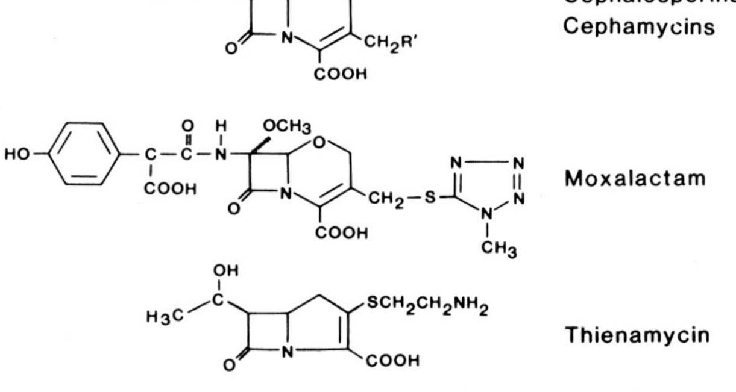

Chromosome- or plasmid-mediated β-lactamase production by gram-negative microorganisms provides the major defense against antibiotics containing the β-lactam ring.[8] In the monobactams investigated to date, antimicrobial activity has varied. The methoxylated monobactam SQ 26,180 showed poor activity, although it showed a high degree of stability to β-lactamases from both gram-negative and gram-positive bacteria.[1,2] This stability is probably because monobactams are poor substrates for the broad-spectrum β-lactamases and tight-binding competitive substrates for the P99 β-lactamase.[1,2,9-16] The desmethoxy derivative of SQ 26,180 was susceptible to β-lactamase hydrolysis and showed poor activity. The substitution of the 3-acyl side chain by an aminothiazolyloximino group increased the activity and broadened the antimicrobial spectrum. The addition of a carboxylic acid group in the oximino moiety and a methyl group at position 4, thus producing aztreonam, destroyed any gram-positive activity but greatly improved gram-negative activity and imparted broad-spectrum, potent β-lactamase stability.[2,9-16] Although the naturally occurring compounds generally have weak antibacterial activity, the synthetic derivative aztreonam proved sufficiently active to warrant further in vitro and in vivo testing.

Mechanism of Action

The bicyclic β-lactam antibiotics (penicillins and cephalosporins) are known to interact with specific penicillin-binding proteins (PBP) in bacterial cell membranes, leading to their physiological effects.[17] The action of the monocyclic aztreonam is also thought to occur through binding to PBP, which induces morphological changes in the bacterium.[2,10,18,19] In all organisms examined, aztreonam at low concentrations has been shown to bind exclusively to PBP 3. Aztreonam is inactive against *Staphylococcus aureus* and *Bacteroides fragilis* and does not bind appreciably to any essential PBP from these strains. Binding of β-lactam antibiotics to essential PBP (i.e., PBP 1, 2, or 3) is responsible for the bactericidal effect.[20,21] Studies have demonstrated that aztreonam binds only to PBP 3 and not to PBP 1a; this indicates that binding to PBP 3 is sufficient to cause cell lysis and death.

Antimicrobial Spectrum

Aztreonam exhibits a narrow spectrum of antimicrobial activity, compared with various penicillins, cephalosporins, and other antimicrobials.[2,7,10-16,22-44] It is active solely against aerobic gram-negative microorganisms. The vast majority of strains of *Escherichia coli*, *Serratia* spp., *Proteus* spp., *Klebsiella* spp., *Enterobacter* spp., *Salmonella* spp., *Shigella* spp., *Providencia* spp., *Haemophilus influenzae*, and *Neisseria gonorrhoeae* are susceptible to aztreonam (that is, minimum inhibitory concentrations are 8 μg/mL or less) irrespective of the organism's ability to produce β-lactamases. Aztreonam is also active against the majority of strains of *Ps. aeruginosa*, including most strains that are resistant to multiple drugs. Aztreonam has little or no activity against gram-positive organisms and anaerobes such as *Clostridium* and *Bacteroides* spp. Addition of clavulanic acid (a β-lactamase inhibitor) did not enhance the activity of aztreonam against *Staphylococcus aureus*, but it sharply lowered the minimum inhibitory concentration (MIC) against *B. fragilis*.[15,23]

Clinically, aztreonam may be useful in combination with other agents, but no useful synergy was found against *Staph. aureus*, *Streptococcus fecalis*, *Streptococcus pneumoniae*, *Ps. aeruginosa*, *Klebsiella* spp., or *E. coli* when the agent was combined in vitro with flucloxacillin, ampicillin, or gentamicin.[15,26,45] Ampel et al.[46] tested the in vitro activity of aztreonam in combination with azlocillin, imipenem, cefoperazone, and gentamicin against five strains each of *Ps. aeruginosa*, *Serratia marcescens*, and *Klebsiella pneumoniae* and in combination with nafcillin, cephalothin, imipenem, and gentamicin against five strains of *Staph. aureus*. The combinations tested against gram-negative organisms generally demonstrated additive or antagonistic (aztreonam plus imipenem) effects, while the combinations tested against *Staph. aureus* demonstrated indifference.

However, opposite results have been reported in other studies. Giamarellou and coworkers[47] demonstrated synergy rates of 83, 97, and 97% for the combination of aztreonam with netilmicin, gentamicin, and tobramycin, respectively, in 30 multiresistant strains of *Ps. aeruginosa*. Stutman and coworkers[45] documented synergy between aztreonam and tobramycin against 62% of 18 isolates of *Ps. aeruginosa*. Buesing and Jorgensen[48] documented synergy between aztreonam and amikacin and between aztreonam and other β-lactams against 71 and 42%, respectively, of 14 multiply resistant isolates of *E. coli*, *Enterobacter cloacae*, *K. pneumoniae*, *S. marcescens*, and *Ps. aeruginosa*. Aronoff and Klinger[49] documented synergy between aztreonam and amikacin against 43% of 44 amikacin-resistant *Ps. aeruginosa* and *Ps. cepacia* isolates from children with cystic fibrosis. Serum bactericidal studies by Van Laethem and coworkers[50] similarly documented the potential for synergy of aztreonam–amikacin and aztreonam–cefoperazone combinations against *E. coli*, *K. pneumoniae*, *S. marcescens*, and *Ps. aeruginosa*. Most investigators have documented indifferent or, at most, additive inhibition by the combination of aztreonam with piperacillin, azlocillin, and ticarcillin.[45,51]

Poor to fair activity has been reported against *Pseudomonas* species other than *Ps. aeruginosa* and against *Acinetobacter* spp., *Achromobacter* spp., *Alcaligenes* spp., *Moraxella* spp., *Bordetella* spp., and some species of *Enterobacter* or *Citrobacter*. MIC data for aztreonam compared with other antimicrobials are summarized in Table 1.

Certain strains of Enterobacteriaceae have consistently defied attack by β-lactams , mainly because they produce chromosomally mediated class I β-lactamase and create barriers to drug penetration.[8] The activity of aztreonam against Enterobacteriaceae that are resistant to other antimicrobials has been excellent,[11-15,23-27,41,44,48,49] indicating a potentially valuable role for the agent in certain institutional settings. However, aztreonam has been reported to induce β lactamase, leading to resistance not only to aztreonam but also to multiple other β-lactam agents. This is a potential problem not limited to aztreonam; its rate of occurrence and clinical importance can only be determined by surveillance studies.[52]

In general, the minimum bactericidal concentration (MBC) is the same as or not more than twice the MIC, although for some species a fourfold or fivefold difference may be seen.[12,13,15,24,34,36-38,40,45,48] Inoculum effects on the MIC are generally small, provided that inoculum size does not exceed an absolute value of 10^6 colony-forming units/mL.[12,15,23,24,28,34-36,38] The presence of serum has little effect on the MIC or MBC.[12,15,23,24,28]

Pharmacokinetics

Aztreonam pharmacokinetic studies have been facilitated by the availability of microbiological, high-pressure liquid chromatographic, and thin-layer radiochromatographic assay procedures.[53-57] Mean pharmacokinetic values for aztreonam in normal volunteers after single i.v. and i.m. doses[53-55,57,58] are given in Table 2. Intravenous data best fit a two-compartment open model, while intramuscular data best fit a one-compartment open model with first-order absorption and elimination. Bioavailability of aztreonam after oral administration is less than 1%.[59]

Aztreonam is widely distributed in the body. The mean volume of distribution is 0.05–0.13 L/kg for the central compartment and 0.11–0.18 L/kg at steady state.[53-55,57,58] Blister fluid studies in volunteers have documented seemingly adequate tissue penetration, with a mean peak fluid concentration of 25.4 μg/mL at 1.8 hours after a single 1.0-g i.v. dose.[53] From three hours after the dose, fluid concentrations exceeded those in serum. Preliminary studies have documented that aztreonam enters the breast milk to a small extent and crosses the placenta and enters the fetal circulation.[60,61]

Madsen et al.[62] documented the prostatic penetration of aztreonam in nine patients after a single 1-g i.m. dose. A mean aztreonam concentration of 7.8 μg/g of tissue was noted 50–180 minutes after dosing, a concentration significantly higher than

Table 1.
MIC[a] Data for Aztreonam and Other Antimicrobial Agents[b] Used against Gram-Negative Pathogens[2,7,10–16,22–44] [c]

Az	Mx	Cft	Ctx	Ctz	Cp	Cx	Pip	G
E. coli								
<0.03–0.25	0.05–0.25	<0.10–0.25	0.05	0.10–0.20	0.10–2	3.10–4	4–75	0.25–1.60
<0.03–8	0.10–1.60	0.05–2	0.05	0.20–0.80	1–>100	8–32	64–>100	0.50–6.30
Klebsiella spp.								
<0.03–0.50	0.10–0.50	≤0.10–0.25	0.10	0.20	0.60–2	2–6.30	8–>100	0.25–0.80
0.10–32	0.20–8	0.20–8	0.25	0.20–1.6	4–>100	4–64	>128–>400	0.50–13
Enterobacter spp.								
<0.03–2.50	0.05–3.12	<0.10–8	3.12	0.20–6.25	0.20–2	6.30–>128	2–12.50	0.25–3.10
0.04–64	0.20–84	0.50–>64	>100	0.50–>100	2.30–100	50–128	32–>100	0.50–6.30
Proteus mirabilis								
<0.005–0.125	0.06–0.25	<0.10	0.05	<0.10	0.10–2	0.80–8	0.50–1.60	0.25–1.60
0.01–0.20	0.10–0.25	<0.10–0.20	0.05	0.05–0.12	1.60–4	0.80–16	64–75	1–3.10
Proteus (+)								
<0.10–0.20	0.10–0.25	<0.03–0.80	0.78	<0.10–8	1.40–3.10	2–12.50	0.50–75	0.12–6.30
<0.015–2	0.20–8	0.10–12.50	>100	<0.10–25	5.80–>100	8–>100	2–>100	1–75
Acinetobacter spp.								
4–128	4–100	1–>100	2–12.50	1–12.50	8–93.80	4–64	. . .	≤0.05
16–200	16–128	4–>100	4–32	4–>100	64–≥128	32–>64	. . .	≤0.05–2
Providencia spp.								
<0.10	0.03–0.10	0.05–1.20	. . .	0.20–1.20	1.20–12.50	0.80–3.40	87	2.50
<0.10	0.10–0.20	0.80–3	. . .	0.80–4.70	4.70–50	12.50	. . .	. . .
Citrobacter spp.								
<0.03–2	0.06–1	0.05–2	0.39	0.10–0.70	0.70–2	1.60–64	8–12.50	0.25–1.60
0.06–32	0.20–6.25	0.10–16	100	0.20–100	0.40–25	3.10–>64	38–64	0.50–3.10
H. influenzae[d]								
0.03–0.10	0.03–0.06	<0.10	. . .	<0.10	<0.10–60.7	. . .	. . .	1
0.12–0.25	0.12	<0.10	. . .	<0.10–0.25	<0.10–>100	. . .	. . .	2
N. gonorrhoeae[e]								
0.032–0.12	0.03–0.06	0.004–<0.10	. . .	0.03–<0.10	<0.10	0.05–0.50	. . .	1
0.063–0.25	0.06–0.25	0.03–<0.10	. . .	<0.10–0.125	0.20	0.50–2	. . .	2
Serratia spp.								
0.07–1	0.30–12.50	0.50–25	. . .	0.40–0.80	4–>100	9–75	12.50	1.50
0.5–6.30	1–50	2–50	. . .	1–3.10	16–>100	>100	25	. . .
Ps. aeruginosa								
2.90–16	8–32	8–32	12.5–16	0.39–4.30	5.60–16	>128–>800	4–32	0.50–128
8–32	16–>100	32–100	32–200	0.78–64	12–400	>128–>800	32–>100	1–>800

[a] Minimum inhibitory concentration, in μg/mL; for each organism and drug, data are given for inhibition of 50% of strains (MIC_{50}, top) and for 90% of strains (MIC_{90}).
[b] Az = aztreonam, Mx = moxalactam, Cft = cefotaxime, Ctx = ceftriaxone, Ctz = ceftazidime, Cp = cefoperazone, Cx = cefoxitin, Pip = piperacillin, G = gentamicin.
[c] Inoculum = 10^4 to 10^6 bacteria/mL.
[d] Includes ampicillin-sensitive and ampicillin-resistant strains.
[e] Includes penicillin-sensitive and penicillin-resistant strains.

the MICs of most members of the Enterobacteriaceae family implicated in chronic prostatitis. The average prostate:serum concentration ratio was 0.25 (range 0.15–0.41). In eight patients with severe renal failure, Watson and coworkers[63] documented aztreonam concentrations in renal parenchymal tissue that were similar to concurrent serum concentrations.

The cerebrospinal fluid (CSF) penetration of aztreonam in patients with and without inflamed meninges was studied by Duma et al.[64] in 34 subjects. Although the CSF aztreonam concentrations in subjects with inflamed meninges were four times higher than in the group without inflamed meninges, all subjects achieved CSF concentrations 5–10 times those necessary to inhibit most Enterobacteriaceae.

Although animal studies indicate adequate aztreonam penetration into ocular tissues,[65] human data will have to be assessed before conclusions can be made. Mean synovial fluid and bone aztreonam concentrations of 102 μg/mL and 41 μg/mL, constituting 116 and 42%, respectively, of simultaneous serum concentrations, have been reported.[66] Bronchial secretion concentrations ranging from 1.9 to 5.2 μg/mL at two to eight hours after a single 2-g i.v. dose have been reported by Bechard and coworkers.[67]

Aztreonam is eliminated predominantly as unchanged drug in the urine (Table 2).[53–55,57,68] Metabolism to a hydrolysis product (SQ 26,992) occurs to a minor extent, accounting for approximately 10% of the 90% of radioactivity recovered from a 144-hour urine and feces collection in normal volunteers.[57] Urine aztreonam concentrations in volunteers have ranged from 1.3 to 9000 μg/mL, de-

Table 2.
Mean Pharmacokinetic Values for Aztreonam in Normal Volunteers[a]

Pharmacokinetic Variable	Dose and Route of Administration							
	0.5 g I.V.[b]	0.5 g I.V.[c]	0.5 g I.M.[d]	1 g I.V.[e]	1 g I.V.[f]	1 g I.M.[g]	2 g I.V.[h]	2 g I.V.[i]
Peak serum concentration (μg/mL)	56.3 ± 3.8 (58.2 ± 3.4)	65.5	21.0 ± 1.3 (22.0 ± 1.8)	72.5 ± 12.6 (125 ± 4)	164	46.5 ± 2.8	. . .	255
Plasma clearance (mL/min/kg)	1.53 ± 0.04 (1.27 ± 0.14)	1.08 ± 0.14	1.46 ± 0.02 (. . .)	1.16 ± 0.09 (1.27 ± 0.14)	0.91 ± 0.06	. . .	1.27 ± 0.14	0.98 ± 0.14
Renal clearance (mL/min/kg)	1.03 ± 0.04 (. . .)	0.60 ± 0.21	0.94 ± 0.03 (. . .)	0.86 ± 0.14 (. . .)	0.59 ± 0.14	. . .	. . .	0.60 ± 0.19
% Excreted unchanged in urine	67.3 ± 2.0 (68 ± 7)	. . .	64.5 ± 1.7 (. . .)	73.7 ± 6.4 (68 ± 7)	. . .	. . .	68 ± 7	. . .
AUC (μg/mL/hr)	. . . (. . .)	109.6 ± 15.5	. . . (. . .)	189.3 ± 16.6 (. . .)	271.2 ± 24.3	. . .	. . .	511.2 ± 91.0
V_1 (L/kg)	0.11 ± 0.01 (0.09 ± 0.02)	0.07 ± 0.02	. . . (. . .)	0.125 ± 0.040 (0.09 ± 0.02)	0.05 ± 0.01	. . .	0.09 ± 0.02	0.08 ± 0.01
V_β (L/kg)	. . . (. . .)	0.23 ± 0.07	. . . (. . .)	0.224 ± 0.040 (. . .)	0.20 ± 0.05	. . .	. . .	0.26 ± 0.01
V_{SS} (L/kg)	0.18 ± 0.00 (0.16 ± 0.02)	0.15 ± 0.03	. . . (. . .)	. . . (0.16 ± 0.02)	0.11 ± 0.01	. . .	0.16 ± 0.02	0.14 ± 0.04
$t_{1/2}\,\alpha$ (hr)	0.23 ± 0.03 (0.20 ± 0.07)	0.33 ± 0.24	. . . (. . .)	. . . (0.20 ± 0.07)	0.22 ± 0.06	. . .	0.20 ± 0.07	0.36 ± 0.14
$t_{1/2}\,\beta$ (hr)	1.59 ± 0.03 (1.66 ± 0.19)	1.98 ± 0.43	1.70 ± 0.09 (1.64 ± 0.21)	1.93 ± 0.14 (1.66 ± 0.19)	1.90 ± 0.21	1.64 ± 0.21	1.66 ± 0.19	2.16 ± 0.38
k_{12}(hr^{-1})	1.19 ± 0.27 (1.44 ± 0.52)	1.89 ± 1.57	. . . (. . .)	. . . (1.44 ± 0.52)	1.46 ± 0.60	. . .	1.44 ± 0.52	0.75 ± 0.36
k_{21}(hr^{-1})	1.64 ± 0.15 (1.78 ± 0.39)	1.48 ± 0.78	. . . (. . .)	. . . (1.78 ± 0.39)	1.21 ± 0.48	. . .	1.78 ± 0.39	1.02 ± 0.44
k_{10} or k_{el}(hr^{-1})	0.85 ± 0.06 (0.87 ± 0.13)	0.97 ± 0.23	0.41 ± 0.02 (0.43 ± 0.06)	. . . (0.87 ± 0.13)	1.05 ± 0.19	0.43 ± 0.06	0.87 ± 0.13	0.70 ± 0.04
Bioavailability (% of i.v. dose)	. . . (. . .)	. . .	101 ± 3 (. . .)	. . . (. . .)	. . .	. . .	. . .	. . .
Time to peak concentration (hr)	. . . (. . .)	. . .	0.88 ± 0.12 (0.94 ± 0.34)	. . . (. . .)	. . .	0.94 ± 0.34	. . .	. . .
Absorption rate constant (hr^{-1})	. . . (. . .)	. . .	2.83 ± 0.87 (2.24 ± 1.10)	. . . (. . .)	. . .	2.24 ± 1.10	. . .	. . .

[a] Data for i.v. adminstration are based on a two-compartment pharmacokinetic model using the following general equations:

$$C = Ae^{-\alpha t} + Be^{-\beta t}$$
$$A = (D/V_1)[(\alpha - k_{21})/(\alpha - \beta)] \text{ and}$$
$$B = (D/V_1)[(k_{21} - \beta)/(\alpha - \beta)]$$

where C is the concentration at time t; D/V_1 is the ratio of the amount of drug administered to the volume of distribution of the central compartment; k_{21} is the distribution rate constant from compartment 2 to compartment 1; V_1 is the volume of distribution of compartment 1; and α and β are composite rate constants of k_{12}, k_{21}, and k_{10} where k_{12} is the distribution rate constant from compartment 1 to compartment 2 and k_{10} is the elimination rate constant from compartment 1.

Data for i.m. adminstration are based on a one-compartment pharmacokinetic model with first-order absorption and elimination, using the following general equations:

$$C = k_a D/V(k_a - k_{el})[e^{-k_{el}t} - e^{-k_a t}]$$
$$t_{pk} = 2.303/k_a - k_{el} \log k_a/k_{el}$$

where C is the concentration at time t; k_a is the apparent first-order absorption rate constant; V is the apparent volume of distribution; k_{el} is the apparent first-order elimination rate constant; and t_{pk} is the time to peak concentration.

[b] Mean ± S.E. for bolus infusion over two minutes[57]; values in parentheses are mean ± S.D. for bolus infusion over three minutes.[54]

[c] Mean or mean ± S.D. for infusion over 30 minutes.[58]

[d] Mean ± S.E.[57]; values in parentheses are mean ± S.D.[54]

[e] Mean ± S.D. for bolus infusion over two minutes[53]; values in parentheses are mean ± S.D. for bolus infusion over three minutes.[54]

[f] Mean or mean ± S.D. for infusion over 30 minutes.[58]

[g] Mean ± S.D.[54]

[h] Mean ± S.D. for bolus infusion over three minutes.[54]

[i] Mean or mean ± S.D. for infusion over 30 minutes.[58]

pending on the dose, route of administration, time after administration, and renal function.[54,55,57,58,69] Biliary concentrations in normal volunteers have not been reported, although only 1.5–3.5% of an i.v. or i.m. dose is excreted in the feces, presumably via the biliary route.[57] The effect of biliary-tract disease on aztreonam biliary excretion was evaluated by Martinez et al.[70] in 10 postcholecystectomy patients with T-tube drainage and 4 patients with obstructive biliary-tract disease with recent placement of external biliary drainage. Maximum biliary concentrations ranged from 9.7 to 88.2 μg/mL (mean 42.9 ± 7.9 μg/mL) and occurred 2.4 hours after injection of a single 1-g i.v. dose. Cumulative 12-hour biliary excretion in the external drainage subset accounted for 0.18 ± 0.06% of the total dose.

Elimination half-life and plasma and renal clearance data for volunteers with normal renal function are detailed in Table 2.[53–55,57,58] Tubular secretion accounted for 45.8% of renal clearance, a finding supported by studies with probenecid.[68] There is no evidence for dose-dependent pharmacokinetics.[54,55,57,58] Renal impairment significantly reduced aztreonam plasma and renal clearances and increased the elimination half-life. Renal impairment was also associated with reduced aztreonam plasma protein binding (58% when creatinine clearance was greater than 80 mL/min and 36% when creatinine clearance was less than 10 mL/min) but with no clinically important changes in volume of distribution.[69,71,72] Four hours of hemodialysis removed approximately 50% of a 1-g aztreonam dose.[71,72] Dialysis clearance of aztreonam during continuous ambulatory peritoneal dialysis (CAPD) represented only 8.8% of total body clearance; 9.7% of a 1-g dose was recovered from the dialysate. However, the bioavailability of aztreonam to the systemic circulation after intraperitoneal administration was 50–70%, indicating a potential role for intraperitoneal administration for the treatment of systemic and peritoneal-cavity infections in peritoneal dialysis patients.[71]

Stable alcoholic cirrhosis, but not primary biliary cirrhosis, was associated with a 20–25% reduction in total body clearance, suggesting the potential for substantial accumulation with prolonged therapy and the need for a modest dose reduction in such patients exposed to high-dose, long-term therapy.[73]

Multiple-dose pharmacokinetic studies in normal volunteers did not demonstrate drug accumulation. In these studies, distribution and elimination half-life, volume of distribution, urinary excretion, and metabolism were consistent with those from single-dose studies.[74] When alterations in renal function are taken into account, the pharmacokinetics of aztreonam is not altered by the presence of gram-negative infection, cancer, or old age.[75–77]

Preliminary pharmacokinetic data in children are available in the single-dose studies of Stutman and coworkers[78] and Reed and coworkers.[79] Stutman et al. demonstrated an inverse correlation of elimination half-life with age (5.71 ± 1.63 hours in newborns less than seven days old weighing less than 2500 g, and 1.67 ± 0.21 hours in children 2–12 years old). Total body clearance values were directly correlated with age, ranging from 0.94 ± 0.14 mL/min/kg to 2.50 ± 0.15 mL/min/kg in these groups. For infants less than one month of age, volume of distribution at steady state (0.26–0.36 L/kg)was somewhat higher than for older children and adults.[78] Reed et al.[79] recently published results of a single-dose pharmacokinetic study of aztreonam in seven patients (8–18 years old) with cystic fibrosis (CF). These results suggest that children with CF may eliminate aztreonam more rapidly than adults (mean total body clearance of 2.51 ± 0.60 mL/min/kg) and display changes in distribution, as evidenced by a larger mean volume of distribution at steady state of 0.24 ± 0.05 L/kg.[79] Further studies, especially with multiple doses, are needed.

Clinical Use

Relatively few clinical studies of aztreonam have been published. Henry and Bendush[80] report that most information about use of this drug has appeared in abstract form or is available in the manufacturer's literature.

Several investigators have conducted open general-use studies of the efficacy of aztreonam in a wide variety of serious gram-negative infections. Dosages have ranged from 250 mg every 12 hours to 2 g every 6 hours, depending on patient weight, renal function, and site and severity of infection. Clinical cure rates of 95,[81] 80,[82] 82,[83] 96,[84] 86,[85] and 90%[86] and microbiological cure rates of 95,[81] 80,[82] 91,[83] 84,[84] 52,[85] and 90%[86] have been noted. Superinfection with *Ps. aeruginosa*, *Pseudomonas maltophilia*, Enterococci, *Staph. aureus*, *Enterobacter aerogenes*, and *Enterobacter cloacae* were noted in two of these studies.[83,84]

Four groups have investigated the efficacy of aztreonam in serious urinary-tract infections (UTI) in comparative, randomized trials.[87–90] Tsouroutsoglou and coworkers[87] compared aztreonam with cefamandole, each in a dosage of 1 g every eight hours i.m. for 5–10 days, in the treatment of serious upper and lower UTIs in 21 patients. There were 13 clinical and bacteriological cures and 1 relapse in the aztreonam group and 5 cures and 2 relapses in the cefamandole group. These results were not assessed statistically. Sattler and coworkers[88] compared aztreonam to gentamicin in 52 patients with serious UTIs. Treatment duration ranged from 5–10 days for nonbacteremic cases to 10–14 days for bacteremic cases. Percentages of unqualified cure, cure with relapse, cure with reinfection, and failure (65.7, 17.1, 17.1, 0.0%, respectively, in the aztreonam group and 52.9, 5.9, 23.5, 17.6% in the gentamicin groups) were not significantly different. In an open study of 11 patients with renal failure (creatinine clearance < 50 mL/min) or gentamicin-resistant isolates, all were cured. However, the authors noted that urinary colonization with enterococci was possible because of the narrow spectrum of aztreonam. Colonization occurred in 30.4% of aztreonam-treated patients, compared with 5.9% of gentamicin-treated patients, a significant difference. However, only 1 of the 14 colonized aztreonam-treated patients required treatment. The issue of gram-positive superinfection requires further study in comparative trials.

Webb and Wyle [89] compared the efficacy of aztreonam and cefamandole, administered in dosages of 1 g every eight hours i.v. (2 g every eight hours i.v. if sepsis was suspected) in 22 patients with serious UTIs. Clinical and bacteriological cure rates were not significantly different for the two drugs (100% in the aztreonam group and 85.7% in the cefamandole group). Similar results were noted by Childs.[90] Type II error caused by small group sizes may have contributed to the lack of significant differences in cure rates in these two studies. In an open study, Childs assessed the efficacy of aztreonam in the treatment of 35 urinary tract infections caused by multiresistant pathogens. Overall organism-specific cure rates were in excess of 87% in all instances.

In a randomized trial comparing aztreonam 2 g every eight hours i.v. with tobramycin 80 mg every eight hours i.v. for the treatment of gram-negative bacillary lower respiratory tract infections in 80 patients, these regimens were equally effective.[91] For the aztreonam group and the tobramycin group, respectively, clinical cure rates were 89.1 and 84.6% and bacteriological cure rates were 92.3 and 94.4%. In contrast, Schentag and coworkers[92] found that aztreonam was superior to tobramycin monotherapy in the treatment of gram-negative pneumonia, despite individualizing tobramycin dosing regimens to achieve peak tobramycin concentrations of 4–10 μg/mL. The clinical cure rate was not significantly different for the two drugs (31% in aztreonam-treated patients and 21% in tobramycin-treated patients). However, comparable figures for clinical cure *or* improvement (93% for aztreonam and 50% for tobramycin) and for bacteriological cure (92% for aztreonam and 57% for tobramycin) were significantly different for the two drugs.

In an open trial of aztreonam in combination with clindamycin in the treatment of 40 women with endometritis, pelvic inflammatory disease, and pelvic cellulitis, Pastorek and coworkers[93] documented clinical cure in 87% of patients. In a randomized trial comparing aztreonam plus clindamycin to gentamicin plus clindamycin in 119 patients with endometritis after cesarean section, clinical cure rates of 91 and 89%, respectively, (not significantly different) were noted.[94]

Pribyl and coworkers[95] examined the efficacy of aztreonam in 17 patients with a variety of orthopedic infections, including osteomyelitis and septic arthritis. Clinical and bacteriological cure rates of 100% were noted, with recurrences developing in 81.3% of patients.

Miller et al.[96] studied the efficacy of aztreonam 1 g i.m. and spectinomycin 2 g i.m. in 112 men with gonococcal urethritis in a prospective, randomized trial. Of the 93 patients who could be evaluated (51 and 42 patients treated with aztreonam and spectinomycin, respectively), both drugs were 100% effective against both penicillin-sensitive and penicillin-resistant strains of gonococci. This may be an important finding in light of the increasing worldwide incidence of spectinomycin-resistant gonococci.[97]

Adverse Reactions and Drug Interactions

No cases of aztreonam overdose have been reported. Because few clinical studies have been published, any conclusions on the incidence or severity of adverse reactions to aztreonam would be premature. A few cases of rashes and asymptomatic rises in serum concentrations of hepatic enzymes (SGOT, SGPT, LDH) have been reported to the manufacturer.[66,80] Phlebitis and pain at the injection site have rarely been reported. Because of its structural similarity to the penicillins and cephalosporins, aztreonam probably has similar adverse effects and a low incidence of nephrotoxicity and ototoxicity.

The potential for immunological cross-reactivity between aztreonam and the penicillin and cephalosporin classes of antibiotics has been explored. A lack of cross-reactivity would be a definite asset for this agent and could expand its potential patient population to include persons who are allergic to penicillins, cephalosporins, or both. Studies in rabbits have documented negligible cross-reactivity between antiaztreonam and antibenzylpenicillin and anticephalothin antibodies.[98] Studies in normal volunteers suggested that aztreonam was only weakly immunogenic in humans.[98] Of 41 subjects who had immunoglobulin E (IgE) antibody to one or more penicillin moieties, none reacted to aztreonam skin tests, suggesting that there is no cross-reactivity between IgE antibodies to penicillin and aztreonam.[99] Although caution is warranted, this study provided a basis for investigating the therapeutic use of monobactams in patients who are allergic to bicyclic β-lactams.

Creasey et al.[100] demonstrated no clinically important pharmacokinetic drug interactions between aztreonam and cephradine, clindamycin, gentamicin, metronidazole, and nafcillin in 48 healthy male volunteers.

Dosage and Administration

The adult dosage range used in study protocols has been 0.5–2 g i.v. or i.m. every 6–12 hours, with dosage adjustments for renal impairment.[69,71,72] Hemodialysis patients should receive a supplemental dose equal to half of their usual maintenance dose immediately after each dialysis session.[71,72] For CAPD patients with peritonitis caused by susceptible organisms, a 1-g i.v. loading dose followed by 0.5 g intraperitoneally every 6 hours has been recommended.[71] For CAPD patients with systemic infections, injection of a loading dose equal to the usual standard dose, followed by one fourth of the standard dose every 6–12 hours, has been recommended.[66] Preliminary dosing recommendations of 30 mg/kg every 4–8 hours in older children and every 8–12 hours in neonates have been proposed, but confirmation in multiple-dose efficacy and safety studies is required before aztreonam use in children and neonates can be advocated.[78,79]

For i.v. administration, each dose should be diluted to 50–100 mL with i.v. fluid and infused over 20–60 minutes. Preliminary compatibility and stability studies have been completed for the intramuscular and intravenous diluents illustrated in Table 3. For each of these diluents, the constituted solutions must be used within 48 hours if stored at room temperature and within seven days if refrigerated at 4 °C.[66] In the first published study of aztreonam stability in i.v. admixtures, the authors have recommended that admixtures containing aztreonam and ampicillin in 0.9% sodium chloride injection should not be stored for longer than 48 hours at 4 °C or 24 hours at 25 °C, and that admixtures of these drugs in 5% dextrose injection should not be stored for longer than eight hours at 4 °C or two hours at 25 °C.[101]

Table 3.
Diluents in Which Aztreonam Is Stable

For Intramuscular Use
Sodium Chloride Injection, USP
Bacteriostatic Sodium Chloride Injection, USP, with benzyl alcohol
Bacteriostatic Sodium Chloride Injection, USP, with methylparaben or propylparaben
Sterile Water for Injection, USP
Bacteriostatic Water for Injection, USP, with benzyl alcohol
Bacteriostatic Water for Injection, USP, with methylparaben or propylparaben
For Intravenous Use
Sterile Water for Injection, USP
Sodium Chloride Injection, USP
Ringer's Injection, USP
Lactated Ringer's Injection, USP
5% Dextrose Injection, USP
10% Dextrose Injection, USP
5% Dextrose and 0.9% Sodium Chloride Injection
5% Dextrose and 0.45% Sodium Chloride Injection, USP
Sodium lactate injection (*M*/6)
Isolyte E Injection (electrolyte solution, McGaw)
Isolyte with 5% Dextrose Injection
Normosol-R Injection (electrolyte solution, Abbott)
Normosol-M with 5% Dextrose Injection
10% Travert (electrolyte solution, Travenol)
5% Mannitol Injection, USP

Formulary Recommendation

The ultimate clinical role of aztreonam is unclear. Potential areas of use include single-drug therapy of gram-negative urinary-tract infections, pneumonias, and orthopedic infections. Aztreonam can also be used in combination with other antibiotics as empiric therapy for respiratory tract, intra-abdominal, skin-structure, and gynecological infections. It would be a useful agent in many patients in whom aminoglycosides are relatively or absolutely contraindicated (e.g., patients with pre-existing otic or renal dysfunction), for long-term therapy when aminoglycoside serum-concentration monitoring cannot be performed, and in the presence of aminoglycoside-resistant gram-negative bacilli. The preservation of aztreonam's bactericidal activity in anaerobic conditions (in contrast to aminoglycoside activity) will have to be evaluated in controlled trials to assess its clinical importance.[13] The ultimate role of aztreonam in relation to the aminoglycosides awaits much further study under general-use conditions and in further controlled, comparative trials.

Theoretical considerations may favor aztreonam over most of the newer broad-spectrum cephalosporins. It is more active in vitro against *Ps. aeruginosa* than any of the third-generation drugs with the exception of ceftazidime. Resistance of previously susceptible *Enterobacter, Serratia* and *Ps. aeruginosa* has developed during therapy with several of the newer cephalosporins.[102] Bacterial resistance has rarely emerged during aztreonam therapy, but final conclusions must await the results of further clinical trials and general use. Superinfection with resistant gram-negative bacilli may be less likely with aztreonam than with the cephalosporins, because aztreonam has no substantial activity against anaerobes and should maintain resistance to gastrointestinal colonization.[103–105] However, this has not yet been evaluated in controlled studies. As with the third-generation cephalosporins, gram-positive superinfection, especially with enterococci, may occur during aztreonam therapy.[106] Preliminary studies indicate a potential role for aztreonam in patients at risk for anaphylaxis with the broad-spectrum bicyclic β-lactam drugs.[98,99]

Although the full clinical role of aztreonam has not been determined, the drug should be added to hospital formularies. Its use should be restricted to patients in whom aminoglycoside therapy should be avoided. As empiric therapy, aztreonam should be used only for serious hospital-acquired infections and in patients whose underlying conditions predispose them to *Ps. aeruginosa* infections. Further delineation of the role of aztreonam awaits the availability of the carbapenems and carboxyquinolones for general use.

Conclusion

Aztreonam, the first of the monocyclic β-lactam antibiotics to be released for general use, is efficacious and safe in the treatment of a wide variety of serious gram-negative infections. Although its role in our antimicrobial armamentarium is not yet fully defined, it should prove useful in the treatment of gram-negative infections in patients in whom aminoglycoside therapy is not desirable, in the treatment of many aminoglycoside-resistant gram-negative infections, and in the treatment of bicyclic β-lactam hypersensitive patients. Full realization of aztreonam's ultimate role in antimicrobial therapy awaits the general arrival of two other new classes of antimicrobial agents, the carbapenems and carboxyquinolones.

References

1. Sykes RB, Cimarusti CM, Bonner DP et al. Monocyclic β-lactam antibiotics produced by bacteria. *Nature.* 1981; 291:489–91.
2. Sykes RB, Bonner DP, Bush K et al. Monobactams—monocyclic β-lactam antibiotics produced by bacteria. *J Antimicrob Chemother.* 1981; 8(Suppl E):1–16.
3. Wells JS, Trejo WH, Principe PA et al. EM 5400, a family of monobactam antibiotics produced by *Agrobacterium radiobacter. J Antibiot.* 1982; 35:295–9.
4. Imada A, Kitano K, Kintaka K et al. Sulfazecin and isosulfazecin, novel β-lactam antibiotics of bacterial origin. *Nature.* 1981; 289:590–1.
5. Aoki H, Sakai H, Kohsaka M et al. Nocardicin A, a new monocyclic β-lactam antibiotic. *J Antibiot.* 1976; 29: 492–500.
6. Parker WL, Cimarusti CM, Floyd DM et al. Monobactams: isolation and structure determination. *J Antimicrob Chemother.* 1981; 8(Suppl E):17–20.
7. Breuer H, Cimarusti CM, Denzel TH et al. Monobactams—structure-activity relationships leading to SQ 26,776. *J Antimicrob Chemother.* 1981; 8(Suppl E):21–8.
8. Sykes RB, Matthew M. The β-lactamases of gram-negative bacteria and their role in resistance to β-lactam antibiotics. *J Antimicrob Chemother.* 1976; 2:115–57.
9. Bush K, Freudenberger JS, Sykes RB. Interaction of azthreonam and related monobactams with β-lactamase from gram-negative bacteria. *Antimicrob Agents Chemother.* 1982; 22:414–20.
10. Sykes RB, Bonner DP, Bush K et al. Azthreonam (SQ 26,776), a synthetic monobactam specifically active against aerobic gram-negative bacteria. *Antimicrob Agents Chemother.* 1982; 21:85–92.
11. Livermore DM, Williams JD. In vitro activity of the monobactam, SQ 26,776, against gram-negative bacteria and its stability to their β-lactamases. *J Antimicrob Chemother.* 1981; 8(Suppl E):29–37.
12. Phillips I, King A, Shannon K et al. SQ 26,776: in vitro antibacterial activity and susceptibility to β-lactamases. *J Antimicrob Chemother.* 1981; 8(Suppl E):103–10.
13. Neu HC, Labthavikul P. Antibacterial activity of a monocyclic β-lactam SQ 26,776. *J Antimicrob Chemother.* 1981; 8(Suppl E):111–22.
14. Russell AD. In vitro studies on SQ 26,776, a new monobactam antibiotic. *J Antimicrob Chemother.* 1981; 8(Suppl E):81–8.
15. Wise R, Andrews JM, Hancox J. SQ 26,776, a novel β-lactam: an in vitro comparison with other antimicrobial agents. *J Antimicrob Chemother.* 1981; 8(Suppl E):39–47.
16. Neu HC, Labthavikul P. In vitro activity and β-lactamase stability of a monobactam, SQ 26,917, compared with those of aztreonam and other agents. *Antimicrob Agents Chemother.* 1983; 24:227–32.
17. Tomasz A. Penicillin-binding proteins in bacteria. *Ann Intern Med.* 1982; 96:502–4.
18. Georgopapadakou NH, Smith SA, Sykes RB. Mode of action of azthreonam. *Antimicrob Agents Chemother.* 1982; 21:950–6.
19. Yourassowsky E, Van der Linden MP, Lismont MJ et al. Growth curve patterns of *Escherichia coli* and *Pseudomonas aeruginosa* submitted to different SQ 26,776 concentrations. *J Antimicrob Chemother.* 1981; 8(Suppl E):89–96.
20. Chase HA, Fuller C, Reynolds PE. The role of penicillin-binding proteins in the action of cephalosporins against *Escherichia coli* and *Salmonella typhimurium. Eur J Biochem.* 1981; 117:301–10.
21. Curtis NAC, Orr D, Ross GW et al. Affinities of penicillins and cephalosporins for the penicillin-binding proteins of *Escherichia coli* K-12 and their antimicrobial activity. *Antimicrob Agents Chemother.* 1979; 16:533–9.
22. Shah PM, Losert-Bruggner B, Stille W. Bactericidal activity of SQ 26,776. *J Antimicrob Chemother.* 1981; 8(Suppl E):77–80.
23. Jacobus NV, Ferreira MC, Barza M. In vitro activity of azthreonam, a monobactam antibiotic. *Antimicrob Agents Chemother.* 1982; 22:832–8.
24. Fainstein V, Weaver S, Bodey GP. Comparative in vitro study of SQ 26,776. *Antimicrob Agents Chemother.* 1982; 21:294–8.
25. Percival A, Thomas E, Hart CA et al. In vitro activity of monobactam, SQ 26,776, against gram-negative bacteria. *J Antimicrob Chemother.* 1981; 8(Suppl E):49–55.
26. Reeves DS, Bywater MJ, Holt HA. Antibacterial activity of the monobactam SQ 26,776 against antibiotic resistant enterobacteria, including *Serratia* spp. *J Antimicrob Chemother.* 1981; 8(Suppl E):57–68.
27. Acar JF, Kitzis MD, Goldstein FW. In vitro activity of SQ 26,776 against multiply-resistant enterobacteria—preliminary results. *J Antimicrob Chemother.* 1981; 8(Suppl E):97–101.
28. Norrby R, Friberg K, Holm SE. In vitro antibacterial activity of SQ 26,776. *J Antimicrob Chemother.* 1981; 8(Suppl E):69–76.
29. Khan MY, Gruninger RP, Nelson SM et al. Comparative in vitro activity of cefodizime, ceftazidime, aztreonam, and other selected antimicrobial agents against *Neisseria gonorrhoeae. Antimicrob Agents Chemother.* 1983; 23:477–8.
30. Strandberg DA, Jorgensen JH, Drutz DJ. Activity of aztreonam and new beta-lactam antibiotics against penicillinase-producing *Neisseria gonorrhoeae. Curr Ther Res.* 1983; 34:955–9.
31. Deforges L, Le Van Thoi J, Soussy CJ et al. Activite in vitro de l'azthreonam sur les bacilles gram negatifs hospitaliers. *Pathol Biol.* 1983; 31:488–91.
32. Appelbaum PC, Tamim J, Pankuch GA et al. Susceptibility of 324 nonfermentative gram-negative rods to 6 cephalosporins and aztreonam. *Chemotherapy.* 1983; 29:337–44.
33. Strandberg DA, Jorgensen JH, Drutz DJ. Activities of aztreonam and new cephalosporins against infrequently isolated gram-negative bacilli. *Antimicrob Agents Chemother.* 1983; 24:282–6.
34. Brumfitt W, Hamilton-Miller JMT, Dixson S et al. Aztreonam, the first of a unique class of β-lactam antibiotics: in vitro activity. *Am J Obstet Gynecol.* 1983; 146:712–4.
35. Lang SDR, McKenzie D. Azthreonam: in vitro activity

against urinary pathogens. *Pathology*. 1983; 15:159–60.
36. Paradelis AG, Tselentis J, Crassaris L et al. In vitro activity of azthreonam (SQ 26,776), a new monobactam antibiotic. *Drugs Exp Clin Res*. 1983; 9:325–9.
37. Cipriani P, Giordano A, Brenciaglia MI et al. In vitro susceptibility test with azthreonam compared with cefotaxime, cefoxitin, cefuroxime, cephalothin, cefoperazone and gentamicin. *Drugs Exp Clin Res*. 1983; 9:275–9.
38. Paradelis AG, Stathopoulos GA, Salpigides GN et al. Antibacterial activity of aztreonam: a synthetic monobactam. A comparative study with thirteen other antibiotics. *Methods Find Exp Clin Pharmacol*. 1983; 5:375–83.
39. Tsouroutsoglou W, Tselentis J, Crassaris L et al. Comparative in vitro activity of azthreonam (SQ 26,776) and cefamandole against gram-negative bacilli. *Drugs Exp Clin Res*. 1983; 9:519–21.
40. Preblud SR, Gill CJ, Campos JM. Bactericidal activities of chloramphenicol and eleven other antibiotics against *Salmonella* spp. *Antimicrob Agents Chemother*. 1984; 25:327–30.
41. Venditti M, Brandimarte C, Santini C et al. Comparative in vitro activity of aztreonam, other beta-lactam antibiotics and aminoglycosides against *Pseudomonas aeruginosa*. *Chemioterapia*. 1984; 3:258–61.
42. Goossens H, DeMol P, Coignau H et al. Comparative in vitro activities of aztreonam, ciprofloxacin, norfloxacin, ofloxacin, HR810 (a new cephalosporin), RU28965 (a new macrolide), and other agents against enteropathogens. *Antimicrob Agents Chemother*. 1985; 27:388–92.
43. Bremner DA. Azthreonam activity against gram-negative bacilli. *Chemotherapy*. 1984; 30:44–8.
44. Thompson KD, O'Keefe JP, Tatarowicz WA. In vitro comparison of amifloxacin and six other antibiotics against aminoglycoside-resistant *Pseudomonas aeruginosa*. *Antimicrob Agents Chemother*. 1984; 26:275–6.
45. Stutman HR, Welch DF, Scribner RK et al. In vitro antimicrobial activity of aztreonam alone and in combination against bacterial isolates from pediatric patients. *Antimicrob Agents Chemother*. 1984; 25:212–5.
46. Ampel NM, Moon-McDermott L, Keating M et al. In vitro activity of aztreonam in combination with four other antibiotics against gram-negative bacilli and *Staphylococcus aureus*. *J Antimicrob Chemother*. 1984; 13:398–9.
47. Giamarellou H, Zissis NP, Tagari G et al. In vitro synergistic activities of aminoglycosides and new β-lactams against multiresistant *Pseudomonas aeruginosa*. *Antimicrob Agents Chemother*. 1984; 25:534–6.
48. Buesing MA, Jorgensen JH. In vitro activity of aztreonam in combination with newer β-lactams and amikacin against multiply resistant gram-negative bacilli. *Antimicrob Agents Chemother*. 1984; 25:283–5.
49. Aronoff SC, Klinger JD. In vitro activities of aztreonam, piperacillin and ticarcillin combined with amikacin against amikacin-resistant *Pseudomonas aeruginosa* and *P. cepacia* isolates from children with cystic fibrosis. *Antimicrob Agents Chemother*. 1984; 25:279–80.
50. Van Laethem Y, Husson M, Klastersky J. Serum bactericidal activity of aztreonam, cefoperazone, and amikacin, alone or in combination, against *Escherichia coli, Klebsiella pneumoniae, Serratia marcescens*, and *Pseudomonas aeruginosa*. *Antimicrob Agents Chemother*. 1984; 26:224–7.
51. Wu DH, Baltch AL, Smith RP et al. Effect of aztreonam in combination with azlocillin or piperacillin on *Pseudomonas aeruginosa*. *Antimicrob Agents Chemother*. 1984; 26:519–21.
52. Dworzack DL, Bartelt MA, Bailey RT Jr et al. Emergence of resistance to aztreonam. *Clin Pharm*. 1984; 3:467, 470. Letter.
53. Wise R, Dyas A, Hegarty A et al. Pharmacokinetics and tissue penetration of azthreonam. *Antimicrob Agents Chemother*. 1982; 22:969–71.
54. Swabb EA, Sugerman AA, Platt TB et al. Single-dose pharmacokinetics of the monobactam azthreonam (SQ 26,776) in healthy subjects. *Antimicrob Agents Chemother*. 1982; 21:944–9.
55. Swabb EA, Leitz MA, Pilkiewicz FG et al. Pharmacokinetics of the monobactam SQ 26,776 after single intravenous doses in healthy subjects. *J Antimicrob Chemother*. 1981; 8(Suppl E):131–40.
56. Pilkiewicz FG, Remsburg BJ, Fisher SM et al. High-pressure liquid chromatographic analysis of aztreonam in sera and urine. *Antimicrob Agents Chemother*. 1983; 23:852–6.
57. Swabb EA, Singhvi SM, Leitz MA et al. Metabolism and pharmacokinetics of aztreonam in healthy subjects. *Antimicrob Agents Chemother*. 1983; 24:394–400.
58. Scully BE, Swabb EA, Neu HC. Pharmacology of aztreonam after intravenous infusion. *Antimicrob Agents Chemother*. 1983; 24:18–22.
59. Swabb EA, Sugerman AA, Stern M. Oral bioavailability of the monobactam aztreonam (SQ 26,776) in healthy subjects. *Antimicrob Agents Chemother*. 1983; 23:548–50.
60. Fleiss PM, Devlin R, Richwald G et al. Aztreonam excretion in human milk. *Clin Pharmacol Ther*. 1984; 35:240. Abstract.
61. Hayashi R, Devlin RG, Frantz M et al. Concentration of aztreonam in body fluids in mid-pregnancy. *Clin Pharmacol Ther*. 1984; 35:246. Abstract.
62. Madsen PO, Dhruv R, Friedhoff LT. Aztreonam concentrations in human prostatic tissue. *Antimicrob Agents Chemother*. 1984; 26:20–1.
63. Watson AJS, Stout RL, Whelton A. The intrarenal distribution of aztreonam in healthy and diseased kidneys: clinical therapeutic implications. *J Infect Dis*. 1984; 150:631–5.
64. Duma RJ, Berry AJ, Smith SM et al. Penetration of aztreonam into cerebrospinal fluid of patients with and without inflamed meninges. *Antimicrob Agents Chemother*. 1984; 26:730–73.
65. Barza M, McCue M. Pharmacokinetics of aztreonam in rabbit eyes. *Antimicrob Agents Chemother*. 1983; 24:468–73.
66. E. R. Squibb & Sons. Aztreonam (Azactam) investigator's brochure. Princeton, NJ; 1985 May.
67. Bechard DL, Hawkins SS, Dhruv R et al. Penetration of aztreonam into human bronchial secretions. *Antimicrob Agents Chemother*. 1985; 27:263–4.
68. Swabb EA, Sugerman AA, Frantz M et al. Renal handling of the monobactam azthreonam in healthy subjects. *Clin Pharmacol Ther*. 1983; 33:609–14.
69. Mihindu JCL, Scheld WM, Bolton ND et al. Pharmacokinetics of aztreonam in patients with various degrees of renal dysfunction. *Antimicrob Agents Chemother*. 1983; 24:252–61.
70. Martinez OV, Levi JU, Devlin RG. Biliary excretion of aztreonam in patients with biliary tract disease. *Antimicrob Agents Chemother*. 1984; 25:358–61.
71. Gerig JS, Bolton ND, Swabb EA. Effect of hemodialysis and peritoneal dialysis on aztreonam pharmacokinetics. *Kidney Int*. 1984; 26:308–18.
72. Fillastre JP, Leroy A, Baudoin C et al. Pharmacokinetics of aztreonam in patients with chronic renal failure. *Clin Pharmacokinet*. 1985; 10:91–100.
73. MacLeod CM, Bartley EA, Payne JA et al. Effects of cirrhosis on kinetics of aztreonam. *Antimicrob Agents Chemother*. 1984; 26:493–7.
74. Swabb EA, Sugerman AA, McKinstry DN. Multiple-dose pharmacokinetics of the monobactam azthreonam (SQ 26,776) in healthy subjects. *Antimicrob Agents Chemother*. 1983; 23:125–32.
75. Janicke DM, Cafarell RF, Parker SW et al. Pharmacokinetics of aztreonam in patients with gram-negative infections. *Antimicrob Agents Chemother*. 1985; 27:16–20.
76. Jones PG, Bodey GP, Swabb EA et al. Clinical pharmacokinetics of aztreonam in cancer patients. *Antimicrob Agents Chemother*. 1984; 26:455–61.
77. Creasey WA, Platt TB, Frantz M et al. Pharmacokinetics of aztreonam in elderly male volunteers. *Br J Clin Pharmacol*. 1985; 19:233–7.
78. Stutman HR, Marks MI, Swabb EA. Single-dose pharmacokinetics of aztreonam in pediatric patients. *Antimicrob*

Agents Chemother. 1984; 26:196–9.
79. Reed MD, Blumer JL, Friedhoff LT et al. Single dose pharmacokinetics of aztreonam in cystic fibrosis. *Clin Pharmacol Ther.* 1985; 37:223. Abstract.
80. Henry SH, Bendush CB. Aztreonam: worldwide overview of the treatment of patients with gram-negative infections. *Am J Med.* 1985; 78(Suppl 2A):57–64.
81. Simons WJ, Lee TJ. Treatment of gram-negative infections with aztreonam. *Am J Med.* 1985; 78(Suppl 2A):27–30.
82. Greenberg RN, Reilly PM, Luppen KL et al. Treatment of serious gram-negative infections with aztreonam. *J Infect Dis.* 1984; 150:623–30.
83. Giamarellou H, Galanakis N, Douzinas E et al. Evaluation of aztreonam in difficult-to-treat infections with prolonged posttreatment follow-up. *Antimicrob Agents Chemother.* 1984; 26:245–9.
84. Torres A, Ramirez-Ronda CH. Aztreonam in the treatment of serious gram-negative infections. *Curr Ther Res.* 1984; 36:875–81.
85. Scully BE, Neu HC. Use of aztreonam in the treatment of serious infections due to multiresistant gram-negative organisms, including *Pseudomonas aeruginosa*. *Am J Med.* 1985; 78:251–61.
86. Hollingsworth JA, Donohoe JF, Hone R et al. Clinical experience with aztreonam in urinary and respiratory tract infections. *Curr Med Res Opin.* 1984; 9:316–22.
87. Tsouroutsoglou W, Sion ML, Stathopoulos GA et al. Comparative study of aztreonam and cefamandole in the treatment of serious urinary tract infections. *Methods Find Exp Clin Pharmacol.* 1983; 5:385–90.
88. Sattler FR, Moyer JE, Schramm M et al. Aztreonam compared with gentamicin for treatment of serious urinary tract infections. *Lancet.* 1984; 2:1315–8.
89. Webb DW, Wyle FA. Randomized comparative study of aztreonam and cefamandole in the treatment of urinary tract infection. *Curr Ther Res.* 1984; 36:113–8.
90. Childs SJ. Aztreonam in the treatment of urinary tract infection. *Am J Med.* 1985; 78(Suppl 2A):44–6.
91. Rodriguez JR, Ramirez-Ronda CH. Efficacy and safety of aztreonam versus tobramycin for aerobic gram-negative bacilli lower respiratory tract infections. *Am J Med.* 1985; 78(Suppl 2A):42–3.
92. Schentag JJ, Vari AJ, Winslade NE et al. Treatment with aztreonam or tobramycin in critical care patients with nosocomial gram-negative pneumonia. *Am J Med.* 1985; 78(Suppl 2A):34–41.
93. Pastorek JG II, Cole C, Aldridge KE et al. Aztreonam plus clindamycin as therapy for pelvic infections in women. *Am J Med.* 1985; 78(Suppl 2A):47–50.
94. Gibbs RS, Blanco JD, Lipscomb KA et al. Aztreonam versus gentamicin, each with clindamycin, in the treatment of endometritis. *Obstet Gynecol.* 1985; 65:825–9.
95. Pribyl C, Salzer R, Beskin J et al. Aztreonam in the treatment of serious orthopedic infections. *Am J Med.* 1985; 78(Suppl 2A):51–6.
96. Miller LK, Sanchez PL, Berg SW et al. Effectiveness of aztreonam, a new monobactam antibiotic against penicillin-resistant gonococci. *J Infect Dis.* 1983; 148:612.
97. Patefield AJ, Westbrook WG III, Johnson NA. Spectinomycin-resistant *Neisseria gonorrhoeae*—worldwide. *Morb Mortal Wkly Rpt.* 1982; 31:632–8.
98. Adkinson NF Jr, Swabb EA, Sugerman AA. Immunology of the monobactam aztreonam. *Antimicrob Agents Chemother.* 1984; 25:93–7.
99. Saxon A, Hassner A, Swabb EA et al. Lack of cross-reactivity between aztreonam, a monobactam antibiotic, and penicillin in pencillin-allergic subjects. *J Infect Dis.* 1984; 149:16–22.
100. Creasey WA, Adamovics J, Dhruv R et al. Pharmacokinetic interaction of aztreonam with other antibiotics. *J Clin Pharmacol.* 1984; 24:174–80.
101. James MJ, Riley CM. Stability of intravenous admixtures of aztreonam and ampicillin. *Am J Hosp Pharm.* 1985; 42:1095–1100.
102. Sanders CC, Sanders WE Jr. Emergence of resistance during therapy with newer β-lactam antibiotics: role of inducible β-lactamases and implications for the future. *Rev Infect Dis.* 1983; 5:639–48.
103. Sykes RB, Bonner DP. Aztreonam: the first monobactam. *Am J Med.* 1985; 78(Suppl 2A):2–10.
104. de Vries-Hospers HG, Welling GW, Swabb EA et al. Selective decontamination of the digestive tract with aztreonam: a study of 10 healthy volunteers. *J Infec Dis.* 1984; 150:636–42.
105. Jones PG, Bodey GP, Swabb EA et al. Effect of aztreonam on throat and stool flora of cancer patients. *Antimicrob Agents Chemother.* 1984; 26:941–3.
106. Chandrasekar PH, Smith BR, LeFrock JL et al. Enterococcal superinfection and colonization with aztreonam therapy. *Antimicrob Agents Chemother.* 1984; 26:280–2.

Product selection criteria for intravascular ionic contrast media

DENNIS P. SWANSON, TERRY J. DICK, STUART M. SIMMS, AND JAMES H. THRALL

Abstract: The chemistry, clinical use, pharmacokinetics, adverse reactions, dosages, and formulary recommendations for intravascular ionic contrast media routinely used in radiologic procedures are reviewed.

The meglumine, sodium, or combined meglumine–sodium salts of triiodinated benzoic acid derivatives, diatrizoic and iothalamic acid, are commonly used as intravascular ionic contrast media for radiographic visualization of blood vessels and the urinary tract. Meglumine salts of iodoxamate and iodipamide are used for intravenous cholangiography. The iodine in the contrast medium is responsible for the absorption of x-rays and the resulting opacification of the organ system or other area under investigation.

Adverse reactions to intravascular ionic contrast media broadly include hypersensitivity and chemotoxic reactions. The incidence of major life-threatening hypersensitivity reactions, such as severe hypotension, cardiac arrhythmias or arrest, pulmonary or laryngeal edema, and convulsions, is estimated at 0.01–0.1% of the population receiving these agents. Dose- and concentration-dependent chemotoxic reactions result from the direct effects of the contrast medium on the blood vessels or organs being perfused. The meglumine salts of diatrizoic acid and iothalamic acid are less toxic in the cerebral circulation than sodium salts; hence, diatrizoate meglumine or iothalamate meglumine are recommended for cerebral angiography. In coronary angiographic examinations, combined meglumine and sodium (6.6 parts meglumine to 1 part sodium) formulations of diatrizoate are recommended because they consist predominantly of the meglumine salt with minimal but adequate amounts of sodium to prevent ventricular fibrillation. Predominantly meglumine salts of diatrizoic and iothalamic acid are also used for peripheral angiography, computerized tomography, and digital subtraction angiography.

The dosages of ionic contrast media vary considerably depending on the nature of the radiological examination, the respective technique employed, and the age and condition of the patient. The cost differences between diatrizoate and iothalamate media are typically minimal. Formulary recommendations regarding the appropriate chemical nature of these media are based on the reported adverse reactions with these agents.

Index terms: Diatrizoate meglumine; Diatrizoate sodium; Dosage; Drugs; Drugs, adverse reactions; Formularies; Iodamide meglumine; Iodaxamate meglumine; Iodipamide meglumine; Iothalamate meglumine; Iothalamate sodium; Pharmacokinetics; Roentgenographic agents; Toxicity
Clin Pharm. 1985; 4:527–38

This article reviews the chemistry, clinical use, pharmacokinetics, adverse reactions, and dosages of intravascular ionic contrast media routinely used for the enhancement of radiological procedures. The review, which includes formulary recommendations, should help pharmacists develop intelligent product selection criteria for these types of drug products.

Chemistry

The ionic contrast media commonly used to enhance the radiographic visualization of blood vessels and the urinary tract are the meglumine, sodium, or combination meglumine and sodium salts of the triiodinated benzoic acid derivatives, diatrizoic acid and iothalamic acid (Figure 1). An additional benzoic acid derivative, iodamide (Figure 2), is available as a meglumine salt for radiologic examination of the kidney. Ionic contrast media for intravenous cholangiography are meglumine salts of the *bis*-triiodinated benzoic acid derivatives, iodoxamate and iodipamide (Figure 3).

Aqueous solutions of these ionic contrast media are clear and colorless to pale yellow. They are stable to heat and cold but sensitive to light. Crystal formation occasionally observed in an ionic contrast medium can usually be resolved by heating the medium to 37 °C.

Solutions of ionic contrast media vary in concen-

DENNIS P. SWANSON, M.S., is Director, Division of Radiology Pharmacy Services, Department of Diagnostic Radiology, Henry Ford Hospital, Detroit, MI; Clinical Associate Professor of Pharmacy, College of Pharmacy, University of Michigan, Ann Arbor; and Adjunct Associate Professor of Pharmacy Practice, School of Pharmacy, Wayne State University, Detroit. TERRY J. DICK is a Pharm.D. candidate, College of Pharmacy, University of Michigan. STUART M. SIMMS, M.D., is Director, Division of Gastrointestinal Radiology; and JAMES H. THRALL, M.D., is Chairman, Department of Radiology, Henry Ford Hospital.

Address reprint requests to Mr. Swanson at the Department of Diagnostic Radiology, Henry Ford Hospital, 2799 W. Grand Boulevard, Detroit, MI 48202.

The assistance of the Iowa Drug Information System in the literature search and Linda Jenkins for her secretarial services is acknowledged.

Figure 1. Chemical structures of diatrizoate and iothalamate contrast media.

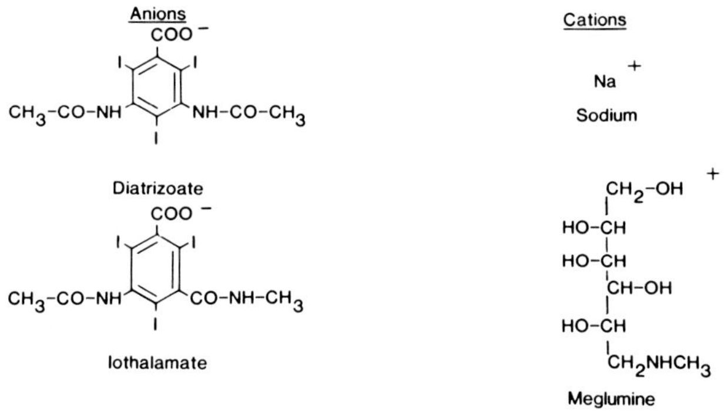

Figure 2. Chemical structure of iodamide.

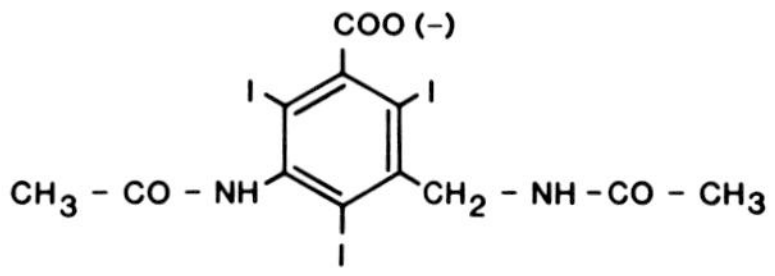

Figure 3. Chemical structures of contrast media used for intravenous cholangiography.

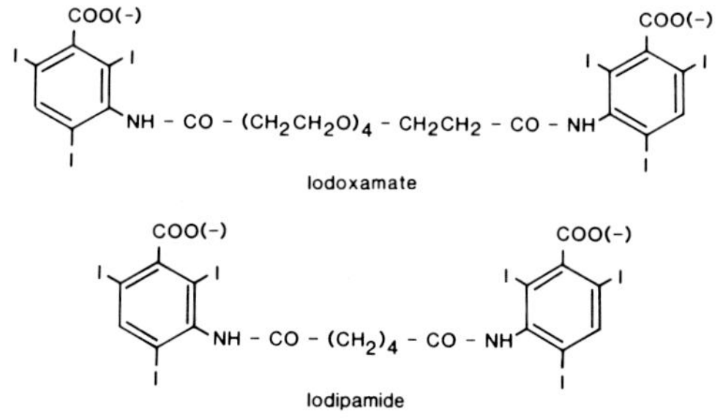

tration and cationic form (e.g., meglumine, sodium, meglumine and sodium) depending on their radiologic indications. Although the concentrations of these contrast media are typically expressed as percent weight of the salt per volume (% w/v), the most important factor is the concentration of iodine, since this component of the medium is responsible for the absorption of radiation and the resulting property of opacification. In this regard, the concentration of iodine in an ionic contrast medium may also be expressed as % w/v or as milligrams of iodine per milliliter (mg I/mL). At an equal salt concentration, meglumine salts of ionic contrast media have a reduced concentration of iodine compared with sodium salts (Table 1). This is because the molecular weight of the meglumine cation (195.2) is approximately 8.5 times the molecular weight of the sodium cation (22.9).

Table 1.
Iodine Concentrations in Meglumine versus Sodium Salt of Diatrizoic Acid

Salt Conc. (% w/v)	Iodine Concentration % (w/v)	Iodine Concentration mg/mL
60% Diatrizoate meglumine	47.1	282
60% Diatrizoate sodium	59.9	358

The osmolality of a radiopaque contrast medium is related to the concentration of osmotically active particles in solution, expressed as osmoles (Osm) of ions/1000 g of water (osmolarity = osmoles of ions/1000 mL of solution). The ionic contrast media currently used for the direct opacification of blood vessels (angiography) and to evaluate the urinary system (intravenous urography) have extremely high osmolalities because they consist of two osmotically active particles (an anion and a cation) in solution for every three atoms of radiopaque iodine (Figures 1 and 2). Depending on the concentration (% w/v) of iodine required to perform the examination, the osmolalities of these media may typically exceed the osmolality of blood (300 mOsm/kg) by factors of approximately two (14% w/v iodine) to seven (40% w/v iodine). Sodium salts of ionic contrast media have higher osmolalities than meglumine salts with equal iodine concentrations, probably because of their greater dissociation in solution (i.e., the number of distinct osmotically active particles in solution increases).

The viscosity of a radiopaque contrast medium is a measure of its resistance to flow expressed in centipoise (cps) units. As the molecular weight of the iodinated chemical salt or the concentration of a given contrast medium increases, so does its viscosity. Hence, at equal iodine concentrations, the viscosity of a meglumine salt of an ionic contrast medium is substantially greater than the respective sodium salt because of its greater molecular weight. The ease and speed at which a viscous contrast medium can be injected is a major problem in radiologic examinations. This problem can be overcome, to a certain degree, by heating the contrast medium to 37 °C before injection, thus substantially decreasing its viscosity (e.g., viscosity of 60% w/v meglumine diatrizoate is approximately 6 cps units at 25 °C and 4 cps units at 37 °C).

Clinical Use and Pharmacokinetics

The clinical use of intravascular ionic contrast media is based upon the ability of these agents to opacify the vasculature of organs being perfused by the media or to opacify organ systems (e.g., urinary, hepatobiliary) that are responsible for excretion of the media. This opacification results from the photoelectric interaction of x-rays with the high-density iodine atoms in these media and the subsequent attenuation of exposure of the radiographic film or alternate radiation-sensitive device. In this regard, the indications for the use of intravascular ionic contrast media are not based on the evaluation of specific disease processes but rather on their application in radiologic procedures. Hence, the diatrizoate or iothalamate ionic contrast media may be indicated for radiologic examinations of the vasculature of the brain (cerebral angiography), heart (coronary angiography), or periphery (peripheral angiography); for enhancement of computed-tomography (CT) procedures, or for evaluation of the urinary system (urography, intravenous pyelography). Similarly, the iodoxamate and iodipamide ionic contrast media are used to evaluate the hepatobiliary system and gallbladder (intravenous cholangiography). Such radiologic procedures are useful in the diagnosis and evaluation of myriad disease processes including tumors, abscesses, vascular abnormalities (such as infarcts or aneurysms), trauma, and excretory dysfunction and obstruction.

In angiographic examinations, maximum opacification of the vessel(s) of interest occurs immediately after bolus injection of the diatrizoate or iothalamate ionic contrast media, followed by a rapid decrease in vascular radiopaque iodine concentration caused by dilution in the intravascular and extravascular (extracellular) fluid compartments and renal excretion. The intravenous use of these media to enhance the evaluation of brain tumors, abscesses, or cerebrovascular abnormalities by computerized tomography is based upon their ability to enter the cerebral extravascular space *only* in those areas associated with lesion-induced alterations in the blood-brain barrier.

These same diatrizoate and iothalamate ionic contrast media are commonly used to evaluate the kidney based upon rapid excretion of the radiopaque anions by glomerular filtration. The amount of these radiopaque anions excreted by the kidney during any period is a function of the product of plasma concentration and the glomerular filtration rate. In normal subjects, the plasma half-life of these radiopaque anions is approximately one hour.[1] Unlike the diatrizoate and iothalamate anions, which are excreted solely by glomerular filtration, iodamide is excreted by a combination of glomerular filtration and active tubular secretion.[2,3] This latter factor results in a more rapid plasma clearance of the iodamide anion.[2]

Following intravenous administration, both the iodoxamate and iodipamide anions are rapidly removed from the blood by the liver and excreted via the organic anion pathway into the bile. Thus, these media may be used to enhance the radiographic visualization of the intrahepatic, hepatic, and common bile ducts, and the gallbladder. The excretion of these agents into the bile may be impaired by poor liver function or high levels of circulating bilirubin, which compete more effectively for the organic-anion excretion pathway.[3] The incidence of major reactions and death associated with the administration of these intravenous cholecystographic agents is greater than the incidence with other contrast media.[4–7] Hence, in view of the efficacy and increased safety of competing diagnostic modalities, including oral cholecystography, ultrasound, and technetium Tc 99m disofenin scintigraphy, the clinical use of these agents should be limited.

The benefit to be gained (i.e., opacification of the organ system, vessel, or disease process under investigation) from the intravascular administration of ionic contrast media is relatively constant and definable as it is directly dependent on the quantity (volume and concentration) of radiopaque iodine administered to the patient. This quantity is determined by the degree of opacification required to perform the respective examination adequately. However, the risk of adverse reactions associated with the intravascular administration of ionic contrast media can vary depending on the chemical and physical environment of these iodine atoms and the site of administration (study indication). Thus, the efficacy of these ionic contrast media can be enhanced by reducing the risk of adverse reactions through appropriate product selection based on a review of the factors responsible for these adverse effects.

Adverse Reactions

Adverse reactions to intravascular ionic contrast media are typically classified according to the severity[4–6,8] of the reaction or the type of reaction. The types of adverse reactions broadly include hypersensitivity (idiosyncratic) and chemotoxic reactions.[6,8,9]

Severity and Incidence. Using a severity classification, mild reactions can be anticipated in approximately 3–8% of patient examinations involving intravascular administration of the currently used ionic contrast media.[4,5,7,8,10] Mild reactions are defined as those that are not life threatening, are of short duration, and require no specific treatment other than supportive measures. Included in this class are nausea, headache, dizziness, and urticaria. The sensations of heat and pain are common following the intravascular administration of ionic contrast media and are not generally classified as adverse reactions. Moderate reactions are also nonlife threatening, but usually have longer durations and require therapeutic intervention. Approximately 1–2% of the patients receiving intravascular ionic contrast media will experience moderate reactions,[4,5,8] including transient hypotension, bronchospasm, and persistent skin reactions. Life-threatening, major reactions have variable durations and require urgent treatment. The incidence of major reactions, such as severe hypotension, cardiac arrhythmias or arrest, pulmonary or laryngeal edema, and convulsions, is estimated at 0.01–0.1% of the population receiving these contrast media.[4–6,8,10] Finally, the reported incidence of death resulting from the intravascular administration of ionic contrast agents ranges from 0.0025% to 0.01%.[4,5,9,10] Although the incidence of major adverse reactions and death associated with these agents does not seem high when presented in percentage terms, the large number of intravascular contrast media studies performed on a daily basis throughout the country must be considered.

Hypersensitivity Reactions. Hypersensitivity reactions to intravascular ionic contrast media tend to be the most perplexing since their occurrence is unpredictable and independent of the dose or concentration of contrast medium administered. Several theories have been proposed on the causative mechanism(s) of these hypersensitivity reactions,[8,10–15] including antibody-antigen reactions,[16,17] basophil and mast-cell release of serotonin and histamine,[18–21] activation of acute complement or coagulation systems,[22–26] and psychologic factors associated with fear of the procedure.[27] The true cause of hypersensitivity reactions may actually be a combination of these events.[6] It is known that a patient history of allergies, asthma, or previous reactions to contrast media increases the likelihood of hypersensitivity reactions by factors of 2, 3, and 4, respectively.[5,7,11,14,28] Hence, the prevention of these reactions may be facilitated by appropriate patient screening and recognition of the individuals at a high risk. If the contrast study remains warranted, such atopic patients, especially previous reactors, should be considered as candidates for pretreatment with antihistamines or corticosteroids.[5,6,8,10,13,14,26,29–31] The use of sensitivity testing to predict contrast-media reactors has fallen into disfavor because of its unreliability in detecting subsequent reactors, its inability to reduce the incidence of major reactions, and the reports of severe adverse reactions to the test dose itself.[5,6–8,10–14,32,33]

Chemotoxic Reactions. Chemotoxic reactions occur as a result of the direct effects of the contrast medium on the blood vessels or the organs being perfused by the medium. These reactions are dose- (volume) and concentration-dependent.[6,8,9,34] Several factors contribute to the chemotoxicity of a radiopaque contrast medium, including its osmolality and viscosity (physical factors), the site and speed of administration, and its chemical properties.

The osmotic effects exerted by the hypertonic ionic contrast media result in cellular diuresis with corresponding chemotoxic effects. The local pain and hemodynamic changes (sensation of warmth, increased blood volume, blood flow, and cardiac output) commonly observed following the intra-

Figure 4. General chemical structures of ionic and low-osmolality contrast agents.

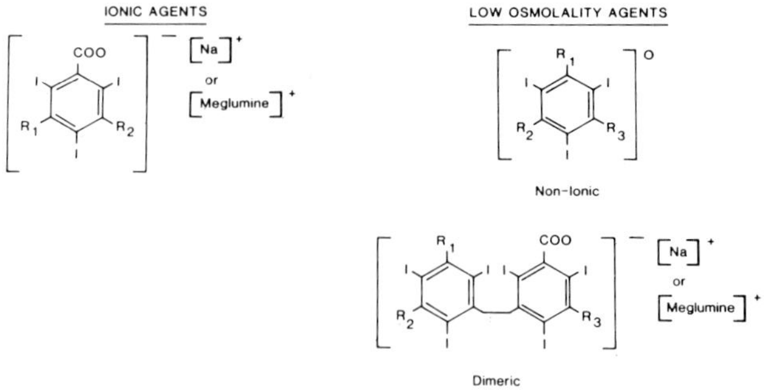

vascular administration of these agents are thought to be primarily associated with their hyperosmolar nature.[6,34–36] In recognition of this, recent developments of radiopaque contrast media have been directed at low-osmolality agents (Figure 4) based on the concept of one osmotically active particle in solution per three iodine atoms (nonionics) or two particles, an anion and a cation, in solution per six iodine atoms (dimeric agents). Both of these configurations reduce the osmolality per given iodine concentration by a factor of approximately two compared to current ionic agents.[37] The synthetic complexity of these low-osmolality agents make them considerably more expensive than the current ionic media and may unfortunately limit their routine clinical use once they have received final approval from the Food and Drug Administration.

Another consideration in regard to adverse reactions is the effect of the viscosity of the ionic contrast medium on the length of time that the sensitive organ or vessel remains exposed to the chemotoxic factors following administration.[38] As previously discussed, the viscosity of an ionic contrast medium can be substantially reduced by preheating the medium to 37 °C before administration.

In regard to the site and speed of administration, the injection of a concentrated radiopaque contrast medium directly into a vessel supplying a sensitive organ such as the heart, brain, or kidney would be expected to produce an increased number and intensity of adverse effects on that organ compared with a systemic intravenous injection. Likewise, a bolus injection would expose the sensitive organ to a high dose and concentration of contrast medium; factors directly associated with chemotoxicity.[4,6,34,39] A tradeoff with lower dose and concentration infusions, however, is the length of time that the sensitive organ is in contact with the contrast medium.

In actuality, the site and speed of administration and the dose and concentration of the contrast medium used are determined by the nature of the radiologic examination and the degree of required opacification. Chemotoxicity factors that can be controlled are the chemical properties of the administered contrast media.[6,40] Various comparative studies have demonstrated that the incidence of patient discomfort and adverse reactions associated with the intravascular administration of ionic contrast media can be reduced by using the appropriate chemical form and concentration of contrast medium as a function of the site of administration and sensitive organ involved.

Product Considerations for Selected Radiologic Procedures

Cerebral Angiography. *Cation Selection.* Meglumine salts of diatrizoic acid and iothalamic acid are less toxic in the cerebral circulation than sodium salts. This specific chemotoxicity factor has been demonstrated in both animal[41–44] and human[45,46] studies following intracarotid administration and in animal models of contrast-media neurotoxicity involving intracisternal[41,47] or spinal-cord-artery[48] injections. The increased neurotoxic effects of the sodium salts may be related to their high osmolalities relative to the meglumine media (at equal iodine concentrations)[43,44] or the direct detrimental effects of sodium on the permeability of the blood-brain barrier with subsequent exposure of the central nervous system to the chemotoxic radiopaque anions or both.[41,44,49] In cerebral angiography, consideration must be given to the presence of even small amounts of sodium in the contrast medium since, at high dosages, the combination meglumine–sodium salt (6.6:1 ratio, 3.76 mg sodium/mL) of diatrizoic acid causes a substantially increased incidence of toxic effects compared with the pure meglumine salt (0.02 mg sodium/mL) of the same diatrizoate anion.[44]

Anion Selection. It is generally believed in radiology circles that the iothalamate anion is safer in the cerebral circulation than the diatrizoate anion.[6] However, in evaluating the comparative data leading to this conclusion, the sodium ion concentrations of the contrast media studied must be considered, especially in view of the previously documented neurotoxicity of sodium. The major animal and clinical studies supporting the superior safety of iothalamate have compared a pure iothalamate meglumine formulation (0.03 mg sodium/mL) with a combination meglumine–sodium salt of diatrizoate (3.76 mg sodium/mL),[41,43,47–52] or with a pure diatrizoate meglumine formulation containing a greater concentration of sodium (0.91 mg/mL) associated with its sequestering and buffering additives.[48,50] In other words, the relative neurotoxicities of the iothalamate and diatrizoate anions were compared using contrast-media formulations that had sodium ion concentrations that differed by factors of 30 to 100.

Unfortunately, there are few comparisons of the relative neurotoxicities of the iothalamate and diatrizoate anion using formulations containing equal sodium ion concentrations, and the results of these limited studies are inconclusive. One such animal study compared equal concentrations of pure sodium iothalamate and pure sodium diatrizoate and demonstrated a greater acute toxicity (mean lethal dose) of the diatrizoate derivative upon direct intracerebral or intracisternal application, and greater injury (brain staining) to the blood-brain barrier following intracarotid injection.[41] In contrast, other animal studies, which compared the intracarotid administration of these pure sodium salts, revealed no major differences between the iothalamate and diatrizoate anions in regard to the incidence or severity of subsequent spasms and convulsions[43] or cardiovascular toxicity.[42,43] Finally, pure meglumine salts of iothalamate and diatrizoate, containing equal concentrations of sodium (0.03 mg/mL and 0.02 mg/mL, respectively), were randomly compared in approximately 300 clinical cerebral angiography examinations.[53] No significant differences between the iothalamate and diatrizoate anions were observed on the basis of subjective patient complaints or objective complications, with the exception of an increased incidence of brachial-artery spasm with the iothalamate derivative.

Coronary Angiography. *Cation Selection.* The cationic nature of a contrast medium injected into vessels directly supplying the heart (i.e., ascending aorta, pulmonary vein, coronary artery) or directly into the cardiac chamber (auriculography, ventriculography) is of extreme importance in preventing the occurrence of adverse reactions. In this regard, the appropriate contrast medium should be predominantly a meglumine salt, but adequate sodium is required to prevent an increased incidence of ventricular fibrillation.

Early experimental studies comparing the myocardial toxicity of sodium and meglumine salts of contrast media demonstrated specific cardiotoxic effects associated with the sodium cation. Following left coronary-artery[54] or ascending-aorta[55,56] injection into dogs, pure sodium salts of diatrizoate or iothalamate produced electrocardiographic changes and decreased myocardial contractility, blood pressure, and heart rate that were substantially more severe and of longer duration than observed with the pure meglumine salts. As the sodium concentration of the contrast media increased, so did its cardiotoxicity. These adverse effects could not be reproduced to the same degree by equivolume injections of isotonic saline (volume effect),[56] equiosmolar solutions of hypertonic dextrose (osmolarity effect),[55,56] or meglumine salts of the same anion (anion and viscosity effects);[54–56] however, they could be reproduced by the administration of 5% sodium chloride solution,[55,56] implicating the sodium cation as the specific causative factor.

On the basis of these observations, the manufacturer of a combination meglumine–sodium (6.6:1 ratio, 4.48 mg sodium/mL) diatrizoate contrast medium altered the cationic composition of the agent to make it predominantly a meglumine salt. However, the clinical use of this "pure" diatrizoate meglumine (0.91 mg sodium/mL associated with sequestering and buffering agents) for coronary angiography unexpectedly resulted in an increased frequency of ventricular fibrillation.[57] Subsequent animal studies, which directly compared the cardiotoxic effects of the combination meglumine–sodium and pure meglumine diatrizoates, confirmed that the complete absence of sodium or its decrease to very low levels significantly increased the incidence of ventricular fibrillation.[57–63] One study demonstrated a significantly decreased incidence of ventricular fibrillation with the addition of sodium chloride (final sodium concentration of 4.5 mg/mL) to the pure meglumine diatrizoate; thus "isolating" the effect of added sodium on cardiotoxicity.[59] Despite the differences in the incidence of ventricular fibrillation, the frequency and severity of hemodynamic and electrocardiographic effects between the combination meglumine–sodium and pure meglumine diatrizoates were relatively equal[57,58,60] indicating that two mechanisms of toxicity may exist in the myocardium.[57] Perhaps the best explanation for the protective effects of added sodium came from the study of Simon et al.[60] in which the measurement of monophasic action potentials from the heart muscle showed that both the combination meglumine–sodium and pure meglumine agents "prolonged the time of cardiac depolarization." As they explained this further:

> The increase in sodium concentration from 0.91 to 4.48 mg/mL was, however, associated with prolongation of the repolarization phase and lengthening of the refractory period (not observed with low-sodium agents). This lengthening of the refractory period displaces the vulnerable period of the myocardial cell temporarily from the prolonged depolarization and, in a manner, probably serves to protect the myocardium from fibrillation.

The exact concentration of sodium required in a contrast medium for coronary angiography has not been determined; however, it is obvious that very low and high concentrations will increase the incidence of cardiotoxicity. The coronary-artery injection of a contrast medium containing a sodium concentration below 1.57 mg/mL resulted in multiple premature ventricular contractions,[60] whereas a combination meglumine and sodium (2:1 ratio) salt of iothalamate, containing 9.4 mg sodium/mL, demonstrated minimal cardiotoxic effects.[61] It is assumed that a combination meglumine–sodium contrast medium containing nearly physiological concentrations of sodium (0.9% sodium chloride = 3.54 mg sodium/mL) would be the most appropriate.[57,59,63]

Anion Selection. No conclusive studies have demonstrated the superiority of the diatrizoate or iothalamate anion for coronary angiography. An early animal experiment, which compared the cardiovascular effects of ascending-aorta injections of 50% w/v sodium diatrizoate and 50% w/v sodium iothalamate, indicated that the iothalamate anion was 3.5 times more cardiotoxic.[55] However, a similar study using coronary-artery injections of the pure sodium and pure meglumine salts of both anions revealed no significant differences in anion toxicity.[54] As previously mentioned, both meglumine and sodium (6.6:1 ratio, 4.48 mg sodium/mL) diatrizoate and meglumine and sodium (2:1 ratio, 9.4 mg sodium/mL) iothalamate demonstrated relatively low toxicity upon the right-coronary artery injection of 0.4-mL doses in rabbits; however, the iothalamate agent did cause arrhythmias at a 0.6-mL dose level versus a 0.9-mL level for the diatrizoate derivative. This may be related to the increased sodium concentration of the iothalamate derivative.

Another important consideration in the selection of a contrast medium for direct injection into the cardiac chambers or vessels supplying these chambers is related to the fact that a major percentage of the cardiac output goes to the brain. As noted in the previous discussion of cerebral angiography, even small concentrations of sodium ions in the cerebral circulation can be associated with neurotoxic effects. Hence, the combination meglumine and sodium contrast medium used for coronary angiography should have an acceptable, but minimal, concentration of sodium. This consideration makes the 6.6:1 meglumine–sodium diatrizoate formulations (76% w/v, 3.6–4.48 mg sodium/mL) more appropriate than the 2:1 meglumine–sodium iothalamate formulation (78% w/v, 9.4 sodium/mL), which is the only combination salt of the iothalamate anion currently available.

Sequestering and Buffering Agents. When a large bolus of a contrast medium is injected in an angiography procedure, it temporarily displaces the blood and deprives the sensitive organ (e.g., heart or brain) of its normal source of physiological ions, oxygen, and nutrients. This factor may explain the requirement for "physiological" concentrations of sodium in the contrast media used for coronary angiography, and it raises additional questions regarding a potential reduction in cardiotoxicity associated with adding other physiological ions or oxygen to these media. Various investigators have demonstrated that the cardiodepressive effects (decreased contractility, conduction delays) of both ionic[64–69] and nonionic[68,70] contrast media could be significantly reduced by the addition of calcium; while the addition of other ions (magnesium, potassium)[64,70] or oxygen[70] provided no advantages. Since calcium ions are important in maintaining the normal contractile and cellular membrane stability of the heart, it has been speculated that contrast media must interfere with the normal transmembrane flux of calcium ions by a direct competition of sodium cations for the transport sites[64,68] or by the direct binding of calcium by the radiopaque anion.[68,71] In 1975, Caulfield et al.[72] implicated an additional factor associated with the cardiotoxic effects of contrast media—the presence of calcium-binding sequestering and buffering agents.

All of the currently available ionic contrast media for intravascular administration have some form of sequestering (edetate disodium, calcium edetate disodium) and buffering (sodium citrate, sodium bicarbonate, monobasic sodium phosphate) agents present in low concentrations to stabilize their solubility characteristics. One combination of these additives, 0.04% edetate disodium and 0.32% sodium citrate, has the ability to directly chelate 13 mmol of calcium per liter.[73] In the study of Caulfield et al.,[72] a contrast medium containing this combination of additives demonstrated extensive in vitro binding of plasma calcium and caused an acute decrease in the coronary sinus concentrations of ionized calcium in normal and arteriosclerotic patients undergoing coronary angiography. In some patients with coronary obstruction, the extent of this calcium decrease was consistent with levels associated with electromechanical dissociation of the heart.

Subsequent studies have isolated the cardiotoxic effects of these 0.04% edetate disodium and 0.32% sodium citrate additives and have stressed the importance of eliminating these agents or neutralizing their calcium-binding properties. The first of these studies documented a significantly greater incidence of ventricular fibrillation in dogs following the coronary-artery administration of meglumine and sodium (6.6:1) diatrizoate containing these sequestering and buffering agents compared with the same medium with 24 mmol/L of calcium chloride added to neutralize the calcium-binding properties of the sequestering and buffering agents.[73] A similar significant increase in the incidence of ventricular fibrillations was observed when a meglumine–sodium (6.6:1) diatrizoate preparation containing 0.04% edetate disodium and 0.32% sodium citrate was compared with an equivalent meglumine and sodium diatrizoate media containing the preneutralized sequestering agent, calcium edetate disodium (0.01%, no other additives).[74,75] In support of these latter studies, the in vitro binding of calcium ions was significantly decreased in contrast media containing calcium edetate disodium versus equivalent media containing edetate disodium and sodium citrate.[71]

In summary, it is apparent that certain cardiotoxic manifestations of contrast media used for coronary angiography are associated with their effect(s) on the normal physiology of calcium ions. There is controversy regarding the appropriate concentration of calcium that should be added to media used for this purpose. The addition of calcium at concentrations of 40–60 meq/L (20–40 mmol/L) to a meglumine and sodium diatrizoate preparation containing 0.04% edetate disodium and 0.32% sodium citrate does abolish its cardiodepressive effects and, in fact, results in an increase in myocardial contractility that could be equally as dangerous in certain compensated patients.[68,69] Nonetheless, all of these studies show that sequestering and buffering agents associated with direct calcium binding should be eliminated or neutralized in contrast media.[68,69,71–76]

Peripheral Angiography, Intravenous Computerized Tomography, Digital Subtraction Angiography, and Urography. *Cation Selection.* Direct measurements of blood flow and pressure have indicated that meglumine salts of ionic contrast media produce less adverse hemodynamic changes (i.e., increased arteriolar vasodilation and decreased peripheral vascular resistance) following intra-arterial administration than their corresponding sodium derivatives.[36] These hemodynamic effects are apparently directly related to the osmolarities of the evaluated agents, since the intra-arterial injection of equiosmolar solutions of sodium chloride, glucose, or urea produced similar effects.[36] Furthermore, clinical studies have documented a reduced incidence of pain with meglumine salts following either intra-arterial[77] or intravenous[78–80] injection. In this regard, it is thought that the pain response may be associated with vascular endothelial changes induced by the contrast medium.[81] Microscopic examinations of exposed vessels have revealed more endothelial damage with sodium contrast media than with meglumine agents.[81–83] Hence, predominantly meglumine salts of the radiopaque anions are the appropriate agents for peripheral angiography and intravenous CT or digital-subtraction angiography (DSA).

Although it is a controversial subject,[84,85] clinical evaluations of urogram quality in patients with both normal and abnormal renal function[80–86] and direct CT measurements of renal contrast density[87] have revealed that greater opacification of the renal medulla, calyces, and pelves can be achieved by using sodium salts of contrast media for urographic examinations than meglumine salts. This phenomenon can possibly be explained by the fact that sodium ions are reabsorbed from the renal tubules whereas meglumine ions are not, thus resulting in an increased osmotic diuretic effect or less reabsorption of water from the kidney with the meglumine agent and, hence, greater dilution of the iodine concentration.[1,86] Apparently, the concentrating effect of the total length of the renal tubules is required before major differences in the degree of opacification can be achieved, since total nephrogram quality[85,86] and renal cortex contrast density[87] do not vary as a function of the nature of the cation. As a related consideration, the bolus administration of a radiopaque contrast medium results in greater urographic opacification than prolonged infusion of the same dose.[87,88] These large-dose, bolus injections are facilitated by the lower viscosities of sodium agents relative to their meglumine counterparts of equal iodine concentration.

A disadvantage of using sodium contrast media for urographic examinations is the expected increase in the incidence of pain and adverse hemodynamic and cardiovascular effects; factors that can be potentiated following bolus versus infusion administration.[89] The high-dose administration of these sodium agents to patients with normal kidney function and pre-existing hypertension or heart disease, especially congestive heart failure, should be an area of concern.[1,90] In contrast to meglumine derivatives, the extensive extravascular distribution and tubular reabsorption of the administered sodium ions increases the extravascular and intravascular osmotic load and, thus, may subject the patient to more severe hypertension or pulmonary edema.[91] In patients with abnormal renal function, the meglumine and the sodium ion would not be excreted or reabsorbed to a great extent, hence both of these cations would contribute equally in the osmotic challenge for a patient with hypertension or heart disease.[1]

Finally, a discussion of relative cation toxicity would not be complete without pointing out that meglumine contrast media have been noted to produce an increased incidence of bronchospasm,[9] perhaps because of a greater degree of histamine release.[19] However, clinical studies designed specifically to evaluate this variable found no significant difference between sodium and meglumine media in regard to the prevalence or magnitude of changes in pulmonary function (forced expiratory volume, maximal expiratory force) in either atopic or nonallergic patients.[92,93] The atopic patients did, however, demonstrate significantly greater decreases in pulmonary function following contrast media (sodium or meglumine) injection compared with the nonallergic patients.

Anion Selection. There are no demonstrated advantages associated with the use of either the diatrizoate or iothalamate anion for peripheral angiography or intravenous CT, DSA, or urography and pyelography examinations.[6] Studies that have evaluated the toxicity of contrast media have indicated that the intravenous LD_{50} of iothalamate exceeds the diatrizoate dose by 20–50% at equivalent cation formulations and concentrations.[41,45,94] However, this difference has apparently insignificant effects upon the incidence of adverse reactions at the dosages routinely used in radiographic procedures.

The combined glomerular filtration and renal tubular excretion of the iodamide anion results in an increase in urinary contrast concentration[2] and improved opacification of the kidneys compared with meglumine derivatives of the diatrizoate and iothalamate anions.[95,96] However, no significant differences in overall urogram density or side effects were observed between equal iodine concentrations and doses of iodamide meglumine versus diatrizoate sodium.[97] Iodamide meglumine has not gained extensive clinical use compared with diatrizoate meglumine or sodium or iothalamate meglumine or sodium, perhaps because of its limited indication, reportedly higher incidence (9.5–13%) of adverse effects,[3] or economic considerations.

Sequestering and Buffering Agents. As discussed under coronary angiography, the combination of sequestering and buffering agents, 0.04% edetate disodium and 0.32% sodium citrate, has the ability to chelate large amounts (13 mmol/L) of calcium ions.[73] The administration of a contrast medium containing this combination of additives in peripheral angiography and intravenous CT procedures significantly reduced systemic calcium concentrations to lower limits of normal; producing a corresponding sharp increase in circulating levels of parathyroid hormone.[98,99] A comparison of a medium containing these edetate disodium and sodium citrate additives with an equivalent medium containing the sequestering agent, calcium edetate disodium with neutralized calcium-binding effects, revealed that both media caused acute changes in the systemic levels of calcium and parathyroid hormone, but the effects of the first agent were significantly greater.[99] Although the clinical importance of these results is unknown, the greater physiological effects induced by the edetate disodium and sodium citrate sequestering and buffering agents should probably be a consideration in the selection of a contrast medium for high-dose peripheral angiography and intravenous CT, DSA, and urography procedures.

Intravenous Cholangiography. *Anion Selection.* A limited number of animal[100] and clinical studies[101,102] have indicated that the iodoxamate anion produces greater opacification of the biliary ducts and gallbladder, especially at higher bilirubin levels, compared with the iodipamide anion. The iodoxamate anion has also demonstrated a reduced number and severity of adverse effects.[3,100–102]

Influence of Concurrent Disease States on Selection of Ionic Contrast Media. A discussion of chemotoxic reactions would not be complete without a brief description of conditions that may predispose patients to these reactions following the intravascular administration of ionic contrast media. As might be expected, the physiological systems of elderly and neonatal patients are less able to compensate for the major hemodynamic changes and direct chemotoxic effects induced by these media.[4,6,91] Similarly, an increased likelihood of severe adverse reactions would be expected in patients with serious illnesses (e.g., heart disease, hypertension, cerebrovascular disease, or renal failure) involving the contrast-media-sensitive organs such as the heart, lung, brain, and kidney.[4,6,39,103,104] Dehydration renders the patients particularly sensitive to the fluid shifts induced by the cellular and osmotic diuretic effects of the hyperosmolar contrast media, and it should be avoided, especially in patients with pre-existing renal dysfunction, including diabetic patients, and in the patients described above.[1,6,90,103–110] Specific contraindications to intravascular ionic contrast media may include multiple myeloma (precipitation of Bence Jones proteins with cast formation leading to renal failure), pheochromocytoma (catecholamine release and hypertensive crisis), and sickle-cell disease (promotion of sickling).[6] Intravascular administration of ionic contrast media should only be performed with extreme caution on these high-risk patients. These patients may present the appropriate indications for using the less chemotoxic, but more expensive, low-osmolality contrast media once final FDA approval has been obtained for these agents.

Dosage

The doses (volumes and concentrations) of ionic contrast media vary considerably depending on the nature of the radiological examination, the respective technique employed, and the age and condition of the patient. In general, the dose is based on the quantity of iodine required to achieve adequate opacification of the area under investigation. This required quantity of iodine is determined by the size and rate of blood flow of the vascular structure(s) to be visualized or the rate and extent of ionic contrast media excretion in the excretory system being studied. Frequently, the patient is given repeat doses of the contrast media to permit adequate or complete evaluation of the total area under investigation.

Cerebral Angiography. As discussed in the section on chemotoxic reactions, increasing the concentration or dose of a contrast medium introduced in the cerebral circulation increases the likelihood of neurotoxic reactions.[42,47] Hence, it is generally recognized that the concentration of ionic contrast media for carotid or vertebral angiography should not exceed 60% w/v of the salt (280 mg iodine/mL).[6,40] Typical adult single doses range from 5 to 12 mL, with total doses (repeat injections) of approximately 30–50 mL.[6]

Coronary Angiography. Ionic contrast media used for coronary angiography procedures require high iodine concentrations (i.e., > 350 mg iodine/mL) because of their rapid dilution by the large volumes and high rates of blood flow at the injection sites. This factor necessitates the administration of meglumine and sodium combinations of diatrizoate or iothalamate with salt concentrations of 76% w/v or greater. The selective evaluation of coronary arteries requires a single adult dose of 5–10 mL with repeat doses, as needed, up to a total dose of 200 mL.[6] Opacification of the cardiac chambers of the right or left heart, pulmonary aorta, or thoracic aorta requires single adult doses of 30–60 mL, with total doses of 200 mL.[6]

Peripheral Angiography. The concentration of an ionic contrast medium used for peripheral angiography is dependent on the route of administration, intravenous versus intra-arterial, and the corresponding volume and rate of flow at the injection site. As with coronary angiography, injections into large, rapid-flow arteries (e.g., translumbar aortography, celiac artery) require high concentrations of iodine (i.e., > 350 mg iodine/mL, 76% w/v salt); whereas injections into more distal, slower-flow arteries (e.g., femoral, renal, hepatic, splenic arteries) require lower concentrations (i.e., ≤ 300 mg iodine/mL, 60% w/v salt). Typical adult, single-dose injections into the large rapid-flow arteries range from 30 to 60 mL, with total doses of approximately 200 mL, if needed. Specific renal arteriography uses a single dose of 8–15 mL (total doses up to 45 mL); whereas femoral, hepatic, or splenic arteriography require single doses of 20–50 mL (total doses up to 200 mL).[6]

Peripheral Phlebography. Direct injection of ionic contrast media into the veins of the extremities requires lower concentrations of iodine because of their small diameter and relatively slow flow rates. In leg phlebography, one study demonstrated that reducing the concentration of a meglumine and sodium (6.6:1 ratio) diatrizoate medium from 60% w/v (salt) to 45% w/v significantly reduced the incidence of immediate pain and the occurrence of delayed, inflammatory reactions.[111] Since these delayed reactions may be associated with the development of thrombophlebitis,[111] the salt concentration of ionic contrast media used for peripheral phlebography should be reduced to 45% w/v or less.[6] Single doses of 30–100 mL are commonly used for peripheral phlebography studies, repeated as necessary.[6]

Intravenous Urography and Computerized Tomography. These radiographic procedures are commonly performed using a bolus injection (30–100-mL single dose) of ionic contrast media containing approximately 300 mg of iodine/mL (i.e., 60% w/v meglumine salts, 50% w/v sodium salts) or by slow infusion (300-mL single dose) of ionic contrast media containing approximately 140 mg of iodine/mL (i.e., 30% w/v meglumine salts). An infusion interval of 3–10 minutes is typically used for urographic procedures and 10–20 minutes for CT. The concentration and dose of ionic contrast media for urography are dependent on the degree of opacification desired and the patient's renal function. Patients with poor renal function

Table 2.
Formulary Recommendations for Intravascular Ionic Contrast Media

Indication	Cation	Anion	Additives	Salt Conc. (% w/v)
Cerebral angiography	Meglumine	Diatrizoate or iothalamate	Calcium edetate disodium	60
Coronary angiography	Meglumine–sodium (6.6:1)	Diatrizoate	Calcium edetate disodium	76
Peripheral angiography				
Large-vessel arteriography	Meglumine–sodium (6.6:1)	Diatrizoate	Calcium edetate disodium	76
Distal arteriography	Meglumine	Diatrizoate or iothalamate	Calcium edetate disodium	60
Phlebography	Meglumine	Diatrizoate or iothalamate	Calcium edetate disodium	≤45
Computerized tomography				
Bolus technique	Meglumine	Diatrizoate or iothalamate	Calcium edetate disodium	60
Infusion technique	Meglumine	Diatrizoate or iothalamate	Calcium edetate disodium	30
Intravenous urography				
Bolus technique	Sodium	Diatrizoate or iothalamate	Calcium edetate disodium	≥50
Infusion technique	Meglumine	Diatrizoate or iothalamate	Calcium edetate disodium	30
Intravenous cholangiography	Meglumine	Iodoxamate	...	9.9

require higher concentrations and doses of iodine (up to 180 mg iodine/kg) than normal subjects because of the lower rate and extent of contrast-media excretion.[1]

Intravenous Cholangiography. The iodipamide meglumine and iodoxamate meglumine media are each available in two concentrations. The higher w/v concentrations (52% and 40.3%, respectively) are intended for rapid intravenous injection (20-mL dose) and the lower concentrations (10.3% and 9.9%, respectively) for intravenous infusion (100-mL dose).[3] It is thought that less patient discomfort (i.e., nausea, vomiting, flushing, and perspiration) occurs with slower infusions.[3,6]

Formulary Recommendations

The formulary recommendations for intravascular ionic contrast media, for various radiologic indications, are summarized in Table 2. The recommendations regarding the appropriate chemical nature (cation, anion, additives) of these media are based on the review and discussion of adverse reactions. The recommendations regarding % w/v salt concentrations may vary depending on the exact nature of the radiologic examination and respective technical variables. The cost differences between diatrizoate and iothalamate media are typically minimal. An attempt to limit the required inventory of these agents should also be taken into consideration in final formulary decisions.

References

1. Talner LB. Urographic contrast media in uremia. *Radiol Clin North Am.* 1972; 10:421–32.
2. Bollerup AC, Hesse B, Steiness E. Renal handling of iodamide and diatrizoate. Evidence of active tubular secretion of iodamide. *Eur J Clin Pharm.* 1975; 9:63–7.
3. E. R. Squibb & Sons, Inc. Squibb radiology reference. Princeton, NJ; 1978–79.
4. Ansell G, Tweedie MCK, West CR et al. The current status of reactions to intravenous contrast media. *Invest Radiol.* 1980; 15:532–9.
5. Shehadi WH. Adverse reactions to intravascularly administered contrast media. *Am J Roentgenol.* 1975; 124:145–52.
6. Committee on Drugs, Commission on Public Health and Radiation Protection. Prevention and management of adverse reactions to intravascular contrast media. Fischer HW, ed. Chicago: American College of Radiology; 1977.
7. Shehadi WH, Toniolo G. Adverse reactions to contrast media. *Radiology.* 1980; 137:299–302.
8. Lasser EC. Adverse reactions to intravascular administration of contrast media. *Allergy.* 1981; 36:369–73.
9. Ansell G. Adverse reactions to contrast agents. *Invest Radiol.* 1970; 5:374–91.
10. Witten DM. Reactions to urographic contrast media. *JAMA.* 1975; 231:974–7.
11. Cogen FC, Zwieman B. Adverse radiographic contrast media reactions. *Compr Ther.* 1978; 4:50–6.
12. Gorevic P, Kaplan AP. Contrast agents and anaphylactic-like reactions. *J Allergy Clin Immunol.* 1979; 63:225–7.
13. Lieberman P, Siegle, RL, Taylor WW. Anaphylactoid reactions to iodinated contrast material. *J Allergy Clin Immunol.* 1978; 62:174–80.
14. Siegle RL, Lieberman P. A review of untoward reactions to iodinated contrast material. *J Urol.* 1980; 119:581–7.
15. Andrews EJ Jr. The vagus reaction as a possible cause of severe complications of radiological procedures. *Radiology.* 1976; 121:1–4.
16. Brasch RC. Allergic reactions to contrast media: accumulated evidence. *Am J Roentgenol.* 1980; 134:797–801.
17. Brasch RC. Evidence supporting the antibody mediation of contrast media reactions. *Invest Radiol.* 1980; 15:529–31.
18. Lasser EC, Walters AJ, Reuter SR et al. Histamine release by contrast media. *Radiology.* 1971; 100:683–6.
19. Rockoff SD, Brasch R. Contrast media as histamine liberators. III. Histamine release and some associated hemodynamic effects during pulmonary angiography in dogs. *Invest Radiol.* 1971; 6:110–4.
20. Arroyave CM. An in-vitro assay for radiographic contrast media idiosyncracy. *Invest Radiol.* 1980; 15:521–5.
21. Ring J, Arroyave CM, Frizler MJ et al. In vitro histamine and serotonin released by radiographic contrast media (RCM). *Clin Exp Immunol.* 1978; 32:105–18.
22. Lang JH, Lasser EC, Kolb WP. Activation of serum complement by contrast media. *Invest Radiol.* 1976; 11:303–8.
23. Kolb WP, Lang JH, Lasser EC. Nonimmunologic complement activation in normal human serum induced by radiographic contrast media. *J Immunol.* 1978; 121:1232–8.
24. Arroyave CM, Schatz M, Simon RA. Activation of complement system by radiographic contrast media: studies in-vivo and in-vitro. *J Allergy Clin Immunol.* 1979; 63:276–80.
25. Lasser EC, Lang JH, Hamblin AE et al. Activation systems

in contrast idiosyncracy. *Invest Radiol.* 1980; 15:52–5.

26. Funk WG, Lasser EC, Lang JH et al. Effect of elevated C1-esterase inhibitor concentrations on white blood cell-endothelium interactions. *Invest Radiol.* 1982; 17:189–92.
27. Lalli AF. Urographic contrast media reactions and anxiety. *Radiology.* 1974; 112:267–71.
28. Witten DW, Hirsh FD, Hartman GW. Acute reactions to urographic contrast medium. *Am J Roentgenol.* 1973; 119:832–40.
29. Dotter CT, Jackson FS. Death following angiocardiography. *Radiology.* 1971; 54:527–33.
30. Greenberger P, Patterson R, Kelly J et al. Administration of radiographic contrast media in high-risk patients. *Invest Radiol.* 1980; 15:540–3.
31. Lasser EC, Lang J, Sovak M et al. Steroids: theoretical and experimental basis for utilization in prevention of contrast media reactions. *Radiology.* 1977; 125:1–9.
32. Pendergrass HP, Tondreaw RL, Pendergrass EP et al. Reactions associated with intravenous urography: historical and statistical review. *Radiology.* 1958; 71:1–12.
33. Fischer HW, Doust VL. An evaluation of pretesting in the problem of serious and fatal reactions to excretory urography. *Radiology.* 1972; 103:497–501.
34. Fischer HW. Hemodynamic reactions to angiographic media: a survey and commentary. *Radiology.* 1968; 91:66–73.
35. Kloster FE, Bustow JD, Porter GA et al. Comparative hemodynamic effects of equiosmolar injections of angiographic contrast materials. *Invest Radiol.* 1967; 2:353–9.
36. Hilal SK. Hemodynamic changes associated with the intra-arterial injection of contrast media. *Radiology.* 1966; 86:615–33.
37. Bettman MA. Angiographic contrast agents: conventional and new media compared. *Am J Roentgenol.* 1982; 139:787-94.
38. Evill CM. Discussion. Digital radiology session. Contrast Material Symposium, San Francisco, CA: Oct. 1984. *Invest Radiol.* 1984; 19(Suppl):S117.
39. Lang EK, Foreman J, Schlegel JU et al. The incidence of contrast medium induced acute tubular necrosis following arteriography. *Radiology.* 1981; 138:203–6.
40. Fischer HW. Contrast media. In: Radiology of the skull and brain: angiography. Newton TH, Potts DG, eds. St. Louis, MO: CV Mosby; 1971.
41. Kodama JK, Butler WM, Tusing TW et al. Iothalamate: a new intravascular radiopaque medium with unusual pharmacotoxic inertness. *Exp Mol Pathol.* 1963;(Suppl 2):65–80.
42. Fischer HW, Cornell SH. The toxicity of sodium and methylglucamine salts of diatrizoate, iothalamate and metrizoate. *Radiology.* 1965; 85:1013–21.
43. Hilal SK. Hemodynamic changes associated with the intra-arterial injection of contrast media. *Radiology.* 1966; 86:615–33.
44. Fischer HW, Redman HC. Comparison of a sodium methylglucamine diatrizoate contrast media of minimal sodium content with a pure methylglucamine preparation. *Invest Radiol.* 1971; 6:115–8.
45. Chase NE, Kricheff II. The comparison of the complication rates of meglumine iothalamate and sodium diatrizoate in cerebral angiography. *Am J Roentgenol.* 1965; 95:852–6.
46. Shealy CN. A comparison of Renografin and Hypaque for carotid arteriography. *J Neurosurg.* 1963; 20:137–8.
47. Melartin E, Tuohimaa PJ, Dabb R. Neurotoxicity of iothalamates and diatrizoates. I. Significance of concentration and cation. *Invest Radiol.* 1970; 5:13–21.
48. Albertson KW, Doppman JL, Ramsey R. Spinal seizures induced by contrast media. *Radiology.* 1973; 107:349–51.
49. Harrington G, Michie C, Lynch PR et al. Blood-brain barrier changes associated with unilateral cerebral angiography. *Invest Radiol.* 1966; 1:431–40.
50. Dempsey PF, Goree JA, Jimenez JP et al. The effect of contrast media on patient motion during cerebral angiography. *Radiology.* 1975; 115:207–9.
51. Bentson JR, Wilson GH. Clinical comparison of three contrast agents used in cerebral angiography. *Invest Radiol.* 1976; 11:602–4.
52. Mani RL, Eisenberg RL. Complications of catheter cerebral angiography: analysis of 5000 procedures. III. Assessment of arteries injected, contrast medium used, duration of procedure and age of patient. *Am J Roentgenol.* 1978; 131:871–4.
53. Kricheff II, Chase NE. Evaluation of complication rates of meglumine diatrizoate and meglumine iothalamate in cerebral angiography. *Radiology.* 1967; 101:220–3.
54. Gensini GG, DiGiorgi S. Myocardial toxicity of contrast agents used in angiography. *Radiology.* 1964; 82:24–34.
55. Brown TG. Cardiovascular actions of angiographic media. *Angiology.* 1967; 18:273–81.
56. Gootman N, Rudolph AM, Buckley NM. Effects of angiographic contrast media on cardiac function. *Am J Cardiol.* 1970; 25:59–65.
57. Paulin S, Adams DF. Increased ventricular fibrillation during coronary arteriography with a new contrast medium preparation. *Radiology.* 1971; 101:45–50.
58. Hildner FJ, Scherlag B, Samet P. Evaluation of Renografin-M-76 as a contrast agent for angiocardiography. *Radiology.* 1971; 100:329–34.
59. Snyder C, Cramer R, Amplatz K. Isolation of sodium as a cause of ventricular fibrillation. *Invest Radiol.* 1971; 6:245–8.
60. Simon AL, Shabetai R, Lang JH et al. The mechanism of production of ventricular fibrillation in coronary angiography. *Am J Roentgenol.* 1972; 114:810–5.
61. Carter AM, Olin T. Toxicity of roentgen contrast media at selective injection into the coronary artery in the rabbit. *Invest Radiol.* 1973; 10:73–8.
62. Refsum H, Passwal M. Arrhythmogenic and cardiodepressive effects of contrast media on isolated rat atria. *Invest Radiol.* 1978; 13:444–9.
63. Snyder CF, Formanek A, Frech RS et al. The role of sodium in promoting ventricular arrhythmia during selective coronary arteriography. *Am J Roentgenol.* 1971; 113:567–71.
64. Salvensen S, Nelsen PL, Holterman H. Ameliorating effect of calcium and magnesium ions on the toxicity of Isopaque sodium. II. Studies on the isolated heart and auricles of the rabbit. *Acta Radiol.* (Scand) [Suppl]. 1967; 270:30–43.
65. Ovitt T, Rizk G, French RS et al. Electrocardiographic changes in selective coronary arteriography: the importance of ions. *Radiology.* 1972; 104:705–8.
66. Tragardh B, Bove AA, Lynch PR. Cardiac conduction abnormalities during coronary arteriography in dogs: reduced effects of a new contrast medium. *Invest Radiol.* 1974; 9:340–5.
67. Frech RS. Toxicity studies of coronary arteriographic media in dogs. *Invest Radiol.* 1975; 10:323–8.
68. Tragardh B, Lynch PR, Vinciguerra T. Cardiac function during coronary arteriography with calcium enriched diatrizoate and metrizamide. *Invest Radiol.* 1976; 11:569–76.
69. Popio KA, Ross AM, Oravec JM et al. Identification and description of separate mechanisms for two components of Renografin cardiotoxicity. *Circulation.* 1978; 58:520–8.
70. Tragardh B, Almen T, Lynch P. Addition of calcium or other cations and of oxygen to ionic and non-ionic contrast media. *Invest Radiol.* 1975; 10:231–8.
71. Wolpers HG, Hunneman DH, Stellway M et al. Calcium binding by arteriographic contrast media. *J Pharm Sci.* 1981; 70:231–2.
72. Caulfield JB, Zir L, Harthorne JW. Blood calcium levels in the presence of arteriographic contrast material. *Circulation.* 1975; 52:119–23.
73. Thomson KR, Violante MR, Kenyon T et al. Reduction in ventricular fibrillation using calcium enriched Renografin-76. *Invest Radiol.* 1978; 13:238–40.
74. Violante MR, Thomson KR, Fischer HW et al. Ventricular fibrillation from diatrizoate with and without chelating agents. *Radiology.* 1978; 128:497–8.
75. Murdock DK, Euler DE, Kozeny G et al. Ventricular fibril-

lation during coronary angiography in dogs: the role of calcium-binding additives. *Am J Cardiol.* 1984; 54:897–901.
76. Fischer HW, Morris TW. Possible factors in intravascular contrast media toxicity. *Invest Radiol.* 1980; 15:S232–8.
77. Holder JC, Dalrymple GV. Choosing a contrast material for aortofemoral runoff angiography. *Radiology.* 1978; 128:787–8.
78. Sommer FG, Laglia A, Goldberg RT. Pain accompanying leg venography: a comparison of sodium and methylglucamine diatrizoates. *Radiology.* 1979; 133:790–1.
79. Friedenberg MJ. Double blind clinical comparison of Conray with Renografin and Hypaque in peripheral angiography. *Am J Roentgenol.* 1964; 91:1371–80.
80. Pearson MC, Gilkes R, Hall JH et al. Sodium or methyglucamine? A comparison of iothalamates in urography. *Br J Radiol.* 1971; 44:55–7.
81. Penry JB, Livingston A. A comparison of diagnostic effectiveness and vascular side effects of various diatrizoate salts used for intravenous pyelography. *Clin Radiol.* 1972; 23:362–9.
82. Fuju K, Grayson T, Margulis AR et al. The effects of intraarterial injection of contrast media on canine intestine. *Am J Roentgenol.* 1963; 89:730–3.
83. Wiedeman MP. Vascular and intravascular responses to various contrast media. *Angiology.* 1963; 14:107–9.
84. Taenzer V, Koeppe P, Samwer KF et al. Comparative pharmacokinetics of sodium and methylglucamine diatrizoate in urography. *Eur J Clin Pharm.* 1973; 6:137–40.
85. McClennon BL, Becker JL. Excretory urography. *Radiology.* 1971; 100:591–6.
86. Dacie JE, Fry IK. A comparison of methylglucamine diatrizoate in clinical urography. *Br J Radiol.* 1971; 44:51–4.
87. Brennan RE, Curtis JA, Pollack HM et al. Computer tomography explorations of renal physiology: contrast excretion by the normal kidney. *Am J Roentgenol.* 1979; 135:206. Abstract.
88. Dure-Smith P. The dose of contrast medium in intravenous urography: a physiologic assessment. *Am J Roentgenol.* 1970; 108:691–7.
89. Standalnik RC, Vera Z, DeSilva O et al. Electrocardiographic response to intravenous urography: prospective evalution of 275 patients. *Am J Roentgenol.* 1977; 129:825–30.
90. Pfister RC, Hutter AM. Cardiac alterations during intravenous urography. *Invest Radiol.* 1980; 15:S239–42.
91. Wood BP, Smith WL. Pulmonary edema in infants following injection of contrast media for urography. *Radiology.* 1981; 139:377–9.
92. Littner MR, Rosenfield AT, Ulreich S et al. Evaluation of bronchospasm during excretory urography. *Radiology.* 1977; 124:17–21.
93. Littner MR, Ulreich S, Putnam CE et al. Bronchospasm during excretory urography. Lack of specificity for the methylglucamine cation. *Am J Roentgenol.* 1981; 137:477–81.
94. Hayes CW, Foster JH, Sewell R et al. Experimental evaluation of concentrated solutions of iothalamic acid derivatives as angiographic contrast media. *Am J Roentgenol.* 1966; 97:755–61.
95. Gerzof SG, Robbins AH, Unger G et al. Double-blind comparison of meglumine iodamide and Renografin-60 for excretory urography. *Am J Roentgenol.* 1977; 128:211–5.
96. Robbins AG, Rosenfield AT, Pizzolato NF et al. Drip infusion urography with meglumine iodamide. *Am J Roentgenol.* 1978; 131:1043–6.
97. Popky GL, Griska LB, Hough JL. Comparison of meglumine iodamide and sodium diatrizoate for excretory urography. *Curr Ther Res.* 1981; 30:786–92.
98. Berger RE, Gomez LS, Mallette LE. Acute hypocalcemic effects of clinical contrast media injections. *Am J Roentgenol.* 1982; 138:283–8.
99. Mallette LE, Gomez LS. Systemic hypocalcemia after clinical injection of radiographic contrast media. Amelioration by omission of calcium chelating agents. *Radiology.* 1983; 147:677–9.
100. Tirone P, Rosati G. Radiopaque contrast media 29. Toxicologic studies with iodoxamic acid, a new intravenous cholegraphic agent. *Farmaco* (Sci). 1973; 28:1011–23.
101. Scholz FJ, Johnston DO, Wise RE. Intravenous cholangiography. *Radiology.* 1975; 114:513–8.
102. Robbins AH, Sargent EN, Vincent ME et al. Double-blind comparison of meglumine iodoxamate (Cholovue) and meglumine iodipamide (Cholografin). *Am J Roentgenol.* 1976; 127:257–60.
103. Cronin RE. Acute renal failure with radiographic contrast media. *Semin Nephrol.* 1981; 1:51–5.
104. Shafi T, Chow SY, Porush JG et al. Infusion intravenous pyelography and renal function. *Arch Intern Med.* 1978; 138:1218–21.
105. Carvallo A, Rakowski TA, Argy WP et al. Acute renal failure following drip infusion pyelography. *Am J Med.* 1978; 65:38–56.
106. Eisenberg RL, Bank WO, Hedgock MW. Renal failure after major angiography can be avoided with hydration. *Am J Roentgenol.* 1981; 136:859–61.
107. D'Elia JA, Gleason RE, Alday M et al. Nephrotoxicity from angiographic contrast material. *Am J Med.* 1982; 72:719–25.
108. Harkonen S, Kjellstrand C. Contrast nephropathy. *Am J Nephrol.* 1981; 1:69–77.
109. Diaz-Buxo JA, Wagoner RD, Hattery RR et al. Acute renal failure after excretory urography in diabetic patients. *Ann Intern Med.* 1975; 83:155–8.
110. Weintraub LA, Healy RW, Leland OS Jr et al. Coronary angiography and acute renal failure in diabetic azotemic nephropathy. *Ann Intern Med.* 1977; 86:56–9.
111. Bettman MA, Paulin S. Leg phlebography: the incidence, nature and modification of undesirable side effects. *Radiology.* 1977; 122:101–4.

Therapy Reviews

Treatment of infectious complications of acquired immunodeficiency syndrome

MELISSA M. FURIO AND CINDY J. WORDELL

Abstract: The infectious complications of the acquired immunodeficiency syndrome (AIDS) are discussed, and the conventional and nonconventional therapies used for these infections are reviewed.

The infections most commonly encounterd in patients with AIDS are *Pneumocystis carinii* pneumonia (58%), *Candida* esophagitis (31%), toxoplasmosis (21%), cytomegalovirus infections (15%), and herpes-simplex virus infections (12%). *Pneumocystis carinii* pneumonia is the most common life-threatening process in these patients. Trimethoprim-sulfamethoxazole (TMP-SMZ) is considered the drug of choice for its treatment. Oral candidiasis often indicates the progression to AIDS in the high-risk populations of homosexual or bisexual men, intravenous drug abusers, and individuals with hemophilia. Nystatin suspension is commonly used to treat oral candidiasis, while *Candida* esophagitis demands systemic therapy with ketoconazole. Toxoplasmosis most commonly manifests itself in patients with AIDS as a cerebral mass lesion. The recommended therapy includes sulfadiazine and pyrimethamine. AIDS patients frequently experience protozoal invasion of the intestinal tract with *Giardia lamblia, Isospora belli,* and *Cryptosporidium muris.* Various drugs have been tried for these infections, including quinacrine hydrochloride, metronidazole, TMP-SMZ, and spiramycin. Cytomegalovirus (CMV) infections commonly involve the lungs, gastrointestinal tract, eyes, brain, and nervous system. Attempts to treat these disseminated CMV infections with antiviral agents, including acyclovir, have not been successful. However, acyclovir has been found beneficial in the treatment of herpes-simplex virus infections.

Multiple infectious complications may occur in patients with AIDS as a result of the cellular-immune deficiency associated with this disease. Until more research is done with AIDS patients, therapy must be based on the data available from the treatment of these infections in immunosuppressed patients without AIDS.

Index terms: Acquired immunodeficiency syndrome; Acyclovir; Anthelmintics; Antifungals; Anti-infective agents; Antiprotozoals; Antivirals; Candidiasis; Herpesvirus infections; Ketoconazole; Metronidazole; Nystatin; Protozoan infections; Pyrimethamine; Spiramycin; Quinacrine hydrochloride; Sulfadiazine; Sulfamethoxazole; Sulfonamides; Trimethoprim; Toxoplasmosis
Clin Pharm. 1985; 4:539–54

In 1981, the acquired immunodeficiency syndrome (AIDS) was first identified and the Centers for Disease Control began recording its occurrence.[1] The populations at highest risk for contracting AIDS appear to be homosexual or bisexual men, intravenous drug abusers, and individuals with hemophilia.

To assist in the identification of AIDS cases, a surveillance definition of the syndrome was developed.[1] Currently, the diagnosis of AIDS requires both of the following:

1. The existence of a diagnosis that predicts a cellular immune deficiency, and
2. The absence of an underlying condition that can be identified as a cause for the cellular immune deficiency.

The diseases associated with a cellular immune deficiency include cancer (Kaposi's sarcoma), protozoal infections (cryptosporidiosis, *Pneumocystis carinii* pneumonia, toxoplasmosis), fungal infections (aspergillosis, candidiasis, cryptococcosis),

MELISSA M. FURIO, PHARM.D., is Clinical Pharmacist in Medical Oncology, and CINDY J. WORDELL, PHARM. D., is Drug Information Coordinator, Thomas Jefferson University Hospital, Philadelphia.

Address reprint requests to Dr. Furio at the Department of Pharmacy, Thomas Jefferson University Hospital, 111 South 11th Street, Philadelphia, PA 19107.

The assistance of Sheila M. Nelson in the preparation of the manuscript is acknowledged.

atypical mycobacteria (*Mycobacterium avium-intracellulare*), and viral infections (*cytomegalovirus, herpes simplex* virus).[1]

The infections most commonly encountered in patients with AIDS are *Pneumocystis carinii* pneumonia (58%), *Candida* esophagitis (31%), cryptococcosis (23%), toxoplasmosis (21%), cytomegalovirus (15%), and herpes simplex virus (12%).[1] These infections frequently occur as multiple infections rather than as a single infection. Since patients with AIDS lack adequate cellular immune function, infections can be difficult to control with conventional therapy. This leads to the use of nonconventional therapy, sometimes with agents that are difficult to find information about and to obtain. The Centers for Disease Control AIDS Task Force indicated that as of April 30, 1985, more than 10,000 cases of AIDS had been documented.[2] As the number of cases increases, many of these less common agents will have to be used to manage the opportunistic infections these patients acquire.

In this paper, the infectious complications of AIDS and the drug therapy for these infections are discussed. We have placed an emphasis on the nonconventional agents since information on these drugs is most difficult to obtain when the need arises. Unfortunately, the literature available to evaluate the management of these infections in AIDS patients frequently consists only of case reports or case series. Many immunosuppressed patients without AIDS have the same infectious complications as patients with AIDS. Until more published experience in patients with AIDS is available, the literature for the non-AIDS immunosuppressed population will have to serve as a guide for therapy selection in patients with AIDS.

Mycobacterial Infections

Mycobacterium avium-intracellulare is actually a complex of two strains of mycobacteria (*M. avium* and *M. intracellulare*) that are very similar in structure, biochemical identification, and serology.[3,4] This complex can be differentiated into several serotypes that vary in their virulence.[3] In the past, *M. avium-intracellulare* resulted in disseminated infection only rarely, with those few cases occurring in immunosuppressed patients or patients with underlying serious illnesses.[4] Since the identification of AIDS, there have been several reports of disseminated *M. avium-intracellulare* infection in this population.[5-12] The organism has been isolated from multiple sites in these patients including the lung, lymph nodes, spleen, bone marrow, brain, adrenal glands, gastrointestinal tract, and blood. Disseminated *M. avium-intracellulare* infections are often fatal in patients with AIDS, and they are frequently not discovered until a postmortem examination.

Antibacterial treatment of disseminated *M. avium-intracellulare* infections has not been very successful, primarily because of its high degree of resistance to standard antitubercular therapy. Therefore, a five- or six-drug regimen is usually used. Davidson[4] recommended the use of a combination of isoniazid, rifampin, ethambutol, streptomycin or capreomycin, ethionamide, and cycloserine for the first year of treatment as long as there is improvement in patient condition and they are tolerated. If drug toxicity develops to one of the agents, pyrazinamide has been suggested as an acceptable alternative. The resistance of *M. avium-intracellulare* infections to conventional drug therapy has led to the use of investigational agents. Following a recent review of 13 cases of disseminated *M. avium-intracellulare* infection in patients without AIDS, Horsburgh et al.[13] recommended a regimen for initial treatment that included isoniazid plus ethambutol, cycloserine, clofazimine, ethionamide, and rifampin or ansamycin.

In reviewing these cases, Horsburgh et al.[13] noted that the patients who received cycloserine had a better response than those who did not. When isoniazid was added to a regimen containing cycloserine, this response was further improved, suggesting an additive effect between these drugs. These investigators also reported that seven of the eight patients receiving clofazimine responded.

Based on our review of the literature, patients in whom a disseminated infection with *M. avium-intracellulare* is suspected should receive initial treatment with ethambutol, streptomycin, clofazimine, ethionamide, and rifampin or ansamycin. The recommended doses and common adverse effects of these agents are shown in Table 1. Cases of disseminated *M. avium-intracellulare* occurring in patients with AIDS that have been reported in the literature have been treated with both clofazimine [6,9] and ansamycin.[6,7,9]

Clofazimine (Lamprene, Ciba-Geigy) is a substituted phenazine quinoneimine dye that is an important drug in the treatment of *M. leprae*, in particular dapsone-resistant strains.[14,15] Davidson et al.[16] provided one of the initial reports of its effectiveness in vivo against *M. avium-intracellulare* infections. In treating nine patients for *M. intracellulare* infections (six with only pulmonary disease and three with disseminated infections), the addition of clofazimine 300 mg daily to a regimen of five or six antitubercular agents led to improvement in all three of the patients with disseminated disease. At this dose, serum clofazimine concentrations reached 1.8 to 3.5 μg/mL after two or more months of starting therapy. Clinical isolates from AIDS patients with disseminated *M. avium-intracellulare* have in vitro minimum inhibitory concentrations (MICs) for clofazimine of 2–5 μg/mL.[5,6] The serum drug concentrations attained with this dose would be adequate for use in a multiple-drug regimen for the managment of disseminated *M. avium-intracel-*

Table 1.
Drugs Used to Treat the Infectious Complications of AIDS and Their Common Adverse Effects

Disease	Drug Regimen	Common Adverse Effects
Mycobacterial Infections		
Mycobacterium avium-intracellulare[a]	Isoniazid 300 mg orally daily	Peripheral neuropathy, central nervous system manifestations
	Rifampin 600 mg orally daily	Gastrointestinal irritation, drug fever, pruritus
	Ethambutol hydrochloride 25 mg/kg/day orally for six weeks then 15/mg/kg/day	Optic neuritis, peripheral neuritis, headache
	Streptomycin 0.75–1.0 g (as the sulfate salt) daily intramuscularly for two months then 2–3 times a week	Vertigo, paresthesias, nausea, tinnitus
	Capreomycin 1 g (as the sulfate salt) daily intramuscularly (alternative to streptomycin)	Nephrotoxicity, ototoxicity, eosinophilia
	Ethionamide 500–1000 mg orally daily in 1–3 divided doses	Gastrointestinal irritation, goiter, rashes
	Cycloserine 750–1000 mg orally daily in 2–4 divided doses	Convulsions, headache, psychoses
	Pyridoxine hydrochloride 100 mg orally daily	
	Pyrazinamide 25 mg/kg/day orally (alternative if toxicity develops)	Arthralgias, hyperuricemia
Resistant *M. avium-intracellulare*[a]	Ansamycin 150–300 mg orally daily (for rifampin-resistant cases)	Minimal information; adverse effects appear similar to rifampin
	Clofazimine 300 mg orally daily in three divided doses	Skin discoloration, pigmentation (skin and ocular), ichthyosis, gastrointestinal
Protozoal Infections		
Pneumocystis carinii pneumonia	Trimethoprim-sulfamethoxazole (TMP-SMZ) Oral: 20 mg/kg/day TMP + 100 mg/kg/day SMZ in four divided doses Intravenous: 15 mg/kg/day TMP + 75 mg/kg/day SMZ in four divided doses	Crystalluria, skin rash, leukopenia, gastrointestinal disorders, fever
	or	
	Pentamidine isethionate 4 mg/kg/day intramuscularly or intravenously	Intramuscular: pain on injection, swelling, sterile abscesses Intravenous: thrombophlebitis, facial flushing, tachycardia, hypotension, metallic taste, nephrotoxicity, glycosuria
Toxoplasma gondii	Sulfadiazine 1 g orally four times daily	Allergy, rash, drug fever, neurotoxicity
	and	
	Pyrimethamine 25 mg orally daily	Bone-marrow suppression, blood dyscrasias
Giardia lamblia	Quinacrine hydrochloride 100 mg orally three times daily	Dizziness, headache, fever, jaundiced appearance
	or	
	Metronidazole 250–500 mg orally three times daily (alternative)	Nausea, headache, metallic taste, disulfiram reactions
Isospora belli	Trimethoprim 160 mg/sulfamethoxazole 800 mg orally four times daily	Anemia, rash, gastrointestinal irritation, central nervous system toxicity
Cryptosporidium muris	Spiramycin 1 g orally three to four times daily	Diarrhea, nausea, vomiting, epigastric pain, giddiness
Fungal Infections		
Candida albicans		
Oral thrush	Nystatin 500,000 units swish in mouth 4–6 times daily	
	or	Nontoxic, rare topical sensitization
	Clotrimazole 10 mg (1 troche) orally five times daily	Nontoxic
Esophagitis	Ketoconazole 400 mg orally daily	Elevated liver function test results, nausea, vomiting, abdominal pain
Transient fungemia	Amphotericin B 0.3 mg/kg/day i.v.	Fever, chills, nausea, thrombophlebitis, anemia, impaired renal function, hypokalemia
Disseminated disease with or without pneumonia	Amphotericin B 0.6 mg/kg/day i.v.	Same effects as listed above
Cryptococcus neoformans		
Meningeal	Amphotericin B 0.3 mg/kg/day i.v.	Same effects as listed above
	plus	
	Flucytosine 150 mg/kg/day orally in four divided doses	Occasional nausea, vomiting, diarrhea, bone marrow depression, elevated liver function tests
Nonmeningeal	Ketoconazole 400 mg orally daily	Same effects as listed above
Histoplasma capsulatum	Amphotericin B 0.6 mg/kg/day i.v.	Same effects as listed above
Petriellidium boydii	Miconazole 600 mg intravenously every eight hours	Frequent phlebitis, nausea, vomiting, fever, chills, pruritus, anemia, and thrombocytosis (dose-related)

Continued on following page

Table 1. *(Continued from previous page)*

Disease	Drug Regimen	Common Adverse Effects
Aspergillus	Amphotericin B 0.6 mg/kg/day i.v.	Same effects as listed above
	or	
	Amphotericin B 0.3 mg/kg/day i.v.	Same effects as listed above
	and	
	Flucytosine 150 mg/kg/day orally in four divided doses	Same effects as listed above
Coccidioides immitis	Amphotericin B 0.6 mg/kg/day i.v.	Same effects as listed above
	Ketoconazole 400 mg orally daily (for the treatment failures)	Same effects as listed above
Viral Infections		
Cytomegalovirus	Acyclovir 500 mg/sq m intravenously every eight hours for seven days[b,c]	Bone-marrow suppression, increased creatinine, increased SGOT and SGPT concentrations, central nervous system manifestations
Herpes simplex	Acyclovir 250 mg/sq m intravenously every eight hours for seven days	Same effects as listed above
	or	
	Vidarabine 15 mg/kg/day intravenously over 12 hours for 10 days	Gastrointestinal (nausea, vomiting, diarrhea), skin rash, hallucinations
Herpes zoster	Acyclovir 500 mg/sq m intravenously every eight hours for seven days[b]	Same effects as listed above
	or	
	Vidarabine 10 mg/kg/day intravenously over 12 hours for 10 days	Same effects as listed above

[a] A five- or six-drug combination is used for disseminated *M. intracellulare* infections. For immunocompromised patients, ansamycin and clofazimine are included in the regimen. Rifampin is not used with ansamycin. Initial regimen for AIDS patients should include ethambutol, streptomycin, clofazimine, ethionamide, and rifampin or ansamycin.

[b] Not approved by FDA for this dose and indication.

[c] Will probably not be effective.

lulare in AIDS patients. These serum concentrations are also well above the in vitro MICs of 0.6 μg/mL and 0.3 μg/mL reported for two laboratory strains of *M. avium-intracellulare*.[17]

Clofazimine is a very lipophilic compound.[14] It has a half-life estimated to be a minimum of 70 days.[15] When administered to volunteers, 0.01–0.41% of a single dose was excreted in the urine in a 24-hour period with 11–59% of a single dose excreted in the feces in three days.[15]

The long history of clofazimine use in the treatment of leprosy has shown that its adverse effects depend on both the dose and duration of treatment. The major adverse effects involve the skin, eyes, and gastrointestinal tract. The most common adverse effect is pigmentation of the skin. This was a complaint in 64.6% of the patients in a review of the side effects noted by patients with leprosy taking clofazimine.[18] This hyperpigmentation appears initially as redness during the first month of treatment. This is probably attributable to the accumulation of the drug in the reticuloendothelial cells and subcutaneous fat of the skin.[19] During the treatment of leprosy, a black-brown color develops in the areas of the lesions.[19] Another troublesome adverse dermatologic effect of clofazimine is dry skin (ichthyosis) reported in 35.4% of the patients.[18] This can be improved through application of urea cream.[20]

Conjunctival pigmentation is the second most common adverse effect of clofazimine.[18] Other ocular toxicities that have been reported include the appearance of fine brown lines in the cornea and deposition of pigment in the macular area of the fundus. These changes may be reversible when therapy is discontinued.[21-23]

The most common gastrointestinal adverse effect is abdominal pain, reported in approximately one third of the leprosy patients treated with clofazimine.[18] Other complaints include nausea, vomiting, and diarrhea,[24,25] which have been accompanied by malabsorption.[26] On radiologic or laparoscopic examination, the serosal surface may be edematous.[24,25] On gross examination, the viscera may be stained an orange-yellow color,[25-27] and crystal deposition has been found in visceral tissue.[25,26,28]

Clofazimine is available from the Ciba-Geigy Corporation for use in immunocompromised patients. The dose used in the literature cases of disseminated *M. avium-intracellulare* was 300 mg daily.[6]

Ansamycin (LM 427) is a rifamycin-S derivative classified as a spiropiperidyl rifamycin that is manufactured by Farmitalia Carlo Erba Research Laboratories in Milan, Italy.[29] Ansamycin has very good in vitro activity against *M. tuberculosis*[30,31] and *M. avium-intracellulare*.[29,30,32]

The in vitro MICs for 12 *M. avium-intracellulare* clinical isolates were determined for both rifampin and ansamycin. All 12 strains were inhibited by ansamycin at a concentration of 2.0 μg/mL. Rifampin at the same concentration inhibited only two strains. When the in vitro susceptibility to ansamycin of 155 *M. avium-intracellulare* clinical isolates was determined, 81.3% of the strains were susceptible at a concentration of 1.0 μg/mL. Only 5.8% of the strains were susceptible to the same concentration of rifampin.[29] A similar in vitro study found that 66 of 68 clinical isolates of *M. avium-intracellulare* were resistant to 1 μg/mL of rifampin. With an increase in the rifampin concentration to a concentration of 5–10 μg/mL, 60% of the isolates were sensitive. Only those isolates resistant to a rifampin concentration of 10 μg/mL were also resistant to ansamycin.[32] In vitro MICs for *M. avium-intracellulare* isolates from patients with AIDS have been 2 μg/mL or less.[5,6,28]

The resistance of *M. avium-intracellulare* to rifampin is probably because of the poor absorption of rifampin by the bacteria. The higher lipophilic nature of ansamycin allows it to be better absorbed into the bacteria, leading to greater sensitivity.[29] Ansamycin is available from the Centers for Disease Control (CDC) after obtaining an investigational new drug (IND) number from FDA. The dosage of ansamycin recommended by CDC for use in disseminated *M. avium-intracellulare* infections is 150–300 mg/day.[a]

Mycobacterium tuberculosis has been reported to occur as an opportunistic infection in patients with AIDS. It has often been the presenting infection seen in Haitian immigrants seeking medical treatment for the initial diagnosis of AIDS.[10,33] The treatment of *M. tuberculosis* infections and disseminated *M. tuberculosis* in the immunocompromised patient involves standard regimens.[34,35] *M. tuberculosis* is not as resistant to the commonly employed antituberculosis agents as *M. avium-intracellulare*. The drug regimens and adverse effects of antitubercular agents are reviewed in detail elsewhere.[34,36]

Mycobacterium xenopi has been isolated from cultures of sputum and liver biopsy specimens obtained from a patient with AIDS.[37] *M. xenopi* has also been isolated from both hot and cold tap water and the water supplies of hospitals. This Mycobacterium is not usually pathogenic but it can be in the immunocompromised host. It has also been frequently isolated from the tonsils during screening.[3] *M. xenopi* is easily eradicated during multiple-drug therapy with commonly used antitubercular agents. It is important to differentiate this Mycobacterium from the more drug-resistant *M. avium-intracellulare*.[37]

Protozoal Infections

Pneumocystis carinii. *Pneumocystis carinii* pneumonia (PCP) is the most common life-threatening process in patients with AIDS. It is one of the two most common initial manifestations of AIDS, along with oral candidiasis. PCP is an initial diagnostic marker in 50% of AIDS patients.[38,39]

PCP is believed to be a protozoan, although the exact taxonomy has not been established. The remarkable feature of this organism, and the disease it causes, is that it remains localized to the lungs with rare exceptions, even in the most severely immunocompromised patients.[40] Early work revealed that the entire life cycle of *P. carinii* occurs extracellularly within the alveoli.[41]

The classic clinical features of PCP include high temperature (38.5 °C) with drenching night sweats, progressive weight loss (10–15 pounds), a dry nonproductive cough, and dyspnea, which may eventually progress to cyanosis and respiratory failure.[38,40] Few rales and other auscultatory findings are noted upon examination. Unexplained diarrhea, either continuous or intermittent, may often precede the pneuomonitis, with or without identification of an enteric pathogen. Other clinical features include frontal alopecia and seborrheic dermatitis over the face and scalp with concurrent facial erythema.

Although the survival rates are relatively similar for patients with AIDS versus non-AIDS PCP (50% versus 57%), there are some striking clinical differences between these two populations.[42] PCP is a more insidious process in patients with AIDS, and drug therapy in these patients is complicated by frequent adverse reactions. Upon diagnosis, the median duration of symptoms for patients with AIDS is 28 days versus 5 days for patients without AIDS. Patients with AIDS have less fever, less tachypnea, and less hypoxemia than patients without AIDS. They also have a lower mean respiratory rate (23.4 versus 30 breaths/min) and a higher median room-air arterial oxygen tension (69 versus 52 mm Hg). Patients without AIDS typically respond faster to drug therapy than patients with AIDS.

Pneumocystis carnii can occasionally be identified in stained sputum, gastric contents, tracheal aspirations, and swabbed specimens from the hypopharynx. The cyst form of the organism is readily identified with Gomori's methenamine-silver or toluidine-blue stains such as Giemsa or Weigert-Gram.[40] An advantage to staining with Giemsa versus methenamine-silver, is that it allows the organism to be identified more quickly.[39] These stains can be used on concentrated lavage fluid or on a tracheal preparation of biopsy tissue.

A typical chest roentgenogram of a patient with PCP shows diffuse bilateral alveolar and interstitial disease beginning in the perihilar areas and lower lung fields and progressing to the lung parenchyma. Changes in the chest roentgenograms are often more subtle in patients with AIDS than in other patients with PCP. Blood gases should be monitored since these measurements reflect any improvement or worsening of disease (and alveolar-capillary block syndrome).

The therapeutic challenge presented by PCP is great since it is virtually exclusive to the immunocompromised host.[43] Early success was seen with trimethoprim-sulfamethoxazole (TMP-SMZ) in the treatment of documented *Pneumocystis* infections complicating childhood neoplasms.[44] In a prospective trial, Hughes et al.[44] found no difference in efficacy between TMP-SMZ and pentamidine isethionate, but the former had fewer side effects. This led to the use of TMP-SMZ as the drug of choice for biopsy-proven disease in adults.[45] Studies in rats have shown no advantage in treating PCP infections with both pentamidine and TMP-SMZ simultaneously, and it is possible that this combination regimen may be more toxic.[43]

TMP-SMZ prevents the biosynthesis of tetrahydrofolic acid, the active metabolite of folic acid. The TMP component reversibly inhibits the enzyme dihydrofolate reductase, and SMZ competes with *p*-aminobenzoic acid in the production of dihydrofolate.[45] There is no significant difference in the survival rates of patients receiving oral versus intravenous TMP-SMZ.[43] Regimens using a combination of intravenous and oral therapy often are less effective and produce intermediate results. The recommended oral dose of TMP-SMZ is 20 mg/kg/day (based on the TMP component) in four divided doses. Because of the low serum concentrations on the first day, a loading dose of one-half of the total daily dose has been suggested.[45]

Since the relapse rates are higher for patients with AIDS treated with oral therapy, intravenous use may be more dependable, especially for the first few days. The recommended intravenous dose of TMP-SMZ is equivalent or 75% of the oral dose (15 mg/kg/day based on TMP) in four divided doses.[46] These recommendations are based on the renal elimination and potential nephrotoxicity of the SMZ component, which is poorly soluble and may cause crystalluria. Intravenous use may also be preferred in more seriously ill patients and in patients who have gastrointestinal disease that precludes oral use. The recommended duration of therapy is 10 to 14 days, or until the infection resolves.

Adverse reactions to TMP-SMZ often resulting in rash and leukopenia are seen in 65% of the patients with AIDS versus 12% of the patients without AIDS.[42] No cause has been found for these idiosyncratic effects on the bone marrow, and patients generally do not respond to empiric therapy with folinic acid.

Common toxicities from TMP-SMZ, occurring at the recommended doses, are skin rashes and gastrointestinal disturbances. The rashes are typically erythematous and maculopapular covering the entire body and are often associated with fevers. The rashes invariably develop after 8 to 12 days of therapy in patients with AIDS.[47] Patients with this reaction develop neutropenia, thrombocytopenia, bleeding, and superinfection that resolve upon discontinuing therapy. Upon rechallenge with the drug, the rash and fever often develop within one hour. AIDS patients seem to have a tenfold increase in the incidence of skin rashes, fever, and hematologic abnormalities over other hospitalized patients receiving TMP-SMZ therapy.[48] This raises a question as to the role of the underlying virus in developing these reactions. In patients with AIDS and Kaposi's sarcoma, one study found that the diffuse maculopapular skin rash developed a median of four days after the initiation of therapy. This occurred in patients with no previous allergy to sulfa or folate antagonists or family history of atopy.[49]

In a recent report of two cases of AIDS patients with PCP, both patients developed hypersensitivity reactions to TMP-SMZ. Both patients remained on intravenous TMP-SMZ therapy and were treated with diphenhydramine and epinephrine if bronchospasm was present. Both patients received a full course of therapy with resolution of their pneumonia. Aggressive use of intravenous diphenhydramine with each dose may be an alternative for patients who experience hypersensitivity reactions.[50]

Because of its renal elimination, doses must be adjusted for renal insufficiency; however, this is not a contraindication to TMP-SMZ therapy.[51] In patients with chronic renal failure, one half to one fifth of the recommended dose is given in three divided doses daily. Therapeutic drug concentration monitoring may be beneficial in this situation, with acceptable SMZ and TMP concentrations of 80–120 μg/mL and 4–10 μg/mL, respectively.[52,53]

When patients do not respond clinically to TMP-SMZ, it is often considered a poor prognostic indicator. Second-line drug therapy for PCP is pentamidine isethionate. Pentamidine interferes with aerobic glycolysis and also inhibits the synthesis of macromolecules by acting as a folic-acid antagonist.[46] This limits the growth and reproduction of *Pneumocystis carinii* by eliminating the supply of exogenous folate sources.

Pharmacokinetic data are limited, but pentamidine appears to be excreted intact in the urine and is bound to tissues, especially the kidney, liver, and lung.[54] Pentamidine isethionate should be administered at doses of 4 mg/kg/day for 10 to 14 days, although it may be continued for as long as 21 days. It may be administered intramuscularly or as a slow intravenous infusion (over 60 minutes) to avoid severe hypotension. The drug should be reconstituted fresh with sterile water for injection. The drug is commercially available from Lypho Med, Inc. and sold as an "orphan drug." It is available as the isethionate salt in 300 mg vials of lyophilized powder.[55] Pentamidine is approved in the United

States only for PCP, although it is used to treat leishmaniasis and trypanosomiasis elsewhere.

Immediate pentamidine toxicities include pain on injection, swelling, sterile abscesses with intramuscular use, and thrombophlebitis with intravenous use. Facial flushing, tachycardia, hypotension, and an unpleasant metallic taste are also common. Occasional delayed toxicities are related to the concentration of pentamidine in the tissues. Most common is renal toxicity in the form of azotemia, tubular toxicity, elevated potassium, and glycosuria. Dosing adjustment must be made if there are changes in renal function.[56] If the glomerular filtration rate drops to less than 50 mL/min, the dosing interval should be adjusted from every 24 hours to every 36 hours; if the rate is less than 10 mL/min, the medication should be given every 48 hours.

Abnormal liver-function test results and hepatotoxicity have been noted, but they do not require dose reduction. Megaloblastic anemia, arrhythmias, thrombocytopenia, hypocalcemia, and confusion and hallucinations have also been reported. The bone-marrow toxicities seen with pentamidine are more gradual in onset than those seen in patients receiving TMP-SMZ; severe neutropenia has been reported.[57] Pancreatitis may be another side effect of pentamidine as a temporal relationship between its administration and elevations in amylase concentrations were seen in a few cases.[58]

Another potentially life-threatening complication of pentamidine is the development of severe fasting hypoglycemia followed by insulin-dependent diabetes mellitus in some cases.[59–61] Blood glucose concentrations ranging from 15 to 41 mg/dL have been reported. It is hypothesized that the drug causes selective toxicity toward the β cells. There is possibly an early cytolytic release of insulin by pentamidine, with subsequent development of diabetes mellitus because of the β-cell destruction and insulin deficiency. One study reported a reversal of the hypoglycemia with oral diazoxide therapy in one patient.[59]

An unapproved third-line agent with some promising results in animal models is dapsone. The drug was used years ago as an antimalarial and is almost exclusively used now to treat dermatitis herpetiformis and leprosy. Because of its similarity to the sulfonamides, it was selected for trial in PCP infections, where it probably acts by affecting folate synthesis.[62] In a rat model, dapsone was tested at doses of 25 mg/kg/day and compared with conventional therapy with TMP-SMZ. For prophylaxis, both regimens prevented PCP-induced infection in all animals. For therapy, the drug was given for 2.5 weeks. At the end of this period, residual pneumonitis was seen in 50% of rats treated with TMP-SMZ, 75% of rats treated with dapsone, and 100% of the rats serving as controls. The authors concluded that dapsone could totally eradicate pneumonitis if treatment was initiated earlier in the course of the infection.

Dapsone was also given in doses of 100 mg daily for six weeks to AIDS patients with Kaposi's sarcoma.[63] After treatment with no other cytostatic medication, re-excision of Kaposi's lesions revealed no histology of sarcoma or fibrosis.

Official dosing recommendations for dapsone from the manufacturer are 100 mg daily (in a minimum of two divided doses) and concurrent TMP therapy of 20 mg/kg/day in four divided doses.[b] The manufacturer also suggests that dividing the dapsone dose into four daily doses may minimize the amount of hemolysis seen with the drug. Patients with glucose-6-phosphate dehydrogenase deficiency should be given dapsone 50 mg daily. Patients should be monitored cautiously for methemoglobulinemia.

Less common adverse effects include leukopenia, agranulocytosis, dermatitis, an infectious mononucleosis-like syndrome, fever, nausea, vomiting, abnormal liver-function test results, and peripheral neuropathy.[64–65]

Protection against recurrent PCP infections may be desirable in patients who have an unusually high risk for the infection. TMP-SMZ therapy at doses of 5 and 25 mg/kg/day orally in two divided doses has been successful.[66] However, the patients are only protected for as long as they take the medication. Unfortunately, prophylaxis is a problem if the patients have had hypersensitivity reactions or other serious side effects from TMP-SMZ. Recently, a combination of pyrimethamine-sulfadoxine (Fansidar) was given to AIDS patients with a history of PCP and hypersensitivity to TMP-SMZ. One tablet each week provided protection against PCP for a median of seven months in 75% of the patients.[67]

Toxoplasma gondii. *Toxoplasma gondii* is a protozoan that infects 20–40% of the adult population in the United States. After infection spread via raw meat or cat feces, the toxoplasma cysts lie dormant in the brain or muscle, contained by the cell-mediated immune response. With severe immune suppression, the cysts become metabolically active, tachyzoites invade the surrounding tissue, and serious disease occurs. Toxoplasmosis most commonly manifests itself in patients with AIDS as a cerebral mass lesion.[68] The organism has emerged as an important opportunistic pathogen in the compromised host that is capable of producing rapidly fatal disseminated infection. Despite its predilection for the central nervous system, the disease may be found in any organ system, including the heart, liver, lung, and spleen.

Clinical symptoms may include lymphadenopathy, hepatosplenomegaly, and persistent fever that is unresponsive to conventional antibiotic therapy. Focal abscess lesions can be seen with computerized tomography, usually in the basal ganglia. Nonspecific neurologic signs include a change in mental status, seizures, motor impairment, headache, and abnormal reflexes that can reflect both diffuse or focal involvement.

A diagnosis can often be made with serology test results for IgG antibodies and elevated antibody titers, and positive histologic findings for tachyzoites on lymph-node biopsy. Elevated protein and low glucose concentrations and no cells are found in the cerebrospinal fluid. Central nervous system lesions in patients with AIDS require a brain biopsy since serology results and cerebrospinal fluid cultures are usually not diagnostic. If the lesions are surgically inaccessible for a diagnosis, long-term empiric therapy is necessary.

The recommended therapy for toxoplasmosis generally is sulfadiazine 1 g orally every six hours and pyrimethamine 25 mg daily (after a 75-mg initial dose), which should be given for a prolonged period depending on the patient's clinical response.[69] If started early, this synergistic regimen provides an 80% response rate. The side effects of sulfa drugs are well known and pyrimethamine causes bone-marrow suppression that may be minimized by adding folinic acid (5 mg daily) therapy to the regimen.

For AIDS-related central nervous system toxoplasmosis, pyrimethamine 25 mg daily and sulfadiazine 1–1.5 g orally every six hours for 6–8 weeks is recommended. Concurrent folinic acid 10 mg orally or intravenously to bypass the folinic-acid blockage may be given. Rashes and bone-marrow suppression are common side effects. Neutropenia may occur, especially in patients receiving phenytoin therapy. In these situations, 50 mg of pyrimethamine alone should be given daily.

When administered for prolonged periods, clindamycin may penetrate the toxoplasma cysts and inhibit growth in chronically infected tissues, especially the spleen and liver. Drug concentrations do not reach the brain.[70] Clindamycin is a second alternative to pyrimethamine use in neutropenic patients.

Recurrent necrotizing retinochoroiditis appears to be attributable to the active multiplication of toxoplasma parasites in the retina.[71] The combination of clindamycin 300 mg (as the hydrochloride or palmitate salt) orally four times daily and sulfadiazine 1 g four times daily for four weeks provides coverage because of the high ocular tissue concentrations provided. Improvement usually results within the first 10 days of therapy.

Giardia lamblia. Another infectious complication for patients with AIDS is protozoal invasion of the intestinal tract. In an immunodeficient patient, eradication of the parasite may be impossible and life-long therapy may be required.

Infections with *Giardia lamblia* are frequently identified in the United States. Homosexual men are at great risk for this infection, and outbreaks are associated with water-borne contamination.[72] The most common symptoms are abdominal distress, diarrhea, and weight loss. A diagnosis is made by stool examination or by duodenal aspiration or small-bowel biopsy, if stool results are consistently negative.

The mainstay of therapy has been quinacrine hydrochloride 100 mg orally three times daily, providing a 95% cure rate in 7–10 days.[73] Expected side effects include dizziness, headache, fever, and yellowing of the urine, skin, and sclera because of distribution in the tissues. More frequently prescribed and equally effective is metronidazole in doses of 250–500 mg orally three times daily. The Centers for Disease Control has recommended its use as an alternative to quinacrine. This is an unlabeled indication by the manufacturer. The advantages of using metronidazole include its availability for injectable use and better patient tolerance than seen with quinacrine. Common side effects are nausea, headache, and lingering metallic taste. Disulfiram-like reactions may occur as well as potentiation of the hypoprothrombinemic activity of warfarin.

Furazolidone 100 mg orally four times a day for seven days provides variable cure rates in 77–92% of the patients. The drug causes brownish discoloration of the urine because of its metabolic degradation. Occasional hypersensitivity reactions occur including hypertension, urticaria, fever, arthralgia, nausea, vomiting, and headaches.[74]

Isospora belli. A rarely diagnosed small-bowel pathogen that may lead to chronic diarrhea, malabsorption, and long-term fever, is *Isospora belli*, also known as intestinal coccidiosis. Recent data suggest that the organism may be sexually transmitted and should be considered in the differential diagnosis of homosexual patients with diarrhea.[75]

Isospora belli may be identified by stool examination. Malabsorption is characterized by a low five-hour D-xylose test and a positive test for fat in the stool. The organism will respond to a prolonged course of TMP-SMZ. Doses of 160 mg (based on TMP) given every six hours orally for 10 days, followed by the same dose twice daily for three weeks are commonly used. A dramatic decrease in the amount of diarrhea can be seen within 48 hours after starting this therapy.[76]

Amprolium is a quarternary organic base used successfully in veterinary medicine as a coccidiostatic drug at doses of 25–66 mg/kg for poultry, calves, and lambs.[77] To date, the use of amprolium in patients with coccidiosis has not been reported, and its potential value in this disease is purely speculative.

Cryptosporidium muris. *Cryptosporidium muris* is an intestinal parasite well known to cause diarrhea in animals. During the past decade, this organism has been implicated in cryptosporidiosis, a chronic opportunistic infection in humans. Closely related to coccidia, these parasites have similar developmental stages in their life cycles. Cryptosporidia attach to the surface of the host cells, multiply and reproduce, and then form oocytes that detach and are passed out of the host in the feces.[78] The oocyst is the infective stage, and infection occurs by ingestion. Cryptosporidia have a predilection for the cells lining the small intestine, but have been isolated from the respiratory tract of birds. A recent report revealed isolation of cryptosporidium species in respiratory secretions and on the mucosal surface of a bronchial biopsy sample.[79] Organ involvement outside of the alimentary tract is not common, and challenges whether the organism is spread to the lungs hematogenously or by aspiration.

Within the intestine, this protozoan attaches to the surface of the mucosa and disrupts the microvilli. This leads to fusion of the villi and degeneration of enterocytes.[80] The spectrum of clinical illness is closely related to the underlying immune competence of the patient. Patients with normal immune function are either asymptomatic or develop self-limiting diarrhea for 1–2 weeks, whereas patients with immune dysfunction often develop chronic diarrhea. The illness is characterized by profuse, watery diarrhea without gross or macroscopic blood. Patients with AIDS with this complication experience enormous fluid losses averaging three liters per day, which is much greater than the amount in patients with normal immune function.[81] Other clinical manifestations of cryptosporidiosis include nausea, vomiting, anorexia, and mild epigastric pain.[81,82]

Routine examination for cryptosporidiosis oocysts in stool samples should be performed in all AIDS patients regardless of gastrointestinal symptoms, since asymptomatic carrier states have been reported.[83] The diagnosis of cryptosporidiosis has been made by histologic examination of small- or large-bowel biopsies or more simply by stool examination.[81] Standard ova and parasite examination are not effective. Cryptosporidia oocysts are small (4–5 μ) and are easily overlooked or confused with yeast. Acid-fast stains have proven useful because they stain most yeast blue-green and cryptosporidia red. Also, iodine "stained" wet mounts have been used. When both are negative, the "cover-slip flotation technique" may be used that has a dense sugar solution (Sheather's sugar) to levitate the oocysts in order to concentrate them.

A new staining method for detecting cryptosporidia oocysts in the feces uses a smear fixed in acid methanol. The smear is stained and heated with safranin and counterstained with methylene blue, which stains the oocysts a vivid orange-pink color.[84]

Because no effective treatment has been found for cryptosporidiosis, treatment must be symptomatic to include nutritional support and rehydration. Fluid and electrolyte replacement is essential to minimize wasting and weight loss.[85] Chronic diarrhea is frequent in patients with AIDS, and most patients need prolonged total parenteral nutrition.[86]

Investigators at the United States Department of Agriculture National Animal Disease Center have tested various drugs for efficacy against cryptosporidium in animals. Neither metronidazole, pentamidine, oxytetracycline, nor quinacrine were found effective.[81,82]

Various therapies have been tried in patients with cryptosporidiosis—TMP-SMZ (25 mg/kg sulfa equivalent four times daily) furazolidone (100 mg orally four times daily), metronidazole (750 mg orally three times daily), pyrimethamine-sulfadiazine (25 mg of pyrimethamine orally every day), diloxanide furoate (500 mg orally three times daily), quinacrine (100 mg orally three times daily), tetracycline (500 mg orally four times daily), and pentamidine (4 mg/kg intramuscularly every day). One study reported that one patient was cured in each of the furazolidone and diloxanide groups.[87] Diloxanide furoate (Furamide) is a substituted acetanilide used to treat mild forms of amoebiasis. It is produced in England and available from the Centers for Disease Control for investigational use. Its most common side effects are excessive flatulence and mild gastrointestinal discomfort.[74] Amprolium was tried in a patient at a dosage of 33 mg/kg daily. The doses were increased to 200 mg/kg, and the patient subsequently developed dyspnea, paralytic ileus, and neurologic sequelae.[77] Therapy was discontinued due to side effects; further investigational data are not available.

Preliminary data from the Centers for Disease Control suggest that some patients may respond to treatment with spiramycin or a combination of clindamycin and quinine. Clindamycin 300 mg and quinine 250 mg were given orally four times daily to six patients.[88] Two had no response after 1–2 weeks, three discontinued therapy because of adverse effects (severe rash, severe vomiting, and thrombocytopenia), and one patient had the diarrhea resolve within two days but persistent oocysts were found in the stools after therapy. If tolerated, this regimen may afford a symptomatic response in a few patients, but it has not provided a cure for cryptosporidiosis to date.

Spiramycin is a macrolide antibiotic with antimicrobial activity similar to clindamycin and erythromycin. It has been used to treat bacterial infections in Europe and Canada for more than 20 years. Given orally, spiramycin has irregular absorption from the gastrointestinal tract and is widely distributed throughout the body.[89] Tissue concentrations remain high for prolonged periods; elimination is primarily in the bile. Serious adverse effects are rare with this drug, although nausea, vomiting, and epigastric pain have been reported. Mild to moderate diarrhea has been reported at various doses. Two patients experienced sweating, giddiness, and paresthesias one hour after a 3-g dose.[88,89]

Three of 13 patients responded to spiramycin 1 g given orally 3 to 4 times daily. These results occurred after three to four weeks of therapy with improved symptoms and negative stools and intestinal biopsy. These patients were still asymptomatic six and seven months after therapy.[88] In another study involving nine patients with AIDS with severely debilitating diarrhea, spiramycin effectively resolved the diarrhea and provided symptomatic improvements.[90] Responses were generally seen within three days, but one patient required therapy for 30 days before a response was seen.

Spiramycin is not commercially available in the United States. The FDA has not approved this agent for routine use; consequently, it must be contacted in order to obtain an IND number so that the drug may be procured. Spiramycin (Rovamycin) is manufactured by Rhone-Poulenc Pharma, Montreal, Quebec, Canada, and it is available as 500-mg capsules. The recommended starting dose is 1 g given orally three times daily. A prolonged course of treatment may be warranted if the patient shows symptomatic improvement but the oocysts persist in the stool.

Fungal Infections

Candida albicans. *Candida albicans* is a member of the indigenous microbial flora of humans that multiplies rapidly to produce disease in immunocompromised patients. Since it is a strict aerobe, infections occur primarily in body cavities where the microorganism is usually found.[91] Patients commonly develop oral thrush before the documentation of Kaposi's sarcoma or a life-threatening opportunistic infection. It also persists after AIDS is documented. Mucocutaneous involvement may include the oral cavity, bronchopulmonary area, or alimentary tract. Systemic disease through lymphatic and hematogenous spread may include the urinary tract, endocarditis, meningitis, and septicemia. Allergic manifestations of candidal infections may occur, such as asthma, gastritis, and uveitis. Therefore, most adults will show a delayed hypersensitivity to *Candida* protein antigens for skin testing.

Oral candidiasis has been shown to indicate the progression to AIDS in at least 59% of the high-risk populations. Although esophageal candidiasis meets the surveillance definition, oral candidiasis currently does not.[92]

Oral candidiasis is characterized by patchy pseudomembranes or ulcers that are painful and debilitating. The therapy for oral thrush is either nystatin suspension 500,000 units to swish and swallow four to six times daily or clotrimazole troches dissolved in the mouth five times daily for 7 to 10 days.[93] Both are equally effective. The use of nystatin vaginal suppositories orally is generally poorly tolerated because of the unpalatability. For refractory cases, ketoconazole may be given in doses of 200–400 mg daily for 10 days.

Prophylaxis against repeated infections caused by candidal overgrowth is desirable in patients who have an especially high-relapse rate, such as patients with AIDS. Nystatin suspension and clotrimazole troches have both been used twice daily with some success.[94]

Candida esophagitis may appear in the presence or absence of oral candidiasis. Patients complain of dysphagia or retrosternal pain, which often mimic herpes infections in symptomatology. Topical therapy alone is not sufficient. Systemic therapy must be implemented with ketoconazole 400 mg daily or a short course of amphotericin B for refractory cases at doses of 100–150 mg intravenously for 5–7 days. If not treated adequately, esophagitis may lead to perforation and hemorrhage.[95]

Ketoconazole is often used to minimize the number of systemic yeast infections. A dose of 200 mg daily provides a tolerable effective prophylactic regimen.[95]

Amphotericin B penetrates well into the peritoneal cavity and peritoneal fluid.[96] The clinical manifestations of Candidal peritonitis include fever, peritoneal inflammation, positive peritoneal cultures, and purulent ascitic fluid. The recommended therapy includes high-dose intravenous amphotericin B (0.6 mg/kg/day) so that the drug may adequately penetrate the abdominal viscera. To minimize the risk of systemic reactions, intraperitoneal amphotericin B 5 mg/L may be given.[97]

Ocular involvement is observed fairly frequently with disseminated candidiasis. Pain or loss of vision or both are common with fundus lesions, while lesions in the peripheral areas are asymptomatic.[98] The local instillation of amphotericin will cause retinal damage, so systemic therapy is recommended with total doses of 500 mg to 1 g usually given for over a month. Regimens must be tailored to clinical regression, patient tolerance, and the extent of disease. Systemic therapy is required because the infection is spread hematogenously.

Another special application for amphotericin B is in *Candida* cystitis.[99] Patients with increased prophylactic antibiotic use and catheters are predisposed to infection. Drug therapy should be started if the patient's clinical condition requires therapy, instead of removing existing intravenous infusion lines and waiting for positive cultures. Alkalinization of the urine with 8–12 g of sodium bicarbonate in divided doses daily decreases the growth potential of *Candida* and will not interact with the amphotericin. Amphotericin bladder irrigations with 5 mg in 1 L of sterile water have been used for an average of 5–15 days.[100] A continuous irrigation administered with a three-way catheter will increase the contact time of the solution with the bladder. Therapy is continued until urine cultures are negative.

Transient candidal fungemia must be treated with low-dose amphotericin B therapy of 0.3 mg/kg/day for 7–14 days. Disseminated candidiasis and *Candida* pneumonia require full-dose amphotericin B therapy and, in cases of endocarditis, surgical intervention as well.

Cryptococcus neoformans. *Cryptococcus neoformans* is a yeast-like organism that forms a large polysaccharide capsule in the tissues. Infections occur through inhalation, thus the primary site of involvement is pulmonary. In immunocompromised hosts, the organism commonly disseminates into the central nervous system to produce meningitis. Roughly 5% of the patients with AIDS are infected with this organism. Although its usual presentation is as meningitis, cryptococcal pneumonia and fungemia may be present simultaneously or may be seen without meningitis. The disseminated disease is characterized by various combinations of fever, pulmonary infiltrates, malaise, and weight loss. Meningitis may initially manifest as insidious personality changes or changes in consciousness, a debilitating illness, or an acute form of the disease.[101]

The treatment of choice for all forms of *Cryptococcus* infections is a combination of amphotericin B 0.3 mg/kg/day and flucytosine 150 mg/kg/day given orally in four divided doses for six weeks. This regimen is less toxic and as effective as amphotericin B alone at a dose of 0.6 mg/kg/day for 10 weeks.[93] Leukopenia in patients with AIDS makes flucytosine therapy difficult to use because of its myelosuppressive qualities. The response to therapy is poor, and relapses are common. A second-line agent for systemic *Cryptococcus* in patients with AIDS is ketoconazole 400 mg daily. In one study of 52 patients, this provided acceptable prophylaxis in approximately two thirds of the AIDS patients.[102]

Histoplasma capsulatum. Histoplasmosis is a disease that appears in many forms in humans and is caused by *Histoplasma capsulatum,* a facultative intracellular parasite.[91,93] It grows in the soil, produces spores, and is spread by inhalation. Thus, a pulmonary presentation is common. In immunocompromised patients, it is seen as disseminated histoplasmosis or structural lung defects from excessive fibrogenesis. Reinfection is prevalent with symptoms appearing soon after exposure (3–4 days) and temperatures as high as 40.6 °C. The disseminated disease may manifest locally as erythema multiforme and granulomas of the skin and mucous membranes. Histoplasmosis has a striking clinical resemblance to mycobacterial infections.

Amphotericin B is the only drug suitable for either pulmonary or extrapulmonary infections. Full doses of 0.6 mg/kg/day are recommended for at least six weeks. Alternate-day therapy at a dose of 0.8 mg/kg is often continued thereafter for a total dose of at least 2.5 g.

Petriellidium boydii. *Petriellidium boydii* is best known as the most common cause of the clinical syndrome mycetoma, which involves the foot.[103] It is increasingly seen in immunocompromised patients, causing pulmonary, prostatic, ophthalmologic, otitic, and disseminated infections. Occasionally central nervous system isolation is detected. Amphotericin B and flucytosine have little therapeutic effect on this organism. Miconazole is recommended as the drug of choice for serious infections.[104] Miconazole has an MIC of 0.08–0.16 μg/mL versus an MIC >2 μg/mL for amphotericin B. The initial treatment of *Petriellidium boydii* pachymeningitis involves administering miconazole 600 mg intravenously every eight hours in combination with ketoconazole in doses up to 800 mg daily. At these high doses, miconazole is expected to maximize any possible central nervous system penetration as a single daily dose. Abscesses require intravenous miconazole doses of 10–15 mg/kg three times daily along with surgical debridement.[105]

Aspergillus. *Aspergillus* is the most common fungi in the environment, found in the soil and decaying vegetation. Its spores become airborne and enter the lower respiratory tract, which is the major portal of entry, after being inhaled or swallowed.[106] *Aspergillus* infections are increasing in frequency and are notoriously refractory to standard antifungal drug therapy.[107,108] Flucytosine and rifampin when added to amphotericin B therapy have been shown to increase in vitro activity of amphotericin B against the *Aspergillus* species. Clinically, synergistic effects have been documented despite the fact that neither of these antimicrobials have any effect independent of amphotericin B. When amphotericin B is given in combination, lower doses (usually half) are required to treat *Aspergillus.* Recent data propose that tetracycline derivatives, especially minocycline, create synergistic activity against *Aspergillus* based on increased permeability to the fungal organism with amphotericin.[109]

Although primarily pulmonary in nature (more than 90% of the cases), two frequent extrapulmonary sites are the kidney and the brain. Pulmonary disease is a major cause of suppuration and hemorrhage.[110] In patients with pre-existing chronic underlying pulmonary damage, drug resistance develops, along with relapse and reinfection.

Coccidioides immitis. *Coccidioides immitis* is a fungus of the soil that produces spores similar to histoplasma. Coccidioidomycosis is transmitted through the air by inhalation. The primary lesion is pulmonary, and incubation periods range from 7 to 28 days.[101] Clinical symptoms include fever, malaise, a slight dry cough, and chest pain. The illness is often self-limited, except in immunocompromised patients where residual cavitary disease, nodules, or pulmonary abscesses develop. Allergic manifestations are commonly seen within a few days to weeks after infection; erythema multiforme and erythema nodosum are most prevalent. Amphotericin B is the only recommended therapy for meningeal involvement. Often intrathecal amphotericin must be administered as well. Pulmonary and extrapulmonary coccidioidomycosis may be treated with amphotericin B. Oral ketoconazole in doses of 400 mg daily is effective in treating about half of patients who did not respond to amphotericin treatment.[111]

Dosing Antifungal Agents. Dosing considerations and administration guidelines for using antifungal agents in patients with renal insufficiency have been published elsewhere.[56,91,93,111] Side effects of therapy and other complications are also addressed in other literature.[112–114]

Viral Infections

Cytomegalovirus. Cytomegalovirus (CMV) infections are common opportunistic infections in patients with AIDS.[1] Previous exposure to CMV was documented by positive antibody titers in 94% of the homosexual men attending a venereal disease clinic. Only 54% of the heterosexual men attending the same clinic had a positive antibody titer. Of a group of male blood donors, not chosen by sexual orientation, 43% had a positive antibody titer. This indicates that homosexual patients have a greater risk of CMV infection.[115] Disseminated CMV infections often occur in patients with AIDS because of their poor immune function. The disseminated disease has involved the lungs,[116–117] gastrointestinal tract,[116–121] eyes,[116,119,122] brain,[116,123] and nervous system.[124]

Attempts to treat CMV infections with antiviral therapy have not been very successful. Vidarabine, cytarabine, and acyclovir have been tried in the treatment of CMV infections and have had poor outcomes.[125] Two patients with AIDS complicated by CMV infection were treated with intravenous vidarabine. A dose of 15 mg/kg of body weight/day for a 10-day course was documented in one of the cases. Both patients had extensive CMV infections on post-mortem examination, indicating little benefit from vidarabine therapy.[116]

Studies evaluating the effect of acyclovir therapy for CMV infections in immunocompromised patients have also shown little benefit.[126] In vitro, CMV requires much higher concentrations of acyclovir for inhibition than the other members of the *herpesvirus* family. While the 50% inhibitory dose of acyclovir for most strains of CMV is >200 μM, it is only 0.1–1.6 μM for herpes simplex types 1 and 2 and 3–4 μM for varicella-zoster.[126] When intravenous acyclovir was administered to AIDS patients with CMV, it did not have a beneficial effect.[123,124] Even with the acyclovir therapy, disseminated CMV infection has been found on post-mortem examination of patients with AIDS.[123,124]

The use of high-dose intravenous acyclovir for treatment of CMV infections in immunocompromised patients without AIDS has met with variable results. Balfour et al.[127] reported that i.v. acyclovir 500 mg/sq m given three times daily for seven days resulted in a substantially faster rate of clinical improvement and decrease in fever. Wade et al.[128] found that i.v. acyclovir in doses of 400–1200 mg/sq m administered every eight hours for 4–31 days resulted in the survival of only one patient in a group of eight with CMV pneumonia. This patient had received a dose of 900 mg/sq m for five days and 1000 mg/sq m for three days. These inconsistent results do not support the use of acyclovir in AIDS patients with CMV infections.

Acyclovir and vidarabine have both been tried in combination with interferon for the treatment of CMV pneumonia in immunocompromised patients without AIDS. These combination therapies did not demonstrate any added benefit over the previously tried regimens.[129,130]

Herpes Simplex. Recurrent herpes simplex virus (HSV) infections have been documented to occur in patients with AIDS.[131–133] Quinnan et al.[133] evaluated the occurrence of *herpesvirus* infections in individuals with or at risk for AIDS. HSV occurred significantly less often than CMV. A risk of disseminated disease exists for patients with deficient cellular immunity and HSV infections.[132]

Acyclovir is a selective antiviral agent that is beneficial in the treatment and prophylaxis of mucocutaneous HSV in immunocompromised patients without AIDS.[125] In placebo-controlled studies, the administration of an intravenous dose of acyclovir 250 mg/sq m body surface area every eight hours for one week, was effective in the treatment of mucocutaneous HSV infection. Acyclovir resulted in less viral shedding, shorter duration of pain, and a shorter time to healing.[134–136] Vidarabine also has been evaluated for the treatment of mucocutaneous HSV infections in immunocompromised patients without AIDS.[137] A dose of 10 mg/kg/day given intravenously for seven days was evaluated in a placebo-controlled, crossover trial. Vidarabine resulted in a significant improvement in duration of pain and fever. No significant improvement occurred in the duration of viral shedding, cessation of new lesion formation, or time to crusting. Unfortunately, acyclovir has not been compared with vidarabine in a controlled trial, but both agents appear to be effective.

The oral preparation of acyclovir may prevent recurrent HSV infections in patients with AIDS. There have been few studies evaluating the effectiveness of oral acyclovir for this purpose. Straus et al.[138] reported four immunocompromised patients without AIDS who experienced fewer recurrences of HSV than were expected during oral acyclovir administration. In this same study, a 200-mg dose of acyclovir given orally five times a day was able to successfully treat HSV infections in immune-deficient patients. Perhaps oral acyclovir is an alternative to intravenous administration for those patients with AIDS and an HSV infection.

Herpes zoster. Herpes zoster (HZ) infections occur less often in patients with AIDS than the other *Herpesviruses*.[133] Although it is less common, the occurrence of herpes zoster in an immune-deficient patient can result in disseminated disease if left untreated. Intravenous vidarabine (10 mg/kg/day for five days) was effective in a placebo-controlled trial designed to evaluate its use to prevent the complications of HZ infections in immunocompromised patients without AIDS.[139]

Acyclovir is also effective in preventing the dissemination of herpes zoster in immunocompromised patients.[140] In a controlled study, a dose of 500 mg/sq m body surface area given intravenously every eight hours for seven days was effective in improving the rate of cutaneous dissemination and visceral zoster in the acyclovir group.[140]

As in HSV infections, acyclovir and vidarabine have not been compared in a controlled trial but both appear to be effective for HZ infections in immunocompromised patients. Acyclovir may be the preferred agent over vidarabine because of a lower incidence of adverse reactions.[125]

Trends in AIDS Research

The etiologic agent of AIDS, the human T-cell leukemia virus (HTLV-III), has been identified.[141] As many as 65% of urban homosexual men and 94% of the individuals with hemophilia in the United States have been infected with HTLV-III according to recent serological studies.[142] The subsequent development of serologic and retrovirus culture techniques are providing measurement devices for studying the AIDS disorder.

While the treatment of specific infectious and neoplastic complications is advancing, there is no successful therapy for the immune defect itself. Attempts to treat this fatal disease have been made with interferons, interleukins, bone-marrow transplantation, thymus transplantation, and other immune-modulatory techniques.[143]

There was no known effective treatment for retrovirus infection until the in vitro work with suramin sodium proved to have anti-HTLV-III activity at clinically achievable concentrations.[144] Suramin sodium is one of the nonmetallic compounds effective in the treatment of trypanosomiasis. A pilot study is currently being performed under the joint auspices of the National Cancer Institute and the National Institute of Allergy and Infectious Diseases. The purposes of this study are to assess the efficacy of suramin against HTLV-III infection and to assess the natural history of the HTLV-III virus.[145]

Suramin interferes with reverse transcriptase, which may inhibit the multiplication of the virus. On a strictly investigational basis, suramin sodium is given in a 10% aqueous solution intravenously over 10 minutes. Currently, a 1-g dose is given weekly for up to 24 months.

Some of the side effects of suramin are weakness, fatigue, kidney damage, skin rashes (worsened by sun exposure), and hepatitis. Other side effects are nausea and vomiting, hypotension, abdominal pain and bloating, hives, and fever. In a pilot trial, the liver and kidney abnormalities resulted in some dosing delays but were not severe enough to require discontinuing therapy. Suramin sodium is available in 1-g ampuls only from the Centers for Disease Control.

Further work at NIH with interleukin-2 and interferon is still in progress. Interferons are known to suppress the replication of animal retroviruses in vivo and in vitro.[146] These effects are thought to be mediated through alterations in viral assembly and release. Recently, recombinant human interferon α A (Hoffman La-Roche) had a dose-related inhibition on HTLV-III replication without toxic effects on target cells.[146] Complete viral inhibition was seen at achievable serum concentrations. This finding may focus studies on the prophylaxis or early treatment of AIDS versus treating AIDS late in its disease course.

Conclusion

Multiple infectious complications may occur in patients with AIDS as a result of the cellular-immune deficiency associated with this disease. Treatment of these infections is difficult, often requiring unconventional agents with substantial adverse effects. Until more research is done with AIDS patients, therapy must be based on the data available from the treatment of these infections in immunosuppressed patients without AIDS.

---

[a] Ford S. Centers for Disease Control Drug Service, CDC. Personal communication. 1985 Jul 17.

[b] Roddenbery T. The Jacobus Company, Inc. Personal communication. 1985 Apr.

References

1. Allen JR. Epidemiology of the acquired immunodeficiency syndrome (AIDS) in the United States. *Semin Oncol*. 1984; 11:4–11.
2. Centers for Disease Control. Update: acquired immunodeficiency syndrome—United States. *MMWR*. 1985; 34:245–8.
3. Wolinsky E. Nontuberculous mycobacteria and associated diseases. *Am Rev Respir Dis*. 1979; 119:107–59.
4. Davidson PT. The treatment of *Mycobacterium avium-intra-*

cellulare complex disease. *Semin Respir Med*. 1981; 2:233–8.
5. Zakowski P, Fligiel S, Berlin GW et al. Disseminated *Mycobacterium avium-intracellulare* infection in homosexual men dying of acquired immunodeficiency. *JAMA*. 1982; 248:2980–2.
6. Greene JB, Sidhu GS, Lewin S et al. *Mycobacterium avium-intracellulare*: a cause of disseminated life-threatening infection in homosexuals and drug abusers. *Ann Intern Med*. 1982; 97:539–46.
7. Elliott JL, Hoppes WL, Platt MS et al. The acquired immunodeficiency syndrome and *Mycobacterium avium-intracellulare* bacteremia in a patient with hemophilia. *Ann Intern Med*. 1983; 98:290–3.
8. Gillin JS, Urmacher C, West R et al. Disseminated *Mycobacterium avium-intracellulare* infection in acquired immunodeficiency syndrome mimicking Whipple's disease. *Gastroenterology*. 1983; 85:1187–91.
9. de Caprariis PJ, Giron JA, Goldstein JA et al. *Mycobacterium avium-intracellulare* infection and possibly venereal transmission. *Ann Intern Med*. 1984; 101:721. Letter.
10. Pitchenik AE, Cole C, Russell BW et al. Tuberculosis, atypical mycobacteriosis, and the acquired immunodeficiency syndrome among Haitian and non-Haitian patients in south Florida. *Ann Intern Med*. 1984; 101:641–5.
11. Poon MC, Landay A, Prasthofer EF et al. Acquired immunodeficiency syndrome with *Pneumocystis carinii* pneumonia and *Mycobacterium avium-intracellulare* infection in a previously healthy patient with classic hemophilia. *Ann Intern Med*. 1983; 98:287–90.
12. Macher AM, Kovacs JA, Gill V et al. Bacteremia due to *Mycobacterium avium-intracellulare* in the acquired immunodeficiency syndrome. *Ann Intern Med*. 1983; 99:782–5.
13. Horsburgh CR, Mason UG III, Farhi DC et al. Disseminated infection with *Mycobacterium avium-intracellulare:* a report of 13 cases and a review of the literature. *Medicine* (Baltimore). 1985; 64:36–48.
14. Feng PCC, Fenselau CC, Jacobson RR. Metabolism of clofazimine in leprosy patients. *Drug Metab Dispos*. 1981; 9:521–4.
15. Levy L. Pharmacologic studies of clofazimine. *Am J Trop Med Hyg*. 1974; 23:1097–109.
16. Davidson PT, Goble M, Fernandez E et al. Clofazimine (B663) for the treatment of *M. intracellulare* infections in man. *Am Rev Respir Dis*. 1979; 119(Suppl):398. Abstract.
17. Collins FM, Klayman DL, Morrison NE. Activity of 2-acetylpyridine and 2-acetylquinoline thiosemicarbazones tested in vitro in combination with other antituberculous drugs. *Am Rev Respir Dis*. 1982; 125:58–60.
18. Moore VJ. A review of side-effects experienced by patients taking clofazimine. *Lepr Rev*. 1983; 54:327–35.
19. Granstein RD, Sober AJ. Drug- and heavy metal-induced hyperpigmentation. *J Am Acad Derm*. 1981; 5:1–18.
20. Caver CV. Clofazimine-induced ichthyosis and its treatment. *Cutis*. 1982; 29:341–3.
21. Ohman L, Wahlberg I. Ocular side-effects of clofazimine. *Lancet*. 1975; II:933–4. Letter.
22. Walinder PE, Gip L, Stempa M. Corneal changes in patients treated with clofazimine. *Br J Ophthalmol*. 1976; 60:526–8.
23. Negrel AD, Chovet M, Baquillon G et al. Clofazimine and the eye: preliminary communication. *Lepr Rev*. 1984; 55:349–52.
24. de Bergeyck E, Janssens PG, de Muynck A. Radiological abnormalities of the ileum associated with the use of clofazimine (Lamprene; B663) in the treatment of skin ulceration due to *Mycobacterium ulcerans*. *Lepr Rev*. 1980; 51:221–8.
25. Belaube P, Devaux J, Pizzi M et al. Small bowel deposition of crystals associated with the use of clofazimine (Lamprene) in the treatment of prurigo nodularis. *Int J Lepr*. 1983; 51:328–30.
26. Harvey RF, Harman RRM, Black C et al. Abdominal pain and malabsorption due to tissue deposition of clofazimine (Lamprene) crystals. *Br J Dermatol*. 1977; 97(Suppl 15):19. Abstract.
27. Jagadeesan K, Visweswaran MK, Iyer KH. Acute abdomen in a patient treated with Lamprene. *Int Surg*. 1975; 60:208–9.
28. McDougall AC, Horsfall WR, Hede JE et al. Splenic infarction and tissue accumulation of crystals associated with the use of clofazimine (Lamprene; B663) in the treatment of pyoderma gangrenosum. *Br J Dermatol*. 1980; 102:227–30.
29. Woodley CL, Kilburn JO. In vitro susceptibility of *Mycobacterium avium* complex and *Mycobacterium tuberculosis* strains to a spiro-piperidyl rifamycin. *Am Rev Respir Dis*. 1982; 126:586–7.
30. Della Bruna C, Schioppacassi G, Ungheri D et al. LM 427, a new spiropiperidylrifamycin: in vitro and in vivo studies. *J Antibiot*. 1983; 36:1502–6.
31. Sanfilippo A, Della Bruna C, Marsili L et al. Biological activity of a new class of rifamycins: spiro-piperidyl-rifamycins. *J Antibiot*. 1980; 33:1193–8.
32. Hawkins JE, Gross WM, Vadney FS. Ansamycin LM 427 activity against mycobacteria in vitro. *Am Rev Respir Dis*. 1984; 129:A187. Abstract.
33. Landesman SH, Vieira J. Acquired immune deficiency syndrome (AIDS): a review. *Arch Intern Med*. 1983; 143:2307–9.
34. National ACCP Consensus Conference on Tuberculosis. Standard therapy for tuberculosis 1985. *Chest*. 1985; 87(Suppl):117S–24S.
35. Glassroth J, Robins AG, Snider DE Jr. Tuberculosis in the 1980s. *N Engl J Med*. 1980; 302:1441–9.
36. Girling DJ. Adverse effects of antituberculosis drugs. *Drugs*. 1982; 23:56–74.
37. Eng RHK, Forrester C, Smith SM et al. *Mycobacterium xenopi* infection in a patient with acquired immunodeficiency syndrome. *Chest*. 1984; 86:145–7.
38. Gottlieb MS. Nonneoplastic AIDS syndromes. *Sem Oncol*. 1984; 11:40–6.
39. Wofsy CB. Opportunistic infections in AIDS. Focus on AIDS. Symposium Proceedings. October 8, 1984:6–10
40. Hughes WT. *Pneumocystis carinii* pneumonitis. *Chest*. 1984; 85:810–3.
41. Campbell WA. Ultrastructure of pneumocystis in human lung. *Arch Pathol*. 1972; 93:312–24.
42. Kovacs JA, Hiemenz JW, Macher AM et al. *Pneumocystis carinii* pneumonia: a comparison between patients with the acquired immunodeficiency syndrome and patients with other immunodeficiencies. *Ann Intern Med*. 1984; 100:663–71.
43. Haverkos HW. Assessment of therapy for *Pneumocystis carinii* pneumonia. *Am J Med*. 1984; 76:501–7.
44. Hughes WT, Feldman S, Chaudhary S et al. Comparison of pentamidine isethionate and trimethoprim-sulfamethoxazole in the treatment of *Pneumocystis carinii* pneumonia. *J Pediatr*. 1978; 92:285–91.
45. Young LS. Trimethoprim-sulfamethoxazole in the treatment of adults with pneumonia due to *Pneumocystis carinii*. *Rev Infect Dis*. 1982; 4:608–12.
46. Johnson JF, Rehder TL, Moore GF. *Pneumocystis carinii* pneumonia: review with a case study. *Drug Intell Clin Pharm*. 1981; 15:732–7.
47. Winston DJ, Lau WK, Gale RP et al. Trimethoprim-sulfamethoxazole for the treatment of *Pneumocystis carinii* pneumonia. *Ann Intern Med*. 1980; 92:762–9.
48. Gordin FM, Simon GL, Wofsy CB et al. Adverse reactions to trimethoprim-sulfamethoxazole in patients with the acquired immunodeficiency syndrome. *Ann Intern Med*. 1984; 100:495–9.
49. Jick H. Adverse reactions to trimethoprim-sulfamethoxazole in hospitalized patients. *Rev Infect Dis*. 1982; 4:426–8.
50. Gibbons RB, Lindauer JA. Successful treatment of *Pneumocystis carinii* pneumonia with trimethoprim-sulfamethoxazole in hypersensitive AIDS patients. *JAMA*. 1985; 253:1259–60. Letter.
51. Mitsuyasu R, Groopman J, Volberding P. Cutaneous reac-

tion to trimethoprim-sulfamethoxazole in patients with AIDS and Kaposi's sarcoma. *N Engl J Med.* 1983; 308:1535. Letter.

52. Bourgault AM, Van Scoy RE, Brewer NS et al. Trimethoprim with sulfamethoxazole for treatment of infections with *Pneumocystis carinii* in renal insufficiency. *Chest.* 1978; 74:91–2.
53. Hughes WT, Feldman S, Sanyal SK. Treatment of *Pneumocystis carinii* pneumonitis with trimethoprim-sulfamethoxazole. *Can Med Assoc J.* 1975; 112(Suppl):47–50.
54. Waalkes TP, Denham C, DeVita VT. Pentamidine: clinical pharmacologic correlations in man and mice. *Clin Pharmacol Ther.* 1970; 11:505–12.
55. Centers for Disease Control. US-manufactured pentamidine isethionate cleared for investigational use. *MMWR.* 1984; 33:270.
56. Bennett WM, Aronoff GR, Morrison G et al. Drug prescribing in renal failure: dosing guidelines for adults. *Am J Kid Dis.* 1983; 3:155–93.
57. Polsky B, Dryjanski J, Whimbey E et al. Severe neutropenia during pentamidine treatment of *Pneumocystis carinii* pneumonia in patients with AIDS. *JAMA.* 1984; 251:1253–4.
58. Murphey SA, Josephs AS. Acute pancreatitis associated with pentamidine therapy. *Arch Intern Med.* 1981; 141:56–8.
59. Fitzgerald DB, Young IS. Reversal of pentamidine-induced hypoglycemia with oral diazoxide. *J Trop Med Hyg.* 1984; 87:15–9.
60. Bouchard P, Sai P, Reach G et al. Diabetes mellitus following pentamidine-induced hypoglycemia in humans. *Diabetes.* 1982; 31:40–5.
61. Sharpe SM. Pentamidine and hypoglycemia. *Ann Intern Med.* 1983; 99:128.
62. Hughes WT, Smith BL. Efficacy of diaminodiphenylsulfone and other drugs in murine *Pneumocystis carinii* pneumonitis. *Antimicrob Agents Chemother.* 1984; 26:436–40.
63. Poulsen A, Hultberg B, Thomsen K et al. Regression of Kaposi's sarcoma in AIDS after treatment with dapsone. Lancet. 1984; I:560. Letter.
64. Graham WR. Adverse effects of dapsone. *Int J Dermatol.* 1975; 14:494–500.
65. De Gowin RL. A review of the therapeutic and hemolytic effects of dapsone. *Arch Intern Med.* 1967; 120:242–8.
66. Hughes WT, Kuhn S, Chaudhary S et al. Successful chemoprophylaxis for *Pneumocystis carinii* pneumonia. *N Engl J Med.* 1977; 297:1419–26.
67. Gottlieb MS, Knight S, Weisman J. Prophylaxis of *Pneumocystis carinii* infection in AIDS with pyrimethamine-sulfadoxine. *Lancet.* 1984; II:398. Letter.
68. Ryning FW, Mills J. *Pneumocystis carinii, Toxoplasma gondii,* cytomegalovirus, and the compromised host. *West J Med.* 1979; 130:18–34.
69. Ruskin J, Remington JS. Toxoplasmosis in the compromised host. *Ann Intern Med.* 1976; 84:193–9.
70. Araujo FG, Remington JS. Effect of clindamycin on acute and chronic toxoplasmosis in mice. *Antimicrob Agents Chemother.* 1974; 5:647–51.
71. Tabbara KF, O'Connor GR. Treatment of ocular toxoplasmosis with clindamycin and sulfadiazine. *Ophthalmology.* 1980; 87:129–34.
72. Most H. Treatment of parasitic infections of travelers and immigrants. *N Engl J Med.* 1984; 310:298–304.
73. Wolfe MS. The treatment of intestinal protozoan infections. *Med Clin North Am.* 1982; 66:707–19.
74. Hallak A, Yust I, Ratan Y et al. Malabsorption syndrome, coccidiosis, combined immune deficiency, and fulminant lymphoproliferative disease. *Arch Intern Med.* 1982; 142:196–7.
75. Whiteside ME, Barkin JS, May RG et al. Enteric coccidiosis among patients with the acquired immunodeficiency syndrome. *Am J Trop Med Hyg.* 1984; 33:1065–72.
76. Westerman EL, Christensen RP. Chronic *Isospora belli* infection treated with co-trimoxazole. *Ann Intern Med.* 1979; 91:413–4.
77. Veldhuyzen Van Zanten SJO, Lange JMA, Sauerwein HP et al. Amprolium for coccidiosis in AIDS. *Lancet.* 1984; 2:345–6. Letter.
78. Collins GH. Cryptosporidiosis—A new disease? *Med J Aust.* 1984; 140:516–7. Editorial.
79. Forgacs P, Tarshis A, Ma P et al. Intestinal and bronchial cryptosporidiosis in an immunodeficient homosexual man. *Ann Intern Med.* 1983; 99:793–4.
80. Bird RG, Smith MD. Cryptosporidiosis in man, parasite life cycle and fine structural pathology. *J Pathol.* 1980; 132:217–33.
81. Navin TR, Juranek DD. Cryptosporidiosis: clinical, epidemiologic, and parasitologic review. *Rev Infect Dis.* 1984; 6:313–27.
82. Soave R, Danner RL, Honig CL et al. Cryptosporidiosis in homosexual men. *Ann Intern Med.* 1984; 100:504–11.
83. Zar F, Geiseler PJ, Brown VA. Asymptomatic carriage of cryptosporidium in the stool of a patient with acquired immunodeficiency syndrome. *J Infect Dis.* 1985; 151:195. Letter.
84. Baxby D. The development and performance of a simple, sensitive method for the detection of cryptosporidiosis oocysts in feces. *J Hyg.* 1984; 93:317–23.
85. Pitlik SD, Fainstein V, Garza D et al. Human cryptosporidiosis: spectrum of disease. *Arch Intern Med.* 1983; 143:2269–75.
86. Modigliani R, Bories C, Le Charpentier Y et al. Diarrhoea and malabsorption in acquired immune deficiency syndrome: a study of four cases with special emphasis on opportunistic protozoan infestations. *Gut.* 1985; 26:179–87.
87. Centers for Disease Control. Cryptosporidiosis: assessment of chemotherapy of males with acquired immunodeficiency syndrome (AIDS) *MMWR.* 1982; 31:589–92.
88. Centers for Disease Control. Update: treatment of cryptosporidiosis in patients with acquired immunodeficiency syndrome (AIDS). *MMWR.* 1984; 33:117–9.
89. Spiramycin. In: Reynolds JEF, Prasad AV, eds. Martindale: The extra pharmacopeia. London: The Pharmaceutical Press; 1982:1212.
90. Portnoy D, Whiteside ME, Buckley E III et al. Treatment of intestinal cryptosporidiosis with spiramycin. *Ann Intern Med.* 1984; 101:202–4.
91. Utz JP. Chemotherapy of the systemic mycoses. Symposium on antimicrobial therapy. *Med Clin North Am.* 1982; 66:221–33.
92. Klein RS, Harris CA, Friedland GH. Oral candidiasis and AIDS. *N Engl J Med.* 1984; 311:1379. Letter.
93. Cohen J. Antifungal chemotherapy. *Lancet.* 1982; II:532–7.
94. Owens NJ, Nightingale CH, Schweizer RT et al. Prophylaxis of oral candidiasis with clotrimazole troches. *Arch Intern Med.* 1984; 144:290–3.
95. Jones PG, Kauffman CA, McAuliffe LS et al. Efficacy of ketoconazole versus nystatin in prevention of fungal infections in neutropenic patients. *Arch Intern Med.* 1984; 144:549–51.
96. Peterson LR, Hall WH, Kelty RH et al. Therapy of *Candida* peritonitis: penetration of amphotericin B into peritoneal fluid. *Postgrad Med J.* 1978; 54:340–2.
97. Bayer AS, Blumenkrantz MJ, Montgomerie JZ et al. *Candida* peritonitis. *Am J Med.* 1976; 61:832–4.
98. Edwards JE. *Candida* endophthalmitis: an overview. *Mycology Observer.* 1985; 5:1–4.
99. Paladino JA, Crass RE. Amphotericin B and flucytosine in the treatment of candidal cystisis. *Clin Pharm.* 1982; 1:349–52.
100. Goldman HS, Littman ML, Oppenheimer GD et al. Monilial cystitis-effective treatment with instillations of amphotericin B. *JAMA.* 1960; 174:359–62.
101. Hermans PE, Keys TF. Antifungal agents used for deep-seated mycotic infections. *Mayo Clin Proc.* 1983; 58:223–31.
102. Dismukes WE, Stamm AM, Graybill JR et al. Treatment of systemic mycoses with ketoconazole: emphasis on toxicity and clinical response in 52 patients. *Ann Intern Med.* 1983;

98:13–20.
103. Schiess RJ, Coscia MF, McClellan GA. *Petriellidium boydii* pachymeningitis treated with miconazole and ketoconazole. *Neurosurgery*. 1984; 14:220–4.
104. Lutwick LI, Galgiani JN, Johnson RH et al. Visceral fungal infections due to *Petriellidium boydii*. *Am J Med*. 1976; 61:632–40.
105. Anderson RL, Carroll TF, Harvey JT et al. *Petriellidium (Allescheria) boydii* orbital and brain abscess treated with intravenous miconazole. *Am J Ophthalmol*. 1984; 97:771–5.
106. Rinaldi MG. Invasive aspergillosis. *Rev Infect Dis*. 1983; 5:1061–6.
107. Codish SD, Tobias JS, Hannigan M. Combined amphotericin B-flucytosine therapy in *Aspergillus* pneumonia. *JAMA*. 1979; 241:2418–9.
108. Utz JP, Garrigues IL, Sande MA et al. Therapy of cryptococcosis with a combination of flucytosine and amphotericin B. *J Infect Dis*. 1975; 132:368–73.
109. Hughes CE, Harris C, Peterson LR et al. Enhancement of the in vitro activity of amphotericin B against *Aspergillus* spp. by tetracycline analogs. *Antimicrob Agents Chemother*. 1984; 26:837–40.
110. Atkinson GW, Israel HL. 5-Fluorocytosine treatment of meningeal and pulmonary aspergillosis. *Am J Med*. 1973; 55:496–504.
111. Medoff G, Kobayashi GS. Strategies in the treatment of systemic fungal infections. *N Engl J Med*. 1980; 302:145–55.
112. Maddux MS, Barriere SL. A review of complications of amphotericin B therapy: recommendations for prevention and management. *Drug Intell Clin Pharm*. 1980; 14:177–81.
113. Butler W, Bennett JE, Aling DW et al. Nephrotoxicity of amphotericin B: early and late effects in 81 patients. *Ann Intern Med*. 1964; 61:175–87.
114. Hume AL, Kerkering TM. Ketoconazole. *Drug Intell Clin Pharm*. 1983; 17:169–74.
115. Drew WL, Mintz L, Miner RC et al. Prevalence of cytomegalovirus infections in homosexual men. *J Infect Dis*. 1981; 143:188–92.
116. Mildvan D, Mathur U, Enlow RW et al. Opportunistic infections and immune deficiency in homosexual men. *Ann Intern Med*. 1982; 96(Part I):700–4.
117. Lerner CW, Tapper ML. Opportunistic infection complicating acquired immune deficiency syndrome: clinical features of 25 cases. *Medicine* (Baltimore). 1984; 63:155–64.
118. Knapp AB, Horst DA, Eliopoulos G et al. Widespread cytomegalovirus gastroenterocolitis in a patient with acquired immunodeficiency syndrome. *Gastroenterology*. 1983; 85:1399–402.
119. Gertler SL, Pressman J, Price P et al. Gastrointestinal Cytomegalovirus infection in a homosexual man with severe acquired immunodeficiency syndrome. *Gastroenterology*. 1983; 85:1403–6.
120. Kram HB, Hino ST, Cohen RE et al. Spontaneous colonic perforation secondary to cytomegalovirus in a patient with acquired immune deficiency syndrome. *Crit Care Med*. 1984; 12:469–71.
121. Blumberg RS, Kelsey P, Perrone T et al. Cytomegalovirus- and cryotosporidium-associated acalculous gangrenous cholecystitis. *Am J Med*. 1984; 76:1118–23.
122. Chou S, Dylewski JS, Gaynon MW et al. Alpha-interferon administration in *Cytomegalovirus* retinitis. *Antimicrob Agents Chemother*. 1984; 25:25–8.
123. Hawley DA, Schaefer JF, Schulz DM et al. Cytomegalovirus encephalitis in acquired immunodeficiency syndrome. *Am J Clin Pathol*. 1983; 80:874–7.
124. Moskowitz LB, Gregorios JB, Hensley GT et al. Cytomegalovirus: induced demyelination associated with acquired immune deficiency syndrome. *Arch Pathol Lab Med*. 1984; 108:873–7.
125. Nicholson KG. Antiviral therapy: varicella-zoster virus infections, *herpes labialis*, and mucocutaneous herpes, and cytomegalovirus infections. *Lancet*. 1984; II:677–82.
126. Laskin OL. Acyclovir: pharmacology and clinical experience. *Arch Intern Med*. 1984; 144:1241–6.
127. Balfour HH, Bean B, Mitchell CD et al. Acyclovir in immunocompromised patients with cytomegalovirus disease: a controlled trial at one institution. *Am J Med*. 1982; 73(Suppl 1A):241–8.
128. Wade JC, Hintz M, McGuffin RW et al. Treatment of cytomegalovirus pneumonia with high-dose acyclovir. *Am J Med*. 1982; 73(Suppl 1A):249–56.
129. Shepp DH, Newton BA, Meyers JD. Intravenous lymphoblastoid interferon and acyclovir for treatment of cytomegaloviral pneumonia. *J Infect Dis*. 1984; 150:776–7.
130. Meyers JD, McGuffin RW, Bryson YJ et al. Treatment of cytomegalovirus pneumonia after marrow transplant with combined vidarabine and human leukocyte interferon. *J Infect Dis*. 1982; 146:80–4.
131. Dotz WI, Berman B. Kaposi's sarcoma, chronic ulcerative Herpes simplex, and acquired immunodeficiency. *Arch Dermatol*. 1983; 119:93–4.
132. Seigal FP, Lopez C, Hammer GS et al. Severe acquired immunodeficiency in male homosexuals manifested by chronic perianal ulcerative Herpes simplex lesions. *N Engl J Med*. 1981; 305:1439–44.
133. Quinnan GV, Masur H, Rook AH et al. *Herpesvirus* infections in the acquired immune deficiency syndrome. *JAMA*. 1984; 252:72–7.
134. Mitchell CD, Bean B, Gentry SR et al. Acyclovir therapy for mucocutaneous Herpes simplex infections in immunocompromised patients. *Lancet*. 1981; I:1389–92.
135. Chou S, Gallagher JG, Merigan TC. Controlled clinical trial of intravenous acyclovir in heart transplant patients with mucocutaneous Herpes simplex infections. *Lancet*. 1981; I:1392–4.
136. Wade JC, Newton B, McLaren C et al. Intravenous acyclovir to treat mucocutaneous Herpes simplex virus infection after marrow transplantation: a double-blind trial. *Ann Intern Med*. 1982; 96:265–9.
137. Whitley RJ, Spruance S, Hayden FG, et al. Vidarabine therapy for mucocutaneous Herpes simplex virus infections in the immunocompromised host. *J Infect Dis*. 1984; 149:1–8.
138. Straus SE, Seidlin M, Takiff H et al. Oral acyclovir to suppress recurring Herpes simplex virus infections in immunodeficient patients. *Ann Intern Med*. 1984; 100:522–4.
139. Whitley RJ, Soong S-J, Dolin R et al. Early vidarabine therapy to control the complications of Herpes zoster in immunosuppressed patients. *N Engl J Med*. 1982; 307:971–5.
140. Balfour HH, Bean B, Laskin OL et al. Acyclovir halts progression of Herpes zoster in immunocompromised patients. *N Engl J Med*. 1983; 308:1448–53.
141. Popovic M, Sarngadhadran MG, Read E et al. Detection, isolation, and continuous production of cytopathic retroviruses (HTLV-III) from patients with AIDS and pre-AIDS. *Science*. 1984; 224:497–500.
142. Centers for Disease Control. Antibodies to a retrovirus etiologically associated with AIDS in populations with increased incidences of the syndrome. *MMWR*. 1984; 33:377–9.
143. Fauci AS. AIDS: epidemiologic, clinical, immunologic, and therapeutic considerations. *Ann Intern Med*. 1984; 100:92–106.
144. Mitsuya H, Popovic M, Yarchoan R et al. Suramin protection of T cells in vitro against infectivity and cytopathic effect of HTLV-III. *Science*. 1984; 226:172–4.
145. Lane HC (Primary Investigator). Trial to determine the efficacy of suramin for AIDS and other HTLV-III related syndromes. Research in Progress. NIH 1985.
146. Ho DD, Rota TR, Kaplan JC et al. Recombinant human interferon alfa-A suppresses HTLV-III relication in vitro. *Lancet*. 1985; I:602–4.

Therapeutic management of cystic fibrosis

ROBERT J. KUHN AND MILAP C. NAHATA

Abstract: The therapeutic management of patients with cystic fibrosis (CF) is reviewed.

CF is an autosomal-recessive genetic disease that affects all exocrine glands. Drug therapy is directed toward the relief of symptoms and prevention of complications. Chronic respiratory tract infections and pancreatic insufficiency are the major manifestations.

The replacement of pancreatic enzymes is best achieved with microencapsulated preparations. The dose of enzymes is increased until a maximum effect on decreasing steatorrhea is observed. *Pseudomonas aeruginosa* and *Staphylococcus aureus* are the most common pathogens in respiratory infections, which usually require 2–3 weeks of intravenous antibiotic therapy. Because patients with CF often have rapid clearance of both penicillins and aminoglycosides and altered apparent distribution volumes of aminoglycosides, individualized dosing is required. The role of prophylactic antibiotic therapy is controversial, since prolonged exposure to antimicrobials may hasten the development of mucoid strains. Aerosolized antibiotics have not been consistently useful in treating these patients, and there is no convincing evidence to support their long-term use. There are also no clear data to support the use of oral or aerosolized mucolytic agents. The inability to deliver the drug to the site of action plus the time and expense of inhalation equipment may only complicate the drug therapy while producing little benefit. Bronchodilators can be useful in improving pulmonary function. Vitamin supplementation with both the fat- and water-soluble vitamins is important in the treatment of CF. Iron supplementation may also be necessary.

Until the basic defect in CF is discovered, the use of antibiotics and replacement of pancreatic enzymes will continue to be the mainstay of therapy.

Index terms: Aerosols; Antibiotics; Bronchodilators; Cystic fibrosis; Mucolytic agents; Pancreatic enzymes; Vitamins
Clin Pharm. 1985; 4:555–65

Cystic fibrosis (CF) is the most common fatal genetic disease in children. It is an autosomal-recessive genetic disease found predominantly in Causasians. It affects all exocrine glands and manifests as complications in the respiratory tract, intestinal tract, and liver. The heterozygous carrier state is quite common in the Caucasian population with a reported frequency of 1 in 20, which accounts for the occurrence of CF in 1 of 1500 to 2000 live births.[1]

Cystic fibrosis was first described clinically in 1938 by Anderson.[2] Since then, intense research efforts have been unable to discover the underlying cellular defect. The introduction of broad-spectrum antibiotic and adjunctive therapy over the past two decades has increased the average life expectancy from three years of age in the late 1950s to the mid-20s at the present time.[3,4]

The specific goal of current therapy for CF is to alleviate the symptoms or to treat its complications, including infections. There are various modalities used in the treatment of CF. Physiotherapy, or postural drainage, is used extensively to help dislodge the thick mucus in the respiratory tract. The patients usually require two or more treatments daily to help loosen mucus plugs and allow them to expectorate sputum. Exercise may also be beneficial in loosening bronchial secretions, as shown in a recent study that demonstrated no difference in sputum production with either physical exercise or postural drainage.[5] In addition, nutritional therapy is often important in the care of these patients. Patients with CF often require higher caloric intakes and the use of nutritional supplements to facilitate growth.[6,7] Pharmacologic intervention is aimed at alleviating gastrointestinal symptoms and preventing possible complications of the disease.

The purpose of this article is to review the current modes of therapy for CF. The pathophysiology and clinical presentation of CF are described briefly. The role of pancreatic enzyme replacement therapy, antibiotics, vitamin supplements, bronchodilators, and aerosols are also discussed to provide a perspective on the optimal management of patients with CF.

Pathophysiology and Clinical Presentation

Cystic fibrosis is a complex condition involving many organ systems of the body. It results in pancreatic, gastrointestinal, respiratory, hepatic, and reproductive abnormalities that occur to varying

ROBERT J. KUHN, PHARM.D., is Assistant Professor of Pharmacy, College of Pharmacy, University of Kentucky, Lexington. At the time of this study, he was Pediatric Pharmacotherapy Fellow, Children's Hospital, Columbus, OH. MILAP C. NAHATA, PHARM.D., is Associate Professor of Pharmacy, College of Pharmacy, and Associate Professor of Pediatrics, College of Medicine, Ohio State University, Columbus.

Address reprint requests to Dr. Nahata at the College of Pharmacy, Ohio State University, 500 West 12th Avenue, Columbus, OH 43210.

degrees in different patients. CF affects exocrine glands in various ways. Mucus-secreting glands become obstructed with thick secretions often referred to as "mucoviscidosis," while serous glands have a defect in the reabsorption of sodium and chloride. Pancreatic involvement, including a pancreatic deficiency of lipase and protease enzymes or pancreatic achylia, occurs in as many as 85% of the patients with CF. Although the underlying defect responsible for pancreatic insufficiency in CF is not known, one study[8] found that patients with CF produced below-normal amounts of pancreatic secretions and that these secretions had a low bicarbonate content, a very high enzyme concentration, and a high viscosity. Hadorn et al.[8] postulated the defect in exocrine function in CF to be a lack of production of a dilute, low-viscosity secretion containing electrolytes to mix with this highly concentrated secretion. Patients with pancreatic involvement usually have a history of passing frequent foul-smelling, oily, floating stools because of their inability to absorb fats. Many patients with CF fail to gain weight or grow normally despite good caloric intake. In addition, 8% of the patients with CF have some defect in the production of insulin and thus have hyperglycemia and glycosuria.[9] Although these patients can be usually managed with insulin therapy, they develop the microvascular complications associated with chronic hyperglycemia. Gastrointestinal symptoms may be present at birth; 7–10% of newborns with CF are unable to pass the thick meconium and develop meconium ileus.[10] Intestinal obstruction, which is commonly referred to as "meconium-ileus equivalent," may occur later in life as the inspissated fecal material becomes impacted at the ileocecal junction. Gastrographic enema may reduce the obstruction, but surgical intervention is often necessary. Steatorrhea and malabsorption of nutrients, particularly fat, are by far the most common gastrointestinal symptoms of CF and can be controlled by the use of pancreatic-enzyme preparations.[1,2,10]

The pulmonary manifestations of CF usually involve the plugging or blockage of airways by thick mucus and respiratory-tract infections. CF pulmonary secretions are relatively dehydrated and have a lower than normal sodium and chloride content, which can lead to airway trapping and mucus plugging. It is often difficult for the patient with CF to expectorate this mucus without the use of physiotherapy or aerosol treatments. Patients with CF often have a decrease in vital capacity and expiratory flow rates as a result of the obstructive nature of their pulmonary disease. When air trapping occurs, hyperinflation can often be seen on chest roentgenogram. As the disease progresses and fibrosis occurs, residual volume increases with little change in lung capacity as occurs in most restrictive lung diseases. Pulmonary infection is one of the most serious complications of CF. No specific cause for the increased susceptibility of CF patients to infection has been found yet, but close clinical and microbiologic observations are needed for the proper treatment of pulmonary infections.

Some patients with CF may have biliary-duct obstruction by eosinophilic material; these patients may develop biliary cirrhosis. Secondary portal hypertension, bleeding esophageal varices, and hypersplenism have also been reported.[10]

There are currently four criteria for a diagnosis of CF. Pilocarpine iontophoresis or "sweat-testing" measures an elevated concentration of chloride in the sweat. Sweat chloride concentrations greater than 60 meq/L are consistent with CF, but it is imperative to obtain a sufficient quantity of sweat (100 mg or more) and perform the analysis in a laboratory that routinely screens for CF. False-positive results have been reported in institutions where routine analyses are not performed. In conjunction with elevated concentrations of chloride in sweat, a history of chronic respiratory-tract infection especially in the first year of life, pancreatic insufficiency, history of foul-smelling stools, failure to thrive, or a family history of CF help to confirm the diagnosis. In addition to this "classical" presentation, patients with CF may also develop symptoms of chronic respiratory disease much later in life, even as adults.

Pancreatic-Enzyme Replacement Therapy

As many as 85% of patients with CF have a deficiency of pancreatic enzymes, resulting in inadequate digestion of food and, ultimately, impairment of growth. Early preparations of pancreatic enzymes were often inactivated or degraded by the acidic pH of the stomach.[11] These preparations contained pancreatin, an extract from swine or ox pancreas that contained varying ratios of amylase, lipase, and protease enzymes because of extraction problems. Later preparations used pancrelipase, an enzyme concentrate derived from porcine pancreas. Pancrelipase has 12 times the lipase activity and 4 times the amylase and protease activity of pancreatin. The acidic pH of the stomach, however, still caused substantial inactivation of these products. Coated products were then introduced, but because of unpredictable dissolution, adequate replacement of pancreatic enzymes was still not achieved.[12,13] With the development of microencapsulated products, enough intact pancreatic enzyme could be delivered to the duodenum, enhancing absorption of nutrients. Microencapsulated products permit better dissolution of enzymes in the duodenum and protect the enzyme preparation from the acid pH of the stomach. In a crossover study[13] comparing microencapsulated and nonmicroencapsulated preparations, microencapsulated products were associated with less stool frequency, less abdominal cramping, and increased growth

Table 1.
Pancreatic-Enzyme Preparations Suitable for Patients with Cystic Fibrosis[14]

Product Name[a] (Manufacturer)	Formulation	Enzyme Activity per Dosage Unit: Lipase	Protease	Amylase
Cotazyme (Organon)	Capsule	8,000	30,000	30,000
	Powder packets (Regular)	16,000	60,000	60,000
	Powder packets (Cherry flavored)	40,000	150,000	150,000
Cotazyme-S (Organon)	Microencapsulated capsule	5,000	20,000	20,000
Ilozyme (Adria)	Tablet	11,000	30,000	30,000
Ku-Zyme HP (Kremers–Urban)	Capsule	8,000	30,000	30,000
Pancrease (McNeil)	Microencapsulated capsule	4,000	25,000	20,000
Viokase (Robins)[b]	Tablets	8,000	30,000	30,000
	Powder[c]	16,800	70,000	70,000

[a] All products listed contain pancrelipase.
[b] The formulation of Viokase was changed in March 1984 to that shown in the table; the product formerly contained pancreatin. (See Berardi RR, Colvin CL. Change in enzyme content and manufacturer of Viokase. *Clin Pharm.* 1985; 4:388. Letter.)
[c] Enzyme activity shown is per 0.7 g (¼ tsp) of powder.

rates as determined by anthropometric measurements. An additional benefit of these preparations is a decrease in the amount of enzymes required and a potential cost savings to the patient. A list of currently available pancreatic-enzyme preparations suitable for patients with CF is presented in Table 1.[14]

Dose titration of pancreatic-enzyme replacements is empiric. The usual starting dose of a microencapsulated preparation is one to three capsules with meals or a snack. Uncoated-enzyme preparations should not be administered in anticipation of meals because if the patient does not eat, severe abdominal cramping and nausea may occur. The dose is increased until the patient has a decrease in steatorrhea and gastrointestinal complaints. Examination of the stools for fat concentration can also be helpful in assessing the titration of pancreatic-enzyme therapy. With proper doses, patients with CF will be able to increase the percentage of fat absorbed, but fat absorption may still be incomplete. Additional enzymes will not increase the percentage of fat absorbed but will add additional expense to the drug therapy. In addition, the administration of increasing doses of pancreatic-enzyme replacement may cause constipation and even fecal impaction.

In an attempt to prevent the problems of pancreatic-enzyme degradation in the stomach, several adjunctive therapies have been used to enhance the efficacy of pancreatic enzymes. With the low bicarbonate content of CF pancreatic secretions, the use of an antacid or H_2-receptor antagonist to raise the pH of the stomach should decrease the degradation of pancreatic enzyme by the acidic environment of the stomach. In a study using adjunctive antacids and bile salts with a conventional pancrelipase preparation,[15] an increase in fat absorption was associated with antacids but not with the preparations containing bile salts. However, this combination therapy is more expensive and inconvenient to administer than the microencapsulated preparations.

Cimetidine has also been studied as an adjunct to pancreatic-enzyme therapy.[16–19] Two studies[16,17] demonstrated some improvement in fat absorption in CF patients using nonmicroencapsulated products plus cimetidine. Hubbard[17] reported a significant gain in weight and reduction in steatorrhea in patients receiving cimetidine 300 mg three times daily in addition to their nonmicroencapsulated pancreatic-enzyme replacement therapy. There is no evidence, however, to suggest that adjunctive cimetidine therapy improves fat absorption or decreases steatorrhea in patients using microencapsulated preparations. A recent double-blind study[20] using various pancreatic-enzyme preparations demonstrated no benefit from additional cimetidine (600 mg/sq m) compared with placebo. This study found no difference in clinical status, weight, or lipoprotein profiles after four months of treatment. In addition, the cimetidine-treated group had an increase in airway resistance after treatment, thought to be caused by possible cimetidine-induced bronchoconstriction, as compared with a decrease in the control group.

Antibiotic Therapy

Chronic pulmonary infections account for most of the morbidity and mortality in patients with CF. The long-term dilation and hypertrophy of the bronchial glands and subsequent mucus plugging provide an excellent environment for the development of infections. Recurrent infection and tissue damage develop, which may progress to bronchiectasis, airflow obstruction, and cor pulmonale. The most common pathogens in respiratory infections are *Pseudomonas aeruginosa* and *Staphylococcus aureus*. Other organisms include *Haemophilus influenzae, Escherichia coli,* and *Klebsiella pneumoniae.*

The epidemiologic pattern of respiratory pathogens has changed over the past two decades; the primary organism is now *Ps. aeruginosa* as compared with *Staph. aureus* in the past.[21] This may be the result of the introduction of antistaphylococcal antibiotics.[1,2] Except for the inability of alveolar macrophages to destroy *Ps. aeruginosa*, no other underlying immunologic defect has been discovered in patients with CF.[21,22] In addition, *Ps. cepacia* has emerged as an important pathogen in CF. This organism is usually very resistant to ticarcillin, piperacillin, and the aminoglycosides, and *Ps. cepacia* infections are associated with a very high mortality rate.[23,24]

Of particular interest is the rapid development of mucoid strains of *Ps. aeruginosa* in patients with CF. The negatively charged exopolysaccharide inhibits the diffusion of the positively charged aminoglycoside[25] and prevents opsonization and phagocytosis.[22] It appears this mucoid phenomenon may not be organism-specific but may be facilitated by the unique environment of the lung tissue of patients with CF. Other organisms have recently shown the development of mucoid strains in patients with CF. In addition, studies have demonstrated a poor correlation between the sensitivity testing of mucoid organism and efficacy.[26] The mucoid strains show excellent in vitro sensitivity to antibiotics while they are often resistant in vivo. This appears to be the result of separation of the mucoid coating from the microorganism that allows for the rapid diffusion of antibiotics into the cell. Furthermore, the bioactivity of aminoglycosides may be altered in the sputum of CF patients. Levy et al.[27] found decreased activity of gentamicin against *Ps. aeruginosa* in CF sputum compared with serum. They attributed this difference to the increased binding of aminoglycoside to the sputum as compared with the serum. Thus, sensitivity testing may be less specific in directing the treatment of pulmonary infections in CF patients with mucoid types of organisms.

Despite some of the problems with culture-and-sensitivity testing in these patients, such tests remain extremely important in determining rational antibiotic therapy in CF. Kulczycki and Weintzen[28] suggested that the continued use of antibiotics in patients with CF may accelerate the colonization of the respiratory tract with *Ps. aeruginosa* and mucoid-*Pseudomonas* species. It has been suggested that the development of mucoid-type *Ps. aeruginosa* is associated with increased morbidity and mortality.[29] Thus, frequent microbiologic monitoring of patients with CF is necessary to devise rational therapy. However, before treatment begins, it is important to distinguish between pulmonary colonization by various microorganisms and pulmonary infection. Although most CF patients are chronically colonized by various possibly pathogenic organisms, antibiotic therapy is indicated only when clinical symptoms occur.[1,2,10]

Pulmonary infections caused by *Staph. aureus* and *H. influenzae* can usually be treated with oral antibiotic therapy. Treatment with a β-lactamase-resistant penicillin, cloxacillin, or dicloxacillin is usually sufficient, although other agents such as cephalexin, ampicillin, erythromycin, and chloramphenicol may be needed.[10] Therapy is usually directed at eradicating these organisms and may need to be continued for as long as 12 weeks.[10] Periodic repeat cultures should be obtained to follow the sensitivity patterns of the organisms and ensure adequate treatment.[1,2,10]

Acute infections usually require 14 to 21 days of intravenous therapy with a ureidopenicillin and an aminoglycoside.[2,4,10] Early in the course of CF, the organisms may be susceptible in vitro to oral antimicrobials such as trimethoprim-sulfamethoxazole, tetracycline, or ampicillin. Even though tetracycline is not recommended for young children, it may be the only oral agent to which the pathogen is sensitive in some young patients with CF. The potential toxicities of tetracycline (such as dental and bone changes) must be weighed against the severity of the pulmonary infection in the patient. Carbenicillin was initially used with aminoglycosides for antipseudomonal therapy in patients with CF. However, given its relatively high minimum inhibitory concentration (MIC) to *Ps. aeruginosa* (>125 μg/mL), carbenicillin 600–800 mg/kg (as the disodium salt) is often needed to treat these infections.[22,30] At our institution in 1984, 39% of the *Ps. aeruginosa* isolates were resistant to carbenicillin, while only 15% of the isolates were resistant to ticarcillin and less than 7% were resistant to azlocillin or piperacillin.[31] Thus, carbenicillin is usually not recommended for the treatment of infections caused by *Ps. aeruginosa* at our hospital.[31] Ticarcillin, mezlocillin, azlocillin,[32,33] and piperacillin[34] have greater activity than carbenicillin against *Ps. aeruginosa*. Although there is some difference in their MICs, one study reported comparable MIC_{90} values against strains of *Ps. aeruginosa* isolated from CF patients.[35] All of these penicillins have a synergistic effect in vitro when used with an aminoglycoside against *Ps. aeruginosa*.[32,35]

First-line therapy for treating *Ps. aeruginosa* infections in CF patients consists of an aminoglycoside, usually gentamicin or tobramycin. Tobramycin has shown greater activity against clinical isolates of *Ps. aeruginosa*[35,36]; however, the selection of an animoglycoside should be based on the microbial-susceptibility patterns of *Ps. aeruginosa* in a given institution. When microbial resistance develops to gentamicin or tobramycin, amikacin is often useful.[35]

Some of the third-generation cephalosporins, particularly ceftazidime, cefoperazone, and cefsulodin, also have activity against *Ps. aeruginosa*.[37–41] Ceftazidime was effective in 15 CF patients with *Ps.*

aeruginosa respiratory-tract infections who did not respond to carbenicillin and aminoglycoside therapy.[40] In addition, ceftazidime demonstrated good activity against 355 strains of *Ps. aeruginosa* from patients with CF.[25] Ceftazidime was shown to be as effective as the combination of ticarcillin and tobramycin in CF patients with acute pulmonary exacerbations.[42] Similar clinical improvement was seen in both treatment groups. Bacterial resistance attributable to *Ps. aeruginosa* was seen in 5% of the patients treated with ceftazidime and in 30% of those treated with ticarcillin and tobramycin. Cefoperazone has been compared with methicillin, ticarcillin, and tobramycin in 25 CF patients.[43] Clinical findings, pulmonary-function test results, and roentgenographic findings were similar in both groups. The bacterial-resistance rate, however, increased from 7% to 17% in the cefoperazone-treated group while all clinical isolates of *Pseudomonas* remained sensitive to tobramycin. Based on limited clinical experience and bacteriologic response, ceftazidime may be preferred over cefoperazone in the treatment of pulmonary exacerbations of CF. Cefsulodin, an investigational cephalosporin, does not have a broad gram-negative spectrum but it has shown good activity against *Ps. aeruginosa*.[44] Clinical studies are needed to determine its efficacy in CF. Further clinical evaluation will help determine the comparative effectiveness of these agents in patients with CF.

Pharmacokinetic Considerations. Shortly after the institution of aggressive antibiotic therapy in CF, it became evident that normal doses of antibiotics were not sufficient to achieve a therapeutic response. Yaffe et al.[45] first described the increased plasma and renal clearance of methicillin in seven patients with CF as compared to normal subjects. Likewise, Jusko et al.[46] demonstrated a 2.5-fold increase in the renal clearance of dicloxacillin in patients with CF. An increase in clearance was thought to be caused by an increased tubular secretion of penicillins. Other investigations have confirmed the increased clearance of cloxacillin,[47] azlocillin,[48] and piperacillin.[34] Spino et al.[47] demonstrated an increase in the total body clearance of cloxacillin and a 2.5-fold increase in nonrenal clearance. Although the source of the nonrenal clearance is unknown, it is postulated that patients with CF may have an increase in drug biotransformation in the liver, kidney, and lungs. Cephalosporins and other antibiotics have not been studied as extensively in CF as penicillins, but a recent study reported a rapid clearance of ceftazidime in CF patients.[49]

Many investigators have examined the pharmacokinetics of aminoglycosides in CF (Table 2).[50-58] Some studies reported a larger apparent volume of distribution (V) of these drugs in patients with CF compared with patients without CF.[50-53] Aminoglycosides are primarily distributed in the extracel-

Table 2.
Aminoglycoside Pharmacokinetics in Patients with Cystic Fibrosis (CF)[a]

Reference	Drug	Number of Patients and Condition	Drug Dose[b] (mg/kg/day)	Clearance (mL/min/1.73 sq m)	Volume of Distribution (L/kg)	Elimination Half-Life (hr)
50	Gentamicin	17 CF	9.89 ± 0.62	73.7 ± 4.09	0.339 ± 0.03	1.62 ± 0.15
	sulfate	17 N	6.82 ± 0.22	40.6 ± 4.74	0.236 ± 0.16	1.98 ± 0.27
51	Tobramycin sulfate	17 CF	8 – 26	180.7 ± 18.1	0.37 ± 0.04	1.2 ± 0.08
52	Amikacin	11 CF	. . .	130.8 ± 27.7	0.288 ± 0.06	1.5 ± 0.5
	sulfate	9 N		107.1 ± 17.8	0.193 ± 0.05	1.6 ± 0.4
53	Tobramycin sulfate	38 CF	11.1 ± 3.9	2.98 ± 0.80[c]	0.33 ± 0.20	1.2 ± 0.5
	Gentamicin sulfate	31 CF	10.3 ± 3.2	2.79 ± 0.75[c]	0.35 ± 0.15	1.4 ± 0.4
54	Gentamicin sulfate	10 CF	. . .	50.35 ± 14.43	0.205 ± 0.06	. . .
55	Tobramycin	12 CF	75.5 ± 10.2[d]	121.2 ± 14.9	0.31 ± 0.08	1.73 ± 0.42
	sulfate	8 N	55.7 ± 14.7[d]	102.2 ± 18.9	0.23 ± 0.07	1.85 ± 0.38
56	Tobramycin	52 CF				
	sulfate	4 < 1 yr	10.30 ± 0.60	82.40 ± 34.70	0.30 ± 0.50	1.50 ± 0.40
		48 ≥ 5 yr	12.5 ± 3.60	127.30 ± 35.90	0.23 ± 0.06	1.10 ± 0.36
57	Tobramycin sulfate	3 CF	14 ± 1.7	3.05 ± 0.88	0.37 ± 0.02	1.4 ± 0.12
58	Netilmicin	8 CF	9.0 ± 0.0	110.3 ± 39.3	0.31 ± 0.11	1.37 ± 0.27
	sulfate	8 N	9.0 ± 0.0	87.6 ± 42.8	0.36 ± 0.16	2.29 ± 0.86

[a] Pharmacokinetic values given as means ± standard deviations.
[b] Dosage expressed in terms of the parent drug.
[c] mL/min/kg.
[d] mg/sq m/day.

lular fluid. With decreased fat stores in many CF patients, a higher *V* (L/kg) might be expected. Kearns et al.[45,50] found no correlation between body weight and *V* in CF patients but did find a correlation in the control group. However, Levy et al.[55] demonstrated a significantly larger *V* in patients with CF than in a control group based on body weight, but no difference existed when these figures were normalized according to body surface area. This study emphasized the need to base the dosage of aminoglycosides in CF patients on body surface area.

In addition to an increased *V*, an increased clearance of gentamicin, tobramycin, and amikacin has been reported also.[50,52] Since aminoglycosides are eliminated primarily by glomerular filtration and are reabsorbed in the proximal renal tubule, a defect in reabsorption or an increase in nonrenal elimination could explain the increased clearance of these agents. No such defect has been identified in patients with CF.

The severity of CF may be another important factor in explaining the increased dosage requirements of aminoglycosides in these patients. In a comparison with normal children, MacDonald et al.[54] found no significant change in the pharmacokinetics of gentamicin in patients with mild disease. This was the first attempt to correlate disease state with dosage requirements. Nahata et al.[59] recently found similar results with cephalexin in CF patients. This may partly explain the substantial variation in the clearance and *V* of aminoglycosides and other antibiotics in CF. As the disease progresses there may be an increase in extracellular fluid and nonrenal elimination pathways, which increase the clearance of antibiotics. Further studies are needed to examine this hypothesis.

Because of the wide variation in pharmacokinetics in CF patients and the need to use aggressive management, routine monitoring and individualization of aminoglycoside doses for these patients is important. There are various recommended starting doses (e.g., 2.5–3 mg/kg every 6–8 hours of tobramycin or gentamicin [as the sulfate salts]),[50,53,60,61] but close monitoring is needed to make dosage adjustments. Peak serum concentrations of 8–12 μg/mL and trough concentrations of less than 2 μg/mL are recommended to permit adequate therapeutic concentrations in the bronchial secretions.[62,63] Clearly, the attainment of effective peak serum concentrations is crucial for optimal therapeutic outcome. Toxicity is usually not a problem in CF patients unless prolonged therapy is required.

Efficacy. The use of intravenous antibiotics to treat acute respiratory-tract infections in CF is quite common. However, because it is often not possible to eradicate the organism from the sputum, therapeutic endpoints are often unclear. Improvement in pulmonary function, arterial-blood gas test results, and global-rating scores (e.g., Schwachman scale),[a] and a decrease in fever have all been used to evaluate therapy.

Hyatt et al.[64] conducted a randomized, double-blind, controlled trial with 24 patients comparing combination therapy with carbenicillin, sisomicin, and oxacillin with oxacillin alone in patients with positive *Ps. aeruginosa* cultures and an acute respiratory exacerbation of their disease. Two of nine patients in the oxacillin group improved clinically, while 12 of 15 in the triple-combination antibiotic group demonstrated improvement. Improvement was seen in the pulmonary-function test results and by a temporary eradication of *Ps. aeruginosa* from sputum samples. Other comparative trials using similar antibiotic regimens have shown similar results.[65] Thus, despite a lack of strong evidence, the aggressive treatment of acute exacerbations with intravenous antibiotic therapy may be necessary in many CF patients.

Prophylactic and Long-Term Therapy. Some CF centers administer oral prophylactic antibiotics, particularly antistaphylococcal penicillins, cephalosporins, or chloramphenicol to prevent the colonization of microorganisms in the sputum. Paporisz et al.[66] evaluated the long-term use (up to 16 weeks) of intramuscular tobramycin therapy in patients with advanced pulmonary disease. Clinically, there was an improvement in the patients treated with tobramycin but *Candida albicans* and *Aspergillus fumigatus* emerged. They could not attribute the clinical improvement of their patients to antibiotic therapy alone. The use of intramuscular therapy, increased awareness of their disease state, and intensified use of adjunctive physiotherapy may have also aided in their clinical improvement.

A 10-year study of patients with CF by Szaff et al.[67] demonstrated increased survival time and decreased morbidity in patients given "maintenance" antipseudomonal therapy every three months. The therapy consisted of tobramycin given in combination with carbenicillin or another β-lactam antibiotic with activity against *Ps. aeruginosa*. The patients received a two-week course of antibiotics every three months and were evaluated monthly. The five-year survival rate increased to 82% compared with a rate of 54% documented for the patients treated in the previous five years. Because of historical controls in this study, it is not possible to reach definitive conclusions about these results. With the risk of side effects from long-term therapy, the emergence of resistant strains (especially mucoid *Ps. aeruginosa*), and the increased cost of therapy, only the patients with the most severe CF should be considered for long-term therapy. Close microbiologic surveillence and aggressive treatment of acute pulmonary exacerbations are imperative in order to decrease the morbidity of this disease.

Antibiotic Aerosols. The respiratory system is

the major site of infection in CF and is often difficult to treat with antibiotic therapy. Because of the systemic toxicity of many of these agents, it would be useful to deliver the antimicrobial directly to the site of infection in the lungs. Aerosolized antibiotic agents that are poorly absorbed should theoretically minimize systemic toxicity while delivering high concentrations of drug to the site of infection and eradicating the causative organism. It has been suggested that aerosol antibiotic therapy should help decrease the inflammatory process of CF in the small airways and decrease morbidity and mortality.[68]

A variety of antibiotic agents have been used as aerosols for the treatment of CF (Table 3).[65–69] However, few clinical studies have demonstrated their effectiveness. Pines et al.[70–71] found no difference in the response rate of patients treated with aerosolized carbenicillin, gentamicin, or colistin and intravenous therapy in a comparison with intravenous therapy alone. If the sputum samples became negative for bacterial growth while the patient was receiving the aerosol therapy, the microorganism soon reappeared after the discontinuation of the therapy. Stephens et al.[72] reported similar findings with tobramycin aerosols. Huang[73] also found no benefit to adjunctive aerosolized carbenicillin in CF treatment.

In a crossover study, Hobson et al.[74] demonstrated an increase in pulmonary function and a decrease in hospital admissions in patients treated with aerosolized carbenicillin 1 g and gentamicin 80 mg twice daily. Resistant organisms developed in four patients, and *Ps. aeruginosa* was not eradicated in any of the patients while receiving this therapy. Hoff et al.[75] also reported an improvement in CF patients treated with aerosolized tobramycin 100 mg twice daily (as the sulfate salt) in addition to intravenous therapy. However, this difference may have been the result of the higher peak serum concentrations of aminoglycosides in those patients being treated with aerosols. The patients treated with aerosolized tobramycin received a higher mean dose of tobramycin and the mean peak serum concentration was higher by 2 μg/mL. Braden et al.[76] demonstrated an increase in the serum concentrations of aminoglycosides when additional drug was given as an aerosol. It is difficult to determine if the benefits from aerosolized aminoglycoside therapy are attributable to the increase in serum concentration or to the route of administration. Furthermore, the administration of high-dose aerosolized aminoglycoside with concurrent intravenous therapy may increase the potential for toxicity. The use of antimicrobial aerosols, especially kanamycin, may cause bronchospasm or irritate hyperactive airways.[77] In addition, the aerosol solutions themselves may become the source for introducing resistant organisms into the respiratory system. In earlier work, Kuhn et al.[78] documented the contamination of aerosolized antibiotics with *Bacillus subtilis*. Without strict aseptic technique, these solutions may exacerbate the pulmonary disease in CF. With the risk of bronchospasm, the unpredictable serum concentrations of aminoglycosides, and being a possible source of contamination, the routine use of antimicrobial aerosols must be questioned.

Table 3.
Aerosolized Antibiotics Used for Patients with Cystic Fibrosis

Drug	Dosage
Ticarcillin[a]	300 mg/kg/day
Tobramycin[b]	60–200 mg/day
Kanamycin[b]	250 mg/day
Polymyxin B[b]	250 mg/day
Neomycin sulfate	25–500 mg/day
Cephaloridine[c]	25 mg/kg/day
Colistin[b]	500,000 units/day
Gentamicin[b]	200 mg/day
Methicillin sodium	1,000 mg/day
Carbenicillin[a]	1,000 mg/day

[a] As the disodium salt.
[b] As the sulfate salt.
[c] No longer marketed.

Mucolytic Therapy

Theoretically, mucolytic agents may help facilitate the expectoration of excessive mucus in patients with CF and therefore improve respiratory function. Compounds such as acetylcysteine (Mucomyst) have often been used as mucolytic agents to degrade the mucus plugs in the bronchioles and small airways. In vitro, acetylcysteine clearly affects the physical properties of the sputum by reducing its viscosity.[68] However, its effectiveness in vivo has been questioned. Waring et al.[79] showed no objective beneficial effects of aerosolized acetylcysteine as a mucolytic in CF patients. Rao et al.[80] also demonstrated no change in pulmonary function after acetylcysteine inhalation. The aerosol administration of acetylcysteine is costly and unpleasant to patients and may cause irritation of the upper airways and precipitate bronchoconstriction.[68]

In addition to the inhalation of acetylcysteine, some investigators have examined its role as a mucolytic after oral administration. Gotz et al.[81] reported no significant differences in pulmonary function or sputum quantity in a crossover study with patients given an average of 9.5 mg/kg/day of oral therapy compared with placebo. Other investigators have compared both the oral and aerosol administration of acetylcysteine in patients with CF.[82,83] Stephan et al.[83] found no deterioration in patients who were switched from aerosol to oral therapy. Of the 126 patients receiving acetylcysteine, the group receiving oral therapy had a significant increase in height and weight. However, this change may have been caused by improvement in the gastrointestinal conditions of the patients, not in their pulmonary status. Based on the data available, the routine use of acetylcysteine cannot be recommended for patients with CF.

Bronchodilator Therapy

Many patients with CF have reactive-airways disease and may require theophylline therapy. Larsen et al.[84] demonstrated a significant improvement in pulmonary function test results as measured by thoracic-gas volume (TGV), residual volume (RV), and maximal-expiratory volume at 60% of total lung capacity ($V_{max60tlc}$) in 10 patients with CF. The patients received aminophylline (4 mg/kg) intravenously over five minutes or 0.9% sodium chloride injection as a placebo. TGV and RV improved from 24% to 37% whereas $V_{max60tlc}$ increased from 35% to 64% over two hours. However, Shapiro et al.[85] showed that theophylline had limited effectiveness in treating the underlying pulmonary disease of CF patients. Compliance problems associated with the outpatient administration of theophylline, insensitive measures of pulmonary function, and limited number of observations make it difficult to extrapolate data from this study.

As with other drugs, altered pharmacokinetic variables have been reported with theophylline in CF patients. Larsen et al.[84] found an apparent volume of distribution of 0.574 L/kg in patients with CF compared with 0.422 L/kg in normal patients. Measurements of clearance and half-life were not significantly different. This may be because of the lower percentage of fat in CF patients compared with normal patients. Other studies[86,87] found wide intersubject variation in the pharmacokinetic variables of theophylline in patients with CF, but the pharmacokinetic values were not significantly different from those of age-matched controls except for the volume of distribution. These studies did not normalize volume of distribution according to body surface area or percentage of body fat. Although only a few trials have been conducted using theophylline, these data suggest that the drug may be beneficial in the management of patients with CF. Because of changes in the volume of distribution and the potential toxicities of theophylline in severely ill patients, serum concentrations must be monitored to maximize efficacy and minimize the potential for toxicity.

In addition to theophylline, other β-adrenergic agents have been used in CF. Terbutaline increases mucociliary transport, which would be beneficial to CF patients, but no clinical trials have demonstrated its superiority to other β-adrenergic agents. Isoproterenol has been used as an aerosol bronchodilator, and it may decrease the side effects of other inhaled products. There are no good studies comparing the use of various β-adrenergic agents in CF patients. However, β-adrenergic medications should theoretically help to improve pulmonary function in these patients just as they help in other types of reactive-airway disease.

Vitamin and Mineral Supplementation

Most patients with CF have some degree of fat malabsorption and are potentially at risk for a fat-soluble vitamin deficiency. Hypoprothrombinemia has been described in these patients because of either a decrease in vitamin K absorption or a decrease in the synthesis of vitamin K clotting factors by the liver.[88] Supplements are usually given to patients with CF at twice the recommended daily allowance for the water-soluble vitamins B and C and the fat-soluble vitamins A and D.[89] Despite this supplementation, deficiencies of vitamin A may occur. Congdren et al.[90] examined the stores of numerous vitamins in 36 CF patients who were supplemented with all vitamins except folic acid and vitamin E. No deficiencies were found in the levels of B vitamins and only two of six patients had low-leucocyte vitamin C concentrations. However, despite supplementation with 400 IU of vitamin D in 25 patients, 4 had low cholecalciferol concentrations. In addition, 43% had low serum vitamin A concentrations despite supplementation that correlated well with global-rating Schwachman scores. Vitamin E concentrations were significantly lower in the patients with CF; 93% of these patients had values two standard deviations lower than the control group. Thus, vitamin E supplementation should be included in the vitamin management of CF patients. Water-miscible forms of vitamin K and E should be used in supplementation therapy for optimal absorption.[91] Although no definite recommendation has been made, doses of 50–100 μg/day orally or 5 mg twice a week of vitamin K and 100–400 IU daily of vitamin E have been used.[89]

In addition to fat-soluble vitamin deficiencies, iron deficiencies have been reported.[92] Despite severe pulmonary disease and periods of hypoxia, CF patients seldom become polycythemic. In fact, many patients have relative anemia and iron deficiency. With iron and vitamin E supplementation, mean hemoglobin concentrations and serum ferritin concentrations increased after treatment with 6 mg/kg/day of elemental iron and 2–3 IU/kg/day of water-miscible vitamin E for four to five weeks. Therefore, careful monitoring of hemoglobin and vitamin E serum concentrations with adequate supplementation may help correct or prevent anemia in patients with CF.

Because of the underlying defect in sodium and chloride reabsorption, patients with CF may require sodium chloride supplementation. Supplementation is not required often, given the high average dietary intake of sodium in the United

States. However, during periods of hot, humid weather or strenuous physical exercise, it may become necessary. The sodium chloride dosage is generally based on weight, but some patients may require up to 5 g/day.[10] When intravenous therapy is required, the maintenance amount of sodium chloride may have to be increased to maintain homeostasis. Although no specific guidelines are available, electrolyte concentrations should be monitored to ensure replacement of losses.

Conclusion

Until the basic underlying pathologic defect in CF is discovered, all therapy will be directed at relieving symptoms and preventing complications of the disease. Drug therapy of CF is indeed complex. Pancreatic-enzyme replacements, antibiotics, aerosolized agents, vitamin preparations, and a host of other adjunctive agents make these regimens complicated and expensive. Studies are needed to examine the role of these agents in minimizing symptoms of CF and preventing complications. The optimal management of patients with CF will continue to be a challenge to all the involved medical personnel and family members.

---

[a] This scoring system evaluates physical findings, nutritional status, activity level, and roentgenographic findings.

References

1. DiSant'Agnese P. Cystic fibrosis (mucoviscodosis). *Am Fam Physician*. 1973; 7:102–11.
2. Anderson DH. Cystic fibrosis of the pancreas and its relation to celiac disease. *Am J Dis Child*. 1938; 56:344–99.
3. Wood RE, Boat TF, Doershuk CF. Cystic fibrosis. *Am Rev Respir Dis*. 1976; 113:833–56.
4. Huang NH. Guide to drug therapy in patients with cystic fibrosis. Atlanta, GA: The Cystic Fibrosis Foundation; 1974.
5. Kerrebijn KF, Veentjer R, Bonzet E et al. The immediate effect of physiotherapy and aerosol treatment on pulmonary function in children with cystic fibrosis. *Eur J Respir Dis*. 1982; 63:35–42.
6. Hodges P, Sauriol D, Man FP. Nutrient intake of patients with cystic fibrosis. *J Am Diet Assoc*. 1984; 84:664–9.
7. Lubin H, Bonner JM. Anthropoemetric evaluation of adolescent and young adults with cystic fibrosis. National Cystic Fibrosis Foundation. Rockville, MD: 1977; 18:17.
8. Hadorn B, Johansen PG, Anderson CM. Pancreozymin secretion test of exocrine pancreatic function in cystic fibrosis and the significance of the result for the pathogenesis of the disease. *Can Med Assoc J*. 1968; 98:377–95.
9. Rodman HM, Matthews LW. Hyperglycemia in cystic fibrosis. In: Uhawich WJ, ed. A review of the lifetime in 1000 years of cystic fibrosis. Minneapolis: University of Minnesota Press; 1981:67–76.
10. Matthews LW, Drotar D. Cystic fibrosis—a challenging long term chronic disease. *Pediatr Clin North Am*. 1984; 31:133–52.
11. Cho YW, Aviado PM. Pancreatic enzyme preparation, with special reference to enterically coated microspheres of pancrelipase. *J Clin Pharmacol*. 1981; 21:224–37.
12. Warwick WJ, Budd JR. Comparison of two forms of enteric-coated pancrelipase in six teenagers with cystic fibrosis. *Clin Ther*. 1982; 5(1):15–20.
13. Khaw KT, Adenniyi-Jones S, Gordon D et al. Comparative effectiveness of Viokase,® Cotazyme® and Pancrease® with cystic fibrosis. National Cystic Fibrosis Foundation. Rockville, MD: 1977; 18:57.
14. Kastrup EK, ed. Facts and comparisons. St Louis: J.B. Lippincott Company; 1982:308–13.
15. Nassif EF, Younoszai MK, Weinberger MM et al. Comparative effects of antacids, enteric coating, and bile salts on the efficacy of oral pancreatic enzyme therapy in cystic fibrosis. *J Pediatr*. 1981; 92:320–3.
16. de B'eville F, Neijens HJ, Fernandes J et al. Cimetidine as an adjunct to oral enzyme in the treatment of malabsorption due to cystic fibrosis. *Acta Pediatr Scand*. 1981; 70(1):33–7.
17. Hubbard VS, Dunn GD, Lester LA. Effectiveness of cimetidine as an adjunct to supplemental pancreatic enzymes in patients with cystic fibrosis. *Am J Clin Nutr*. 1980; 33(11):2281–6.
18. Durie PR, Bell L, Linton W et al. Effect of cimetidine and sodium bicarbonate on pancreatic replacement therapy in cystic fibrosis. *Gut*. 1980; 21(9):778–86.
19. Schoni M, Kraemer R, Rossi E. Cimetidine and fat malabsorption in children with cystic fibrosis. *Helv Pediatr Acta*. 1981; 36:359–69.
20. Schoni M, Kraemer R, Ruedeberg A et al. Long-term cimetidine in children with cystic fibrosis: a randomized double-blind study. *Pediatr Res*. 1984; 18:66–70.
21. Means MB, Hunt GH, Rushworth R. Bacterial flora of the respiratory tract in patients with cystic fibrosis. *Arch Dis Child*. 1972; 47:902–27.
22. Marks MI. The pathogenesis and treatment of pulmonary infections in patients with cystic fibrosis. *J Pediatr*. 1981; 98:173–9.
23. Isles A, Maclusky I, Corey M et al. *Pseudomonas cepacia* infection in cystic fibrosis: an emerging problem. *J Pediatr*. 1984; 104:206–10.
24. McKevit A, Woods P. Characterization of *Pseudomonas cepacia* isolates from patients with cystic fibrosis. *J Clin Micro*. 1984; 19:291–3.
25. Slack MD, Nicholas WV. The penetration of antibiotics through sodium alginate and through the exopolysaccharide of a mucoid strain of *Pseudomonas aeruginosa*. *Lancet*. 1981; 2:502–3.
26. Dernko CA, Thomasson MJ. Effect of mucoid property on antibiotic susceptibility of *Pseudomonas aeruginosa*. *Curr Microbiol*. 1980; 4:69–73.
27. Levy J, Smith A, Kenney MA et al. Bioactivity of gentamicin in purulent sputum from patients with cystic fibrosis or bronchiectasis: comparison with activity in serum. *J Infect Dis*. 1983; 148:1069–75.
28. Kulcyzycki LL, Weintzen R. The use and abuse of antibiotics, including in management of pulmonary manifestations in cystic fibrosis. *Monogr Paediatr*. 1979; 10:27–30.
29. Kulczycki LL, Murphy TM, Bellanti JA. *Pseudomonas* colonization in cystic fibrosis. *JAMA*. 1978; 240:30–4.
30. Nelson JD. Carbenicillin therapy of systemic infections due to *Pseudomonas*. *J Infect Dis*. 1970; 122(Suppl 48–58):57–79.
31. Antimicrobial susceptibility profile. Microbiology Section, Department of Laboratory Medicine. Columbus, OH: Columbus Children's Hospital; 1984.
32. Huang NN, Palmer J, Keith H et al. Comparative efficacy and tolerance study of azlocillin and carbenicillin in patients with cystic fibrosis: a double blind study. *J Antimicrob Chemother*. 1983; 11(Suppl B):205–14.
33. McLaughlin FJ, Matthews WJ, Strieder DJ et al. Randomized, double blind evaluation of azlocillin for the treatment of pulmonary exacerbations of cystic fibrosis. *J Antimicrob Chemother*. 1983; 11(Suppl B):195–203.
34. Reed MD, Bertino JS, Aronoff SC et al. Efficacy and pharmacokinetics of piperacillin in patients with cystic fibrosis. Paper presented to 21st Interscience Conference on Antimicrobial Agents and Chemotherapy. Chicago: Nov 1981.
35. Scribner RK, Marks MI, Weber AH et al. Activities of various beta-lactams and aminoglycosides, alone and in combi-

nation against isolates of *Pseudomonas aeruginosa* from patients with cystic fibrosis. *Antimicrob Agents Chemother.* 1982; 21:939–43.
36. Pennington JE, Reynolds HY. Tobramycin in bronchial secretions. *Antimicrob Agents Chemother.* 1973; 4:299–301.
37. Padoan R, Brienza A, Crossignani RM et al. Ceftazidime in the treatment of acute pulmonary exacerbations in patients with cystic fibrosis. *J Pediatr.* 1983; 103(2):320–4.
38. Dodge J, Zamiri I, Goodchila M et al. Experience with ceftazidime in cystic fibrosis. *J Antimicrob Chemother.* 1983; 12(Suppl A):325–9.
39. Strandvik B, Malmborg AS, Alfredson H et al. Clinical results and pharmacokinetics of ceftazidime in patients with cystic fibrosis. *J Antimicrob Chemother.* 1983; 12(Suppl A):283–7.
40. Permin H, Koch C, Hoiby N et al. Ceftazidime treatment of chronic *Pseudomonas aeruginosa* tract infections in cystic fibrosis. *J Antimicrob Chemother.* 1983; 12(Suppl):313–23.
41. Mastella G, Agostini M, Barlocco G et al. Alternative antibiotics for the treatment of *Pseudomonas* infections in cystic fibrosis. *J Antimicrob Chemother.* 1983; 12(Suppl):297–311.
42. Gold R, Overmyer A, Knie B et al. Controlled trial of ceftazidime vs ticarcillin and tobramycin in the treatment of acute respiratory exacerbations in patients with cystic fibrosis. *Pediatr Infect Dis.* 1985; 4:172–7.
43. Jewett CV, Ledbetter J, Lyrene RK et al. Comparison of cefoperazone sodium vs methicillin, ticarcillin and tobramycin in treatment of pulmonary exacerbations in patients with cystic fibrosis. *J Pediatr.* 1985; 106:669–72.
44. Cabezudo I, Thompson RL, Selden RF et al. Cefsulodin sodium therapy in cystic fibrosis patients. *Antimicrob Agents Chemother.* 1984; 25:4–6.
45. Yaffe S, Gerbracht LM, Mosovich LL et al. Pharmacokinetics of methicillin in patients with cystic fibrosis. *J Infect Dis.* 1977; 135(5):828–31.
46. Jusko W, Mosovich LL, Gerbracht LM et al. Enhanced renal excretion of dicloxacillin in patients with cystic fibrosis. *J Pediatr.* 1975; 56:1038–44.
47. Spino M, Chai RP, Isles AF et al. Cloxacillin absorption and disposition in cystic fibrosis. *J Pediatr.* 1984; 105:829–35.
48. Malmborg AS, Alfredsson H, Kusoffsky E et al. Azlocillin and gentamicin in respiratory tract infections with *Pseudomonas aeruginosa* in patients with cystic fibrosis. *Scand J Infect Dis.* 1981; 29(Suppl):64–9.
49. Leeder LS, Spino M, Isles AF et al. Ceftazidime disposition in acute and stable cystic fibrosis. *Clin Pharmacol Ther.* 1984; 36:355–62.
50. Kearns GL, Hilman BC, Wilson JT. Dosing implications of altered gentamicin disposition in patients with cystic fibrosis. *J Pediatr.* 1982; 100(2):312–8.
51. Kelly HB, Menendez RM, Fan L et al. Gentamicin and tobramycin pharmacokinetics in patients with cystic fibrosis. *J Pediatr.* 1982; 100(2):318–21.
52. Vogelstein B, Kowarski AA, Lietman PS et al. Pharmacokinetics of amikacin in children. *J Pediatr.* 1977; 91:331–3.
53. Bauer L, Piecoro JJ, Wilson HD et al. Gentamicin and tobramycin pharmacokinetics in patients with cystic fibrosis. *Clin Pharm.* 1983; 2:262–4.
54. MacDonald NE, Anas NG, Peterson RG et al. Renal clearance of gentamicin in cystic fibrosis. *J Pediatr.* 1983; 103.
55. Levy J, Smith AL, Koup JR et al. Disposition of tobramycin in patients with cystic fibrosis: a prospective controlled study. *J Pediatr.* 1984; 105:117–24.
56. Hsu J, Aquila HA, Schmidt VL et al. Individualization of tobramycin dosage in patients with cystic fibrosis. *Pediatr Infect Dis.* 1984; 3:526–9.
57. Fraser G, Grimes GR, Valenti AJ. Applied pharmacokinetics in acute exacerbations of *Pseudomonas aeruginosa* pneumonia in cystic fibrosis. *J Pediatr.* 1982; 101:792.
58. Michalsen H, Bergin T. Pharmacokinetics of antibiotics in children with cystic fibrosis with particular reference to netilmicin. *Acta Pediatr Scand.* 1982; 30(Suppl):101–5.
59. Nahata MC, Lubin AH, Visconti JA. Cephalexin pharmacokinetics in patients with cystic fibrosis. *Dev Pharmacol Ther.* 1984; 7:221–8.
60. Hendeles L, Stillwell P, Mangos J et al. Gentamicin dosage requirements for cystic fibrosis. *Drug Intell Clin Pharm.* 1981; 15:479. Abstract.
61. Kelly HW, Lavato C. Antibiotic use in cystic fibrosis. *Drug Intell Clin Pharm.* 1984; 18:772–83.
62. McCrae WM, Raeburn JA, Hanson EJ et al. Tobramycin therapy of infections due to *Pseudomonas aeruginosa* in patients with cystic fibrosis: effect of dosage and concentration of antibiotic in sputum. *J Infect Dis.* 1976; 134(Suppl): 191–3.
63. Alexander MR, Schoell J, Hicklin G et al. Bronchial secretion concentrations of tobramycin. *Am Rev Respir Dis.* 1982; 125:208–9.
64. Hyatt AC, Chipps BE, Kumor KM et al. A double-blind controlled trial of anti-*Pseudomonas* chemotherapy of acute respiratory exacerbations in patients with cystic fibrosis. *J Pediatr.* 1981; 99(2):307–11.
65. Hoiby N, Friis B, Jensen K et al. Antimicrobial chemotherapy in cystic fibrosis patients. *Acta Paediatr Scand.* 1982; 301(Suppl):82.
66. Paporisz C, Posselt HG, Wonne R et al. Evaluation of long term tobramycin therapy in patients with cystic fibrosis and advanced pulmonary disease. *Eur J Pediatr.* 1979; 130:259–69.
67. Szaff M, Hoiby N, Flensborg EW et al. Frequent antibiotic therapy improves survival of cystic fibrosis patients with chronic *Pseudomonas aeruginosa* infection. *Acta Paediatr Scand.* 1983; 72:651–7.
68. Wanner A, Rao A. Clinical indications for and effects of blind, mucolytic and antimicrobial aerosols. *Am Rev Respir Dis* 1980; 122:79–103.
69. Gough P, Schuddekopt N. A review of the therapeutic efficacy of aerosolized and endotracheally instilled antibiotics. *Pharmacotherapy.* 1982; 2:367–77.
70. Pines A, Raafat H, Plucinski. Gentamicin and colistin in chronic purulent bronchial infections. *Br Med J.* 1967; 2:543–5.
71. Pines A, Raafat H, Siddigui GM et al. Treatment of severe *Pseudomonas* infections of the bronchi. *Br Med J.* 1970; 1:663–5.
72. Stephens D, Garey N, Isles A et al. Efficacy of inhaled tobramycin in the treatment of pulmonary exacerbations in children with cystic fibrosis. *Pediatr Infect Dis.* 1983; 2(3):209–11.
73. Huang HN, Hiller GT, Macni CM et al. Carbenicillin in patients with cystic fibrosis: clinical pharmacology and therapeutic evaluation. *J Pediatr.* 1971; 78:338–45.
74. Hodson ME, Wingfield HJ, Baten JC. Tobramycin and carbenicillin compared with gentamicin and carbenicillin in the treatment of infection with *Pseudomonas aeruginosa* in adult patients with cystic fibrosis. *Br J Dis Chest.* 1983; 77(1):71–7.
75. Hoff GE, Schiotz PO, Paulsen J. Tobramycin treatment of *Pseudomonas aeruginosa* infections in cystic fibrosis. *Scand J Infect Dis.* 1974; 6:333–7.
76. Braden NJ, Jones PR, Greiner GE. Systemic absorption of aerosolized tobramycin in a patient with cystic fibrosis. Paper presented to 19th Annual ASHP Midyear Clinical Meeting. Dallas, TX: Dec 1984.
77. Biludeau M, Roy JC Girojx M. Studies of absorption of kanamycin by aerosolization. *Ann NY Acad Sci.* 1966; 132:870–8.
78. Kuhn RJ, Lubin HL, Jones PR et al. Bacterial contamination of aerosol solution used to treat cystic fibrosis. *Am J Hosp Pharm.* 1982; 39:308–9.
79. Waring WN. Current management of cystic fibrosis. *Adv Pediatr.* 1976; 23:401–38.
80. Rao S, Wilson DB, Brooks RC et al. Acute effects of nebulization of n-acetylcysteine on pulmonary mechanics and gas exchange. *Am Rev Respir Dis.* 1970; 102:17–22.
81. Gotz M, Kraemer R, Kerrebijn KF et al. Oral acetylcysteine in cystic fibrosis. A co-operative study. *Eur J Respir Dis.* 1980; (Suppl)111:122–6.

82. Ribeiro TM, Cunha LG, Santos M et al. Treatment of bronchial disease in pediatrics. Results of the use of oral acetylcysteine in 80 cases. *Eur J Respir Dis*. 1980; (Suppl 111):136–8.
83. Stephan U, Bowing B, Goering U et al. Acetylcysteine in the oral mucolytic treatment of cystic fibrosis. *Eur J Respir Dis*. 1980; (Suppl)111:127–31.
84. Larsen GL, Barron RJ, Landay RA et al. Intravenous aminophylline in patients with cystic fibrosis. *Am J Dis Child*. 1980; 134:1143–8.
85. Shapiro GG, Rauman J, Kanarek P et al. The paradoxical effect of adrenergic and methylxanthine drugs in cystic fibrosis. *Pediatrics*. 1976; 58:740–3.
86. Isles A, Spino M, Tabachnik E et al. Theophylline disposition in cystic fibrosis. *Am Rev Respir Dis*. 1983; 127(4):417–21.
87. Valet SB, Schwartz RH, Brooks JG et al. Pharmacokinetics of theophylline and bioavailability of a sustained release preparation in patients with cystic fibrosis. *Ann Allergy*. 1983; 50(3):161–5.
88. Tortstenson OL, Humphrey GB, Edson JR et al. Cystic fibrosis presenting with severe hemorrhage due to vitamin K malabsorption: a report of three cases. *Pediatrics*. 1970; 45:857–61.
89. Chase HP, Long MA, Lavin MH. Cystic fibrosis and malnutrition. *J. Pediatr*. 1979; 95:337–47.
90. Congden PJ, Bruce G, Rothburn MM et al. Vitamin status in treated patients with cystic fibrosis. *Arch Dis Child*. 1981; 56(9):708–14.
91. Harrigs JT, Mullen DPR. Absorption of different doses of fat soluble and water miscible preparations of vitamin E in children with cystic fibrosis. *Arch Dis Child*. 1971; 46: 341–4.
92. Ater JL, Herbst JJ, Landaw SA et al. Relative anemia and iron deficiency in cystic fibrosis. *Pediatrics*. 1983; 71:810–4.

Grand Rounds

Papers in the Grand Rounds section are patient case reports and literature review combined in a way that gives them high educational value. The papers lead off with a well-documented case report of an unusual drug experience (e.g., adverse drug reaction or other unexpected drug response, experimental use of a drug). The case generally deals with a difficult therapeutic problem or dilemma that is commonly encountered but may be overlooked or misunderstood. (Esoteric or rare occurrences of minor importance do not make good Grand Rounds material.) A literature review puts the case in perspective with previously reported similar cases and alternative treatments. The review is integrated with related discussions of the new case being reported.

CP readers are encouraged to use Grand Rounds for educational group discussions. For this purpose, discussion questions are printed at the end of Grand Rounds papers.

Recognition and management of acute suppurative parotitis

RICHARD S. PERRY

Abstract: Acute suppurative parotitis (ASP) is a rare infectious process occurring after surgery or in debilitated patients. This case describes a 41-year-old man who was hospitalized initially for acute bacterial endocarditis. Late in the hospital course his recovery was complicated by the development of ASP. Subsequent cultures of blood and parotid-fluid samples grew *Pseudomonas aeruginosa*. Despite early empiric antibiotic therapy followed by more specific therapy with an aminoglycoside, the patient continued to experience severe pain, swelling, and facial-nerve palsy. Surgical incision and drainage of the parotid gland was accomplished on the ninth day after onset of ASP, and the patient experienced a rapid resolution of the disease process.

Acute suppurative parotitis was originally attributed to infection with gram-positive organisms, primarily *Staphylococcus aureus* and *Streptococcus* species. More recently, reports of ASP caused by gram-negative and anaerobic bacteria have been published. This review describes the etiology, pathogenesis, microbiology, and clinical features of ASP. Nonpharmacologic, pharmacologic, and surgical management of the disease is discussed.

Although ASP is a rare occurrence in the hospital setting, early recognition and appropriate management are important in avoiding serious morbidity and mortality.

Index terms: Aminoglycosides; Antibiotics; Clindamycin phosphate; Gentamicin sulfate; Parotitis; *Pseudomonas aeruginosa*; Resistance; Tobramycin sulfate; Vancomycin hydrochloride
Clin Pharm. 1985; 4:566–71

Acute suppurative parotitis (ASP) occurs uncommonly in hospitalized patients; however, the seriousness of the disease may adversely affect the patient's hospital course and outcome. It often occurs postoperatively but may also be seen in debilitated or severely ill patients.[1,2] *Staphylococcus aureus* is the most common organism isolated from the parotid gland; however, gram-negative and anaerobic bacteria are also frequently found in glandular secretions.[1-3] This report describes a case of ASP caused by *Pseudomonas aeruginosa* and reviews the epidemiology, pathogenesis, clinical presentation, and management of ASP.

Case Report

A 41-year-old white man was admitted to our hospital for neurosurgical evaluation. He had been

RICHARD S. PERRY, PHARM.D., is Assistant Professor of Pharmacy Practice, College of Pharmacy, North Dakota State University; and Clinical Pharmacist, St. Luke's Hospitals, Fargo, ND.
Address reprint requests to Dr. Perry at the Department of Pharmacy Practice, College of Pharmacy, North Dakota State University, Fargo, ND 58105.

well with no acute or chronic illnesses until three weeks before admission when he developed an acute onset of flu-like symptoms, nausea, vomiting, and generalized weakness. Two days later the patient became semiresponsive and was admitted to another hospital. The evaluation at this time included lumbar puncture (LP), computed tomography (CT) of the head, and blood cultures. The LP was abnormal with a cell count revealing 90% polymorphonuclear leukocytes, and blood cultures were positive for *Staphylococcus aureus* sensitive to nafcillin (MIC < 0.25 $\mu g/ml$) and chloramphenicol (MIC < 4.0 $\mu g/mL$). The patient was treated with nafcillin 2 g i.v. (as the sodium salt) every four hours and chloramphenicol 1 g i.v. (as the sodium succinate salt), every six hours; however, progressive central nervous system (CNS) symptoms developed with the rapid onset of aphasia and right hemiparesis. A repeat CT scan revealed an area consistent with brain abscess, and an echocardiogram showed an aortic-valve vegetation consistent with endocarditis. Because of his deteriorating clinical condition, the patient was transferred to our hospital for further care. His problems included acute infective endocarditis with septic emboli, cerebritis, and abscess formation.

Upon admission the patient was semi-responsive, aphasic, and disoriented. Chloramphenicol therapy was stopped, nafcillin was continued at the same dosage, and rifampin 600 mg orally each day was added. Cardiology, cardiovascular surgery, infectious disease, and neurology consultations were obtained. Their recommendations included continuing intravenous antibiotic therapy for four to six weeks followed by aortic-valve replacement when the patient's condition stabilized. Serum bactericidal titers on hospital day 3 were greater than 1:64 at peak and trough antibiotic concentrations. The next two weeks of hospitalization were unremarkable; however, on the day 16 after this admission the patient complained of fever and headache. His temperature had increased to 40.4 °C, and swelling was observed in the left parotid area. Acute parotitis was suspected, and the infectious disease service suggested performing bacterial cultures of parotid fluid samples. The white blood cell (WBC) count had decreased to 1800 cells/cu mm, and nafcillin and rifampin were discontinued because of suspected drug-induced leukopenia. Vancomycin 1 g i.v. (as the hydrochloride salt) every 12 hours was begun for treatment of the endocarditis. Also, clindamycin 900 mg i.v. (as the phosphate salt) every eight hours and gentamicin 100 mg i.v. (as the sulfate salt) every eight hours were begun as empiric therapy for acute suppurative parotitis. On day 17 the patient experienced a shaking chill, increasing pain and swelling in the left parotid area, and a temperature elevation to 40.6 °C. On day 19 cultures of the parotid gland and blood samples revealed *Pseudomonas aeruginosa* sensitive to tobramycin (MIC 1 $\mu g/mL$) and resistant to gentamicin. Clindamycin and gentamicin were discontinued, and tobramycin 100 mg i.v. (as the sulfate salt) every eight hours was begun. The patient became afebrile on day 20 and remained stable, and the WBC count had increased to 15,600 cells/cu mm by day 21. On day 22 a left facial-nerve palsy was noted, and the patient was unable to close his left eye. Peak and trough serum bactericidal titers on day 23 were reported as $>$ 1:64. On day 27, peak and trough serum tobramycin concentrations were 5.4 and 0.5 $\mu g/mL$, respectively.

Parotid swelling and facial-nerve palsy persisted through day 31 when incision and drainage of the parotid gland was performed. Cultures of parotid fluid samples taken at this time subsequently revealed *Pseudomonas aeruginosa* sensitive to tobramycin but resistant to gentamicin. Repeat serum tobramycin concentrations on day 31 were reported at peak to be 6.1 $\mu g/mL$ and at trough, 0.5 $\mu g/mL$. Vancomycin concentrations determined on day 36 revealed a peak of 27.0 $\mu g/mL$ and a trough of 4.0 $\mu g/mL$. The patient continued to improve with less pain, no fever, and improving speech and ambulation. On day 42 cultures of blood and parotid fluid samples were negative, and tobramycin was discontinued. Vancomycin was discontinued on day 49, and the patient was discharged from the hospital to return for aortic-valve replacement at a future date.

Discussion

Acute suppurative parotitis, also referred to as pyogenic, postoperative, or nosocomial parotitis, occurs as an acute infectious process involving the parotid gland and adjacent anatomic structures.[4-7] In the pre-antibiotic era, ASP was recognized as a rare but serious complication of surgery.[7-10] With knowledge of the etiology of this disease and improvements in nursing care, ASP has become a less frequent complication of surgical procedures. Instead, it has been recognized more commonly, albeit rarely, in the medical patient.[5,6,11]

Etiology. The overall incidence of this disease has been reported to be 0.01–0.02% of all hospital admissions and 0.002–0.04% of postoperative patients.[3,4,8,9] The epidemiology of ASP has been reviewed in several large series of patients.[4,8,9,12] Typically, the patient is elderly and debilitated, often with a severe underlying disease. Before the 1950s, the majority of cases of ASP were reported to occur during the postoperative period.[8-10] Subsequent reports by Spratt[4] and Krippaehne et al.[12] found that only 30–40% of the patients in their series were in the postoperative period. These figures were confirmed by reports in two smaller series of patients where 7 of 22 and 3 of 7 subjects, respectively, were in the postoperative period when ASP developed.[5,11] Other conditions that

Figure 1. Anatomic location of the salivary glands.

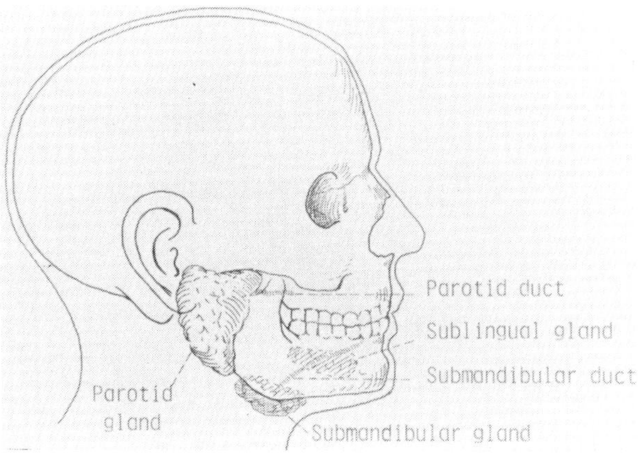

have been associated with ASP include cancer, other sites of infection, and the presence of a tracheostomy.[4,5,11,12]

In an attempt to identify factors that would predispose a patient to develop ASP, several authors analyzed the data from their series of patients.[4,6,11,12] Factors associated with an increased incidence of ASP include diuretic therapy, treatment with anticholinergic drugs, prior antibiotic therapy, poor oral hygiene, malnutrition, and dehydration.[4–6,11–13] Lundgren et al.[5] noted that 19 of 22 patients were receiving diuretics or drugs with anticholinergic properties at the time of onset of ASP. Similarly, 25% of the patients described by Krippaehne et al.[12] were receiving drugs with potent anticholinergic properties. Power[13] reported on five patients who developed parotitis after potent diuretic therapy. Several authors have also described an association between previous antibiotic therapy and the occurrence of ASP.[5,10,11] The patient described here had been receiving antibiotics for three weeks before the onset of ASP.

Pathogenesis. The parotid glands are located in the subcutaneous area of the cheeks anterior and inferior to the ears.[14] They are one of three pairs of salivary glands located in the neck region. The parotid duct extends in an anterior direction from the gland and opens into the oral cavity beyond the second molar (Figure 1). Parasympathetic stimulation causes the parotid gland to secrete a clear, watery secretion, which is emptied from the parotid duct into the oral cavity. Parotid secretions aid in the hydrolysis of dietary starch. Saliva also provides lubrication and moistening of food and exerts a cleansing action on teeth that helps maintain oral hygiene.

Under normal conditions, salivary flow protects against bacterial infection of the glands.[1] However, in the presence of reduced salivary flow resulting from dehydration or drugs, obstruction of the duct, or increased viscosity of the saliva, bacteria normally present in the oral cavity may invade the duct and spread to the gland, producing ASP. Once the inflammatory process has begun, invasion of glandular and surrounding tissues may develop.[12] Without proper treatment, the infectious process may invade facial and neck tissues and the auditory canal. Dissemination of the infection into surrounding tissues may cause airway obstruction, bacteremia, or other serious complications.[1,7] The potential for a fulminant course requires prompt diagnosis and treatment.

Microbiology. The oropharyngeal cavity serves as a reservoir for a wide variety of bacterial organisms. Predominant flora include facultative aerobes, such as *Streptococcus, Neisseria, Lactobacillus,* and *Corynebacterium* species.[15] Equally important are obligate anaerobic bacteria, often accounting for more than half of the organisms cultured from normal healthy subjects. Obligate anaerobes usually found in the oral cavity include *Peptostreptococcus, Actinomyces, Veillonella, Fusobacterium,* and *Bacteroides* species. *Bacteroides fragilis* is a common pathogen in the lower abdomen; however, it is rarely recovered from the oral cavity. Enteric facultative gram-negative organisms are generally thought to be a rare finding in normal oropharyngeal flora. However, careful culture techniques have isolated enteric gram-negative organisms in to 18% of healthy subjects; these organisms include *Klebsiella* sp., *Escherichia coli, Enterobacter* sp., *Acinetobacter,* and *Pseudomonas aeruginosa*.[16–18]

In contrast to healthy subjects, hospitalized patients often exhibit a different spectrum of bacterial flora.[16,19] Routine culturing of the oropharyngeal cavity in various patient populations has revealed increasing colonization with gram-negative enteric aerobes as the level of care increases.[18,20] Various explanations have been provided for the increase in gram-negative colonization.[16,18,19] Valenti et al.[18] found that gram-negative colonization of the oropharyngeal area was associated with increasing age, severity of illness or underlying disease, deterioration of clinical status, loss of functional abilities, and reduced ambulation. In addition, impaired clearance of bacteria from the pharyngeal area secondary to reduced salivary flow and decreased swallowing may be a contributing factor.[16,18,19] Others have identified an increased adherence of gram-negative bacteria to oral epithelial cells in hospitalized patients through nonspecific binding to cell walls.[21–24] Anaerobes also are increasingly recognized as pathogens, particularly with respect to infections of the oral cavity.[25,26] Sabiston et al.[27] found that 66% of dental infections were caused by anaerobic bacteria. Regardless of the mechanism, the incidence of gram-negative and anaerobic infections in hospitalized patients has increased in recent years.[16,20]

The changing spectrum of oropharyngeal bacteria may be reflected in recent literature describing patients with ASP. Early reports of ASP indicated a predominance of gram-positive bacteria, particularly *Staphylococcus aureus* and *Streptococcus* spp.[4,5,11,12] However, it must be noted that Spratt[4] and Krippaehne et al.[12] were unable to isolate an organism in the majority of ASP patients. A likely explanation for the early predominance of gram-positive bacteria was the lack of sophisticated culture techniques for anaerobic and gram-negative bacteria.[4–12,16] Increasingly, gram-negative and anaerobic bacteria have been isolated from patients with ASP reflecting the recent change in the spectrum of nosocomial infections.[16] Recently, Pruett and Simmons[6] and others[28,29] have reported cases in which gram-negative or anaerobic organisms were the only isolates from parotid fluid. The wide array of bacteria implicated in ASP highlights the need for broad-spectrum antibiotic therapy. Appropriate empiric therapy with antibiotics having a spectrum of activity broad enough to treat gram-positive, gram-negative, and possibly anaerobic bacteria should be selected.

Clinical Features. The typical patient with ASP is elderly, debilitated, and usually has been hospitalized for some other disease process. In the postoperative patient the onset of symptoms usually occurs within two weeks of surgery, while in the nonsurgical patient symptoms often occur later in the hospital course and may coincide with deterioration in the patient's condition.[4,5]

In most patients with ASP, the disease is unilateral, but up to 17% may have it bilaterally.[4] The patient typically exhibits an acute onset of pain, swelling, and tenderness in the area of the parotid gland.[1,3,5] The affected area is found to be warm, firm, indurated, erythematous, and tender.[3,5] With external pressure on the gland, pus may be expressed from the parotid duct in up to 75% of patients.[3] The temperature may be as high as 40.5 °C, and the WBC count may increase above 40,000 cells/cu mm.[3] Petersdorf et al.[11] reported an average WBC count of 33,000 cells/cu mm in their seven patients. Some patients may experience a spontaneous resolution of the infectious process with complete healing at this point, but most remain symptomatic and require definitive treatment.[4–6]

Management. Acute suppurative parotitis occurs predominantly in the hospitalized patient and, consequently, prevention represents the most important step in management. Early recognition of the patient at risk (elderly, debilitated, dehydrated) is a vital first step in prevention. Emphasis should be given to maintaining adequate hydration, and special attention should be directed toward the patient's oral hygiene.[4–6,8,11] Ice chips or stimulants to salivary flow, such as hard candy or chewing gum, may be used in the patient who complains of xerostomia.[4,5,7] One author suggests cautious use of drugs that suppress salivation and the removal of dentures as important preventative measures.[5] Judicious attention to preventive measures should be a priority when poor oral hygiene has been identified in the patient at risk.

When ASP does develop, prompt treatment is important. The patient should be adequately rehydrated if necessary, and specimens of pus should be obtained from the parotid duct for culture and sensitivity testing.[4,7] Initiation of empiric antibiotic therapy is recommended pending culture and sensitivity results.[4,5,11,12] The choice for initial antibiotic therapy should include agents that provide coverage of *Staphylococcus aureus*, *Streptococcus*, and gram-negative bacilli.[6] Although anaerobic bacteria may cause ASP, anaerobes isolated on culture are almost always normal oropharyngeal bacteria and are usually highly susceptible to penicillin.[15,27–29] Some authors report that because of the obligate nature of these anaerobes, adequate treatment of the aerobic bacteria will successfully eradicate anaerobes from the infected site.[15]

Appropriate empiric therapy for ASP should consist of an aminoglycoside antibiotic plus a penicillinase-resistant penicillin or first-generation cephalosporin. In penicillin-allergic patients, clindamycin, vancomycin, or a cephalosporin are acceptable alternatives. After culture and sensitivity results are obtained, antibiotic therapy can be adjusted if necessary. The patient's response should be rapid, and improvement in signs and symptoms should be observed within 48 to 72 hours of initiating therapy.[3] An optimal duration of therapy for ASP has not been determined; however, the patient should be asymptomatic and have no signs of suppuration present before therapy is stopped. Two aspects of the disease should be considered when planning antibiotic therapy. First, the presence of fibrous septae in the gland may impair antibiotic penetration; second, the inflammatory process may affect the response to antibiotics. If the patient fails to respond, reevaluation of antibiotic therapy should be considered and other approaches to therapy should be explored. Antibiotic therapy does not obviate the need for surgical drainage if complications develop or localization of the infection occurs.

Surgical Therapy. Prompt incision and drainage remains the primary treatment for most infectious processes involving abscess formation. Before the availability of effective antimicrobials, early reports of ASP described nonspecific medical management with early surgical intervention.[8,9,11] However, the anatomic strucure of the parotid gland with its fibrous nature and multiple septae make surgical incision a difficult procedure.[11,14] Early incision may disrupt natural tissue barriers and promote spread of the infectious process.[1,11] It is important that surgical drainage of the gland be delayed until localization of the process occurs.[11,12] The advent of safe and effective antibiotics has relegated surgical incision and drainage to a secondary role in management of this disease.[4,5,11,12]

Within 48 to 72 hours after initiation of antibiotics the patient should experience an improvement in pain, fever, and swelling, and the WBC count should begin to decrease. Early drainage may be indicated if the patient exhibits a very rapidly progressive or rapidly deteriorating disease course, or if intolerable pain accompanies the process.[4,5,12] Surgical drainage may be indicated after the initial 72 hours if complications of ASP develop or symptoms persist despite appropriate antibiotic therapy.[4,5,12] Spratt[4] recommended late drainage of the gland when edema leading to airway obstruction, extreme pain, or extension of the infection was present. This viewpoint is shared by other authors.[1,2,13,14] Inadvertent damage to the facial nerve may result in permanent facial-nerve palsy; therefore, caution is necessary when using surgical drainage.[4]

Adjunctive Therapy. Various forms of adjunctive therapy may be used to provide patient comfort in ASP. Analgesics may be necessary for the patient experiencing severe pain, and salivary stimulants may be useful to reestablish or increase salivary flow.[3,5,6] Continued attention to good oral hygiene and the use of a mouthwash and mechanical cleansing may be useful.[4–6]

In the past low-dose irradiation of the parotid gland was used as a therapeutic modality to relieve pain and decrease glandular secretions.[4,7,12] Lary[7] advocated early use of irradiation and found no benefit when used late in the disease process. Krippaehne et al.[12] suggested that irradiation was most effective when used within 24 hours of the onset of symptoms, and Petersdorf et al.[11] observed a poor response in their group of patients treated with irradiation. Spratt,[4] after reviewing the literature, concluded that the lack of controlled trials and the inconsistent response observed with irradiation raise questions about the value of this form of therapy. Because patients may be at risk from the adverse effects of radiation, this form of therapy is best avoided.

Complications of ASP may occur despite appropriate antibiotic therapy. Abscess formation and gangrene may develop at the site of infection.[3,5,12] The abscess may rupture into adjacent structures such as the ear, mastoid, pharynx, and neck, and swelling may become severe enough to obstruct the airway and affect respiratory function.[1,3,7] Other complications reported with ASP include osteomyelitis of facial bones, empyema formation, infection at distant sites, sepsis, facial-nerve palsy, and death.[3,4,6,7] The development of complications indicates the need for surgical drainage despite antibiotic therapy.

Prognosis. The course of the disease may be mild and uncomplicated with good response to therapy. A more fulminant course associated with a high incidence of death has been described by some authors.[4,5,9,11] Robinson[9] reported 14 deaths in 32 surgical patients with ASP. Spratt[4] implicated ASP as the cause of death in 31% of 178 cases. Two of seven patients with ASP described by Petersdorf et al.[11] died; more recently, Lundgren et al.[5] reported that 6 of 22 patients with ASP died during hospitalization. Mortality rates as high as 45–50% have been reported despite antibiotic therapy and surgical drainage, although antibiotic therapy was less than optimal in some of the earlier reports.[9] The most recent series of reports describes a mortality rate of 25%.[5,6] These reports accentuate the potential for an adverse outcome and the need for early, aggressive therapy. Table 1 summarizes the outcomes reported by several authors in patients with ASP.

Table 1.
Mortality in Reported Cases of Acute Suppurative Parotitis

Reference	No. Patients Studied	Type of Therapy	No. Patients Receiving Indicated Therapy[a]	Total Mortality (%)
12	161	Antibiotics	115	29.8
		Radiation	40	
		Surgical drainage	47	
5	22	Antibiotics		27
		Radiation		
4	178	Antibiotics	60	19
		Radiation	44	
		Surgical drainage	78	
		Nonspecific	69	
9	32	Nonspeciic		44
7	16	Radiation	11	19
		Antibiotics	11	
		Surgical drainage	10	
11	7	Surgical drainage	2	29
		Radiation	2	
		Antibiotics	7	
8	80	Surgical drainage		NR[b]
		Radiation		
		Nonspecific		

[a] Some patients received more than one form of therapy.
[b] Not reported.

Conclusion

Acute suppurative parotitis is a rare condition occurring almost exclusively in the hospitalized patient. This case describes a patient who, although not elderly, was typical of the patient who develops ASP. Because of the potential for a fulminant course and adverse outcome, the clinician should be aware of the epidemiology, clinical features, and management of ASP. In patients who may be at high risk prevention should be the major goal, but early recognition and treatment are essential to prevent complications. Empiric antibiotic therapy providing broad coverage of gram-positive and gram-negative bacteria should be instituted immediately. Surgical drainage may be necessary if response to antibiotics is not observed. With appropriate therapy, most patients with ASP will recover uneventfully.

Discussion Questions

1. How might the patient who is at risk for ASP be identified? What precautions could be instituted to prevent its development?
2. What would constitute an initial antibiotic regimen for empiric treatment of ASP? What alternatives could be suggested in the patient with side effects or hypersensitivities?
3. What should be the duration of antibiotic therapy for a patient with ASP? What criteria could be used to determine when to stop antibiotics?
4. When would surgical incision and drainage be most useful and when would its value be limited?

References

1. Schwartz SI. Complications. In: Schwartz SI, ed. Principles of surgery. New York: McGraw-Hill; 1984:458–9.
2. Adams GL. Infections of the head and neck. In: Simmons RL, Howard RJ, eds. Surgical infectious diseases. New York: Appleton-Century-Crofts; 1984:593–628.
3. McAnally T. Parotitis—clinical presentation and management. *Postgrad Med.* 1982; 71(2):87–99.
4. Spratt JS. The etiology and therapy of acute pyogenic parotitis. *Surg Gynecol Obstet.* 1961; 112:391–405.
5. Lundgren A, Kylen P, Odkvist LM. Nosocomial parotitis. *Acta Otolaryngol.* 1976; 82:275–8.
6. Pruett TL, Simmons RL. Nosocomial gram-negative bacillary parotitis. *JAMA.* 1984; 251:252–3.
7. Lary BG. Postoperative suppurative parotitis. *Arch Surg.* 1964; 89:653–5.
8. Gustafson JR. Acute parotitis. *Surgery.* 1951; 29:786–801.
9. Robinson JR. Surgical parotitis: a vanishing disease. *Surgery.* 1955; 39:703–7.
10. Perzik SL. Surgical management of acute parotitis. *Arch Surg.* 1962; 85:247–51.
11. Petersdorf RG, Forsyth BR, Bernanke D. Staphylococcal parotitis. *N Engl J Med.* 1958; 259:1250–4.
12. Krippaehne WW, Hunt TK, Dunphy JE. Acute suppurative parotitis: study of 161 cases. *Ann Surg.* 1962; 156:251–7.
13. Power L. Parotitis after diuretic therapy. *N Engl J Med.* 1959 260:1059.
14. Hightower NC, Janowitz HD. Salivary secretion. In: Brobeck JR, ed. Best and Taylor's physiological basis of medical practice. Baltimore: Williams & Wilkins; 1979; 2:24–2:37.
15. Chow AW, Roser SM, Brady FA. Orofacial odontogenic infections. *Ann Intern Med.* 1978; 88:392–402.
16. Johanson WG, Pierce AK, Sanford JP. Changing pharyngeal bacterial flora of hospitalized patients. *N Engl J Med.* 1969; 281:1137–40.
17. Rosenthal S, Tager IB. Prevalence of gram-negative rods in the normal pharyngeal flora. *Ann Intern Med.* 1975; 83:355–7.
18. Valenti WM, Trudell RG, Bentley DW. Factors predisposing to oropharyngeal colonization with gram-negative bacilli in the aged. *N Engl J Med.* 1978; 298:1108–11.
19. Johanson WG, Pierce AK, Sanford JP et al. Nosocomial respiratory infections with gram-negative bacilli. *Ann Intern Med.* 1972; 77:701–6.
20. Tillotson JR, Finland M. Bacterial colonization and clinical superinfection of the respiratory tract complicating antibiotic treatment of pneumonia. *J Infect Dis.* 1969; 119:597–24.
21. Johanson WG, Woods DE, Chaudburi T. Association of respiratory tract colonization with adherence of gram-negative bacilli to epithelial cells. *J Infect Dis.* 1979; 139:667–73.
22. Woods DE, Straus DC, Johanson WG et al. Factors influencing the adherence of *Pseudomonas aeruginosa* to mammalian buccal epithelial cells. *Rev Infect Dis.* 1983; 5(Suppl): S846-51.
23. Van Houte J. Bacterial adherence in the mouth. *Rev Infect Dis.* 1983; 5(Suppl):S659–69.
24. Gibbons RJ, Van Houte J. Bacterial adherence in oral microbial ecology. *Ann Rev Microbiol.* 1975; 29:19–44.
25. Busch DF. Anaerobes in infections of the head and neck and ear, nose and throat. *Rev Infect Dis.* 1984; 6(Suppl):S115-22.
26. Newman MG. Anaerobic oral and dental infection. *Rev Infect Dis.* 1984; 6(Suppl):S107-14.
27. Sabiston CB, Grigsby WR, Segerstrom N. Bacterial study of pyogenic infections of dental origin. *Oral Surg.* 1976; 41:430–5.
28. Brook I, Finegold SM. Acute suppurative parotitis caused by anaerobic bacteria: report of two cases. *Pediatrics.* 1978; 62:1019–20.
29. Anthes WH, Blaser MJ, Reller LB. Acute suppurative parotitis associated with anaerobic bacteremia. *Am J Clin Pathol.* 1981; 75:260–2.

Drug Experience

Straightforward reports of unusual drug experiences are included in this section. These may be confirmations of previously reported drug experiences or brief apparent first reports. While selected references may be cited, the purpose of a Drug Experience report is not to present an extensive review of the literature.

A related section, Grand Rounds, includes papers that are well-documented patient case reports with a thorough review of the important literature to help put the case in perspective.

Failure of creatinine clearance to predict gentamicin half-life in a renal transplant patient with diabetes mellitus

KATHERINE A. MICHAEL, JAMES L. MOHLER, ROBERT A. BLOUIN, BRUCE A. LUCAS, AND ROBERT P. RAPP

Clin Pharm. 1985; 4:572–5

Gram-negative septicemia is a major cause of morbidity and mortality in immunosuppressed renal-transplant patients.[1-4] Aminoglycoside antibiotics are reliable for treating these infections in these patients, but it is particularly important to individualize dosage regimens because of the suggested relationships between serum drug concentrations, therapeutic efficacy, and the incidence of nephrotoxicity.[5,6]

Several predictive methods have been developed for individualizing aminoglycoside dosing regimens according to age, sex, lean body weight, and renal function.[7-10] These methods are useful in many situations; however, they cannot be applied to all patient populations. These methods are based on a one-compartment model and generally assume that the patient's volume of distribution is constant and that the relationship between elimination rate constant and creatinine clearance is linear.[5] Sawchuk and Zaske[11,12] proposed an alternate method that allows individual pharmacokinetic variables to be calculated using three postinfusion serum samples. Although this method is more accurate than previous methods, it may not be practical for all patients.

In some patients, aminoglycoside pharmacokinetics cannot be predicted by creatinine clearance methods. We describe a renal-transplant patient with diabetes mellitus in whom gentamicin half-life could not be predicted from measurements of creatinine clearance, despite stable renal function and continuous collection of urine for measurement of creatinine clearance.

Case Report. A 35-year-old black man with end-stage renal disease secondary to juvenile-onset diabetes mellitus underwent a cadaveric kidney transplant on July 1, 1983. By the fourth postoperative day, his urine output exceeded 2 L/day and his serum creatinine was 2.0 mg/dL. After the transplant he received traditional therapy with azathioprine and glucocorticoids. Approximately one week after his transplant, the patient experienced an episode of acute rejection; his temperature increased to 101 °F, and his serum creatinine concentration increased to 7.0 mg/dL. Cultures of blood, urine, and sputum indicated no infection. The patient was treated successfully with lymphocyte immune globulin, antithymocyte globulin (equine) (ATG) and methylprednisolone.

On August 2, the patient's temperature increased to 104 °F, and his serum creatinine concentration was 3.1 mg/dL. The results of a kidney biopsy showed severe, acute rejection, and blood cultures indicated a moderate growth of penicillin-sensitive *Listeria monocytogenes*. A seven-day course of ATG was started along with penicillin G potassium

KATHERINE A. MICHAEL, PHARM. D., is Assistant Professor of Pharmacy, College of Pharmacy, Medical University of South Carolina, Charleston, SC; at the time of this study she was Resident in Hospital Pharmacy, Albert B. Chandler Medical Center, University of Kentucky, Lexington. JAMES L. MOHLER, M.D., is Research Fellow, Brady Urological Institute, The Johns Hopkins Hospital, Baltimore, MD; at the time of this study he was Chief Resident in Urology, Department of Surgery, Albert B. Chandler Medical Center, University of Kentucky, Lexington. ROBERT A. BLOUIN, PHARM.D., is Associate Professor, College of Pharmacy, University of Kentucky. BRUCE A. LUCAS, M.D., is Associate Professor and Surgical Director, Kidney Transplant Program, Department of Surgery, Albert B. Chandler Medical Center. ROBERT P. RAPP, PHARM.D., is Professor, College of Pharmacy, University of Kentucky.

Address reprint requests to Dr. Michael at the Department of Clinical and Institutional Pharmacy, College of Pharmacy, Medical University of South Carolina, Charleston, SC 29425-0810.

Presented at the 19th Annual ASHP Midyear Clinical Meeting, Dallas, TX, December 6, 1984.

2.5 million units administered intravenously every four hours. One week later, the serum creatinine concentration had decreased to 2.0 mg/dL and blood cultures showed no growth, but intermittent temperature elevations to 102 °F continued. At this time gentamicin was added to the antibiotic regimen for its synergistic effect.[13,14]

The Dettli method[9] was used for all predictions of elimination rate constant from creatinine clearance and for estimations of volume of distribution. Equations derived by Sawchuk and Zaske[11,12] were then used to develop a gentamicin dosing regimen that would give the desired maximum and minimum concentrations. After each dosage adjustment, peak and trough concentrations were measured, and individual pharmacokinetic values were calculated using a two-point modification of the Sawchuk and Zaske method. All serum gentamicin concentrations were determined by EMIT (Syva Company, Palo Alto, CA).

The patient weighed 90 kg (approximately his ideal body weight for his height of 203 cm), and his fluid status was stable. Volume of distribution (V) was estimated at 22.5 L. Measured creatinine clearance was 61.5 mL/min/1.73 sq m, giving an estimated elimination rate constant (k) of 0.199 hr^{-1} with a resultant half-life ($t_{1/2}$) of 3.5 hours. Based on these values, the patient was given a loading dose of gentamicin sulfate 2 mg/kg i.v. and was then started on a maintenance dose of 150 mg (1.67 mg/kg) i.v. every 12 hours to give predicted peak and trough serum concentrations of 7.0 and 1.0 μg/mL, respectively.

Just before the second maintenance dose was administered (24 hours after the loading dose), the serum gentamicin trough concentration was 4.9 μg/mL, and the peak concentration after this dose was 7.7 μg/mL. The next scheduled dose was not given, and 24 hours after the second maintenance dose, the gentamicin concentration was 2.1 μg/mL, indicating that the previous trough concentration of 4.9 μg/mL was obtained at an appropriate time. Using values calculated from these concentrations, the regimen was changed to gentamicin sulfate 150 mg i.v. every 24 hours. This gave a predicted peak serum concentration of 7.3 μg/mL and a predicted trough concentration of 1.6 μg/mL. After administration of the second maintenance dose of the new regimen, the measured peak gentamicin concentration was 4.3 μg/mL and the trough concentration was 0.9 μg/mL. The measured creatinine clearance remained stable throughout this period at 57.0 mL/min/1.73 sq m. Because of problems with predicting the half-life from the patient's creatinine clearance, gentamicin concentrations were determined in serial blood samples to characterize the disposition of gentamicin in this patient more accurately.

On the patient's fifth day of gentamicin therapy (the fourth day at a regimen of 150 mg i.v. every 24 hours), he appeared to be at steady state with two consecutive trough concentrations of 0.9 μg/mL. Drug concentrations were determined at 1, 4.5, 8.5, 14, and 23.5 hours after the dose (Figure 1). The peak concentration was 4.93 μg/mL and the trough was 0.9 μg/mL, which was consistent with previous concentrations obtained with this dose. The measured creatinine clearance during the same 24-hour period was basically unchanged at 54.5 mL/min/1.73 sq m.

Log linear least-squares regression analysis of the serum concentration–time curve was used to calculate individual pharmacokinetic values, which were then compared with values predicted from the measured creatinine clearance (CL_{cr}) over the same time period (Table 1). Total body clearance (CL) was calculated from the volume of distribution and the elimination rate constant and expressed as a ratio of total body clearance to creatinine clearance (CL/CL_{cr}). Creatinine clearance

Figure 1. Measured serum gentamicin concentrations (■) and gentamicin concentrations predicted from creatinine clearance (▲).

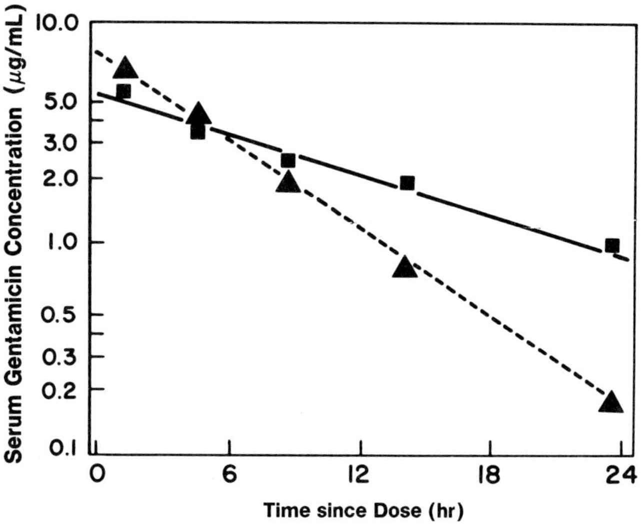

Table 1.
Pharmacokinetic Values Calculated from Serum Concentrations and Predicted from Creatinine Clearance

Variable	Value Calculated from Serum Concentration	Value Predicted from Creatinine Clearance[a]
Elimination rate constant (hr^{-1})	0.091	0.165
Half-life (hr)	7.6	4.23
Volume of distribution (L)	35.5 (0.39 L/kg)	22.5 (0.25 L/kg)
Total body clearance (mL/min)	53.8	61.6
CL/CL_{cr}[b]	1.04	0.94

[a] Measured creatinine clearance was 51.7 mL/min/1.73 sq m.
[b] Ratio of total body clearance of gentamicin to creatinine clearance.

continued to be a poor predictor of half-life in this patient. The source of error appeared to be an unusually large volume of distribution, rather than fluctuating renal function. Although the patient was receiving prednisone, his weight remained stable and he had no clinical evidence of fluid-status changes that may have increased his apparent volume of distribution. The observed total body clearance was similar to the predicted value.

Discussion. Tofte et al.[15] compared the nomogram of Sarubbi and Hull (group 1) with the method of Sawchuk and Zaske (group 2) for predicting serum amikacin concentrations in a series of 27 renal-transplant patients. Patients in group 2 had significantly more peaks in the therapeutic range, whereas patients in the nomogram group (group 1) had twice as many subtherapeutic peaks as those in group 2. Similar results were noted when patients were grouped according to pretreatment serum creatinine concentrations. Serum trough concentrations were not significantly different between the two groups irrespective of renal function before treatment. The authors concluded that problems associated with the nomogram method (Sarubbi and Hull) may have resulted from an overestimation of creatinine clearance during periods when serum creatinine and renal function were changing rapidly.

This study confirmed the findings of Noone et al.,[16] who found that nomograms based on serum creatinine concentrations were of little value in adjusting aminoglycoside dosage in a group of patients who had recently received renal transplants. Maintenance doses required to attain desired serum drug concentrations varied greatly between patients and were unrelated to serum creatinine concentrations. This finding was again attributed to widely fluctuating serum creatinine concentrations in patients with unstable renal function.

Rush et al.[17] retrospectively reviewed the charts of 2000 patients who received either gentamicin or tobramycin on a dosage schedule that was monitored by measuring serum aminoglycoside concentrations. Of the 2000 patients with initially appropriate serum concentrations, 17 demonstrated aminoglycoside accumulation and a decrease in renal function later in therapy. None of these patients had previously diagnosed renal disease or experienced events that would have added to the risk of developing nephrotoxicity. Of the 17 patients, 12 were known diabetics whose blood glucose concentrations had been elevated repeatedly during therapy. The five remaining patients were not diagnosed as having diabetes but experienced hyperglycemia during aminoglycoside therapy. Hypertension was a common factor in 11 patients; no other common risk factors were identified. The authors postulated that diabetic patients with associated microvascular disease may accumulate excessive aminoglycoside intrarenally while exhibiting controlled serum concentrations. In contrast to these findings, another retrospective analysis conducted by Moore et al.[18] showed that diabetes was not a risk factor in the development of aminoglycoside nephrotoxicity.

In the absence of changes in plasma protein binding, changes in tissue binding may affect volume of distribution but not total body clearance. Furthermore, since the elimination rate constant is a dependent variable, changes in volume of distribution or total body clearance will alter the value of the elimination rate constant.[19] Aminoglycosides are bound to plasma proteins in negligible amounts, and tissue accumulation of these drugs has been widely demonstrated.[20–24]

In 1976, Matas et al.[25] reported a "pseudorejection" phenomenon in diabetic renal-transplant patients. In these patients hyperglycemia resulted in elevations in serum creatinine but there was no other indication of decreasing renal function or graft rejection. Creatinine values returned to baseline when serum glucose concentrations were controlled. "False" elevation of serum creatinine secondary to hyperglycemia could make creatinine clearance an unreliable predictor of renal function and would result in overestimation of aminoglycoside half-life. However, in our patient there was no correlation between serum creatinine and serum glucose, and half-life was underestimated (rather than overestimated) by creatinine clearance.

Changes in serum glucose with resultant fluctuations in osmolarity cause fluid shifts between intracellular and extracellular compartments. These intercompartmental shifts could alter the volume of distribution of the aminoglycoside in the absence of apparent changes in total-body fluid balance.

In our patient, changes in tissue binding or intercompartmental fluid shifts may have contributed to the large volume of distribution. This would explain the inability to predict half-life from conventional creatinine-clearance methods that assume a standard volume of distribution. As expected, total body clearance could be predicted from creatinine clearance regardless of the relationship between renal function and the elimination rate constant.

Conclusion. Until the effects of diabetes mellitus on aminoglycoside pharmacokinetics are better understood, gentamicin dosing in diabetic patients should be based on careful monitoring of serum drug concentrations instead of solely on predictions based on creatinine clearance.

References

1. Hill RB Jr, Dahrling BE, Starzl TE. Death after transplantation. An analysis of sixty cases. *Am J Med*. 1967; 42:327.
2. Murphy FJ, McDonald FD, Dawson M et al. Factors affecting the frequency of infection in renal transplant recipi-

ents. *Arch Intern Med.* 1976; 136:670.
3. Nielson HE, Korsager B. Bacteremia after renal transplantation. *Scand J Infect Dis.* 1977; 9:111.
4. Tapia HR, Holley KE, Woods JE et al. Cause of death after renal transplantation. *Arch Intern Med.* 1975; 131:204.
5. Yee GC, Evans WE. Reappraisal of guidelines for pharmacokinetic monitoring of aminoglycosides. *Pharmacotherapy.* 1981; 1:55–75.
6. Burkle WS. Comparative evaluation of aminoglycoside antibiotics for systemic use. *Drug Intell Clin Pharm.* 1981; 15:847–62.
7. Hull JH, Sarubbi FA. Gentamicin serum concentrations: pharmacokinetic predictions. *Ann Intern Med.* 1976; 85:183–9.
8. Sarubbi FA, Hull JH. Amikacin serum concentrations: prediction of levels and dosage guidelines. *Ann Intern Med.* 1978; 89:612–8.
9. Dettli LC. Drug dosage in patients with renal disease. *Clin Pharmacol Ther.* 1974; 16:274–80.
10. Chan RA, Benner EJ, Hoeprich RD. Gentamicin therapy in renal failure: a nomogram for dosage. *Ann Intern Med.* 1978; 76:775–8.
11. Sawchuk RJ, Zaske DE. Pharmacokinetics of dosing regimens which utilize multiple intravenous infusions: gentamicin in burn patients. *J Pharmacokinet Biopharm.* 1976; 4:183–95.
12. Sawchuk RJ, Zaske DE, Cipolle RJ. Kinetic model for gentamicin dosing with the use of individual patient parameters. *Clin Pharmacol Ther.* 1977; 21:362–9.
13. Moellering RC Jr, Medoff G, Leech I et al. Antibiotic synergism against *Listeria monocytogenes. Antimicrob Agents Chemother.* 1972; 1:30–4.
14. Wiggins GL, Albritton WL, Feeley JC. Antibiotic susceptibility of clinical isolates of *Listeria monocytogenes. Antimicrob Agents Chemother.* 1978; 13:854–60.
15. Tofte RW, Canafax DM, Simmons RL et al. Aminoglycoside dosing in renal transplant patients. *Ann Surg.* 1982; 195:287–93.
16. Noone P, Beale DF, Pollock SS et al. Monitoring aminoglycoside use in patients with severely impaired renal function. *Br Med J.* 1978; 2:470–3.
17. Rush DS, DiPiro JT, Record KE et al. Diabetes: a risk factor in aminoglycoside nephrotoxicity. *Curr Surg.* 1982; 39:244–7.
18. Moore RD, Smith CR, Lipsky JJ, et al. Risk factors for nephrotoxicity in patients treated with aminoglycosides. *Ann Intern Med.* 1984; 100:352–7.
19. Gibaldi M, Koup JR. Pharmacokinetic concepts: drug binding, apparent volume of distribution and clearance. *Eur J Clin Pharmacol.* 1981; 20:299–305.
20. Schentag JJ, Jusko WJ, Vance JW et al. Gentamicin disposition and tissue accumulation on multiple dosing. *J Pharmacokinet Biopharm.* 1977; 5:599–677.
21. Schentag JJ, Jusko WJ, Plaut ME et al. Tissue persistence of gentamicin in man. *JAMA.* 1977; 237:327–9.
22. Schentag JJ, Jusko WJ. Renal clearance and tissue accumulation of gentamicin. *Clin Pharmacol Ther.* 1977; 22:364–70.
23. Schentag JJ, Lasezkay G, Cumbo TJ et al. Accumulation pharmacokinetics of tobramycin. *Antimicrob Agents Chemother.* 1978; 13:649–56.
24. Colburn WA, Schentag JJ, Jusko WJ et al. A model for the prospective identification of the prenephrotoxic state during gentamicin therapy. *J Pharmacokinet Biopharm.* 1978; 6:179–86.
25. Matas JA, Simmons RL, Goetz FG et al. Hyperglycemic pseudorejection in the diabetic transplant patient. *Surgery.* 1976; 79:132–6.

CP Continuing Education

The ASHP Continuing Education system gives readers a self-assessment mechanism for selected articles in Clinical Pharmacy *and the* American Journal of Hospital Pharmacy. *It also allows readers to obtain continuing-education credit for these articles.*

For the purpose of CE-credit enrollment a blank answer sheet is published at the end of each installment of the column for the CE articles in that issue. An enrollee accumulates these answer sheets until the enrollment is submitted, using the form that is published in the May–June and November–December issues of Clinical Pharmacy *and in the June and December issues of the* American Journal of Hospital Pharmacy. *Any combination of tests within a 12-month period, from both* Clinical Pharmacy *and* American Journal of Hospital Pharmacy, *may be included in an enrollment. More complete details about enrollment in the system will appear in the semiannual enrollment form.*

All education aspects of the program are directed by Warren E. McConnell, Ph.D., Special Assistant in the ASHP Executive Office.

Article 680-204-8515 (see page 507)
Qualifies for 1.0 hour of CE credit

Pentamidine isethionate in the treatment of *Pneumocystis carinii* pneumonia

Learning Objectives

After studying this article, the reader should be able to

1. Describe the development of pentamidine leading to its current availability as an orphan drug.
2. Identify the spectrum and mechanism of antiprotozoal activity of pentamidine.
3. Identify the host responses to *Pneumocystis carinii* pneumonia (PCP) and describe the mortality associated with each before and after the availability of pentamidine therapy.
4. Identify the criteria for therapeutic success with pentamidine (including dosage, duration of therapy, and risk factors).
5. List the major adverse reactions associated with the use of pentamidine and describe their impact on therapy.

Self-assessment Questions

For each question there is one best answer only.

1. Pentamidine is structurally related to synthalin, an agent whose antiprotozoal effects were noted secondary to its use in
   a. Hyperthyroidism.
   b. Diabetes mellitus.
   c. Toxoplasmosis.
   d. Malaria.
2. Pentamidine has been used effectively in all of the following protozoal infections *except*
   a. Chagas disease.
   b. Leishmaniasis.
   c. *Pneumocystis carinii* pneumonia.
   d. African sleeping sickness.
3. When used in the treatment of PCP in adults and children with underlying immunodeficiencies, pentamidine lowers the mortality rate by
   a. 0–25%.
   b. 15–30%.
   c. 25–50%.
   d. 40–70%.
4. The lack of therapeutic success with pentamidine in certain early case reports of PCP was attributed to
   a. Inappropriate dosing.
   b. Intolerance of adverse reactions caused by pentamidine.
   c. Substantial disease progression before beginning therapy.
   d. Prior use of pyrimethamine–sulfadiazine.
5. Which of the following was a major factor in the high success rates with pentamidine in PCP noted by various researchers?
   a. Pentamidine was administered for at least 14 days.
   b. Pentamidine was administered early in the course of the disease.
   c. Pentamidine was administered intramuscularly rather than intravenously.
   d. Patients receiving pentamidine had good renal function.
6. When compared with trimethoprim–sulfamethoxazole (TMP–SMX) in children with PCP, pentamidine is
   a. The preferred agent.
   b. Less effective and more toxic.
   c. Equally effective and less toxic.
   d. Equally effective and more toxic.
7. The most commonly reported adverse reaction to pentamidine is

a. Pain at the injection site.
b. Nephrotoxicity.
c. Hypotension.
d. Hypoglycemia.

8. Based on the side-effect profile, pentamidine should be used cautiously in patients with

a. Hypotension.
b. Diabetes mellitus.
c. Renal impairment.
d. All of the above.

9. An appropriate dose of pentamidine isethionate for a patient with a glomerular filtration rate of 5 mL/min is

a. 4 mg/sq m every 36 hours.
b. 4 mg/kg every 48 hours.
c. 4 mg/sq m every 48 hours.
d. 2 mg/kg every 48 hours.

10. Which of the following is true concerning drug therapy of PCP in patients with acquired immunodeficiency syndrome (AIDS)?

a. Pentamidine is the drug of choice.
b. Pentamidine is associated with a higher incidence of adverse reactions in AIDS patients than in other patients with PCP.
c. TMP–SMX is associated with a higher incidence of adverse reactions in AIDS patients than in other patients with PCP.
d. Animal studies have shown that the combination of pentamidine and TMP–SMX results in a lower incidence of mortality in patients with PCP.

Article 680-204-8516 (see page 516)
Qualifies for 1.0 hour of CE credit

Aztreonam, a new monobactam antimicrobial

Learning Objectives

After studying this article, the reader should be able to

1. Identify the antimicrobial spectrum of aztreonam and compare it with those of other currently available β-lactam and aminoglycoside antimicrobials.
2. Describe the pharmacokinetic characteristics of aztreonam with respect to main route of elimination and dosage adjustment in disease states.
3. Identify tissues into which aztreonam penetrates in therapeutic concentrations.
4. On the basis of the clinical trials presented, name the types of infections for which aztreonam has been shown to be clinically useful.
5. Describe the dosing recommendations and the adverse reaction profile of aztreonam.

Self-assessment Questions

For each question, there is one best answer only.

1. Aztreonam is not active against which of the following bacteria?

a. *Escherichia coli.*
b. *Pseudomonas aeruginosa.*
c. *Klebsiella pneumoniae.*
d. *Bacteroides fragilis.*
e. *Serratia marcescens.*

2. The total body clearance of aztreonam is

a. Not altered by renal dysfunction.
b. Altered by aging.
c. Altered by the presence of gram-negative infection.
d. Altered by the presence of cancer.
e. Altered by the presence of cirrhosis.

3. Which of the following would be safest to use in a patient with a *Pseudomonas* bacteremia who also had a history of penicillin anaphylaxis?

a. Aztreonam.
b. Cefsulodin.
c. Piperacillin.
d. Netilmicin.
e. Ceftazidime.

4. Which of the following would be expected to cause the least perturbation of bowel flora?

a. Cefoperazone.
b. Piperacillin.
c. Cefoxitin.
d. Aztreonam.
e. Moxalactam.

5. Which of the following statements concerning the pharmacokinetics of aztreonam is not true?

a. The serum elimination half-life is approximately two hours.
b. The biliary-tract penetration of aztreonam is low.
c. Probenecid reduces the renal clearance of aztreonam.
d. The volume of distribution of aztreonam is not altered by renal failure.
e. All of the above statements are true.

6. Aztreonam may be administered

a. Orally only.
b. Intravenously only.
c. Intramuscularly only.
d. Intravenously and intramuscularly only.
e. Orally, intramuscularly, and intravenously.

7. Which of the following minimum inhibitory concentrations is considered the "threshold" for sensitivity?

a. 2 μg/mL.
b. 4 μg/mL.
c. 8 μg/mL.
d. 16 μg/mL.
e. 32 μg/mL.

8. Aztreonam has been demonstrated effective in the treatment of which of the following infections?

a. Skin and skin-structure infections.
b. Intra-abdominal infections.
c. Urinary-tract infections.
d. All of the above alternatives are correct.
e. Alternatives b and c only are correct.

9. Which of the following is generally most potent in vitro against *Pseudomonas aeruginosa?*

   a. Cefoperazone.
   b. Ceftazidime.
   c. Aztreonam.
   d. Cefonicid.
   e. Cefotaxime.

10. In vivo pharmacokinetic interaction has been documented between aztreonam and which of the following antimicrobials?

   a. Clindamycin.
   b. Metronidazole.
   c. Gentamicin.
   d. Nafcillin.
   e. None of the above alternatives is correct.

Answer sheet

September–October 1985 *Clinical Pharmacy*

Note: An enrollment form for the ASHP Continuing-Education System appears in the May–June and November–December issues. Please accumulate all the answer sheets you wish to use in one enrollment and submit them at one time with a completed enrollment form.

Place an X in the box(es) at the top of the column(s) corresponding to the test(s) you are taking. Darken the boxes corresponding to the correct answers.

□ 680-204-8515 1.0 hour	a b c d	□ 680-204-8516 1.0 hour	a b c d e
1.	□□□□	1.	□□□□□
2.	□□□□	2.	□□□□□
3.	□□□□	3.	□□□□□
4.	□□□□	4.	□□□□□
5.	□□□□	5.	□□□□□
6.	□□□□	6.	□□□□□
7.	□□□□	7.	□□□□□
8.	□□□□	8.	□□□□□
9.	□□□□	9.	□□□□□
10.	□□□□	10.	□□□□□

ASHP Use Only
(1.0)8515________(3)
(1.0)8516________(3)

Current Literature

Book Reviews

The Aging Process: Therapeutic Implications

Edited by Robert N. Butler and Alexander G. Bearn.
Published by Raven Press, 1140 Avenue of the Americas, New York, NY 10036, 1985. xii + 337 p. Price $45.00.

As geriatric clinicians will attest, a lamentable poverty of drug information specifically devoted to our growing geriatric clientele exists. Editors Robert Butler, M.D., a former first director of the NIH Institute on Aging, and Alexander Bearn, M.D., a senior vice president at Merck Sharp & Dohme, have admirably undertaken the challenge to fill the gap. They have compiled an interconnecting series of essays by international multidisciplinary experts examining various aspects of aging relative to medicine and pharmacotherapy. In addition, the text begins and ends with their own insightful discourse. Perhaps the best explanation of their objectives is summarized by Bearn's reflection that "... many of the infirmities of old age, traditionally regarded as untreatable, are ... amenable to therapy ...."

Each chapter is followed by references, a content summary, and a discussion segment featuring conversation between the chapter's author and members of the multinational Medical Advisory Council (MEDAC). Chapter authors appear to have been meticulously chosen for their expertise in the topic and for their firsthand knowledge. Among the excellent chapters are "Patterns of Prescribing and Drug Use," "Adverse Drug Reactions in the Elderly," and a series of articles examining the different chronic problems common to aging—such as, hypertension, Alzheimer's disease, rheumatic diseases—with associated aspects of drug treatment. These chapters will provide rare treats for the practitioner in geriatrics in that the associated pharmacokinetics and adverse drug reactions are written with specific regard to geriatric physiology. This brings up the one basic flaw of this project—a repetition of geriatric-based information such as demographic trends, adverse drug reaction material, and pharmacokinetic changes. Probably this problem is largely unavoidable in such undertakings that attempt a comprehensive focus with multiple contributors. Style overlap, however, is not a problem—the text is quite readable; tables and equations are plentiful and appropriate.

One common thread found throughout the book is the appeal for rational, safe prescribing and drug testing (including postmarketing surveillance) in the elderly. In particular, the pharmaceutical industry is called upon to assume a leadership role in adapting to the coming demographic changes while valuing and preserving the quality of our prolonged life spans. While *The Aging Process* has specifically addressed aspects of aging in need of acknowledgment by the pharmaceutical industry, including pharmacologists, researchers, and regulatory officials, others who may benefit from such a resource include consultant pharmacists, students of medicine and pharmacy, and hospital pharmacists, because of the startling growth of geriatric patients in the acute-care setting. The reference listings after each chapter are overwhelming and will provide an exhaustive wealth of resources for the ambitious reader interested in further reading. Considering the influx of survivors over the age of 60, aptly referred to as the "longevity revolution" by Butler in his chapter on demographics, this book has arrived at an opportune time.

Reviewed by Judi B. Shor, Pharm.D., Shor Associates, Chester, NJ 07930.

Beta Blockers in the Treatment of Cardiovascular Disease

Edited by John B. Kostis and Eugene A. De Felice.
Published by Raven Press, 1140 Avenue of the Americas, New York, NY 10036, 1984. x + 307 p. Price $40.00.

Since the availability of the first beta-adrenoreceptor blocking agent nearly two decades ago, knowledge about this class of drugs has undergone tremendous expansion. As additional beta-blockers become available, the selection of appropriate agents for individual patients presents a challenge to the clinician. Kostis and De Felice have attempted to provide a "state of the art" review of the vast amount information about the use of β blockers for the practitioner involved in the management of cardiovascular diseases. At first glance, it appears that the editors have compiled material from notable researchers and practitioners regarding the pharmacologic, hemodynamic, and metabolic effects of β blockers and their clinical utility in a variety of disorders. However, upon closer examination, some important areas are not discussed, and there is an obvious emphasis on selected aspects of β-blocker pharmacology underlying the entire text—specifically the importance of intrinsic sympathomimetic activity (ISA). This emphasis is made at the expense of a balanced discussion of other aspects of β-blocker pharmacology, such as cardioselectivity, membrane-stabilizing activity, and α-adrenoreceptor blocking activity or vasodilating properties.

The first chapter reviews the clinical pharmacology of the β-blocking agents, with consideration given to structure-activity relationships as they relate to properties of ISA and cardioselectivity. The metabolic effects of these agents and their effects on peripheral resistance and blood flow to selected regional vascular beds are also discussed. Several chapters are devoted to the use of β

Continued on page 588

Continued from page 583

blockers in the treatment of hypertension, angina pectoris, arrhythmias, myocardial infarction, stress and anxiety, and chronic autonomic failure. The underlying theme in each of these chapters emphasizes those β blockers having ISA, to the extent that in some instances the β blockers are categorized according to whether or not they possess ISA—not a usual method of classifying these drugs.

In view of the great concern for the metabolic consequences of antihypertensive therapy, the effects of β blockers on carbohydrate and lipid metabolism are discussed, with recommendations for the practical application of this data to patient management. Although based on small numbers of studies, definitive conclusions are made about the advantages of β blockers with ISA.

A final chapter reviews the clinical importance of ISA in β-blocking agents. While it is stated that ISA may prove to be an important property upon which to differentiate and select these drugs for particular patients, it should be noted that Frishman et al. state on page 253 of the text that "whether the presence of ISA in a β blocker constitutes an advantage or disadvantage in cardiac therapy is currently being debated."

Topics receiving limited coverage in this text include pharmacokinetic differences among β blockers and the role of β blockers with α-adrenoreceptor blocking properties and vasodilating properties.

In conclusion, *Beta-Blockers in the Treatment of Cardiovascular Disease*, though attempting to provide an up-to-date review of the subject, has some serious omissions. More important, it overemphasizes the importance of a single pharmacologic property—ISA—suggesting that it constitutes a well-accepted, clinically important advantage over other pharmacologic factors in the evaluation and therapeutic use of this class of drugs. Currently, the presence of ISA in a β-blocking agent represents a more important academic, rather than practical, consideration of limited value to the general practitioner.

Reviewed by Renee P. Tannenbaum, Pharm.D., Professional Information, Merck Sharp & Dohme, Division of Merck & Co., Inc., West Point, PA 19486.

Clinical Guide to Parenteral Micronutrition

Edited by Thomas B. Baumgartner.
Published by Educational Publications, Ltd., 2020 Ruby Street, Melrose Park, IL 60160, 1984. xii + 388 p. Price $29.95.

Clinical Guide to Parenteral Micronutrition is a welcome resource for the practicing clinician involved in providing nutritional support services. It is intended to serve as a point of reference that provides the clinician with practical information about micronutrient requirements. It offers a concise overview of parenteral micronutrients, addressing product information, professional implications, and patient considerations encountered in the metabolic support of hospitalized patients.

The book is divided into three primary sections. Section I, entitled "Electrolytes," discusses seven electrolytes routinely monitored, including the cations sodium, potassium, calcium, and magnesium, as well as the anions chloride, bicarbonate and its precursors, and phosphate. Section II includes a comprehensive review of the trace minerals iron, zinc, copper, chromium, manganese, fluoride, iodide, molybdenum, and selenium. Section III covers both fat and water soluble vitamins. The sections are organized to address each micronutrient individually, providing a thumbnail review of its clinical relevance in nutritional support. Each section briefly summarizes the chemistry, pharmacology, commercial availability, and therapeutic considerations in a clear and comprehensive fashion. In fact, the consistent format throughout the book expedites the pursuit of specific clinical inquiries encountered in daily practice. It is this feature which makes the text so useful.

In addition, there is a brief review of carnitine and its role in nutrition. Finally, there are four appendices, which summarize specific characteristics of parenteral micronutrients essential to successful nutritional management.

The text contains contributions from individuals who have significant experience and interest in micronutrition. Each has been able to present information clearly within the standard format of the text.

In summary, *Clinical Guide to Parenteral Micronutrition* is presented in a clear and concise format that facilitates ready access to specific information. It is a well-referenced text that should be considered a valuable addition to the libraries of pharmacists and associated clinicians involved in the nutritional management of hospitalized patients.

Reviewed by David F. Driscoll, Nutrition Support Service, New England Deaconess Hospital, 185 Pilgrim Road, Boston, MA 02215.

Evaluation and Treatment of Chronic Pain

Edited by Gerald M. Aronoff.
Published by Urban & Schwarzenberg, Inc., 7 E. Redwood Street, Baltimore, MD 21202, 1985. xliv + 684 p. Price $65.00.

Chronic pain is among the major unsolved medical problems and is most likely the top medically based socioeconomic burden in the United States. This is very unfortunate since methods exist for alleviating much of the suffering that has, until now, been accepted as part of the human condition. In addition, many recent advances have been made in the treatment of pain. The stated purpose of *Evaluation and Treatment of Chronic Pain* is to provide a concise and up-to-date treatise on the subject. The text is intended primarily for physicians involved in the management of patients with chronic pain; at the same time, it is multidisciplinary in its scope and authorship. However, pharmacists are not included as authors nor are they recognized as having a role in the multidisciplinary approach to the management of patients with chronic pain.

The book is composed of 39 chapters written by a number of authorities in specialty areas such as pain physiology, painful neurological disorders, headache, facial pain, back pain, physical therapy, joint pain, and painful metabolic bone disorders. There are specific chapters on control of pain associated with malignancy and the pharmacologic management of chronic pain. In addition, several chapters are devoted to the concept of multidisciplinary pain centers.

As anyone who has dealt with such patients knows, these are among the most difficult patients to interact with. This text provides a very useful framework for approaching this patient population. My only major disappointment with the book is that, throughout, the discussion of the drug therapy of chronic pain is very shallow and is not objective. Rather, the discussion of drug therapy is opinionated and anecdotal.

Overall, the book is easy to read. Case presentations and discussions are used throughout. The tables and illustrations are easy to comprehend. The references are, in general, current and appropriate. An appendix entitled "Listen to Your Patients" gives five case histories written by patients actually treated by the Boston Pain Center.

Pharmacists who are actively involved in the management of patients with chronic pain or who practice in neurosurgical or neurology settings would find this text useful because of its discussion of various chronic pain syndromes. However, I cannot recommend this text as a comprehensive source of information on drug therapy for chronic pain syndromes because of the limited information provided.

Reviewed by Stephen J. Bollish, Pharm.D., IMED Corporation, 9925 Carroll Canyon Road, San Diego, CA 92131

Pediatric Medications: An Emergency and Critical Care Reference

By Carolyn M. Stewart and Linda B. Stewart.

Published by Aspen Systems Corporation, 1600 Research Boulevard, Rockville, MD 20850, 1984. xxv + 453 p. Price $45.00.

Information on pediatric drug doses and drug use is often hard to find. Company literature is void of experience reported about drug use in pediatric patients where FDA approval for children under 12 years of age has not been given. Other references may include pediatric doses but fail to distinguish pediatric responses to a drug from adult responses. Stewart and Stewart have collected information on drug use in pediatric patients and compiled this information into an easy-to-use reference book.

The purpose of this book is to provide health professionals with important information on drugs given to children in emergency settings. Discussions on pharmacology are scattered throughout the book. They provide an introduction to drug use in children and background information on various classes of pharmacologic agents. Topics include administration of medications to children, developmental pharmacology, the central nervous system, and the coagulation system. These discussions are simple and brief but provide rationale for the use of drugs that are subsequently discussed.

Most of the book is dedicated to drug monographs. The drugs are grouped according to pharmacologic activity. For each drug, the administration, indications, actions, contraindications, precautions, side effects and adverse reactions, drug incompatibilities, drug interactions, and antidotes are discussed. The list of drugs is extensive and includes much more than emergency medications. In addition to the expected classes of drugs, such as adrenergics, antiarrhythmics, antihypertensives, anticonvulsants, bronchodilators, and antibiotics, this book also provides information on oral rehydrating solutions, colloid plasma expanders, antidotes, antivenins, and antiserums. Notably missing from the anti-infective medications are vidarabine, cefuroxime, and ceftriaxone. The latter two cephalosporins are gaining popularity among pediatricians but were released after this book was published. The quality of the information provided is quite good. Most useful were the suggestions for monitoring therapy and antidotes if too much drug is administered. On rare occasions I disagreed with a dosage recommendation—their dose being less aggressive than mine. My only criticism about the information provided in the monographs concerns the lack of pharmacokinetic data. Digoxin pharmacokinetics are discussed briefly, and desired serum concentrations are listed for some other drugs. Inclusion of more of this material would greatly enhance the value of this book for pharmacists. The appendix of this book is loaded with excellent tables and the "how to" of important calculations. Examples of topics covered are immunizations, pediatric doses of emergency medications, pediatric fluid requirements, drug compatibility in syringes, and i.v. drip calculations.

The book concludes with a bibliography and an index. The bibliography is made up of an equal number of textbooks and articles from the primary literature. Unfortunately, the monographs are not referenced individually. The index is easy to use and gives both the brand names and the generic names of drugs.

The strengths of this book are its ease of use and the practicality of the information provided. The weaknesses for pharmacists are the lack of depth of discussions and the failure to relate the information given to the primary literature. Although the book is designed primarily for nursing personnel, I feel that the ready availability of important information on pediatric drug use also makes it a good addition to a pharmacy library.

Reviewed by Kathleen M. Reilly, Pharm.D., University of South Carolina, Columbia, SC 29203

Books Received

Books are listed as received; selected books may be reviewed in Book Reviews in subsequent issues.

The Cancer Pharmacology Annual 3, edited by B. A. Chabner and H. M. Pinedo. Published by Elsevier Science Publishers B.V., Amsterdam, The Netherlands, 1985. Distributed by Elsevier Science Publishing Co., Inc., 52 Vanderbilt Ave., New York, NY 10017. xi + 216 p. Price $33.25; Dfl. 90.00.

The Chemistry of Natural Products, edited by R. H. Thomson. Published by Blackie & Son Limited, Glasgow and London, 1985. Distributed in the United States by Chapman and Hall in association with Methuen, Inc., 733 Third Ave., New York, NY 10017. xii + 467 p. Price $75.00.

Interpretation of Clinical Laboratory Tests, edited by Gérard Siest, Joseph Henry, Françoise Schiele et al. Published by Biomedical Publications, P.O. Box 8209, Foster City, CA 94404, 1985. xvi + 459 p. Price $47.50.

Introduction to Pharmaceutical Dosage Forms, Fourth Edition, by Howard C. Ansel. Published by Lea & Febiger, 600 Washington Square, Philadelphia, PA 19106-4198, 1985. viii + 405 p. Price $29.75 (U.S.), $39.50 (Canada).

Manual of Drug Therapy, edited by David A. Scheinberg and Labe Scheinberg. Published by Raven Press, 1140 Avenue of the Americas, New York, NY 10036, 1985. xiii + 386 p. Price $17.50.

Optimization of Drug Delivery, Proceedings of the Alfred Benzon Symposium 17, edited by Hans Bundgaard, Anne Bagger Hansen, and Helmer Kofod. Published by Munksgaard International Publishers Ltd., Copenhagen, Denmark, 1982. Distributed by Raven Press, 1140 Avenue of the Americas, New York, NY 10036. 434 p. Price $39.00.

Pharmacokinetics: A Modern View, edited by Leslie Z. Benet, Gerhard Levy, and Bobbe L. Ferraiolo. Published by Plenum Press, 233 Spring St., New York, NY 10013, 1984. xvi + 531 p. Price $65.00.

Premenstrual Syndrome: A Clinic Manual, by H. Jane Chihal. Published by Creative Infomatics, Inc., P.O. Box 1607, Durant, OK 74702-1607, 1985. 150 p. Price $7.95/single copy; multiple copies discounted.

A Primer of Drug Action (Fourth Edition), by Robert M. Julien. Published by W. H. Freeman and Company, 41 Madison Ave., New York, NY 10010, 1985. xiii + 305 p. Price $22.95 (cloth), $14.95 (paper).

Principal Drugs: An Alphabetical Guide to Modern Therapeutic Agents, by S. J. Hopkins. Published by Faber and Faber, 39 Thompson St., Winchester, MA 01890, 1985. 208 p. Price $4.95.

Selective Toxicity: The Physico Chemical Basis of Therapy (Seventh Edition), by Adrien Albert. Published by Chapman and Hall, 733 Third Ave., New York, NY 10017, 1985. xii + 750 p. Price $69.95 (cloth), $34.95 (paper).

Side Effects of Drugs Annual 9 — 1985, edited by M.N.G. Dukes and L. Beeley. Published by Elsevier Science Publishers B. V., P.O. Box 1126, 1000 BC Amsterdam, The Netherlands, 1985. Distributed in the U.S. and Canada by Elsevier Science Publishing Co., Inc., 52 Vanderbilt Ave., New York, NY 10017. xxiii + 476 p. Price $70.25, Dfl. 190.00.

Thymic Hormones and Lymphokines: Basic Chemistry and Clinical Applications, edited by Allan L. Goldstein. Published by Plenum Press, 233 Spring St., New York, NY 10013, 1984. xiii + 669 p. Price $75.00.

The Women's Drugstore, by Harold M. Silverman. Published by Dell Publishing Co., Inc., 1 Dag Hammarskjold Plaza, New York, NY 10017, 1985. xii + 403 p. Price $9.95 (U.S.), $12.50 (Canada).

Advertising Index

Advanced Therapeutics Communications
Positions Available, 485
American College of Clinical Pharmacy
Call for Papers, 575
American Critical Care, A Division of American Hospital Supply Corporation
Hespan, 492–494
American Society of Hospital Pharmacists
Clinical Pharmacy, 590A, 590B, inside back cover
Clinical Research Forum, 506
Bristol-Myers Oncology Division
Mexate, 483–484
Burroughs Wellcome Company
Zovirax, 472–474
Edlaw Preparations, Inc.
Colyte, 501–502
The Johns Hopkins Hospital
Position Available, 485
Lederle Laboratories, A Division of American Cyanamid Company
Maxzide, 477–478
Midland Hospital Center
Position Available, 486
Mount Sinai Medical Center
Position Available, 578
National Council on Patient Information and Education
Institutional, 565
Pfipharmecs, Division of Pfizer Corporation
Vibramycin, 503–504
Roche Laboratories, Division of Hoffmann-La Roche Inc.
Coactin, 579–582
Institutional, 584–585
Rocephin, 495–500
Smith Kline & French Laboratories
Ancef, 487, 586–587
Cefizox, inside front cover
Monocid, 490–491
E.R. Squibb & Sons
Institutional, 471
Stuart Pharmaceuticals, Division of ICI Americas, Inc.
Institutional, outside back cover
University of Michigan
Positions Available, 489
The Upjohn Company
Micronase, 480–482
Veterans Administration
Positions Available, 578

News

Conference outlines challenges in the treatment of cocaine abuse

Drug abuse makes for catchy headlines, whether the story involves a celebrity's acknowledged drug use, a cracked drug ring, or the emergence of a new abused substance, like "ecstasy." Cocaine abuse recently drew attention in the press—not as a new problem but as a large one with more serious consequences than previously thought.[1,2]

The treatment of cocaine abuse poses challenges for health practitioners—challenges outlined at a two-day symposium in Brookfield, Wisconsin, last April featuring nationally known experts in the field. The conference, sponsored by the Wisconsin Institute on Drug Abuse and cosponsored by the National Institute on Drug Abuse (NIDA), focused on the cocaine problem and potential solutions.[3,4]

The successful treatment of cocaine abuse currently commands high priority because of the large number of individuals using the drug and because of cocaine's adverse health consequences. According to Edgar H. Adams, M.S., of NIDA's Division of Epidemiology and Statistical Analysis, the number of current cocaine users in the United States (individuals who used cocaine within the last month) increased from 1.6 million in 1977 to 4.3 million in 1979 and remained relatively steady since then. While NIDA officials take some solace in the leveling-off trend, they are alarmed at the increasing number of users who are encountering serious problems with the drug.

For instance, primary or secondary cocaine problems accounted for only 10% of all patients admitted to publicly funded treatment programs in 1977, and only 17% in 1981. The most recent figures for 1984 indicated that 29% of all treatment clients reported to NIDA have a problem with cocaine. Similarly, the number of cocaine-related emergency-room mentions reported through NIDA's Drug Abuse Warning Network jumped from 2981 to 8510 annually between 1980 and 1984. At the same time, the number of deaths associated with cocaine reported by a sample of medical examiners increased from 169 in 1980 to 548 four years later.

William Pollin, M.D., former Director of NIDA, told conference participants that these morbidity and mortality trends reflect more destructive patterns of cocaine use. While snorting continues as the predominant mode of cocaine administration (representing 57% of treatment admissions during the first half of 1984), 16% of clients with a primary cocaine problem in 1984 reported freebasing the drug. (Freebasing involves inhaling the free cocaine base, which is prepared from cocaine hydrochloride and then vaporized with heat.) That is up from 5% in 1981. Another 25% of all primary cocaine admissions in 1984 used injection as the principal route of administration. Aggravating the situation both in terms of adverse health consequences and treatment is the fact that most cocaine users also use other drugs.

Pathway of Cocaine Users. Sidney Cohen, M.D., Ph.D., internationally recognized expert on cocaine, characterized the challenge of treating cocaine abusers:

> We are finding that cocaine addiction is a difficult condition to treat. It requires a continuing resolve by the patient never to use it again, a devotion by the caregiver to be available for impending relapses, and considerable family support if one still exists. Some patients remain disabled physically, mentally, and socially, unable to live without cocaine and unable to live with it. Some die.

Cohen noted, though, that only 20% of all cocaine users encounter such serious problems with the drug. The remaining 80% are so-called social users, meaning that they are infrequent or low-level consumers who experience no perceptible social or health problems. According to Cohen, the 20% of users with serious problems "... come from the large group of social users, who after weeks, months, or years of modest use, slipped into a pattern of incessant consumption whenever cocaine was available."

There is no way to predict who will fall into this 20%. Cohen attributes the slippage to some "misfortune," like inheriting money, getting a raise, or acquiring a free source of cocaine. Likewise, substantial stress or loss of self-confidence may be the turning point.

The stereotype of cocaine abusers as being narcissistic reflects the characteristics of abusers who sought treatment during the early phases of the current cocaine epidemic, said J. Fred E. Shick, M.D., Medical Director of the Substance Abuse Treatment Unit at Chicago Lakeshore Hospital. These individuals typically were affluent, well-educated, white men holding responsible jobs, who frequently demanded special treatment. "While cocaine abusers often are grandiose individuals, their psychopathology is frequently more complex," said Shick. He believes that perhaps as many as 30–50% of the cocaine users now seeking treatment have some discernible psychopathology that persists long after detoxification. He was quick to add, though, that a person need not be psychopathologic to get into serious trouble with the drug.

According to Herbert E. Kleber, M.D., Director of the Substance Abuse Treatment Unit at Connecticut Mental Health Center, only two published studies applied the axis I (psychiatric diagnosis) criteria of the *Diagnostic and Statistical Manual of Mental Disorders*[5] (DSM-III) to cocaine abusers.[6,7] Both studies found some axis I diagnosis relating to depression in almost 50% of the sample. One

Continued on page 601

Continued from page 595

of the studies also found a high proportion of DSM-III, axis II diagnoses (personality disorders and specific developmental disorders) of borderline, narcissistic, and histrionic disorders.[6]

Kleber and Shick agreed that differential diagnosis is important for selecting an appropriate treatment for each individual cocaine user. In the past, only psychological treatment approaches were used, probably because cocaine abuse was considered a psychological problem. Recently, however, various drug therapies have been tried, some with promising results. All treatment approaches—psychological and pharmacological alike—share a common goal: stopping the cocaine use and then maintaining abstinence.

While proponents of the various treatment approaches claim great success, Kleber explained that no consensus on the optimal treatment strategy exists. Lacking, he said, are double-blind, controlled studies that account for extent of cocaine use, previous treatments, and presence of other psychiatric illnesses.

Psychological Approaches. Kleber categorized the psychological treatment approaches as three types: behavioral, supportive, and psychodynamic.

Contingency contracting is the best known of the behavioral approaches, said Kleber, and it consists of two parts: "The patient agrees to participate in a urine-monitoring program, and some aversive contingency is attached to producing a urine sample positive for cocaine or failing to produce a scheduled urine sample." The aversive contingency, which is specific for each patient (e.g., relinquishing a medical license if the patient is a physician), is scheduled to occur at the very next use of cocaine.

"Contingency contracting focuses the patient's attention on the aversive consequences of using cocaine," said Kleber. "Even without a formal contingency contract, . . . asking the patient to write down all the negative things that will occur if the patient continues using cocaine . . . can be a powerful tool . . . for focusing attention on the price of continued cocaine use." Urinalysis is important even when therapy does not involve a contingency contract. Kleber explained: "If urinalysis is not done and the patient 'gets away with drug use,' the patient tends to think of the therapist as just another person who can be fooled." Because cocaine's major metabolite, benzoylecgonine, is present in the urine for only 27 hours, Kleber recommends doing a urinalysis at least weekly.

Supportive therapy aims at helping the cocaine user develop strategies for dealing with his or her cocaine use. Kleber and his colleagues do this by focusing a patient's attention on six points:

- High-risk situations,
- Conditioning factors,
- Early warning signals,
- The opponent-process theory of addiction (i.e., the cycle of the user accumulating negative reasons for using the drug until finally the drug use stops, and then forgetting those reasons and just remembering the positive effects of the drug),
- Abstinent violation effect (i.e., the recognition that one instance of drug use does not constitute a relapse), and
- Stress reduction and lifestyle changes.

Because alcohol and other drugs are often conditioned cues for using cocaine, Kleber advises his patients to abstain from all mind-altering substances even if they do not have previous problems with those substances. Most often patients relapse, however, before believing the need for total abstinence, explained Kleber.

Psychodynamic approaches aim at helping cocaine users understand the roles of cocaine in their lives and helping them find alternative ways of fulfilling those roles without drugs.

Pharmacological Approaches. Various drugs have been tried in the treatment of cocaine abuse: tricyclic antidepressants, phenelzine, lithium carbonate, methylphenidate, pemoline, tyrosine, and tryptophan. Of these, the tricyclics and lithium carbonate show the most promise.

In one open clinical study conducted by Kleber and his colleagues, patients were treated with desipramine or lithium carbonate as adjuncts to psychotherapy.[7] Kleber explained, "The rationale for using the tricyclic antidepressant [in this case, desipramine] in the treatment of cocaine abusers is based on animal studies showing that the tricyclic antidepressants have opposite effects to those of chronic cocaine on catecholamine receptors and on intracranial self-stimulation." By the end of week 1, no changes in cocaine use or craving were seen in the six patients receiving desipramine; a small effect was apparent by week 2. By week 5, however, cocaine use stopped and craving markedly decreased in five of the six patients, and this pattern continued for at least three months.

The results for lithium carbonate showed a bimodal effect, said Kleber. The three patients who had a diagnosis of bipolar or cyclothymic disorder stopped using cocaine right away, and they continued cocaine free throughout the three-month study. On the other hand, the other three patients in the lithium group without such a diagnosis continued using cocaine as before the study.

One rationale for using lithium carbonate in the treatment of cocaine abusers, said Kleber, is that lithium reportedly blocks stimulant euphoria in animals. But the three patients in his study who continued using cocaine while receiving lithium reported no such blockade. Cohen stated that he knew of no controlled study documenting lithium's general usefulness as an anticraving agent in humans.

Because the tricyclic antidepressants have a delayed onset of action, one group of researchers has used phenelzine in treating cocaine abusers.[8] While their results have been good, Kleber warned against this therapy because patients could develop hypertensive crisis if they ingested cocaine along with the monoamine oxidase inhibitor.

The most controversial drug therapy for treating cocaine abusers involves methylphenidate. Methylphenidate has been tried both for the general treatment of cocaine abusers and specifically for cocaine abusers diagnosed as having attention deficit disorders (ADDs). According to Kleber, the rationale for trying methylphenidate as a general agent was to determine whether it could serve as a maintenance drug for cocaine abusers just as methadone is for heroin addicts. After all, methylphenidate seemingly offers the same characteristics as methadone: more orally effective and longer acting than

Continued on page 604

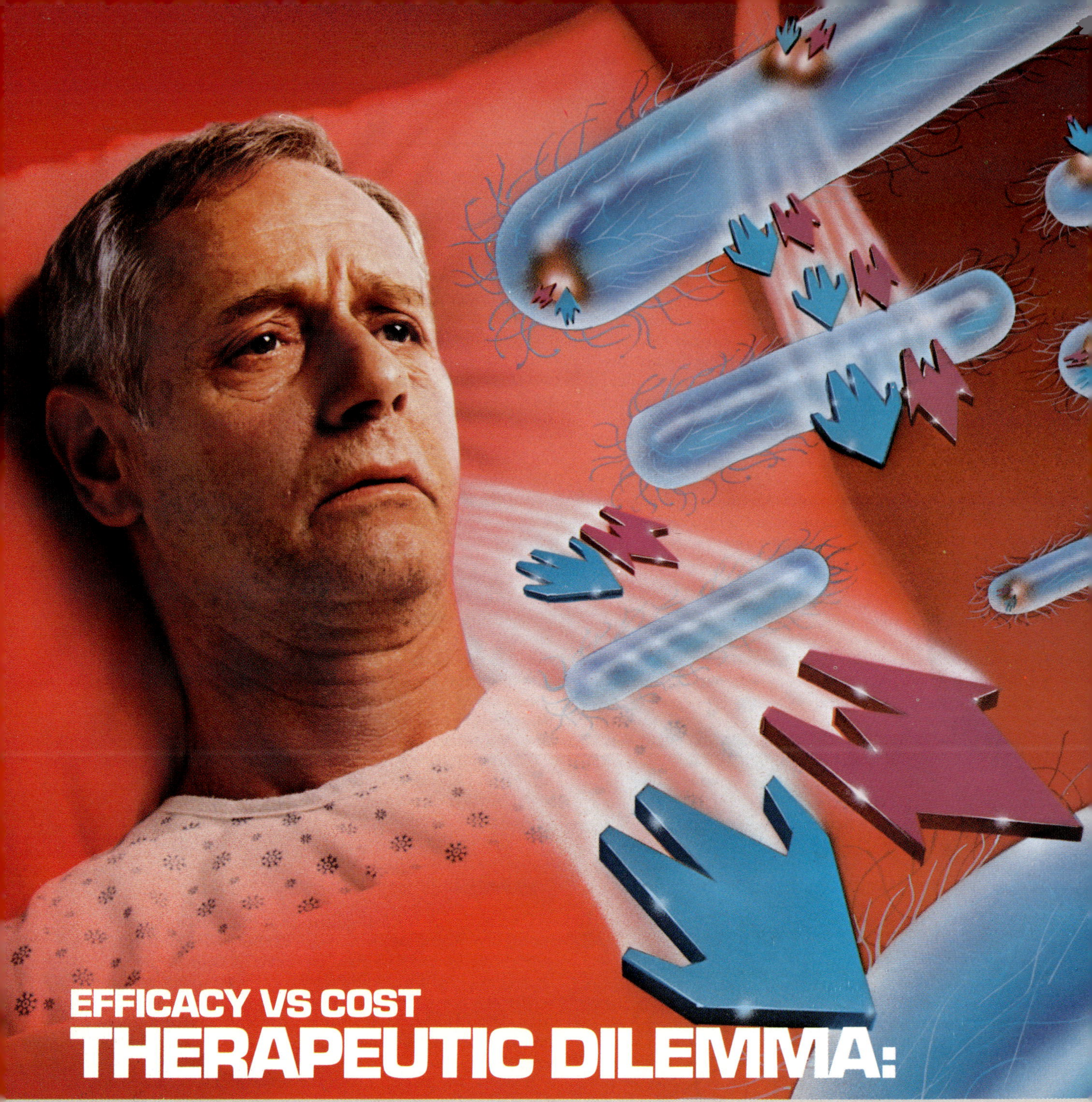

When choosing which antipseudomonal penicillin to pair with an aminoglycoside for *Pseudomonas* in immunocompromised patients, consider:

- Decisions must take into account mounting pressure to control antibiotic costs
- Cost-containment need not be attained at the expense of clinical efficacy and safety
- Important differences exist among the antipseudomonal penicillins

TICAR® TICARCILLIN DISODIUM
PLUS AN AMINOGLYCOSIDE

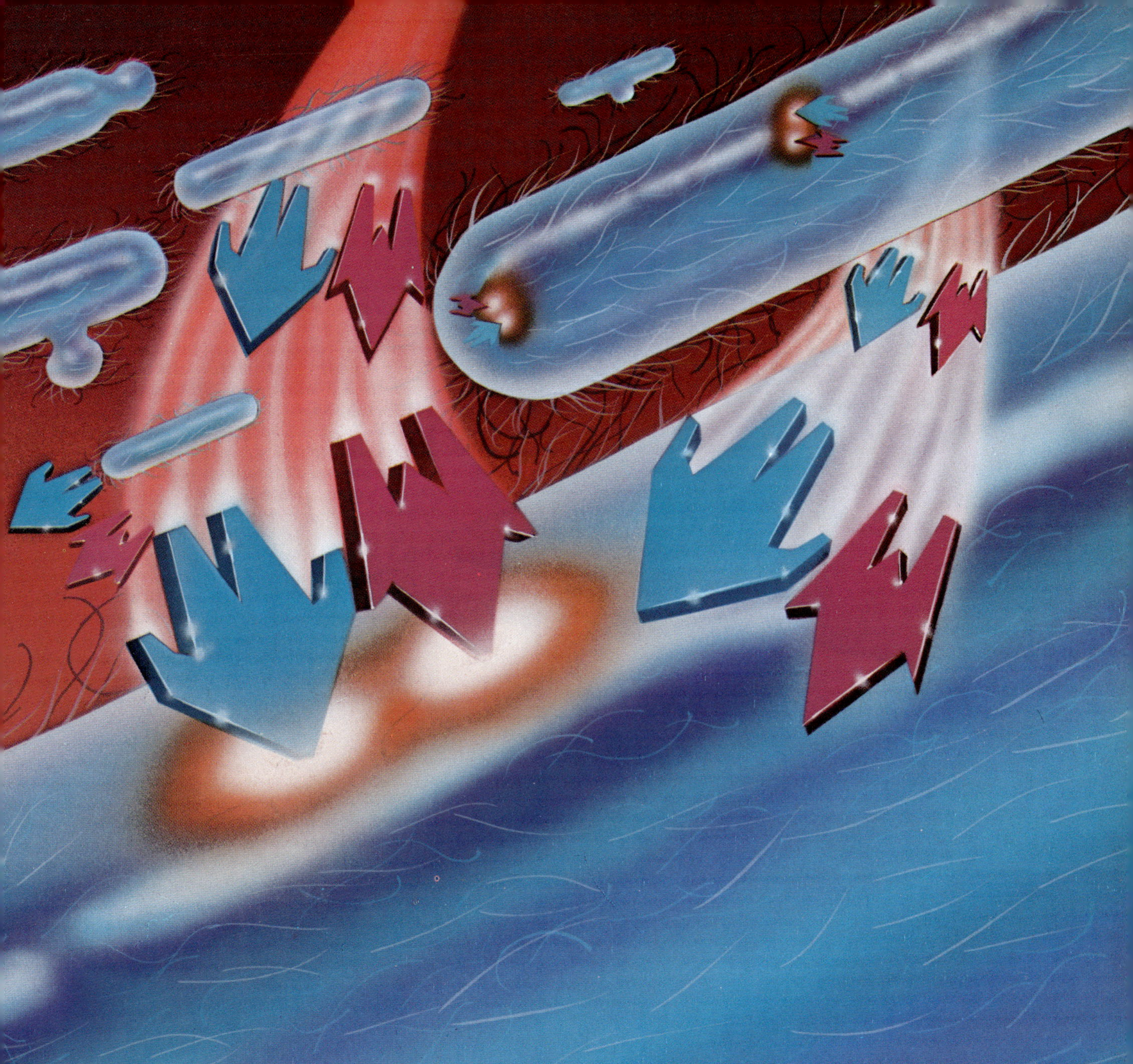

THERAPEUTIC DISTINCTION:

TICAR® (TICARCILLIN DISODIUM) **is distinguished as**
THE PROVEN STANDARD against which the others are judged.

- Efficacy documented over 12 years of widespread use[1]
- Clinical performance unsurpassed by any other antipseudomonal penicillin[2]
- Superior track record of safety contrasts with emerging toxicity concerns about other penicillins[3]
- The newer antibiotics are generally more expensive[2]

TICAR® TICARCILLIN DISODIUM
PLUS AN AMINOGLYCOSIDE
THE PROVEN STANDARD IN ANTIPSEUDOMONAL
THERAPY FOR IMMUNOCOMPROMISED PATIENTS

Beecham
laboratories
BRISTOL, TENNESSEE 37620

PLEASE SEE NEXT PAGE FOR BRIEF SUMMARY OF PRESCRIBING INFORMATION.

News *Continued from page 601*

the primary drug of abuse, but producing much less euphoria. Kleber and his colleagues tried this with a group of patients and found they were wrong.[9] Methylphenidate hydrochloride 10 mg twice daily decreased cocaine craving for several days, but then the effect wore off and patients requested an increased dose. The cycle continued until the patients one month later were receiving 100 mg of methylphenidate hydrochloride daily and using cocaine. Explained Kleber, "Methylphenidate not only did not take away craving, but we think it even stimulated craving." He added, however, that several case reports have described success in treating cocaine abusers with pemoline, a stimulant with less abuse potential than methylphenidate.

Methylphenidate has been used successfully by Kleber and others in treating cocaine abusers diagnosed as having attention-deficit disorders of the residual type.[10] According to Kleber, these patients tend to use cocaine in a self-medicating fashion (regularly spaced, small doses), which is in stark contrast to the bingelike pattern cocaine abusers generally exhibit. While Kleber advocated caution in prescribing methyphenidate only after a careful diagnosis of ADD is made, Cohen adamantly opposed its use. He argued:

> Anybody who is on cocaine has an attention-deficit disorder. Cocaine users are so disorganized that they cannot attend, and therapists cannot make the diagnosis until the patient has been off cocaine for a while. Except in the rare instance in which a patient really has an attention-deficit disorder, I would not prescribe a stimulant. There have been some terrible instances of Ritalin [methylphenidate hydrochloride] dependency.

A final category of drugs tried in the treatment of cocaine abuse is the neurotransmitter precursors, tyrosine and tryptophan. The rationale for their use is that tyrosine (as a precursor for dopamine and norepinephrine) and tryptophan (as a precursor for serotonin) replace neurotransmitters depleted by cocaine. Preliminary reports suggest that these precursors ameliorate the cocaine "crash" and cocaine craving; however, no controlled studies have documented their effectiveness.

Integrated Approach. How does all of this fit together? Considering the heterogeneity of cocaine users seeking treatment, Dorynne Czechowicz, M.D., Assistant Director of Medical and Clinical Affairs at NIDA, advocated using an integrated approach to treatment. So, too, did Kleber, who presented a possible schema for integrating the various approaches based on severity of the cocaine abuse (see table).[11]

Cohen advocated treating severely depressed cocaine users with a course of a tricyclic antidepressant, the choice of agent being the one with which the physician is most familiar. Likewise, he recommended treating patients diagnosed as being manic with lithium.

Because of scarce treatment and monetary resources, outpatient treatment of cocaine abusers is preferred, said Cohen. He noted, however, that some patients definitely should be treated on an inpatient unit for several weeks—patients with severe psychological illness (e.g., schizophrenia or severe depression), heart problems made worse by cocaine, convulsions, or loss of one third or more of body weight. He also advised hospitalization for cocaine abusers who are dealers or who repeatedly failed in outpatient treatment programs.

Possible Future Guidelines for Cocaine Abuse Treatment[a]

Cocaine Abuse Severity	Psychotherapeutic Approach	Pharmacotherapeutic Approach
Mild	Behavioral with or without psychodynamic	None
Moderate	Supportive and psychodynamic with or without behavioral	Only if psychiatric diagnosis is present. Choice of agent based on symptoms. If no treatable diagnosis exists, general treatment (desipramine) may be usefully tried in difficult cases
Severe	Supportive with or without hospitalization for acute phase; then as in "moderate"	General treatment (desipramine) indicated unless diagnosis dictates another treatment choice

[a] Reprinted from reference 11, page 123.

Long-term supportive therapy in groups such as Narcotics Anonymous or Cocaine Anonymous was deemed important for continued abstinence.

What Forgiveness. While more research is needed on the optimal methods for treating cocaine abusers, Pollin was optimistic about the level of success already seen among cocaine abusers referred to appropriate treatment programs. Still, challenges remain, and Kleber aptly concluded his talk—and, as the last speaker, the conference—by reminding participants of cocaine's addiction potential:

> Whenever people ask whether I have ever tried cocaine, my answer is no and I give them the quote from T. S. Eliot: 'After such knowledge, what forgiveness.' I really do not want to know how good cocaine feels. When I am in stressful situations, I do not want that memory. I think there is some knowledge one is better off not acquiring. Given the problems I described in treating cocaine abusers, it is clearly more prudent not to get started.

1. Pollin W. The danger of cocaine. *JAMA.* 1985; 254:98.
2. Bozarth MA, Wise RA. Toxicity associated with long-term intravenous heroin and cocaine self-administration in the rat. *JAMA.* 1985; 254:81–3.
3. Brink CJ, ed. Cocaine: a symposium. Madison, WI: Wisconsin Institute on Drug Abuse; 1985.
4. Brink CJ. Wisconsin conference dispels myths about cocaine. *Am J Hosp Pharm.* 1985; 42:1454–5, 1459–60, 1469. News.
5. American Psychiatric Association. Diagnostic and statistical manual of mental disorders, 3rd ed. Washington, DC: American Psychiatric Association; 1980.
6. Weiss RD, Mirin SM, Michael JL. Psychopathology in chronic cocaine abusers. Paper presented at the 136th annual meeting of the American Psychiatric Association. New York: 1983 May 4.
7. Gawin FH, Kleber HD. Cocaine abuse treatment: an open pilot trial with lithium and desipramine. *Arch Gen Psychiatry.* 1984; 41:903–10.
8. Resnick RB, Resnick E. Psychological issues in the treatment of cocaine abusers. Presented at a meeting entitled Cocaine abuse: new treatment approaches. Columbia University, New York: 1985 Jan 5.
9. Gawin FH, Kleber HD. Methylphenidate treatment of non-ADD cocaine abusers. *Am J Drug Alcohol Abuse.* In press.
10. Khantzian EJ, Gawin FH, Riordan C et al. Methylphenidate treatment of cocaine dependence—a preliminary report. *J Subst Abuse Treat.* 1984; 1:107–12.
11. Kleber HD, Gawin FH. Cocaine abuse: a review of current and experimental treatments. In: Grabowski J, ed. Cocaine: pharmacology, effects, and treatment of abuse. National Institute on Drug Abuse research monograph 50. DHHS publication no. (ADM)84-1326. Washington, DC: U.S. Government Printing Office; 1984:111–29.

CARLA J. BRINK, M.S.
Clinical Pharmacy Correspondent

New NIH recommendations for adjuvant therapy for breast cancer

Adjuvant endocrine therapy will benefit many older women with breast cancer, according to an NIH Consensus Development Conference panel that considered the role of adjuvant cytotoxic and endocrine therapy for breast cancer. The conference was held in Bethesda, MD, on September 9–11. Specifically, the panel recommended that tamoxifen should be regarded as standard therapy in postmenopausal patients with histologically positive axillary lymph nodes and positive hormone-receptor status. In reporting the panel's findings, chairman John H. Glick, M.D., director of the University of Pennsylvania Cancer Center, noted that previously "there was no agreement, nationally or internationally, as to what constituted a standard of care for the postmenopausal woman" with cancer limited to the breast and axillary lymph nodes.

This conference was the second NIH Consensus Development Conference to address the role of adjuvant therapy for breast cancer. In 1980, the panel recommended adjuvant cytotoxic therapy for premenopausal patients with positive axillary lymph nodes. Specific treatment guidelines were not extended to other subgroups of patients. Continued evaluation of adjuvant regimens in controlled clinical trials and the application of new techniques for tumor analysis led to the need for reevaluating the relative benefits and toxicities of cytotoxic and endocrine therapies, criteria for selection of patients to receive adjuvant therapy, and directions for future research.

An estimated 120,000 cases of breast cancer will have been diagnosed in the United States this year. It is estimated that the disease will be limited to the breast and axillary lymph nodes in 90% of these patients. More than one third of women with limited disease (involvement of breast and lymph nodes) at diagnosis will ultimately develop systemic disease and die. The goal of adjuvant therapy is eradication of occult metastatic disease that

Continued on page 611

The Only First-Generatio

ANCEF
ANCEF
ANCEF

brand of sterile

CEFAZOLIN SODIUM IV/IM

(LYOPHILIZED) Injection: 500 mg. and 1 gram vials

The following is a brief summary of prescribing information. For complete prescribing information, please see SK&F literature or *PDR*.

INDICATIONS

Bone and joint infections due to *Staphylococcus aureus* and other indicated infections due to susceptible organisms. See complete prescribing information for a complete list of indications.

CONTRAINDICATIONS

'ANCEF' IS CONTRAINDICATED IN PATIENTS WITH KNOWN ALLERGY TO THE CEPHALOSPORIN GROUP OF ANTIBIOTICS.

WARNINGS

BEFORE CEFAZOLIN THERAPY IS INSTITUTED, CAREFUL INQUIRY SHOULD BE MADE CONCERNING PREVIOUS HYPERSENSITIVITY REACTIONS TO CEPHALOSPORINS AND PENICILLIN. CEPHALOSPORIN C DERIVATIVES SHOULD BE GIVEN CAUTIOUSLY IN PENICILLIN-SENSITIVE PATIENTS.

SERIOUS ACUTE HYPERSENSITIVITY REACTIONS MAY REQUIRE EPINEPHRINE AND OTHER EMERGENCY MEASURES.

There is some clinical and laboratory evidence of partial cross-allergenicity of the penicillins and the cephalosporins. Patients have been reported to have had severe reactions (including anaphylaxis) to both drugs.

Any patient who has demonstrated some form of allergy, particularly to drugs, should receive antibiotics cautiously. No exception should be made with regard to 'Ancef'.

Pseudomembranous colitis has been reported with the use of cephalosporins (and other broad-spectrum antibiotics); therefore, it is important to consider its diagnosis in patients who develop diarrhea in association with antibiotic use.

Treatment with broad-spectrum antibiotics alters normal flora of the colon and may permit overgrowth of clostridia. Studies indicate a toxin produced by *Clostridium difficile* is one primary cause of antibiotic-associated colitis. Cholestyramine and colestipol resins have been shown to bind the toxin *in vitro*.

Mild cases of colitis may respond to drug discontinuance alone.

Moderate to severe cases should be managed with fluid, electrolyte and protein supplementation as indicated.

When the colitis is not relieved by drug discontinuance or when it is severe, oral vancomycin is the treatment of choice for antibiotic-associated pseudomembranous colitis produced by *C. difficile*. Other causes of colitis should also be considered.

PRECAUTIONS

General—Prolonged use of 'Ancef' may result in the overgrowth of non-susceptible organisms. Careful clinical observation of the patient is essential.

When 'Ancef' is administered to patients with low urinary output b of impaired renal function, lower daily dosage is required (see Dos and Administration).

'Ancef', as with all cephalosporins, should be prescribed with caut individuals with a history of gastrointestinal disease, particularly cc

Drug Interactions—Probenecid may decrease renal tubular secret cephalosporins when used concurrently, resulting in increased anc prolonged cephalosporin blood levels.

Drug/Laboratory Test Interactions—A false positive reaction for g in the urine may occur with Benedict's solution, Fehling's solution with Clinitest® tablets, but not with enzyme-based tests such as C and Tes-Tape®.

Positive direct and indirect antiglobulin (Coombs) tests have occur these may also occur in neonates whose mothers received cephalosporins before delivery.

Carcinogenesis/Mutagenesis—Mutagenicity studies and long-terr studies in animals to determine the carcinogenic potential of 'Ance not been performed.

Continued from page 605

would not be eliminated by primary treatment with surgery, radiation therapy, or both. The efficacy of adjuvant drug regimens is measured by effect on overall survival, disease-free survival, and quality of life.

Treatment of Postmenopausal Patients. The decision to use tamoxifen in the treatment of postmenopausal women with breast cancer involving the axillary lymph nodes should be based on analysis of the estrogen- and progesterone-receptor content of the primary tumor. Numerous studies of tamoxifen in patients with hormone-receptor-positive tumors have demonstrated significant prolongation of disease-free survival. However, most of these clinical trials involve limited numbers of patients and have not shown significant increases in overall survival. However, an overview of tamoxifen clinical trials, reported by Richard Peto, a cancer study statistician from Oxford University, showed "a highly significant and substantial improvement in overall survival" with the five-year mortality reduced from 30 to 25%. Tamoxifen therapy is generally regarded as ineffective in the treatment of postmenopausal patients with estrogen-receptor-negative, node-positive tumors.

Cytotoxic therapy may offer patients who have receptor-negative, node-positive tumors "a small advantage in disease-free and overall survival," the panel concluded. However, benefits have not been consistently reported when results of clinical trials are analyzed by receptor status. The panel concluded that chemotherapy cannot be considered standard care; relative benefits and toxicities must be considered on an individual basis.

Treatment of Premenopausal Patients. The panel stated that adjuvant cytotoxic therapy has resulted in "a highly significant increase in disease-free survival and a significant reduction in mortality" in premenopausal women with histologically positive axillary lymph nodes. The panel concluded that combination chemotherapeutic regimens of proven efficacy should be considered standard care in this group of patients regardless of hormone receptor status. Numerous chemotherapeutic agents have been studied; frequently used regimens contain the combination of cyclophosphamide, methotrexate, and fluorouracil (alone or with other cytotoxic drugs) and combination regimens containing doxorubicin. The optimal drug regimen has not been identified. In recommending cytotoxic therapy, the panel emphasized that treatment outside a clinical trial should involve drug regimens of proven efficacy and should conform to the dose intensity and treatment schedule specified in the study protocol. Survival is not prolonged by adjuvant endocrine therapy, alone or in combination with chemotherapy.

Treatment of Node-Negative Patients. Little progress has been made in defining the role of adjuvant therapy in premenopausal or postmenopausal patients with histologically negative lymph nodes. The panel suggested that chemotherapy may be considered on a case-by-case basis for high-risk patients who are ineligible for enrollment in clinical trials.

Toxicity of Adjuvant Therapy. The acute toxicities of the chemotherapeutic drugs used to treat breast cancer are well known and include leukopenia, nausea and vomiting, fatigue, and alopecia. Amenorrhea develops frequently and is rarely reversible in women over 40 years of age. In a review of long-term toxicity in more than 8000 women participating in the National Surgical Adjuvant Project for Breast Cancers (NSABP clinical trials), Bernard Fisher, M.D., of the University of Pittsburgh, reported the 10-year cumulative risk of leukemia in chemotherapy recipients to be 1.7% compared with 0.3% in women treated by surgery alone. Current data suggest that the risk of developing a second solid tumor is not increased by adjuvant chemotherapy.

Tamoxifen is generally well tolerated, although side effects caused by estrogen deprivation are common. Late complications appear to be minimal, but long-term follow-up data are limited.

Participation in Clinical Trials. In establishing these guidelines for adjuvant therapy for breast cancer, the panel urged patients and physicians to participate in ongoing clinical trials. Although substantial advances have been made, optimal therapy has not been defined. Establishment of a regimen as the standard of practice when the gains are modest or restricted to subgroups of patients requires the participation of large numbers of patients. Demonstration of even moderate effects on survival may translate into substantial public-health benefits because of the large number of women who have breast cancer.

JANE L. MILLER

Leuprolide approved for palliative treatment of advanced prostatic cancer

Leuprolide acetate (Lupron), a synthetic nonapeptide analog of luteinizing-hormone-releasing hormone (gonadotropin-releasing hormone), was marketed in April by TAP Pharmaceuticals for the palliative treatment of advanced prostatic cancer. Leuprolide appears to be as effective as diethylstilbestrol (DES) in suppressing testicular steroidogenesis and is better tolerated; however, the relative expensiveness of the drug may limit its widespread use.

Subcutaneous administration of single daily doses of leuprolide results in an initial increase in circulating levels of luteinizing hormone (LH) and follicle-stimulating hormone (FSH) with a corresponding increase in serum concentrations of testosterone and dihydrotestosterone. However, continuous daily administration results in decreased levels of LH and FSH, and within two to four weeks testosterone and dihydrotestosterone concentrations fall to castrate levels.

Leuprolide offers an alternative treatment of prostatic cancer when orchiectomy or estrogen administration are either not indicated or unacceptable to the patient. In a randomized controlled trial in 199 patients with previously untreated advanced prostatic cancer, the objective response rates and survival rates after one year were comparable for the group treated with leuprolide and the group treated with DES. Leuprolide is much less effective in patients previously treated with orchiectomy or DES.

The recommended dose of leuprolide is 1 mg (0.2 mL) administered as a single daily subcutaneous injection.

Continued on page 614

When a type II diabetic patient
needs more than diet,
unique MICRONASE® Tablets (glyburide)
are a logical first choice.

Choosing antidiabeti

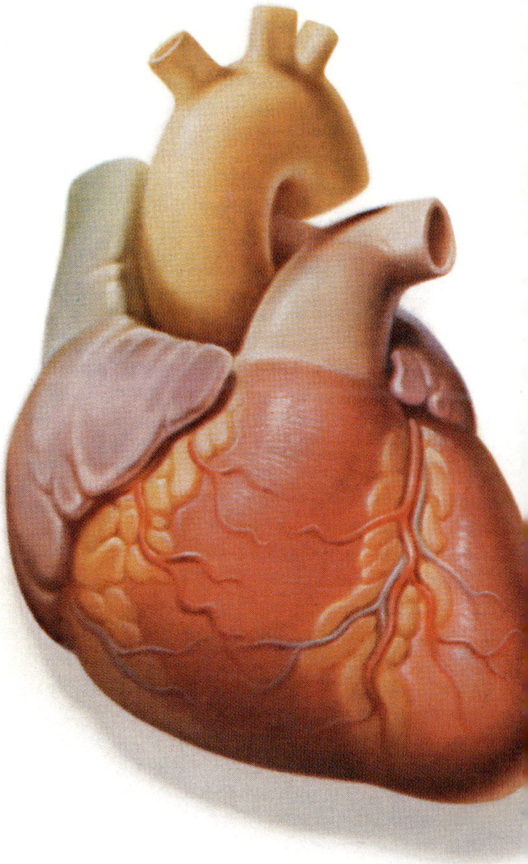

1. Micronase—a rational choice in type II diabetes

Insulin levels are normal or elevated in most patients with type II diabetes, although insulin action is markedly impaired. MICRONASE helps normalize the tissue response to endogenous insulin.

Initially, MICRONASE helps lower serum glucose in responsive patients by stimulating the release of additional insulin. As therapy continues, MICRONASE is believed to promote peripheral glucose metabolism by helping to correct defects at the cellular receptor and postreceptor levels.

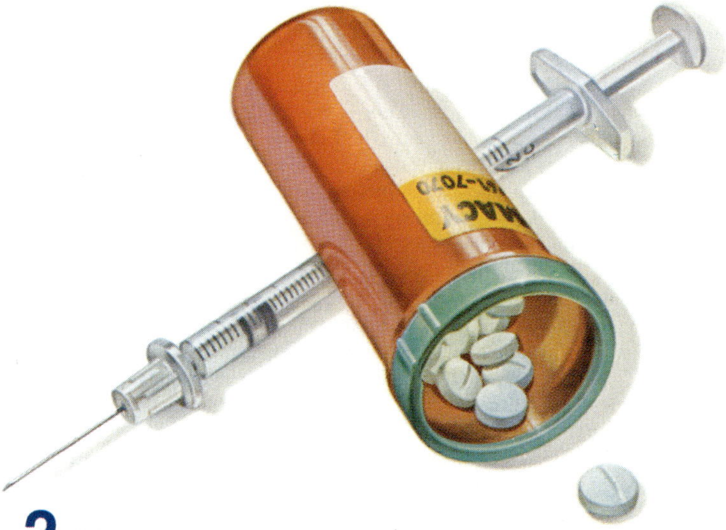

2. Micronase—a single, daily dose provides 24-hour glycemic control

MICRONASE provides 24-hour control of blood glucose with a single, daily, low-milligram dose. MICRONASE may be taken with food, since food intake does not appear to affect its bioavailability.

3. Micronase—for the type II diabetic patient who is also hypertensive: Control without risk of water retention

This may also be significant for the type II diabetic p
with congestive heart failure. MICRONASE actually ca
mild diuresis.

herapy today

Micronase—an important consideration in type II diabetic patient with renal impair-nt: Control plus unique dual excretion... 6 urine, 50% bile

nation of MICRONASE equally in bile and urine reduces the of drug accumulation, which may result in hypoglycemia. CONASE should be used with caution in patients with renal irment; however, in a single-dose study, plasma clearance of ONASE was prolonged only in patients with severe renal irment.

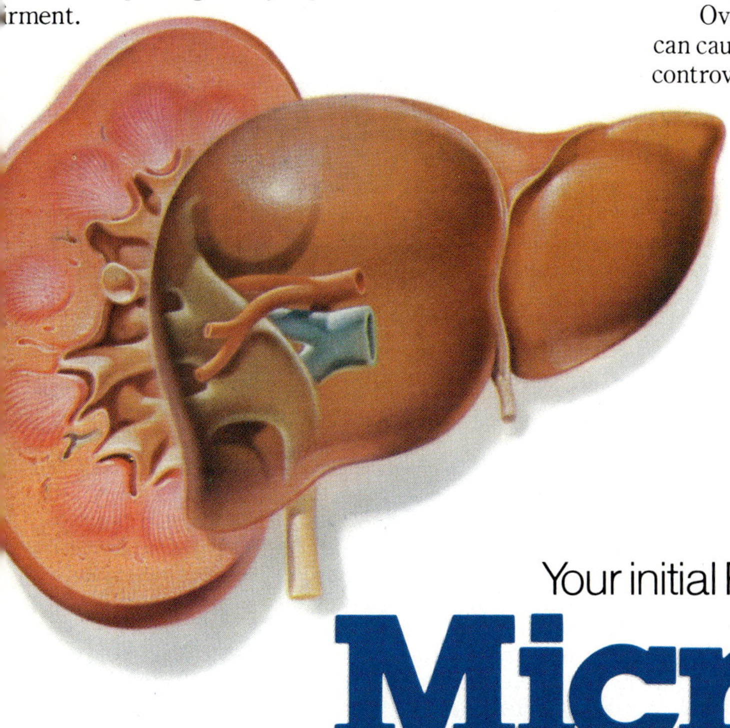

5. Micronase—for the patient who fails on other diabetic therapy: Potency and dosage flexibility

MICRONASE may prove effective when other drugs fail. Five mg of MICRONASE is approximately equivalent to 250 mg of chlorpropamide or 500 mg of acetohexamide in its ability to lower blood glucose. The dosage range of MICRONASE allows for greater dosage flexibility than other agents.

Overdosage of sulfonylureas, including MICRONASE, can cause hypoglycemia. Although the interpretations are controversial, the UGDP study reported in 1970 that the use of tolbutamide, an oral hypoglycemic drug, was associated with increased cardiovascular mortality.

Upjohn The Upjohn Company
Kalamazoo, MI 49001

Your initial Rx in type II diabetes

Micronase®

glyburide, **5 mg** Tablets

For brief summary of prescribing information, please turn page.

News *Continued from page 611*

The transient increase in testosterone concentrations during the first week of therapy may be associated with a temporary worsening of signs and symptoms, usually manifested by an increase in bone pain.

Leuprolide is supplied as a sterile solution in a 2.8-mL multiple-dose vial. The suggested wholesale price to pharmacists is $131.25 per vial.

New β blocker for glaucoma approved by FDA

Betaxolol hydrochloride (Betoptic, Alcon Laboratories, Inc., Fort Worth, TX 76101), a β_1-adrenergic receptor blocking agent, was approved by the FDA in September for use in the treatment of ocular hypertension and chronic open-angle glaucoma. When instilled in the eye as a 0.5% ophthalmic solution, betaxolol reduces elevated as well as normal intraocular pressure but has minimal effect on pulmonary or cardiovascular function.

The results of clinical studies in nearly 1000 patients in U.S. medical centers indicate that betaxolol reduces mean intraocular pressure 25% from baseline. In one long-term study involving 250 patients, no reduction in efficacy was seen after a mean period of two years of continuous treatment.

Betaxolol can be used alone or in combination with other antiglaucoma drugs. Betaxolol is contraindicated in patients with sinus bradycardia, greater than a first-degree atrioventricular block, cardiogenic shock, or overt cardiac failure and should be used with caution in patients with severe reactive airway disease.

The usual dose of betaxolol is one drop in the affected eye or eyes twice daily. The onset of action occurs within 30 minutes with maximal effect at two hours after a dose is administered.

Betaxolol is supplied as a sterile, isotonic ophthalmic solution in 5- and 10-mL plastic dropper containers. Alcon has priced Betoptic at $7.40 per 5-mL bottle and $10.60 per 10-mL bottle.

Studies of bepridil in use against arrhythmias halted

McNeil Pharmaceutical has halted studies of bepridil, an experimental calcium-channel-blocking agent, in use against arrhythmias after officials in the United Kingdom voiced concern about deaths in patients using the drug in clinical trials in Europe. The company plans to continue testing bepridil for its primary use in treating angina.

Both McNeil and Carter-Wallace Inc. are seeking to market bepridil in the United States. If approved for marketing, bepridil would be the only calcium-channel-blocking agent available for single daily dosing. A spokesman for Carter-Wallace would not indicate whether the company also was halting its tests.

A spokesman for McNeil was quoted as saying that the company is not certain why deaths have been reported only in patients under study for arrhythmias, but added that the patients were sicker than those being studied for angina.

Letters

The Letters *column is a forum for rapid exchange of ideas among readers of* CP. *Liberal criteria are applied in the review of submissions to encourage contributions to this column.*

The Letters *column includes the following types of contributions: (1) comments, addenda, and minor updates on previously published work, (2) alerts on potential problems related to drug therapy or clinical research, (3) observations or comments on trends in drug therapy or clinical research, and (4) brief expressions of opinion about controversies in drug therapy or clinical research.*

Letters need not be submitted with the journal's manuscript checklist. The following conditions, however, must be adhered to: (1) the body of the letter must be no longer than two typewritten pages, (2) the use of references, tables, and illustrations should be minimized, (3) the authors' names, affiliations, and mailing addresses must be typed at the end of the letter in the format used by CP, *and (4) the entire letter (including references, tables, and authors' names) must be typed double spaced on plain white paper (not letterhead). Following acceptance of a letter, the authors are required to sign an exclusive publication statement and a copyright-transferral form.*

Successful treatment of cerebellar tremor with clonazepam

Static and proximal kinetic tremors are frequent symptoms of cerebellar disease.[1] These tremors can be exceedingly disabling, often making routine daily living activities impossible. Unfortunately, however, there is little physiological or biochemical understanding of their mechanism. Moreover, there is no current established pharmacologic therapy for these types of tremors. In essential tremor, administration of beta blockers such as propranolol has been shown to be beneficial in some patients.[2] Sabra et al.[3] recently reported that in an open trial isoniazid, a putative gamma aminobutyric acid (GABA) agonist, produced marked improvement of cerebellar tremors associated with multiple sclerosis. The rationale for using isoniazid was related to the fact that GABA appears to be the inhibitory neurotransmitter used by the Purkinje cells of the cerebellum.[4]

The following report concerns two patients with intention tremor in whom clonazepam caused marked and sustained amelioration of the tremor. The first patient was a 27-year-old woman with multiple sclerosis who was handicapped by severe intention tremor of the upper limbs. Because of her cerebellar deficit, she was unable to feed herself without support and was put into an institution. The severity of the tremor was rated 3 (on a scale of 0 to 4 of increasing severity). Clonazepam 4 mg daily administered in four divided doses produced marked amelioration of the tremor. The severity of the tremor was rated 1 a week after initiation of therapy. As a result of clonazepam administration, she regained the ability to hold objects and feed herself without support and was discharged.

The second patient was a 54-year-old man who sustained a head injury in 1979 following a motorcycle accident. He was comatose for 10 days after the injury. His residual neurologic deficit included a mild sixth and seventh nerve palsy on the left, a bilateral corticospinal-tract lesion, marked truncal ataxia, and a bilateral but predominantly right-sided intention tremor (2–3 on clinical rating scale). A computed-tomography scan of the brain was normal except for some dilatation of the fourth ventricle and cisterna magna, indicating cortical cerebellar atrophy. Because of his cerebellar deficit, particularly the intention tremor of the upper limbs, he was severely handicapped in his daily activities and was dependent on constant nursing care. Clonazepam 8 mg daily in four divided doses noticeably decreased the severity of the intention tremor, which was rated 0–1 after one week of therapy. In both patients clonazepam was well tolerated except for mild and temporary sedation experienced by the second patient.

Beta-adrenergic blocking agents have been shown to be beneficial in the management of essential tremor of both the static and the kinetic types.[2] These agents, however, are of no value in the treatment of cerebellar tremor.[5]

Clonazepam has been shown to have a broad spectrum of activity against various types of epilepsy, specifically myoclonus epilepsy.[6] The antimyoclonic properties of clonazepam have been attributed to its ability to enhance serotonergic transmission.[7] Moreover, clonazepam has been shown to act through potentiation of GABA transmission.[8] Reduction in cerebrospinal fluid GABA con-

Continued on page 618

As safe as albumin or PPF

In comparative clinical studies, platelet counts, hematocrits, serum fibrinogen levels, prothrombin times (PT), and partial thromboplastin times (PTT) seen with Hespan were comparable to those seen with albumin or plasma protein fraction (PPF).[1,2]

Other studies demonstrate that when any reduction in platelet count or prolongation of PT or PTT does occur with Hespan, no increased bleeding results, even in patients with multiple trauma.[3-5] As with any volume expander, patients should be monitored for excessive hemodilution of coagulant factors or circulatory overload when large volumes are administered.

When Hespan-treated patients were monitored to detect localized or systemic sepsis, there was no evidence of a decrease in their ability to ward off infection or combat an established infection.[5]

Hespan is nonantigenic and, as with blood-derived colloids, any risk of allergic reaction is minimal. Hespan also has a negligible effect on subsequent blood typing or crossmatching.[6]

As effective as albumin or PPF

Comparative clinical studies have repeatedly demonstrated that Hespan is as effective as albumin or PPF in postoperative myocardial revascularization,[1-3] and hemorrhagic, traumatic, or septic shock.[4,5,7]

No significant differences between Hespan and albumin or PPF were noted in any efficacy parameter.[1-5,7] Hespan effectively maintained colloid osmotic pressure, restored plasma volume, and improved cardiac output and renal function in hypovolemic patients.[1-5,7] And, the volume-expanding effect of a single infusion of Hespan can persist for 24 hours or longer.

Half the price of albumin or PPF

Hespan offers a potential savings to your hospital of tens of thousands of dollars a year.

double the price.

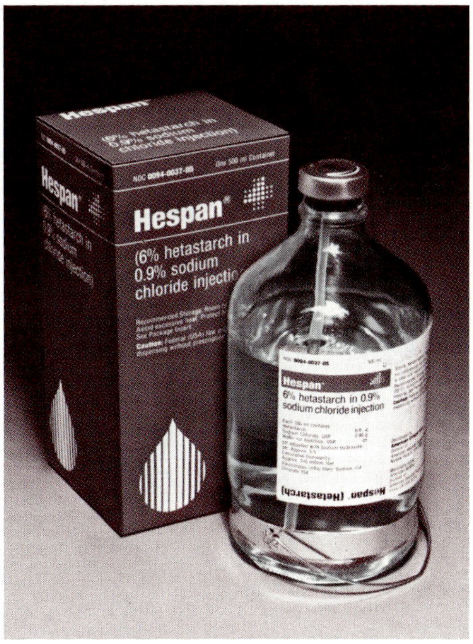

For additional information, contact the Medical Services Department, American Critical Care, 1600 Waukegan Road, McGaw Park, IL 60085. Phone 1-800-323-4980.

Lifesaving, moneysaving

HESPAN®
(hetastarch)

American Critical Care

American Hospital Supply Corporation

Please see references and brief summary of prescribing information on following page.

Letters *Continued from page 615*

centrations has been noted in a variety of CNS disorders, including multiple sclerosis and cerebellar cortical atrophy.[9] In the patients reported here, clonazepam ameliorated cerebellar tremor, an effect possibly related to the GABA-facilitatory effect of clonazepam. Sedation is a known side effect of clonazepam and other benzodiazepines. However, when the drug is administered at slow increments, sedation may be avoided.

This report suggests that clonazepam may be a useful agent in the management of severe and incapacitating cerebellar tremor. This drug should be considered for patients in whom other agents have failed to produce amelioration of cerebellar tremor.

1. Gilman S, Bloedel JR, Lechtenberg R. Disorders of the cerebellum. Philadelphia: F. A. Davis Co.; 1981:171–3.
2. Young RR, Shahani BT. Pharmacology of tremor. In: Klawans HL, ed. Clinical neuropharmacology, vol. 4. New York: Raven Press; 1980:139–57.
3. Sabra AF, Hallett M, Sudarsky L et al. Treatment of action tremor in multiple sclerosis with isoniazid. *Neurology.* 1982; 32:912–4.
4. Defeadis FV. Amino acids as central neurotransmitters. *Ann Rev Pharmacol Toxicol.* 1975; 15:105–30.
5. Koller WC. Pharmacologic trials in the treatment of cerebellar tremor. *Arch Neurol.* 1984; 41:280–1.
6. Chadwick D, Harris R, Jenner P et al. Manipulations of brain serotonin in the treatment of myoclonus. *Lancet.* 1981; ii:434.
7. Jenner P, Chadwick D, Reynolds EH et al. Altered 5-HT metabolism with clonazepam, diazepam and diphenylhydantoin. *J Pharm Pharmacol.* 1975; 27:707–10.
8. Trelles L, Trelles JO, Castro C et al. Successful treatment of two cases of intention tremor with clonazepam. *Ann Neurol* 1984; 16:621.
9. Neophytides AN, Suria A, Chase TN. Cerebrospinal fluid GABA in neurologic disease. *Neurology.* 1978; 28:359–64.

R. Sandyk, M.D., M.S.
The University of Arizona Health Sciences Center
Tucson, AZ 85724

Phenytoin injection precautions

There have been several recent reports within our institution of severe local reactions when phenytoin (Dilantin) is administered via intravenous push into a vein in the back of the hand. These reactions have occurred in elderly women and consist of erythema, edema, and a pronounced discoloration of the hand described as a "purple glove." Extravasation and rate of administration have been ruled out as possible causes of the reactions.

A review of the literature disclosed a report that described similar reactions in nine patients at another hospital.[1] As with our cases, most of the patients were elderly women with friable veins. However, the reaction also occurred in one 18-year-old man. In most cases, resolution of the described symptoms occurred within three weeks; however, one patient required limb amputation. In all cases, it was suspected that the reaction was the result of a local irritant effect of the drug or its vehicle on small veins.

As a result of the above-reported problems and our case review, our pharmacy and therapeutics committee issued a policy statement that phenytoin is not to be administered via i.v. push into veins in the back of the hand. The committee recommends that injectable phen-

Continued on page 620

Continued from page 618

ytoin be given only as an i.v. push medication into larger veins at a rate not exceeding 50 mg per minute.

Inasmuch as this type of adverse drug reaction to phenytoin has been reported infrequently and because of the seriousness of the reaction, we suggest that physicians, pharmacists, and nurses be made aware of this potential drug administration problem. In fact, the subject may be appropriate for pharmacy and therapeutics committee consideration or more intense study through a drug-use review. Also, reports of such reactions should be made to the manufacturer and to the Food and Drug Administration.

1. Kilarski DJ, Buchanan C, Von Behren L. Soft-tissue damage associated with intravenous phenytoin. *N Engl J Med.* 1984; 311:1186–7. Letter.

PETER D. REEME, PHARM. D., Director of Pharmacy Services
DAVID L. DAY, M.S., Assistant Director of Pharmacy Services
Bethesda Hospital, Inc.
Cincinnati, OH 45206

Drug clearance in patients undergoing continuous arteriovenous hemofiltration

It was with both interest and relief that I read the paper by Lehman and Kolb[1] describing gentamicin pharmacokinetics in a patient undergoing continuous arteriovenous hemofiltration (CAVH). The fact that someone in the United States is studying the effects of this new method of dialysis on the clearance of drugs is gratifying since the literature on the subject is sparse. However, there are a few other articles, albeit from foreign publications, that describe the use of drugs, including gentamicin, during CAVH.

Rumpf et al.[2] investigated the use of several drugs during CAVH in patients with renal insufficiency. Gentamicin was administered as a single dose with plasma, and filtrate measurements were obtained at 30-minute intervals for five hours. The results illustrated that as the CAVH process continued, the ratio of drug in the filtrate to drug in the plasma increased over time. The authors suggested that this phenomenon may have been attributable to the adherence of the gentamicin molecule to the filter, which may explain the lack of correlation between protein binding and filtrate-to-plasma ratio.

Kraft and Lode[3] administered gentamicin 1 mg/kg and ampicillin 2 g as single doses to nine patients during CAVH. Blood and filtrate samples were taken several times after administration. Serum half-life of ampicillin appeared to be similar to that reported for this drug during hemodialysis; however, the gentamicin clearance was considerably more rapid than that observed during conventional hemodialysis. Again, gentamicin binding to the hemofilter may be responsible for the unexpected differences in the elimination pharmacokinetics between the two types of dialysis.

There are at least two other papers that examine the use of antibiotics during CAVH.[4,5] After a review of these articles it becomes apparent that interpretation of results is difficult because of the variety of methods used in the CAVH process. For example, the type of hemofilter used in Europe differs from that used in the United States, which may explain the binding phenomenon. The presence or absence of suction during the process would obviously change the flow rates and, therefore, the elimination of the drug. Finally, prefilter versus postfilter dilution may be important in the calculation of drug elimination through the hemofilter.

There is an obvious need to investigate drug pharmacokinetics in patients requiring CAVH. The changes in drug disposition in patients undergoing hemodialysis and peritoneal dialysis have been the subject of much research. Perhaps reports such as that of Lehman and Kolb will stimulate similar interest in studying the pharmacokinetic alterations of many drugs during a procedure that will probably become a popular alternative to traditional methods of dialysis.

1. Lehman ME, Kolb KW. Gentamicin elimination in a patient undergoing continuous ultrafiltration. *Clin Pharm.* 1985; 4:327–30.
2. Garcia MJ, Dominguez-Gil A, Tabernero JM et al. Pharmacokinetics of cefoxitin during hemofiltration. *Eur J Clin Pharmacol.* 1983; 25:345–8.
3. Rumpf KW, Rieger J, Doht B et al. Drug elimination by hemofiltration. *J Dialysis.* 1977; 1:677–88.
4. Gravert C, Schulz E, Sack K. Ceftazadime in intensive care medicine and hemofiltration. *J Antimicrob Chemother.* 1983; 12 (Suppl A):177–80.
5. Gouyette A, LeMoine R, Adhemar JP et al. Kinetics of cisplatin in an anuric patient undergoing hemofiltration dialysis. *Cancer Treat Rep.* 1981; 65:665–8.

MICHAEL RUBINO, M.S., Assistant Director of Pharmacy
University of Connecticut Health Center
Farmington, CT 06032

Effect of warfarin on activated partial thromboplastin time

Having read the fine review article by Carter et al.[1] for the second time, I found one statement that concerned me. The authors mention, appropriately, that warfarin administration will affect the activated partial thromboplastin time (aPTT). The point with which I find difficulty is their statement, "Some increase in the aPTT may be anticipated when warfarin is begun." It appears that they attribute only a minor effect on the aPTT to warfarin therapy, and this is probably not the case.

The aPTT test screens for deficiencies in factors II, V, VII, IX, X, XI, and XII and in fibrinogen and is sensitive, therefore, to substances that modify these factors.[2] Since warfarin affects the production of two factors in the "common" pathway (II, X) and one in the "intrinsic" pathway (IX), it can cause considerably more than "some" increase in the aPTT. As it turns out, full anticoagulation with warfarin may, besides elevating the prothrombin time (PT), also increase the aPTT into what would be considered a therapeutic range.[3] Perhaps this fact is not appreciated, since monitoring of warfarin anticoagulation is performed with the PT test and simultaneous aPTT is not often obtained.

The authors are certainly correct that there is some interaction and that the extent of the effect may be difficult to quantify. Factor IX has a disappearance half-time of approximately 24 hours,[4] and therefore the effect on aPTT, though dependent on individual rates of metabolism, will not be immediate. However, since the current method of management suggests starting warfarin very early in the anticoagulation course, it is quite likely that the effect on aPTT will become evident. Indeed, this may be one reason for the observation[5] that after several days of therapy, heparin dosage may need to be decreased to avoid excessive prolongation of the aPTT.

The practitioner should be aware that warfarin may have a pronounced effect on the aPTT. Whether this affects the management of patients receiving both heparin and warfarin is not readily apparent except for the previously mentioned suggestion that heparin dosage be reduced. However, not to realize that warfarin may produce an increase in the aPTT may cause unnecessary interventions or repeat laboratory tests if it does.

1. Carter BL, Jones ME, Waickman LA. Pathophysiology and treatment of deep-vein thrombosis and pulmonary embolism. *Clin Pharm.* 1985; 4:279–96.
2. Hougie C. Recalcification time test and its modifications. In: Williams WJ, Beutler E, Erslev AJ et al., eds. Hematology. 3rd ed. New York: McGraw-Hill; 1983:1662–5.
3. Ravel R. Clinical laboratory medicine: clinical application of laboratory data. 3rd ed. Chicago: Year Book Medical Publishers; 1978:68.
4. Williams WJ. Life-span of plasma coagulation factors. In: Williams WJ, Beutler E, Erslev AJ et al., eds. Hematology. 3rd ed. New York: McGraw-Hill; 1983:1230–7.
5. White TM, Bernene JL, Marino AM. Continuous heparin infusion requirements: diagnostic and therapeutic implications. *JAMA.* 1979; 241:2717–20.

THOMAS G. BURNAKIS, PHARM.D., Coordinator, Clinical Pharmacy Services
Wyandotte General Hospital
Wyandotte, MI 48192

We appreciate the comments of Dr. Burnakis concerning the effect of warfarin on the activated partial thromboplastin time (aPTT). Our statements were not intended to diminish the potential influence warfarin may have on the aPTT, but rather to indicate that this effect has not been studied thoroughly. Of course, the aPTT has occasionally been used to monitor warfarin therapy. However, during the first few days of therapy when the prothrombin time has increased only slightly, the effect of warfarin on the aPTT is unpredictable.

As Dr. Burnakis points out, once warfarin is initiated the heparin dosage frequently must be reduced, which may reflect the influence of warfarin. However, it has been observed that heparin dose requirements may be greater with active thromboembolism.[1-3] Another proposed explanation for the lower heparin requirements is the cessation of the active thromboembolic process.

1. White TM, Bernene JL, Marino AM. Continuous heparin infusion requirements: diagnostic and therapeutic implications. *JAMA.* 1979; 241:2717–20.
2. Simon TL, Hyers TM, Gaston JP et al. Heparin pharmacokinetics: increased requirements in pulmonary embolism. *Br J Haematol.* 1978; 39:111–20.
3. Hirsh J, van Aken WG, Gallus AS et al. Heparin kinetics in venous thrombosis and pulmonary embolism. *Circulation.* 1976; 53:691–5.

BARRY L. CARTER, PHARM.D.
MARK E. JONES, PHARM.D.
College of Pharmacy
University of Iowa
Iowa City, IA 52242

Drug Review

Nomifensine maleate: A new second-generation antidepressant

JANET L. KINNEY

Abstract: The pharmacology, pharmacokinetics, clinical efficacy, adverse effects, drug interactions, dosage, and formulary recommendations for nomifensine maleate are reviewed.

Nomifensine is a potent inhibitor of norepinephrine but has little effect on serotonin. It is unique in that it is a potent reuptake inhibitor of dopamine. Nomifensine is rapidly and completely absorbed and is widely distributed throughout the body. The major route of elimination is through the kidneys. Because of its short half-life and resultant lack of accumulation, nomifensine is usually given in divided doses.

Nomifensine is approved for the treatment of depression. In clinical trials with imipramine, amitriptyline, nortriptyline, maprotiline, and various investigational antidepressant drugs, it has been found to be as effective as the standard antidepressant agents. In general, nomifensine has been well tolerated by patients and has caused few side effects. It also has not been associated with serious toxic effects in overdose situations. The usual effective dose of nomifensine maleate is 100–200 mg daily given in divided doses. It appears to be a good choice for patients with profoundly retarded depression and for those who cannot tolerate the side effects of traditional antidepressant drugs. Nomifensine should not be used alone in patients with schizoaffective disorders or in patients with agitated depression.

Nomifensine is a safe and effective antidepressant with a fairly unique pharmacological profile. Because the drug is relatively safe and causes little sedation, it may offer substantial advantages over the more traditional antidepressants and should be considered for formulary addition.

Index terms: Absorption; Antidepressants; Contraindications; Depression; Dosage; Drug interactions; Drugs, body distribution; Half-life; Mechanism of action; Nomifensine maleate; Pharmacokinetics; Toxicity
Clin Pharm. 1985; 4:625–36

Nomifensine maleate is a tetrahydroisoquinaline derivative antidepressant with the chemical formula 8-amino-1,2,3,4-tetrahydro-2-methyl-4-phenylisoquinoline maleate. It is marketed by Hoechst-Roussel as Merital in the United States and as Alival outside the United States. Nomifensine was originally introduced into the European market in 1976–1977 and since then has been marketed in at least 70 countries. It was first marketed in the United States in July 1985. Chemically, nomifensine is unrelated to the tricyclic or tetracyclic antidepressants, monoamine oxidase inhibitors, or other available antidepressants. Its structure is shown in Figure 1.

Figure 1. Chemical structure of nomifensine maleate.

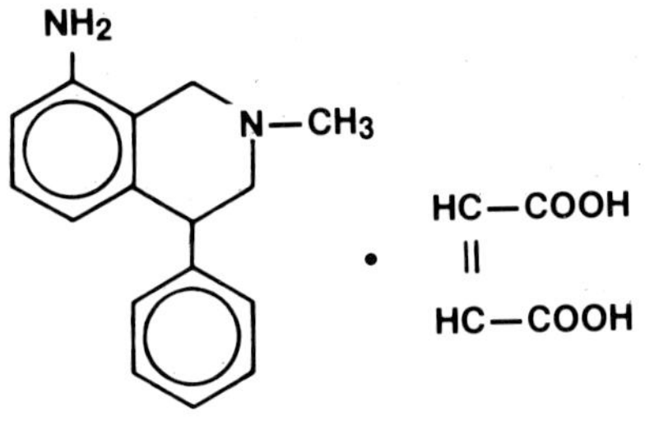

This article reviews the pharmacology, pharmacokinetics, clinical efficacy, adverse effects, and

JANET L. KINNEY, PHARM. D., is Clinical Assistant Professor of Pharmacy Practice and Psychiatry, Colleges of Pharmacy and Medicine, University of Arizona, and Unit Coordinator, Pharmacy Programs, Southern Arizona Mental Health Center, Tucson.

Address reprint requests to Dr. Kinney at the Department of Pharmacy Practice, College of Pharmacy, University of Arizona, Tucson, AZ 85721.

The assistance of Edward P. Armstrong, Pharm.D., is acknowledged.

This is **article 680-204-8517** in the **ASHP Continuing Education System.** See page 692 for learning objectives and test questions.

dosage of nomifensine maleate. In addition, formulary recommendations are made.

Pharmacology

In animal tests that are indicative of antidepressant activity, nomifensine demonstrated good efficacy and tolerability when compared with other antidepressants.[1-4] Nomifensine proved to be more effective than imipramine in blocking reserpine-induced hypothermia in mice and in influencing reserpine and tetrabenazine-induced catalepsy in mice and rats.[1-3]

In tests of yohimbine toxicity, behavioral despair syndrome, and internal capsule lesions, nomifensine was as effective as reference antidepressants.[1] Antidepressant drugs are known to depress mice-killing aggression in rats. In tests with both spontaneous and *p*-chloro-phenylalanine-induced killers, nomifensine significantly reduced killing activity.[4]

At least part of the therapeutic action of antidepressants is thought to be caused by an increased availability of the neurotransmitters norepinephrine and serotonin, resulting from the drugs' inhibition of reuptake mechanisms. Recent investigations have led to the modification of this biogenic-amine hypothesis, and the therapeutic action of antidepressants is now believed to be closely related to the desensitization of postsynaptic-receptor sites, primarily β-adrenoreceptors.[5]

Similar to some of the traditional tricyclic antidepressants, nomifensine is a potent reuptake inhibitor of norepinephrine. Its potency is similar to that of desipramine and is more pronounced than that of imipramine.[6] Serotonin-reuptake inhibition for nomifensine is approximately the same as for desipramine but is weaker than for imipramine or chlorimipramine.[1] It has little, if any, effect on histamine-H_1 receptors.[7] In accordance with the modifications of the biogenic-amine hypothesis, nomifensine has also been found to reduce the density of β-adrenoreceptors with long-term therapy.[1]

However, unlike the more traditional tricyclic antidepressants, nomifensine is also a potent reuptake inhibitor of dopamine and is, in fact, the first marketed antidepressant to have a major effect on dopamine reuptake. Its potency is similar to that of benztropine and slightly greater than that of methylphenidate or D-amphetamine.[6] Although it is a controversial subject, nomifensine or its metabolites may have a dopamine-releasing action[8] or a direct effect on postsynaptic-dopamine receptors[9] in addition to the major effect on reuptake inhibition. The potencies of several antidepressants in inhibiting the reuptake of norepinephrine, serotonin, and dopamine are shown in Table 1.[10]

Recent studies have suggested that depression is neurochemically heterogenous and that there may be a subgroup of depressed patients who have a relative lack of dopamine in central synapses. In particular, patients with a predominant condition of psychomotor inhibition, retardation, and apathy may have lowered dopamine turnover. In one study, these patients responded better to nomifensine, with its strong dopamine-potentiating activity, than to clomipramine, a drug with little effect on dopamine.[11]

Amphetamine-like drugs are divided into two classes, the amphetamine group and the methylphenidate group, according to the inhibition of stereotypic behavior by reserpine and α-methyltyrosine. Based on the results of these tests, nomifensine belongs to the methylphenidate group of amphetamine-like drugs.[8] This similarity to methylphenidate has raised the concern that nomifensine may also share its addictive properties. It has been shown that both naive rats and rats conditioned to self-administer cocaine will self-administer intravenous nomifensine and work to maintain relatively constant serum concentrations.[12] However, to date, there have been no clinical reports of abuse by humans. In one study, subjects given amphetamine, nomifensine, and placebo had no preference for nomifensine over placebo.[13]

To date, there is no evidence for dysmorphogenic or carcinogenic effects with nomifensine. Nomifensine was studied for one year in 32 rhesus monkeys at doses of 0, 5, 20, or 80 mg/kg per day orally. No tissue damage attributable to nomifensine was found in the histological studies.[14] Rat and mice studies have also shown no evidence of tumorigenic potential.[15] In rats, a slight increase in in utero deaths and a decrease in fetal weight were noted when nomifensine was given in doses of 1, 8, or 64 mg/kg daily after mating. No drug-induced deformities were found in these offspring.[14] Because there are no well-controlled studies of nomifensine in pregnant women, the drug should only be given if the potential benefit justifies the risk to the fetus. Nomifensine has a pregnancy category B

Table 1.
In Vitro Inhibition of the Reuptake of Norepinephrine, Serotonin, and Dopamine by Several Antidepressants[a,b]

Drug	Norepinephrine	Serotonin	Dopamine
Amitriptyline	++	++	+
Amoxapine	+++	++	−
Desipramine	++++	+	0/+
Doxepin	++	+	+
Imipramine	+++	++	0/+
Maprotiline	+++	0/+	+
Nomifensine	++++	0/+	+++
Nortriptyline	+++	+	+
Protriptyline	++++	+	+
Trimipramine	+	+	+
Trazodone	Weak	++	Weak

[a] Each cross represents a gross comparative difference of 10-fold.
[b] Adapted with permission from a table in reference 10.

rating.[15]

Because of its effect on inhibiting the reuptake of dopamine, a role for nomifensine in the differential diagnosis of hyperprolactinemia caused by prolactinomas versus pituitary deafferentation has been suggested. To date, the results of investigations have been contradictory and it cannot be stated that nomifensine provides a definitive diagnostic tool.[16] Roles for nomifensine in the treatment of attention deficit disorder[1] and Parkinson's disease[9] have also been suggested.

Pharmacokinetics

The early pharmacokinetic data collected on nomifensine are questionable because of problems with the assay that had not yet been clarified. Nomifensine is known to exist in serum primarily as an acid-labile conjugate. Less than 5%, and probably less than 1.5%, of the parent drug is present in the unconjugated form.[17,18] However, when plasma is allowed to stand at room temperature, the conjugated nomifensine quickly decomposes to free nomifensine. Dawling et al.[19] demonstrated that after five hours the free nomifensine plasma concentration had doubled and that after one week it had increased 16-fold; total nomifensine concentration did not change. This phenomenon does not occur when samples are immediately frozen at −20 °C, and thus this is now the recommended procedure.[19] Additionally, the conjugated nomifensine easily hydrolyzes at a pH less than 7.1 so urine must be alkalinized for urine studies.[17]

Nomifensine is rapidly and completely absorbed. Comparison of the mean areas under the curve for intravenous and oral formulations are identical, indicating complete absorption.[20] Maximum serum concentrations are reached in one to two hours after administration.[18] In contrast to the pharmacokinetic data, pharmacodynamic data obtained from quantitative pharmacoelectroencephalogram and psychometric testing suggest a maximum effect four to six hours after administration.[20] The authors suggested that this delay in psychodynamic effect may be attributable to a slowly formed active metabolite, the drug acting on deep-compartment receptors, or both of these factors.

Animal studies have indicated that nomifensine is widely distributed and concentrates in the liver, kidney, and lungs.[21] In humans, the apparent β volume of distribution (V_β) for unconjugated nomifensine ranges from 8.8 to 99.4 L/kg and for total nomifensine it ranges from 0.79 to 1.52 L/kg.[22] The large V_β for unconjugated nomifensine suggests that the drug is extensively distributed throughout body tissues and fluids in humans and in animals. Protein binding is approximately 60% regardless of drug concentration.[18] It is not known whether the drug is excreted in breast milk. Because other antidepressants are found in breast milk, nomifensine should be administered with caution to nursing mothers.[15]

Three principal metabolites of nomifensine have been identified—4′-hydroxy-nomifensine (M1); 4′-hydroxy 3′-methoxy-nomifensine (M2); and 3′-hydroxy-4′-methoxy-nomifensine (M3). They are found in a ratio of 1:1:1 in both blood and urine and account for 22% of the radiolabeled drug that is excreted in urine. In addition to the three main metabolites, four other metabolites have been identified that together make up less than 1% of total radioactivity administered.[17,18] M2 and M3 have little or no pharmacological activity. In contrast, M1 has shown some antidepressant activity in animal studies, although it is less potent than nomifensine. Additionally, M1 is equipotent with nomifensine in inhibiting the reuptake of dopamine, twice as active in inhibiting norepinephrine, and also potent as an inhibitor of serotonin reuptake. Despite the apparent antidepressant activity of M1, its contribution to the effectiveness of nomifensine is most likely minimal since it only accounts for 7% of excreted radioactivity.[3] Elimination is primarily renal; 88% of the drug is excreted in the first 24 hours. Animal studies have shown that there is no enterohepatic circulation and that only conjugated drug is detected in the bile.[14] Less than 1% of the administered radioactivity is present in expired air.[20]

Nomifensine best fits a two-compartment, open kinetic model with first-order absorption. In a study by Lassman et al.,[22] the α half-life ($t_{1/2\alpha}$) for total nomifensine averaged 0.6 hours and the β half-life ($t_{1/2\beta}$) averaged 2.7 hours. McIntyre et al.[23] found the mean plasma half-life for unconjugated nomifensine was 1.9 hours and for total nomifensine was 4.1 hours. Heptner et al.[24] and Chamberlain and Hill[25] found elimination half-lives of 1.9 hours and 1–2 hours, respectively. Because of the short half-life (an average of two hours) and resultant lack of accumulation, nomifensine is usually given in divided doses. This differs substantially from the traditional tricyclic antidepressants that tend to accumulate and are administered in single daily doses.

In one study of 10 patients with variable degrees of renal failure, the half-life of nomifensine was prolonged from 1.5 to 46 hours.[26] The concentration of nomifensine was unchanged after three hours[26] in three patients on hemodialysis. Because the half-life is prolonged and the drug accumulates in patients with renal failure, these authors suggested that nomifensine should not be given to patients with a glomerular filtration rate of less than 25 mL/min. Although no data are available, it might be prudent to decrease the dose or extend the dosing interval in patients with renal dysfunction.

As with other antidepressants, plasma concentrations of nomifensine exhibit substantial interpatient variability, making it difficult to correlate plasma concentration with clinical response. A further difficulty in correlating clinical response and plasma concentration is that it is not known whether unconjugated, conjugated, or total nomifensine concentrations should be measured. One study[20] suggested that unconjugated nomifensine concentrations may correlate more closely with pharmacodynamic effects than total nomifensine concentrations. One early study[14] reported a possible correlation between plasma concentrations and clinical response, but this has not been substantiated by more recent studies. Three recent studies[27-29] found no correlation between plasma concentration and clinical response or adverse effects. At this time, there is no rationale for routinely measuring nomifensine concentrations.

Clinical Trials

When the antidepressant properties of a new drug are investigated, two questions are important: (1) does the drug have antidepressant efficacy or is it any better than placebo? and (2) how does the drug compare with other antidepressant drugs? Both of these questions are difficult to answer for numerous reasons. Placebo studies in severely depressed patients are difficult to justify ethically because of the risks, such as suicide, incurred by withholding efficacious treatment. Yet placebo-drug differences may not be evident in patients with the more neurotic types of depression. Another major difficulty is that it is almost impossible to compare different studies because of differences in diagnostic criteria and rating scales. Other problems include fairly high rates of spontaneous remission and placebo response. In addition, the crossover design is not feasible because the first treatment may induce a lasting change.

To date, several thousand patients have been treated with nomifensine in open trials. The New Drug Application filed for nomifensine included reports of studies by 78 investigators under 39 protocols in 2303 patients.[30]

Double-Blind, Placebo-Controlled Studies. Nomifensine has been compared with placebo in several double-blind studies. In 1974, a study was conducted that compared nomifensine with placebo in 30 hospitalized patients who were treated with either placebo or 75 mg of nomifensine maleate daily for eight days and then crossed over to the comparative treatment.[31] Despite the extremely short treatment period, improvement with nomifensine and no improvement with placebo were found most frequently. In 1976, 24 hospitalized patients were treated with 75 mg of nomifensine maleate daily in a crossover study with a 14-day treatment period, and it was found that the efficacy of nomifensine may be differentiated from placebo.[31]

Three more recent studies have also demonstrated the efficacy of nomifensine over placebo in a noncrossover design.[32-34] Goldstein et al.[34] and Feighner et al.[32] evaluated a total of 241 outpatients aged 18 to 65 years old with a diagnosis of primary affective disorder and depression according to the Feighner criteria. Additionally, patients were required to have a total score of at least 20 on the Hamilton depression rating scale (HDRS) and a score of at least 14 on the Beck depression inventory. Patients were randomly assigned to receive either 150–200 mg of nomifensine maleate or placebo for 28 days. Evaluations were performed weekly. In both studies, nomifensine was significantly more effective than placebo in reducing the severity of symptoms on HDRS and clinical global impressions (CGI). Georgia,[33] in a similar design, also found that nomifensine demonstrated greater efficacy than placebo on HDRS and CGI.

Double-Blind, Controlled Trials with Active Reference Drugs. The results from 20 double-blind studies comparing nomifensine with amitriptyline, imipramine, nortriptyline, a fluphenazine–nortriptyline combination, maprotiline, zimelidine, or mianserin are summarized in Table 2.[35-53] In general, these trials showed that nomifensine is as effective as the reference antidepressants in treating various types of depression. Although none of the studies demonstrated a statistically significant difference between nomifensine and the reference antidepressant, three suggested a trend favoring nomifensine over imipramine[46] or nortriptyline.[48,49] Six studies suggested that nomifensine may be less effective than amitriptyline,[36] imipramine,[28,41,42] a fluphenazine–nortriptyline combination,[50] or mianserin.[53]

Most of the studies were not structured to assess the rapidity of drug onset, but three studies[35,45,47] concluded that nomifensine may possibly have an earlier onset of action than amitriptyline, imipramine, or nortriptyline. It is difficult to give these studies much weight since there are 17 studies that conclude that there is no difference in the onset of action of nomifensine.

Five studies have evaluated the effectiveness and safety of nomifensine in the elderly.[54-58] In these double-blind studies, nomifensine was compared with amitriptyline, imipramine, or placebo. All patients were 60 years of age or older and had a diagnosis of depression. Jansen et al.,[56] Cohn et al.,[54] Goldstein et al.,[55] and Merideth et al.[57] studied patients who met the Feighner criteria for primary affective disorder depression. Dosages of nomifensine maleate ranged from 75 to 200 mg per day according to the patients' clinical condition. They each found that nomifensine caused significantly more improvement than placebo and was no different from the reference antidepressant. Montgomery et al.[58] used doses of 75, 75, and 30 mg per day for imipramine, nomifensine, and mianserin,

Table 2.
Double-Blind, Controlled Trials of Nomifensine for Depression

Reference Number	Diagnosis	Drug	No. of Patients	Average Dose (mg)	Length of Study	Results[a]	Comments[b]
35	Primary depression outpatients	Nomifensine Amitriptyline	12 12	50–200 50–225	8 weeks	At 8 weeks, 7 nomifensine and 5 amitriptyline patients considerably improved by HDRS. The authors suggested that nomifensine may have a more rapid onset.	Variable dose hard to evaluate. No placebo.
36	Depressive neurosis, depressive psychosis, or mixed depression outpatients	Nomifensine Amitriptyline	20 17	150 150	4 weeks	Both groups improved by HDRS at 4 weeks. There was a trend favoring amitriptyline.	Only evaluated pretreatment and at 4 weeks. More patients with endogenous depression in nomifensine group. No placebo.
37	Depressive neurosis, manic-depressive outpatients	Nomifensine Amitriptyline	10 7	75 75	9 weeks	No difference in effect after one week.	Dosing probably too low. HRDS used. No placebo.
38	Major depressive disorders (by RDC criteria) inpatients	Nomifensine Amitriptyline	15 14	150 150	6 weeks	Amelioration of 50% or more in 9 nomifensine and 10 amitriptyline patients. Fatigue more improved by amitriptyline.	CPRS used. No placebo.
39	Depressed outpatients	Nomifensine Imipramine	16 18	75–150 75–150	4 weeks	Both effective, no differences. Nomifensine more rapid improvement of anxiety.	Dosing not clearly outlined. BECK and HDRS used. No placebo.
40	Endogenous depression, reactive depression outpatients and one inpatient	Nomifensine Imipramine	5 6	147.9 158.3	6 weeks	Both effective, no differences.	BPRS, HDRS, and CGI data inadequately detailed. Half the patients withdrawn. No placebo.
41	Depression outpatients and inpatients	Nomifensine Imipramine	8 12	146.4 141.6	6 weeks	Significant improvement with both. More patients improved with imipramine.	HDRS, BPRS, and CGI used. No clear diagnostic criteria and no placebo.
42	"Depressed" inpatients	Nomifensine Imipramine	30	150 150	30 days	Imipramine group better at 30 days.	HDRS used. No placebo. Data not presented in detail. Older patients and patients with longer duration of illness in nomifensine group.
43	Primary affective depression outpatients	Nomifensine Imipramine	13 7	150–200 150–200	4 weeks	Mean differences between scores on HDRS significant for both groups. No differences between groups.	HDRS and CGI used. No placebo.

Continued on following page

Table 2. *(Continued from previous page)*

Reference Number	Diagnosis	Drug	No. of Patients	Average Dose (mg)	Length of Study	Results[a]	Comments[b]
44	Endogenous depression outpatients	Nomifensine Imipramine	18 21	250 283.3	4 weeks	Both demonstrate significant reduction in symptoms. No differences noted between groups.	HDRS and BECK used. No placebo washout period.
45	Depressive neurosis, manic-depressive, involutional melancholia outpatients	Nomifensine Imipramine Placebo	49 51 46	175 159 181	6 weeks	Nomifensine may have earlier onset. Significant difference on HDRS total score for active drug versus placebo.	Met criteria for major depressive disorder. HDRS and HSCL used. When separated into exogenous and endogenous, difference between active and placebo became significant for endogenous depression.
28	Primary affective disorder inpatients	Nomifensine Imipramine Mianserin	14 13 14	150 150 90	6 weeks	No significant overall differences between groups. Imipramine better than nomifensine at 6 weeks.	HDRS and MADRS used. Imipramine group had older patients. Placebo washout period.
46	Primary affective disorder depression outpatients (by Feighner criteria)	Nomifensine Imipramine	110 56	180 175	4 weeks	Nomifensine equal or superior to imipramine. In each group 90% of patients improved.	Imipramine group older. HDRS and CGI used.
47	Depressive neurosis inpatients	Nomifensine Imipramine	16 20	220 200	4 weeks	Both showed improvement with no significant differences. Nomifensine possibly had earlier onset.	HDRS, CGI, and BPRS used. Placebo washout period.
48	Endogenous depression, psychogenic depression, mixed depression outpatients	Nomifensine Nortriptyline	20 20	150 150	21 days	Both showed improvement with no significant difference. Nomifensine may have been better.	Study may not have been long enough. No placebo or washout period.
49	Endogenous depression, reactive depression, mixed depression outpatients	Nomifensine Nortriptyline	20 20	150 150	21 days	No significant difference. There was a trend favoring nomifensine.	Of the 20 original patients, 14 stopped treatment. More patients in nortriptyline group. Duration of study may not have been long enough. No placebo or washout period.
50	Mixed anxiety-depression outpatients	Nomifensine Fluphenazine/ Nortriptyline	29 28	75–150 1.5/30	4 weeks	Both treatments effective. Fluphenazine nortriptyline patients did better especially early in treatment.	Dosing may not have been appropriate. Rating scales not standard. Mixed diagnosis.

Continued on following page

Table 2. *(Continued from previous page)*

Reference Number	Diagnosis	Drug	No. of Patients	Average Dose (mg)	Length of Study	Results[a]	Comments[b]
51	Endogenous depression (by DSM criteria) outpatients; some hospitalized for part of study	Nomifensine Maprotiline	14 14	100 100	4 weeks	Significant drop on HDRS for both drugs at week 1, 82% improvement for nomifensine and 71% improvement for maprotiline group.	HDRS used. Dose may have been low.
52	Endogenous or reactive depression (by RDC criteria) inpatients	Nomifensine Zimelidine	21 21	166.6 233	6 weeks	Zimelidine gave greater than 50% reduction of CPRS in 75% of patients. Nomifensine gave greater than 50% in 70% of patients. No overall difference.	CPRS and CGI used. Placebo washout.
53	Moderate to severe primary affective disorder (by Feighner criteria) outpatients	Nomifensine Mianserin	40 40	150 60	4 weeks	Study showed a 39% reduction in HDRS for mianserin group, 28% for nomifensine group. There was a trend favoring mianserin.	HDRS, BECK, and CGI used. Nomifensine group had more women.

[a] HDRS = Hamilton depression rating scale. CPRS = comprehensive psychopathological rating scale.

[b] Rating scales used and limitations of the study. BECK = Beck depression inventory, CGI = clinical global impressions, BPRS = brief psychiatric rating scale, HSCL = Hopkins symptom checklist, and MADRS = Montgomery and Asberg depression rating scale.

respectively, and found that imipramine was significantly more effective than nomifensine. In each of the studies, nomifensine was well tolerated and no patients in the nomifensine groups dropped out because of side effects, as they did in the amitriptyline and imipramine groups.

Adverse Effects

During the years of clinical experience with antidepressant drugs, several areas of concern have developed including the drugs' anticholinergic effects, sedative properties, effects on psychomotor function, cardiac effects, and epileptogenic potential. In part, the development of newer antidepressants has been attributable to the search for an effective antidepressant with fewer problems in these areas. The safety and tolerability of nomifensine in each of these areas must be evaluated.

Anticholinergic Effects. Both animal and human studies have demonstrated that nomifensine has very little anticholinergic effect. Nomifensine has an antagonistic influence on oxotremorine-induced hypothermia but not tremor and has a very slight effect on carbachol-induced contractions of isolated guinea pig ileum.[3] In single-dose studies with human volunteers receiving nomifensine maleate in 150-mg doses, Clemmesen et al.[59] found that the level of salivation inhibition is probably below the level of clinical importance. Richelson[60] examined the affinity (in units of $10^{-7} \times 1/Kb$, where Kb is the equilibrium dissociation constant expressed in molarity) of several antidepressants for muscarinic-acetylcholine receptors in human brain caudate nucleus. He found that trazodone and nomifensine had very little affinity, 0.00031 and 0.00040, respectively, whereas drugs like amitriptyline and imipramine had significant affinity, 5.5 and 1.1, respectively, for these receptors.

Cardiac Effects. Minimal cardiac effects in both humans and animals have been observed with nomifensine administration. Biamino[61] administered nomifensine to seven patients with angina pectoris or following myocardial infarction. The drug produced no significant effects on heart rate, cardiac output, mean arterial pressure, pulmonary artery pressure, or end-diastolic left-ventricular pressure. No changes were noted on electrocardiograms.

Several other authors have investigated the effects of nomifensine in depressed patients without a history of cardiac abnormalities. Burrows et al.[62] found no significant effect on heart rate or blood pressure (supine and standing). No ST–T wave abnormalities or changes in QRS width or Q-T interval were noted. In a study of 10 patients, McIntyre et al.[63] found that 7 had an increase in heart rate that did not reach statistical significance and 1 had an increased P-R interval. There were no significant changes in A-H interval, H-V interval, corrected Q-T interval, or supine and standing blood pressure. Bethge et al.[64] also found an increase in heart rate with nomifensine but no significant changes in electrocardiogram with 10-hour monitoring.

Sedation and Psychomotor Function. Sedating drugs such as amitriptyline and imipramine tend to impair cognitive and psychomotor function in healthy volunteers. Nomifensine is reported to have drive-enhancing or activating properties and should, therefore, have little effect on psychomotor function. This has been confirmed in tests with normal volunteers.[65] Nomifensine maleate in doses of 75–100 mg either did not affect flicker-fusion threshold or increased it significantly, indicating a rise in central nervous system arousal and alertness. Perceptual flexibility and memory function are not altered by nomifensine. Nomifensine, either does not change or significantly improves attentional behavior and concentration and performance on psychomotor coordination, speed, and car-driving abilities.

Epileptogenic Properties. In vitro techniques assessing the epileptogenic potential of antidepressant drugs have demonstrated that low concentrations (25–100 ng/mL) of nomifensine increase neuronal excitability but higher concentrations (200 ng/mL) stop it completely.[66] In animal studies, nomifensine does not appear to induce seizures or lower seizure threshold, and it may actually have a protective mechanism.[67] Dopamine agonists are known to have antiepileptic properties, and nomifensine's dopamine-agonist properties may be responsible for these effects. Nomifensine has been used safely in several groups of depressed epileptic patients with no changes in seizure frequency.[68] However, there have been reports of seizures occurring in patients receiving nomifensine,[69,70] so caution is indicated.

Miscellaneous Adverse Effects. In general, nomifensine has been well tolerated by patients. Side effects, when they occur, are generally mild to moderate in severity and do not often require discontinuation of the drug. The most common side effects of nomifensine are dry mouth or bad taste, nervousness or restlessness, insomnia or sleep disturbances, headaches, nausea and vomiting, drowsiness, and constipation. Table 3 lists the common side effects and their incidences as reported by three separate sources.[14,15,69] In contrast to most antidepressants, nomifensine appears to produce an anorexigenic effect although appetite increases have also been reported with long-term use.[15,69] This should be considered when nomifensine is prescribed for patients who have weight loss as a part of their depression symptomatology. Rarely, hemolytic anemia,[71,72] paranoid symptoms,[73] a lupus-like syndrome,[74] dyskinesias,[75,76] increased sexual function,[77] liver impairment,[61] and febrile reactions[61,78] have been reported. Twenty-six of the 27 people who developed fever recovered without sequelae. Fever usually occurs within the first month of therapy and resolves within a day or two of discontinuing the drug.[15]

Overdosage

There is evidence that an overdose of nomifensine will not cause the serious complications of seizures, cardiac arrhythmias, and respiratory arrest caused by the tricyclic antidepressants. Three cases of nomifensine overdosage have been reported. Montgomery et al.[79] described a 28-year-old woman who ingested 1.5 g of nomifensine maleate. On admission, she was conscious; pulse, blood pressure, respiration, and neurological signs were normal. During hospitalization, she developed a sinus tachycardia that rapidly resolved; no other symptoms were noted. Vohra et al.[80] reported a case involving a 43-year-old woman who ingested 3.5 g of nomifensine maleate, 20 g of nitrazepam, and 200 mg of chlorpromazine. Although her speech was slurred, she was alert and showed no serious cardiac changes. In a case described by Prescott et al.[81] a 25-year-old woman who had ingested 2 g of nomifensine maleate, 100 mg of nitrazepam, and 300 mg of chlordiazepoxide developed acute intravascular hemolysis two days following the overdose. Two months after the overdose, laboratory results for hemoglobin, platelet count, plasma urea, and plasma creatinine were all normal.

Two series documenting overdose cases have been published. The Paris Poison Center evaluated 119 cases of which 35 involved nomifensine alone.[61] Of these 35, 20 patients were asymptomatic and the remaining patients had one or more mild symptoms, i.e., somnolence, sinus tachycardia, and ventricular extrasystoles. Seventy-four cases have been evaluated by the London Centre of the National Poison Information Service at Guy's Hospital.[61] Of these 74, 28 patients ingested nomifensine alone. The most common symptoms in these 28

Table 3.
Incidence (%) of Common Side Effects According to Three Sources

Side Effect	Yakabow et al.[69] $n = 1319$	Brogden et al.[14] $n = 938$	Package Insert[15] $n = 578$
Dry mouth	13	0.56	12.8
Constipation	6	0.34	5.2
Sweating	3	0.45	1.7
Blurred vision	3	. . .	2.6
Drowsiness	7	0.68	5.2
Dizziness	5	. . .	3.6
Nervousness or restlessness	11	2.93	11.4
Tremors	3	. . .	2.4
Insomnia or sleep disturbances	11	5.87	10.7
Headaches	11	0.68	8.1
Gastrointestinal	3	. . .	1.6
Nausea and vomiting	8	0.68	7.3
Cardiorespiratory	6	0.90	1.7
Alterations in sensation	5	. . .	1.2
Alterations in emotional tone	3	. . .	1.0
Skin reaction	4	0.34	4.5

patients included drowsiness, tremor, sinus tachycardia, transient hypertension, coma, and dilated or constricted pupils. Convulsions, cardiac arrhythmias, and other electrocardiographic abnormalities were not reported. These findings suggest that when nomifensine is taken alone the incidence of serious side effects is likely to be low.

Drug Interactions

Three studies have been designed to determine the likelihood of drug interactions with nomifensine. Rupp et al.[82] found that there was no pharmacokinetic interaction between nomifensine and clobazam, an investigational 1,5-benzodiazepine that is not hydroxylated at the 3-position as are 1,4-benzodiazepines. Whether these results can be extrapolated to 1,4-benzodiazepines is unknown.

Taeuber[83] examined the pharmacodynamic effects of alcohol alone and in combination with nomifensine. He found that there were no significant differences in physiological and behavioral variables between alcohol alone or in combination with nomifensine. He therefore concluded that nomifensine, unlike most other antidepressants, will not potentiate the effects of alcohol.

The pharmacokinetics of nomifensine were evaluated in patients taking anticonvulsant combinations of phenytoin and phenobarbital or phenytoin and carbamazepine by Nawishy et al.[84] They found that the plasma concentrations of nomifensine were significantly reduced in patients receiving anticonvulsant medications compared with controls and postulated that the clearance of nomifensine is increased by the hepatic-enzyme induction by the anticonvulsant drugs.

Because nomifensine inhibits the reuptake of norepinephrine, nomifensine may antagonize the hypotensive effects of adrenergic-neuron-blocking agents such as bethanidine, debrisoquin, or guanethidine as do tricyclic antidepressant agents.[14] Also because of this pharmacological action, nomifensine should generally not be given concomitantly with monoamine oxidase inhibitors. It is further recommended that monoamine oxidase inhibitors be discontinued two weeks before beginning nomifensine therapy.[15] Nomifensine may have the capacity to potentiate the effects of sympathomimetics such as those found in decongestants or local anesthetics.[15]

FDA-Labeled Indications

The FDA has approved nomifensine for the treatment of depression. In the clinical trials to date, the diagnoses of the patients most closely correspond to the condition of major depressive disorder described in the *Diagnostic and Statistical Manual of Mental Disorders*.[85] The symptoms of a major depressive disorder include prominent and persistent depressed or dysphoric mood lasting at least two weeks, sleep disturbance, appetite disturbance, psychomotor retardation or agitation, decreased energy, anhedonia, decreased cognitive abilities, feelings of guilt or worthlessness, and suicidal ideation. The effectiveness of nomifensine in the treatment of hospitalized depressed patients has not been demonstrated.

Dosage and Availability

The usual effective dose of nomifensine maleate is 100–200 mg daily. This should be administered in divided doses, usually in the morning and early afternoon. Dosing should be initiated with 50 mg twice daily and increased as necessary with additions to the morning dose. The maximum FDA-approved dose is 300 mg daily, but it is not known whether doses greater than 200 mg daily increase the drug's efficacy. Because there are no data available on the effects of food on the absorption of nomifensine, the drug should be taken on an empty stomach or at least one hour after eating. Although alcohol has not been shown to interact with nomifensine, patients are advised not to drink alcohol while taking nomifensine.[15]

In general, the elderly tolerate nomifensine well. Many of the clinical trials involving elderly patients used normal doses with no ill effects. One author[14] recommended that a lower initial dose, 25 mg twice daily, be used. Because 25-mg capsules are not available in this country, it might be prudent to start with a single daily dose of 50 mg and increase as tolerated. The efficacy of single daily dosing has been demonstrated in at least one study.[86] Few data are available on the effectiveness of nomifensine in children. In one study, nomifensine was found to be effective and safe to use in children aged 5–15 years in doses of 1–2 mg/kg daily.[14]

Nomifensine maleate is available as 50-mg brown- and orange-banded capsules supplied in bottles of 100 for oral administration. The 1985 average wholesale price was $35 per bottle of 100.

Patient Instructions

Patients should be told to take their medication as directed, usually in morning and early afternoon doses, not increasing or decreasing the dosage without first talking with their physicians. Patients who forget to take a dose should be instructed to take it as soon as they remember. If it is close to the next dose, the missed dose should not be taken. Nomifensine should be taken on an empty stomach. Patients should be reminded that it may take 2–4 weeks before they will begin to notice the effects of the drug.

Although alcohol does not appear to interact with nomifensine, patients should be warned against using alcohol while taking the drug. They should also be cautioned against driving or using heavy machinery until they see how the drug affects them.

Patients should be instructed to talk with their physicians if they are breast-feeding, pregnant, planning to become pregnant, or taking any other prescription or nonprescription medications and if they develop a fever or have any medical problems. They should be informed that the common side effects include dry mouth or bad taste, restlessness or nervousness, sleep disturbances, headache, nausea or vomiting, and constipation.

Formulary Recommendations

Nomifensine is an antidepressant with a unique clinical profile. Unlike other antidepressants, it is a potent reuptake inhibitor of dopamine and so it may have a different spectrum of activity. It causes very few side effects (e.g., sedation, anticholinergic effects, cardiovascular effects, or epileptogenic effects) and appears to be relatively safe when taken in an overdose. For these reasons, it should be considered for formulary addition. In particular, nomifensine appears to be a good choice for patients with a profoundly retarded depression or for those who cannot tolerate the side effects of traditional antidepressants.

Conclusion

Nomifensine is a safe and effective antidepressant with a fairly unique pharmacological profile. In addition to being a potent inhibitor of the reuptake of norepinephrine, it also inhibits the reuptake of dopamine, which means it causes little sedation. Because of its amphetamine-like effects, the drug may cause increased alertness and insomnia; nomifensine does not impair cognition or psychomotor function and may cause less lowering of the seizure threshold than other antidepressants. However, because of its dopaminergic effects, two precautions are necessary: (1) nomifensine should not be given alone to patients with a schizoaffective disorder since it may revive or exaggerate psychotic features; and (2) nomifensine should not be used in patients with agitated depression since it may increase agitation.

The pharmacokinetic profile of nomifensine is also different from most antidepressants. It has a very short half-life and must be given in divided doses. Dosing adjustments should be made for patients with renal failure. Side effects with nomifensine have generally been mild to moderate. Although it is difficult to accurately measure relative incidences of side effects, nomifensine appears to cause a decreased incidence of side effects compared with the tricyclic antidepressants. It also appears to cause fewer toxicities in overdose.

Thus, nomifensine is an effective antidepressant that may offer substantial advantages over the more traditional antidepressants in the areas of side effects and safety in overdose.

References

1. Fielding S, Szewczak MP. Pharmacology of nomifensine: a review of animal studies. *J Clin Psychiatry*. 1984; 45(4, Sec 2):12–20.
2. Hoffman I. A comparative review of the pharmacology of nomifensine. *Br J Clin Pharmacol*. 1977; 4:69S–75S.
3. Hoffman I. Pharmacology of nomifensine. *Int Pharmacopsychiatry*. 1982; 17(Suppl 1):4–20.
4. Kostowski W, Valzelli L, Kozak W et al. Activity of desipramine, fluoxetine and nomifensine on spontaneous and *p*-CPA-induced muricidal aggression. *Pharmacol Res Commun*. 1984; 16:265–71.
5. Frazer A, Conway P. Pharmacologic mechanisms of action of antidepressants. *Psychiatr Clin North Am*. 1984; 7:575–86.
6. Schacht U, Leven M, Gerhards HJ et al. Recent investigations on the mechanism of action of nomifensine. *Int Pharmacopsychiatry*. 1982; 17(Suppl 1):21–34.
7. Hall H, Ogren SO. Effects of antidepressant drugs on histamine-H_1 receptors in the brain. *Life Sci*. 1984; 34:597–605.
8. Braestrup C, Scheel-Kruger J. Methylphenidate-like effects of the new antidepressant drug nomifensine (HOE 984). *Eur J Pharmacol*. 1976; 38:305–12.
9. Gianutsos G, Morrow G, Light S et al. Dopaminergic properties of nomifensine. *Pharmacol Biochem Behav*. 1982; 17(5):951–4.
10. Baldessarini RJ. Overview of recent advances in antidepressant pharmacology: part II. *McLean Hosp J*. 1982; 7:1–27.
11. Van Scheyen JD, Van Praag HM, Korf J. Controlled study comparing nomifensine and clomipramine in unipolar depression, using the probenecid technique. *Br J Clin Pharmacol*. 1977; 4:179S–184S.
12. Spyraki C, Fibiger HC. Intravenous self-administration of nomifensine in rats: implications for abuse potential in humans. *Science*. 1981; 212:1167–8.
13. Taeuber K, Zapf R, Rupp W et al. Pharmacodynamic comparison of the acute effects of nomifensine, amphetamine and placebo in healthy volunteers. *Int J Clin Pharmacol Biopharm*. 1979; 17:32–7.
14. Brogden RN, Heel RC, Speight TM et al. Nomifensine: a review of its pharmacological properties and therapeutic efficacy in depressive illness. *Drugs*. 1979; 18:1–24.
15. Hoechst-Roussel Pharmaceuticals, Inc. Merital package insert. Somerville, NJ: 1985 Jan.
16. Minuto F, Barbarino A, Baviera G et al. Multicentric experience on the acute effect of nomifensine in hyperprolactinemic women. *J Endocrinol Invest*. 1984; 7:137–40.
17. Heptner W, Hornke I, Cavagna F et al. Metabolism of nomifensine in man and animal species. *Arzneimittelforsch*. 1978; 28:58–64.
18. Heptner W, Hornke I, Uihlein M. Kinetics and metabolism of nomifensine. *J Clin Psychiatry*. 1984; 45(4, Sec 2):21–5.
19. Dawling S, Braithwaite R. The stability of the antidepressant agent nomifensine in human plasma. *J Pharm Pharmacol*. 1980; 32:304–5.
20. Saletu B, Grunberger J, Linzmayer L et al. The pharmacokinetics of nomifensine: comparison of pharmacokinetics and pharmacodynamics using computer pharmaco-EEG. *Int Pharmacopsychiatry*. 1982; 17(Suppl 1):43–72.
21. Kellner HM, Baeder C, Christ O et al. Kinetics and metabolism of nomifensine in animals. *Br J Clin Pharmacol*. 1977; 4:109S–16S.
22. Lassman HB, Puri SK, Ho I et al. The pharmacokinetics and bioavailability of nomifensine maleate in healthy men. *J Clin Psychiatry*. 1984; 45(4, Sec 2):26–32.
23. McIntyre IM, Norman TR, Burrows GD et al. Pharmacokinetics of nomifensine after a single oral dose. *Br J Clin*

Pharmacol. 1982; 13:740–3.
24. Heptner W, Badian MJ, Baudner S et al. Determination of nomifensine by a sensitive radioimmunoassay. *Br J Clin Pharmacol.* 1977; 4:123S–7S.
25. Chamberlain J, Hill HM. A simple gas chromatographic method for the determination of nomifensine in plasma and a comparison of the method with other available techniques. *Br J Clin Pharmacol.* 1977; 4:117S–121S.
26. Ringoir S, Lameire N, Munche M et al. Pharmacokinetics of nomifensine in impaired renal function. *Br J Clin Pharmacol.* 1977; 4:129S–34S.
27. McIntyre IM, Burrows GD, Norman TR et al. Plasma nomifensine concentration, cardiological effects and clinical response. *Int Pharmacopsychiatry.* 1980; 15:325–33.
28. Montgomery SA, Roy D, Wynne-Willson S et al. Plasma levels and clinical response with imipramine in a study comparing efficacy with mianserin and nomifensine. *Br J Clin Pharmacol.* 1983; 15:205S–11S.
29. Syvalahti E, Lindberg R, Iisalo E. Clinical effects and serum levels of nomifensine in depressive patients. *J Int Med Res.* 1983; 11:259–62.
30. Gillings D, Grizzle J, Koch G et al. Pooling 12 nomifensine studies for efficacy generalizability. *J Clin Psychiatry.* 1984; 45(4, Sec 2):78–84.
31. Taeuber K. Comparison of nomifensine and placebo. *Br J Clin Pharmacol.* 1977; 4:209S–13S.
32. Feighner JP, Merideth CH, Claghorn JL. Multicenter placebo-controlled evaluation of nomifensine treatment in depressed outpatients. *J Clin Psychiatry.* 1984; 45(4, Sec 2):47–51.
33. Georgia EH. Double-blind comparison of the efficacy and safety of nomifensine maleate versus placebo in depressed outpatients. *J Clin Psychiatry.* 1984; 45(4, Sec 2):43–6.
34. Goldstein BJ, Brauzer B, Kentsmith D et al. Double-blind, placebo-controlled, multicenter evaluation of the efficacy and safety of nomifensine in depressed outpatients. *J Clin Psychiatry.* 1984; 45(4, Sec 2):52–5.
35. Grof P, Saxena B, Daigle L et al. Dopaminergic agonist nomifensine compared with amitriptyline: a double-blind clinical trial in acute primary depression. *Br J Clin Pharmacol.* 1977; 4:221S–5S.
36. McClelland HA, Kerr TA, Little JC. A clinical comparison of nomifensine and amitriptyline. *Br J Clin Pharmacol.* 1977; 4:233S–6S.
37. Ong SBY, Lee CT. A double-blind comparison of nomifensine and amitriptyline in the treatment of depression. *Acta Psychiatr Scand.* 1981; 63:198–207.
38. Wistedt B, Agren H, Bjaring B et al. Nomifensine and amitriptyline in the treatment of depression. *Acta Psychiatr Scand.* 1983; 68:212–20.
39. Forrest A, Hewett A, Nicholson P. Controlled randomized group comparison of nomifensine and imipramine in depressive illness. *Br J Clin Pharmacol.* 1977; 4:215S–20S.
40. Amin MM, Ban TA, Lehmann HE. Nomifensine in the treatment of depression: a report on the Canadian part of a transcultural study. *Psychopharmacol Bull.* 1978; 14:35–7.
41. Amin MM, Ban TA, Pecknold JC. Nomifensine in the treatment of depression: a standard-controlled clinical study. *Psychopharmacol Bull.* 1978; 14:37–9.
42. Woggon B, Angst J. Comparative efficacy of nomifensine and imipramine. *Psychopharmacol Bull.* 1979; 15:29–31.
43. McCawley A. A double-blind evaluation of nomifensine and imipramine in depressed outpatients *Am J Psychiatry.* 1979; 136:841–3.
44. Dencker SJ, Lundin L, Jensen K et al. Nomifensine and imipramine in endogenous depression: a double-blind Scandinavian multicenter study. *Int Pharmacopsychiatry.* 1982; 17(Suppl 1):116–44.
45. Rickels K, Weise CC, Sandler K et al. Nomifensine, imipramine and placebo in depressed outpatients. *Int Pharmacopsychiatry.* 1982; 17(Suppl 1):73–88.
46. Bremner JD, Abrahams LM, Crupie JE et al. Multicenter double-blind comparison of nomifensine and imipramine for efficacy and safety in depressed outpatients. *J Clin Psychiatry.* 1984; 45(4, Sec 2):56–9.
47. Fann WE, Lyle FA, Higginbotham W. Nomifensine vs imipramine in depressed inpatients. *J Clin Psychiatry.* 1984; 45(4, Sec 2):60–2.
48. Poldinger W, Gammel G. Differences in effect between nomifensine and nortriptyline. *Int Pharmacopsychiatry.* 1978; 13:58–68.
49. Poldinger W, Streichenwein SM. A clinical trial comparing nomifensine and nortriptyline. *Int Pharmacopsychiatry.* 1982; 17(Suppl 1):106–15.
50. Valle-Jones JC, Craven JR, Wallis TD et al. Mixed anxiety/depressive illness in general practice: a therapeutic comparison of nomifensine with fluphenazine/nortriptyline. *Acta Psychiatr Scand.* 1983; 68:494–500.
51. Levin A. Nomifensine and maprotiline in endogenous depression: comparative efficacy and side effects. *Int Pharmacopsychiatry.* 1982; 17(Suppl 1):89–96.
52. Knudsen P, Bjørndal N, Johnsen T et al. Zimeldine versus nomifensine: a double-blind study of depressed patients. *Neuropsychobiology.* 1984; 11:236–42.
53. Hamouz W, Van Dorth R, Pinder RM et al. A double-blind trial of mianserin and nomifensine in depressed outpatients. *Br J Clin Pharmacol.* 1983; 15:219S–25S.
54. Cohn JB, Varga L, Lyford A. A two-center, double-blind study of nomifensine, imipramine and placebo in depressed geriatric outpatients. *J Clin Psychiatry.* 1984; 45(4 Sec 2):68–72.
55. Goldstein SE, Birnbom F, LaLiberte R. Nomifensine in the treatment of depressed geriatric patients. *J Clin Psychiatry.* 1982; 43:287–9.
56. Jansen W, Siegfried K. Nomifensine in geriatrics: a placebo-controlled study. *J Clin Psychiatry.* 1984; 45(4, Sec 2):63–7.
57. Merideth CH, Feighner JP, Hendrickson G. A double-blind comparative evaluation of the efficacy and safety of nomifensine, imipramine and placebo in depressed geriatric outpatients. *J Clin Psychiatry.* 1984; 45(4, Sec 2):73–7.
58. Montgomery S, Roy D, Montgomery DB. Supersensitivity and nomifensine in depressed patients. In: Costa E, Racagni G, eds. Typical and atypical antidepressants: clinical practice. New York: Raven Press; 1982:105–11.
59. Clemmesen L, Mikkelsen PL, Lund H et al. Assessment of the anticholinergic effects of antidepressants in a single-dose crossover study of salivation and plasma levels. *Psychopharmacology.* 1984; 82:348–54.
60. Richelson E. The newer antidepressants: structures, pharmacokinetics, pharmacodynamics and proposed mechanisms of action. *Psychopharmacol Bull.* 1984; 20:213–23.
61. Stonier PD. A review of the clinical safety and tolerability of nomifensine. *J Clin Psychiatry.* 1984; 45(4, Sec 2):89–95.
62. Burrows GD, Vohra J, Dumovic P et al. Cardiological effects of nomifensine, a new antidepressant. *Med J Aust.* 1978; 1:341–3.
63. McIntyre IM, Burrows GD, Norman TR et al. Plasma nomifensine concentration, cardiological effects and clinical response. *Int Pharmacopsychiatry.* 1980; 15:325–33.
64. Bethge KP, Godt U, Blanco-Cruz E et al. Incidence of cardiac arrhythmias during antidepressant therapy with maprotiline or nomifensine. *J Cardiovasc Pharmacol.* 1982; 4:142–8.
65. Siegfried K, Taeuber K. Pharmacodynamics of nomifensine: a review of studies in healthy subjects. *J Clin Psychiatry.* 1984; 45(4, Sec 2):33–8.
66. Luchins DJ, Oliver AP, Wyatt RJ. Seizures with antidepressants: an *in vitro* technique to assess relative risk. *Epilepsia.* 1984; 25:25–32.
67. Trimble MR, Meldrum BS, Anlezark G. Effect of nomifensine on brain amines and epilepsy in photosensitive baboons. *Br J Clin Pharmacol.* 1977; 4:101S–7S.
68. Trimble MR. Epilepsy, antidepressants and the role of nomifensine. *J Clin Psychiatry.* 1984; 45(4, Sec 2):39–42.
69. Yakabow AL, Hardiman S, Nash RJ. An overview of side effects and long-term experience with nomifensine from United States clinical trials. *J Clin Psychiatry.* 1984; 45(4, Sec

2):96–9.
70. Gillman MA, Sandyk R. Nomifensine exacerbates depression and seizures in an epileptic patient. *Neurology*. 1984; 34:1620–1. Letter.
71. Bournerias F, Habibi B. Nomifensine-induced immune haemolytic anaemia and impaired renal function. *Lancet*. 1979; 2:95–6. Letter.
72. Lylloff K, Jersild C, Bacher T et al. Massive intravascular haemolysis during treatment with nomifensine. *Lancet*. 1982; 2:41. Letter.
73. Katona C. Paranoid symptoms after nomifensine. *Lancet*. 1982; 384–5. Letter.
74. Garcia-Morteo O, Maldonado-Cocco JA. Lupus-like syndrome during treatment with nomifensine. *Arthritis Rheum*. 1983; 26:936. Letter.
75. Gibson AC. Nomifensine and dyskinesia. *Br J Psychiatry*. 1981; 138:439. Letter.
76. Sandyk R, Gillman MA. Nomifensine exacerbates orofacial dyskinesia in hypothyroidism. *Neurology*. 1985; 35:282. Letter.
77. Freed E. Increased sexual function with nomifensine. *Med J Aust*. 1983; 2:551. Letter.
78. Nielsen JL, Lund NO. Drug fever due to nomifensine treatment in patients with endogenous depression. *Int Pharmacopsychiatry*. 1981; 16:66–8.
79. Montgomery S, Crome P, Braithwaite R. Nomifensine overdose. *Lancet*. 1978; 15:828–9. Letter.
80. Vohra JK, Burrows GD, McIntyre I et al. Cardiovascular effects of nomifensine. *Lancet*. 1978; 2:902–3. Letter.
81. Prescott LF, Illingworth RN, Critchley JA et al. Acute haemolysis and renal failure after nomifensine overdosage. *Br Med J (Clin Res)* 1980; 281:1392–3.
82. Rupp W, Heptner W, Uihlein M et al. Kinetic interaction of nomifensine with a 1,5-benzodiazepine (clobazam). *Br J Clin Pharmacol*. 1977; 4:143–6S.
83. Taeuber K. Dynamic interaction of nomifensine with alcohol. *Br J Clin Pharmacol*. 1977; 4:147S–51S.
84. Nawishy S, Hathway N, Turner P. Interactions of anticonvulsant drugs with mianserin and nomifensine. *Lancet*. 1981; 2:871–2. Letter.
85. Diagnostic and statistical manual of mental disorders. 3rd ed. Washington, DC: American Psychiatric Association; 1980:210–8.
86. Hanks GW, Magnus RV, Myskova I et al. Antidepressants in single daily doses: studies with nomifensine. In: Stonier PD, Jenner FA, eds. *Nomifensine*. Proceedings of the International Congress and Symposium. London, December, 1979. New York: Grune & Stratton, 1980:87–94.

“

Adequate and Well Controlled

Clinicians have long recognized the value of clinical observations, but tend to accept them uncritically. This may result in unjustified and incorrect conclusions, with sometimes diastrous consequences. In contrast, and partly in reaction, the scientific community had developed a generally skeptical attitude toward evaluations based on clinical experience and nonexperimental studies, particularly as sources of information about drug efficacy. A similar prejudice at the FDA has led to an interpretation of the statutory requirement for "adequate and well-controlled investigations" as meaning [randomized clinical trials] RCTs and only RCTs. These prejudices, together with ethical and logistical limitations in the applicability of RCTs, have led to otherwise unnecessary gaps in the available clinical information. Clearly, clinical experience and nonexperimental studies must be examined critically and used very carefully in evaluating drug efficacy; the RCT is still the standard with which other techniques must be compared. Yet, although these other techniques are unlikely to be as powerful or as convincing as RCTs, they can be useful in many settings, particularly those in which an experimental study is either unnecessary, infeasible, or too costly relative to the benefits expected from the results.

. . . Proper recognition of the potential utility of clinical experience and nonexperimental studies, along with appropriate skepticism about them, could permit the updating of drug labeling after marketing, based on *all* the valid information available at the time of the update. Such a new perspective might also encourage researchers and manufacturers to address questions of efficacy that currently remain unanswered even after marketing because RCTs are felt to be unethical or prohibitively costly.

—Strom BL, Melmon KL, Miettinen OS. *Arch Intern Med*. Postmarketing studies of drug efficacy. 1985; 145:1791–4. Editorial.

”

Therapy Reviews

Preventing *Haemophilus influenzae* type b disease

DANIEL T. CASTO AND DEBORAH L. EDWARDS

Abstract: The pathogenesis of *Haemophilus influenzae* type b (Hib) disease and methods for limiting spread of outbreaks of Hib disease are reviewed.

Many strains of *H. influenzae* are surrounded by an outer polysaccharide capsule; of the six antigenically distinct capsular types, Hib is the predominant cause of such serious infections as meningitis, especially among children younger than five years of age. The age-specific incidence of Hib disease appears to be related to the relatively small concentrations of anti-Hib antibody present in young children. Children younger than 48 months of age who reside in the same house or attend the same day-care center as a child who develops Hib disease appear to be at increased risk for contracting systemic Hib infections.

Prophylactic administration of rifampin 20 mg/kg once daily for four days can substantially decrease asymptomatic carriage of Hib in household contacts of the index patient and reduce the incidence of secondary Hib disease. The index patient should also receive prophylactic rifampin therapy before discharge from the hospital; i.v. antibiotics may cure the systemic infection but allow nasopharyngeal colonization to persist. A vaccine formulated from purified Hib capsular polysaccharide confers protection to more than 90% of children vaccinated at a minimum age of 24 months. Other candidates for vaccination include children between the ages of two and five years who attend day-care centers and children with anatomic or functional asplenia or malignancies. The vaccine is not effective in children younger than 18 months of age (who account for 60% of Hib disease in the U.S.); methods to increase vaccine immunogenicity in young infants are being evaluated.

Reduction of Hib disease in the U.S. may be possible through widespread use of the new vaccine.

Index terms: Age; Antibiotics; *Haemophilus* b polysaccharide vaccines; *Haemophilus influenzae*; Immunization; Pediatrics; Rifampin; Toxicity, environmental; Vaccines
Clin Pharm. 1985; 4:637–46

Although *Haemophilus influenzae* has been recognized as a major pathogen in pediatric patients for a number of years, epidemiologic findings concerning *H. influenzae* type b (Hib) infections in children have only recently indicated that the organism is contagious. Antimicrobial chemoprophylaxis can reduce the rate of carriage of Hib in high-risk populations, and two influential groups have published recommendations for the prophylactic use of rifampin.[1-3] Although these recommendations are followed by many clinicians, acceptance is not universal and selection of the best measures for containing a potential outbreak of Hib infections remains a public health issue of considerable controversy.

Until early this year, attempts to develop an effective Hib vaccine had been largely unsuccessful. The recent marketing of such a vaccine now offers hope of immunologic protection to a substantial portion of the population at high risk for developing serious Hib infection.

The goal of this review is to characterize the problem of Hib disease, summarize some of the important data concerning measures used to limit the development of both primary and secondary cases, and identify important factors for consider-

DANIEL T. CASTO, PHARM.D., is Clinical Assistant Professor of Pharmacy, Pharmacology, and Pediatrics, The University of Texas at Austin and The University of Texas Health Science Center at San Antonio. DEBORAH L. EDWARDS, M.S., is Pediatric Clinical Pharmacist, The University of Michigan Hospitals, Ann Arbor, and Clinical Instructor, College of Pharmacy, The University of Michigan, Ann Arbor.

Address reprint requests to Dr. Casto at Clinical Pharmacy Programs, Department of Pharmacology, University of Texas Health Science Center at San Antonio, 7703 Floyd Curl Drive, San Antonio, TX 78284.

The secretarial assistance of Virtena M. Rainer in preparing this manuscript is acknowledged.

This is **article 680-204-8518** in the **ASHP Continuing Education System.** See page 692 for learning objectives and test questions.

ation when attempts are made to limit the spread of Hib infections.

Clinical Importance of *Haemophilus influenzae*

Haemophilus influenzae organisms are small, pleomorphic, gram-negative microorganisms that are common inhabitants of the upper respiratory tract in children and adults.[4] Many, but not all, strains of *H. influenzae* are surrounded by an outer polysaccharide capsule for which a serotyping system has been developed and to which virulence appears to be related. Of the six antigenically distinct capsular types that have been identified and designated a through f,[5] *H. influenzae* type b is the predominant cause of serious illness.[6] Although common as a cause of otitis media in children and chronic bronchitis in adults, untypable (nonencapsulated) strains of *H. influenzae* are rarely responsible for invasive (bacteremic) disease. Of the typable strains, types a, c, d, e, and f also do not commonly cause serious illness. The prevalence and pathogenicity of various strains of *H. influenzae* are summarized in Table 1.

Although Hib can cause disease in adults,[7-8] it is often considered a pediatric pathogen because of the frequent occurrence of Hib infections in children younger than five years of age.[9] This high incidence of infection reflects the low serum concentration of anti-Hib antibody typically found in young children.[10,11] The importance of Hib as a pathogen in infants and children was demonstrated by Dajani et al.,[6] who reported that approximately 1% of general medical admissions to a pediatric hospital in Detroit during a four-year period were attributable to Hib disease, with meningitis accounting for more than half of all Hib infections (Figure 1). The overall peak incidence for these infections was seen in infants 6–12 months of age, with the exception of epiglottitis, which occurred most often in children between the ages of two and four years.

Because meningitis is the most common of Hib infections, it is also the most thoroughly studied. Hib currently is the leading cause of bacterial meningitis in the United States, accounting for an estimated 10,000 to 12,000 cases annually.[12-14] Infants and young children are most susceptible to the disease; more than half of the cases occur in patients younger than one year of age, and more than 90% occur in children younger than five years of age.[13] It is estimated that approximately 1 in 500 children younger than five years of age will contract Hib meningitis.

Fortunately, the nearly 100% case-fatality rate of the pre-antibiotic era has been reduced to less than 10%, largely because of the availability of effective antimicrobial agents and sensitive diagnostic methods that allow appropriate therapy to begin soon after diagnosis. However, as more patients have survived the primary illness, the morbidity of Hib meningitis has emerged as a major problem. Up to 50% of patients experience at least minor neurologic sequelae[15-17]; serious long-term handicaps, such as hearing impairment, vision impairment, learning disorders, mental retardation, seizures, and cerebral palsy, afflict approximately 20–30% of survivors.

Hib meningitis is not only a disease of substantial mortality and morbidity; it also appears to be highly contagious. Suspected spread of the disease among family members has been reported on numerous occasions,[18-22] and recent information from a national study indicates that individuals residing in the same household as a patient with meningitis are at substantial risk for contracting the disease.[23] Family members younger than six years of age have a risk of infection that is 585 times

Table 1.
Nasopharyngeal Carriage Rate and Pathogenicity of Various Strains of *Haemophilus influenzae*

Strain	Nasopharyngeal Carriage Rate (%)	Common Manifestations of Pathogenicity
Nonencapsulated (nontypable)	50–90	Chronic bronchitis, otitis media, sinusitis, conjunctivitis (Patients commonly adults; bacteremic infections rare)
Encapsulated type b	2–4	Meningitis, epiglottitis, pneumonia, septic arthritis, cellulitis, osteomyelitis, pericarditis (Patients commonly young children; bacteremic infections common)
Encapsulated types a, c, d, e, and f	1–2	Uncommon as pathogens

Figure 1. Distribution of *Haemophilus influenzae* infections among 292 pediatric patients.[6]

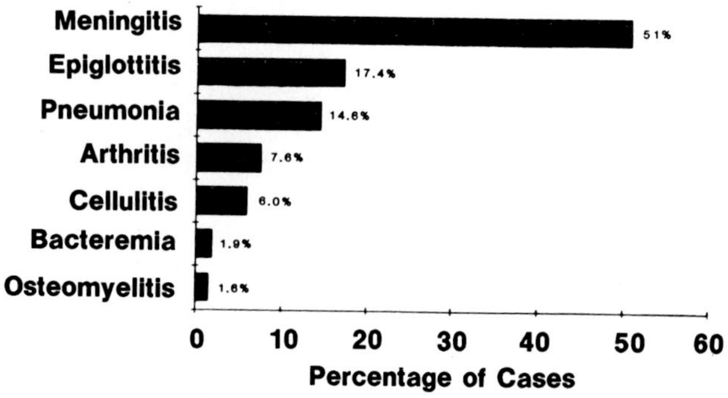

greater than that of the general population. Outbreaks among children attending day-care centers[24,25] or living in institutional settings[26,27] have also been reported, suggesting that an increased risk of infection may exist for individuals in these environments.

Susceptibility to *Haemophilus influenzae* type b Disease

In the United States, the incidence of Hib meningitis is highest in autumn, with a secondary peak in spring. Most population studies have shown that the disease occurs with approximately the same frequency in boys and girls. Although differences in the incidence of Hib meningitis have not been apparent in all studies, the results of most studies suggest that blacks develop the disease more frequently than whites, that the incidence of Hib disease among Navajo Indians is considerably greater than the incidence among most blacks, and that Eskimos from southwest Alaska develop Hib disease more frequently than any other racial group. Socioeconomic factors, such as family size and structure, crowding of living quarters, educational level, and annual income, have at times been related to the incidence of Hib meningitis, but additional data are needed in order to appropriately assess their influence on the risk of this disease.[28]

Perhaps the most striking feature of Hib disease is its age-related susceptibility. An explanation of this phenomenon was first suggested in 1933 by Fothergill and Wright[10]; their experiments demonstrated that the blood from children in the age group most commonly afflicted with Hib meningitis was significantly deficient in its ability to kill Hib in vitro, and that a fairly good inverse relationship existed between bactericidal activity in the blood from individuals of varying age groups and the age-specific incidence of Hib disease. Subsequent investigations generally confirmed these findings. The bactericidal effect was attributed to a serum anti-Hib antibody because passive immunization with rabbit antiserum offered protection against Hib infection in both an animal model and humans[29] and gamma globulin administered to patients with X-chromosome-linked agammaglobulinemia was also of prophylactic value.[30]

The antibody that confers protection from Hib infections is thought to be directed against polyribosyl ribose phosphate (PRP), the polysaccharide component of the capsule of *H. influenzae* type b organisms.[31] Other components of the organism, such as outer membrane proteins, are also antigenic.[32-34] However, the anticapsular antibody has been identified as the protective element in rabbit antiserum,[35] and in humans the serum concentration of anti-PRP antibody varies directly with age in the same manner that bactericidal activity does (Table 2).[36-38]

During the first few months of life, infants have substantial serum concentrations of transplacentally acquired anticapsular antibody that is predominantly of the IgG class. This transplacentally acquired antibody, along with small amounts of IgA and IgM that nursing infants may derive from colostrum and milk, is responsible for the low incidence of Hib infections in young infants. As serum concentrations of maternally derived anticapsular antibody decline, the infants become dependent on exposure to an immunogenic stimulus to produce their own antibody for continued protection. However, the ability to respond to polysaccharide antigenic challenge develops slowly. Whereas immunologic response to proteins can be elicited in infants as young as two to three months of age, response to polysaccharides is generally poor throughout the first year of life or longer.[39] Therefore, despite exposure to capsular PRP, many infants remain highly susceptible to Hib infection until an age at which they are capable of mounting an immunologic response.

Human antibodies to PRP increase substantially following Hib infection or administration of the purified capsular polysaccharide.[36,37,39-41] However, studies have consistently indicated that immunologic response to purified PRP is much lower among infants and young children than in older subjects.[38,40,42-45] Persistence of antibody also appears to be age dependent.[45] The concentration of anticapsular antibody that confers immunity against Hib infection is not known, but based on concentrations found to be protective in agammaglobulinemic patients who were receiving replacement immunoglobulin therapy and the results of a field trial of a Hib vaccine, a concentration of 0.15 μg/mL has been suggested.[46]

Secondary *Haemophilus influenzae*

Although Hib has been recognized as a major pathogen of early childhood for many years, it has not always been considered a highly contagious one. Occasional reports suggested that Hib infections were sufficiently contagious to warrant prophylactic measures among contacts of patients,[19,20]

Table 2.
Mean Serum Anti-Polyribosyl-Ribose-Phosphate Concentrations According to Patient Age[a]

Age (mo)	No. Samples	Geometric Mean Concentration (μg/mL)
Newborn–4	111	0.063
5–12	18	0.014
13–24	39	0.041
25–36	27	0.100
37–48	46	0.120
49–59	11	0.400

[a] Adapted from reference 38 with permission.

but this concept was not widely accepted until the mid-1970s. Reports of clusters of Hib cases among household contacts,[21,47] in long-term-care institutional settings,[26,48] and in day-care centers[24,25] strongly suggested that transmission of Hib infection among individuals in close contact was common. These reports stimulated a great deal of interest in identifying methods that would limit the spread of Hib disease.

At least five studies have examined the epidemiology of Hib disease among household contacts of patients with documented Hib infections (generally meningitis).[9,21-23,49] "Household contact" can be defined in a variety of ways but is generally accepted to be an individual who either resides in the same house as the index patient or is a nonresident who has contact with the index patient for a minimum of four hours daily for five of the seven days before the index patient is hospitalized.[2] The increased risk to household contacts of developing invasive Hib disease during the month following diagnosis of the index case has been demonstrated consistently (Table 3). The risk of secondary disease is greatest for children younger than two years of age; the incidence of secondary attacks in this age group is approximately 4%. Children six years of age or older have a risk equivalent to that of the adult population. The overall risk for all household contacts younger than six years of age is 0.3%—a risk approximately 585 times greater than the risk for the general population.[23]

The onset of secondary disease in household contacts occurs soon after detection of the primary case. The majority (75%) of secondary cases develop within seven days of the index case (Figure 2).[3] Some reports indicate that disease may develop in contacts as late as several months later[50]; however, whether this represents transmission of disease from the index case or acquisition from another source is debatable.

The risk for young children outside the home setting to develop secondary Hib disease is less well defined. Numerous outbreaks have been reported in day-care centers and nurseries,[24,25,51] indicating that these environments may promote Hib transmission. As in the home setting, children younger than two years of age make up the majority of secondary cases. However, these cases develop more slowly than do household cases, sometimes occurring weeks to months after the index case.

Whether the attack rate in day-care centers equals that in households is questionable. Band et al.[52] reported an attack rate of 0.7% in 161 day-care contacts compared with a rate of 0.5% in 604 household contacts and suggested that the risk is similar in both groups. However, Osterholm et al.[53] found no secondary cases of Hib disease in 406 day-care contacts and suggested that the day-care environment posed less risk of secondary disease than did the home environment. Recent studies have suggested that among children younger than 4 years of age, a greater risk of Hib infection associated with day-care attendance exists,[54,55] but the risk may be for primary rather than secondary disease.

The presumed pathogenesis of secondary cases of Hib disease involves transmission of the organism by respiratory droplets or oral secretions, nasopharyngeal colonization of the new host, and development of bacteremia via lymphatic drainage or direct invasion of the bloodstream.[56] Nasopharyngeal carriage of Hib is generally less than 5% in the general population; however, colonization rates in enclosed populations (such as household or day-care centers) in which a primary case of Hib has been identified are generally much higher, with a range of 13–85% of contacts of the index case.[24,27,48,57,58] The high rate of carriage and frequent contact between members of households and day-care center attendees probably contribute

Table 3.
Age-Related Percent Risk of the Occurrence of *Haemophilus influenzae* type b Disease in Household Contacts of a Primary Case[a]

Reference No.	Age of Contact (yr) ≤1	2–3	4–5	≥6	All Ages
9	4.2	0	0	0	0.3
21	7.9	2.0	0	0	0.4
22	5.7	3.5	0	0	0.7
23	3.7	1.2	0.1	0	0.2
49	3.4	0	0	0	0.4

[a] Percent risk calculated as (number of associated cases/number of household contacts in age group) × 100.

Figure 2. Interval between diagnosis of index case of *Haemophilus influenzae* type b (Hib) disease and onset of secondary disease in household contacts for 24 pairs of patients.[3] Each pair consisted of a patient with primary disease and a patient who developed secondary disease as a result of contact with the primary patient. The numbers on the bars represent the percentage of all pairs of patients in which secondary disease developed during the specified time interval.

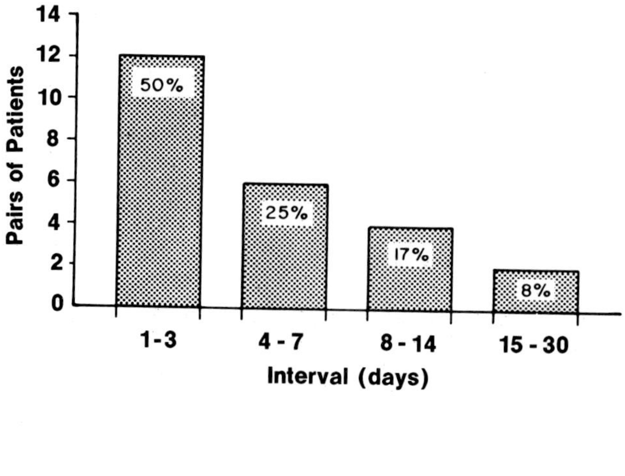

heavily to the high rate of secondary disease. Young, uncolonized members of the population who encounter *H. influenzae* readily develop invasive disease because of their low level of circulating anti-PRP antibody. Two strategies have been used to disrupt this sequence of events: (1) treatment of the entire contact population with antibiotics to eliminate the carrier state within the population, and (2) immunization of high-risk individuals to decrease their susceptibility to infection.

Chemoprophylaxis of *Haemophilus influenzae* type b Disease

The prophylactic administration of antimicrobial agents to close contacts of patients with Hib disease is directed at decreasing carriage of the invasive organism and thereby limiting spread of the disease. Such an approach has been used to prevent *Neisseria meningitidis* infections for some time. The high prevalence of asymptomatic Hib carriage among contacts of primary cases, coupled with the findings of Ward et al.[23] that no secondary disease occurred (by history) in any children younger than 10 years of age who had received antibiotics during the month following diagnosis of the index case, suggest that chemoprophylaxis might be useful in reducing outbreaks of Hib disease.

Agents considered for use in chemoprophylaxis should meet two criteria: They should possess good in vitro activity against the offending organism and they should achieve inhibitory (or bactericidal) concentrations at the site of colonization. Hoeprich[59] suggested that comparing the achievable concentration of a drug in saliva with the minimum inhibitory concentration of *Neisseria meningitidis* was useful in predicting the chemoprophylactic value of that drug. This model appears to be applicable at least for screening purposes in Hib disease.[60] The ideal chemoprophylactic agent should also have a low incidence of side effects, should not promote the rapid development of resistance, and should be readily available in a dosage form easily administered to infants and children.

Several antimicrobial agents, each of which is less than ideal in some category, have been evaluated for their chemoprophylactic value in Hib disease. Ampicillin, despite being relatively safe and convenient to administer, has several shortcomings. The prevalence of β-lactamase-producing strains of Hib has increased dramatically over the past decade and an ampicillin resistance rate of 30% among Hib isolates is not uncommon.[61] No data concerning salivary penetration are available; however, a report that nasopharyngeal colonization persisted following even high-dose i.v. ampicillin therapy for Hib infections suggests that penetration may be poor.[62] Four courses of ampicillin therapy at doses of 75–100 mg/kg/day in 32 colonized patients eradicated the Hib carrier state in only 21 patients, indicating that efficacy is unacceptably low.[24–26,57]

Erythromycin in combination with sulfisoxazole is available for pediatric use. This combination is recommended for the treatment of a variety of *H. influenzae* infections and produces relatively few adverse reactions. The combination has been studied for its chemoprophylactic value in 10 patients colonized with Hib, but eradication of nasopharyngeal carriage was not accomplished in a single individual.[63] This may be attributable to the fact that salivary concentrations of erythromycin do not exceed the minimum inhibitory concentration for Hib.[64]

Cefaclor, which is frequently used to treat pediatric infections, has very good activity against *H. influenzae* and was initially reported to penetrate saliva readily.[65] However, a five-day course of cefaclor at a dosage of 45 mg/kg/day eliminated Hib carriage in only 21 of 36 patients; dosages of 60 mg/kg/day administered for five days resulted in eradication of the carrier state in only 5 of 25 cases.[63] A follow-up study suggested that the initial report of good salivary concentrations may have been attributable to residue of the orally ingested dose and concluded that true penetration of cefaclor into saliva is minimal.[64]

Although the ability of the combination of trimethoprim–sulfamethoxazole to penetrate saliva has not been reported, the chemoprophylactic value of this combination has been evaluated in at least three studies on the basis of its in vitro activity against *H. influenzae*.[48,66,67] Various doses of the combination given for 5–15 days resulted in elimination of Hib carriage in 0–100% of subjects in these investigations. Combined results indicate that eradication was accomplished in only 48 of 78 carriers.

Rifampin penetrates saliva well and has good in vitro activity against *H. influenzae*.[60] To date, rifampin has been the most effective of any of the agents used to eliminate nasopharyngeal carriage of Hib (Table 4). Initial reports indicated that eradication of Hib from the nasopharynx would be unlikely if the minimum inhibitory concentration of rifampin for the colonizing organism was 0.5 μg/mL or greater.[68] However, subsequent studies demonstrated that successful eradication of Hib depends on the dosage regimen employed; 20 mg/kg of rifampin given once daily for four doses consistently results in eradication rates of 90% or greater. Because of this high degree of efficacy, rifampin has gained popularity as a chemoprophylactic agent despite the facts that it is not available in a convenient dosage form and its use as a single agent has historically resulted in rapid development of resistance.[72]

Although data concerning the influence of antibiotics on Hib carriage are useful, the question that

Table 4.
Efficacy of Rifampin in Eradicating Carrier State in Contacts of Patients with Invasive *Haemophilus influenzae* type b Disease

Reference No.	Study Design and Population	Rifampin Dosage (duration in days)	No. Contacts Treated	Eradication Rate (%)
68	Open, institution	10 mg/kg/day (3)	7	29
69	Open, institution and household	10 mg/kg b.i.d. (2)	15	87
58	Prospective randomized, household and institution	10 mg/kg b.i.d. (2)	121	63.6
70	Prospective randomized, household	10 mg/kg b.i.d. (2)	44	64
58	Prospective randomized, household and institution	10 mg/kg b.i.d. (4)	18	83
64	Open, institution	10 mg/kg b.i.d. (4)	13	100
58	Prospective randomized, household and institution	20 mg/kg/day (4)	52	96
71	Prospective randomized, institution	20 mg/kg/day (4)	39	95
57	Prospective randomized, institution	20 mg/kg/day (4)	15	100
27	Prospective randomized, institution	20 mg/kg/day (4)	25	96
67	Nonrandomized, institution	20 mg/kg/day (4)	25	88

must ultimately be answered is whether chemoprophylaxis will reduce the incidence of Hib disease in high-risk populations. Data concerning this question have been reported only recently and indicate that chemoprophylaxis may indeed reduce the incidence of secondary Hib disease.[52] In a multicenter placebo-controlled study of household and day-care center contacts of patients with invasive Hib disease, secondary disease developed in 4 of 765 contacts who received placebo and none of 1112 contacts who were treated with rifampin; this difference was significant. Attack rates among household and day-care center contacts younger than 48 months of age were not significantly different for patients who received placebo or rifampin, although a trend favoring rifampin was noted in both groups. Side effects consisting primarily of gastrointestinal disturbances, dizziness, and headache occurred in 22% of rifampin recipients versus 11% of placebo recipients, and no rifampin-resistant Hib strains were isolated. Nasopharyngeal carriage was eliminated in 97% of contacts who received rifampin at a dose of 20 mg/kg/day for four days, compared with an eradication rate of 28% in placebo recipients.

Based on the preceding information, both the Centers for Disease Control[3] and the American Academy of Pediatrics[1,2] have issued recommendations concerning antimicrobial chemoprophylaxis in contacts of patients with Hib disease. A summary of their recommendations is as follows:

1. Contacts who develop symptoms that are commonly associated with Hib disease (such as fever and headache) should be evaluated by a physician as soon as possible. Families of all contacts should be notified of the occurrence of the index case and educated about the risk of developing secondary disease. The need for education and the importance of careful observation of household and day-care center contacts recently have been re-emphasized.[2] If the index patient attended a day-care class and had classmates younger than four years of age, written notification to all parents concerning the circumstances of the outbreak of Hib disease and the potential benefit of prophylactic therapy with rifampin is advisable.
2. All household contacts (young and old, resident and nonresident) of a patient with systemic Hib disease should receive rifampin 20 mg/kg/day

(maximum 600 mg/day) once daily for four days if at least one of the contacts is younger than four years of age. Rifampin therapy is not necessary if all contacts are older than four years of age because they are not at increased risk of developing Hib disease[25] and recurrence of disease in the index patient is exceedingly rare.[73] The recommended dosage of rifampin for contacts younger than one month of age is 10 mg/kg/day, but this reduced dosage apparently has not been evaluated. Rifampin can be administered to children in a mixture with applesauce or as a 1% suspension in simple syrup.[60]

Definitive recommendations concerning rifampin use in day-care center contacts cannot be made because the efficacy of rifampin in preventing secondary disease in this setting is still not well defined. Most authorities recommend that only careful observation of contacts is necessary in centers in which a single case of Hib disease has been identified. If two cases from the same center occur within 60 days of each other, all attendees and staff members should receive prophylactic therapy with rifampin.[50] It is unlikely that chemoprophylaxis will be of much benefit unless strict compliance is achieved in at least 75% of contacts.[3]

3. Chemoprophylaxis should be instituted in the appropriate contacts as soon as possible following the onset of symptoms in the index case because most secondary cases occur within seven days. The benefit of antibiotic administration after seven days will probably be less than if given earlier. If the time lapse has been greater than one week, chemoprophylaxis probably is not indicated.
4. Nasopharyngeal cultures should not be used as a guide to chemoprophylaxis. Awaiting culture results would only delay implementation of prophylactic therapy. Furthermore, *H. influenzae* can persist in the nasopharynx for long periods of time,[62,74] and its presence does not constitute a risk for developing disease. Colonization has actually been associated with a decreased risk of disease, and data from animal models suggest that uncolonized individuals are probably at highest risk of developing Hib disease because bacteremia and invasive Hib disease occur rapidly following nasopharyngeal introduction of the organism.
5. The index patient should also receive prophylactic rifampin therapy before discharge from the hospital, since treating invasive Hib disease with i.v. ampicillin or chloramphenicol may cure the systemic infection but allow nasopharyngeal colonization to persist.[62,75] Rifampin chemoprophylaxis in index cases should prevent reintroduction of the invasive organism into the high-risk population of close contacts. Although one group of investigators suggests that rifampin should be given to the index patient soon after admittance to the hospital,[76] there apparently are no data to suggest that patients receiving treatment for Hib disease represent a special risk to hospital contacts. Furthermore, coadministration of rifampin to patients receiving chloramphenicol can lower serum chloramphenicol levels[77] (presumably by enzyme induction) and could potentially contribute to treatment failure. Therefore, rifampin therapy should be withheld until therapy for the primary infection has been completed. Information on persistent colonization in the index case following treatment with agents such as the newer cephalosporins is scant; until more data are available, rifampin therapy should be administered before the patient is discharged from the hospital,[78] although official recommendations do not address this point.
6. Rifampin should not be used in pregnant women because it has been shown to be teratogenic in laboratory animals.

Although these recommendations are followed by many clinicians, they are the topic of great debate.[73,79–82] The wisdom of recommending such widespread use of chemoprophylaxis on the basis of a single study that barely achieved statistical significance in demonstrating the efficacy of rifampin in reducing secondary disease has been questioned.[82] It has also been suggested that the large number of day-care center contacts who received rifampin and the large number of household contacts who received placebo biased the study in favor of demonstrating rifampin efficacy.[83] The feasibility of widespread use of prophylaxis in day-care centers has been questioned; in most instances, prophylaxis of all contacts of a single case will involve numerous physicians, whose cooperation in implementing prophylaxis will not be uniform.[82] Also of concern is the issue of who should be responsible for coordinating prophylactic efforts during an outbreak and whether such efforts can be instituted sufficiently early to be of benefit.[81] Practical problems, such as the lack of an appropriate rifampin dosage form for infants, inadequate supply of rifampin, and the expense of the drug, have been identified as obstacles to an effective prophylaxis program. Whether rifampin-resistant strains of Hib will become common remains to be seen,[84] as does whether chemoprophylaxis and eradication of nasopharyngeal carriage will impede the development of anti-Hib antibody.

Despite these concerns, prophylactic use of rifampin to prevent secondary Hib disease likely will (and already has in some areas) become a standard practice. However, it has been estimated that chemoprophylaxis will prevent only about 180 cases annually, thus reducing endemic disease by only 1.2%.[52] Therefore, the development of an effective vaccine for high-risk individuals is of paramount importance.

Vaccine Prophylaxis for *Haemophilus influenzae* type b Disease

After years of search for a vaccine that would be effective against Hib disease and appropriate for widespread use, *Haemophilus* b polysaccharide vaccine was recently marketed in the United States as b-Capsa I Vaccine. The vaccine is manufactured by Praxis Biologics, Inc. (Rochester, NY) and distributed by Mead Johnson Nutritional Division (Evansville, IN). The active component of the lyophilized vaccine is purified Hib capsular polysaccharide; the product also contains lactose 2.5 mg per 0.5-mL dose to increase its stability and, when reconstituted, contains thimerosal in a 1:10,000 concentration and sodium chloride. Each dose of vaccine delivers 25 μg of capsular PRP.[85]

Trials of the efficacy of the newly marketed vaccine consist primarily of studies conducted in Finland using *Haemophilus* b polysaccharide vaccine prepared by scientists from Praxis Biologics.[42,44,46] In these studies, approximately 49,000 children between the ages of three months and five years received Hib vaccine and approximately an equal number of children received a meningococcal vaccine and served as a control group; the two groups were evaluated during a four-year follow-up period. Antibody concentrations measured three weeks following vaccination were equal to or greater than 0.15 μg/mL in 9% of children aged 3–5 months, 52% of children aged 6–11 months, and 80% of children aged 12–17 months. Despite the development of this concentration of antibody in a significant portion of children younger than 18 months of age, bacteremic Hib infections occurred with the same frequency in the vaccinated and control groups (Table 5). However, children immunized with Hib vaccine at 18–71 months of age had significantly fewer infections than similar children in the control group. Although a serum antibody concentration of 0.15 μg/mL had been proposed as the minimal effective antibody concentration, closer analysis of the data revealed that a concentration of 1.0 μg/mL or greater three weeks after immunization correlated better with protective effect over the following year (Figure 3).[86] This is not surprising, since antibody concentrations decline from their peak levels fairly rapidly in younger patients; following an initial rise, the antibody concentration in children immunized at 18–23 months of age will decline by about 78% over the ensuing 18 months.[45,87] Therefore, it has been suggested that the three-week postimmunization concentration be referred to as the "protective response correlate" that will likely provide a continuing protective level.[85] Because the method of determining antibody concentration can influence results substantially, use of the protective response correlate for predictive purposes should be restricted only to the radioimmunoassay method employed in the Finnish studies.

Estimates suggest that immunizing Finnish children at 18 months of age could prevent approximately 60% of systemic Hib disease in Finland (Figure 3). Because the age distribution of Hib infections in the United States is slightly different (Table 6),[14] immunizing all children in the United States at 18 months of age would prevent 40% of Hib disease (assuming the vaccine offered protection to all recipients). However, it is not known what percentage of children would develop immunity if vaccinated at exactly 18 months of age; approximately 75% of children immunized between 18 and 23 months of age will mount a protective response.[44] Protection is conferred to over 90% of children vaccinated at a minimum age of 24 months; therefore, about one fourth of all Hib disease in our country would be preventable through a widespread immunization program for children of this age.

The American Academy of Pediatrics[14] and the Centers for Disease Control[88] now recommend that all children receive *Haemophilus* b polysaccharide vaccine at 24 months of age. For children older than 24 months of age, the risk of Hib disease decreases with increasing age and the benefit derived from vaccination diminishes. Because day-care center attendance has been identified as a risk factor for Hib disease,[54,55] all attendees between two and five years of age should be considered candidates for vaccination. Children between 18 and 24 months of age should also be considered candidates if they attend day-care centers, but efficacy of the vaccine is lower in this age group and parents should be counseled accordingly. Children

Table 5.
Incidence of Bacteremic *Haemophilus influenzae* Infections in Two Age Groups of Children Vaccinated with the *H. influenzae* type b (Hib) Polysaccharide Vaccine or a Group A Meningococcal (Men A) Vaccine[a]

	No. of Infections			
	Vaccinated at 18–71 Months of Age		Vaccinated at 3–17 Months of Age	
No. Years After Vaccination	Hib Group (n = 37,393)	Men A Group (n = 38,431)	Hib Group (n = 11,584)	Men A Group (n = 10,864)
1	0	11	7	1
2	2	5	1	3
3	0	2	2	1
4	0	2	0	0
Total	2[b]	20[b]	10	5

[a] Reprinted from reference 44 with permission.
[b] Significantly different at a level of $p < 0.001$.

Figure 3. The protective potential of *Haemophilus influenzae* type b (Hib) vaccine in Finnish children. The left-hand axis represents the age-specific incidence of invasive *H. influenzae* disease per 100,000 children per year. The arrow indicates the earliest suggested age of vaccination (18 months); 40% of meningitis and other *H. influenzae* infections occur before this age and 60% occur after this age. The shaded area represents the 60% of meningitis and other *H. influenzae* infections that might be preventable if all children were vaccinated at 18 months of age. The stepped lines indicate the percentage of children at each age who had titers of anti-Hib antibody ≥1.0 μg/mL before or after vaccination (right-hand axis); the black bars represent the corresponding percentages among adults and neonates (reproduced from reference 44 with permission).

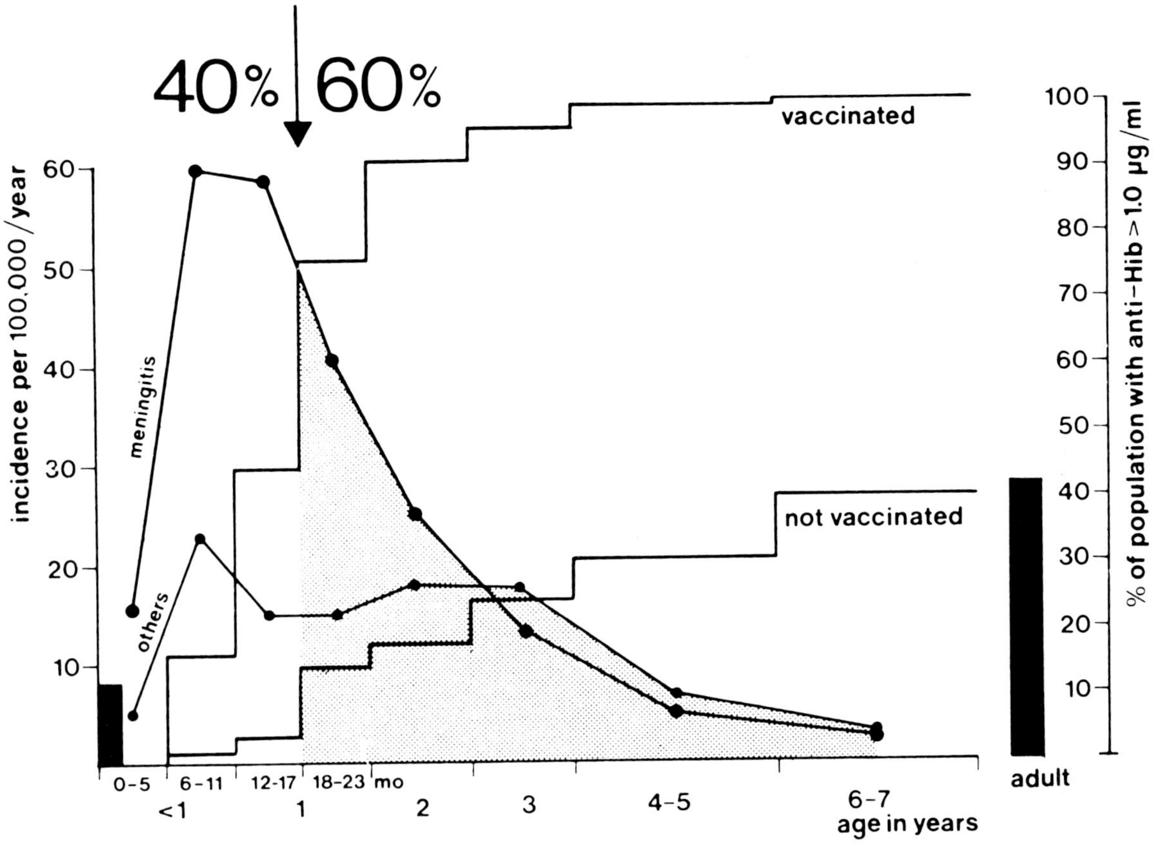

Table 6.
1984 Incidence of *Haemophilus influenzae* type b Disease in U.S. Children Younger than Five Years of Age

Patient Age (mo)	Meningitis: Attack Rate[b]	Meningitis: No. Cases	Other: Attack Rate	Other: No. Cases	Total: Attack Rate	Total: No. Cases
0–5	112	2,099	41	768	153	2,867
6–11	192	3,579	106	1,983	298	5,562
12–17	113	2,088	49	896	162	2,984
18–23	59	1,083	63	1,152	122	2,235
24–35	33	1,222	23	832	56	2,054
36–47	17	597	30	1,088	47	1,684
48–59	8	272	16	576	24	848
Total	60	10,940	40	7,295	100	18,235

[a] Reprinted from reference 14 with permission.
[b] Number of cases per 100,000 children younger than five years of age per year.

younger than 24 months of age at the time of vaccination probably should receive a second dose of vaccine within 18 months of the initial dose to increase the likelihood of protection; however, the most appropriate timing for this second dose is not known at present. Repeat doses of vaccine do not produce the T-cell memory response and booster effect that is typically observed with protein antigens; instead, the response is an increase in anti-PRP antibody concentration similar to that observed in children of the same age who have not previously received the vaccine. Simultaneous administration of diphtheria–pertussis–tetanus (DPT) and Hib vaccines at different sites does not impair immunologic response to either and can be considered safe.[42]

Children with anatomic or functional asplenia (splenectomy, sickle cell disease) and those with malignancies and immunosuppression should receive the vaccine because they are considered to be at high risk for developing Hib infections.[89,90] However, data supporting the protective effect of the vaccine in these children are lacking at this time and further studies are needed to define the usefulness of the vaccine. Administering the vaccine to adults who have chronic conditions that might render them susceptible to Hib infection cannot be recommended at this time because of a lack of data. Children younger than 18 months of age should not be given the vaccine even though they are at high risk of infection because of lack of efficacy in this age group.

The administration of more than 60,000 doses of *Haemophilus* b polysaccharide vaccine to children and several hundred doses to adults has been accomplished with remarkable safety.[38,42,43,91] Anaphylaxis responsive to epinephrine developed in one patient and is the only serious reaction that has been noted.[42] Fever and such local side effects as erythema and induration at the injection site occurred in about half of vaccine recipients in the Finnish study, but these effects were mild and generally resolved within 24 hours.[42] A temperature greater than or equal to 38.3 °C (101 °F) 24 hours after vaccination was noted in 13% of children. Data about the vaccine available in the United States indicate that fewer than 2% of recipients experienced high fever or local reactions 24 hours after vaccine administration.[85] Whether this lower incidence is attributable to a more refined product than the one used in the early field trials or to the smaller number of patients studied (267) is unclear. Administration of Hib vaccine at the same time as DPT vaccine produces the same incidence of side effects observed when DPT vaccine is given alone, so 18-month-old infants can safely receive both vaccines simultaneously.[42]

The availability of the new vaccine offers hope for substantially reducing the occurrence of Hib infections in young children, but the optimal strategy for providing maximal benefit is not well defined at this time. Cochi et al.[92] have suggested that, despite lower efficacy of the vaccine in children 18–23 months old than in children older than 24 months, universal vaccination of children at 18 months of age represents the most cost-effective use of the vaccine. Vaccination of all children at 18 months, with repeat vaccination for day-care center attendees, would substantially increase effectiveness of the program with minimal increase in cost.[92]

Even with the marketing of the new vaccine, children younger than 18 months of age (who account for 60% of the Hib disease in our country and who do not respond immunologically to PRP) will remain at risk for developing serious infections. Efforts to develop a vaccine that is effective in young infants are continuing. Various methods to increase vaccine immunogenicity in young infants, such as combining PRP with DTP vaccine[91] or whole pertussis cells[93] or conjugating it with various proteins,[94,95] are being evaluated and look promising. However, until such time that a vaccine suitable for use in children of all ages is available, the development and spread of Hib disease will remain a major public health issue.

Conclusion

Prophylactic administration of rifampin to close contacts of patients with invasive Hib disease is an effective method for eradicating asymptomatic carriage of the organism and may reduce secondary spread of disease. However, because secondary cases represent only a small percentage of all Hib infections that occur annually, prevention of primary disease through an effective immunization program is highly desirable. The recently marketed polysaccharide vaccine appears to be safe and is very effective at preventing Hib disease in children at least 24 months of age. Although the product is of little or no benefit to the very young children who are at highest risk for developing Hib disease, substantial reduction of Hib disease in the United States may be possible through widespread use of the vaccine.

References

1. American Academy of Pediatrics. Report of the Committee on Infectious Diseases. Evanston, IL: American Academy of Pediatrics; 1982.
2. American Academy of Pediatrics Committee on Infectious Diseases. Revision of recommendation for use of rifampin prophylaxis of contacts of patients with *Haemophilus influenzae* infection. *Pediatrics.* 1984; 74:301–2.
3. Centers for Disease Control. Prevention of secondary cases of *Haemophilus influenzae* type b disease. *Morb Mortal Wkly Rep.* 1982; 32:672–80.
4. Box QT, Cleveland RT, Willard CY. Bacterial flora of the upper respiratory tract. *Am J Dis Child.* 1961; 102:293–301.
5. Pittman M. Variation and type specificity in the bacterial species *Haemophilus influenzae. J Exp Med.* 1931; 53:471–93.
6. Dajani AS, Asmar BI, Thirumoorthi MC. Systemic *Haemophilus influenzae* disease: an overview. *J Pediatr.* 1979; 94:355–64.
7. Plouffe JF, Powell DA. Serious infections in adults exposed to children with *Haemophilus influenzae* type b meningitis. *Ann Intern Med.* 1981; 94:785–6.
8. Glode MP, Halsey NA, Murray M et al. Epiglottitis in adults: association with *Haemophilus influenzae* type b colonization and disease in children. *Pediatr Infect Dis.* 1984; 3:548–51.
9. Granoff DM, Basden M. *Haemophilus influenzae* infections in Fresno, California: a prospective study of the effects of age, race, and contact with a case on incidence of disease. *J Infect Dis.* 1980; 141:40–6.
10. Fothergill L, Wright J. Influenzal meningitis: the relation of age incidence to the bactericidal power of blood against the causal organism. *J Immunol.* 1933; 24:273–84.
11. Peter G, Smith DH. *Haemophilus influenzae* meningitis at the Children's Hospital Medical Center in Boston, 1958 to 1973. *Pediatrics.* 1975; 55:523–30.

12. Fraser DW, Geil CC, Feldman RA. Bacterial meningitis in Bernalillo County, New Mexico: a comparison with three other American populations. *Am J Epidemiol.* 1974; 100:29–34.
13. Parke JC Jr, Schneerson R, Robbins JB. The attack rate, age incidence, racial distribution, and case fatality rate of *Haemophilus influenzae* type b meningitis in Mecklenberg County, North Carolina. *J Pediatr.* 1972; 81:765–9.
14. American Academy of Pediatrics Committee on Infectious Diseases. *Haemophilus* type b polysaccharide vaccine. *Pediatrics.* 1985; 76:322–4.
15. Ferry PC, Culbertson JL, Cooper JA et al. Sequelae of *Haemophilus influenzae* meningitis: preliminary report of a long-term follow-up study. In: Sell SH, Wright PF, eds. *Haemophilus influenzae.* New York: Elsevier Science Publishing Co., Inc. 1982:111–6.
16. Tejani A, Dobias B, Sambursky J. Long-term prognosis after *H. influenzae* meningitis: prospective evaluation. *Dev Med Child Neurol.* 1982; 24:338–42.
17. Taylor HG, Michaels RH, Mayur PM et al. Intellectual, neuropsychological, and achievement outcomes in children six to eight years after recovery from *Haemophilus influenzae* meningitis. *Pediatrics.* 1984; 74:198–205.
18. Hertzhog AJ, Cameron SL, Karlstrom AE. Influenzal meningitis in brothers. *JAMA.* 1944; 124:502–3.
19. Rothman M, Nabil FJ. Prophylaxis in meningitis due to type b *Haemophilus influenzae. N Engl J Med.* 1955; 253:653.
20. Kline AM. *Haemophilus* influenzal meningitis: is prophylaxis indicated? *Am J Dis Child.* 1962; 104:595–7.
21. Filice GA, Andrews JC, Hudgins MP et al. Spread of *Haemophilus influenzae:* secondary illness in household contacts of a patient with *H. influenzae* meningitis. *Am J Dis Child.* 1978; 132:757–9.
22. Glode MP, Daum RS, Goldmann DA et al. *Haemophilus influenzae* type b meningitis: a contagious disease of children. *Br Med J.* 1980; 2:899–901.
23. Ward JI, Fraser DW, Baraff LJ et al. *Haemophilus influenzae* meningitis: a national study of secondary spread in household contacts. *N Engl J Med.* 1979; 301:122–6.
24. Ginsburg CM, McCracken GH, Rae S et al. *Haemophilus influenzae* type b disease: incidence in a day-care center. *JAMA.* 1977; 238:604–7.
25. Ward JI, Gorman G, Phillips C et al. *Haemophilus influenzae* type b disease in a day-care center: report of an outbreak. *J Pediatr.* 1978; 92:713–7.
26. Glode MP, Schiffer MS, Robbins JB et al. An outbreak of *Haemophilus influenzae* type b meningitis in an enclosed hospital population. *J Pediatr.* 1976; 88:36–40.
27. Shapiro ED, Wald ER. Efficacy of rifampin in eliminating pharyngeal carriage of *Haemophilus influenzae* type b. *Pediatrics.* 1980; 66:5–8.
28. Fraser DW. *Haemophilus influenzae* in the community and the home. In: Sell SH, Wright PF, eds. *Haemophilus influenzae.* New York: Elsevier Science Publishing Co., Inc.; 1982:11–22.
29. Alexander HE. Treatment of type b *Haemophilus influenzae* meningitis. *J Pediatr.* 1944; 25:517–32.
30. Rosen FS, Janeway CA. The gammaglobulin: III. The antibody deficiency syndromes. *N Engl J Med.* 1966; 275:709–15.
31. Zamenhof S, Leidy G, Fitzgerald PL et al. Polyribophosphate, the type-specific substance of *Haemophilus influenzae* type b. *J Biol Chem.* 1953; 203:695–704.
32. Anderson P, Johnston RB Jr, Smith DH. Human serum activities against *Haemophilus influenzae* type b. *J Clin Invest.* 1972; 51:31–8.
33. Insel RA, Anderson P, Loeb MR et al. A polysaccharide-protein complex from *Haemophilus influenzae* type b: II. Human antibodies to its somatic components. *J Infect Dis.* 1981; 144:521–9.
34. Hansen EJ, Frisch CF, McDade RL et al. Identification of immunogenic outer membrane proteins of *Haemophilus influenzae* type b in the infant rat model system. *Infect Immun.* 1981; 32:1084–92.
35. Alexander HE, Heidelberger M, Leidy G. The protective or curative element in type b *H. influenzae* rabbit serum. *Yale J Biol Med.* 1944; 16:425–34.
36. Schneerson R, Rodrigues LP, Parke JC et al. Immunity to disease caused by *Haemophilus influenzae* type b: II. Specificity and some biological characteristics of "natural" infection-acquired and immunization induced antibody to the capsular polysaccharide of *Haemophilus influenzae* type b. *J Immunol.* 1971; 107:1081–10.
37. Anderson P, Smith DH, Ingram DL et al. Antibody to polyribophosphate of *Haemophilus influenzae* type b in infants and children: effect of immunization with polyribophosphate. *J Infect Dis.* 1977; 136(Suppl):S57–S62.
38. Smith DH, Peter G, Ingram DL et al. Responses of children immunized with the capsular polysaccharide of *Haemophilus influenzae* type b. *Pediatrics.* 1973; 52:637–44.
39. Robbins JB. Vaccines for the prevention of encapsulated bacterial diseases: current status, problems and prospects for the future. *Immunochemistry.* 1978; 15:839–54.
40. Robbins JB, Parke JC, Schneerson R et al. Quantitative measurement of "natural" and immunization-induced *Haemophilus influenzae* type b capsular polysaccharide antibodies. *Pediatr Res.* 1973; 7:103–10.
41. Anderson P, Peter G, Johnston RB Jr. et al. Immunization of humans with polyribophosphate, the capsular antigen of *Haemophilus influenzae* type b. *J Clin Invest.* 1972; 51:39–44.
42. Peltola H, Kayhty H, Sivonen A et al. *Haemophilus influenzae* type b capsular polysaccharide vaccine in children: a double-blind field study of 100,000 vaccinees 3 months to 5 years of age in Finland. *Pediatrics.* 1977; 730–7.
43. Park JC Jr., Schneerson R, Robbins JB et al. Interim report of a controlled field trial of immunization with capsular polysaccharides of *Haemophilus influenzae* type b and group C *Neisseria meningitidis* in Mecklenberg County, North Carolina (March 1974–March 1976). *J Infect Dis.* 1977; 136(Suppl):S51–6.
44. Peltola H, Kayhty H, Virtanen M et al. Prevention of *Haemophilus influenzae* type b bacteremic infections with the capsular polysaccharide vaccine. *N Engl J Med.* 1984; 310:1561–6.
45. Kayhty H, Karanko V, Peltola H et al. Serum antibodies after vaccination with *Haemophilus influenzae* type b capsular polysaccharide and responses to reimmunization: no evidence of immunologic tolerance or memory. *Pediatrics.* 1984; 74:857–65.
46. Makela PH, Peltola H, Kayhty H et al. Polysaccharide vaccine of group A *Neisseria meningitidis* and *Haemophilus influenzae* type b: a field trial in Finland. *J Infect Dis.* 1977; 136:S43–S50.
47. Tejani A, Dobias B, Nangia BS et al. Intrafamily spread of *Haemophilus influenzae* type b infections. *Am J Dis Child.* 1977; 131:778–81.
48. Yogev R, Lander HB, Davis AT. Effect of TMP-SMX on nasopharyngeal carriage of ampicillin-sensitive and ampicillin-resistant *Haemophilus influenzae* type b. *J Pediatr.* 1978; 93:394–7.
49. Campbell LR, Zedd AJ, Michaels RH. Household spread of infection due to *Haemophilus influenzae* type b. *Pediatrics.* 1980; 66:115–7.
50. Granoff DM, Daum RS. Spread of *Haemophilus influenzae* type b: recent epidemiologic and therapeutic considerations. *J Pediatr.* 1980; 97:854–60.
51. Band JD. Chemoprophylaxis of *Haemophilus influenzae* type b disease: a strategy for preventing secondary cases. In: Sell SH, Wright PF, eds. *Haemophilus influenzae.* New York: Elsevier Science Publishing Co., Inc.; 1982:309–15.
52. Band JD, Fraser DW, Ajello G et al. Prevention of *Haemophilus influenzae* type b disease. *JAMA.* 1984; 251:2381–6.
53. Osterholm MT. The risk of secondary transmission of *Haemophilus influenzae* type b disease in day care: results of a statewide surveillance system. Paper presented at the 23rd Interscience Conference on Antimicrobial Agents and Chemotherapy. Las Vegas, NV: 1983 Oct 26.
54. Redmond SR, Pichichero ME. *Haemophilus influenzae* type b

disease. An epidemiologic study with special reference to day-care centers. *JAMA*. 1984; 252:2581–4.
55. Istre GR, Conner JS, Broome CV et al. Risk factors for primary invasive *Haemophilus influenzae* disease. Increased risk from day-care attendance and school-aged household members. *J Pediatr*. 1985; 106:190–5.
56. Moxon ER. Experimental studies of *Haemophilus influenzae* infection in a rat model. In: Sell SH, Wright PF, eds. *Haemophilus influenzae*. New York: Elsevier Science Publishing Co., Inc.; 1982:59–71.
57. Gessert C, Granoff DM, Gilsdorf J. Comparison of rifampin and ampicillin in day-care contacts of *Haemophilus influenzae* type b disease. *Pediatrics*. 1980; 66:1–4.
58. Golde MP, Daum RS, Halsey NA et al. Rifampin alone and in combination with trimethoprim in chemoprophylaxis for infections due to *Haemophilus influenzae* type b. *Rev Infect Dis*. 1983; 5(Suppl):S549–55.
59. Hoeprich PD. Prediction of antimeningococcic chemoprophylactic efficacy. *J Infect Dis*. 1971; 123:125–33.
60. McCracken GH, Ginsburg CM, Zweighaft TC et al. Pharmacokinetics of rifampin in infants and children: relevance of prophylaxis against *Haemophilus influenzae* type b disease. *Pediatrics*. 1980; 66:17–21.
61. Istre GR, Conner JS, Glode MP et al. Increasing ampicillin-resistance rates in *Haemophilus influenzae* meningitis. *Am J Dis Child*. 1984; 138:366–9.
62. Michaels RH, Norden CW. Pharyngeal colonization with *Haemophilus influenzae* type b: a longitudinal study of families with a child with meningitis or epiglottitis due to *H. influenzae* type b. *J Infect Dis*. 1977; 136:222–8.
63. Horner DB, McCracken GH Jr, Ginsburg CM et al. A comparison of three antibiotic regimens for eradication of *Haemophilus influenzae* type b from the pharynx of infants and children. *Pediatrics*. 1980; 66:136–8.
64. Ginsberg CM, McCracken GH. Salivary penetration of antibiotics after oral administration. Paper presented at the 21st Interscience Conference on Antimicrobial Agents and Chemotherapy. Chicago, IL: 1981 Nov 4.
65. McCracken GH, Ginsberg CM, Clahsen JC et al. Pharmacokinetics of cefaclor in infants and children. *J Antimicrob Chemother*. 1978; 4:515–21.
66. Melish ME. Epidemic spread of *H. influenzae* type b in a day-care center. *Pediatr Res*. 1976; 10:348. Abstract.
67. Granoff D, Gilsdorf J, Gessert C et al. *Haemophilus influenzae* type b disease in a day care center: eradication of carrier state by rifampin. *Pediatrics*. 1979; 63:397–401.
68. Yogev R, Lander HB, Davis AT. Effect of rifampin on nasopharyngeal carriage of *Haemophilus influenzae* type b. *J Pediatr*. 1979; 94:840–1.
69. Yogev R, Melick C. Persistance of nasopharynx carriage of *Haemophilus influenzae* type b following cefaclor therapy. *Pediatr Res*. 1980; 1:567. Abstract.
70. Daum RS, Golde MP, Goldmann DA et al. Rifampin chemoprophylaxis for household contacts of patients with invasive infections due to *Haemophilus influenzae* type b. *J Pediatr*. 1981; 98:485–91.
71. Cox F, Trincher R, Rissing P et al. Rifampin prophylaxis for contacts of *Haemophilus influenzae* type b disease. *JAMA*. 1981; 245:1043–5.
72. Weidmer CE, Dunkel TB, Pettyjohn FS et al. Effectiveness of rifampin in eradicating the meningococcal carrier state in a relatively closed population. Emergence of resistant strains. *J Infect Dis*. 1971; 124:172–8.
73. Shapiro ED. Prophylaxis for contacts of patients with meningococcal or *Haemophilus influenzae* type b disease. *Pediatr Infect Dis*. 1982; 1:132–8.
74. Turk DC. Nasopharyngeal carriage of *Haemophilus influenzae* type b. *J Hyg*. 1963; 61:247–56.
75. Shapiro ED. Persistent pharyngeal colonization with *Haemophilus influenzae* type b after intravenous chloramphenicol therapy. *Pediatrics*. 1981; 64:435–7.
76. Alpert G. Persistent upper airway colonization in *Haemophilus influenzae* type b meningitis. *Pediatr Res*. 1985; 19:285A. Abstract.
77. Prober CG. Effect of rifampin on chloramphenicol levels. *N Engl J Med*. 1985; 312:788–9.
78. Casto DT, Gal P, McCue J et al. Salivary penetration of moxalactam. *Clin Pharm*. 1985; 4:67–70.
79. Glode MP. Commentary: what price orange urine? *Pediatr Infect Dis*. 1982;1:140–1.
80. Fulginiti VA. Point: red book committee recommendations for rifampin prophylaxis. *Pediatr Infect Dis*. 1982; 1:377–8.
81. Daum RS, Halsey NA. Counterpoint: the red blood opts for red urine. *Pediatr Infect Dis*. 1982; 1:378–81.
82. Mann JM, Hull HF. New *Haemophilus influenzae* type b control strategy: premature commitment to prophylaxis? *Pediatrics*. 1983; 72:118–21.
83. Osterholm MT, Murphy T. Does rifampin prophylaxis prevent disease caused by *Haemophilus influenzae* type b? *JAMA*. 1984; 251:2408–9.
84. Murphy TV, McCracken GH Jr., Zqeighaft TC et al. Emergence of rifampin-resistant *Haemophilus influenzae* after prophylaxis. *J Pediatr*. 1981; 99:406–9.
85. Mead Johnson Nutritional Division. b-Capsa I package insert. Evansville, IN; 1985 April.
86. Kayhty H, Peltola H, Karanko V et al. The protective level of serum antibodies to the capsular polysaccharide of *Haemophilus influenzae* type b. *J Infect Dis*. 1984; 149:1034.
87. Anderson P. The protective level of serum antibodies to the capsular polysaccharide of *Haemophilus influenzae* type b. *J Infect Dis*. 1984; 149:1034.
88. Anon. Polysaccharide vaccine for prevention of *Haemophilus influenzae* type b disease. *Morbid Mortal Wkly Rep*. 1985; 34:201–5.
89. Ward J, Smith AL. *Haemophilus influenzae* bacteremia in children with sickle cell disease. *J Pediatr*. 1976; 88:261–3.
90. Siber GR. Bacteremias due to *Haemophilus influenzae* and *Streptococcus pneumoniae:* their occurrence and course in children with cancer. *Am J Dis Child*. 1980; 134:668–72.
91. Pincus DJ, Morrison D, Andrews C et al. Age-related response of two *Haemophilus influenzae* type b vaccines. *J Pediatr*. 1982; 100:197–201.
92. Cochi SL, Broome CV, Hightower AW. Immunization of U.S. children with *Haemophilus influenzae* type b polysaccharide vaccine: a cost-effectiveness model of strategy assessment. *JAMA*. 1985; 253:521–9.
93. Kuo JSC, Monji N, McCoy DW. Development of *Haemophilus influenzae* type b vaccine: a combined vaccine consisting of the capsular polysaccharide, polyribosyl ribitol phosphate, and *Bordetella pertussis*. In: Sell SH, Wright PF, eds. *Haemophilus influenzae*. New York: Elsevier Science Publishing Co., Inc.; 1982:243–53.
94. Lepow ML, Samuelson JS, Gordon LK. Safety and immunogenicity of type b-polysaccharide diphtheria toxoid conjugate vaccine in infants 9 to 15 months of age. *J Pediatr*. 1985; 106:185–90.
95. Schneerson R, Barrera O, Sutton A et al. Preparation, characterization, and immunogenicity of *Haemophilus influenzae* type b polysaccharide-protein conjugates. *J Exp Med*. 1980; 152:361–76.

Use of antihypertensive agents in patients with glucose intolerance

JAMES M. MCKENNEY, ROBERT P. GOODMAN, AND JACKSON T. WRIGHT, JR.

Abstract: The selection, use, and potential adverse effects of antihypertensive agents in patients with glucose intolerance are reviewed.

Thiazide diuretics frequently impair glucose tolerance, but this deterioration is usually modest and should not preclude use of these agents in most patients with glucose intolerance. The loop diuretics furosemide and ethacrynic acid have also been associated with decreased glucose tolerance. The β-adrenergic blocking agents may inhibit insulin secretion, but few patients will experience clinically important elevations in blood glucose. Rather than producing glucose intolerance, these agents may delay recovery from hypoglycemic episodes and may mask catecholamine-induced symptoms of hypoglycemia. In certain cases, use of cardioselective β blockers or avoidance of β-blocker therapy may be indicated, especially in insulin-dependent diabetics. The calcium-channel blocking agents nifedipine and verapamil have been reported to produce diabetogenic effects in a few studies, but further investigations are needed to define the extent of these effects. Available evidence indicates that sympatholytic agents such as guanethidine and reserpine, α_2-adrenergic agonists such as methyldopa and clonidine, the α_1-blocking agent prazosin, and the vasodilators captopril and hydralazine produce few, if any, clinically important changes in glucose tolerance.

While no antihypertensive agents are abolutely contraindicated in patients with glucose intolerance, patients with glucose intolerance who are receiving thiazide diuretics, β blockers, and calcium-channel blocking agents should be monitored with extra care for hyperglycemia or deterioration in glucose tolerance.

Index terms: Clonidine; Contraindications; Diuretics; Ethacrynic acid; Furosemide; Glucose intolerance; Guanethidine; Hypotensive agents; Methyldopa; Nifedipine; Prazosin; Reserpine; Sympatholytic agents; Sympathomimetic agents; Thiazides; Toxicity; Vasodilating agents; Verapamil
Clin Pharm. 1985; 4:649–56

Population surveys suggest that 40–60% of patients with diabetes mellitus also have hypertension.[1-3] Hypertension occurs about 50% more often in a diabetic population than in a nondiabetic population.[4] The incidence of glucose intolerance in hypertensive populations is estimated to be between 25 and 35%.[3,5]

Each of these conditions represents an independent risk factor for cardiovascular disease and death.[4] The Framingham data have demonstrated that carbohydrate intolerance is an additive risk in hypertensive patients.[6] In addition, Christlieb et al., after following a large group of type I diabetics for 40 years or until death, reported that hypertension had been present commonly in those who died (the cause of death most frequently being coronary heart disease) but was rarely observed in survivors.[7]

Hypertension appears to be related to many of the complications associated with diabetes.[8-10] For example, noninsulin-dependent diabetics with systolic blood pressures of less than 145 mm Hg experience half the incidence of retinopathy seen in diabetics with systolic blood pressures greater than 145 mm Hg.[9] Further, antihypertensive treatment may alter these complications. For example, the rate of decline in glomerular filtration rate and renal plasma flow has been shown to be slowed when antihypertensive therapy is administered to diabetic hypertensives with proteinuria.[9-10] Thus, aggressive treatment of the hypertensive diabetic is indicated.

Many commonly prescribed antihypertensive agents have the potential for adversely affecting insulin secretion and glucose homeostasis and thus compromising optimal diabetic control. This paper reviews the selection and use of antihypertensive agents in hypertensive patients with glucose intolerance, with particular emphasis on the potential adverse effects of these agents on glucose tolerance.

Diuretics

Diuretics remain the mainstay of antihypertensive therapy. Their low cost, effectiveness, and synergism with other antihypertensive agents make them the most commonly preferred first-step

JAMES M. MCKENNEY, PHARM.D., is Associate Professor, Department of Pharmacy and Pharmaceutics, School of Pharmacy, Medical College of Virginia–Virginia Commonwealth University (MCV–VCU), Richmond. ROBERT P. GOODMAN, M.D., is Assistant Professor, and JACKSON T. WRIGHT, JR., M.D., PH.D., is Assistant Professor, Department of Internal Medicine, School of Medicine, MCV–VCU.

Address reprint requests to Dr. McKenney at Box 581, MCV Station, Medical College of Virginia, Richmond,VA 23298–0001.

This is article **680-204-8519** in the **ASHP Continuing Education System.** See page 693 for learning objectives and test questions.

agents.[11,12] However, diuretics can cause a wide range of metabolic derangements, including hypokalemia, hyperkalemia, hyperuricemia, hypercalcemia, hypomagnesemia, hyponatremia, and adverse changes in total cholesterol and high-density-lipoprotein cholesterol.[13,14] Diuretic therapy also has been associated with altered glucose metabolism; this occurs most commonly in patients with preexisting impaired glucose tolerance but is also observed in nondiabetics.[15,16] (Table 1).

The thiazides are frequently associated with impaired glucose tolerance.[16-20] Elevations in fasting serum glucose concentrations of 10% in the nondiabetic hypertensive patient[15,16] and up to 50% in the diabetic hypertensive patient[17,18] have been reported. No clear evidence has been presented to confirm that this is a dose-related effect. Several mechanisms of thiazide-induced hyperglycemia have been suggested. A decrease in insulin release by the pancreatic β cell has been demonstrated in vitro using isolated pancreatic islet cells and in vivo by measuring insulin release after glucose loading or sulfonylurea administration.[21-24] Diazoxide, a nondiuretic antihypertensive structurally related to the thiazides, has also been shown to be a potent inhibitor of insulin release.[25]

Thiazides may also decrease tissue sensitivity to insulin.[22-24] This has been observed in animal studies of insulin-stimulated glucose use in skeletal muscle and adipose tissue and in human studies using the glucose-clamp and tolbutamide-response techniques.[15,22]

At least some of the hyperglycemic action of the thiazides may be attributable to the hypokalemia caused by these agents. Potassium supplementation in patients taking thiazide diuretics has been shown to prevent the hyperglycemic effects of the drug.[26,27] Patients with nondiuretic-induced hypokalemia (e.g., resulting from primary or secondary hyperaldosteronism or therapy with potassium-binding resins) exhibit impaired glucose tolerance, which is reversed or prevented with potassium supplementation.[27-29] Like thiazide-induced hyperglycemia, the hypokalemia-induced hyperglycemia is associated with both decreased insulin release and decreased tissue sensitivity to insulin.

Table 1.
Antihypertensive Drug Effects in Glucose-Intolerant Patients

Antihypertensive Drug Type	Demonstrated Effect	Proposed Mechanism of Action	Clinical Importance
Thiazide diuretics[15-29]	Elevated serum glucose, decreased glucose tolerance	Reduced insulin secretion from pancreatic β cells and reduced tissue sensitivity to insulin, possibly associated with hypokalemia	Changes occur in about one third of treated patients, are usually modest (i.e., 10% increase in fasting glucose) and infrequently require a change in hypoglycemic therapy
Peripheral sympatholytics[45-48]	Improved glucose tolerance	Reduced catecholamine release on nerve stimulation and thus glucose-stimulated insulin secretion is unopposed	This is a minor effect that is probably unimportant clinically
β Blockers[52-60]	Elevated serum glucose (rare), delayed recovery from hypoglycemia and masked hypoglycemic symptoms (nonselective > selective agents)	Reduced insulin secretion, inhibition of catecholamine release subsequent to hypoglycemia and bradycardia secondary to β blockade	Delayed recovery from hypoglycemia and masking of associated symptoms are clinically important, especially in diabetics prone to hypoglycemia; close monitoring is advised
α_2 Agonists[65-74] (clonidine)	Elevated serum glucose, decreased insulin levels, and blunted recovery during the first 15 minutes after hypoglycemia	Reduced insulin secretion through a direct agonist effect on α_2 receptors in pancreatic cells	These are minor effects that are probably unimportant clinically
α_1 antagonist[75-76]	None	...	...
Calcium-channel blockers[78-92]	Elevated serum glucose, decreased glucose tolerance	Reduced calcium influx into pancreatic β cell, decreased cytosolic calcium concentration and thereby reduced insulin secretion	Changes have been reported in a minority of clinical investigations but have been of a magnitude that cannot be ignored; close monitoring is advised
Vasodilators (hydralazine)[76]	None	...	...
Angiotensin-converting enzyme inhibitors (Captopril)[93,94]	Increased rate of glucose disposal	Reduced circulating catcholamines may increase insulin resistance	This is probably not a clinically important effect

Although the potassium-sparing diuretics have been reported to have an adverse effect on glucose tolerance, this effect appears to be uncommon and has been reported only in patients with severe diabetes.[30-33]

Indapamide, a more recently developed benzothiadizine drug, thus far has not been reported to affect glucose tolerance at the recommended antihypertensive doses.[34,35] However, relatively low (nondiuretic) doses of this drug have usually been studied. When higher doses are used (>2.5 mg/day), metabolic abnormalities typically seen with thiazides (including hypokalemia and hyperuricemia) are observed.[36] Further, since a disturbance in carbohydrate metabolism may appear only during long-term drug administration,[35,37] more experience with indapamide is needed to confirm that this drug does not affect glucose tolerance.

Other nonthiazide diuretics have also been reported to impair glucose tolerance. Decreased glucose tolerance has been reported in patients receiving the loop diuretics furosemide and ethacrynic acid.[38-40] Pancreatitis has also been reported in patients receiving these drugs, suggesting a possible direct pancreatotoxic effect.[41,42] The possible contribution of hypokalemia to the diabetogenic effects of these agents has not yet been investigated.

When managing the glucose-intolerant hypertensive patient, it is not necessary to avoid the use of thiazide diuretics. The deterioration in glucose tolerance that may occur is usually modest and should not present a major management problem. Further, the alternatives among the nonthiazide diuretics are less acceptable. In comparison with thiazide diuretics, loop diuretics appear to cause a similar worsening of glucose tolerance and are not as effective in lowering blood pressure. Potassium-sparing diuretics may not cause an alteration in glucose status, but they are inferior hypotensive agents. Indapamide doses that achieve a hypotensive effect similar to that of thiazides may not affect glucose tolerance, but indapamide is much more expensive.

Blood glucose concentrations should be monitored carefully because some of the glucose-intolerant patients who receive a thiazide diuretic will experience a worsening of glucose status. A fasting glucose measurement within one to two weeks after initiation of thiazide therapy is recommended; thereafter, interval measurements should be made as dictated by clinical circumstances. In patients who demonstrate substantial deterioration in glucose status, home glucose monitoring may be helpful to follow the degree of change.

If glucose tolerance is seriously compromised after the initiation of a thiazide diuretic, the patient's potassium status should be evaluated and corrected, if needed, since maintenance of eukalemia may improve glucose tolerance. Any correction of potassium deficiency should be made carefully, however, because of the increased risk of hyperkalemia in diabetics.[10] If potassium therapy fails to correct the problem, more stringent caloric restriction or a modest adjustment in the dose of an oral hypoglycemic agent or insulin may be required.

Adrenergic-Blocking Agents

Insulin secretion is regulated by several mechanisms including the adrenergic nervous system. Stimulation of the α_2-adrenergic receptor inhibits insulin secretion, while stimulation of the β_2-adrenergic receptor promotes insulin secretion.[43] The β_2 effect predominates at the low catecholamine concentrations found under normal physiologic conditions, whereas high catecholamine concentrations activate α_2 receptors and inhibit insulin secretion. Antihypertensive agents that affect adrenergic activity have the potential for altering insulin secretion and interfering with glucose homeostasis.

Peripheral Sympatholytic Agents. Theoretically, agents such as guanethidine and reserpine that deplete presynaptic norepinephrine stores could remove the adrenergic component of control of insulin secretion, leaving other mechanisms that regulate insulin release unopposed. Thus, an antidiabetic or even a hypoglycemic effect may be anticipated with these agents. There is evidence that this may occur (Table 1). Several authors have reported hypoglycemia,[44] reduced insulin requirements,[45] and improved glucose tolerance[46] in diabetic patients taking guanethidine. Reserpine has also been reported to improve glucose tolerance in rats.[47] Kansel et al.[48] compared the effect of reserpine and guanethidine in six healthy men volunteers and found glucose tolerance was better during reserpine therapy but not during guanethidine administration.[48]

The scarcity of literature on the effects of these agents makes it difficult to draw conclusions. However, the evidence suggests the antidiabetic effects of reserpine and guanethidine are modest and clinically unimportant. These agents can be employed in the management of glucose-intolerant hypertensive patients without concern that the patients' glucose status will be compromised.

β-Blocking Agents. The β-adrenoceptor blocking agents are currently widely used in the therapy of hypertension, and are, in some circumstances, recommended as step-1 therapy.[11] However, because of the potentially adverse effects of these drugs on endogenous glucose homeostasis and on the symptomatic response to hypoglycemia (Table 1), questions have been raised about the use of these drugs in patients with diabetes.

One basis for the concern over the use of β blockers is the demonstration in vitro that the pancreatic islet is innervated by the autonomic nervous system and that β-receptor blockade inhibits insulin secretion induced by direct nerve stimulation.[43] In humans, direct stimulation of the β receptor (especially β_2) causes insulin release and also augments glucose-stimulated insulin release.[49] Thus, β blockers would be expected to inhibit insulin secretion and further impair glucose tolerance in diabetics.

Concern over the use of β blockers in diabetics is also related to a potential for interference with recovery from hypoglycemia. Stimulation of β receptors (again primarily β_2) by endogenous epinephrine elevates blood glucose by stimulating hepatic gluconeogenesis. Catecholamine secretion, along with glucagon secretion, serves as the major counterregulatory system for protection from hypoglycemia in normal humans.[50] Many patients with diabetes, however, lack the glucagon component to their response and become totally dependent upon endogenous catecholamines for counterregulation.[51] Accordingly, any interruption of the adrenergic pathway in diabetics might greatly affect glucose homeostasis.

Concern has been expressed that β blockers will disrupt the endogenous catecholamine secretion that is responsible for the clinical signs and symptoms of hypoglycemia: tachycardia, diaphoresis, palpitations, anxiety, tremor, and the elevation of systolic pressure and decrease in diastolic pressure. Thus, recognition of the hypoglycemic state in its early stages might be masked by administration of β blockers.

The influence of β blockers on glucose tolerance has been examined in epidemiologic studies and in clinical trials monitoring plasma insulin and glucose concentrations in response to a defined glucose load. In one crossover study involving 20 patients (16 receiving oral hypoglycemic agents), both metoprolol and propranolol raised fasting, noon, and midafternoon blood glucose concentrations 10–20%.[52] However, the increase was clinically important in only a few of the patients. In another study, the nonselective antagonist alprenolol was compared with metoprolol; alprenolol significantly elevated fasting blood glucose levels and reduced glucose tolerance in response to standard injectable and oral glucose loads.[53] Again, this difference was particularly pronounced in only a few patients.

An interesting issue has been raised by the finding that D-propranolol, which has no appreciable β-adrenoreceptor blocking activity, suppresses glucose-stimulated insulin release as effectively as D,L-propranolol.[54] This suggests that some other property of the molecule, such as membrane stabilization, may be important and that thinking only in terms of β-receptor activity may be an oversimplification.

Published data demonstrating potentiation of hypoglycemia are based on prospective and epidemiologic surveys examining symptomatic episodes in diabetic patients receiving β blockers as well as on controlled trials examining the response to insulin-induced hypoglycemia in diabetics. In one study, Barnett et al.[55] compared 50 insulin-dependent diabetics receiving β blockers (cardioselective agents in seven patients, nonselective agents in the remainder) with 100 matched diabetic controls. The incidence of hypoglycemic symptoms and episodes was the same in both groups. In a larger survey by the British Diabetic Association, none of 152 subjects receiving propranolol were found to suffer a hypoglycemic episode.[56]

Recovery from insulin-induced hypoglycemia has been evaluated in several studies.[57,58] The nonselective β antagonists (propranolol was most frequently examined) consistently delayed recovery from hypoglycemia but did not consistently alter the absolute concentration of glucose at its nadir. The selective antagonists (e.g., metoprolol, atenolol) had less effect on these variables than did the nonselective agents. In some instances, the selective antagonists caused effects that were no different from placebo. Neither the nonselective nor the selective agents affected fasting blood glucose concentrations.

The fear that β blockers might mask the warning symptoms of hypoglycemia has also been closely examined. As noted above, Barnett et al.[55] found no increase in unconsciousness from hypoglycemia in diabetics receiving β-blockade therapy. In patients made hypoglycemic by insulin, treatment with propranolol was found to be associated with significant bradycardia and elevated diastolic blood pressure when compared with placebo, whereas metoprolol had intermediate effects. A number of cases describing increased blood pressure during hypoglycemia in patients receiving propranolol have been reported,[59] including one report of the development of hypertensive crisis.[60] Diaphoresis, a classic symptom of hypoglycemia, is not altered by nonselective β blockade and has actually been noted to be more pronounced with propranolol than with placebo or metoprolol.[57]

In the management of the glucose-intolerant hypertensive patient, β-blocker therapy need not be avoided, although caution should be exercised. With β blockers alone, few patients will experience a clinically important deterioration in glucose status. Combined use of a thiazide diuretic and a β blocker may increase the risk of hyperglycemia, although evidence supporting or refuting this is scarce. Whenever β-blockade therapy is used, careful monitoring of the patient's glucose status is indicated. Measurements one week after initiating therapy and as frequently as clinically indicated thereafter are recommended. On the rare occasion that the elevation in the patient's blood glucose concentration is substantial, the problem should be managed with an alteration in the oral hypoglycemic or insulin dose or, if necessary, discontinuation of the β blocker.

When β blockers are given to insulin-dependent diabetics, especially those prone to hypoglycemia, unique problems may be encountered. If hypoglycemia should occur in these patients, the rate of recovery may be delayed and typical symptoms masked. In these circumstances, cardioselective β blockers are preferred, since they seem to have less effect on blood glucose recovery time and masking of hypoglycemic symptoms. It is advisable that these patients monitor glucose concentrations daily at home and be carefully instructed on ways to identify hypoglycemia. If the diabetic is prone to frequent hypoglycemic episodes, it is best to avoid β-blocker therapy entirely.

α_2 Agonists. Drugs in this class (i.e., clonidine, methyldopa, and guanabenz) might be expected to impair glucose homeostasis in the diabetic hypertensive by inhibiting insulin release. Peripherally, α_2 adrenergic stimulation has been demonstrated to reduce insulin secretion and cause hyperglycemia.[61,62] Studies show that clonidine causes a slight increase in plasma glucose and decrease in insulin concentrations.[63–67] (Table 1).

In a study of tissue from rat pancreas, clonidine had a higher affinity for pancreatic receptors than prazosin, suggesting that these receptors are primarily of the α_2 type.[68] In humans, administration of phentolamine, an α-receptor antagonist, reverses the effect of clonidine on insulin and glucose, lending further support to the presence of an α-adrenergic-mediated mechanism.[65] Clonidine therapy has also been reported to elevate blood glucose in two patients with cervical spinal cord transsections; this suggests a peripheral, rather than a central, mechanism.[65] These data support the hypothesis that clonidine may inhibit insulin secretion and cause hyperglycemia by a direct effect on the α_2 receptors that innervate pancreatic cells.

The effect of clonidine on glucose homeostasis is modest and probably not of clinical importance in most diabetics. In single-dose evaluations, basal plasma glucose increased a mean of 12 mg/dL approximately one hour after clonidine administration and returned to predose levels over the next three hours.[65] After multiple doses, increases of up to 10% in fasting and postprandial glucose concentrations have been reported by some investigators,[65–67] although others have been unable to demonstrate any change.[68–70] The combination of clonidine with a diuretic may cause a further (although still clinically unimportant) increase in fasting concentrations.[69] These effects of clonidine on glucose tolerance have been reported in both normal[65,66] and diabetic hypertensive populations.[67] Whether these effects of clonidine on glucose concentrations are dependent on dose or on duration is not known, since doses greater than 0.4 mg daily and therapy for longer than 10 weeks have not been evaluated.

The fact that clonidine inhibits catecholamine release from adrenergic nerve terminals raises the possibility that recovery of a clonidine-treated diabetic patient from an insulin-induced hypoglycemic episode may be altered. Studies have demonstrated that clonidine markedly delays the catecholamine response in this situation and may blunt the glucose recovery observed during the first 15 minutes after the nadir.[71–72] Thereafter, there is no difference in recovery; return of plasma glucose to baseline levels is usually complete within two hours regardless of whether the patient is pretreated with clonidine.

Methyldopa, which has been inadequately studied, causes either no change in plasma glucose[73] or only a modest elevation.[74] There are no reports of the effect of guanabenz on glucose homeostasis.

Given this evidence, there is no reason to withhold α_2-agonist therapy from glucose intolerant hypertensives or to expect any compromise in glucose status with these agents.

α_1-Blocking Agents. Prazosin, a selective α_1-adrenoreceptor antagonist, is currently the only agent of its class used in the treatment of hypertension. Although published data on this drug in patients with diabetes are not extensive, the available data do not support the occurrence of adverse effects in diabetics.[75] The α_1 receptor does not appear to be involved with insulin secretion or glucose homeostasis.[43] Thus, it is not surprising to find that prazosin did not interfere with glucose control in a diabetic hypertensive population nor alter the response to insulin-induced hypoglycemia in nondiabetic hypertensive subjects.[76] Further, rigorously designed studies, however, are necessary to confirm these favorable observations.

Calcium-Channel-Blocking Agents

The calcium-channel-blocking agents diltiazem, nifedipine, and verapamil are under study for the treatment of hypertension and will probably play increasingly important roles in hypertension management. Preliminary evidence suggests that these drugs have the potential to interfere with insulin secretion and thus may present problems in the management of hypertensives with glucose intolerance (Table 1).

Pancreatic β cells possess voltage-sensitive and voltage-insensitive channels that, when stimulated by glucose or other insulinotropic agents, cause an increased calcium influx across the cell membrane. Insulin secretion from these cells is dependent on a cytosolic accumulation of this cation through stimulus secretion coupling.[77] Drugs that interfere with the passage of calcium into the pancreatic cell, such as calcium-channel-blocking agents, may decrease insulin release and contribute to the development of hyperglycemia. However, because the currently available calcium-channel blockers are chemically dissimilar, there may be differences between these agents and their effects on glucose homeostasis. A number of in vitro investigations support this possibility. For example, studies with isolated pancreatic islet cells in rats demonstrated that verapamil, at very high concentrations, interferes with calcium influx and insulin secretion.[78-79] In vivo animal studies demonstrated that verapamil, at high therapeutic concentrations, caused a 30% reduction in insulin secretion but, at low therapeutic concentrations, caused no change in insulin secretion or glucose levels.[80]

Studies of the effects of calcium-channel blockers on glucose homeostasis in normal humans and in diabetic patients have produced variable results. After up to three months of therapy with the three available calcium-channel blockers in usual therapeutic doses, most studies have shown no changes in fasting glucose concentrations or in blood glucose concentrations after a glucose load.[81-87]

A few studies, however, have demonstrated a substantial diabetogenic effect with nifedipine and verapamil in humans.[88-92] Giugliano et al.,[92] for example, showed that plasma glucose concentrations two hours after a glucose load were approximately 20% higher and insulin concentrations were correspondingly reduced in patients with "chemical diabetes" who were given 30 mg of nifedipine for 10 days. Charles et al.[88] also reported that nifedipine increased plasma glucose concentrations approximately 60% above control values at 60, 90, and 120 minutes and decreased insulin concentrations substantially below control at 30 and 60 minutes in five of six nondiabetic volunteers given a glucose load. The nifedipine dose in this study (60 mg per day), was higher than the doses used in the studies with negative results. This suggests a dose-related effect. In addition, measurements were made after only three days of nifedipine administration, whereas measurements were obtained in most of the other studies after a longer period of time (7, 10, and 30 days). This may indicate that the effect on glucose tolerance occurs with short-term, rather than long-term therapy.

Additional evaluations are required to define the nature and extent of the diabetogenic effect of calcium-channel blockers and to characterize the dose and duration relationships. Until more information is available, the calcium-channel blockers need not be avoided in glucose-intolerant hypertensive patients. A change in glucose tolerance, if it occurs at all, would probably be modest. Monitoring of a patient's glucose status is advised soon after a calcium-channel blocker is initiated (one week) as well as later in the course of therapy (one month). Since tolerance may develop to initial changes in glucose status, no change in the patient's management other than close monitoring of glucose concentrations is recommended when hyperglycemia is seen soon after the initiation of calcium-channel-blocker therapy (as long as the patient is not adversely affected by these initial changes). In the occasional patient who develops a marked and sustained elevation in glucose concentrations, the problem may be managed with an alteration in oral hypoglycemic or insulin doses or possibly by downward titration of calcium-channel-blocker doses.

Other Agents

On the basis of the known mechanisms of insulin secretion and glucose homeostasis, other antihypertensive agents are not expected to interfere with glucose control in the diabetic. This is true for hydralazine, which has been found to cause no change in either baseline plasma glucose or the response to insulin-induced hypoglycemia.[76]

However, captopril has been linked in preliminary reports with an alteration in carbohydrate metabolism. Even though an efficacy and safety investigation of captopril in hypertensive patients has shown no change in plasma glucose,[93] Ferriere et al.[94] reported four cases of unexplained hypoglycemia in diabetics receiving captopril. A subsequent investigation using the euglycemic glucose-clamp technique showed no difference in average blood glucose concentrations before or during captopril therapy but revealed a higher rate of glucose disposal during captopril therapy. Although no mechanisms for the findings were demonstrated, it was speculated that a decrease in circulating catecholamines with captopril decreases insulin resistance. Until more information is available, this should not deter the use of captopril in the management of the glucose-intolerant hypertensive.

Conclusion

Peripheral sympatholytics, α_2 agonists, α_1 antagonists, angiotensin-converting enzyme inhibitors, and vasodilators do not cause clinically important adverse changes in insulin secretion or glucose homeostasis and may be used without concern about compromising the glucose status of most patients. Thiazide and loop diuretics, β blockers, and calcium-channel blockers can cause statistically significant changes in glucose tolerance, but they only rarely cause clinically important alterations. It is unusual for the fasting glucose concentrations to increase more than 20% with any of these agents, and in most instances the change is much less. However, use of these agents together may cause an additive effect and produce a larger elevation in glucose concentrations.

While none of these antihypertensive drugs are

absolutely contraindicated in glucose-intolerant hypertensive patients, in a few patients these agents may cause substantial deterioration in glucose tolerance or increased risk if hypoglycemia should occur. Therefore, clinicians should have a fundamental understanding of the mechanisms of insulin secretion and glucose homeostasis, should be aware that certain drugs may adversely affect this balance, and should be prepared to monitor and manage the patient if problems occur.

References

1. Root HF, Sharkey TP. Arteriosclerosis and hypertension in diabetes. *J Intern Med.* 1936; 9:873–82.
2. Christlieb AR. Diabetes and hypertensive vascular disease. *Am J Cardiol.* 1973; 32:592–606.
3. Hamet P. Metabolic aspects of hypertension. In: Genest S, Kuchel O, Hamet P et al., eds. Hypertension. New York: McGraw-Hill Book Company; 1983; 408–27.
4. Pell S, D'Alonzo CA. Some aspects of hypertension in diabetes mellitus. *JAMA.* 1967; 202:104–10.
5. Tcherdaroff P, Aiach M, Greze M et al. Troubles de la glycoregulation chez 96 hypertendus—etude systematique. *Presse Med.* 1971; 79:2363–6.
6. Kannel WB. Diabetes and cardiovascular disease: the Framingham study: 18 year follow-up. *Cardiol Digest.* 1976; 11:11–5.
7. Christlieb AR, Warram JH, Krolewski AS et al. Hypertension: the major risk factor in juvenile-onset insulin-dependent diabetics. *Diabetes.* 1981; 30(Suppl 2):90–6.
8. Knowler WB, Bennett PH, Ballintine EJ. Increased incidence of retinopathy in diabetics with elevated blood pressure. *N Engl J Med.* 1980; 302:645–50.
9. Mogensen CE. High blood pressure as a factor in the progression of diabetic nephropathy. *Acta Med Scand.* 1970; 602 (Suppl):29–32.
10. Mogensen CE. Renal function changes in diabetics. *Diabetes.* 1976; 25:872–9.
11. The 1984 Report of the Joint National Committee on Detection, Evaluation and Treatment of High Blood Pressure. *Arch Intern Med.* 1984; 144:1045–57.
12. Baum C, Kennedy DL, Forbes MB et al. Drug use in the United States in 1981. *JAMA.* 1984; 251:1293–7.
13. McMahon FC. Management of essential hypertension: the new low-dose era. 2nd ed. Mt. Kisco, NY: Futura Publishing Company, Inc.; 1984.
14. Weidmann P, Gerber A, Mordnini R. Effects of antihypertensive therapy on serum lipoproteins. *Hypertension.* 1983; 5(Suppl III):120–31.
15. European Working Party on Hypertension in the Elderly. Glucose intolerance during diuretic therapy. *Lancet.* 1978; 1:681–3.
16. Shapiro AP, Benedek TG, Small JL. Effect of thiazides on carbohydrate metabolism in patients with hypertension. *N Engl J Med.* 1961; 265:1023–33.
17. Goldner MG, Zarowitz H, Akgun S. Hyperglycemia and glycosuria due to thiazide derivatives administered in diabetes mellitus. *N Engl J Med.* 1960; 262:403–5.
18. Runyan JW. Influence of thiazide diuretics on carbohydrate metabolism in patients with mild diabetes. *N Engl J Med.* 1962; 267:541–3.
19. Hollis WC. Aggravation of diabetes mellitus during treatment with chlorothiazide. *JAMA.* 1961; 176:947–9.
20. Wolff FW, Parmley WW, White K et al. Drug induced diabetes. *JAMA.* 1963; 185:568–74.
21. Barzune LS, Seltzer HS. Impingement of various diabetogenic agents upon beta cell repsonsiveness. *Clin Res.* 1968; 16:32A.
22. Fajans SS, Floyd JC, Knopf RF et al. Benzothiadiazine suppression of insulin release from normal and abnormal islet cell tissue in man. *J Clin Invest.* 1966; 45:481–93.
23. Weller JN, Borondy PE. Effects of benzothiadiazide drugs on carbohydrate metabolism. *Metabolism.* 1965; 14:708–14.
24. Barnett CA, Whitney JE. The effect of diazoxide and chlorothiazide on glucose uptake in-vitro. *Metabolism.* 1966; 15:88–93.
25. Okun R, Russell RP, Wilson WR. Use of diazoxide with trichlormethiazide for hypertension. *Arch Intern Med.* 1963; 112:882–8.
26. Helderman JH, Elahi D, Anderson DK et al. Prevention of glucose intolerance of thiazide diuretics by maintenance of body potassium. *Diabetes.* 1983; 32:106–11.
27. Conn JW. Hypertension, the potassium ion and impaired carbohydrate tolerance. *N Engl J Med.* 1965; 273:1135–43.
28. Rowe JW, Tobin JD, Rosa RM et al. Effects of experimental potassium deficiency on glucose and insulin metabolism. *Metabolism.* 1980; 29:498–502.
29. Gardner LI, Talbot NB, Cook CD et al. The effect of potassium deficiency on carbohydrate metabolism. *J Lab Clin Med.* 1950; 35:592–602.
30. Lowenthal DT, Gould A, Shirk J et al. Effects of amiloride on oral glucose loading, serum potassium, renin and aldosterone in diet controlled diabetes. *Clin Pharmacol Ther.* 1980; 27:671–6.
31. Falch DK, Schreinen A. The effect of spironolactone on lipid, glucose, and uric acid levels in blood during long-term administration in hypertensives. *Acta Med Scand.* 1983; 213:27–30.
32. Spiekerman RE. Potassium sparing effects of triamterene in the treatment of hypertension. *Circulation.* 1966; 34:524–31.
33. Walker BR. Hyperkalemia after triamterene in diabetic patients. *Clin Pharmacol Ther.* 1972; 13:643–51.
34. Royer RJ. Progress in the treatment of hypertension: a multicenter study of indapamide in 442 patients. *Curr Med Res Opin.* 1977; 5 (Suppl 1):151–2.
35. Harrower ABD, McFarlane G, Donnelly T et al. Blood pressure and diabetic control. Results of indapamide treatment. *Practitioner.* 1984; 228:602–3.
36. Furman BL, Razak TBA. A further examination of the possible effects of indapamide on glucose tolerance and insulin secretion in the rat and mouse. *J Pharm Pharmacol.* 1981; 33:735–57.
37. Lewis PJ, Kohner EM, Petrie A et al. Deterioration of glucose tolerance in hypertensive patients on prolonged diuretic treatment. *Lancet.* 1976; 1:564–6.
38. Greenblatt DJ, Duhme DW, Allen MD et al. Clinical toxicity of furosemide in hospitalized patients. *Am Heart J.* 1977; 94(1):6–13.
39. Lowe J, Gray J, Henry D et al. Adverse reactions to furosemide in hospital inpatients. *Br Med J.* 1979; 2:360–2.
40. Tasker PRW, Mitchel-Heggs PF. Non-ketotic diabetic precoma associated with high dose furosemide therapy. *Br Med J.* 1976; 1:626–7.
41. Jones PE, Oelbaum MH. Furosemide induced pancreatitis. *Br Med J.* 1975; 1:133–4.
42. Wilson AE, Mehra SK, Gomersall CR et al. Acute pancreatitis associated with furosemide therapy. *Lancet.* 1967; 1:105.
43. Mahen RE. Pancreatic neuroendocrinology: peripheral neural mechanisms in the regulation of the islets of Langerhans. *Endocrine Rev.* 1981; 2:471–94.
44. Gupta KK. The anti-diabetic actions of guanethidine. *Postgraduate Med J.* 1969; 45:455–7.
45. Gupta KK, Lillicrap CA. Guanethidine and diabetes. *Br Med J.* 1968; 2:697–8.
46. Gupta KK. Guanethidine and glucose tolerance in diabetics. *Br Med J.* 1968; 3:697.
47. Neuvonen PJ, Vapaatolo HI, Torsti P. Tissue catecholamines, blood glucose and plasma free fatty acids after combined treatment with reserpine and diuretics. *Eur J Pharmacol.* 1969; 7:180–5.
48. Kansel PC, Buse J, Durling FC et al. Effect of guanethidine and reserpine on glucose tolerance. *Curr Ther Res.* 1971; 13:517–22.

49. Harns HH, Gouren I, Spoelstra AJG et al. Blockade of isoprenaline-induced changes in plasma free fatty acids, immunoactive insulin levels and plasma renin activity in healthy human subjects by propranolol, pindolol, practolol, atenolol, metoprolol and acebutolol. *Br J Clin Pharmacol.* 1978; 5:19–26.
50. Cryer PE. Glucose counterregulation in man. *Diabetes.* 1981; 30:261–4.
51. Popp DA, Shah SD, Cryer PE. Role of epinephrine-mediated β-adrenergic mechanisms in hypoglycemic glucose counterregulation and posthypoglycemic hyperglycemia in insulin-dependent diabetes mellitus. *J Clin Invest.* 1982; 69:315–26.
52. Wright AD, Barber SG, Kendall MJ et al. Beta-adrenoceptor-blocking drugs and blood sugar control in diabetes mellitus. *Br Med J.* 1979; 1:159–61.
53. Holm G, Johansson S, Vedin A et al. The effect of beta-blockade on glucose tolerance and insulin release in adult diabetes. *Acta Med Scand.* 1980; 208:187–91.
54. Myers MG, Hope-Gill HG. Effect of *d* and *dl*-propranolol on glucose-stimulated insulin release. *Clin Pharmacol Ther.* 1979; 25:303–8.
55. Barnett AH, Leslie D, Watkins PJ. Can insulin-treated diabetics be given beta adrenergic blocking drugs. *Br Med J.* 1980; 280:976–8.
56. Fitzgerald JD. Effects of propranolol on blood sugar, insulin, and free fatty acids. *Diabetologia.* 1968; 5:339.
57. Lager I, Blohme G, Smith U. Effect of cardioselective and non-selective β-blockade on the hypoglycemic response in insulin-dependent diabetics. *Lancet.* 1979; 1:458–61.
58. Ostman J, Arner P, Haglund K et al. A cardio-selective beta blocker (Metoprolol) in hypertensive, insulin-dependent diabetics. *Acta Med Scand* [*Suppl*]. 1980; 639:29–32.
59. Waal-Manning HJ. Can β-blockers be used in diabetic patients? *Drugs.* 1979; 17:157–60.
60. McMurry RL. Propranolol, hypoglycemia and hypertensive crisis. *Ann Intern Med.* 1974; 80:669–70.
61. Robertson RP, Porte D Jr. Adrenergic modulation of basal insulin secretion in man. *Diabetes.* 1973; 22:108.
62. Robertson RP, Halter JB, Porte D Jr. A role for alpha-adrenergic receptors in abnormal insulin secretion in diabetes mellitus. *J Clin Invest.* 1976; 57:791–5.
63. Metz SA, Halter JB, Robertson RP. Induction of defective insulin secretion and impaired glucose tolerance by clonidine. *Diabetes.* 1978; 27:554–62.
64. Saibene V, Martinelli G, Fiammetta V et al. Clonidine effect on insulin secretion and lipolysis in man. *Acta Diabetologia Latina.* 1978; 15:192–7.
65. Guthrie GP, Miller RE, Rotcher TA et al. Clonidine in patients with diabetes and mild hypertension. *Clin Pharmacol Ther.* 1983; 34:713–7.
66. Webster WB, McConnaughey MM. Clonidine and glucose intolerance. *Drug Intell Clin Pharm.* 1982; 16:325–8.
67. Sung PK, Samet P, Yeh BIC. Effects of clonidine and chlorthalidone on blood pressure and glucose tolerance in hypertensive patients. *Curr Ther Res.* 1971; 13:280–5.
68. Raftos J, Bauer GE, Lewis RG et al. Clonidine in the treatment of severe hypertension. *Med J Aust.* 1973; 1:786–93.
69. Kramer VD, Krause W, Renner H. Bericht uber eine langzeitpufuny mit 2-(2,6-dichlorphenyl amino)-2-imidazolin-hydrochlorid. *Arzneimittelforsch.* 1970; 20:519–21.
70. Mroczek WJ, Davidov M, Finnerty FA. Prolonged treatment with clonidine. Comparative antihypertensive effects alone and with a diuretic agent. *Am J Cardiol.* 1972; 30:536–41.
71. Metz SA, Halter JB. Effects of clonidine on hormone and substrate responses to hypoglycemia. *Clin Pharmacol Ther.* 1980; 28:441–8.
72. Hedeland H, Dymling JF, Horfelt B. The effect of insulin induced hypoglycemia on plasma renin activity and urinary catecholamines before and following clonidine (Catapresan) in man. *Acta Endocrinol.* 1972; 71:321–30.
73. Verhiest W, Croonenberghs J, Devos P et al. Double blind cross-over study comparing prazosin and methyldopa in the treatment of mild hypertension. *Acta Cardiol.* 1974; 24:217–33.
74. Benfield GFA, Hunter KR. Oxprenolol, methyldopa and lipids in diabetes mellitus. *Br J Clin Pharmacol.* 1982; 13:219–22.
75. Lipman LG. Special problems in treatment of hypertension in the patient with diabetes mellitus. *Arch Intern Med.* 1984; 144:1829–31.
76. Buzzo LA, Steele JM, Lowenstein J. Unimpaired beta adrenergic responses during prazosin administration. *J Pharmacol Exp Ther.* 1979; 21:345–9.
77. Lebron P, Malaisse WJ, Herchuetz A. Evidence for two distinct modalities of Ca^{+2} influx into pancreatic B cell. *Am J Physiol.* 1982; 242:E59–66.
78. Malaisse WJ, Pipeleers DG, Malaisse-Lagae F et al. Effect of a verapamil derivative (D 600) on calcium uptake and insulin release by isolated islets. *Diabetologia.* 1973; 9:80.
79. Devis G, Somer G, VanObberghen E et al. Calcium antagonists and islet function I. Inhibition of insulin release by verapamil. *Diabetes.* 1975; 24:547–51.
80. Dominiz JA, Miller RE, Anderson J et al. Pharmacology of verapamil II. Impairment of glucose tolerance by verapamil in the conscious dog. *Pharmacology.* 1980; 20:196–202.
81. Donnelly T, Harrower ADB. Effect of nifedipine on glucose tolerance and insulin secretion in diabetic and non-diabetic patients. *Cur Med Res Opin.* 1980; 6:690–3.
82. Greenwood RH. Hyperglycemic effect of nifedipine. *Br Med J.* 1982; 284:50.
83. Anderson DEH, Rojdmark S. Improvement of glucose tolerance by verapamil in patients with non-insulin-dependent diabetes mellitus. *Acta Med Scand.* 1981; 210:27–33.
84. DeMartnis LD, Barbarino A. Calcium antagonists and hormone release I. Effects of verapamil on insulin release in normal subjects and patients with islet-cell tumor. *Metabolism.* 1980; 29:599–604.
85. Segrestaa JM, Caulin C, Dahan R et al. Effects of diltiazem on plasma glucose, insulin and glucagon during an oral glucose tolerance test in healthy volunteers. *Eur J Clin Pharmacol.* 1984; 26:481–3.
86. Abadie E, Gauville C, Brisson C. Nifedipine and endocrine status in diabetic patients. *Br J Clin Pharmacol.* 1984; 18:648–50.
87. Vessby B, Abelin J, Finnson M et al. Effects of nifedipine treatment on carbohydrate and lipoprotein metabolism. *Curr Ther Res.* 1983; 33:1075–81.
88. Charles S, Ketelslegers JM, Guyschaert M et al. Hyperglycemic effect of nifedipine. *Br Med J.* 1980; 283:19–20.
89. Anderson DEH, Rojdmark S, Hed R et al. Effect of verapamil on glucose response to glucagon during intravenous infusion of somatostatin. *Horm Metab Res.* 1980; 12:554–5.
90. Rojdmark S, Anderson DEH, Hed R et al. Effect of verapamil on glucose response to intravenous injection of glucagon and insulin in healthy subjects. *Horm Metab Res.* 1980; 12:285–90.
91. Anderson DEH, Rojdmark S. Effect of verapamil on blood glucose and serum insulin in patients with hyper- and hypothyroidism. *Acta Med Scand.* 1980; 208:375–9.
92. Giugliano D, Torella R, Cacciapuoti F et al. Impairment of insulin secretion in man by nifedipine. *Eur J Clin Pharmacol.* 1980; 18:395–8.
93. Liedtke R, Riedl L. Comparative monitoring of biochemical parameters during treatment with captopril and other antihypertensive agents. *Drug Dev Eval.* 1980; 4:107–22.
94. Ferriere M, Lachkar H, Richard J et al. Captopril and insulin sensitivity. *Ann Intern Med.* 1985; 102:134–5.

Drug-induced systemic lupus erythematosus

MARK A. STRATTON

Abstract: Systemic lupus erythematosus (SLE) induced by drugs, primarily hydralazine and procainamide, is reviewed and compared with idiopathic SLE, and the use of these drugs in patients with idiopathic SLE is discussed.

The etiology of SLE is unclear, but genetic predisposition is an important factor. Although more than 25 drugs have been suggested as causes of SLE, the majority of confirmed cases of drug-induced SLE involve hydralazine or procainamide. Parts of these chemical compounds apparently interact with nucleoproteins, causing stimulation of antinuclear antibody (ANA) production. The average age of patients with drug-induced SLE is nearly twice that of patients with idiopathic SLE. Approximately half the patients with drug-induced SLE are women, compared with 92% of patients with idiopathic SLE. For SLE induced by hydralazine or procainamide, musculoskeletal symptoms (especially arthritis in the hands and wrists) are the most common clinical manifestation. In patients with SLE induced by these drugs, ANAs and LE cells are present, erythrocyte sedimentation rate is often elevated, and a false-positive serologic test for syphilis is seen more frequently than in idiopathic SLE.

Baseline ANA status should be determined before therapy with these drugs, and patients should be observed carefully for signs and symptoms of SLE. Hydralazine-induced SLE may be dose related; limiting the daily dose to 200 mg is recommended. Some drugs have been shown to exacerbate idiopathic SLE; these include estrogen-containing oral contraceptives and ibuprofen. Hydralazine and procainamide are probably safe for use in patients with idiopathic SLE, but alternative therapy should be considered.

The clinical and laboratory manifestations of drug-induced SLE are similar to those of idiopathic SLE, but central nervous system and renal involvement are rare in drug-induced SLE.

Index terms: Age; Cardiac drugs; Dosage; Drugs, adverse reactions; Hydralazine; Hypotensive agents; Lupus; Mechanism of action; Pharmacogenetics; Procainamide; Sex; Toxicity
Clin Pharm. 1985; 4:657–63

The first report of a drug-related syndrome resembling systemic lupus erythematosus (SLE) was published in 1945 and implicated sulfadiazine.[1] More than 25 drugs have since been suggested as causes of an SLE syndrome. However, few large prospective studies have been published; information for most of the agents has been in the form of case reports. Additionally, the patterns described are often labeled "lupus-like" because evidence is insufficient to support a diagnosis of SLE.

Hydralazine and procainamide are the agents most clearly associated with drug-induced SLE.[2] This paper compares the patient characteristics and clinical and laboratory manifestations of SLE caused by hydralazine and procainamide with those of idiopathic SLE and reviews several other drugs less commonly implicated as causes of SLE. The use of these drugs in patients with idiopathic SLE and the monitoring and treatment of drug-induced SLE are discussed.

Etiology and Diagnosis

The causes of SLE remain unknown; genetic, hormonal, viral, and environmental influences have been described.[3] Genetic factors, manifested as defects in B-lymphocyte function, in T-lymphocyte regulation, or both, seem to play the most important role in SLE pathogenesis (Figure 1).[3] According to the proposed mechanism, if the genetic predisposition exists in a particular patient there is excessive B-lymphocyte activation that is initially seen as B-lymphocyte proliferation, possibly from excessive stem-cell activity. The abnormality in B-

Figure 1. Pathogenic factors in systemic lupus erythematosus; ADCC = antibody-dependent cellular cytotoxicity (used with permission of A. Steinberg and the American College of Physicians).

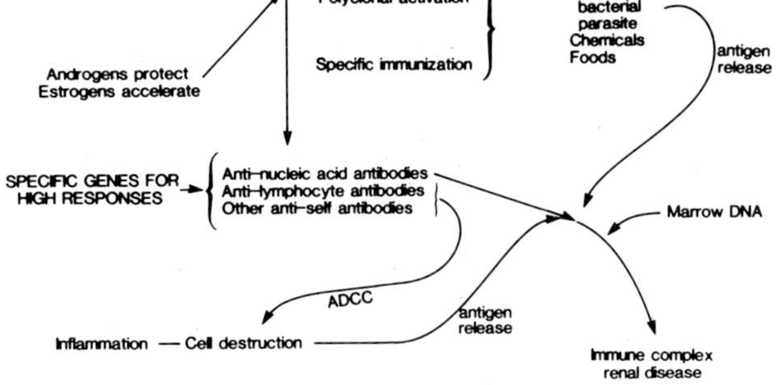

MARK A. STRATTON, PHARM.D., is Associate Professor of Pharmacy and Assistant Professor of Family, Community, and Emergency Medicine, University of New Mexico, Albuquerque, NM 87131.

The assistance of Leslie McCament-Mann, Michael T. Reed, Pharm.D., and William G. Troutman, Pharm.D., is acknowledged.

Presented at the 18th Annual ASHP Midyear Clinical Meeting, Atlanta, Georgia, December 5, 1983.

cell activation may be attributed to several causes, including a defect in regulatory T cells. Eventually, the proliferating B cells differentiate into antibody-forming cells that are responsible for expression of the disease.

Although numerous hypotheses have been proposed to explain the etiology of drug-induced SLE, the exact etiology has not been determined because there is no acceptable animal model that can be used in extensive studies.[2] Early hypotheses suggested that drugs either activated latent SLE or activated an SLE-inducing virus.[4,5] A more recent hypothesis proposes that in genetically susceptible individuals (i.e., slow acetylators) drugs such as procainamide and hydralazine accumulate in their parent form. These compounds have either an amino or a hydrazine group, both of which are highly reactive with nucleoproteins. Because these compounds are capable of freely interacting with sections of DNA, histones, or other nucleoproteins, they can cause these proteins to be antigenic and to stimulate the production of antinuclear antibodies. T lymphocytes may be evoked to help B cells produce the antinuclear antibodies, or B cells may be altered in some other way to allow them to make these antibodies.[5–8]

According to the 1982 revised criteria for the diagnosis of idiopathic SLE,[9] 4 or more of the 11 criteria listed in Table 1 must be present serially or simultaneously during any interval of observation for a diagnosis of SLE to be established. The same criteria should be used for the diagnosis of drug-induced SLE; in addition, it must be established that therapy with the suspected offending agent was initiated before the onset of signs and symptoms and that complete reversal of all clinical and laboratory evidence occurred when the agent was discontinued.[10]

Table 1.
1982 Revised Criteria for Diagnosis of Systemic Lupus Erythematosus

1. Malar rash
2. Discoid rash
3. Photosensitivity
4. Oral ulcers
5. Arthritis (nondeforming; involving two or more joints)
6. Serositis (pleuritis or pericarditis)
7. Renal disorder (proteinuria >0.5 g/day or cellular casts)
8. Neurologic disorder (seizures or psychosis)
9. Hematologic disorder
   - Hemolytic anemia or
   - Leukopenia (<4000 leukocytes/cu mm on two or more occasions) or
   - Lymphopenia (<1500 lymphocytes/cu mm on two or more occasions) or
   - Thrombocytopenia (<100,000 thrombocytes/cu mm in the absence of offending drugs)
10. Immunologic disorder
    - Positive LE cell preparation or
    - Anti-DNA (antibody against native DNA) in abnormal titers or
    - Anti-Sm (antibody against Smith nuclear antigen) in abnormal titers or
    - False-positive test for syphilis
11. Antinuclear antibody in abnormal titers

Demographic Characteristics

Idiopathic SLE occurs at a much earlier age (average of 29 years[11]) than SLE induced by hydralazine (53 years[12]) or procainamide (62 years[13]). These age differences are probably related to the long-term use of these drugs by older patients.[12] Although 89% of patients with idiopathic SLE are women,[11] women compose 64% and 41%, respectively, of patients with SLE induced by hydralazine[12] and procainamide.[14] The underpresentation of men in the idiopathic SLE population may reflect the proposed protective effect of androgens[3]; however, in drug-induced SLE this protective effect is apparently lost. Of patients with idiopathic SLE, 64% are white,[11] but the percentages of drug-induced SLE patients who are white are much higher (86–95% for hydralazine[15] and 95% for procainamide[14]). There is no clear explanation for this observation.

Clinical Manifestations of SLE Associated with Hydralazine and Procainamide

Most reports of drug-induced SLE concern hydralazine or procainamide.

Hydralazine. By 1955, 10 reports of a syndrome resembling SLE associated with hydralazine had appeared in the literature, and by 1975 this number exceeded 150.[10,16] In prospective studies of hydralazine-induced SLE, as many as 54% of patients receiving the drug had positive antinuclear antibody (ANA) test results, and 2–21% of these patients developed signs and symptoms consistent with SLE.[10]

There is a positive relationship between the daily dose of hydralazine and the likelihood of developing ANA positivity, symptoms of SLE, or both. Other predisposing factors for hydralazine-induced SLE include slow-acetylator phenotype, positive personal or family history of other autoimmune diseases, and HLA-DRw4 phenotype.[2,10] For these reasons, a maximum daily hydralazine dose of 200 mg for long-term therapy is recommended, especially in slow acetylators.[17] Although this recommendation has led to a reduction in the incidence of hydralazine-induced SLE,[18–20] the syndrome has been reported in patients receiving daily hydralazine doses of less than 200 mg.

The most common symptoms associated with hydralazine-induced SLE involve the musculoskeletal system (Table 2). The arthritis is usually symmetrical and nondeforming, beginning in the small joints of the hands and wrists and then progressing to the larger joints.[12]

Malaise and fever occur in hydralazine-induced SLE less frequently than in idiopathic lupus. The fever follows no particular temporal pattern and can be associated with sweating and chills.[12]

Pleuropulmonary involvement is also seen less commonly in hydralazine-induced SLE than in idiopathic SLE. In drug-induced SLE the chest roentgenogram often reveals pleural effusions and pleural thickening.[4] Cardiac manifestations are unusual but pericarditis can occur, and pericardial tamponade has been reported.[21,22]

In comparison with idiopathic SLE, renal involvement in hydralazine-induced SLE is unusual, and central nervous system involvement has not been reported.[12,23] The low incidence of renal involvement may be a reflection of the fact that complement levels are usually unchanged in drug-induced SLE and thus deposition of complement with immunoglobulins in the kidney does not occur. However, of all the drug-induced SLE syndromes, that associated with hydralazine probably causes the highest incidence of renal dysfunction.[2]

Procainamide. Procainamide was first reported as a cause of lupus erythematosus by Ladd in 1962.[24] Since this initial report, procainamide has been recognized as the greatest cause of drug-induced SLE and the most potent stimulator of antinuclear antibodies.[4] Antinuclear antibodies are found in 50–100% of all patients receiving procainamide.[2,25] Of these patients, 5–30% develop signs and symptoms of SLE.[2]

As with hydralazine, the most important predisposing factor for the development of procainamide-induced SLE is slow-acetylator phenotype, which was first recognized in 1968.[25] It is clear that the slow-acetylating patient receiving procainamide will develop ANA positivity and symptoms of the SLE syndrome more quickly and at a lower total dose of drug than will the fast acetylator.[2,26] The most comprehensive study to date, published in 1978, revealed that slow acetylators receiving procainamide developed ANA positivity in an average of 2.9 months with a cumulative dose of 1.5 gm/kg and developed symptoms of SLE after one year of drug ingestion.[27] Fast acetylators developed ANA positivity at an average of 7.3 months after a cumulative dose of 6.1 gm/kg and developed symptoms of SLE after four years of drug ingestion.

Acetylation of the primary amine group of procainamide to form *N*-acetylprocainamide apparently results in a lower risk of developing antinuclear antibodies or the lupus syndrome. This issue was first described in a case report of a patient whose lupus symptoms and ANA positivity disappeared when the patient was switched from procainamide to *N*-acetylprocainamide.[28] A more recent prospective study revealed a significantly lower incidence of ANA positivity in patients receiving *N*-acetylprocainamide compared with those receiving procainamide. The few patients who did develop positive ANA tests while receiving *N*-acetylprocainamide did so after a longer course of therapy than with procainamide.[29] To date there have been no case reports of SLE induced by *N*-acetylprocainamide.

As with hydralazine-induced SLE, musculoskeletal complaints are the most common clinical features of SLE induced by procainamide (Table 2).[14] The arthritis is symmetrical and nondeforming, beginning in the small joints of the hands and wrists.

The next most frequent, but the most serious, clinical manifestation is pleuropulmonary involvement, with pleuritis and pleural effusions reported in a slightly greater percentage of patients than with idiopathic lupus (Table 2).[4,14,30]

Pericarditis is reported less frequently than in idiopathic lupus.[4,14,30] Cardiac tamponade and constrictive pericarditis have been reported rarely.[31-33]

In contrast with idiopathic lupus, renal and CNS involvement are rare with procainamide-induced lupus (Table 3).[14,15] There have been at least seven case reports of renal involvement in patients with procainamide-induced lupus,[34,35] fewer reports of renal involvement than with hydralazine.[4] Skin involvement and adenopathy are much less common in procainamide-induced SLE than in idiopathic SLE (Table 2).

Table 2.
Clinical Manifestations of Idiopathic and Drug-Induced SLE[a]

Problem	Idiopathic[11]	Hydralazine[15]	Procainamide[14]
Arthralgias	91.6	92–93	77
Arthritis	. . .	57–76	18
Malaise	. . .	24–37	. . .
Fever	83.6	14–27	45
Skin changes	71.5	24–34	5
Adenopathy	58.6	5–12	9
Myalgias	48.2	. . .	48
Renal involvement	46.1	2–20	
Pleuritis or pleural effusion	45.0	14–25	52
Pericarditis	30.5	. . .	14
CNS involvement	25.5	0	2
Hepatomegaly	. . .	3–45	20
Joint deformity	26	0	0
Splenomegaly	9	8–20	5

[a] Percentage of patients with each type of systemic lupus erythematosus (SLE) in whom the problem has been reported.

Laboratory Findings in SLE Associated with Hydralazine and Procainamide

Hydralazine. Antinuclear antibody positivity is found in virtually all clinically evident cases of hydralazine-induced SLE (Table 3).[7,15,26] A review of available cases did not reveal any particular pattern in elevation of ANA titers. The antinuclear antibodies are directed primarily against dena-

Table 3.
Laboratory Manifestations of Idiopathic and Drug-Induced SLE[a]

Indicator	Idiopathic[11]	Hydralazine[15]	Procainamide[4,14,20,30]
Positive antinuclear antibody test	100%	98%	100%
Presence of LE cells	75.7%	47–80%	77%
Elevated erythrocyte sedimentation rate	. . .	80%	46%
Positive VDRL[b] test	11%	5–41%	28%
Increased immunoglobulin levels	Yes	Slight	Slight
Complement level	Decreased	Usually normal	Usually normal
Anemia	56.5%	6–46%	9–21%
Leukopenia	42.6%	10–24%	2–33%

[a] Percentage of patients with each type of systemic lupus erythematosus (SLE) in whom these laboratory findings have been reported.
[b] Venereal Disease Research Laboratories.

tured or single-stranded DNA, not against native or double-stranded DNA as in idiopathic SLE.[6] Antinuclear antibodies directed against histones are also commonly found.[2]

Other common laboratory findings in hydralazine-induced SLE include elevated erythrocyte sedimentation rate, presence of LE cells, and false-positive serologic test for syphilis (Table 3).[15] Immunoglobulin levels (IgG and IgM) are also commonly elevated, but no consistent pattern of elevation has become evident.[12] Complement levels are almost always normal, but the quantity of complement can be decreased, more often with hydralazine than with other drugs.[2,15] Prolonged coagulation times have been reported rarely, suggesting the presence of circulating antibodies to clotting factors.[12]

The anemia commonly encountered is normocytic and normochromic and is caused by hemolysis.[15] Mild leukopenia is also frequently seen, mild thrombocytopenia is seen rarely.[25]

Procainamide. Antinuclear antibodies are present in 100% of all symptomatic cases of procainamide-induced SLE (Table 3).[14] As with hydralazine-induced SLE, these antibodies are directed against single-stranded DNA and not against double-stranded DNA.[14] Antibodies to ribonucleoprotein and histones are also found.[14] A review of the literature did not reveal any pattern in the elevation of ANA titers.

Other common serologic findings (Table 3) include elevated erythrocyte sedimentation rate, presence of LE cells[3,14] positive rheumatoid factor in 32% of cases,[14] and up to 28% incidence of a false-positive test for syphilis.[14]

Hypergammaglobulinemia occurs in 4% of cases.[4] Normal complement levels are the general rule, but eight cases of hypocomplementemia have been reported.[36] Prolonged coagulation times have been reported rarely, again suggesting the presence of circulating antibodies directed against various clotting factors.[37,38]

The anemia of procainamide-induced SLE is normochromic and normocytic and is thought to be caused by hemolysis.[4,14,30] Mild leukopenia is common, and mild thrombocytopenia occurs in 2–4% of cases.[4,14,30]

Resolution of SLE Induced by Hydralazine or Procainamide

The clinical manifestations of drug-induced SLE resolve in a matter of days to a few weeks after drug withdrawal.[15,30] Aspirin or other nonsteroidal anti-inflammatory agents may help to relieve musculoskeletal problems. More serious pleuropulmonary or pericardial manifestations warrant short-term therapy with prednisone beginning at 40 mg per day.[2]

Laboratory manifestations are much slower to resolve. LE cells may remain for up to 10 months after procainamide withdrawal.[30] ANA positivity can take up to two years to resolve after procainamide[14] and usually several months after hydralazine, but in one case of hydralazine-induced SLE, ANA positivity remained for nine years.[15]

Other Drugs Associated with SLE

Reports have associated several other drugs with the development of SLE.

Isoniazid. SLE caused by isoniazid has been documented in 15–20 cases.[10,39,40] A slow-acetylator phenotype may be an important predisposing factor in the development of ANA positivity and symptoms of SLE.[10,41]

The limited information available on isoniazid-induced SLE suggests that arthritis, arthralgias, and fever are the most common clinical symptoms.[40] Pleuritis and pericarditis have been reported, as has one case of pericardial tamponade.[40]

Antinuclear antibody positivity occurs in about one fourth of patients receiving isoniazid; the antibodies are directed against single-stranded DNA.[10] In patients with symptoms of SLE induced by isoniazid, anemia and an elevated erythrocyte sedimentation rate are quite common, but LE cell positivity is relatively uncommon.[2,39]

Phenothiazines. Chlorpromazine is the most frequently implicated phenothiazine to induce

ANA positivity or the SLE syndrome. One study suggested that ANA positivity could occur in about 25% of patients receiving chlorpromazine.[42] The antibodies are directed against single-stranded DNA.[43] Despite the high incidence of ANA positivity with chlorpromazine use, only a handful of potential cases of chlorpromazine-induced lupus have been reported,[43–45] and only five of these patients meet the criteria for SLE.[43,44]

Anticonvulsants. Since 1945, many case reports have suggested that various anticonvulsants cause an SLE syndrome. Trimethadione, ethosuximide, and the hydantoins have been implicated most frequently.[2,10] A single case of primidone-induced SLE has been reported.[46]

Many of the reports of anticonvulsant-induced SLE are inconclusive. When prospective studies were conducted in children receiving anticonvulsants, ANA positivity was found more frequently than in the control group in two studies,[47,48] and no difference in incidence was found in another study.[49] One of the factors that makes interpretation of reports of anticonvulsant-induced SLE difficult is that seizures may be the initial manifestation of idiopathic SLE. Therefore, while anticonvulsants may induce ANA positivity, their causative role in SLE is inconclusive.

β Blockers. Practolol (which is no longer marketed) was the first β blocker reported to induce a lupus-like syndrome.[50] Pindolol,[51] labetalol,[52] propranolol,[53] and acebutolol[54] have been reported as possible causes of SLE in one patient each. A critical review of these cases reveals that only the patient receiving pindolol met the criteria for a diagnosis of SLE. In a 1980 review of antinuclear antibodies and cardiac drugs, Wilson[26] reported ANA positivity in 25.5% of patients receiving acebutolol, 19.6% receiving labetalol, 9.1% receiving pindolol, and 9.4% receiving propranolol. More recently, in a study comparing the antihypertensive effects of acebutolol and propranolol, ANA positivity was reported in 11% and 5%, respectively, of patients receiving these drugs.

Quinidine. Eleven cases of a quinidine-induced lupus-like syndrome have been described in the literature,[56–61] but only one of these reports meets the criteria for the diagnosis of lupus.[60]

Sulfasalazine. Four possible cases of sulfasalazine-induced SLE have been reported in patients with Crohn's disease, ulcerative colitis, and Sjögren's syndrome[62–65]; only two of these patients fit the criteria for SLE.[64,65] Furthermore, these patients had other autoimmune disorders that may have affected the serologic test results.

Trimethoprim-Sulfamethoxazole. One report has been published of a patient who developed SLE while receiving trimethoprim–sulfamethoxazole.[66] While the patient meets the criteria for lupus, it is difficult to assess the causal role of the antibiotic because the patient had Sjögren's syndrome and was also being treated with isoniazid.

Tetracycline. Three cases of tetracycline-induced SLE were reported in 1959.[67] None of the patients in that report meet the criteria for lupus.

Nitrofurantoin. In 1975, Selroos and Edgren[68] reported that three patients who had chronic pulmonary reactions to nitrofurantoin also developed signs and symptoms of SLE.[68] None of these patients meet the criteria for SLE.

Penicillamine. There has been considerable debate about whether penicillamine is an important cause of an SLE syndrome, which has been reported in 0.4–2.0% of patients receiving this drug.[69] Chalmers et al.[69] described six patients with rheumatoid arthritis; five of these patients clearly developed signs and symptoms consistent with a diagnosis of SLE after penicillamine was initiated. Hypocomplementemia and antibodies to native DNA were present. The issue of penicillamine-induced SLE is complicated because penicillamine is used to treat other autoimmune disorders, which suggests that considerable overlap in serologic tests could occur.

Methyldopa and Levodopa. Both of these agents have been clearly shown to induce positive ANA and Coombs's tests. ANA positivity can be found in 18.5% of patients receiving methyldopa.[2] Two cases of methyldopa-induced SLE have been reported to date,[70,71] but only one of these patients actually meets the criteria for SLE.[70] No conclusive reports of a levodopa-induced SLE have been published.

Lithium. Despite a reported 18% incidence of ANA positivity, no conclusive reports have been published of an SLE syndrome caused by lithium.[72]

Others. One possible case of SLE has been attributed to each of the following agents: propylthiouracil,[73] aminoglutethimide,[74] clofibrate,[75] and phenylbutazone.[76] An assessment of each of these reports revealed that none of the patients fit the criteria for the diagnosis of SLE.

Drug-Induced Exacerbation of Idiopathic SLE

Several authors have studied the effects of drugs in patients with idiopathic SLE. Exacerbation of idiopathic SLE by oral contraceptives was first reported in 1966.[77] Subsequently, worsening of SLE after ingestion of estrogen-containing oral contraceptives has been described.[78–80] A retrospective study by Junger et al.[81] described exacerbation of idiopathic SLE symptoms in 9 of 26 patients receiving estrogen-containing contraceptives.

Estrogens appear to have a deleterious effect on the immune system, while androgenic substances may have a protective effect.[3] Interestingly, none of the 11 patients evaluated prospectively by Junger et al. who received oral contraceptives containing only progestogens experienced worsening of their SLE symptoms. These authors recommended that women with idiopathic SLE use a progestogen-only oral contraceptive if a nonhormonal method of contraception is not acceptable.[81]

Ibuprofen has been reported to exacerbate SLE symptoms.[82,83] In a review of seven cases of SLE, four patients had abnormal liver-function tests with abdominal pain, nausea, and vomiting, in addition to fever and worsening rash.[83] An unusual reaction reported in a patient with SLE who received ibuprofen was aseptic meningitis.[84] This has also been reported in one patient each receiving sulindac[85] and tolmetin.[86]

It is not clear whether agents such as hydralazine or procainamide can safely be used in patients with idiopathic SLE. In a single published report addressing this issue, seven patients with idiopathic SLE were treated with hydralazine for a mean duration of 21 months.[87] None of these patients experienced worsening of their SLE, either clinically or serologically. However, all the patients were also receiving immunosuppressive therapy. Since the pathogenesis for drug-induced SLE is probably different from that for idiopathic SLE, it is probably safe to use hydralazine or procainamide in patients with idiopathic SLE if there is no other acceptable alternative.

Conclusion

The clinical and laboratory manifestations of drug-induced SLE are similar to those of idiopathic SLE. However, central nervous system and renal involvement are rare in drug-induced SLE.

Hydralazine and procainamide are the drugs that pose the most serious threat of inducing SLE. Before initiation of therapy with procainamide or hydralazine, patients' baseline ANA status should be determined. Because subsequent development of ANA positivity does not necessitate the discontinuance of a suspected agent, regularly scheduled testing for ANA is not recommended. However, the patient should be monitored more closely for the development of signs or symptoms of SLE, and the minimum effective dose of the suspected agent should be determined. Should signs or symptoms of SLE develop in patients receiving procainamide or hydralazine, the drug should be discontinued.

References

1. Huffman BJ. Sensitivity to sulfadiazine resembling acute disseminated lupus erythematosus. *Arch Dermatol Syph.* 1945; 51:190–2.
2. Weinstein A. Drug-induced systemic lupus erythematosus. *Prog Clin Immunol.* 1980; 4:1–21.
3. Steinberg AD, Raveche ES, Laskin CA et al. Systemic lupus erythematosus: insights from animal models. *Ann Intern Med.* 1984; 100:714–27.
4. Alarcon-Segovia D. Drug induced lupus syndrome. *Mayo Clin Proc.* 1969; 44:664–81.
5. Holm G. Immunological side-effects of antihypertensive drugs. *Acta Med Scand (Suppl).* 1978; 628:85–8.
6. Tan EM. Drug-induced autoimmune disease. *Fed Proc.* 1974; 33:1894–7.
7. Shoen RT, Trentham DE. Drug-induced lupus: an adjuvant disease? *Am J Med.* 1981; 71:5–8.
8. Parker CW. Hapten immunology and allergic reactions in humans. *Arthritis Rheum.* 1981; 24:1024–36.
9. Tan EM, Cohen AS, Fries JF et al. The 1982 revised criteria for the classification of systemic lupus erythematosus. *Arthritis Rheum.* 1982; 25:1271–7.
10. Lee SL, Chase PH. Drug-induced systemic lupus erythematosus. A critical review. *Semin Arthritis Rheum.* 1975–6; 5:83–103.
11. Dubois EL. The clinical picture of systemic lupus erythematosus. In: Dubois EL, ed. Lupus erythematosus. Los Angeles: University of Southern California Press; 1976; 232–379.
12. Alarcon-Segovia D, Wakim KG, Worthington SW et al. Clinical and experimental studies on the hydralazine syndrome and its relation to SLE. *Medicine.* 1967; 46:1–31.
13. Muna W, Osterman FA, Stevens MB et al. Procainamide-induced lupus. *Johns Hopkins Med J.* 1976; 138:289–95.
14. Blomgren SE, Condem JS, Vaughan JH. Procainamide-induced lupus erythematosus. *Am J Med.* 1972; 52:338–48.
15. Perry HM. Late toxicity to hydralazine resembling systemic lupus erythematosus or rheumatoid arthritis. *Am J Med.* 1973; 54:58–73.
16. Henn MJ, Parkin TW, Hargraves MM et al. Acute systemic lupus erythematosus from hydralazine hydrochloride. *Arch Intern Med.* 1955; 95:857–62.
17. American hospital formulary service–drug information 85. McEvoy GK, ed. Hydralazine hydrochloride. Bethesda, MD: American Society of Hospital Pharmacists; 1985:660–3.
18. Berkowitz HS. Disseminated lupus erythematosus. *S Afr Med J.* 1976; 50:797. Letter.
19. Ramsay LE, Silas J, Freestone S. Hydralazine antinuclear antibodies and the lupus syndrome. *Br Med J.* 1982; 284:1711. Letter.
20. Chisholm JC. Acute low-dose hydralazine induced lupus syndrome. *J Natl Med Assoc.* 1981; 73:278–80.
21. Aylward PE, Tonkin AM. Cardiac tamponade in hydralazine induced systemic lupus erythematosus. *Aust NZ J. Med.* 1982; 12:546–9.
22. Carey RM, Coleman M, Feder A. Pericardial tamponade: a major presenting manifestation of hydralazine induced lupus syndrome. *Am J Med.* 1973; 54:84–7.
23. White AB. Hydralazine lupus with fatal renal failure. *J Am Geriatr Soc.* 1966; 14:361–5.
24. Ladd AT. Procainamide-lupus erythematosus. *N Engl J Med.* 1962; 267:1357–8.
25. Lappat ES, Cowan MJ. A familial study of procainamide-induced systemic lupus erythematosus. *Am J Med.* 1968; 45:846–52.
26. Wilson JD. Antinuclear antibodies and cardiovascular drugs. *Drugs.* 1980; 19:292–305.
27. Woosley RL, Drayer DE, Reidenberg MM et al. Effect of acetylator phenotype on the rate at which procainamide induces antinuclear antibodies and the lupus syndrome. *N Engl J Med.* 1978; 298:1157–9.
28. Stec GP, Lertova JJL, Atkinson AS et al. Remission of procainamide-induced lupus erythematosus with *N*-acetylprocainamide therapy. *Ann Intern Med.* 1979; 90:799–801.
29. Lahita R, Kluger J, Drayer DE et al. Antibodies to nuclear antigens in patients treated with procainamide or acetylprocainamide. *N Engl J Med.* 1979; 301:1382–5.
30. Dubois EL. Procainamide induction of a systemic lupus erythematosus-like syndrome. *Medicine.* 1969; 48:217–28.
31. Donlan CJ, Forker AD. Cardiac tamponade in procainamide-induced lupus erythematosus. *Chest.* 1972; 61:685–6.
32. Ghose MK. Pericardial tamponade: a presenting manifestation of procainamide-induced lupus erythematosus. *Am J Med.* 1975; 58:581–5.
33. Sunder SK, Shah A. Constrictive pericarditis in procainamide-induced lupus erythematosus syndrome. *Am J Cardiol.* 1975; 36:960–2.

34. Whittle TS, Ainsworth SK. Procainamide-induced systemic lupus erythematosus. *Arch Pathol. Lab Med.* 1976; 100:469–74.
35. Zech P, Colon S, Labeeur M et al. Nephrotic syndrome in procainamide-induced lupus nephritis. *Clin Nephrol.* 1979; 11:218–21.
36. Mohan-Rao KVR, Diaz R, Quigley TJ. Procainamide-induced systemic lupus erythematosus with hypocomplementemia. *J Amer Geriatr Soc.* 1977; 25:230–1.
37. Bell WR, Boss GR, Wolfson JS. Circulating anticoagulant in the procainamide-induced lupus syndrome. *Arch Intern Med.* 1977; 137:1471–3.
38. Edwards RL, Rick ME, Wakem CJ. Studies on a circulating anticoagulant in procainamide-induced lupus erythematosus. *Arch Intern Med.* 1981; 141:1688–90.
39. Siegel M, Lee SL, Peress NS. The epidemiology of drug-induced systemic lupus erythematosus. *Arthritis Rheum.* 1967; 10:407–15.
40. Greenberg JH, Lutcher CL. Drug-induced systemic lupus erythematosus. *JAMA.* 1972; 222:191–3.
41. Reidenberg MM. The chemical induction of systemic lupus erythematosus and lupus-like illnesses. *Arthritis Rheum.* 1981; 24:1004–9.
42. Berglund S, Gottfries CG, Gottfries I et al. Chlorpromazine-induced antinuclear factors. *Acta Med Scand.* 1970; 187:67–74.
43. Dubois EL, Tallman E, Wonka RA. Chlorpromazine-induced systemic lupus erythematosus. *JAMA.* 1972; 221:595–6.
44. Fabius AJM, Gaulhofer WK. Systemic lupus erythematosus induced by psychotropic drugs. *Acta Rheum Scand.* 1971; 17:137–47.
45. Goldman LS, Hudson JI, Weddington WW. Lupus-like illness associated with chlorpromazine. *Am J Psychiatry.* 1980; 137:1613–4.
46. Ahuja GK, Schumacher GA. Drug-induced SLE: primidone as a possible cause. *JAMA.* 1966; 198:201–3.
47. Beernink DH, Miller JJ. Anticonvulsant-induced antinuclear antibodies and lupus-like disease in children. *Pediatr Pharmacol.* 1973; 88:113–7.
48. Singsen BH, Fishman L, Hanson V. Antinuclear antibodies and lupus-like syndrome in children receiving anticonvulsants. *Pediatrics.* 1976; 57:529–34.
49. Anderson P, Mosekilde L. Immunoglobulin levels and autoantibodies in epileptics on long term anticonvulsant therapy. *Acta Med Scand.* 1977; 201:69–74.
50. Raferty EB, Denman AM. Systemic lupus erythematosus induced by practolol. *Br Med J.* 1973; 2:452.
51. Bensaid J, Aldigier JC, Gaulde N. SLE syndrome induced by pindolol. *Br Med J.* 1979; 1:1603–4.
52. Brown RC, Cooke J, Losowsky MS. SLE syndrome, probably induced by labetalol. *Postgrad Med J.* 1981; 57:189–90.
53. Harrison T, Siscats J, Wood WH. Propranolol-induced lupus syndrome. *Postgrad Med.* 1976; 59:241–4.
54. Record NB. Acebutolol-induced pleuropulmonary lupus syndrome. *Ann Intern Med.* 1981; 95:326.
55. Wahl J, Turlapaty P, Singh BW. Comparison of acebutolol and propranolol in essential hypertension. *Am Heart J.* 1985; 109:313–21.
56. Kendall MJ, Hawkins CF. Quinidine-induced systemic lupus erythematosus. *Postgrad Med J.* 1970; 46:729–31.
57. Anderson FP, Wanerka GR. Drug induced systemic lupus erythematosus due to quinidine. *Conn Med.* 1972; 36:84–5.
58. Donoho CR, Pascual E. Quinidine induced lupus erythematosus. *Arthritis Rheum.* 1974; 17:322. Abstract.
59. Yudis M, Meehan JJ. Quinidine-induced lupus nephritis. *JAMA.* 1976; 235:2000.
60. West SG, McMahon M, Portanora JP. Quinidine-induced lupus erythematosus. *Ann. Intern Med.* 1984; 100:840–2.
61. Lavie CJ, Biundo J, Quinet RJ et al. Systemic lupus erythematosus (SLE) induced by quinidine. *Arch Intern Med.* 1985; 145:446–8.
62. Griffiths ID, Kane SP. Sulphasalazine-induced lupus syndrome in ulcerative colitis. *Br Med J.* 1977; 2:1188–9.
63. Rafferty P, Young AC, Haeney MR. Sulphasalazine-induced cerebral lupus erythematosus. *Postgrad Med J.* 1982; 58:88–99.
64. Crisp AJ, Hoffbrand BI. Sulphasalazine-induced SLE in a patient with Sjögrens syndrome. *J R Soc Med.* 1980; 73:60–1.
65. Carr-Locke DL. Sulfasalazine-induced lupus in a patient with Crohn's disease. *Am J Gastroenterol.* 1982; 77:614–5.
66. Grennan DM, Bell G, Rooney PJ et al. SLE precipitated by antibodies in a patient with Sjögrens syndrome and rheumatoid arthritis. *Br Med J.* 1977; 2:1188–9.
67. Domz CA, McNamara DH, Holzapfel HF. Tetracycline provocation in lupus erythematosus. *Ann Intern Med.* 1959; 50:1217–26.
68. Selroos O, Edgren J. Lupus-like syndrome associated with pulmonary reaction to nitrofurantoin. *Acta Med Scand.* 1975; 197:125–9.
69. Chalmers A, Thompson D, Stein HE et al. Systemic lupus erythematosus during penicillamine therapy for rheumatoid arthritis. *Ann Intern Med.* 1982; 97:659–63.
70. Dupont A, Six R. Lupus-like syndrome induced by methyldopa. *Br Med J.* 1982; 285:693–4.
71. Harrington TM, Davis DE. Systemic lupus-like syndrome induced by methyldopa therapy. *Chest.* 1981; 79:696–7.
72. Presley AP, Kahn A, Williamson W. Antinuclear antibodies in patients taking lithium carbonate. *Br Med J.* 1976; 2:280–1.
73. Amrhein JA, Kenny FM, Ross D. Granulocytopenia, lupus-like syndrome and other complications of propylthiouracil therapy. *J Pediatr.* 1970; 76:54–63.
74. McCraken M, Benson EA, Hickling P. SLE induced by aminoglutethimide. *Br Med J.* 1980; 281:1254.
75. Howard EJ, Brown SM. Clofibrate induced antinuclear factor and lupus-like syndrome. *JAMA.* 1973; 226:1358–9. Letter.
76. Farid N, Anderson J. SLE-like reaction after phenylbutazone. *Lancet.* 1971; 1:1022–3. Letter.
77. Primstone B. Systemic lupus erythematosus exacerbated by oral contraceptives. *S Afr J Obstet Gynecol.* 1966; 462–3.
78. Chapel TA, Burns RE. Oral contraceptives and exacerbation of lupus erythematosus. *Am J Obstet Gynecol.* 1971; 110:366–9.
79. Elias PM. Erythema nodosum and serological lupus erythematosus: simultaneous occurrence in a patient using oral contraceptives. *Arch Dermatol.* 1973; 108:716–8.
80. Garovich M, Agudelo C, Pisko E. Oral contraceptives and systemic lupus erythematosus. *Arthritis Rheum.* 1980; 23:1396–8.
81. Jungers P, Dougados M, Pelissier C et al. Influence of oral contraceptive therapy on the activity of systemic lupus erythematosus. *Arthritis Rheum.* 1982; 25:618–21.
82. Shoenfeld Y, Livni E, Shaklaim C et al. Sensitization to ibuprofen in systemic lupus erythematosus. *JAMA.* 1980; 244:547–8. Letter.
83. Sonnenblick M, Abraham AS. Ibuprofen hypersensitivity in systemic lupus erythematosus. *Br Med J.* 1978; 1:619–20.
84. Widener HL, Lihman BH. Ibuprofen-induced meningitis in systemic lupus erythematosus. *JAMA.* 1978; 239:1062–4.
85. Ballas ZK, Donta ST. Suldinac-induced aseptic meningitis. *Arch Intern Med.* 1982; 142:165–6.
86. Ruppert GB, Barth WF. Tolmetin-induced aseptic meningitis. *JAMA.* 1981; 245:67–8.
87. Reza MJ, Dornfeld L, Goldberg LS. Hydralazine therapy in hypertensive patients with idiopathic systemic lupus erythematosus. *Arthritis Rheum.* 1975; 18:335–8.

Research

Pharmacokinetics of high-dose azlocillin sodium in patients with cystic fibrosis

ROGER A. WOOLF, JEFFREY R. KOUP, ARNOLD L. SMITH, BETTINA C. HILMAN, DONALD GOLDMANN, AND JUDY WILLIAMS-WARREN

Abstract: The pharmacokinetics of high-dose azlocillin sodium was studied in 18 patients with cystic fibrosis.

Nine male and nine female patients with a mean age of 14.7 years (range 3 to 29 years) participated in the study. They received azlocillin 450 mg/kg/day (as the sodium salt) in six divided doses. During a steady-state dosing interval, a dose of azlocillin was coadministered with a 10-mg/kg dose of iothalamate sodium as a 30-minute infusion. Serum concentrations of azlocillin and iothalamate were determined by high-pressure liquid chromatography assay. The data were analyzed using model-independent methods.

The mean elimination rate constant for azlocillin was 0.64 ± 0.22 hr^{-1} and the mean serum half-life was 1.22 ± 0.39 hr. Total clearance of azlocillin, calculated by noncompartmental analysis, was 77.2 ± 26.4 mL/min/sq m. Glomerular filtration rate, as estimated by measuring iothalamate clearance, was 79.6 ± 21.9 mL/min/sq m. The total clearance of azlocillin correlated with iothalamate clearance.

Patients with cystic fibrosis appear to eliminate azlocillin more rapidly than healthy individuals. This rapid elimination warrants the use of high doses to maintain high serum concentrations.

Index terms: Azlocillin; Azlocillin sodium; Blood levels; Cystic fibrosis; Dosage; Excretion; Half-life; Iothalamate; Iothalamate sodium; Penicillins; Pharmacokinetics; Roentgenographic agents
Clin Pharm. 1985; 4:664–9

Azlocillin sodium is a new ureidopenicillin, a class of antibiotics that also includes mezlocillin sodium and piperacillin sodium. These penicillins have a broad spectrum of antimicrobial activity and also some unusual pharmacokinetic properties. One unique property is that these agents clearly exhibit dose-dependent pharmacokinetics.[1–4] This phenomenon appears to be most pronounced for azlocillin,[4] but it is also seen with mezlocillin and piperacillin. Altered pharmacokinetics have been described with β-lactam antibiotics in patients with cystic fibrosis.[5] Disease-associated pharmacokinetic differences consist of higher plasma clearance values and lower serum concentrations. The recommended adult dosage of azlocillin for serious infections is 200–300 mg/kg (as the sodium salt) per day. Only limited data are available on the use of high-dose azlocillin in patients with cystic fibrosis. Since azlocillin exhibits dose-dependent pharmacokinetics and cystic fibrosis patients appear to eliminate β-lactam antibiotics differently, we studied the pharmacokinetics of high-dose azlocillin sodium in these patients.

Methods

Patients. Eighteen patients with cystic fibrosis were evaluated. Nine male and nine female pa-

ROGER A. WOOLF, PHARM.D., is a resident in pharmacy administration, University of California, San Francisco. At the time of this study, he was a Pharm.D. candidate, School of Pharmacy, University of Washington. JEFFREY R. KOUP, PHARM.D., is Associate Professor of Pharmacy Practice and Pediatrics, University of Washington. ARNOLD L. SMITH, M.D., is Professor of Pediatrics, University of Washington, and Head, Division of Infectious Disease, Childrens Orthopedic Hospital and Medical Center, Seattle. BETTINA C. HILMAN, M.D., is Professor of Pediatrics, Louisiana State University, Shreveport. DONALD GOLDMANN, M.D., is Associate Professor of Pediatrics, Harvard Medical School, Childrens Hospital and Medical Center, Boston. JUDY WILLIAMS-WARREN is Research Nurse, Division of Infectious Disease, Childrens Orthopedic Hospital and Medical Center, Seattle.

Address reprint requests to Dr. Koup at the Department of Pharmacy Practice, SC-69, University of Washington, Seattle, WA 98105.

Presented at the 20th Annual ASHP Midyear Clinical Meeting, New Orleans, LA, December X, 1985.

tients made up the study population with a mean age of 14.7 years (range 3 to 29 years). All patients had a Shwachman score[6] between 40 and 75 and a Taussig score[7] between 50 and 90.[a,b] Additional patient information is listed in Table 1. The study was approved by the Institutional Review Board of our institution, and informed consent was obtained from all of the participants.

Drug Therapy. The patients received azlocillin (supplied by Miles Pharmaceuticals) 450 mg/kg/day (as the sodium salt) in six divided doses. All but two patients also received tobramycin 5.0–11.2 mg/kg/day (as the sulfate salt) in three or four divided doses. Tobramycin was administered as a 30-minute intravenous infusion that was completed at least 30 minutes before the azlocillin infusion was initiated.

The azlocillin dose was dissolved in sterile water and then diluted to 100 mL with 5% dextrose injection in 0.9% sodium chloride. Just before administration, a 10-mg/kg dose of iothalamate sodium was added (Conray 400, Mallinckrodt Chemical Corp., St. Louis, MO), and the solution was mixed by inversion. In a preliminary study that we conducted, azlocillin and iothalamate showed no interactions in solution when mixed at room temperature and frozen; these solutions were stable for up to a week. The azlocillin and iothalamate were administered in a 30-minute infusion at a constant rate using a Harvard infusion pump.

Serum samples were collected immediately before the infusion was started and at 30, 60, 90, 180, and 240 minutes after the infusion began. The blood was allowed to clot, and the serum was removed and stored at −70 °C until time of assay.

Serum concentrations of azlocillin were determined by a high-pressure liquid chromatography (HPLC) assay.[8] This method correlates well with the microbiological assay and is sensitive to 0.4 μg/mL of azlocillin. The precision was reflected by coefficients of variation of 4.2% and 5.6% at 50 μg/mL and 10 μg/mL, respectively. Iothalamate concentrations were also determined by an HPLC assay developed in our laboratory.[9]

Pharmacokinetic Analysis. The data were analyzed using model-independent methods. The terminal elimination rate constant (β) was estimated using a nonlinear regression-analysis program.[10] Data were weighted as one divided by the concentration squared, and a simplex-fitting algorithm was employed.

The total clearance was calculated by a noncompartmental analysis of all the serum concentration data.[11] The relationship assumed by this technique is that total clearance is equal to dose divided by the area under the serum concentration curve from time zero to infinity (AUC). The log trapezoidal rule was used to estimate AUC from time zero to the last sampling point. The AUC from the last sampling point to time infinity was estimated by dividing the last concentration value by the elimination rate constant.

The apparent volume of distribution at steady state (V_{ss}) was calculated from the following equation[11]:

$$V_{ss} = [D\,(\mathrm{AUMC})/(\mathrm{AUC})^2] - [D\,(T)/2(\mathrm{AUC})]$$

where D is the dose, AUMC is the total area under

Table 1.
Characteristics of Patients in the Study

Patient Number	Age (yr)	Sex (M/F)	Weight (kg)	BSA[a] (sq m)	Serum Creatinine (mg/dL)	Dose (mg)
1	19	M	47.5	1.49	0.8	3600
2	8	F	29.5	1.05	0.6	2200
3	4	F	13.5	0.61	0.5	1013
4	29	F	45.0	1.37	0.6	3400
5	21	M	66.5	1.81	0.9	5000
6	4	M	11.7	0.55	0.3	900
7	13	F	21.4	0.88	0.5	1600
8	13	M	34.5	1.19	0.6	2820
9	16	F	39.0	1.25	0.6	3066
10	18	M	37.1	1.25	0.6	2821
11	29	F	57.2	1.63	1.1	4300
12	15	F	37.7	1.27	0.6	2850
13	13	M	35.2	1.19	0.5	2650
14	15	F	40.4	1.33	0.5	3100
15	3	F	16.3	0.68	0.6	1140
16	13	M	29.0	1.07	0.5	2200
17	18	M	56.4	1.61	0.9	4200
18	13	M	48.7	1.52	0.9	3653
Mean ± S.D.	14.7 ± 7.1		37.0 ± 14.9	1.21 ± 0.35	0.64 ± 0.19	2806 ± 1122

[a] Body surface area (BSA) calculated using the method described by Haycock et al.[13]

the first moment curve, and T is the duration of infusion.

The apparent volume of the terminal slope (V_β) was also determined for comparison with the results of previous studies. V_β was calculated by dividing the total body azlocillin clearance by the elimination rate constant, assuming $V_\beta = CL_\beta/\beta$.

Values for the glomerular filtration rate (GFR) were estimated in 14 patients by measuring the plasma iothalamate clearance. This clearance was calculated using the noncompartmental analysis described above. This method provides an estimate of GFR that correlates well with that measured by standard inulin-infusion methods.[12]

Since creatinine clearance (CL_{cr}) is generally reported after there has been a correction made for body surface area (L/min/sq m) we corrected the volume of distribution and all the clearance values to surface area. Body surface was calculated using the method of Haycock et al.[13]

Least-squares, linear-regression analysis was used to determine the correlation between azlocillin and iothalamate clearances. The level of significance was set at $p < 0.05$.

Results

The mean azlocillin serum concentrations (±S.D.) are presented in Figure 1. For all patients, the trough concentrations taken just before the dose averaged 50 ± 40 μg/mL and the mean peak concentration at the end of infusion averaged 381 ± 100 μg/mL.

The pharmacokinetic values for azlocillin and estimates of glomerular filtration rate are shown in Table 2. For all patients, the average azlocillin clearance was 77.2 ± 26.4 mL/min/sq m, the apparent volume of distribution at steady state was 7.1 ± 2.1 L/sq m, and the elimination half-life was 1.22 ± 0.39 hr.

The mean iothalamate clearance was 79.6 ± 21.9 mL/min/sq m. This correlated with the mean azlocillin clearance (Figure 2). Regression analysis of iothalamate clearance (X) versus azlocillin clearance (Y) resulted in the following regression equation: $Y = -12.14 + 1.15X$. The 95% confidence interval of the intercept for this regression analysis was from −40.3 to 15.75. The mean estimated creatinine clearance value also correlated with the azlocillin clearance value.

Figure 1. Mean (±S.D.) serum azlocillin concentration versus time (n = 18).

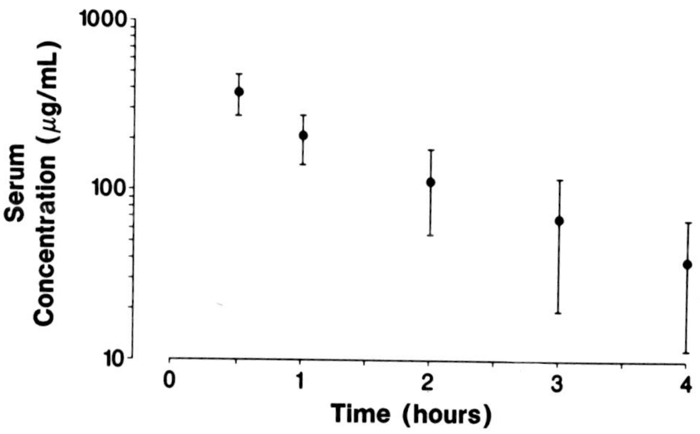

Table 2.
Pharmacokinetic Variables

Patient Number	Peak Concentration[a] (μg/mL)	β (hr^{-1})	$t_{1/2}$ (hr)	V_β (L/sq m)	V_{ss} (L/sq m)	Total Body Clearance (mL/min/sq m) Azlocillin	Iothalamate	Creatinine[b]
1	302	0.39	1.76	12.3	11.0	80.6	78.6	68.0
2	279	1.12	0.62	5.5	6.0	102.6	84.6	72.6
3	416	1.03	0.68	3.8	3.3	64.2	74.6	63.0
4	420	0.47	1.48	8.8	7.7	68.4	83.0	80.0
5	390	0.40	1.74	8.7	8.2	57.5	57.6	63.2
6	190	0.85	0.82	11.3	9.4	159.0	136.0	98.0
7	250	0.68	1.01	8.4	8.0	95.6	104.6	85.2
8	420	0.86	0.81	5.8	5.2	82.6	91.5	80.0
9	460	0.55	1.25	7.4	6.7	68.5	71.4	76.3
10	460	0.46	1.50	8.4	7.6	64.3	62.5	82.1
11	445	0.41	1.68	6.2	6.6	42.4	. . .[c]	48.4
12	478	0.77	0.90	5.9	4.8	75.0	. . .[c]	82.7
13	250	0.72	0.97	9.0	9.6	106.8	93.4	94.1
14	542	0.54	1.28	5.2	4.5	46.9	71.1	102.1
15	434	0.76	0.92	4.0	4.0	50.8	42.0	53.2
16	295	0.56	1.23	9.4	7.4	88.2	. . .[c]	92.2
17	497	0.51	1.37	8.0	6.8	67.8	. . .[c]	58.3
18	326	0.37	1.88	11.4	10.7	68.6	63.9	62.2
Mean ± S.D.	381 ± 100	0.64 ± 0.22	1.22 ± 0.39	7.7 ± 2.4	7.1 ± 2.1	77.2 ± 26.4	79.6 ± 21.9	75.6 ± 15.2

[a] Samples for peak concentrations drawn at the end of a 30-minute infusion.
[b] Creatinine clearance was estimated using the method described by Schwartz et al.[26]
[c] Iothalamate clearance was not determined.

Discussion

The pharmacokinetic characteristics of the ureidopenicillins are similar to those of other penicillins. They have a small distribution volume producing high peak serum concentrations and high plasma clearance values seen in the rapid elimination from the plasma. These antibiotic agents are eliminated by both renal and nonrenal routes.[14] Ureidopenicillins are unique in that they exhibit dose-dependent pharmacokinetics. This was first demonstrated for mezlocillin[1] and later for azlocillin[2,4] and piperacillin.[3] Azlocillin pharmacokinetics have been described for normal patients and patients with cystic fibrosis, and dose-dependent kinetics have been found in both populations.[15–18]

Bergan et al.[4] described the pharmacokinetics of azlocillin in healthy adult individuals after a single intravenous bolus dose of 5.0 g (approximately 75 mg/kg). They reported a serum half-life of 1.53 hr and a total clearance of 1.57 mL/min/kg in these individuals. The comparison of these data with our results (Table 3) supports the theory that azlocillin is more rapidly eliminated in patients with cystic fibrosis. We used a similar dose on a milligram per kilogram basis and found the half-life (1.22 hr) shorter and the total clearance (2.76 mL/min/kg) substantially greater in our patients with cystic fibrosis compared with their healthy adult patients.

Figure 2. Correlation of azlocillin clearance with iothalamate clearance for 14 patients. Solid line represents the least-squares regression line ($Y = -12.14 + 1.15X$; $r = 0.90$, $p < 0.001$).

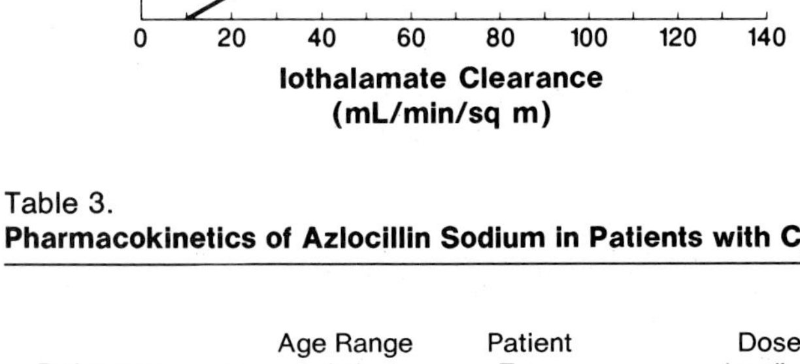

In the study by Bosso et al.,[18] the pharmacokinetic characteristics of azlocillin were described in 10 patients with cystic fibrosis after they received 350 mg/kg/day in four to six divided doses. Eight of the patients received 87.5 mg/kg every six hours. The calculated mean values for peak serum concentration, half-life, and total clearance were 389 μg/mL, 1.74 hr, and 2.05 mL/min/kg, respectively. The shorter half-life and higher clearance values in our patients suggested slightly more rapid elimination. However, comparison of these studies is difficult because of the small number of patients in each study and the small differences in the amounts of the administered doses.

The differences in the pharmacokinetic values may be explained by variations in the patient characteristics alone. The difference in results may also be explained by the different methods and data analysis used by the various investigators. First, Bosso et al.[18] used a nonspecific microbiologic assay. Although they attempted to remove the aminoglycoside, a positive interference could have occurred that would have caused the variation in the clearance values derived by the two studies. They also collected samples over a longer period of time, which could have produced a longer elimination half-life estimate.

The elimination pharmacokinetics of a number of β-lactam antibiotics have been demonstrated to be different in patients with cystic fibrosis compared with the normal population. This difference has been described most clearly for the penicillins. Jusko et al.[19] first demonstrated the increased clearance of dicloxacillin in patients with cystic fibrosis. Higher clearance values and consequently lower serum concentrations have also been demonstrated for methicillin,[20] azlocillin,[16,18] cloxacillin,[21] and piperacillin.[22] The reason for the increased clearances is still unclear. Many authors have speculated that increased active secretion is responsible for the increased clearance of these drugs in cystic fibrosis patients. However, nonrenal routes of elimination may also be involved.[21]

We administered isothalamate with the azlocillin test dose in order to measure glomerular filtration rate simultaneously with the assessment of azlocillin clearance. In subjects with relatively nor-

Table 3.
Pharmacokinetics of Azlocillin Sodium in Patients with Cystic Fibrosis and in Normal Adult Patients

Reference	*n*	Age Range (yr)	Patient Type	Dose (mg/kg)	Peak Concentration[a] (μg/mL)	V_β[b] (L/kg)	$T_{1/2}$	Total Body Clearance mL/min/sq m	Total Body Clearance mL/min/kg
Bergan et al.[4]	10	21–36	Normal adults	73[c]	771	0.21	1.53	63.7	1.57
Bosso et al.[18]	8	11–28	Cystic fibrosis	87.5 every six hours	389	0.29	1.87	. . .	1.81
This study	18	3–29	Cystic fibrosis	75 every four hours	366	0.27	1.22	77.2	2.76

[a] Peak concentrations determined at the end of a 30-minute infusion.
[b] Drug administered by intravenous bolus over 4–5 minutes.
[c] Volume of distribution during the β-elimination phase (V_β).

mal renal function, approximately 99% of a dose of iothalamate is excreted unchanged in the urine.[23] As with inulin or creatinine clearance values, iothalamate renal clearance values determined during constant infusion[24] or plasma clearance values determined after an intravenous bolus[25] can also be used as accurate estimates of glomerular filtration rate.

A linear correlation between the plasma clearance of azlocillin and the estimated glomerular filtration rate was observed. This correlation was not unexpected since azlocillin has considerable renal elimination.

Urine samples were not collected, and therefore renal clearance could not be calculated directly. The intercept of azlocillin (Y) and iothalamate clearance (X) as determined by linear regression was not significantly different from zero, suggesting little or no nonrenal elimination. However, this impliction must be viewed cautiously. It has been shown that azlocillin has substantial nonrenal elimination and that the capacity of this pathway to eliminate drug is limited.[15] The amount eliminated renally as compared with nonrenal routes is highly dependent on the amount of the dose. Urinary recovery of 59.4% has been reported following a 1-g dose compared with 74.7% following a 5-g dose.[4]

The high dose of azlocillin used in our study would be expected to result in a high degree of renal elimination. Nonrenal clearance would be relatively small in terms of total clearance. Based on the confidence interval for the intercept in our regression analysis, the nonrenal clearance could be as high as 15.75 mL/min/sq m or 20% of the total clearance.

The correlation between azlocillin clearance and glomerular filtration rate as estimated by iothalamate clearance provides a good estimate of the dosing requirements in cystic fibrosis patients with relatively normal renal function. However, since the mean iothalamate clearance in our patients was almost 80 mL/min/sq m and none of the patients had iothalamate clearances less than 40 mL/min/sq m, extrapolation of these data to patients with impaired renal function must be done cautiously.

Conclusion

Patients with cystic fibrosis appear to eliminate azlocillin sodium more rapidly than healthy individuals. This rapid elimination warrants the use of high doses (450 mg/kg/day) to maintain high serum concentrations. Further evaluations of high-dose regimens are needed to assess clinical outcomes.

---

[a] Shwachman and Taussig scores classify patients with cystic fibrosis on the basis of clinical tests, manifestations, and complications of the disease.

[b] Taussig score is also an indicator of prognosis. Patients with scores of 81–90, 71–80, 61–70, and <60 are considered to have very good, good, fair, and poor prognoses, respectively.

References

1. Bergan T. Pharmacokinetics of mezlocillin in healthy volunteers. *Antimicrob Agents Chemother.* 1978; 14:801–6.
2. Leroy A, Humbert G, Godin M et al. Pharmacokinetics of azlocillin in subjects with normal and impaired renal function. *Antimicrob Agents Chemother.* 1980; 17:344–9.
3. Bergan T, Williams JD. Dose dependence of piperacillin pharmacokinetics. *Chemotherapy.* 1982; 28:153–9.
4. Bergan T, Thorsteinsson SB, Steingrimsson O. Dose-dependent pharmacokinetics of azlocillin compared to mezlocillin. *Chemotherapy.* 1982; 28:160–70.
5. Kelly WH, Lovato C. Antibiotic use in cystic fibrosis. *Drug Intell Clin Pharm.* 1984; 18:772–83.
6. Shwachman H, Lucas L, Kulczycki. Long-term study of one hundred five patients with cystic fibrosis. *Am J Dis Child.* 1958; 96:6–15.
7. Taussig LM, Kattwinkel J, Friedewald WT et al. A new prognostic score and clinical evaluation system for cystic fibrosis. *J Pediatr.* 1973; 82:380–90.
8. Weber A, Opheim KE, Wong K et al. High-pressure liquid chromatographic quantitation of azlocillin. *Antimicrob Agents Chemother.* 1983; 24:750–3.
9. Weber AF, Lee DW, Opheim K et al. Quantification of iothalamate in serum and urine by high-pressure liquid chromatography. *J Chromatogr.* 1985; 337:434–40.
10. Yamaoka K, Tanigawara Y, Nakagawa T et al. A pharmacokinetic analysis program (MULTI) for microcomputer. *J Pharm Dyn.* 1981; 4:879–85.
11. Gibaldi M. Biopharmaceutics and clinical pharmacokinetics. 3rd ed. Philadelphia: Lea & Febiger; 1984:17–28.
12. Silkalns GI, Jeck D, Earon J et al. Simultaneous measurement of glomerular filtration rate and renal plasma flow using plasma disappearance curves. *J Pediatr.* 1973; 83:749–57.
13. Haycock GB, Chir B, Schwartz GJ et al. Geometric method for measuring body surface area: a height-weight formula validated in infants, children and adults. *J Pediatr.* 1978; 93:62–6.
14. Wilson CB, Koup JR. Comparative pharmacology, safety and efficacy of the expanded spectrum penicillins in children. *J Pediatr.* 1985; 106:1049–56.
15. Bergan T. Overview of acylureidopenicillins pharmacokinetics. *Scand J Infect Dis.* 1981; 29:33–48.
16. Malmborg A, Alfredsson H, Kusoffsky E et al. Azlocillin and gentamicin in respiratory tract infections with *Pseudomonas aeruginosa* in patients with cystic fibrosis. *Scand J Infect Dis.* 1981; 29:64–9.
17. Bergan T, Michalsen H. Pharmacokinetics of azlocillin in children with cystic fibrosis. *Arzneimittelforsch.* 1979; 29:1955–7.
18. Bosso JA, Saxon BA, Herbst JJ et al. Azlocillin pharmacokinetics in patients with cystic fibrosis. *Antimicrob Agents Chemother.* 1984; 25:630–2.
19. Jusko WJ, Mosovich LL, Gerbracht LM et al. Enhanced renal excretion of dicloxacillin in patients with cystic fibrosis. *Pediatrics.* 1975; 56:1038–44.
20. Yaffe SJ, Gerbracht LM, Mosovich LL et al. Pharmacokinetics of methicillin in patients with cystic fibrosis. *J Infect Dis.* 1977; 135:828–31.
21. Spino M, Chai RP, Isles AF et al. Cloxacillin absorption and disposition in cystic fibrosis. *J Pediatr.* 1984; 105:829–35.
22. Prince AS, Neu HC. Use of piperacillin, a semi-synthetic penicillin, in the therapy of acute exacerbations of pulmonary disease in patients with cystic fibrosis. *J Pediatr.* 1980; 97:148–51.
23. Talner LB. Urographic contrast media in uremia; physiology and pharmacology. *Radiol Clin North Am.* 1972; 10:421–32.
24. Elwood CM, Sigman EM. The measurement of glomerular

filtration rate and effective renal plasma flow in man by iothalmate ^{125}I and iodopyracet ^{131}I. *Circulation*. 1967; 36:441–8.
25. Groth T, Tengstrom B. A simple method for the estimation of glomerular filtration rate. *Scand J Lab Invest*. 1977; 37:39–47.
26. Schwartz GJ, Haycock GB, Edelmann CM et al. A simple estimate of glomerular filtration rate in children derived from body length and plasma creatinine. *Pediatrics*. 1976; 58:259–63.

Research Note

Clearance of procainamide and *N*-acetylprocainamide in patients undergoing continuous ambulatory peritoneal dialysis

CYNTHIA L. RAEHL, A. VISHNU MOORTHY, GREGORY J. BEIRNE, AND MICHAEL E. PITTERLE

Clin Pharm. 1985; 4:669–72

During the past decade, continuous ambulatory peritoneal dialysis (CAPD) has developed as a suitable alternative to hemodialysis for patients with end-stage renal disease. The clearance of antiarrhythmic agents during CAPD has not been studied sufficiently, despite the narrow therapeutic range of these agents.

Procainamide undergoes both renal and nonrenal elimination.[1] In patients with normal renal function, approximately half of an absorbed procainamide dose is excreted unchanged in the urine. The remaining procainamide is cleared nonrenally, primarily by acetylation to the cardioactive metabolite *N*-acetylprocainamide (NAPA). The biological half-life of procainamide is two to four hours in patients with normal renal function; in patients with severe renal impairment, the half-life increases to approximately 11 hours, necessitating dosage reduction.[2] NAPA is cleared almost entirely by the kidney; however, the half-life of NAPA is two to three times longer than the half-life of the parent drug.[3]

Two case reports have suggested that CAPD is not an efficient process for removing procainamide and NAPA.[3,4] The purpose of our study was to assess the clearance of procainamide and NAPA after administration of a single 500-mg oral dose of procainamide hydrochloride to patients undergoing routine CAPD treatment.

Methods. All CAPD patients receiving medical care in the renal clinic of our hospital were asked to participate in this study, which was approved by the University of Wisconsin Human Subjects Committee. Patients were not eligible for participation in the study if they exhibited any of the following: (1) New York Heart Association class IV heart failure, (2) second- or third-degree atrioventricular heart block, (3) concomitant antiarrhythmic therapy, (4) known or suspected hypersensitivity or previous adverse reaction to procainamide, or (5) clinically important hepatic disease (as evidenced by a serum bilirubin concentration greater than twice the normal value or serum transaminase concentrations greater than the normal values). Six men volunteered to participate. None of the patients had peritonitis at the time of the study or was receiving medications known to interfere with peritoneal dialysis clearance determinations.

Each patient received a single 500-mg oral dose of procainamide hydrochloride (Pronestyl 250 mg, E. R. Squibb & Sons, Inc., Princeton, NJ 08540, lot 11019-2). Although food does not alter the rate or extent of absorption of an oral procainamide dose,[1] all but one patient (patient 3) fasted for at least 12 hours before ingesting the dose.

Dialysis was carried out with a Tenckhoff peritoneal catheter using Dianeal 137 solutions (Travenol Laboratories, Inc.) containing varying amounts of dextrose. Because patients continued their usual dialysis therapy, dialysis regimens varied among patients. Baseline peritoneal creatinine clearance was measured in each patient during the dialysis exchange immediately preceding inges-

CYNTHIA L. RAEHL, PHARM.D., is Clinical Assistant Professor, School of Pharmacy, University of Wisconsin, Madison, and Clinical Pharmcist, William S. Middleton Memorial Veterans Hospital, Madison, WI. A. VISHNU MOORTHY, M.D., is Associate Professor, School of Medicine, University of Wisconsin, and Assistant Chief, Renal Section, William S. Middleton Memorial Veterans Hospital. GREGORY L. BEIRNE, M.D., is Associate Professor, School of Medicine, University of Wisconsin, and Chief, Renal Section, William S. Middleton Memorial Veterans Hospital. MICHAEL E. PITTERLE, M.S., is Clinical Assistant Professor, School of Pharmacy, University of Wisconsin.
Address reprint requests to Dr. Raehl at the School of Pharmacy, University of Wisconsin, 425 N. Charter Street, Madison, WI 53706.

Table 1.
Patient Characteristics

Patient No.	Race[a]	Age (yr)	Weight (kg)	BSA[b] (sq m)	Diagnosis	Duration of CAPD (mo)	Residual Creatinine Clearance (mL/min)	Peritoneal Creatinine Clearance[c] (mL/min)
1	C	68	90.7	2.10	Nephrosclerosis	16	5.1	5.6
2	C	56	70.5	1.85	Bilateral renal artery stenosis	8	2.2	6.7
3	C	53	71.4	1.83	Nephrosclerosis	24	0	10.0
4	C	69	98.2	2.04	Diabetic nephropathy	7	0	10.4
5	NA	35	58.2	1.58	Chronic pyelonephritis	42	0	6.8
6	NA	58	85.0	1.96	Nephrosclerosis	1	3.2	5.1

[a] C = Caucasian, NA = Native American.
[b] Body surface area as determined by nomogram from Documenta Geigy Scientific Tables.[5]
[c] Measured for four- or five-hour exchange periods.

tion of the procainamide dose.

Each patient had an indwelling intravenous catheter to facilitate blood collection. Serial 5-mL blood samples were collected for 20–38 hours after administration of procainamide hydrochloride. Sampling times were coordinated to accommodate patients' dialysis schedules and to ensure that mid-exchange blood samples were obtained during each dialysis exchange. Samples were drawn into plastic syringes and transferred to heparinized Vacutainer tubes (avoiding contact of blood with the stopper). The samples were centrifuged immediately and the plasma was stored at −70 °C for up to 12 months pending analysis by high-performance liquid chromatography (see appendix). Previous stability studies (unpublished data) performed in our laboratory demonstrated that procainamide and NAPA are stable in plasma for up to 18 months when stored at −70 °C.

After each dialysis exchange, the volume of dialysate was determined and an aliquot was frozen for later analysis. Throughout the study, 24-hour urine samples were collected daily; the volume of each sample was noted and specimens were frozen for later analysis.

The peritoneal dialysis clearances of procainamide and NAPA were calculated using the following equation:

$$CL_{PD} = (V_{dialysate})(C_{dialysate})/(C_{midpoint})(t)$$

where CL_{PD} is the peritoneal dialysis clearance of procainamide or NAPA, $C_{dialysate}$ is the concentration of procainamide or NAPA in the dialysate, $V_{dialysate}$ is the measured volume of dialysate for a dialysis exchange lasting t hours, and $C_{midpoint}$ is the plasma drug concentration at the midpoint of the exchange. Each patient's residual creatinine clearance was calculated for a 24–48 hour urine-collection period using a modified version of this equation.

Results. The mean (± standard deviation) age of study patients was 56.5 ± 12 years (Table 1). Three patients were able to produce urine; however, residual creatinine clearance was less than 5.1 mL/min in all patients. Mean baseline peritoneal creatinine clearance was 7.4 ± 2 mL/min for a dialysis exchange lasting four or five hours.

Table 2.
Peritoneal Dialysis Clearance Rates for Procainamide and *N*-Acetylprocainamide

Patient No.	Clearance Rate (mL/min) During Indicated Dialysis Exchange[a] 1	2	3	4	5	6	7
Procainamide							
1	6.3	8.0	2.3[b]	7.8	9.3	8.7	2.2[b]
2	7.2	8.2	8.2	1.9[b]	23.9[c,d]	7.6[e]	. . .[f]
3	7.3	6.9	2.5[b]	8.0	8.4	2.7	. . .
4	10.8[d]	6.0[e]	1.8[d,g]	5.8[e]	. . .	. . .	. . .
5	6.8[e]	7.3[e]	6.2[e]	6.4[e]	3.4[e,h]	. . .	. . .
6	1.5	8.3[e]	0.8[h]	3.8[e]	. . .	. . .	. . .
N-*Acetylprocainamide*							
1	8.1	11.4	4.3[b]	8.5	10.0	8.0	3.2[b]
2	6.8	9.2	7.8	3.2[b]	27.9[c,d]	9.0[e]	. . .[f]
3	5.8	4.7	3.3[b]	5.8	7.0	1.9	. . .
4	18.8[d]	7.9[e]	2.5[d,g]	7.0[e]	. . .	. . .	. . .
5	9.8[e]	8.1[e]	6.1[e]	6.5[e]	4.7[e,h]	. . .	. . .
6	4.2	7.8[e]	0.4[h]	5.8[e]	. . .	. . .	. . .

[a] All exchanges were performed using Dianeal 137 solution with 1.5% dextrose for four or five hours except as indicated.
[b] 12-hour exchange.
[c] 90-minute exchange.
[d] Dianeal 137 with 4.25% dextrose.
[e] Dianeal 137 with 2.5% dextrose.
[f] No dialysis exchange performed.
[g] 10-hour exchange.
[h] 8-hour exchange.

Peritoneal dialysis clearance rates for all dialysis exchanges studied are listed in Table 2. Most exchanges were performed after a four- or five-hour dialysate dwell time; the mean peritoneal dialysis clearances of procainamide and NAPA for all four- or five-hour exchanges were 7.0 ± 2 mL/min and 7.8 ± 3 mL/min, respectively. Except for patient 6, the peritoneal dialysis clearances of procainamide and NAPA were fairly constant for a given patient, if exchange times were constant.

Dialysate clearance rates were inversely proportional to dwell time and dialysate flow rate. As the dwell time increased, the peritoneal dialysis clearances of both procainamide and NAPA decreased, reflecting the change in duration of dialysis (t) in the denominator of the equation. Long dwell times (8, 10, or 12 hours) were encountered during the evening hours. One patient (patient 2) experienced a very short dwell time (90 minutes) during exchange 5 because of difficulties with the Tenckhoff catheter; increases in the peritoneal dialysis clearance rates of both procainamide and NAPA were observed.

CAPD apparently did not preferentially remove either procainamide or NAPA, as indicated by a ratio of dialysate clearance rates approximately equal to one for all exchanges. In the three patients who produced urine during the study, less than 1% of the total administered procainamide dose was recovered in the urine as either procainamide or NAPA (Table 3).

Discussion. As peritoneal dialysis gains acceptance as a therapeutic modality for end-stage renal disease, its potential effect on concomitant drug therapy is receiving increased attention. Before this study, a single case report described the use of procainamide in a CAPD patient recovering from a myocardial infarction.[3] In this patient, the peritoneal dialysis clearances of procainamide and NAPA during one dialysis exchange were 6.5 and 5.3 mL/min, respectively. The estimated elimination half-life of procainamide was 11.5 hours, essentially unchanged from the half-life observed previously in patients with end-stage renal disease.[2]

In our study, peritoneal dialysis clearance of procainamide and NAPA was usually about 7 mL/min. To simulate clinical conditions closely, we did not alter patients' dialysis regimens. Our study revealed little interpatient or intrapatient variation in the peritoneal dialysis clearance of either procainamide or NAPA, provided dialysis times were held constant. CAPD did not shorten the prolonged procainamide half-life common in end-stage renal disease, as evidenced by the observed procainamide half-life of 11.7 ± 4 hours. Peritoneal dialysis consistently represented a small fraction (less than 5%) of total body clearance of procainamide. Similarly, CAPD did not cause rapid reductions in plasma procainamide concentrations that might make maintenance of therapeutic plasma concentrations of procainamide difficult.

Our study was limited by such methodologic problems as a small number of patients, variable dialysis regimens, oral dosing, and sampling times insufficient to characterize NAPA pharmacokinetic variables. However, our results suggest that further clarification of the effect of CAPD on procainamide or NAPA pharmacokinetics may be unnecessary. Because NAPA is not removed substantially, it accumulates in CAPD patients just as it does in patients with end-stage renal disease. Careful monitoring of serum concentrations of both procainamide and NAPA is recommended.

Conclusion. The amount of procainamide or N-acetylprocainamide removed by CAPD is not clinically important. Because CAPD does not cause rapid decreases in plasma procainamide concentrations, it does not increase the risk of arrhythmias in patients receiving procainamide therapy.

References

1. Lima JJ. Procainamide. In: Evans WE, Schentag JJ, Jusko WJ, eds. Applied pharmacokinetics: principles of therapeutic drug monitoring. San Francisco: Applied Therapeutics, Inc.;1980:404–35.
2. Gibson TP, Lowenthal DT, Nelson HA et al. Elimination of procainamide in end-stage renal failure. *Clin Pharmacol Ther.* 1975; 17:321–9.
3. Kroboth PD, Mitchum K, Puschett JB. Use of procainamide in chronic ambulatory peritoneal dialysis: report of a case. *Am J Kidney Dis.* 1984; 1:78–9.
4. Villalba-Pimental L, Epstein LM, Sellers EM et al. Survival after massive procainamide ingestion. *Am J Cardiol.* 1973; 32:727–30.
5. Diem K, Lentner C, eds. Documenta Geigy Scientific Tables. New York: Geigy Pharmaceuticals; 1970:537.

Appendix—Stability-Indicating High-Performance Liquid Chromatographic Assay for Procainamide and N-Acetylprocainamide

Procainamide and N-acetylprocainamide (NAPA) were analyzed by reverse-phase high-performance liquid chromatography (HPLC). Chromatographic analysis was performed on a Beckman model 332 system (Beckman Instruments, Berkeley, CA 94710) with the following components: model 110A solvent delivery system, model 420 controller, and model 160 detector equipped for ultraviolet detection at 280 nm. An HP85 computer (Hewlett Packard, Palo Alto, CA 94304) was coupled with a

Table 3.
Urinary Recovery of Procainamide and N-Acetylprocainamide in CAPD Patients with Some Renal Function

Patient No.	Collection Time (hr)	Urine Volume (mL)	Procainamide Concentration (μg/mL)	N-Acetylprocainamide Concentration (μg/mL)	Amount of Drug in Urine (mg) Procainamide	Amount of Drug in Urine (mg) N-Acetylprocainamide
1	0–24	710	3.9	1.6	2.8	1.1
	24–44	730	1.1	1.8	0.8	1.3
2	0–32	205	6.6	3.0	1.4	3.3
5	0–20	325	4.1	5.6	1.3	1.8

software package (Nelson Analytical, Cupertino, CA 95015) as an electronic integrator. A 10-μm, reverse-phase octadecyl C-18 bonded column (4.6 mm × 25 cm; model 600RPA, Alltech Associates, Inc., Deerfield, IL 60015) was used with a precolumn.

Plasma extraction was performed with the Baker-10 extraction system (Baker Co., Inc., Sanford, ME 04073) using 1-mL disposable C-18 extraction columns (model 326342, American Scientific Products, McGaw Park, IL 60085). Sample mixtures, prepared in glass conical tubes, contained 250 μL of standard (procainamide and NAPA at equal concentrations) or sample plasma, 250 μL of 0.1 *M* sodium carbonate, and 150 μL of internal standard solution containing 10.0 μg/mL of the dipropyl analog of procainamide (E. R. Squibb & Sons, Inc., Princeton, NJ 08540, lot SQ 2510). The extraction columns were conditioned with two column-volumes of methanol followed by two column-volumes of deionized distilled water. After addition of 520 μL of the sample mixture, the extraction columns were washed with three column-volumes of 10% methanol in deionized distilled water. Samples were eluted with two 200-μL aliquots of 100 m*M* acetic acid and 50 m*M* triethylamine in methanol. Samples were evaporated to dryness at room temperature under nitrogen and reconstituted in 50 μL of deionized distilled water immediately before HPLC analysis.

Figure 1. Chromatogram of procainamide (3 μg/mL) and *N*-acetylprocainamide (3 μg/mL) in plasma showing separation of procainamide (A), *N*-acetylprocainamide (B), and internal standard (C). Associated peak heights were 5357, 3260, and 3718 for peaks A, B, and C, respectively.

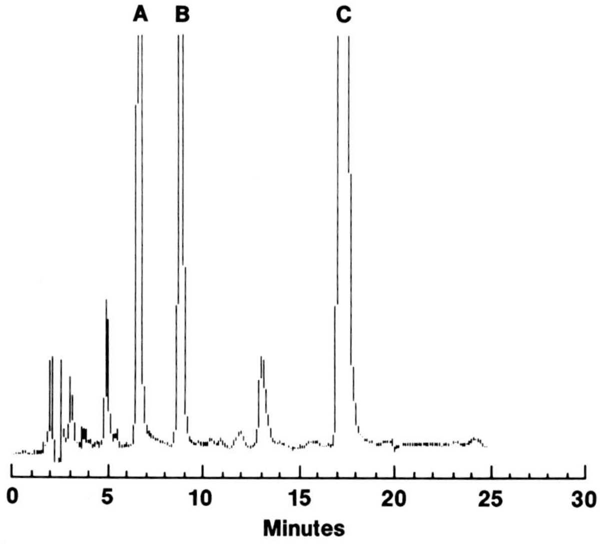

A 20-μL aliquot of the reconstituted sample was injected onto the analytical column. The mobile phase consisted of sodium acetate 4 g, glacial acetic acid 30 mL, acetonitrile 150 mL, and triethylamine 1 mL brought to a volume of 1000 mL with deionized distilled water (final pH 4.5). Analytical conditions included a flow rate of 1.5 mL/min (2000 psi), ambient column temperature, and detection at 280 nm at 0.01 absorbance units full scale. Retention times under these conditions were 6.7, 8.9, and 17.4 minutes, respectively, for procainamide, NAPA, and internal standard (Figure 1). Recoveries were 98% and 85%, respectively.

Calibration curves prepared in plasma, dialysate, and urine were linear for procainamide and NAPA concentrations of 0.1–5.0 μg/mL with correlation coefficients of 0.990–0.997 for procainamide and 0.981–0.990 for NAPA. The slopes of the standard lines were similar for all three media. Both day-to-day and within-day precision studies at 0.5, 2, and 5 μg/mL of procainamide and NAPA showed coefficients of variation less than 5%. Analysis of predose plasma samples from each patient showed no evidence of compounds that might interfere with analysis of procainamide, NAPA, or the internal standard.

“

Drug Treatment for Alzheimer's Disease

About 10% of people over 65 years of age suffer from dementia, the prevalence increasing to about 22% for those over 80 years of age. As the percentage of the total population over age 65 is steadily increasing in the developed countries of the world (with those aged 75 years or over increasing more than twice as fast as the general population), one can anticipate an imminent quiet epidemic of dementia. One of life's greatest disasters, to the afflicted person as well as to the family, is the onset of severe mental impairment in the elderly person. The course is often one of long term decline toward death, with loss of humanity.

Many drug treatments for senile dementia of the Alzheimer type have been tried, but most have been found wanting. The problems in evaluating drug therapy are considerable, for one is often dealing with a complex interplay of psychosocial, brain and general physical disorders. Some of these factors may fluctuate, while others are progressive. The contribution of each of these multiple factors to the total degree of disability is difficult to gauge. Many studies to evaluate drug therapy are performed in patients so deteriorated that it would take a miracle to show much positive benefit. In any case, gains are likely to be small and may take a while to become apparent.

—Hollister LE. Alzheimer's disease: Is it worth treating? *Drugs*. 1985; 29:483–8.

”

Editorial

Nomifensine: An antidepressant with a difference?

The most recently marketed antidepressant, a structurally and pharmacologically unique tetrahydroisoquinoline derivative, nomifensine maleate (Merital, Hoechst-Roussel), reviewed in this issue of *Clinical Pharmacy*,[1] is a potent blocker of norepinephrine and dopamine reuptake in the central nervous system. Although new to the United States market, it has been used for over eight years in 14 million patients in 60 countries. With the continued introduction of "new and improved" antidepressant agents, an overview, comparing many of these agents with nomifensine and focusing on pharmacologic and formulary issues, is appropriate.

During the past five years, four structurally unique antidepressants (amoxapine, maprotiline, trazodone, and trimipramine) have been marketed in the United States. The triazolobenzodiazepine, alprazolam, also may possess antidepressant activity. Unfortunately, the ideal antidepressant does not exist. Specific benefits from some (but not all) newer agents include greater safety in overdose, a possibly more rapid onset of action, and perhaps, diminished adverse effects. Specific agents can cause seizures at therapeutic doses, mild to moderate orthostatic blood pressure changes, anticholinergic effects, behavioral disinhibition, physical dependence and withdrawal, priapism, or extrapyramidal symptoms. Additionally, the full potential of these newer antidepressants for causing rare adverse effects remains undetermined. Nomifensine appears to possess significant advantages over other therapies in selected depressed patients. Moreover, with an extensive track record in Europe, this new antidepressant should live up to its potential advantages with few, if any, surprises to the clinician.

Clinically important side effects occurring with both the standard and second-generation antidepressants are readily explained by their pharmacologic actions on in vitro receptor systems.[2] Orthostatic hypotension results from peripheral α_1 blockade and central serotonergic and adrenergic augmentation. Blockade of the histamine H_1- and α_1-adrenergic receptors centrally correlates with sedation. Potential increases in myocardial oxygen consumption in patients with ischemic heart disease are related to anticholinergic and adrenergic mechanisms. Additionally, the likelihood of iatrogenic myocardial conduction disturbances and dysrhythmias is partially related to these drugs' widely differing effects on the phase 0 slope of the action potential.

Therefore, based on its pharmacologic dissimilarities, nomifensine would be expected to display a "cleaner" side-effect profile.[1-4] The pharmacologic data, when taken in combination with the clinical findings, suggest that toxic ingestion of nomifensine is unlikely to be fatal and that therapeutic doses are unlikely to cause cardiac conduction disturbances or orthostatic hypotension.[2] The absence of tachycardia or hypertension with nomifensine (except rare transient effects) suggests that central adrenergic mechanisms mediating vasomotor control are modifying peripheral adrenergic stimulation (if present) for most patients. Nomifensine represents a valuable therapeutic alternative in the patient intolerant of orthostatic blood pressure changes. Nevertheless, patients who are recovering from myocardial infarction and individuals with severe ischemic heart disease should not be treated with nomifensine until additional safety data are available. One might consider using alprazolam or trazodone for patients in whom catecholamine-induced changes in cardiac function are contraindicated.

Nomifensine is the least sedating of the recently marketed antidepressants.[2] Those agents possessing mild to high sedative effects can be useful therapeutically in the anxious patient with insomnia, but for a large number of patients they are undesirable. In patients with psychomotor retardation or poor ability to concentrate, nomifensine could acutely worsen their incapacitation. Nomifensine's lack of sedation makes it an excellent choice for the anergic, withdrawn, depressed patient. However, overactivation of the central nervous system is a bothersome problem for some patients, and nomifensine should be administered in the morning and afternoon, not evening. The condition of patients who are agitated or psychotic might be exacerbated by nomifensine's dopaminergic potentiation. Trazodone or amoxapine might be considered in these individuals.

Nomifensine has a number of rare adverse effects not commonly associated with standard tricyclic antidepressant therapy. Nausea and vomiting might be the direct result of dopamine receptor activation in the medullary chemoreceptor trigger zone. Weight loss and normal to lowered prolactin concentrations, instead of the usual weight gain and hyperprolactinemia associated with tricyclic antidepressant agents, also are caused by dopaminergic augmentation. Exacerbation of orofacial dyskinesia has been reported.[3] Iatrogenic hyperpyrexia, liver enzyme elevations, and hemolytic anemia are thought to be caused by immune or hypersensitivity reactions.[2] However, hyperpyrexia is also mechanistically possible via disruption of central dopaminergic temperature-regulation processes.

Based on nomifensine's pharmacologic profile, the issue of abuse and dependence must be addressed. Nomifensine originally was classified as methylphenidate-like, especially when given by the intravenous route.[4] However, therapeutic efficacy of nomifensine in depression is not tied to euphoria. Similarly, cocaine and other dopamine stimulants are only partially effective in treating major affective disorders. Based on foreign experience and clinical investigations to date, abuse does not appear to be a substantial problem with oral nomifensine. However, no systematic study involving high-dose escalation and sudden withdrawal has been performed.

Nomifensine, consistent with the adrenergic dysregulation hypothesis for depression, downregulates β-adrenergic receptors by decreasing their density.[1,5,6] Additionally, nomifensine is unique in its ability to block the reuptake of dopamine centrally. The role of dopamine in depression is more equivocal. Whether nomifensine-induced dopamine autoreceptor subsensitivity is linked to adrenergic receptor changes is unclear.[7] Serotonergic effects also have been described for nomifensine.[8] This pharmacologic profile for nomifensine suggests that it might be useful in patients refractory to standard tricyclic antidepressant therapy.

A unique aspect of nomifensine's pharmacokinetics is its apparent dependence on renal mechanisms for elimination. Special dosing guidelines in severe renal insufficiency (<25 mL/min creatinine clearance) probably are needed.[1] Despite an extremely short apparent elimination half-life (~2 hours), patients can receive nomifensine in fewer divided doses than the pharmacokinetics might suggest. Efficacy has been demonstrated with once-daily dosing in geriatric patients.[9] Although peak concentrations after oral dosing occur within one to two hours, pharmacodynamic effects appear to peak at four to six hours after the dose and last for more than eight hours.[10] This possibly might be explained by the production of three different hydroxy metabolites that may possess pharmacologic effects.[11] Plasma concentration monitoring of both free and conjugated nomifensine has not demonstrated a meaningful relationship with response.[12]

Nomifensine should be added to formularies despite its increased cost. Analogous to the situation with new and earlier generations of cephalosporins, however, many of the less expensive generic tricyclic antidepressant agents are still drugs of choice in the young, physically healthy patient. All formulary antidepressants should be evaluated critically to determine which ones are no longer first-line agents. Redundancy in product selection for agents with similar profiles (e.g., amitriptyline, trimipramine, and doxepin) should be reconsidered. Clinical decision making and formulary selection should also reflect the most recent data on adverse experiences and considerations for monitoring therapeutic plasma concentrations.[13] In contrast to the new-generation antidepressants that have only poor correlations between plasma levels and response, nortriptyline, desipramine, and imipramine plasma concentration values can expedite the dosing and response of patients.

Nomifensine is an important new alternative for the treatment of depression with psychomotor retardation or in those who are refractory to standard therapy. Additionally, the absence of orthostatic hypotension, the mild anticholinergic effects, and safety in overdose suggest that nomifensine be considered as a first-choice agent for geriatric patients who do not have severe renal insufficiency, for suicidal outpatients, and for those with a concomitant medical illness. Nomifensine clearly has a niche in our pharmacologic armamentarium for depression. As appropriate for any new drug, careful patient monitoring and prompt adverse-experience reporting are essential.

1. Kinney JL. Nomifensine maleate: a new second-generation antidepressant. *Clin Pharm.* 1985;4:
2. Coccaro EF, Siever LJ. Second generation antidepressants: a comparative review. *J Clin Pharmacol.* 1985; 25:241–60.
3. Sankyk R, Gillman MA. Nomifensine exacerbates orofacial dyskinesia in hypothyroidism. *Neurology.* 1985; 35:282.
4. Braestrup C, Scheel-Kruger J. Methylphenidate-like effects of the new antidepressant drug nomifensine. *Eur J Pharmacol.* 1976; 38:305–12.
5. Bryant SG, Ereshefsky L. Antidepressant properties of trazodone. *Clin Pharm.* 1982; 1:406–17.
6. Siever LF, Davis KL. Overview: toward a dysregulation hypothesis of depression. *Am J Psychiatry.* 1985; 142:1017–31.
7. Sulser F. Mode of action of antidepressant drugs. *J Clin Psychiatry.* 1983; 44:14–20.
8. Fielding S, Szeqczak MR. Pharmacology of nomifensine: a review of animal studies. *J Clin Psychiatry.* 1984; 45(sec 2):12–20.
9. Jansen W, Siegfried K. Nomifensine in geriatric inpatients: a placebo-controlled study. *J Clin Psychiatry.* 1984; 45(sec 2):63–7.
10. Siegfried K, Taeuber D. Pharmacodynamics of nomifensine: a review of studies in healthy subjects. *J Clin Psychiatry.* 1984; 45(sec 2):33–8.
11. Heptner W, Uihlein M. Kinetics and metabolism of nomifensine. *J Clin Psychiatry.* 1984; 45(sec 2):21–5.
12. Syvalahti E, Lindberg R, Iisalo E. Clinical effects and serum levels of nomifensine on depressive patients. *J Int Med Res.* 1983; 11:259–62.
13. Task force on the use of laboratory tests in psychiatry. Tricyclic antidepressants-blood level measurements and clinical outcome: an APA task force report. *Am J Psychiatry.* 1985; 142:155–62.

LARRY ERESHEFSKY, PHARM.D.
Program Director, Psychiatric Pharmacy
Associate Professor, Pharmacy
The University of Texas at Austin
Associate Professor, Pharmacology and Psychiatry
The University of Texas Health Science Center
7703 Floyd Curl Drive
San Antonio, TX 78284

Grand Rounds

Drug-induced torsade de pointes

CYNTHIA L. RAEHL, ASHVIN K. PATEL, AND MARIE LEROY

Abstract: Three patients who developed torsade de pointes associated with antiarrhythmic or psychotropic drugs are described, and the electrocardiographic characteristics, clinical presentation, predisposing factors, and management of this form of ventricular tachycardia are reviewed.

The first patient was a 56-year-old schizophrenic man receiving thioridazine hydrochloride, trifluoperazine hydrochloride, and benztropine mesylate who was admitted to a hospital after a syncopal episode. Subsequently, the patient experienced several episodes of ventricular tachycardia combined with multifocal premature ventricular contractions (PVCs) and torsade de pointes; the arrhythmias were attributed to antipsychotic therapy. The second patient was a 69-year-old man who experienced ventricular tachycardia that progressed to ventricular fibrillation 41 days after surgery. Quinidine sulfate probably induced the ventricular tachycardia, which was identified as torsade de pointes. The third patient was a 71-year-old man admitted to the hospital for treatment of refractory ventricular arrhythmias. Previous drug therapy with quinidine sulfate and procainamide hydrochloride had been associated with torsade de pointes. Despite unsuccessful treatment of ventricular ectopy, the patient was discharged on maintenance therapy with pindolol, topical nitrates, and phenytoin. No additional episodes of torsade de pointes have been observed.

Torsade de pointes is characterized by polymorphous electrocardiographic appearance and delayed repolarization (prolonged QT interval). It may occur in association with a number of disease states and also as a complication of treatment with therapeutic doses of drugs that affect repolarization (quinidine, disopyramide, procainamide, and phenothiazines). Clinical outcomes range from asymptomatic, self-terminating arrhythmias to ventricular fibrillation resulting in cardiac arrest. The definitive emergency therapy for torsade de pointes is overdrive pacing; cautious isoproterenol administration can also be used. Lidocaine and bretylium are often ineffective in treating this form of ventricular tachycardia. Potassium and magnesium repletion appear to be essential in abolishing drug-induced torsade de pointes.

Drug-induced torsade de pointes is best prevented by avoiding agents known to induce arrhythmias in patients with a pre-existing prolonged QT interval. Periodic serum electrolyte assessment is warranted, and new drugs that prolong the QT interval should be considered potential causative agents of torsade de pointes.

Index terms: Benztropine mesylate; Bretylium tosylate; Cardiac drugs; Drugs, adverse reactions; Isoproterenol hydrochloride; Lidocaine; Procainamide hydrochloride; Psychotherapeutic agents; Quinidine sulfate; Sympathomimetic agents; Thioridazine hydrochloride; Toxicity; Trifluoperazine hydrochloride
Clin Pharm. 1985; 4:675–90

Dessertenne et al.[1] described and named torsade de pointes in 1966 as a peculiar form of ventricular tachycardia with a twisting QRS axis and polymorphous appearance. The electrocardiogram (ECG) observed in an 80-year-old woman with complete heart block showed cycles of alternating polarity in which the QRS complexes appeared to be twisting around the isoelectric baseline.[2] Although Desser-

CYNTHIA L. RAEHL, PHARM.D., is Clinical Assistant Professor, University of Wisconsin School of Pharmacy, and Clinical Pharmacist, William S. Middleton Memorial Veterans Hospital, Madison, WI. ASHVIN K. PATEL, M.D., is Director, Coronary-Care Unit, William S. Middleton Memorial Veterans Hospital, and Associate Professor, School of Medicine, University of Wisconsin, Madison. MARIE LEROY, M.S., is Clinical Coordinator, Pharmacy Department, University of Wisconsin Hospital and Clinics, Madison.

Address requests to Dr. Raehl at the School of Pharmacy, University of Wisconsin, 425 North Charter Street, Madison, WI 53706.

This is **article 680-204-8520** in the **ASHP Continuing Education System**. See page 694 for learning objectives and test questions.

Papers in the Grand Rounds section are patient case reports and literature review combined in a way that gives them high educational value. The papers lead off with a well-documented case report of an unusual drug experience (e.g., adverse drug reaction or other unexpected drug response, experimental use of a drug). The case generally deals with a difficult therapeutic problem or dilemma that is commonly encountered but may be overlooked or misunderstood. (Esoteric or rare occurrences of minor importance do not make good Grand Rounds material.) A literature review puts the case in perspective with previously reported similar cases and alternative treatments. The review is integrated with related discussions of the new case being reported.

CP readers are encouraged to use Grand Rounds for educational group discussions. For this purpose, discussion questions are printed at the end of Grand Rounds papers.

tenne popularized the term torsade de pointes, other authors have since described similar unusual-appearing forms of ventricular tachycardia and assigned to them a variety of names, including atypical ventricular tachycardia,[3] paroxysmal ventricular fibrillation,[4] transient recurrent ventricular fibrillation,[5] cardiac ballet,[6] ventricular fibrilloflutter,[7] polymorphous ventricular tachycardia,[8-10] and delayed repolarization syndrome.[11]

Much confusion exists regarding interpretation of the term torsade de pointes.[12] Torsade de pointes is a type of paroxysmal ventricular tachycardia that meets certain morphologic and electrophysiologic criteria.[13] It is similar to polymorphic ventricular tachycardia in electrocardiographic appearance, yet it can be distinguished from polymorphic ventricular tachycardia by considering etiology, precipitating factors (drugs or electrolyte imbalance), initiation by a premature ventricular contraction late in diastole, prolongation of the QT interval or presence of a prominent U wave, and type of therapeutic intervention (Table 1). Differentiation between torsade de pointes and polymorphous ventricular tachycardia is critical in designing therapeutic regimens. During the last several years, the number of drugs reported to cause torsade de pointes has increased steadily. This article reviews drug-induced torsade de pointes and provides diagnostic and therapeutic guidelines. A glossary of relevant electrocardiographic terms is included at the end of the article.

Case Reports

Case 1. A 56-year-old white man with a long history of schizophrenia who "slumped over while eating lunch" was examined at a local emergency room and was transferred to our hospital. Physical examination on admission revealed a thin man with a blood pressure of 80/50 mm Hg, heart rate 60, temperature 99 °F, and respiratory rate 24/min. The patient's maintenance medications included thioridazine hydrochloride 200 mg orally twice a day, trifluoperazine hydrochloride 20 mg orally twice a day, and benztropine mesylate 2 mg orally daily. The only abnormal finding of a cardiac examination was a grade II/VI systolic ejection murmur. Neurologic examination revealed tangential thought processes; however, the patient was alert and oriented to person, place, and time. Laboratory test values were within normal limits except for a white blood cell count of 12,000/cu mm and a hematocrit of 40%. The patient's serum electrolyte values and results of an arterial blood gas analysis were normal. ECG revealed a normal sinus rhythm, and the cardiac monitor showed rare premature ventricular con-

Table 1.
Differentiation of Polymorphous Ventricular Tachycardia and Torsade de Pointes[a]

Variable	Polymorphous Ventricular Tachycardia	Torsade de Pointes
Etiology	Coronary-artery disease, cardiomyopathy	Congenital, pharmacologic, or metabolic abnormality
QT interval	Normal	Prolonged (≥ 0.50 sec)
Preceding ECG events	Increased ventricular ectopy, no long–short initiating sequence	Increased ventricular ectopy, long–short initiating sequence, prominent U wave
Morphology	QRS complex alternating in polarity, yielding an undulating baseline	QRS complex alternating in polarity, yielding an undulating baseline
Ventricular rate	150–300 beats/min	150–300 beats/min
Termination	Usually nonsustained but may degenerate into ventricular fibrillation	Usually nonsustained but may degenerate into ventricular fibrillation
Therapeutic intervention	Class Ia antiarrhythmics useful, isoproterenol therapy should be avoided	Avoid class Ia antiarrhythmics; treat with pacing, isoproterenol, or electrolyte replacement
Prognosis	Poor	Usually good with correction of underlying factors

[a] Information in table was adapted from references 1, 11, and 13.

tractions (PVCs) and occasional pairs of PVCs. The patient was thought to have experienced a vasovagal reaction. All psychotropic medications were discontinued.

By the following morning the patient's blood pressure had stabilized at 90–100/60–70 mm Hg. At 1000, during transfer from the coronary-care unit, he experienced a six-second episode of ventricular tachycardia, for which he received a bolus of lidocaine hydrochloride 50 mg intravenously and a 2-mg/min lidocaine hydrochloride infusion. Over the next 30 minutes, three more episodes of ventricular tachycardia required 200 mg of i.v. lidocaine plus a 4-mg/min lidocaine infusion, two direct-current cardioversions, and bretylium tosylate 500 mg i.v. followed by a 2 mg/min infusion. Throughout this period the patient exhibited a variety of ventricular arrhythmias, including multifocal PVCs, ventricular tachycardia, and torsade de pointes associated with a QT interval of 0.58–0.64 second (Figure 1).

Phenothiazine-induced torsade de pointes was first recognized after a total of 150 mg of i.v. lidocaine hydrochloride was infused. Lidocaine hydrochloride 3 mg/min and bretylium tosylate 2 mg/min were continued. Vital signs were as follows: blood pressure 102/70 mm Hg, heart rate 60 (sinus rhythm with QT interval 0.60 second), temperature 100.2 °F rectally, and respiratory rate 20/min. Laboratory data revealed a serum potassium concentration of 3.8 meq/L, for which a total of 40 meq of potassium chloride was infused over four hours. Cardiac isoenzyme concentrations were within normal limits. A central venous pressure catheter was inserted into the left subclavian vein to facilitate possible placement of a temporary pacemaker.

Over the next several hours, the patient maintained sinus rhythm with a heart rate of 65–70 without ectopy. At 1730 on the following day, the lidocaine infusion was discontinued because of lidocaine toxicity (somnolence, nausea, vomiting). During the night, the patient's heart rate ranged from 50 to 65 without ventricular ectopy, and associated QT intervals were 0.58–0.60 second. Because serum potassium concentrations were low, the patient was given periodic intravenous potassium chloride supplementation. At 0600 on the next day the patient developed a junctional rhythm (heart rate 45) and systolic blood pressure fell to 70 mm Hg. Bretylium was discontinued and isoproterenol hydrochloride was started at a rate of 1 μg/min. An isoproterenol infusion of 1–1.5 μg/min maintained heart rate between 70 and 90. By the fourth day after admission, the arrhythmias resolved and isoproterenol therapy was stopped. Despite a low heart rate (40–50), the QT interval normalized to 0.45 second. Ambulatory Holter monitoring revealed no further ventricular ectopy. Before discharge, haloperidol therapy was instituted at 5 mg orally twice daily. The primary-care physician was advised to avoid phenothiazine therapy in this patient.

Case 2. A 69-year-old white man underwent surgical repair of a perforated colonic diverticulum. He had a history of chronic obstructive pulmonary disease, inferior-wall myocardial infarction, congestive heart failure, two-vessel coronary-artery bypass graft, left bundle-branch block, ventricular ectopy, type IV hyperlipidemia, and pancreatitis. His hospital course was complicat-

Figure 1. Two episodes of phenothiazine-induced torsade de pointes. Panel A shows the characteristic long–short ventricular sequence that often precedes onset of torsade de pointes. A premature ventricular beat (left arrow) was followed by a long compensatory pause (RR interval 1120 msec) and a nodal escape beat (center arrow). Another premature ventricular beat (right arrow) (RR interval of 600 msec) is followed by the torsade de pointes episode with a cycle length of 300 msec. Panel B shows another torsade de pointes episode in the same patient.

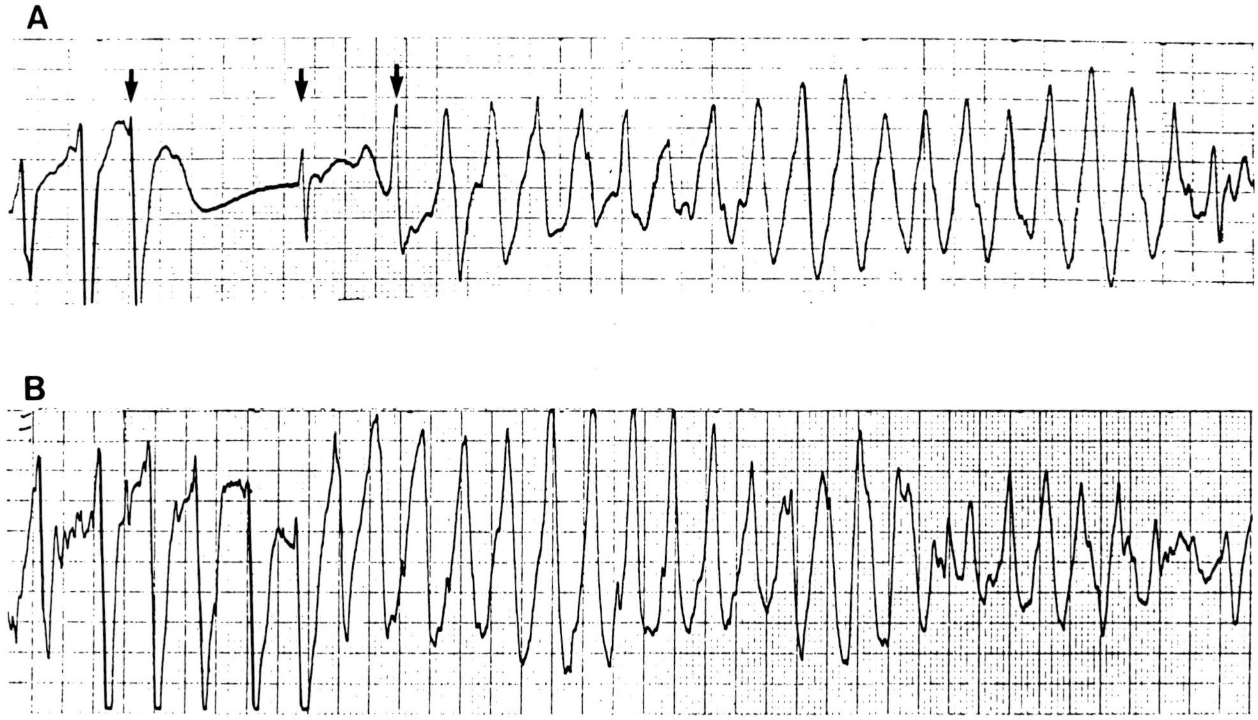

ed by fungal septicemia and respiratory failure. Forty-one days after surgery, he became unresponsive. Ventricular tachycardia was observed, which degenerated to ventricular fibrillation after one minute. Defibrillation resulted in sinus rhythm with frequent premature atrial contractions. Postresuscitation ECG revealed a heart rate of 90 (atrial bigeminy) with an associated QT interval of 0.56 second. Medications at the time of ventricular fibrillation included digoxin, furosemide, acetazolamide, and quinidine sulfate (200 mg orally every eight hours). Trough serum digoxin and quinidine concentrations 24 hours before ventricular fibrillation were 0.9 ng/mL and 3.6 μg/mL, respectively; serum potassium, magnesium, and calcium concentrations were within normal limits.

Therapy with lidocaine hydrochloride was started for multifocal PVCs; the patient was given a 100-mg i.v. bolus dose followed by a 3-mg/min infusion. Blood pressure was stable at 110/70 mm Hg, and heart rate was 100. Seven hours later, the patient again experienced ventricular tachycardia; this was identified as torsade de pointes (Figure 2), which responded to a precordial thump. Quinidine and lidocaine were discontinued, and bretylium tosylate was administered as a 300-mg i.v. bolus dose followed by an infusion of 2 mg/min. Despite bretylium therapy, the patient experienced three additional torsade de pointes episodes that required treatment with 400 watt-sec defibrillation. Lidocaine therapy was reinstituted, bretylium was discontinued, and a dopamine hydrochloride infusion was started to support blood pressure. The patient remained in atrial bigeminy, and an infusion of isoproterenol hydrochloride was started at a rate of 2 μg/min to maintain a heart rate of 120–130. In addition to isoproterenol and lidocaine therapy, a temporary atrial pacemaker was inserted. Over the next eight hours, the infusion rates of isoproterenol and lidocaine were decreased to 1 μg/min and 1 mg/min, respectively. A serum potassium concentration of 3.9 meq/L prompted intravenous potassium chloride supplementation.

The QT interval normalized to 0.44 second 24 hours after discontinuation of quinidine therapy. Administration of isoproterenol and lidocaine continued for 48 and 72 hours, respectively. The temporary pacemaker was removed after 96 hours. The patient died of pneumonia with acute respiratory insufficiency 72 days after admission.

Case 3. A 71-year-old white man was referred to this hospital for treatment of refractory ventricular arrhythmias. The patients' history of cardiac problems dated back to 1976, when hypertension and vague nonexertional chest pain were noted. One year later, asymptomatic bradycardia with first-degree heart block and frequent PVCs were noted. In 1982, the patient experienced a syncopal episode, and, on arrival in an emergency room, was noted to have a serum potassium concentration of 2.9 meq/L; his ECG showed quadrigeminy and a prolonged QT interval (0.48 second). The patient's ventricular ectopy persisted despite potassium repletion.

Therapy with quinidine sulfate 300 mg orally four times daily produced a trough serum quinidine concentration of 3.3 μg/mL but did not suppress ventricular ectopy. An increase in the dosage of quinidine sulfate to 400 mg four times daily (producing serum peak and trough concentrations of 8.5 and 5.5 μg/mL, respectively) resulted in an episode of torsade de pointes (QT interval 0.60 second, Figure 3), which spontaneously resolved. Ventricular ectopy persisted after quinidine therapy was discontinued. Attempts to control ectopy with propranolol hydrochloride were complicated by sinus bradycardia (heart rate 38–60). Although cardiac pacing therapy might have permitted continued β-blocker therapy and arrhythmia control, the patient refused pacemaker placement. He was discharged with prescriptions for methyldopa 500 mg orally twice daily and hydrochlorothiazide 25 mg with triamterene 50 mg once daily and instructed to return if the symptoms recurred.

Nine months later, on July 19, 1983, the patient again complained of palpitations. The results of 24-hour Holter monitoring revealed greater than 1000 PVCs per hour. A second trial with quinidine sulfate and propranolol hydrochloride therapy controlled the PVCs, despite prolongation of the QT interval to 0.64 second.

Two months later, the patient was again admitted for symptomatic ventricular arrhythmias. A trial with procainamide hydrochloride resulted in torsade de pointes associated with a QT interval of 0.60 second (Figure 4). Serum procainamide and *N*-acetylprocainamide concentrations were 11.5 and 18.5 μg/mL, respectively. He was

Figure 2. Quinidine-induced torsade de pointes. Panel A depicts torsade de pointes occurring in spite of antiarrhythmic therapy with lidocaine. The QT interval was prolonged to 0.50 second in the hour preceding this episode. Panel B depicts another torsade de pointes episode occurring three hours later despite bretylium therapy.

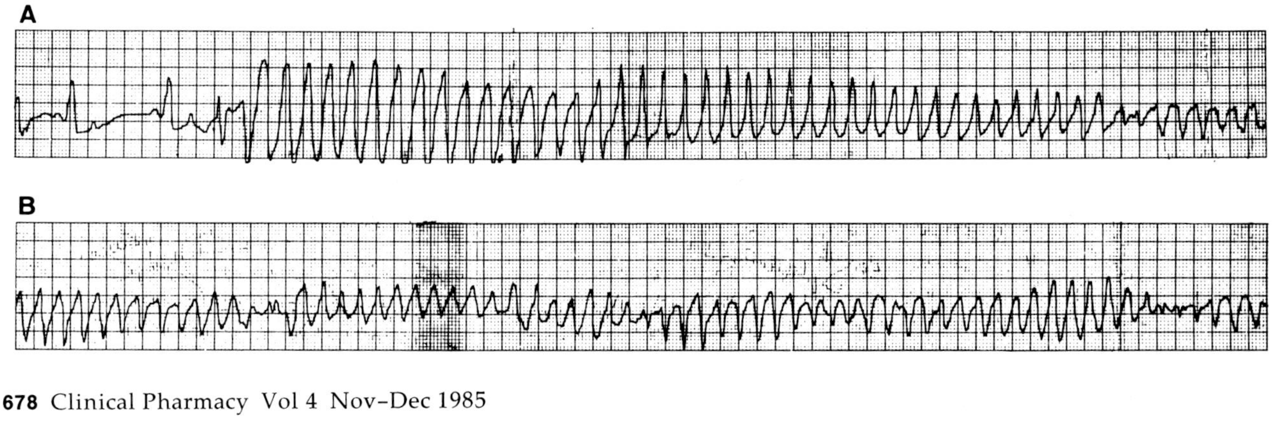

then referred to our hospital on September 16, 1983.

Except for a serum potassium concentration of 3.6 meq/L, admission laboratory test results were within normal limits. Potassium chloride 120 meq was infused during the first 24 hours. Ventricular ectopy was controlled with a 24-hour infusion of lidocaine hydrochloride; serum lidocaine concentration at steady state was 5.7 μg/mL. Three days later, a temporary pacemaker was inserted. Polymorphous ventricular tachycardia occurred shortly thereafter despite a normal serum potassium concentration and a QT interval of 0.32 second. Attempts to control additional ventricular arrhythmias with ventricular pacing resulted in severe hypotension, presumably because of loss of atrial contraction.

On September 20, 1983, an atrioventricular sequential pacemaker was inserted, but it failed to suppress ventricular ectopy. Intravenous lidocaine hydrochloride was administered for two days while the patient received oral loading doses of phenytoin sodium. Despite a high serum phenytoin concentration (20.5 μg/mL), ectopy persisted. Trial therapy with pindolol 10 mg orally twice daily and correction of borderline hypomagnesemia (serum magnesium concentration 2.1 meq/L) did not suppress the ectopy.

The patient was not considered a candidate for either cardiac catheterization or electrophysiologic study. He continues therapy with pindolol 30 mg orally three times a day, topical nitrates, and phenytoin sodium. The patient's QT interval ranges from 0.34 to 0.38 second. Asymptomatic ventricular ectopy persists; however, no additional episodes of torsade de pointes have been observed.

Electrocardiographic Characteristics of Torsade de Pointes

QT Prolongation. Prolonged ventricular repolarization, as evidenced by QT-interval prolongation or a prominent U wave, or both, is the most striking ECG feature associated with torsade de pointes.[1,13,14] Reports of drug-induced torsade de pointes routinely cite the presence of QT prolongation.[15,16] An analysis of 61 episodes of torsade de pointes in 32 patients revealed prolongation of corrected QT interval (QT_c) in all patients, with a mean QT_c interval of 0.59 second.[17] A mean QT_c interval of 0.45 second was observed in patients who were receiving no cardiac medications and had no metabolic abnormalities. Patients who exhibit repolarization abnormalities before drug therapy is started are particularly prone to develop further QT prolongation and torsade de pointes.[8] Other patients may exhibit transient repolarization alterations that may be secondary to fluctuating autonomic, metabolic (electrolyte imbalance, ischemia), or drug status. Finally, there are patients who appear to have an idiosyncratic response to therapy with drugs such as quinidine. In these

Figure 3. Quinidine-induced torsade de pointes with characteristic long–short initiating sequence. A premature ventricular beat (left arrow) was followed by a long compensatory pause (RR interval 1560 msec). The conducted beat (center arrow) is followed by another premature ventricular beat (right arrow) (RR interval of 680 msec) that initiated the torsade de pointes with a cycle length of 320 msec.

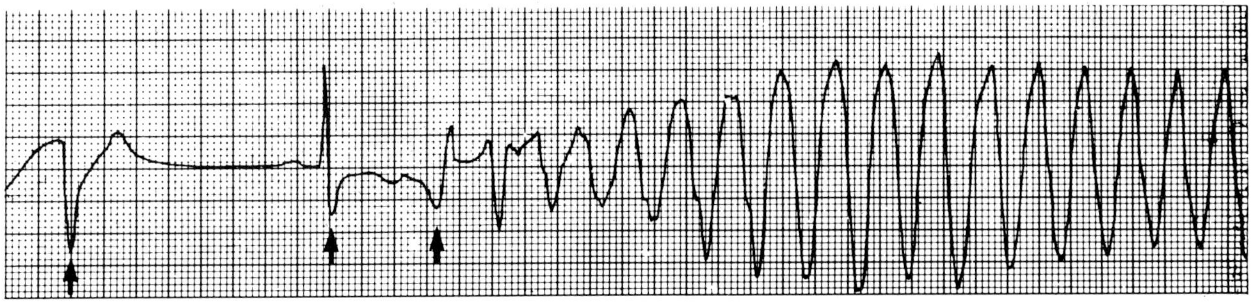

Figure 4. Procainamide-induced torsade de pointes (ECG tracing retouched for clarity).

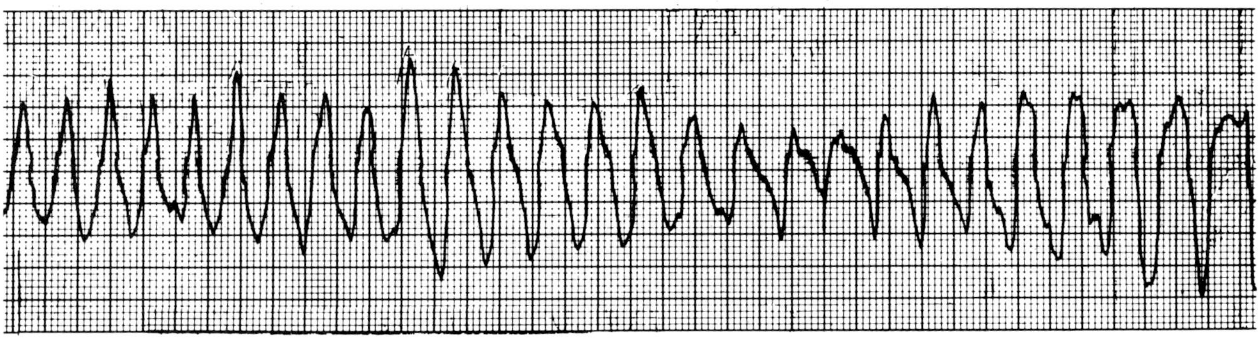

patients, the QT interval is prolonged despite the presence of a normal metabolic state and a nontoxic serum drug concentration.

Correct diagnosis of torsade de pointes requires identification of the prolonged QT interval. The numerical criterion for QT prolongation is arbitrary. Tzivoni[8] chose 0.60 second as a minimum reference value for QT prolongation. However, we favor less stringent criteria: a QT_c interval greater than 0.44 second or an uncorrected QT interval greater than 0.50 second.[11]

Long-Short Initiating Sequence. The torsade de pointes rhythm is usually initiated by premature ventricular beats exhibiting a long-short cycle length (Figures 1 and 3). Kay et al.[17] identified the long-short ventricular cycle-length sequence in 41 of 44 observed torsade de pointes episodes and in 115 of 131 (87.8%) previously published cases. This electrocardiographic feature, which was present in two of our patients, helps distinguish torsade de pointes from polymorphous ventricular tachycardia. Others have noted the emergence of a large slow wave in the ECG minutes before an episode of torsade de pointes.[18] The slow wave begins near the end of the T wave and may represent increased amplitude of the normal U wave.

R-on-T Phenomenon. Although the R-on-T phenomenon remains controversial as a cause of ventricular tachycardia, it appears to be important in the initiation of torsade de pointes. Kay et al.[17] observed the R-on-T initiation cycle in 38 of 44 torsade de pointes episodes. Nikolic et al.[19] demonstrated a similar arrhythmogenic potential of R-on-T events. Of 21 cardiac arrests documented by ambulatory ECG monitoring, 7 were preceded by torsade de pointes. Of the seven fatal torsade de pointes episodes, five were initiated by the R-on-T phenomenon.

Morphology. Electrocardiographic diagnosis of torsade de pointes is based on characteristic changing QRS complexes and polarity. A more precise definition of the torsade de pointes morphology includes complete reversal of the QRS-complex and T-wave deflections. These changes occur progressively, yielding an undulating baseline on the ECG. The QRS complexes at the portion of the curve with the least amplitude may appear normal. However, if only a single ECG lead is monitored, torsade de pointes morphology may appear uniform, thus complicating recognition.[12,18] In addition to the standard extremity leads, lead V_2 or V_3 should be examined. Polymorphous ventricular tachycardia is similar to torsade de pointes in morphologic appearance. Therefore, relying solely on ECG appearance is dangerous because its precludes rational therapeutic decision making.

Duration and Termination. Individual episodes of torsade de pointes vary in length but generally last for 5–20 beats.[16] Torsade de pointes attacks may be brief and may recur repetitively if underlying factors are not corrected.[3,18] Most attacks terminate spontaneously and result in no adverse hemodynamic effects. However, torsade de pointes is a potentially malignant arrhythmia that may deteriorate to ventricular fibrillation.[20]

Precursors. Torsade de pointes most often follows a period of enhanced ventricular ectopy. Lewis et al.[16] evaluated the ambulatory electrocardiographic recordings of 12 patients who experienced either ventricular fibrillation or torsade de pointes (3 patients) and syncope. Data from this report permit identification of premonitory ECG features in patients about to experience either ventricular fibrillation or torsade de pointes. One to three hours preceding the episode of ventricular fibrillation or torsade de pointes, the frequency of total hourly PVCs, total hourly couplets, and ventricular tachycardia episodes was significantly increased compared with earlier monitoring results in 11 of the 12 patients. The length and duration of episodes of monomorphic ventricular tachycardia also increased. Repetitive short runs of ventricular tachycardia often preceded torsade de pointes or ventricular fibrillation. Thus, the complexity of ventricular ectopy increases dramatically in patients about to experience torsade de pointes. This observation has been substantiated in recent studies by Kempf et al.[21] and Panidis et al.[22]

Clinical Presentation and Predisposing Factors

Torsade de pointes may result from any disease process that causes QT prolongation.[18] It frequently occurs in association with severe bradycardias or complete heart block; both of these arrhythmias are associated with prolonged QT intervals.[2,23] Torsade de pointes is also associated with metabolic abnormalities, including hypokalemia,[6] hypomagnesemia,[24–26] and perhaps localized cellular hypocalcemia.[27] Electrolyte abnormalities with subsequent torsade de pointes probably contributed to the fatal events observed in patients on liquid-protein diets.[28]

Prolongation of the QT interval and torsade de pointes have been identified in a number of cardiovascular conditions in addition to bradycardias: acute myocardial infarction,[29,30] congenital QT-prolongation syndrome,[31–33] mitral-valve prolapse,[34] coronary-artery vasospasm,[35] and myocarditis.[2] Other diseases or conditions rarely associated with torsade de pointes include hypothyroidism[36] and subarachnoid hemorrhage.[37,38] Drug-induced torsade de pointes has been attributed to more than 20 agents. Most drugs reported to precipitate torsade de pointes are antiarrhythmic or psychotropic agents (Table 2), both of which affect myocardial repolarization.

Lack of a uniform definition for torsade de pointes complicates interpretation of previously published case reports and studies of drug-induced torsade de pointes; we examined the reports cited in the remainder of this article using the criteria outlined in Table 1.

Classification of Antiarrhythmic Drugs

Vaughan Williams[39] classified antiarrhythmic agents based on electrophysiologic effects. Class I antiarrhythmic drugs reduce the initial rate of increase (phase 0) of cardiac action potentials. Because these drugs have varying effects on other action potential characteristics (QRS width, conduction, effective refractory period, and action potential duration), they are further subdivided. The effects of antiarrhythmic agents may be to lengthen (class Ia), shorten (class Ib), or produce little change (class Ic) in action potential duration.

Class Ia drugs (quinidine, procainamide, disopyramide) are most likely to cause torsade de pointes. Class Ib agents (lidocaine, tocainide, mexiletine, and phenytoin) are attractive alternate antiarrhythmic agents because they shorten action potential duration and pose little risk of inducing torsade de pointes. Class Ic drugs (encainide, flecainide, and lorcainide) do not greatly affect action potential duration. Encainide, for example, causes little or no QT prolongation after i.v. or short-term oral administration. However, the accumulation of active metabolites after long-term oral administration may result in QT prolongation.[40] Flecainide possesses both class I and class III activity; thus, it is associated with QT prolongation.[41] Torsade de pointes has not been reported as a complication of therapy with class Ic agents, although these agents may induce other forms of ventricular tachycardia.[42]

Table 2.
Drugs Reported To Induce Torsade de Pointes

Cardiovascular Agents
Ajmaline
Amiodarone
Aprindine
Bepridil
Disopyramide
Encainide
Lidoflazine
Moxaprindine
N-acetylprocainamide
Prenylamine
Procainamide
Propranolol
Quinidine
Sotalol
Psychotropic Agents
Amitriptyline
Imipramine
Maprotiline
Thioridazine
Trifluoperazine
Other Agents
Vasopressin
Diuretics

Class II agents with sympatholytic activity include bretylium and most β blockers. These drugs pose little risk of inducing torsade de pointes. Class III antiarrhythmic drugs prolong action potential duration. Some β blockers, most notably sotalol, lengthen action potential duration and cause torsade de pointes.[43] Amiodarone is the prototype class III agent, and it lengthens action potential duration but has little class I or sympatholytic effect.[39] Torsade de pointes sometimes complicates amiodarone therapy.[44] The class IV agents are the calcium-channel blockers, which differ widely in chemical structure, tissue selectivity, and electrophysiologic activity. Unless these drugs also lengthen the QT interval (e.g., lidoflazine, bepridil), they are unlikely to cause torsade de pointes.[45]

Specific Cardiac Drugs

Quinidine. Quinidine is the most common cause of drug-induced torsade de pointes. It was a precipitating factor in the development of the arrhythmias in patients 2 and 3. Recognized as a potential hazard for decades,[46] quinidine syncope varies in incidence between 1 and 8%.[47] When Sclarovsky et al.[10] retrospectively analyzed 34 episodes of polymorphous ventricular tachycardia meeting torsade de pointes criteria, quinidine therapy was cited as the causative factor in 22 cases. Most patients had severe underlying organic heart disease and were receiving quinidine therapy for suppression of ventricular ectopy. The authors noted that there was no relationship between amount or duration of quinidine prescribed and the appearance of torsade de pointes. Because metabolic and electrolyte data were not provided in this report, the potential role of multiple precipitating factors is unknown.

The electrocardiographic characteristics of quinidine-induced torsade de pointes in 5 patients were evaluated by Denes et al.[48] in a retrospective review of 3307 patients undergoing Holter monitoring. Characteristics common to the patients included severe congestive heart failure (New York Heart Association class III or IV), recent introduction of quinidine therapy (4–12 days duration), QT-interval prolongation (range, 0.48–0.68 second), and complex ventricular ectopy (couplets and bigeminy). Quinidine therapy was prescribed to control ventricular arrhythmias in four of the five patients; doses ranged from 0.8 to 2.6 g/day. Serum quinidine concentrations obtained one hour after dosing ranged from 1.24 to 5.18 μg/mL. One patient was receiving concurrent procainamide therapy (peak serum concentration 16.4 μg/mL). No patient was thought to have either digitalis toxicity or electrolyte imbalances. All patients with torsade de pointes suffered a syncopal attack. Two of the five patients had spontaneous termination of torsade de pointes. Three required resuscitation, and only one of the three patients survived.

Similar electrocardiographic and clinical features were observed by Kay et al.[17] Quinidine was the agent cited most often as responsible for torsade de pointes; the drug was prescribed for 19 of 32 patients. Serum quinidine concentrations exceeded generally accepted effective concentrations in only 4 of the 17 patients for whom drug concentration values were available. Four patients exhibited concomitant hypokalemia (serum potassium concentration less than 3.5 meq/L). One of these patients developed torsade de pointes only when serum potassium concentration fell to 2.7 meq/L. After potassium supplementation, this patient was successfully maintained with the same quinidine dose prescribed before the development of torsade de pointes. Hypomagnesemia may have contributed to the development of torsade de pointes, because serum magnesium concentrations were less than 2.2 meq/L in five of the seven patients for whom serum magnesium was measured. The ECG recorded immediately before torsade de pointes developed in patients receiving quinidine showed a mean QT_c interval of 0.62 second (range, 0.47–0.79 second). The long–short ventricular cycle-length sequence preceded torsade de pointes in all cases; the R-on-T phenomenon was observed in all but three patients.

Bauman et al.[47] reviewed the records of 31 patients who developed torsade de pointes that was caused by quinidine. Of the patients studied, 71% were receiving quinidine to control atrial fibrillation or atrial flutter. The duration of quinidine therapy was less than one week in 23 patients (74%) and less than three months in 28 patients (90%). For most of the patients, serum quinidine concentrations were within generally accepted effective values. Although 90% of the patients were receiving concomitant digoxin therapy, no patient had serum digoxin concentrations in the range that is considered potentially toxic. Hypokalemia, evidenced by a serum potassium concentration of less than 3.5 meq/L within 24 hours before the onset of torsade de pointes, was observed in 5 (24%) of 21 patients whose data were available. Two patients whose serum magnesium concentrations were obtained were hypomagnesemic with values of 1.5 and 1.9 meq/L, respectively. Serum calcium values were normal in the nine patients for whom this determination was made. ECG rhythm strips preceding torsade de pointes were available for 11 of the 31 patients. Of the 10 patients in sinus rhythm, all exhibited the long–short ventricular sequence immediately before developing torsade de pointes. Quinidine therapy was discontinued for most patients. However, torsade de pointes recurred in 18 (58%) of 31 patients[47]; 14 patients (45%) required one or more direct-current cardioversions, 1 died, and 2 patients who were rechallenged with quinidine had nonfatal torsade de pointes recurrences. Eight patients received other class Ia antiarrhythmic agents (disopyramide and procainamide). In five of the eight patients torsade de pointes recurred, resulting in one death.

Several concepts emerge from these published observations. Quinidine-induced torsade de pointes often occurs at quinidine doses that produce serum quinidine concentrations within the generally accepted effective range (case 2).[16,47–49] Interpretation of a dose–response relationship is difficult when nonspecific quinidine assays are used.[50] Variations in protein binding may yield very high free quinidine concentrations in spite of normal total serum concentrations.[51]

While torsade de pointes may occur at any time during quinidine therapy, most patients first exhibit this arrhythmia shortly after beginning therapy. When torsade de pointes appears later, it probably occurs because of an increased dosage of drug or because of the development of exacerbating factors such as hypokalemia. Concomitant electrolyte disturbances, particularly hypokalemia and hypomagnesemia, contribute to quinidine-induced torsade de pointes, as observed in cases 2 and 3 in this paper. Prolongation of the QT interval is universal. The long–short ventricular sequence often immediately precedes the onset of torsade de pointes. Clinical outcomes of quinidine-induced torsade de pointes range from an asymptomatic self-terminating episode to cardiac arrest and death.

Disopyramide. Disopyramide, a class Ia antiarrhythmic agent, is a predictable precipitator of torsade de pointes. Nicholson[52] reported three cases of disopyramide-induced torsade de pointes in 1979. Electrocardiograms showed markedly prolonged QT intervals in two patients and a prolonged QU interval in the remaining patient. The arrhythmias occurred in spite of normal serum potassium concentrations and "therapeutic" disopyramide doses (150 mg orally every four or six hours). In one patient torsade de pointes terminated spontaneously, while another patient required overdrive pacing. The third patient suffered cardiopulmonary arrest but was successfully resuscitated.

In another study, therapy with oral disopyramide resulted in torsade de pointes with QT prolongation in a patient receiving disopyramide for maintenance of sinus rhythm after cardioversion from atrial fibrillation.[53]

Disopyramide at low therapeutic doses was an apparent causative factor in the development of torsade de pointes in three patients described by Kay[17] and in one patient described by Soffer.[9] Like quinidine, disopyramide exhibits variations in protein binding (concentration-dependent) that make total plasma concentration determinations difficult to interpret.[54] Riccioni et al.[55] described disopyramide-induced torsade de pointes that disappeared only after an intravenous infusion of 10 mL of 10% calcium gluconate.

Procainamide and *N*-acetylprocainamide. Although early investigators assumed that procainamide could induce torsade de pointes through a quinidine-like mechanism,[2,4,10] detailed reports of this did not appear until 1981. Strasberg et al.[56] described seven cases of procainamide-induced torsade de pointes associated with a prolonged QT interval (0.48–0.78 second). Four patients experienced the disorder after intravenous administration of 200–400 mg procainamide hydrochloride for sustained ventricular tachycardia; the remaining three patients received oral procainamide hydrochloride 3–4 g daily for chronic ventricular ectopy or atrial flutter. Four patients experienced no morbidity, while two died from irreversible ventricular fibrillation. The remaining patient had a permanent pacemaker inserted, and torsade de pointes did not recur despite continued procainamide therapy.

In 1982, Soffer et al.[9] described development of torsade de pointes in a 68-year-old man after intravenous administration of 500 mg of procainamide hydrochloride. Kay et al.[17] cited procainamide as a precipitating factor in the development of torsade de pointes in seven patients. Serum procainamide concentrations measured in five of the seven patients ranged from 2.8 to 7.5 μg/mL. In only two of these patients (serum procainamide concentrations 2.8 and 5.2 μg/mL, respectively) was procainamide the sole precipitating factor of the arrhythmia. The other patients had multiple precipitating factors including electrolyte imbalances (hypokalemia and hypocalcemia) and therapy with a drug known to induce torsade de pointes (disopyramide and quinidine).

In another study by Lewis,[16] a 68-year-old woman with three-vessel coronary-artery disease and a history of anterior myocardial infarction developed torsade de pointes or ventricular fibrillation (rhythm not specified) after receiving procainamide for 120 days and digoxin for nine years. This patient exhibited a profoundly lengthened QT interval (0.70 second) immediately before the arrhythmia. No information about procainamide dose, serum drug concentrations, or electrolyte balance was provided.

N-acetylprocainamide (NAPA), a pharmacologically active metabolite of procainamide that is classified as a class III antiarrhythmic agent, has also been implicated in causing torsade de pointes.[57] NAPA accumulation may have contributed to the torsade de pointes episodes we observed in patient 3.

Recently, Chow et al.[58] reported the first well-documented case of torsade de pointes induced by NAPA. A 72-year-old woman with recurrent ventricular tachycardia and a procainamide-induced lupus syndrome was evaluated while receiving NAPA therapy alone. She had experienced previous episodes of torsade de pointes while receiving quinidine or disopyramide. Before NAPA administration, her QT_c interval (0.45 second) and serum electrolyte concentrations were within normal limits. Intravenous infusion of NAPA produced a plasma drug concentration of 36.3 μg/mL and a corresponding increase in the QT_c interval to 0.50 second. Because of favorable arrhythmia suppression with this trial of NAPA, the patient was started on oral NAPA therapy at 1.5 g every eight hours, and this dose was subsequently increased to 2 g every eight hours. The patient soon developed torsade de pointes, with the characteristic long-short cycle sequence, which degenerated to ventricular fibrillation requiring direct-current cardioversion and lidocaine therapy. The serum NAPA concentration was 32.4 μg/mL, and the QT_c interval was prolonged at 0.60 second. The patient was discharged without further antiarrhythmic therapy.

Procainamide, like quinidine, may precipitate torsade de pointes at nontoxic doses. More often procainamide-induced torsade de pointes occurs in the presence of multiple precipitating factors, such as concurrent quinidine therapy or electrolyte imbalance. NAPA, which is known to prolong action potential duration, may contribute to the procainamide-induced torsade de pointes syndrome.[59,60] NAPA as a single agent also produces torsade de pointes. The experiences cited with NAPA therapy indicate that acute antiarrhythmic drug testing may not always predict subsequent drug-induced torsade de pointes.

Amiodarone. Amiodarone, a class III antiarrhythmic agent, is useful in treating life-threatening ventricular arrhythmias. The drug's electrophysiologic and pharmacokinetic properties distinguish it from currently marketed antiarrhythmic agents.[61,62] Amiodarone prolongs atrial and ventricular action potential duration without altering resting membrane potential. Its clinical use is characterized by a delayed onset of action and a prolonged elimination half-life (estimated at 30–45 days).[62]

Amiodarone, like quinidine, procainamide, and disopyramide, prolongs the QT (QTU) interval. However, amiodarone's observed effect on the QT interval, which is apparent after four days of oral therapy, may not be fully reached until 4–5 weeks of therapy.[61] Intravenous administration of amiodarone may cause marked prolongation of the QT interval within 12 hours.[63] The effects of amiodarone on the QT interval persist for a long period after the drug is discontinued.

Sclarovsky et al.[44] presented five cases of amiodarone-induced torsade de pointes associated with a prolonged QT interval (0.58–0.60 second) and recurrent syncope or dizziness. In two patients, torsade de pointes persisted despite correction of simultaneous hypokalemia. Standard treatment of torsade de pointes (electrolyte correction, administration of isoproterenol, or ventricular pacing) was successful in all five patients. However, prolonged amiodarone elimination half-life made it necessary to treat patients for 5–10 days.

Santinelli et al.[64] described the development of torsade de pointes in a 49-year-old woman receiving long-term amiodarone therapy. The disorder was associated with a QT interval of 0.60 second and was controlled by treatment with intravenous mexiletine and a potassium infusion. The QT interval did not return to normal until 10 days after the amiodarone was discontinued.

Torsade de pointes developed within 2–5 days after the addition of amiodarone 800 mg/day in two patients who had been treated previously with disopyramide 600 mg/day for three and six months.[65] In both patients, the QT interval did not return to normal until five days after the drug was discontinued. Torsade de pointes did not recur after cessation of amiodarone therapy and continued disopyramide therapy. Thus, amiodarone-induced torsade de pointes may occur alone or with other contributing disease states and medications.[66] Caution must be exercised if amiodarone is used concurrently with class Ia antiarrhythmic drugs. Also, because amiodarone has a long elimination half-life, amiodarone-induced torsade de pointes requires prolonged therapy.[67]

Aprindine. Aprindine, an experimental class I antiarrhythmic agent, may also precipitate torsade de pointes. Scagliotti et al.[68] described five patients with aprindine-induced torsade de pointes. In these patients, the QT interval returned to predrug levels after aprindine withdrawal. Interestingly, three of these patients had developed torsade de pointes previously while receiving other class I antiarrhythmic agents (quinidine or disopyramide). Two of the patients who developed aprindine-induced torsade de pointes required direct-current cardioversion; one patient received intravenous isoproterenol. The remaining patient required an atrial pacemaker. Moxaprindine, a pharmacologically similar aprindine derivative, has also been associated with torsade de pointes.[69]

Lidocaine Congeners. Two lidocaine congeners mexiletine and tocainide are sometimes recommended for treating torsade de pointes,[18,64,70] but have also been implicated in causing this arrythmia. However, electrocardiographic criteria consistent with true torsade de pointes are lacking in these reports.[71,72]

Sotalol. Sotalol, a nonselective β-blocking agent with no intrinsic sympathomimetic activity or membrane-stabilizing properties, prolongs the action potential and effective refractory period in ventricular muscle and Purkinje fibers.[73] Sotalol is a class III antiarrhythmic drug and is used to treat both supraventricular and ventricular arrhythmias. In 1982, Tötterman et al.[74] described four patients with sotalol-induced torsade de pointes who were successfully treated with overdrive pacing. Three of the four patients did not respond to lidocaine therapy. Sotalol-induced torsade de pointes in association with marked QT prolongation and sinus bradycardia may occur during treatment with a low daily dose of sotalol (320 mg/day).[75]

McKibbin et al.[43] described 13 patients who developed syncope and a prolonged QT_c interval while receiving therapeutic sotalol doses. Of the 13 patients studied, 11 exhibited polymorphous ventricular tachycardia that met the criteria for torsade de pointes. In all patients, torsade de pointes was initiated by a premature ventricular beat occurring on the preceding T wave. Hypokalemia appeared to play a role in the development of torsade de pointes in most of these patients. Four patients were also receiving other drugs known to prolong the QT interval (disopyramide and tricyclic antidepressants). Thus, sotalol should be administered cautiously with other drugs known to prolong repolarization or cause hypokalemia.

Calcium-Channel-Blocking Agents. Torsade de pointes is most often induced by drugs known to affect myocardial repolarization. The introduction of calcium-channel blockers that prolong the QT interval (lidoflazine and bepridil) prompts concern that torsade de pointes may be induced by calcium-channel blocking agents. Lidoflazine is an antianginal calcium blocker with coronary vasodilator effects that has been implicated in causing torsade de pointes.[2] Bepridil, an antianginal calcium blocker undergoing clinical study in the United States, prolongs the action potential duration substantially and therefore prolongs the QT_c interval.[45] Bepridil-induced torsade de pointes has been reported in studies of European patients.[18]

Of the three calcium-channel blockers currently marketed in the United States, only nifedipine has been reported to induce torsade de pointes.[76] However, the cause-and-effect relationship between nifedipine and torsade de pointes in this single case report is suspect. The patient had several contributing factors that included hypokalemia, doxepin therapy within the preceding 24 hours, and underlying coronary-artery disease. Furthermore, the QT interval was only slightly prolonged at 0.44 second.

Psychotropic Agents. Cardiovascular effects of phenothiazines and tricyclic antidepressants are well documented. Thioridazine and other phenothiazines exhibit quinidine-like electrophysiologic effects including depression of the following: action potential duration, action potential amplitude, maximal rate of rise during phase 0 of the action potential, and duration and amplitude of phase 2, along with a prolonged phase 3 repolarization.[77] Electrocardiographic effects of phenothiazines are primarily ventricular repolarization abnormalities, such as QT interval prolongation, depression of T-wave amplitude, and increased U-wave amplitude. About 5% of patients receiving 200–400 mg/day of thioridazine hydrochloride exhibit ECG abnormalities. Torsade de pointes is one of many ventricular arrhythmias associated with phenothiazine therapy.[78]

Kemper et al.[79] described a patient treated with progressively increasing thioridazine hydrochloride doses reaching a maximum of 1500 mg/day who experienced a cardiopulmonary arrest. Postarrest ECG showed characteristic ST-segment flattening, prominent U wave, and QT_c prolongation (0.56 second). While thioridazine-induced torsade de pointes is associated most often with high daily doses, such as 2100–3000 mg/day,[8–10] it may also occur at low doses. The patient described in case 1 received chronic thioridazine and trifluoperazine therapy and later developed torsade de pointes requiring isoproterenol therapy.

Tricyclic antidepressants such as imipramine and desipramine also exhibit electrophysiologic effects similar to quinidine, including prolongation of the PR, QRS, and QT intervals.[80] These agents are known to precipitate arrhythmias including torsade de pointes.[16] Interestingly, they are also under investigation for their antiarrhythmic potential.[81] Maprotiline, a tetracyclic anthracene-derivative antidepressant, has been linked with torsade de pointes.[82]

Miscellaneous Drugs That Induce Torsade de Pointes. Several other drugs have been reported to cause torsade de pointes. Prenylamine is a coronary vasodilator that has been implicated.[2,83] Ajmaline,[10] propranolol,[16] and encainide[16] are rarely associated with the development of torsade de pointes. Vasopressin apparently provoked torsade de pointes in a patient without known heart disease.[84] Diuretic agents and hypokalemia, hypomagnesemia, and hypocalcemia induced by these agents are common causes of torsade de pointes.[1–17,85] Torsades de pointes also occurred following the ingestion of 31 mg/kg (total of 2.5 g) of amantadine hydrochloride.[86]

Mechanisms Causing Torsade de Pointes

The electrophysiologic mechanisms causing torsade de pointes remain unclear. Effects on both reentry and automaticity may be responsible, especially in the presence of a marked and uneven delay in myocardial repolarization. When Dessertenne et al.[1] described torsade de pointes in 1966, they postulated that abnormal automaticity was the mechanism causing the disorder. Recent work suggests that re-entry may be the dominant mechanism in patients with intrinsic heart disease.[13,87–92] In these patients, torsade de pointes may be induced by programmed stimulation. Unfortunately, electrophysiologic studies are less informative when torsade de pointes is drug induced. If the causative drug is removed, the disorder is rarely induced by programmed stimulation. Repeat challenge with the offending drug does not always induce torsade de pointes.[12]

Class Ia antiarrhythmic drugs may prevent reentrant arrhythmias by making refractoriness uniform in both normal and ischemic regions, by converting a unidirectional block to a complete (bidirectional) block, or by promoting homogeneous propagation.[93] As previously mentioned, these also prolong the QT interval and thus have the potential to prolong refractoriness. Therefore, class Ia antiarrhythmics may create new areas of re-entry or worsen existing re-entrant circuits. These mechanisms correspond with the observed clinical effect of these drugs: either suppression or induction of ventricular arrhythmias. Torsade de pointes, initiated by a premature ventricular beat occurring late in diastole, probably results from an excessive increase in refractory periods as evidenced by marked prolongation of the QT interval.

In early studies, torsade de pointes was thought to be a transitional form of ventricular fibrillation.[2] The morphologic appearance of torsade de pointes may be produced by phasic stimulation of the right and left ventricles.[89,93] Epicardial-mapping studies in dogs demonstrated that each change in QRS morphology was associated with a change in the site of epicardial breakthrough of the impulse.[93] The observed QRS complexes were actually a composite representing competition between two or more activating sequences. The characteristic undulating pattern followed changes in epicardial activation. The QRS complex changed slightly if the next site of epicardial breakthrough was near the previous site. However, if the sites were distant from one another, the change in morphology was noticeable. A more dramatic shift of the epicardial activation site caused the polarity of the QRS complex to change on the surface ECG.

Torsade de pointes usually terminates spontaneously. If, however, the sites of activation differ, torsade de pointes may degenerate into ventricular fibrillation. Similarly, if one activation site dominates, torsade de pointes may convert to a sustained ventricular tachycardia. By increasing refractoriness, administration of a class Ia antiarrhythmic agent during an episode of torsade de pointes may permit one dominant exit site, thus converting torsade de pointes to typical sustained ventricular tachycardia.

One paradox is that antiarrhythmic agents intended to suppress ventricular arrhythmias actually aggravate them in about 11% of patients.[94] Antiarrhythmic therapy may be a possible cause of out-of-hospital cardiac arrests.[94–96] Some of these deaths are undoubtedly caused by torsade de pointes.[21,22] Because torsade de pointes most often occurs without warning, studies that mimic the clinical conditions associated with this arrhythmia are difficult to design. Often a combination of precipitating factors must be present, such as concomitant drug therapy, electrolyte abnormality, and myocardial ischemia. Animal models and clinical studies have successfully reproduced the major criteria for torsade de pointes, including undulating QRS morphology, QT prolongation, and spontaneous termination.[87-89,97] However, caution must be used in extrapolation of these results to common clinical settings.

Therapeutic Management of Torsade de Pointes

Management of ventricular tachycardia with a polymorphic appearance depends on the presence or absence of QT prolongation. Torsade de pointes is characterized by the typical ECG pattern occurring in the setting of a prolonged QT interval or a prominent U wave. Polymorphous ventricular tachycardia that is not associated with QT prolongation is not torsade de pointes and may therefore respond to class Ia antiarrhythmic drugs.[11] In contrast, torsade de pointes is exacerbated by class Ia antiarrhythmic agents. Treatment of torsade de pointes is directed at shortening and unifying the prolonged and nonuniform repolarization underlying the disorder or at suppressing enhanced automaticity.[98]

Emergency Intervention. Torsade de pointes is a potentially fatal ventricular arrhythmia. Class I quinidine-like antiarrhythmic agents should be avoided at all costs in patients with torsade de pointes. Offending agents should be discontinued immediately. If the disorder is associated with hemodynamic deterioration or degeneration to ventricular fibrillation (exemplified in case 2), defibrillation is warranted.[18]

Cardiac Pacing. The definitive therapy of torsade de pointes is overdrive pacing from either the atrium or the ventricle.[99,100] Integrity of the atrioventricular (AV) conduction system determines selection of the pacing mode.[98] If AV conduction is intact, atrial pacing is ideal because it results in maximal shortening of the QT interval and is less likely to induce arrhythmias than is ventricular pacing.[9] If it is difficult to obtain or maintain stable atrial pacing, right-ventricular pacing is an alternative.[9,98] Pacing should be performed at the lowest rate (usually 90–110 beats/min) that will effectively stop torsade de pointes.[18] Breakthrough development of torsade de pointes during temporary pacing is rare. Pacing should probably be continued until the QT_c interval has normalized.

Isoproterenol. Isoproterenol is the drug most commonly used to treat torsade de pointes.[1-3,9-12,20,47,65,100] However, it is not always as effective as overdrive pacing.[13] The isoproterenol infusion rate is titrated to optimally increase the heart rate, thus shortening the QT interval. The patients we described required isoproterenol in doses ranging from 1 to 2 μg/min. The risks associated with the use of isoproterenol in these patients are high and the drug should be avoided in patients with serious ischemic or hypertensive cardiovascular disease. Isoproterenol is especially hazardous if drug-induced torsade de pointes develops in a patient who has recently suffered an acute myocardial infarction.

Isoproterenol may be used temporarily until pacing is instituted (cases 1 and 2), or it may be continued cautiously until repolarization abnormalities have resolved. In patients with amiodarone-induced torsade de pointes, isoproterenol and pacing may need to be continued for 5–10 days because of amiodarone's long elimination half-life. However, in most patients with drug-induced torsade de pointes, this therapy is required for approximately 24–48 hours.

Bretylium and Lidocaine. Bretylium may suppress drug-induced torsade de pointes.[2,9-11,17,20,47] Because of its differential effect on ischemic and normal tissue, bretylium may minimize the disparity in action potential duration caused by quinidine-like drugs.

Like the efficacy of bretylium, that of lidocaine depends on differential effects on normal versus abnormal tissue. However, lidocaine shortens refractory periods primarily at normal or border sites and not in damaged tissue.[86] Lidocaine, in contrast to bretylium, may sometimes increase the disparity in refractoriness between normal and damaged tissue. Therefore, lidocaine is often ineffective in treating torsade de pointes,[9,10,17,56,57,65,77,79] whereas bretylium may be effective. Two of the patients (described in cases 1 and 2) did not respond to bretylium and lidocaine therapy. In the third patient (case 3) torsade de pointes apparently was suppressed with lidocaine therapy, although ventricular ectopy persisted.

Correction of Electrolyte Imbalance. Each patient who develops torsade de pointes should have a thorough assessment of serum electrolytes. Hypokalemia, hypomagnesemia, and perhaps hypocalcemia are often present; if not corrected, these conditions may prevent abolition of the arrhythmia (case 1 and 3). While serum potassium concentrations are usually monitored, hypomagnesemia often is not detected.[101,102] In a recent study,[17] serum magnesium concentrations were obtained in only 11 of 32 patients, and 8 of these 11 patients had hypomagnesemia.

Many electrolyte disorders are interrelated. Hypokalemia, hypophosphatemia, hyponatremia, and hypocalcemia should all alert the clinician to possible magnesium depletion.[103,104] Clinical conditions associated with both magnesium depletion and torsade de pointes include acute myocardial infarction, diuretic therapy, malnutrition, and liquid protein diets.[105,106] Routine serum magnesium determinations are warranted for these patient populations.[102]

Recent reports suggest that intravenous administration of magnesium sulfate is effective in treating torsade de pointes regardless of serum magnesium concentration.[107] Iseri et al.[108] described two patients with recurrent ventricular tachycardia or ventricular fibrillation or torsade de pointes who had normal serum magnesium concentrations but did not respond to treatment with potassium chloride, lidocaine, or bretylium tosylate. Both patients were receiving prolonged diuretic therapy that may have resulted in cellular hypomagnesemia not reflected by low serum magnesium concentrations. Both patients were also receiving quinidine sulfate. After four hours of magnesium therapy, serum magnesium concentrations rose from 2.6 to 3.7 meq/L, with abolition of arrhythmias.

Tzivoni et al.[26] reported success with the use of 1–2 g of intravenous magnesium sulfate in three consecutive patients with torsade de pointes. The disorder was induced in these patients by therapy with a combination of quinidine and amiodarone, procainamide therapy, and imipramine overdose, respectively. Each patient exhibited a prolonged QT interval before receiving magnesium sulfate. In two patients, magnesium sulfate therapy did not alter measured serum magnesium concentrations, which were within normal limits before magnesium supplementation. None of the three patients demonstrated an immediate shortening of the QT interval after receiving magnesium sulfate.

Magnesium sulfate therapy appears attractive for treating drug-induced torsade de pointes, although clinical experience with its use is limited. Some advantages to magnesium sulfate are that it is easily administered and poses less risk to the patient than isoproterenol infusion. Magnesium sulfate therapy is not associated with worsening of arrhythmias or ischemic heart disease. Mild hypotension induced by magnesium sulfate therapy is not life threatening if proper drug-administration precautions are followed.

Ramee et al.[107] have proposed guidelines for magnesium replacement in patients with torsade de pointes. According to Ramee, magnesium replacement should begin with an initial infusion of 16 meq over one minute, followed by 1 meq/kg during the first 24 hours and 0.5 meq/kg daily for three days. However, oliguric renal failure may be an absolute contraindication to magnesium therapy. Also, because potassium depletion and magnesium depletion often occur simultaneously, detection of either abnormality may warrant repletion of both ions. Magnesium supplementation deserves additional study as treatment for torsade de pointes.

Prevention. Prevention of drug-induced torsade de pointes is best achieved by recognizing the predisposing factors. Before initiating drugs with known potential to induce torsade de pointes, the QT interval should be measured. If the QT interval is prolonged, class Ia and class III antiarrhythmic agents, phenothiazines, and tricyclic and tetracyclic antidepressant agents should be avoided. There does not appear to be a critical degree of QT prolongation or a critical drug dose that can predict the onset of torsade de pointes.[109,110]

Patients receiving long-term diuretic therapy should be assessed periodically for potassium, magnesium, and calcium imbalances. Care should also be taken to avoid simultaneous hypokalemia, hypocalcemia, or hypomagnesemia with class I and class III antiarrhythmic therapy. Any new therapeutic agent that is associated with QT prolongation should be suspected of causing torsade de pointes.

Conclusion

Drug-induced torsade de pointes is a potentially lethal arrhythmia. Although the electrophysiologic mechanisms underlying drug-induced torsade de pointes have not been fully identified, any drug that prolongs the QT interval is suspect. The definitive emergency therapy is overdrive pacing. Isoproterenol infusion offers a reasonable but sometimes risky alternative. Preliminary reports suggest that intravenous magnesium sulfate supplementation may be safe and efficacious. Traditional antiarrhythmic therapy with lidocaine or bretylium is only occasionally effective in abolishing drug-induced torsade de pointes.

Although it is difficult to predict which patients will experience drug-induced torsade de pointes, patients with a pre-existing prolonged QT interval are at greater risk. Concomitant hypokalemia and hypomagnesemia are synergistic with QT-prolonging drugs in producing torsade de pointes.

Discussion Questions

1. In each of the three cases described, magnesium sulfate therapy was not tried as a treatment modality. What specific dose and administration recommendations would you provide if this drug were used in the acute management of drug-induced torsade de pointes? What patient-monitoring criteria would you employ, and how would you define the therapeutic endpoints?
2. The numerical criteria for QT prolongation observed during torsade de pointes are arbitrary. Do you think the criteria outlined in this paper are appropriate? How is the QT interval measured and what are its normal limits?
3. Discuss the relationship between hypokalemia and hypomagnesemia. Recommend appropriate diuretic therapy if both potassium-sparing and magnesium-sparing properties are desired.
4. The development of generally accepted plasma concentrations for antiarrhythmic agents has sometimes relied on older analytical methods. Discuss your institution's current analytical methods for

measuring antiarrhythmic concentrations. Focus on the limitations of each assay.

5. The electrophysiologic effects of intravenously and orally administered amiodarone differ. Is i.v. amiodarone likely to cause torsade de pointes? If so, what might be the time course of the onset and disappearance of the arrhythmia?

References

1. Dessertenne F, Fabiato A, Coumel P. Les variations progressives de l' amplitude de l' electrocardiogramme. *Actual Cardiol Angeiol Int.* 1966; 15:241–58.
2. Smith WM, Gallagher JJ. "Les torsades de pointes": an unusual ventricular arrhythmia. *Ann Intern Med.* 1980; 93:578–84.
3. Krikler DM, Curry PVL. Torsade de pointes, an atypical ventricular tachycardia. *Br Heart J.* 1976; 38:117–20. Editorial.
4. Loeb HS, Pietras RJ, Gunnar RM et al. Paroxysmal ventricular fibrillation in two patients with hypomagnesemia. Treatment by transvenous pacing. *Circulation.* 1968; 37:210–5.
5. Tamura K, Tamura T, Yoshida S et al. Transient recurrent ventricular fibrillation due to hypopotassemia with special note on the U wave. *Jpn Heart J.* 1967; 8:652–60.
6. Smirk FH, Ng J. Cardiac ballet: repetitions of complex electrocardiographic patterns. *Br Heart J.* 1969; 31:426–34.
7. Ranquin R, Parizel G. Ventricular fibrillo-flutter ("torsade de pointe"): an established electrocardiographic and clinical entity. *Angiology.* 1977; 28:115–8.
8. Tzivoni D, Keren A, Stern S. Torsades de pointes versus polymorphous ventricular tachycardia. *Am J Cardiol.* 1983; 52:639–40.
9. Soffer J, Dreifus LS, Michelson EL. Polymorphous ventricular tachycardia associated with normal and long Q-T intervals. *Am J Cardiol.* 1982; 49:2021–9.
10. Sclarovsky S, Strasberg B, Lewin RF et al. Polymorphous ventricular tachycardia: clinical features and treatment. *Am J Cardiol.* 1979; 44:339–44.
11. Schweitzer P, Mark H. Delayed repolarization syndrome. *Am J Med.* 1983; 75:393–401.
12. Horowitz LN, Greenspan AM, Spielman SR et al. Torsades de pointes: electrophysiologic studies in patients without transient pharmacologic or metabolic abnormalities. *Circulation.* 1981; 63:1120–8.
13. Horowitz LN, Josephson ME. Torsades de pointes. In: Surawicz B, Reddy CP, Prystowsky EN, eds. *Tachycardias.* Boston: Martinus Nijhoff Publishing; 1984:283–91.
14. Zipes DP. Specific arrhythmias: diagnosis and treatment. In: Braunwald E, ed. Heart disease: a textbook of cardiovascular medicine. Philadelphia: W. B. Saunders Company; 1984; 725–6.
15. Fisch C. Electrocardiography and vectorcardiography. In: Braunwald E, ed. Heart disease: a textbook of cardiovascular medicine. Philadelphia: W. B. Saunders Company; 1984; 203–4.
16. Lewis BH, Antman EM, Graboys TB. Detailed analysis of 24 hour ambulatory electrocardiographic recordings during ventricular fibrillation or torsade de pointes. *J Am Coll Cardiol.* 1983; 2:426–36.
17. Kay GN, Plumb VJ, Arciniegas JG et al. Torsade de pointes: the long-short initiating sequence and other clinical features: observations in 32 patients. *J Am Coll Cardiol.* 1983; 2:806–17.
18. Jackman WM, Clark M, Friday KJ et al. Ventricular tachyarrhythmias in the long QT syndrome. *Med Clin North Am.* 1984; 68:1079–1109.
19. Nikolic G, Bishop RL, Singh JB. Sudden death recorded during Holter monitoring. *Circulation.* 1982; 66:218–25.
20. Bigger JT. Definition of benign versus malignant ventricular arrhythmias. *Am J Cardiol.* 1983; 52:47C–54C.
21. Kempf FC, Josephson ME. Cardiac arrest recorded on ambulatory electrocardiograms. *Am J Cardiol.* 1984; 53:1577–82.
22. Panidis IP, Morganroth J. Sudden death in hospitalized patients: cardiac rhythm disturbances detected by ambulatory electrocardiographic monitoring. *J Am Coll Cardiol.* 1983; 2:798–805.
23. Bissett JK, Watson JW, Scovil JA et al. Sudden death in cardiomyopathy: role of bradycardia-dependent repolarization changes. *Am Heart J.* 1980; 99:625–9.
24. Topol EJ, Lerman BB. Hypomagnesemic torsades de pointes. *Am J Cardiol.* 1983; 52:1367–8.
25. Levine SR, Crowley TJ, Hai HA. Hypomagnesemia and ventricular tachycardia. *Chest.* 1982; 81:244–7.
26. Tzivoni D, Keren A, Cohen AM et al. Magnesium therapy for torsades de pointes. *Am J Cardiol.* 1984; 53:528–30.
27. Doroghazi RM, Childers R. Time-related changes in the Q-T interval in acute myocardial infarction: possible relation to local hypocalcemia. *Am J Cardiol.* 1978; 41:684–8.
28. Singh BN, Gaarder TD, Kanegae T et al. Liquid protein diets and torsade de pointes. *JAMA.* 1978; 240:115–9.
29. Griffin J, Most AS. Torsade de pointes complicating acute myocardial infarction. *Am Heart J.* 1984; 107:169–70.
30. Grenadier E, Alpan G, Maor N et al. Polymorphous ventricular tachycardia in acute myocardial infarction. *Am J Cardiol.* 1984; 53:1280–3.
31. Jervell A, Lange-Nielsen F. Congenital deaf-mutism, functional heart disease with prolongation of the Q-T interval and sudden death. *Am Heart J.* 1957; 54:59–68.
32. Ward OC. A new familial cardiac syndrome in children. *J Ir Med Assoc.* 1964; 54:103–6.
33. Andersson P, Lundkvist L. The Q-T syndrome—a family description. *Acta Med Scand.* 1979; 206:73–6.
34. Puddu PE, Pasternac A, Tubau JF et al. QT interval prolongation and increased plasma catecholamine levels in patients with mitral valve prolapse. *Am Heart J.* 1983; 105:422–8.
35. Przybojewski JZ. Multiple coronary vasopasm: a cause of repeated myocardial infarction and symptomatic 'torsade de pointes' (atypical ventricular tachycardia). *S Afr Med J.* 1983; 63:103–12.
36. Fredlund BO, Olsson SB. Long QT interval and ventricular tachycardia of "torsade de pointe" type in hypothyroidism. *Acta Med Scand.* 1983; 213:231–5.
37. Sen S, Stober T, Burger L et al. Recurrent torsade de pointes type ventricular tachycardia in intracranial hemorrhage. *Intensive Care Med.* 1984; 10:263–4.
38. Hust MH, Nitsche K, Hohnloser S et al. QT prolongation and torsades de pointes in a patient with subarachnoid hemorrhage. *Clin Cardiol.* 1984; 7:44–8.
39. Vaughan Williams EM. A classification of antiarrhythmic actions reassessed after a decade of new drugs. *J Clin Pharmacol.* 1984; 24:129–47.
40. Pottage A. Clinical profiles of newer class I antiarrhythmic agents—tocainide, mexiletine, encainide, flecainide, lorcainide. *Am J Cardiol.* 1983; 52:24C–31C.
41. Lui HK, Lee G, Dietrich P et al. Flecainide-induced QT prolongation and ventricular tachycardia. *Am Heart J.* 1982; 103:567–9.
42. Sellers TD, DiMarco JP. Sinuosoidal ventricular tachycardia associated with flecainide acetate. *Chest.* 1984; 85:647–9.
43. McKibbin JK, Pocock WA, Barlow JB et al. Sotalol, hypokalemia, syncope, and torsade de pointes. *Br Heart J.* 1984; 51:157–62.
44. Sclarovsky S, Lewin RF, Kracoff O et al. Amiodarone-induced polymorphous ventricular tachycardia. *Am Heart J.* 1983; 105:6–12.
45. Somberg J, Torres V, Flowers D et al. Prolongation of QT interval and antiarrhythmic action of bepridil. *Am Heart J.* 1985; 109:19–26.
46. Reynolds EW, VanderArk CR. Quinidine syncope and the delayed repolarization syndromes. *Mod Concepts Cardio-*

vasc Dis. 1976; 45:117–22.
47. Bauman JL, Bauernfeind RA, Hoff JV et al. Torsade de pointes due to quinidine: observations in 31 patients. *Am Heart J.* 1984; 107:425–30.
48. Denes P, Gabster A, Huang SK. Clinical, electrocardiographic and follow-up observations in patients having ventricular fibrillation during Holter monitoring. Role of quinidine therapy. *Am J Cardiol.* 1981; 48:9–16.
49. Jenzer HR, Hagemeijer F. Quinidine syncope: torsade de pointes with low quinidine plasma concentrations. *Eur J Cardiol.* 1976; 4:447–51.
50. Holford NHG, Coates PE, Guenteral TW et al. The effect of quinidine and its metabolites on the electrocardiogram and systolic time intervals: concentration effect relationships. *Br J Clin Pharmacol.* 1981; 11:187–95.
51. Woosley RL, Siddoway LA, Thompson K et al. Potential applications of free drug level monitoring in cardiovascular therapy. *Clin Pharmacokinet.* 1984 (Suppl 4); 9:79–83.
52. Nicholson WJ, Martin CE, Gracey JG et al. Disopyramide-induced ventricular fibrillation. *Am J Cardiol.* 1979; 43:1053–5.
53. Commerford PJ, Beck W. Ventricular tachycardia with torsade de pointes morphology induced by oral disopyramide. *S Afr Med J.* 1980; 58:447–8.
54. Giacomini KM, Blaschke TF. Effect of concentration-dependent binding for plasma proteins on the pharmacokinetics and pharmacodynamics of disopyramide. *Clin Pharmacokinet.* 1984; 9 (Suppl 1):42–8.
55. Riccioni N, Castiglioni M, Bartolomei C. Disopyramide-induced QT prolongation and ventricular tachyarrhythmias. *Am Heart J.* 1983; 105:870–1.
56. Strasberg B, Sclarovsky S, Erdberg A et al. Procainamide-induced polymorphous ventricular tachycardia. *Am J Cardiol.* 1981; 47:1309–14.
57. Olshansky B, Martins J, Hunt S. N-acetylprocainamide causing torsades de pointes. *Am J Cardiol.* 1982; 50:1439–41.
58. Chow MJ, Piergies AA, Bowsher DJ et al. Torsade de pointes induced by n-acetylprocainamide. *J Am Coll Cardiol.* 1984; 4:621–4.
59. Herre JM, Thompson JA. Polymorphic ventricular tachycardia and ventricular fibrillation due to N-acetylprocainamide. *Am J Cardiol.* 1985; 55:227–8.
60. Stratmann HG, Walter KE, Kennedy HL. Torsade de pointes associated with elevated NAPA levels. *Am Heart J.* 1985; 109:375–7.
61. Saksena S, Rothbart ST, Shah Y et al. Clinical efficacy and electropharmacology of continuous intravenous amiodarone infusion and chronic oral amiodarone in refractory ventricular tachycardia. *Am J Cardiol.* 1984; 54:347–52.
62. Latini R, Tognoni G, Kates RE. Clinical pharmacokinetics of amiodarone. *Clin Pharmacokinet.* 1984; 9:136–56.
63. Bertholet M, Dubois C, Materne P et al. Sudden marked QT prolongation after intravenous administration of amiodarone. *Am J Cardiol.* 1983; 52:1361.
64. Santinelli V, Chiariello M, Condorelli M. Amiodarone-induced ventricular tachyarrhythmias. *Am J Cardiol.* 1984; 107:610–1. Letter.
65. Keren A, Tzivoni D, Gavish D et al. Etiology, warning signs and therapy of torsade de pointes: a study of 10 patients. *Circulation.* 1981, 64:1167–74.
66. Forfar JC, Gribbin B. Torsade de pointes after amiodarone withdrawal; effects of mild hypokalemia on repolarization. *Eur Heart J.* 1984; 5:510–2.
67. Bhandari AK, Quock C, Sung RJ. Polymorphous ventricular tachycardia associated with a marked prolongation of the Q–T interval induced by amiodarone. *PACE.* 1984; 7:341–5.
68. Scagliotti D, Strasberg B, Hai HA et al. Aprinidine-induced polymorphous ventricular tachycardia. *Am J Cardiol.* 1982; 49:1297–1300.
69. Waleffe A, Guillaume D, Mary-Rabine L et al. The efficacy of intravenous moxaprindine on ventricular ectopic activity. *Acta Cardiol.* 1980; 35:257–68.
70. Shah A, Schwartz H. Mexiletine for treatment of torsade de pointes. *Am Heart J.* 1980; 170:589–91.
71. Cocco G, Strozzi C, Chu D et al. Torsades de pointes as a manifestation of mexiletine toxicity. *Am Heart J.* 1980; 100:878–90.
72. Engler RL, LeWinter M. Tocainide-induced ventricular fibrillation. *Am Heart J.* 1981; 101:494–6.
73. Laakso M, Pentikainen PJ, Lampainen E. Sotalol, prolonged Q–T interval, and ventricular tachyarrhythmias. *Ann Clin Res.* 1981; 13:439–40.
74. Tötterman KJ, Turto H, Pellinen T. Overdrive pacing as treatment of sotalol-induced ventricular tachyarrhythmias (torsade de pointes). *Acta Med Scand* (Suppl). 1982; 668:28–33.
75. Kuck KH, Kunze KP, Roewer N et al. Sotalol-induced torsade de pointes. *Am Heart J.* 1984; 107:179–80.
76. Grayson HA, Kennedy JD. Torsades de pointes and nifedipine. *Ann Intern Med.* 1982; 97:144 Letter.
77. Fowler NO, McCall D, Chou TC et al. Electrocardiographic changes and cardiac arrhythmias in patients receiving psychotropic drugs. *Am J Cardiol.* 1976; 37:223–30.
78. Liberatore MA, Robinson DS. Torsade de pointes: a mechanism for sudden death associated with neuroleptic drug therapy. *J Clin Psychopharmacol.* 1984; 4:143–6.
79. Kemper AJ, Dunlap R, Pietro DA. Thioridazine-induced torsade de pointes. *JAMA.* 1983; 249:2931–4.
80. Cassem N. Cardiovascular effects of antidepressants. *J Clin Psychiatry.* 1982; 43:22–8.
81. Connolly SJ, Mitchell B, Swerdlow CD et al. Clinical efficacy and electrophysiology of imipramine for ventricular tachycardia. *Am J Cardiol.* 1984; 53:516–21.
82. Herrmann HC, Kaplan LM, Bierer BE. Q–T prolongation and torsades de pointes ventricular tachycardia produced by the tetracyclic antidepressant agent maprotiline. *Am J Cardiol.* 1983; 51:904–6.
83. Abinader EG, Shahar J. Possible female preponderance in prenylamine-induced 'torsade de pointes' tachycardia. *Cardiology.* 1983; 70:32–40.
84. Klein GJ. Vasopressin, "Torsades de pointes," and QT syndrome. *Ann Intern Med.* 1980; 93:511–2. Letter.
85. Rowlands DB, Littler WA. Ventricular fibrillation induced by indapamide. *Br Med J.* 1982; 284:1407. Letter.
86. Sartori M, Pratt CM, Young JB. Torsade de pointe: malignant cardiac arrhythmia induced by amantidine poisoning. *Am J Med.* 1984; 77:388–91.
87. Evans TR, Curry PVL, Fitchett DH et al. "Torsade de pointes" initiated by electrical ventricular stimulation. *J Electrocardiol.* 1976; 9:255–8.
88. Wellens HJJ. Value and limitations of programmed electrical stimulation of the heart in the study and treatment of tachycardias. *Circulation.* 1978; 57:845–53.
89. D'Alnoncourt CN, Zierhut W, Lüderitz B. "Torsade de pointes" tachycardia: re-entry or focal activity? *Br Heart J.* 1982; 48:213–6.
90. Sasyniuk BI. Concept of reentry versus automaticity. *Am J Cardiol* 1984; 54:1A–6A.
91. Han H, Moe GK. Nonuniform recovery of excitability in ventricular muscle. *Circ Res.* 1964; 14:44–60.
92. Kinoshita S, Kato Y, Kawasaki T et al. Ventricular tachycardia initiated by late-coupled ventricular extrasystoles: the concept of longitudinal dissociation in the microentry pathway. *Am Heart J.* 1982; 103:1090–5.
93. Bardy GH, Ungerleider RM, Smith WM et al. A mechanism of torsades de pointes in a canine model. *Circulation.* 1983; 67:52–9.
94. Velebit V, Podrid P, Lown B et al. Aggravation and provocation of ventricular arrhythmias by antiarrhythmic drugs. *Circulation.* 1982; 65:886–94.
95. Ruskin JN, McGovern B, Garan H et al. Antiarrhythmic drugs: a possible cause of out-of-hospital cardiac arrest. *N Engl J Med.* 1983; 21:1302–6.
96. Torres V, Flowers D, Somberg JC. The arrhythmogenicity of antiarrhythmic agents. *Am Heart J.* 1985; 109:1090–7.

97. Brachmann J, Scherlag BJ, Rosenshtraukh LV et al. Bradycardia-dependent triggered activity: relevance to drug-induced multiform ventricular tachycardia. *Circulation.* 1983; 68:846–56.
98. Khan MM, Logan KR, McComb JM et al. Management of recurrent ventricular tachyarrhythmias associated with Q-T prolongation. *Am J Cardiol.* 1981; 47:1301–8.
99. Kowey PR, Engel TR. Overdrive pacing for ventricular tachyarrhythmias: a reassessment. *Ann Intern Med.* 1983; 99:651–6.
100. Inoue H, Matsuo H, Mashima S et al. Effects of atrial pacing, isoprenaline, and lignocaine on experimental polymorphous ventricular tachycardia. *Cardiovasc Res.* 1984; 18:538–47.
101. Wong ET, Rude RK, Singer FR. A high prevalence of hypomagnesemia in hospitalized patients. *Am J Clin Pathol.* 1983; 79:348–52.
102. Whang R, Aikawa JK, Oei TO et al. Routine serum magnesium determination: an unrecognized need. In: Cantin M, Seelig MS, eds. Magnesium in health and diseases. New York: SP Medical and Scientific Books; 1980:1–5.
103. Whang R, Oei TO, Aikawa JK et al. Predictors of clinical hypomagnesemia. *Arch Intern Med* 1984; 144:1794–6.
104. Dyckner T, Wester PO. Relation between potassium, magnesium and cardiac arrhythmias. *Acta Med Scand.* (Suppl): 1981; 647:163–9.
105. Whang R, Oei TO, Aikawa JK et al. Magnesium and potassium interrelationships: experimental and clinical. *Acta Med Scand.* (Suppl): 1981; 647:139–44.
106. Flink EB. Magnesium deficiency. Etiology and clinical spectrum. *Acta Med Scand.* (Suppl): 1981; 647:125–37.
107. Ramee SR, White CJ, Svinarich JT et al. Torsade de pointes and magnesium deficiency. *Am Heart J.* 1985; 109:164–6.
108. Iseri LT, Chung P, Tobis J. Magnesium therapy for intractable ventricular tachyarrhythmias in normomagnesemic patients. *West J Med.* 1983; 138:823–8.
109. Surawicz B, Knoebel SB. Long QT: good, bad, or indifferent? *J Am Coll Cardiol.* 1984; 4:398–413.
110. Somberg J, Tepper D, Wynn J. Prolonged repolarization: a historical perspective. *Am Heart J.* 1985; 109:395–8.

Glossary

Long–short initiating sequence: a premature ventricular contraction that occurs late in diastole (Figure 1).

Morphology: electrocardiographic configuration.

Overdrive pacing: Electrical pacing at a rate more rapid than that of inherent cardiac pacemaker.

R-on-T: an extrasystole that interrupts a T wave; the importance of this pattern is thought to be associated with sudden death caused by cardiac arrhythmias.

QT interval: the time elapsing from the beginning of the QRS complex to the end of the T wave; it reflects, within limitations, the duration of depolarization and repolarization.

QT_c interval: the QT interval corrected for heart rate.

U wave: a positive wave following the T wave of the electrocardiogram; its origin may be repolarization of Purkinje fibers and diastolic relaxation of the myocardium.

Statement of Ownership Management and Circulation (Required by 39 U.S.C. 3685) 1. Title of publication, Clinical Pharmacy. 1A. Publication No. 02782677. 2. Date of filing, October 1, 1985. 3. Frequency of issue, Bimonthly, 3A. No. issues published annually, 6. 3B. Annual subscription price, $35.00. 4. Location of known office of publication, 4630 Montgomery Avenue, Bethesda, Montgomery County, MD 20814. 5. Location of the headquarters or general business offices of the publishers, 4630 Montgomery Avenue, Bethesda, MD 20814. 6. Publisher, American Society of Hospital Pharmacists, Inc., 4630 Montgomery Avenue, Bethesda, MD 20814. Editor, William A. Zellmer, 4630 Montgomery Avenue, Bethesda, MD 20814. Managing Editor, C. Richard Talley. 7. Owner, American Society of Hospital Pharmacists, Inc., 4630 Montgomery Avenue, Bethesda, MD 20814. 8. Known bondholders, mortgagees, and other security holders owning 1% or more of total amount of bonds, mortgages or other securities, None. 9. For completion by nonprofit organizations authorized to mail at special rates (Section 132.122, PSM). The purpose, function, and nonprofit status of this organization and the exempt status for federal income tax purposes have not changed during preceding 12 months. 10. Extent and nature of circulation, A. Total no. copies printed, 8,468/8,670*; B. Paid circulation, 1. Sales through dealers and carriers, street vendors and counter sales, 500/200. 2. Mail subscriptions, 7,050/7,123; C. Total paid circulation, 7,550/7,323; D. Free distribution by mail, carrier or other means, samples, complimentary and other free copies, 515/560; E. Total distribution, 8,065/7,883; F. Copies not distributed, 1. Office use, left over, unaccounted, spoiled after printing, 403/787. Returns from news agents, 0,0. G. Total, 8,468/8,670. I certify that the statements made by me are correct and complete, signed William A. Zellmer.
*First figure, average no. copies each issue during preceding 12 months; second figure, actual no. of copies single issue published nearest to filing date.

ASHP Report

Acknowledgment to reviewers—October 1, 1984, to September 30, 1985

This year, 179 manuscripts were submitted for publication consideration to *Clinical Pharmacy*, including papers solicited by the editors. Approximately 50% of the papers received were ultimately accepted. During this same period, we received critiques from 263 reviewers who evaluated the merit of *Clinical Pharmacy* submissions. Readers are indebted to these reviewers, who contributed their time in this advisory capacity. Their efforts have helped maintain the high standards of *CP*. Several referees reviewed more than one paper during the year, and their extra contributions are especially appreciated.

Marie A. Abate
Michael R. Alexander
Majorie C. Allan
Ron Ballentine
George Banister
Joseph A. Barone
Steven L. Barriere
Sharyn R. Batey
Larry A. Bauer
Jay H. Bauman
Jerry L. Bauman
Steven F. Bauwens
J. Edward Bell
Richard C. Berchou
Joseph S. Bertino, Jr.
Robert A. Blouin
Stephen J. Bollish
William S. Bond
Dan Bonner
John A. Bosso
Bradley A. Boucher
Talmadge A. Bowden, Jr.
J. Chris Bradberry
Gilbert J. Burckart
Wayne S. Burkle
Michael E. Burton
Henry I. Bussey
R. Keith Campbell
Daniel M. Canafax
Barry L. Carter
Sandra Chase
Frank C. Chenella
Nelly M. Childress
Moses S. S. Chow
Robert J. Cipolle
Geoffrey E. Clark
Jordan L. Cohen
James H. Coleman
Thomas J. Comstock
Brian L. Crabtree
Burke A. Cunha
Peter A. Czajka
Larry H. Danziger
Robert J. Davis
Edward L. Decker
Francine Dela Cruz
Jeffrey C. Delafuente
James Dice
David M. DiPersio
Joseph T. DiPiro
Joel H. Dobbs
Paul L. Doering
Alvin Donner
Robert T. Dorr
Michael N. Dudley
James E. Dugas
George E. Dukes, Jr.
Bruce R. Ellinoy
Larry Ereshefsky
Ronald P. Evens
Kenneth H. Falchuk
William R. Finch
Jack Fincham
John M. Fischer
Michael S. Flagstad
Richard J. Fleck
Donald G. Floriddia
Elizabeth Forrence
Gary N. Foulks
Dennis M. Fruin
Peter Gal
John G. Gambertoglio
John A. Gans
Susan K. Gardner
William R. Garnett
Elwyn A. Garrard
Thomas P. Gibson
Mark A. Gill
Jamie T. Gilman
Thomas Gilman
James Goodwin
Bruce M. Gordon
John D. Grabenstein
David A. Graves
Barbara L. Greenberg
Rachel Griffith
Ashok K. Gumbhir
Ernest L. Gurwich
Peter R. Gwilt
Charles E. Halstenson
Philip D. Hansten
James Hanyok
Thomas C. Hardin
Guy R. Hasegawa
Peggy E. Hayes
Richard Helms
Herbert R. Henney III
Donald M. Hilligoss
Richard P. Hoffmann
Linda C. Hogan
Mark J. Hogan
Alan W. Hopefl
John R. Horn
Denise Howrie
Robert Hyndiuk
Martha L. Hyneck
R. Peter Iafrate
Robert J. Ignoffo
Thomas E. Imhoff
Kathleen Ingalls
Judith Jaeger
Ann L. Janer
Michael W. Jann
Paul Jeffrey
John W. Jenne
Martin Job
Matthew H. Johnson
Steven M. Johnson
E. Maurice Jones
P. K. Jones
Randy P. Juhl
Mitchell V. Kaminski, Jr.
Alan F. Kaul
Gregory L. Kearns
Donald J. Kellerman
H. William Kelly
P. K. Kenney
Karen J. Klamerus
Michael L. Kleinberg
Thomas Klotz
Steven F. Kowalsky
Edward P. Krenzelok
James J. Kresel
Cynthia A. Kristoff
Peggy G. Kuehl
Richard L. Lalonde
Victor Lampasona
Jeffrey R. Latts
Timothy Lesar
James H. Lewis
Martin Lipschutz
Elaine Long
Richard R. Lorber
Rex S. Lott
Virgil S. Lucas, Jr.
Thomas M. Ludden
David E. Magnuson
Thomas C. Majerus
Richard J. Mangini
Edwina Marks
Michael A. Marr
William D. Mason
Marc Massanari
Earl Matthews
Gary R. Matzke
Charles N. May
Jonathan E. McDermed
James M. McKenney
Steven Meisel
Frederick L. Meister
David M. Melikian
Steve Mendel
Glenda Meneilly
Donald Miller
Lucinda G. Miller
Carol H. Millette
John F. Mitchell
Catherine D. Momjian
Michael A. Montwill
Jerome S. Morrow
Dennis R. Mungall
John E. Murphy
Jean Nappi
Thomas R. Navin
Richard W. Nelson
David E. Nix
Paul E. Nolan, Jr.
Gary M. Oderda
John Opsahl
Rapin Osathanondh
John Ostrosky
Norma J. Owens
Glen D. Park
Michael D. Parr
Thomas W. Paton
Vaughn W. Payne
Mitchell Pelter
Tim Peltier
Curlee-lyn Petty
Thomas E. Platek
Ron E. Polk
Timothy L. Pruett
W. Nathan Rawls
Carolyn M. Rayment
Michael D. Reed
Donald P. Reitberg
William J. Rietscha
J. Daniel Robinson
Michael B. Robinson
John H. Rodman
Joseph Roney
Kathleen R. Rosenberry
Sal J. Rubino
Ronald J. Ruggiero
William J. Rusho
Steven L. Russell
Patrick B. Ryan
Stephen R. Saklad
Donald J. Salberg
Fred J. Salter
William T. Sawyer
Jerome J. Schentag
Gerald E. Schumacher
Terry L. Schwinghammer
Steven L. Sheaffer
Richard L. Slaughter
Gary E. Sloskey
Ralph E. Small
Bruce R. Smith
Gary H. Smith
Catherine A. Sohn
Walter Soja
John C. Somberg
William J. Spruill
Peter W. Stacpoole
Christopher Stock
Gary Stoehr
Robert Straka
Kim J. Sveska
Richard Sykes
Robert L. Talbert
Renee P. Tannenbaum
Teresa A. Tartaglione
Kathryn A. Taubert
Jerry W. Taylor
Kathleen McNeil Teasley
Francis J. Tedesco
Sharon Ternullo
Charles Thayer
James Thorp
Theodore Tong
Frank L. Tornatore
Glenda Treadway
Lawrence A. Trissel
Elaine Tuomanen
Donald L. Uden
Peter H. Vlasses
Nicholas A. Votolato
Bill Wade
Elaine S. Waller
Michael E. Ward
I. N. Weinstein
Hugh Wilson
James E. Wilson
Michael E. Winter
Constance B. Wofsy
J. W. Wohltmann
Bradley G. Wulf
Pamela Y-F Yih
Gary C. Yee
Jen Yeh
Sharon L. Young
Darwin E. Zaske
Karen E. Zenk

CP Continuing Education

Article 680-204-8517 (see page 625)
Qualifies for 1.0 hour of CE credit

Nomifensine maleate: A new second-generation antidepressant

Learning Objectives

As a result of studying this article, the reader should be able to

1. Describe the effects of nomifensine on brain neurotransmitters and receptors.
2. Outline the pharmacokinetics of nomifensine compared with that of standard tricyclic antidepressants.
3. Outline the most common symptoms associated with nomifensine overdose.
4. Recommend a dosing regimen given a specific patient.
5. Decide whether or not a specific patient would be a good candidate for nomifensine therapy.

Self-assessment Questions

For each question there is one best answer only.

1. Nomifensine is a unique antidepressant in that it
   a. Does not inhibit the reuptake of serotonin.
   b. Desensitizes postsynaptic β receptors.
   c. Inhibits the reuptake of dopamine.
   d. Blocks postsynaptic dopamine receptors.
2. Pharmacokinetic and pharmacodynamic times of maximum effect for nomifensine are, respectively,
   a. 1–2 hours, 1–2 hours.
   b. 1–2 hours, 4–6 hours.
   c. 4–6 hours, 4–6 hours.
   d. 4–6 hours, 6–8 hours.
3. Clinical studies have clearly demonstrated that nomifensine is
   a. Less effective than nortriptyline.
   b. More effective than imipramine.
   c. More effective than desipramine.
   d. As effective as amitriptyline.
4. Which one of the following does not describe a true difference between nomifensine and imipramine?
   a. Nomifensine has very little, if any, anticholinergic activity.
   b. Nomifensine does not lower the seizure threshold.
   c. Nomifensine does not impair cognitive abilities.
   d. Nomifensine causes frequent ECG changes.
5. The most common side effects of nomifensine include all of the following except
   a. Weight gain.
   b. Dry mouth.
   c. Headaches.
   d. Nervousness.
6. Which one of the following is not commonly associated with nomifensine overdose?
   a. Sinus tachycardia.
   b. Seizures.
   c. Drowsiness.
   d. Tremor.
7. Which one of the following drug interactions can be expected with nomifensine?
   a. Nomifensine will antagonize the effects of guanethidine.
   b. Nomifensine will antagonize the effects of pseudoephedrine.
   c. Nomifensine blood concentrations will be increased when given with phenytoin and phenobarbital.
   d. Nomifensine will potentiate the effects of alcohol.
8. Which one of the following patients would be a good candidate for nomifensine therapy?
   a. A woman who is breast-feeding.
   b. A patient with symptoms of agitation and nervousness.
   c. A patient with a diagnosis of schizoaffective disorder.
   d. A patient with symptoms of hypersomnia and retardation.
9. Which one of the following is the appropriate dose of nomifensine for a young, healthy, adult male?
   a. 50 mg in the morning and early afternoon, increasing to 200 mg as tolerated.
   b. 50 mg in the morning, increasing as tolerated.
   c. 50 mg in the morning and 100 mg at bedtime.
   d. 150 mg at bedtime.
10. Patients should be given which of the following dietary instructions when taking nomifensine?
    a. Take with food to decrease stomach upset.
    b. Food will not affect the absorption of nomifensine.
    c. Take one hour before or two hours after a meal.
    d. Avoid taking it with dairy products.

Article 680-204-8518 (see page 637)
Qualifies for 1.0 hour of CE credit

Preventing *Haemophilus influenzae* type b disease

Learning Objectives

As a result of studying this article the reader should be able to

1. Describe the magnitude of the problem of *Haemophilus influenzae* type b (Hib) disease in pediatric-aged patients.
2. Explain the age-related susceptibility to Hib infections.
3. Identify which contacts of patients with Hib infection are at greatest risk for developing secondary Hib disease.
4. Explain the rationale for using prophylactic antimicrobial therapy to prevent outbreaks of Hib disease and outline an appropriate strategy for chemoprophylaxis.
5. Describe the benefits and limitations of using *Haemophilus* b polysaccharide vaccine to prevent Hib disease.

Self-assessment Questions

1. In the United States, *Haemophilus influenzae* type b (Hib) annually causes approximately 10,000 cases of
   a. Bacteremia.
   b. Epiglottitis.
   c. Meningitis.
   d. Septic arthritis.
   e. None of the above alternatives is correct.
2. The majority of Hib disease in the United States occurs in children between the ages of
   a. 0 and 2 months.
   b. 2 and 18 months.
   c. 18 and 24 months.
   d. 2 and 5 years.
   e. 5 and 9 years.
3. Young children are more susceptible to invasive Hib disease than adults because they have
   a. More respiratory tract infections.
   b. Lower serum titers of anti-Hib antibody.
   c. A higher incidence of *H. influenzae* otitis media.
   d. Alternatives b and c are both correct.
   e. None of the above alternatives is correct.
4. Which of the following would be considered a close contact of a patient hospitalized for Hib meningitis?
   a. The patient's 29-year-old mother.
   b. The patient's one-year-old brother.
   c. The admitting physician.
   d. A dinner guest who visited the patient's family two days before the patient's illness was diagnosed.
   e. Alternatives a and b are both correct.
5. Which of the following household contacts of a patient with Hib meningitis is at greatest risk for developing secondary Hib illness?
   a. A 2-year-old sibling.
   b. A 79-year-old grandmother.
   c. A 7-year-old sibling.
   d. A 16-year-old babysitter.
   e. All of the above alternatives are correct.
6. Antimicrobial prophylaxis of Hib disease is directed at
   a. Stimulating immunity in high-risk contacts of patients with Hib disease.
   b. Protecting individuals colonized with Hib from developing systemic disease.
   c. Reducing the Hib colonization level in a defined population.
   d. Alternatives b and c are both correct.
   e. None of the above alternatives is correct.
7. If two children from the same day-care class develop Hib meningitis within a 10-day period, who of the following should receive prophylactic rifampin therapy?
   a. All children in the class older than 48 months of age.
   b. All children in the class younger than 48 months of age.
   c. All adult day-care center personnel.
   d. Family members of all children in the class.
   e. Alternatives a, b, and c are all correct.
8. Nasopharyngeal Hib colonization within a defined population is best reduced by which of the following antibiotic regimens?
   a. Rifampin 20 mg/kg given once daily for four days.
   b. Rifampin 20 mg/kg/day given in two divided doses for two days.
   c. Rifampin 20 mg/kg/day given in two divided doses for three days.
   d. Rifampin 20 mg/kg given once daily for seven days.
   e. None of the above alternatives is correct.
9. What is the approximate efficacy of *Haemophilus* b polysaccharide vaccine when administered to children between the ages of 18 and 24 months?
   a. 100%.
   b. 90%.
   c. 75%.
   d. 50%.
   e. 25%.
10. Which of the following groups would not benefit from vaccination with *Haemophilus* b polysaccharide vaccine?
    a. Healthy children between the ages of 6 and 12 months.
    b. Healthy children between the ages of 24 and 36 months.
    c. Healthy children between the ages of 60 and 72 months.
    d. Alternatives a and c are both correct.
    e. Alternatives b and c are both correct.

Article 680-204-8519 (see page 649)
Qualifies for 2.0 hours of CE credit

Use of antihypertensive agents in patients with glucose intolerance

Learning Objectives

As a result of studying this article, the reader should be able to

1. Identify antihypertensive agents that may adversely affect basal glucose control, tolerance to a glucose load, and response to hypoglycemia.
2. Define a mechanism for these adverse drug effects.
3. Characterize the adverse effect of antihypertensive drugs on glucose tolerance in terms of the degree of change in glucose levels, incidence of the problem, clinical sequelae, and implicated drugs.
4. Characterize the adverse effect of β blockers on response to hypoglycemia in terms of the nadir in

glucose levels, symptomatology, and recovery.
5. Describe how these adverse drug effects can be managed.

Self-assessment Questions

For each question there is one best answer only.

1. Which one of the following drugs does *not* adversely affect glucose tolerance?
   a. Propranolol.
   b. Furosemide.
   c. Nifedipine.
   d. Reserpine.
2. Which one of the following drugs alters glucose tolerance through a reduction in cytosolic calcium?
   a. Captopril.
   b. Metoprolol.
   c. Verapamil.
   d. Guanethidine.
3. Propranolol causes a deterioration in glucose tolerance by
   a. Blockade of α_2 receptors.
   b. Reduction in insulin release via β_2 stimulation.
   c. Reduction in calcium influx.
   d. Altering glucose sensitivity.
4. The average elevation in fasting serum glucose seen in nondiabetic hypertensive patients receiving thiazide therapy is
   a. 10%.
   b. 30%.
   c. 50%.
   d. 70%.
5. Clonidine causes a clinically important glucose elevation
   a. Rarely.
   b. Occasionally.
   c. Often.
   d. Always
6. Altered recovery from a hypoglycemic episode does not occur with
   a. Propranolol.
   b. Metoprolol.
   c. Atenolol.
   d. Reserpine.
7. The hypoglycemic symptom *not* masked with a nonselective β blocker is
   a. Tremor.
   b. Diaphoresis.
   c. Palpitations.
   d. Hypotension.
8. If a diabetic patient developed mild, asymptomatic deterioration in fasting glucose levels while receiving hydrochlorothiazide, it would be best to
   a. Switch to furosemide.
   b. Switch to triamterene.
   c. Switch to indapamide.
   d. Leave on hydrochlorothiazide.
9. In the above patient, which of the following initial management steps would be best?
   a. Start an oral hypoglycemic agent.
   b. Evaluate and correct (if needed) the serum potassium.
   c. Increase the dose of insulin.
   d. Lower the dose of the diuretic.
10. In the case of the "brittle" insulin-dependent diabetic patient who is receiving propranolol and experiences a hypoglycemic episode every day for a week, it would be best to
    a. Change the β blocker to metoprolol.
    b. Lower the dose of propranolol.
    c. Discontinue propranolol.
    d. Relax the diabetic control to the point of hyperglycemia.

Article 680-204-8520 (see page 675)
Qualifies for 2.0 hours of CE credit

Drug-induced torsade de pointes

Learning Objectives

As a result of studying this article, the reader should be able to

1. Compare and contrast torsade de pointes and polymorphic ventricular tachycardia.
2. List the electrocardiographic characteristics of torsade de pointes.
3. Estimate the probability that an investigational drug will cause torsade de pointes, given its electrophysiologic profile.
4. Recommend therapeutic intervention in patients who develop torsade de pointes associated with life-threatening hemodynamic deterioration.
5. Outline a patient-specific course for prevention of recurrent torsade de pointes including recommendations for drug and electrolyte therapy and monitoring.

Self-assessment Questions

For each question there is one best answer only.

1. Torsade de pointes (TdP) is differentiated from polymorphous ventricular tachycardia (PVT) by
   a. QT interval prolongation present in TdP, not PVT.
   b. Long–short initiating sequence before TdP, not PVT.
   c. Class Ia antiarrhythmics useful in treating TdP, not PVT.
   d. All of the above are correct.
   e. Alternatives a and b only are correct.
2. Factors that predispose to the development of torsade de pointes include
   a. Severe bradycardias.
   b. Acute myocardial infarction
   c. Subarachnoid hemorrhage.
   d. All of the above alternatives are correct.
   e. Alternatives a and c only are correct.
3. All of the following are true regarding quinidine-induced torsade de pointes except
   a. Quinidine-induced TdP occurs only at doses producing serum concentrations usually considered toxic.
   b. Most patients first exhibit quinidine-induced TdP shortly after beginning therapy.
   c. Quinidine-induced TdP may be precipitated by addition of a potassium-wasting diuretic.
   d. QT prolongation is a universal marker of quini-

dine-induced TdP.

e. The clinical outcome of quinidine-induced TdP may include death.

4. Which calcium-channel-blocking agent or agents are likely to precipitate torsade de pointes?
   a. Nifedipine.
   b. Verapamil, diltiazem.
   c. Lidoflazine, bepredil.
   d. None of the above agents will precipitate TdP.
   e. All of the above agents will precipitate TdP.
5. The acute definitive therapy of torsade de pointes associated with deterioration in hemodynamic status not requiring defibrillation is
   a. Overdrive pacing.
   b. Bretylium.
   c. Lidocaine.
   d. Isoproterenol.
   e. Haloperidol.
6. All of the following are true regarding magnesium supplementation in torsade de pointes except
   a. Magnesium-sulfate therapy appears useful only if serum magnesium concentration is below normal limits.
   b. Cellular hypomagnesemia is not always reflected in low serum magnesium concentrations.
   c. Mild hypotension induced by magnesium-sulfate therapy should not pose a problem.
   d. Hypokalemia is a predictor of hypomagnesemia.
   e. I.V. magnesium sulfate is effective in treating TdP regardless of serum magnesium concentration.
7. Drugs reported to cause torsade de pointes include
   a. Quinidine, procainamide, and disopyramide.
   b. Amiodarone.
   c. Tricyclic antidepressants.
   d. All of the above alternatives are correct.
   e. Alternatives b and c only are correct.
8. Which of the following is a reasonable guideline for identification of the QT interval in torsade de pointes?
   a. QT interval greater than 0.40 second.
   b. QT interval greater than 0.50 second.
   c. QT_c interval greater than 0.44 second.
   d. Alternatives a and b are both correct.
   e. None of the above alternatives is correct.
9. A patient has a history of quinidine-induced torsade de pointes and requires suppression of chronic premature ventricular contractions. Which one of the following is the most appropriate therapy?
   a. Quinidine gluconate.
   b. Procainamide.
   c. Disopyramide.
   d. Amiodarone.
   e. Tocainide.
10. A patient requires drug therapy for schizophrenia and has a history of quinidine-induced torsade de pointes. Which one of the following is the most appropriate initial therapy?
    a. Haloperidol.
    b. Thioridazine.
    c. Trifluoperazine.
    d. Chlorpromazine.
    e. All of the above drugs should be avoided.

Answer sheet

November–December 1985 ***Clinical Pharmacy***

Note: An enrollment form for the ASHP Continuing-Education System appears in the May–June and November–December issues. Please accumulate all the answer sheets you wish to use in one enrollment and submit them at one time with a completed enrollment form.

Place an X in the box(es) at the top of the column(s) corresponding to the test(s) you are taking. Darken the boxes corresponding to the correct answers.

	☐ 680-204-8517 1.0 hour a b c d	☐ 680-204-8518 1.0 hour a b c d e
1.	☐☐☐☐	☐☐☐☐☐
2.	☐☐☐☐	☐☐☐☐☐
3.	☐☐☐☐	☐☐☐☐☐
4.	☐☐☐☐	☐☐☐☐☐
5.	☐☐☐☐	☐☐☐☐☐
6.	☐☐☐☐	☐☐☐☐☐
7.	☐☐☐☐	☐☐☐☐☐
8.	☐☐☐☐	☐☐☐☐☐
9.	☐☐☐☐	☐☐☐☐☐
10.	☐☐☐☐	☐☐☐☐☐

	☐ 680-204-8519 1.0 hour a b c d	☐ 680-204-8520 2.0 hours a b c d e
1.	☐☐☐☐	☐☐☐☐☐
2.	☐☐☐☐	☐☐☐☐☐
3.	☐☐☐☐	☐☐☐☐☐
4.	☐☐☐☐	☐☐☐☐☐
5.	☐☐☐☐	☐☐☐☐☐
6.	☐☐☐☐	☐☐☐☐☐
7.	☐☐☐☐	☐☐☐☐☐
8.	☐☐☐☐	☐☐☐☐☐
9.	☐☐☐☐	☐☐☐☐☐
10.	☐☐☐☐	☐☐☐☐☐

ASHP Use Only

(1.0)8517______(3)
(1.0)8518______(3)
(1.0)8519______(3)
(2.0)8520______(3)

The ASHP Continuing Education system gives readers a self-assessment mechanism for selected articles in Clinical Pharmacy *and the* American Journal of Hospital Pharmacy. *It also allows readers to obtain continuing-education credit for these articles.*

All education aspects of the program are directed by Warren E. McConnell, Ph.D., Special Assistant in the ASHP Executive Office.

ASHP CE instructions and enrollment form

Instructions

1. The system is flexible. You may, within a 12-month period, select any combination of tests from the *American Journal of Hospital Pharmacy* and *Clinical Pharmacy* to give you the number of credits you need.
2. An Answer Sheet is published at the end of each installment of the CE column. An Enrollment Form is published in the May–June and November–December issues of *CP* and in the June and December issues of *AJHP*.
3. Complete only one Enrollment Form, but note on the form all the tests you are taking. Staple together all answer sheets for one enrollment.
4. Tests included in one enrollment must have been published within the past 24 months. Once a particular test is included in an enrollment, it may not be included in a subsequent enrollment.
5. The passing score on each test is 70%. Within four weeks of receiving your enrollment, ASHP will mail you a CE certificate or notify you that certain tests were failed. Failed tests may be retaken only one time, without additional cost. There are no refunds for failed tests.
6. ASHP is approved by the American Council on Pharmaceutical Education as a provider of continuing pharmaceutical education (Provider Number 680-204). (The following states recognize ACPE-approved providers: AK, AR, AZ, FL, IA, ID, IN, KS, KY, LA, MA, ME, MI, MS, MT, NE, NH, NM, NV, OH, OR, SD, WA, and WY [also Puerto Rico].) Most states that recognize ACPE-approved providers will accept credit earned through journal CE programs; however, since some states have restrictions on the number of credit hours or CE units they will accept toward the total requirement, it is advised that readers check with their respective state board of pharmacy if they are uncertain about the board's regulations.
7. Send your Enrollment Form, Answer Sheet(s), and check (made payable to ASHP) to:

ASHP CE
American Society of Hospital Pharmacists
4630 Montgomery Avenue
Bethesda, MD 20814

Enrollment Form

Name____________________

Address____________________

City__________ State__________ Zip__________

Tests included in this enrollment:

Test Number	*Hours of Credit*

(Write additional numbers and hours on a separate sheet and attach it to this form.)

Total hours __________

Total fee($) enclosed __________

Fee Schedule
$3.50/hour
$15.00 minimum/enrollment

Current Literature

Book Reviews

AMA Handbook of Poisonous and Injurious Plants

By Kenneth F. Lampe and Mary Ann McCann.

Published by the American Medical Association, Chicago, IL 60610, 1985. Available from Chicago Review Press, 213 West Institute Place, Chicago, IL 60610. xi + 432 p. Price $18.95 + $2.50 shipping and handling.

Determining whether a given plant is potentially toxic or not can sometimes be difficult. The *AMA Handbook of Poisonous and Injurious Plants* is a welcome addition to the poisonous plant literature. It contains information on a broader variety of plants than do most previous publications. Indigenous and cultivated plants found in Canada, the United States, the West Indies, Mexico, and Guam are included. There is considerable information on plants found in the most tropical areas of these countries.

The book is arranged in three major sections along with an introductory portion on the general management of plant poisoning and botanical nomenclature. Section I, "Systemic Plant Poisoning," details the toxicity of some 148 genera of plants and numerous species. Each genus is detailed as to scientific name, trivial or common name, description of the plant, geographical distribution, toxic part, toxin involved, symptoms, and management of the exposure. Section II, "Plant Dermatitis," includes discussion of the various types of plant dermatitis, including mechanical or irritant chemical injury, contact urticaria, photodermatitis, and allergic contact dermatitis. Following this discussion are tables listing the plants that fall within each category. These tables list both the scientific names and the common names of the plants and, in most cases, refer the reader to a color picture of the plant. Section III, "Mushroom Poisoning," contains a differential diagnosis of mushroom poisoning followed by a management section categorized by presenting symptoms.

Following the text portion of the book are 437 color plates. These pictures illustrate all but one of the systemically toxic plants, more than two thirds of those producing dermatitis, and 15 mushrooms. (There is one figure mixup, which ought to be explained by an errata slip in each copy: the pictures in 378 and 379 are reversed.) The quality of the color plates is excellent, and they are of considerable assistance in helping to identify the plants. The comprehensive index lists both the scientific and the common names of the included plants and mushrooms.

The authors have done an excellent job in providing a well-written, concise, authoritative, and beautifully illustrated text. Each entry is well referenced and is presented in an easily readable format. This text should be of great interest to any pharmacist, nurse, physician, or toxicologist who has an interest in poisonous plants. It should also prove to be an excellent reference for those who simply want to know about the toxicity of the plants in their own yards.

Reviewed by Michael D. Ellis, M.S., Texas State Poison Center, The University of Texas Medical Branch, Galveston, TX 77550

Blue Book of Pharmacologic Therapeutics

By Gordon E. Johnson.

Published by W. B. Saunders Company, West Washington Square, Philadelphia, PA 19105, 1985. xxi + 713 p. Price $24.95.

This publication is one in a series of Saunders Blue Books published in soft-cover, spiral-bound, pocket-sized formats. At a thickness of 1-1/2 inches, it is oversized and cumbersome to carry but would do well on a reference shelf. The subject matter is directed toward students or the novice in drug pharmacology. The book is divided into two distinct parts—the "white" pages and the "blue" pages.

The white pages (pages 1–241) begin with a chapter on "General Principles of Pharmacology" and are followed by 16 chapters dealing with the treatment principles and pharmacologic properties of drugs for specific disease states. Within each section the drugs are classified in groups, with three, very brief, descriptive paragraphs—mechanism of action and pharmacologic effects, therapeutic uses, and adverse effects. At the end of each chapter is a short list of recommended reading. This portion of the book is very superficial in its discussion of agents and even duplicates material that is found later in the blue pages.

The blue pages are actually the primary focus of the book and consist of 62 tables. These tables are ordered in the same sequence as are the disease states briefly discussed in the white pages and are entitled "Drugs for the Treatment of ...." The format for each table is to list first the generic and trade names for the first group of drugs to be discussed in that table. Next the page is divided into two columns—Therapeutic Uses, which lists the dosage forms and dosages for each drug, and Adverse Effects. Dosages for adults are given primarily, with dosages for children or elderly patients provided in some cases.

Information on dosage adjustments for renal dysfunction is limited. Following this section, the page is again divided into two columns—Contraindications and/or Precautions, and Drug Interactions. Under Drug Interactions, the name of the class of an interacting drug is given with a sentence or two about the exact effect. The reader is sometimes referred to another table if the full description is listed under the other drug of the interaction. The table then repeats this format for another group of drugs used to treat the disease state under consideration. For example, "Drugs for the Treatment of Hypertension" begins with the thiazides and continues with the loop diuretics, beta blockers, and so on.

A major difficulty is in identifying where the description of one group of drugs ends and the next begins. Another is the fact that information on groups of drugs used in more than one disease is repeated under each disease state almost word for word in some cases. Again, the reader is sometimes referred to another table to obtain a portion of information. Still another problem is the fact that some information listed for a group of drugs under one disease heading may be omitted under a different disease heading, which can be frustrating. For example, the drug interaction between beta-blockers and antidiabetic agents is listed under hypertension but omitted under angina.

The index is alphabetized according to drug name (trade or generic) with subcategories for the drug's use in each disease state.

Overall, one must do a lot of page flipping to obtain all the information included on a specific agent. The format of the blue pages was designed to minimize page flipping by placing information on a drug group under each disease state. However, the flaw is that complete incorporation of material on each drug was not repeated. Also, handling the book is difficult because the pages are printed in two different directions; to read the blue pages it is necessary to turn the book sideways. The index is also printed sideways.

If one is interested in a quick overview of drug information, this handbook would be useful. However, to the knowledgeable reader or specialty clinician with a specific drug problem, other resources may be necessary.

Reviewed by Karen J. Klamerus, Pharm.D., College of Pharmacy, University of Illinois at Chicago, Chicago, IL. 60612.

Interpretation of Clinical Laboratory Tests

Edited by Gérard Siest, Joseph Henry, Françoise Schiele et al.

Published by Biomedical Publications, P.O. Box 8209, Foster City, CA 94404, 1985. xvi + 459 p. Price $47.50.

This book is a compilation and review of laboratory tests used to monitor disease states. It provides information on the interpretation of abnormal values with respect to clinical findings and a thorough review of the factors causing variation in these values. The text is written by 27 clinical scientists (two pharmacists) associated with the Center for Preventive Medicine, Vandoeuvre-les-Nancy, France, and one clinical scientist from the Mayo Clinic, Rochester, Minnesota.

At the beginning of the book is a listing of laboratory abbreviations and an explanation of the units of concentration used throughout the text. The book is divided into three parts. The first part consists of one chapter, which discusses the theory of reference values. It is devoted to the concept and use of reference values by the clinician. Both analytical and biological sources of variation are covered extensively. This chapter is a very good review for pharmacy students or practitioners preparing to review a patient's laboratory results as part of their clinical pharmacy services. A general bibliography is included at the end of this section.

The second part (Chapters 2–6) describes how reference values can be obtained for a general population. The detailed description of the collection of clinical data, quality control of analysis, physiologic and demographic characteristics of the reference population, and statistical methods used to analyze the data complement Chapter 1 but would be of more benefit to clinical chemists employed within laboratories than to clinical pharmacists doing therapeutic evaluations.

Part 3 (Chapters 7–33) covers biological variations of blood constituents and their reference values for 27 clinical chemistry analyses. Each chapter includes a review of the metabolism and pathophysiology of these constituents, the major analytical methods employed, the preanalytical factors that affect the variation of these methods, the known causes of biological variation (including the effects of drugs and other xenobiotics), the correlation with other biological variables, and the establishment of reference values. (It must be kept in mind that the reference limits will differ from laboratory to laboratory and should not be considered identical to those published in the text.) This is the most useful part of the text for a pharmacy student to learn or for a practicing pharmacist to review regarding the use of a clinical laboratory test.

At the end of each chapter, there is a table of the reference limits obtained at the Center for Preventive Medicine. They are categorized by age and sex of the patients. A convenient figure that summarizes the known biological and pathological causes of variation for the analysis is also published. Following this is a list of references. It includes a good compilation of work done up to about 1980 but seems to have eliminated any studies published within the last five years.

Throughout the text, the reader will find many tables and figures related to biological variations, as well as descriptions of clinically significant drug–laboratory interactions. This type of material can be very beneficial to those reviewing patient profiles during routine clinical pharmacy services.

Clinical laboratory test values have both a diagnostic and a prognostic role. The values are considered together with clinical findings. If the two are not in agreement, most clinicians give preference to the clinical information, which usually is more relevant. This problem may be magnified in the area of prevention of chronic diseases, since most credence is lent to the laboratory test results in distinguishing those patients suffering from diseases from those who are in good health. If medications that may influence the laboratory test results are being used, improper conclusions regarding the presence of disease may be formulated. It is important to be aware of these clinically relevant interactions, as well as those laboratory indices that are necessary for proper monitoring of the use of medications. This text explains these causes of variation, in addition to others, which makes it an invaluable reference book for clinical chemists, clinical pharmacists, and physicians.

Reviewed by Ralph E. Small, Pharm.D., Department of Pharmacy and Pharmaceutics, Medical College of Virginia, Virginia Commonwealth University, Richmond, VA 23298-0001.

Books Received

Books are listed as received; selected books may be reviewed in Book Reviews in subsequent issues.

α-Adrenoceptor Blockers in Cardiovascular Disease, edited by Helge Refsum and Ole D. Mjøs. Published by Churchill Livingstone Inc., 1560 Broadway, New York, NY 10036, 1985. 328 p. Price $42.00.

A Companion to Medical Statistics, by Edmond A. Murphy. Published by The Johns Hopkins University Press, 701 West 40th St., Baltimore, MD 21211, 1985. xv + 303 p. Price $27.50.

The Encyclopaedia of Medical Ignorance: Exploring the Frontiers of Medical Knowledge, edited by Ronald Duncan and Miranda Weston-Smith. Published by Pergamon Press Ltd., Oxford, England, 1984. Available from Pergamon Press Inc., Maxwell House, Fairview Park, Elmsford, NY 10523, 1984. vii + 253 p. Price $17.95.

Guide to Parenteral Administration of Drugs, by C. E. Hipwell, M. L. Mashford, and M. B. Robertson. Published by ADIS Health Science Press, Sydney, Australia, 1984. Distributed by Williams & Wilkins, 428 E. Preston St., Baltimore, MD 20202. xv + 163 p. Price $28.00.

Melloni's Illustrated Medical Dictionary, Second Edition, William R. Hensyl, editor. Published by Williams & Wilkins, 428 East Preston St., Baltimore, MD 21202, 1985. li + 533 p. Price $22.50.

Surgical Pharmacology of the Eye, edited by Marvin L. Sears and Ahti Tarkkanen. Published by Raven Press, 1140 Avenue of the Americas, New York, NY 10036, 1985. xiii + 592 p. Price $59.50.

New Periodical

The American Journal of Alzheimer's Care, edited by Stacey Wiley. Published quarterly by Prime National Publishing Corporation, 470 Boston Post Road, Weston, MA 02193. First issue, Winter 1986. Price $25.00 per year.

This journal, a professional journal devoted exclusively to Alzheimer's disease and related disorders, will share information and ideas on how to provide better professional and community care for Alzheimer's patients. As a reference tool for all health professionals, it will promote understanding of the disease by disseminating results of research and knowledge gleaned from a variety of Alzheimer's-related disciplines.

Advertising Index

American Critical Care, Division of American Hospital Supply Corporation
Hespan, 616–618
American Lung Association
Christmas Seals, 704
American Society of Hospital Pharmacists
Clinical Pharmacy, 624
Positions Available, 621
Appalachian Regional Hospitals
Positions Available, 704
Beecham Laboratories
Ticar, 602–604
Bristol-Myers Oncology Division
Mexate, 593–594
Burroughs Wellcome Company
Zovirax, 608–610
Emory University Hospital
Residency Training Programs, 705
Lederle Laboratories, A Division of American Cyanamid Company
Maxzide, 599–600
LyphoMed, Inc.
Institutional, 622–623
Pfipharmecs, Division of Pfizer Corporation
Institutional, 619, inside back cover
Roche Laboratories, Division of Hoffmann-La Roche, Inc.
Rocephin, 697–702
Smith Kline & French Laboratories
Ancef, inside front cover, 606–607
Monocid, 596–598
Stuart Pharmaceuticals, Division of ICI Americas, Inc.
Institutional, outside back cover
The Upjohn Company
Micronase, 612–614
Veterans Administration
Positions Available, 705

Index to Volume 4

The index to Volume 4 is composed of three parts: a subject index, an author index, and an advertising index.

The subject index is made up mainly of terms constructed by *International Pharmaceutical Abstracts*. The *IPA* index is an alphabetical, open-ended, controlled-vocabulary index that makes use of standardized headings. (The primary index terms for major articles are listed routinely in *Clinical Pharmacy* as "index terms" following abstracts.) *IPA* covers all authored papers and editorials in *Clinical Pharmacy* as well as selected letters and news reports. The subject index also notes all regular columns, and, under the respective column headings, the titles of items in the "Editorials," and "Book Reviews" sections and the titles of individual stories in "News." The subject index also contains, under the heading "Correction Notices," the title and issue of publication of items for which corrections were printed, as well as the page numbers on which the corrections appear.

Issue	*Pages*	*Issue*	*Pages*
January–February	1–118	July–August	355–468
March–April	119–240	September–October	469–590
May–June	241–354	November–December	591–716

Subject Index

A

Absorption
digitoxin; interactions, review, 404
digoxin; interactions, review, 404
nomifensine maleate; review, 625
procainamide; rate constants, 186
testosterone propionate; interactions, warfarin, 332
warfarin; short-bowel syndrome, 325
Acecainide; clearance; peritoneal dialysis, 669
Acetylcysteine; atelectasis; therapy, infants, 255
Acquired immunodeficiency syndrome
infections; therapy, review, 539
therapy, 475
Acyclovir
herpesvirus infections; therapy, AIDS, review, 539
pharmacokinetics; peritoneal dialysis, 320
Acyclovir sodium; pharmacokinetics; peritoneal dialysis, 320
Adrenergic agents, see **Sympathomimetic agents**
Adsorbents; charcoal activated; and cathartics, GI transit time, 446; antidotes, trazodone poisoning, 97
Adverse reactions, see **Drugs, adverse reactions**
Advertising Index, 118, 240, 354, 468, 590, 706
Aerosols
antibiotics; cystic fibrosis therapy, review, 555
bitolterol mesylate; therapy, review, 393
drug administration; reservoirs, systems, 452
fenoterol hydrobromide; therapy, review, 393
Age
patients; drug-induced systemic lupus erythematosus, review, 657; effects, metoclopramide toxicity, 102
pediatrics; *H. influenzae* type b, risks, 637
AIDS, see **Acquired immunodeficiency syndrome**
α-Interferon; acquired immunodeficiency syndrome; therapy, 475
Albuterol; and steroids, cortico-; viral bronchiolitis therapy, 297
Allergies
carbamazepine; pediatrics, 19
isosulfan blue; anaphylaxis, 219
streptokinase; vasculitis, 383
theophylline anhydrous; sustained-action, pruritus, 334
Alopecia; cimetidine; toxicity, 145
Alprazolam; structure–activity relationships; triazolo derivatives, 258
Aluminum; toxicity; osteomalacia, review, 434
Amantadine sulfate; intravenous; Parkinson's disease therapy, 146
Ambulatory care; self-medication; dobutamine injections, 195
American Society of Hospital Pharmacists; *Clinical Pharmacy;* journals, history, 82
Amikacin; pharmacokinetics; obesity, effects, surgery, 70
Amikacin sulfate; pharmacokinetics; obesity, effects, surgery, 70
Aminoglycosides
amikacin sulfate; pharmacokinetics, obesity, surgery, 70
gentamicin sulfate; and antibiotics, parotitis therapy, 566; and clindamycin, prophylaxis, 316; arteriovenous ultrafiltration, 327; half-life predictions, diabetes, 572; pharmacokinetics, effects; surgery, 182
tobramycin sulfate; and antibiotics, parotitis therapy, 566
Aminophylline; metabolism; theophylline excretion, 59; theophylline pharmacokinetics, paraplegics, 448
Amiodarone; interactions; digoxin, review, 404
Amitriptyline; alone and with anticonvulsants or phenothiazines; postherpetic neuralgia therapy, 170
Analgesics and antipyretics
aspirin; overdose poisoning, 97
baclofen and carbamazepine; trigeminal neuralgia therapy, 93
carbamazepine; trigeminal neuralgia therapy, 93
diacetylmorphine; pain therapy, 80
ibuprofen; combined therapy, cancer pain, 53
morphine sulfate; i.m., i.v., 48; patient-controlled analgesia, 41
neuralgia; postherpetic, therapy, 170
Analysis; interference; digoxin blood levels, 81
Anaphylaxis; isosulfan blue; adverse reactions, 219
Androgens; testosterone propionate; interactions, warfarin, 332
Anesthetics; dentistry; NIH recommendations, 357
Ansamycin; acquired immunodeficiency syndrome; therapy, 475
Antacids; toxicity; aluminum-related osteomalacia, 434
Anthelmintics; quinacrine hydrochloride; protozoan infection therapy, AIDS, review, 539
Antiarrhythmic agents, see **Cardiac drugs**
Antibiotics
aztreonam; therapy, review, 516
bacitracin; enterocolitis therapy, review, 304
clindamycin phosphate; and aminoglycosides, parotitis therapy, 566; and gentamicin, prophylaxis, 316
cystic fibrosis; therapy, review, 555
moxalactam; and piperacillin, therapy, 327
moxalactam disodium; comparison, prophylaxis, 316; saliva levels, 67
rifampin; *H. influenzae* prophylaxis, review, 637
toxicity; enterocolitis, 304
vancomycin; enterocolitis therapy, review, 304
vancomycin hydrochloride; dosage prediction methods, 311
vancomycin sulfate; and aminoglycosides, parotitis therapy, 566
Antibodies; influenza; vaccines, interactions, phenytoin, 191
Anticoagulants
heparin; interactions, digitoxin, digoxin, review, 404; i.v. therapy, 325; therapy, review, 279
warfarin; interactions, testosterone ointment, 332; therapy, review, 279
warfarin sodium; absorption, short-bowel syndrome, 325; dosage prediction methods, 440
Anticonvulsants
and amitriptyline; postherpetic neuralgia therapy, 170
carbamazepine; allergies, pediatrics, 19; toxicity, 221
clonazepam; cerebellar tremor therapy, 615
phenytoin; interactions, influenza vaccines, 191
phenytoin sodium; toxicity; i.v., administration sites, 618
Antidepressants
interactions; carbamazepine, review, 425
nomifensine maleate; therapy, 673; therapy review, 625
trazodone hydrochloride; overdose poisoning, 97
triazolam; structure–activity relationships, 258
tricyclic; postherpetic neuralgia therapy, 170
Antidiarrhea agents; therapy; travelers' diarrhea, 141
Antidotes; charcoal activated; trazodone poisoning, 97
Antiemetics; metoclopramide hydrochloride; toxicity, 102
Antifungals
ketoconazole; candidiasis therapy, AIDS, review, 539
nystatin; candidiasis therapy, AIDS, review, 539
Anti-infective agents
metronidazole; enterocolitis therapy, review, 304
pyrimethamine; toxoplasmosis therapy, AIDS, review, 539
trimethoprim, combination, sulfamethoxazole; infection therapy, AIDS, review, 539
trimethoprim, combination, sulfamethoxazole; gonococcal urethritis therapy, 455
Anti-inflammatory agents
indomethacin; patent ductus arteriosus, neonates, 248
interactions; digoxin, review, 404
Antilipemic agents; and diet; coronary disease prevention, 123
Antimanic agents
lithium; dosage prediction methods, 77; interactions, carbamazepine, review, 425
lithium carbonate; overdose poisoning, 97
Antineoplastic agents
and radiation; osteogenic sarcoma therapy, 485
doxorubicin; toxicity, myocardial diseases, 502
plicamycin; effects, etidronate, hypercalcemia, 204
tamoxifen; postmenopausal breast neoplasm therapy, 605
toxicity; enterocolitis, 304
Antiparkinson agents; amantadine sulfate; i.v. therapy, 146
Antiprotozoals
metronidazole; therapy, AIDS, review, 539
pentamidine isethionate; *P. carinii* pneumonia therapy, review, 507
spiramycin; therapy, AIDS, review, 539
Antithyroid drugs; interactions; digoxin, review, 404
Antivirals
acquired immunodeficiency syndrome; therapy, 475
acyclovir; therapy, AIDS, review, 539
acyclovir sodium; peritoneal dialysis, 320
ribavirin; bronchiolitis therapy, pediatrics, 297
Anxiolytics, sedatives and hypnotics
alprazolam; structure–activity relationships, 258
dentistry; NIH recommendations, 357
flurazepam hydrochloride; opiate withdrawal therapy, 100
pentobarbital sodium; seizure therapy, neonate, 330
triazolam; structure–activity relationships, 258
Aspirin; poisoning; overdose, 97
Ataxia; carbamazepine; toxicity, 93
Atelectasis; acetylcysteine; therapy, infants, 255
Atropine sulfate; combination, diphenoxylate hydrochloride; travelers' diarrhea therapy, 141
Availability, drugs, see **Drugs, availability**

Azlocillin; pharmacokinetics; high dose, cystic fibrosis, 664
Azlocillin sodium; pharmacokinetics; high dose, cystic fibrosis, 664
Aztreonam; therapy, review, 516

B

Bacitracin; enterocolitis; therapy, review, 304
Baclofen; and carbamazepine; trigeminal neuralgia therapy, 93
Benztropine mesylate; toxicity; tachycardia, review, 675
Bioavailability, see **Drugs, availability**
Bismuth subsalicylate; diarrhea; travelers', therapy, 141
Bitolterol mesylate; aerosols; therapy, review, 393
Blood levels
acecainide; peritoneal dialysis, 669
acyclovir; peritoneal dialysis, 320
amikacin; obesity, effects, surgery, 70
azlocillin; high dose, cystic fibrosis, 664
carbamazepine; toxicity, review, 425
ceftriaxone; kidney failure, 177
digoxin; relation, effects, toxicity, 81
gentamicin; arteriovenous ultrafiltration, 327; effects, surgery, 182; prediction, 74; predictions, diabetes, 572
glucose; lack, effects, ceftazidime, 72
iothalamate; cystic fibrosis, 664
lithium; overdose poisoning, 97
monitoring; drug therapy, limitations, 3
morphine; patient-controlled analgesia, 41
moxalactam; lack, effects, *H. influenzae* b meningitis, 67
pentobarbital; neonate, 330
phenytoin; interactions, influenza vaccines, 191
procainamide; peritoneal dialysis, 669; prediction, 186
pseudoephedrine hydrochloride; availability, sustained-action suspensions, 199
ranitidine; relation, lactation, 322
salicylates; overdose poisoning, 97
sampling; time, 84
testosterone; interactions, warfarin 332
tetracycline; relation, metallic taste, 455
theophylline; effects, excretion, 59; overdose poisoning, 97; spinal cord injuries, 448
trazodone; overdose poisoning, 97
vancomycin; relation, creatinine clearance, 311
warfarin; short-bowel syndrome, 325
Body surface area; patients; amikacin pharmacokinetics, obesity, 70
Book reviews, 113, 228, 342, 468, 583, 703
AMA Handbook of Poisonous and Injurious Plants, 703
The Aging Process: Therapeutic Implications, 583
Antacids and Other Drugs in Gastrointestinal Diseases, 113
Antimicrobial Prescribing, Second Edition, 113
Antimicrobial Therapy, 342
Beta Blockers in the Treatment of Cardiovascular Disease, 583
Blue Book of Pharmacologic Therapeutics, 703
A Clinical Companion to Biochemical Studies, Second Edition, 114
Clinical Guide to Parenteral Micronutrition, 588
Clinical Pharmacy and Therapeutics, Third Edition, 228
Critical Care: A Comprehensive Approach, 342
Evaluation and Treatment of Chronic Pain, 588
Guide for Adult Immunization, 704
Guide to Clinical Studies and Developing Protocols, 235
Interpretation of Clinical Laboratory Tests, 704
Manual of Antibiotics and Infectious Diseases, Fifth Edition, 114
New Drugs Annual: Cardiovascular Drugs (Volume 2), 238
Pediatric Medications: An Emergency and Critical Care Reference, 589
Practice of Critical Care Pharmacy, 468
Side Effects of Drugs, Annual 8, 1984, 117
The Psychopharmacology of Lithium, 347
Books Received, 118, 240, 350, 468, 589, 706
Breast neoplasms; tamoxifen; postmenopausal combined therapy, 605
Bretylium tosylate; tachycardia; therapy, drug-induced, review, 675
Bronchial spasm
bitolterol mesylate; aerosols, therapy, review, 393
fenoterol hydrobromide; aerosols, therapy, review, 393
Bronchiolitis; therapy; viral, pediatrics, 297
Bronchodilators; cystic fibrosis; therapy, review, 555

C

Calcium antagonists; interactions; digoxin, review, 404
Calcium regulators; etidronate disodium; effects, plicamycin dosage, 204
Calculations
dosage; gentamicin pharmacokinetics, 74
dosage; lithium, prediction, 77
excretion; theophylline, 59
Cancer; obesity; relation, 367
Cancer drugs, see **Antineoplastic agents**
Candidiasis; therapy; AIDS, review, 539
Captopril; and hydrochlorothiazide; dosage, hypertension therapy, 65
Carbamazepine
adverse reactions; allergies, pediatrics, 19
alone and with baclofen; trigeminal neuralgia therapy, 93
and amitriptyline; postherpetic neuralgia therapy, 170
mental disorders; therapy, review, 425
toxicity; thrombocytopenia, 221
Cardiac drugs
bretylium tosylate; tachycardia therapy, review, 675
digitoxin; interactions, review, 404
digoxin; blood levels, effects, 81; interactions, review, 404
levodopa; myocardial diseases therapy, 502
lidocaine; tachycardia therapy and toxicity, review, 675
procainamide; toxicity, systemic lupus erythematosus, review, 657
procainamide hydrochloride; blood level prediction, 186; peritoneal dialysis clearance, 669; toxicity, hypotension, 504
quinidine; interactions, digoxin, review, 404
toxicity; tachycardia, review, 675
Cathartics and laxatives
combination, charcoal activated; GI transit time, 446
magnesium citrate; therapy, overdose poisoning, 97
Ceftazidime; effects; glucose blood levels, 72
Ceftriaxone; pharmacokinetics; kidney failure, 177
Ceftriaxone sodium; pharmacokinetics; kidney failure, 177
Cephalosporins
ceftazidime; lack, effects, glucose blood levels, 72
ceftriaxone sodium; pharmacokinetics, kidney failure, 177
Charcoal activated
alone and with cathartics and laxatives; GI transit time, 446
antidotes; trazodone poisoning, 97
combination, sorbitol; GI transit time, 446
Cimetidine
interactions; digoxin, review, 404
toxicity; alopecia, 145
Clearance, see **Excretion**
Clinical Pharmacy
Acknowledgment to reviewers, 691
journals; ASHP, history, 82
Procedure for submission of manuscripts to journals published by the American Society of Hospital Pharmacists, 105
Statement of ownership, management, and circulation, 690
Clindamycin phosphate
and gentamicin sulfate; comparison, moxalactam, prophylaxis, 316
gentamicin sulfate or tobramycin sulfate and vancomycin hydrochloride; parotitis therapy, 566
Clonazepam; tremor; cerebellar, therapy, 615
Clonidine
effects; glucose intolerance, 649
Gilles de la Tourette's disease; and opiate withdrawal therapy, 494
Clonidine hydrochloride; and naloxone hydrochloride; opiate withdrawal therapy, 100
Cocaine; abuse; therapy, 595
Combined therapy
antineoplastic agents and radiation; osteogenic sarcoma, 485
baclofen and carbamazepine; trigeminal neuralgia, 93
captopril and hydrochlorothiazide; dosage, hypertension, 65
carbamazepine and baclofen; trigeminal neuralgia, 93
clonidine hydrochloride and naloxone hydrochloride; opiate withdrawal, 100
cyclophosphamide; bone marrow transplantation, review, 149
etidronate disodium and plicamycin; hypercalcemia, 204
hydrochlorothiazide and captopril; dosage, hypertension, 65
ibuprofen and opiates; cancer pain, 53
naloxone hydrochloride and clonidine hydrochloride; opiate withdrawal, 100
opiates and ibuprofen; cancer pain, 53
plicamycin and etidronate disodium; hypercalcemia, 204
radiation and antineoplastic agents; osteogenic sarcoma, 485
tamoxifen, postmenopausal breast neoplasms, 605
Contraceptives, oral; ethinyl estradiol, combination, norethindrone; triphasic, 24
Contraindications
hypotensive agents; glucose intolerance, 649
nomifensine maleate; depression therapy, review, 625
Coronary disease; prevention; diet, 123
Correction Notices, 25; Dietary interaction with phenytoin (Mar–Apr 1984, Letters), 25
Costs
clindamycin phosphate and gentamicin sulfate; comparison, prophylaxis, 316
gentamicin; blood level prediction, 74
gentamicin sulfate and clindamycin phosphate; comparison, prophylaxis, 316
heparin; lock, 488
moxalactam disodium; comparison, prophylaxis, 316
vancomycin; enterocolitis therapy, review, 304
warfarin sodium; dosage prediction methods, 440
Creatinine; clearance; gentamicin half-life predictions, 572
CP Continuing Education, 111, 224, 336, 463, 576, 692
Current Literature, 113, 228, 342, 468, 583, 703
Cyclophosphamide; combined therapy; bone marrow transplantation, review, 149
Cystic fibrosis
azlocillin sodium; pharmacokinetics, high dose, 664
therapy; review, 555
Cytotoxic agents, see **Antineoplastic agents**

D

Deferoxamine; osteomalacia; therapy, review, 434
Dentistry
anesthetics; NIH recommendations, 357
anxiolytics, sedatives and hypnotics; NIH recommendations, 357
Depression
nomifensine maleate; therapy, 673; therapy review, 625
propranolol hydrochloride; toxicity, review, 214
Devices
drug administration; reservoir aerosols, 452
infusion pumps; dobutamine injections, 195
Diabetes mellitus
gentamicin; half-life predictions, errors, 572
obesity; relation, 367
Diacetylmorphine; pain; therapy, regulations, 80
Dialysis
hemo-; gentamicin pharmacokinetics, 74
peritoneal; acyclovir pharmacokinetics, 320; acecainide and procainamide clearance, 669
Diarrhea; therapy; travelers', 141
Diatrizoate meglumine; roentgenographic agents; intravascular, review, 527
Diatrizoate sodium; roentgenographic agents; intravascular, review, 527
Digestants
pancreatin; Viokase reformulation, pancrelipase, 388
pancrelipase; reformulation, powders, tablets, 388
Digitoxin; interactions; review, 404
Digoxin
blood levels; relation, effects, toxicity, 81
concomitant therapy; myocardial diseases, 502
interactions; review, 404
Diphenoxylate hydrochloride; combination, atropine sulfate; travelers' diarrhea therapy, 141
Diuretics
hypotensive agents; effects, glucose intolerance, 649
interactions; digoxin, review, 404
Dobutamine hydrochloride; heart failure; congestive, therapy, 195
Dosage
acyclovir sodium; peritoneal dialysis, 320
amikacin sulfate; pharmacokinetics, obesity, surgery, 70
anticoagulants; therapy, review, 279
azlocillin sodium; high, pharmacokinetics, cystic fibrosis, 664
baclofen and carbamazepine; trigeminal neuralgia therapy, 93
carbamazepine; trigeminal neuralgia therapy, 93
ceftriaxone sodium; pharmacokinetics, kidney failure, 177

cyclophosphamide; bone marrow transplantation, review, 149
dobutamine hydrochloride; congestive heart failure therapy, 195
drugs; sampling, blood levels, 84
enalapril maleate; therapy, review, 27
gentamicin; blood level prediction, 74
gentamicin sulfate; effects, surgery, 182; half-life predictions, diabetes, 572
globulin immune; high, thrombopenic purpura therapy, 206
hydralazine; toxicity, systemic lupus erythematosus, review, 657
lithium; prediction methods, 77
morphine sulfate; patient-controlled analgesia, 41
nomifensine maleate; review, 625
pentamidine isethionate; *P. carinii* pneumonia therapy, review, 507
pentobarbital sodium; seizure therapy, neonate, 330
roentgenographic agents; intravascular, review, 527
theophylline; effects, excretion, 59
thrombolytic agents; therapy, review, 279
vancomycin hydrochloride; prediction methods, 311
warfarin; interactions, testosterone ointment, 332
warfarin sodium; prediction methods, 440

Dosage forms
nitroglycerin; transdermal, efficacy, 453
pancrelipase; reformulation, powders, tablets, 388
procainamide hydrochloride; blood level prediction, 186
pseudoephedrine hydrochloride; sustained-action suspensions, 199

Dosage schedules
captopril; hypertension therapy, 65
nitroglycerin; transdermal, efficacy, 453
phenytoin; interactions, influenza vaccines, 191
plicamycin; effects, etidronate, hypercalcemia, 204

Doxorubicin; toxicity; myocardial diseases, 502
Doxycycline; diarrhea; travelers', therapy, 141

Drug abuse
cocaine; therapy, 595
morphine sulfate; lack, patient-controlled analgesia, 41

Drug administration
self-medication; dobutamine injections, 195; i.v. morphine, 48; i.v. morphine injections, 41
sodium chloride; indwelling injection sites, 488

Drug administration rate
irrigating solutions; bowel cleansing, review, 414
phenytoin sodium; toxicity, i.v. sites, 618
procainamide hydrochloride; toxicity, hypotension, 504

Drug administration routes
morphine sulfate; i.m., i.v., 48
nitroglycerin; transdermal, efficacy, 453

Drug administration sites
injections; indwelling, flushing, 488
phenytoin sodium; toxicity, i.v. injections, 618

Drug administration systems; aerosols; reservoirs, 452

Drug interactions
baclofen and carbamazepine; trigeminal neuralgia therapy, 93
carbamazepine and baclofen; trigeminal neuralgia therapy, 93
carbamazepine and lithium; review, 425
digoxin; and metabolites, blood levels, 81
influenza vaccines and phenytoin, 191
lithium and carbamazepine; review, 425
nomifensine maleate; review, 625
phenytoin and influenza vaccine, 191
smoking and theophylline; spinal cord injuries, 448
testosterone propionate and warfarin; potentiation, 332
theophylline and smoking; spinal cord injuries, 448
warfarin and testosterone propionate; potentiation, 332

Drugs; selection; intravascular roentgenographic agents, review, 527

Drugs, adverse reactions
carbamazepine; allergies, pediatrics, 19
iatrogenic diseases; systemic lupus erythematosus, review, 657; 675
isosulfan blue; anaphylaxis, 219
roentgenographic agents; intravascular, review, 527
theophylline anhydrous; sustained-action, pruritus, 334

Drugs, availability; pseudoephedrine hydrochloride; sustained-action suspensions, 199

Drugs, body distribution
acecainide; peritoneal dialysis, 669
amikacin; obesity, effects, surgery, 70
digitoxin; interactions, review, 404
digoxin; interactions, review, 404
gentamicin; effects, surgery, 182; prediction, 74; predictions, diabetes, 572
moxalactam; lack, effects, *H. influenzae* b meningitis, 67
nomifensine maleate; review, 625
procainamide; peritoneal dialysis, 669
theophylline; spinal cord injuries, 448

Drug use
anesthetics; dentistry, NIH recommendations, 357
anxiolytics, sedatives and hypnotics; dentistry, NIH recommendations, 357

Drug withdrawal; opiates; relation, Tourette's disease, therapy, 494; therapy, 100
Ductus arteriosus; indomethacin; patent, i.v. therapy, neonates, 248
Dystonia; metoclopramide hydrochloride; toxicity, 102

E

Editorials, 80, 355, 452, 673
How reliable are serum digoxin assays? 82
Nomifensine: an antidepressant with a difference? 673
Progress and problems with pain, 80
Reservoir aerosol delivery systems, 452
Transdermal nitroglycerin patches, 453
Volume 4, 82

Electrolytes; irrigating solutions; oral, bowel cleansing, review, 414
Elimination, see **Metabolism**
Enalaprilat; metabolites; enalapril, review, 27
Enalapril maleate; hypertension; therapy, review, 27
Enterocolitis; therapy; review, 304
Equations; dosage; lithium, prediction, 77
Equivalency; pseudoephedrine hydrochloride; sustained-action suspensions, 199

Errors
blood levels; digoxin analysis, 81
dosage; gentamicin half-life predictions, 572
drug administration rate; procainamide, toxicity, hypotension, 504

Ethacrynic acid; effects; glucose intolerance, 649
Ethinyl estradiol; combination, norethindrone; triphasic oral contraceptives, 24
Etidronate disodium; and plicamycin; hypercalcemia therapy, neoplasms, 204

Excretion
acecainide; peritoneal dialysis, 669
amikacin; obesity, effects, surgery, 70
azlocillin; high dose, cystic fibrosis, 664
aztreonam; review, 516
charcoal activated; fecal, effects, cathartics, 446
creatinine; gentamicin half-life predictions, 572
digitoxin; interactions, review, 404
digoxin; interactions, review, 404
drugs; arteriovenous hemofiltration, 620
gentamicin; arteriovenous ultrafiltration, 327; prediction, 74; rate constants, 182
iothalamate; cystic fibrosis, 664
procainamide; peritoneal dialysis, 669; rate constants, 186
theophylline; factors affecting, 59; spinal cord injuries, 448
trazodone; overdose poisoning, 97
vancomycin; relation, creatinine, 311
warfarin; short-bowel syndrome, 325

F

Fenoterol hydrobromide
aerosols; therapy, review, 393

Filtration
hemo; drugs, arteriovenous, 620
ultra; gentamicin, arteriovenous, 327

Flow
irrigating solutions; bowel cleansing, review, 414
rates; peritoneal dialysis, procainamide clearance, 669

Flurazepam hydrochloride; therapy; opiate withdrawal, 100
Fluids; bronchiolitis; viral, therapy, pediatrics, 297
Food and Drug Administration (U.S.); indomethacin; regulations, patent ductus arteriosus, 248

Formularies
pentamidine isethionate; *P. carinii* pneumonia therapy, review, 507
roentgenographic agents; intravascular, review, 527

Formulations
pancrelipase; powders, tablets, 388
pseudoephedrine hydrochloride; sustained-action suspensions, 199

Foscarnet sodium; acquired immunodeficiency syndrome; therapy, 475
Furosemide; effects; glucose intolerance, 649

G

Gastric emptying; charcoal activated; effects, cathartics, 446
Gastric lavage; irrigating solutions; oral, review, 414

Gastrointestinal drugs
cimetidine; interactions, digoxin, review, 404; toxicity, alopecia, 145
maldigestion; therapy, review, 161
ranitidine hydrochloride; lactation, 322

Gentamicin
blood levels; prediction, 74
excretion; arteriovenous ultrafiltration, 327
half-life; predictions, diabetes, 572
pharmacokinetics; effects, surgery, 182

Gentamicin sulfate
and clindamycin phosphate; comparison, moxalactam, prophylaxis, 316
and piperacillin; therapy, ultrafiltration, 327
clindamycin phosphate and vancomycin hydrochloride; parotitis therapy, 566
dosage; half-life predictions, diabetes, 572
pharmacokinetics; effects, surgery, 182

Geriatrics
phenytoin sodium; toxicity, i.v. sites, 618
tamoxifen; postmenopausal breast neoplasm therapy, 605

Gilles de la Tourette's disease
clonidine; therapy, 494
pentazocine; therapy, 494

Globulin immune; purpura; thrombopenic, therapy, 206
Glucose intolerance; hypotensive agents; contraindications, 649
Guanethidine; effects; glucose intolerance, 649

H

***Haemophilus* b polysaccharide vaccines**
immunization; pediatrics, review, 637

Haemophilus influenzae
moxalactam disodium; type b, lack, effects, 67
type b; prevention, review, 637

Half-life
aztreonam; excretion, review, 516
ceftriaxone; kidney failure, 177
acyclovir; peritoneal dialysis, 320
azlocillin; blood levels, cystic fibrosis, 664
drugs; sampling time, 84
gentamicin; prediction, 74; predictions, diabetes, 572
nomifensine maleate; review, 625
ranitidine; lactation, 322
trazodone; excretion, 97
warfarin; short-bowel syndrome, 325
theophylline; spinal cord injuries, 448

Health; patients; obesity, risks, 367
Heart diseases; obesity, relation, 367

Heart failure
dobutamine hydrochloride; congestive, therapy, 195
enalapril maleate; congestive, therapy, review, 27

Heavy metal antagonists; deferoxamine; osteomalacia therapy, review, 434
Hematologic diseases; therapy; bone marrow transplantation, review, 149

Heparin
concomitant therapy; pulmonary embolism, 383
interactions; digitoxin, digoxin, review, 404
lock; sodium chloride irrigations, 488
therapy; anticoagulants, 325
thrombophlebitis; and pulmonary embolism therapy, review, 279

Herpes zoster
acyclovir sodium; therapy, 320
therapy, 170

Herpesvirus infections; therapy; AIDS, review, 539
History; *Clinical Pharmacy;* ASHP journals, 82
Hospitals; length of stay; warfarin dosage prediction, 440
HPA-23; acquired immunodeficiency syndrome; therapy, 475
Hydralazine; lupus; erythematosus, systemic, toxicity, review, 657
Hydrochlorothiazide; alone and with captopril; hypertension therapy, 65
Hypercalcemia; etidronate disodium; therapy, plicamycin dosage, 204
Hypercholesterolemia; therapy, diet, 123
Hyperlipidemia; obesity; relation, 367

Hypertension
captopril and hydrochlorothiazide; therapy, dosage, 65
enalapril maleate; therapy, review, 27

hydrochlorothiazide and captopril; therapy, dosage, 65
obesity; relation, 367
Hypotension; procainamide hydrochloride; toxicity, rapid i.v., 504
Hypotensive agents
captopril and hydrochlorothiazide; hypertension therapy, 65
contraindications; glucose intolerance, 649
enalapril maleate; therapy, review, 27
hydralazine; toxicity, systemic lupus erythematosus, review, 657
hydrochlorothiazide and captopril; hypertension therapy, 65
propranolol hydrochloride; toxicity, review, 214

I

Iatrogenic diseases, see **Drugs, adverse reactions**
Ibuprofen; and opiates; cancer pain therapy, 53
Immunization
Haemophilus influenzae; type b, vaccines, review, 637
influenza; vaccines, interactions, phenytoin, 191
Immunosuppressive agents
cyclophosphamide; bone marrow transplantation, review, 149
Immunotherapy; interleukin-2; AIDS, 475
Indomethacin
intravenous; patent ductus arteriosus, neonates, 248
Influenza vaccines; interactions; phenytoin, 191
Inhalation therapy; aerosols; drug administration systems, 452
Injections
amikacin sulfate; pharmacokinetics, obesity, surgery, 70
phenytoin sodium; toxicity, i.v., administration sites, 618
sodium chloride; irrigations, indwelling sites, 488
Interleukin-2; acquired immunodeficiency syndrome; therapy, 475
Intracranial pressure; pentobarbital sodium; therapy, neonate, 330
Iodamide meglumine; roentgenographic agents; intravascular, review, 527
Iodipamide meglumine; roentgenographic agents; intravascular, review, 527
Iodoxamate meglumine; roentgenographic agents; intravascular, review, 527
Iothalamate; pharmacokinetics; cystic fibrosis, 664
Iothalamate meglumine; roentgenographic agents; intravascular, review, 527
Iothalamate sodium
pharmacokinetics; cystic fibrosis, 664
roentgenographic agents; intravascular, review, 527
Irrigating solutions
oral; bowel cleansing, review, 414
sodium chloride; indwelling injection sites, 488
Isoproterenol hydrochloride; tachycardia; therapy, drug induced, review, 675
Isosulfan blue; anaphylaxis; adverse reactions, 219
Isotretinoin; toxicity; short term, 142

J

Journals; *Clinical Pharmacy;* ASHP, history, 82

K

Keratolytic agents; isotretinoin; toxicity, 142
Ketoconazole; candidiasis; therapy, AIDS, review, 539
Kraurosis vulvae; testosterone propionate; therapy, 332

L

Labeling; pancrelipase; reformulation, powders, tablets, 388
Lactation; ranitidine; pharmacokinetics, 322
Letters, 19, 145, 255, 370, 488, 615
Acetylcysteine for severe atelectasis in premature infants, 255
Beneficial hemodynamic effects of oral levodopa in a patient with cardiomyopathy, 502
Change in enzyme content and manufacturer of Viokase, 388
Cimetidine-induced alopecia, 145
Drug clearance in patients undergoing continuous arteriovenous hemofiltration, 620
Effect of warfarin on activated partial thromboplastin time, 620
Hypersensitivity vasculitis associated with streptokinase, 383
I.V. amantadine sulfate for extrapyramidal crisis, 146
The opioid–noradrenergic link in Gilles de la Tourette's syndrome, 494
Oral acyclovir pharmacokinetics, 370
Origins of aztreonam resistance, 23
Pharmacologic effects of the triazolo group, 258
Phenytoin injection precautions, 618
Potentiation of opiate analgesia with ibuprofen, 505
Procainamide-induced hypotension during CPR, 504
Putting amoxicillin–potassium clavulanate in perspective, 145
Severe hypersensitivity secondary to extended carbamazepine administration, 19
Successful treatment of cerebellar tremor with clonazepam, 615
Update on the new triphasic oral contraceptives, 24
Use of 0.9% sodium chloride injection without heparin for maintaining indwelling intermittent injection sites, 488
Venoconstriction by angiotensin II, 266
Levodopa; myocardial diseases; oral, therapy, 502
Lidocaine; tachycardia; therapy and toxicity, review, 675
Lithium
dosage; prediction methods, 77
interactions; carbamazepine, review, 425
Lithium carbonate; poisoning; overdose, 97
Liver diseases; ceftazidime; lack, effects, glucose blood levels, 72
Loperamide hydrochloride; diarrhea; travelers', therapy, 141
Lupus
hydralazine; erythematosus, systemic, toxicity, review, 657
procainamide; erythematosus, systemic, toxicity, review, 657

M

Magnesium citrate
antidotes; trazodone poisoning, 97
combination, charcoal activated; GI transit time, 446
Magnesium sulfate; combination, charcoal activated; GI transit time, 446
Maldigestion; therapy; review, 161
Manufacturers; pancrelipase; Viokase reformulation, 388
Mechanism of action
clonazepam; cerebellar tremor therapy, 615
contraceptives, oral; triphasic, 24
enalapril maleate; therapy, review, 27
hydralazine; toxicity, systemic lupus erythematosus, review, 657
indomethacin; patent ductus arteriosus, neonates, 248
nomifensine maleate; depression therapy, review, 625
pentobarbital sodium; seizure therapy, neonate, 330
phenytoin sodium; toxicity, i.v. sites, 618
procainamide; toxicity, systemic lupus erythematosus, review, 657
trazodone; overdose poisoning, 97
Meetings; National Institutes of Health; anesthetics and sedative use, dentistry, 357
Meningitis; moxalactam disodium; *H. influenzae* b, therapy, 67
Mental disorders; carbamazepine; therapy, review, 425
Metabolism
aminophylline; theophylline excretion, 59; theophylline pharmacokinetics, paraplegics, 448
digoxin; effects, blood levels, 81
digitoxin; interactions, review, 404
enalapril maleate; review, 27
procainamide hydrochloride; peritoneal dialysis clearance, 669
Methodology
dosage; lithium, prediction, 77; vancomyin, prediction, 311; warfarin, prediction, 440
excretion; theophylline, prediction, 59
gentamicin; blood level prediction, 74
pharmacokinetics; procainamide blood levels, 186
Methyldopa; effects; glucose intolerance, 649
Metoclopramide hydrochloride; toxicity; dystonic reactions, 102
Metronidazole
enterocolitis; therapy, review, 304
protozoan infections; therapy, AIDS, review, 539
Mithramycin see Plicamycin
Models
blood levels; gentamicin, prediction, 74
pharmacokinetics; procainamide blood levels, 186
Morphine; blood levels; patient-controlled analgesia, 41
Morphine sulfate
administration routes; i.m., i.v., postoperative pain, 48
pain; therapy, patient-controlled, 41
Moxalactam
and piperacillin; therapy, ultrafiltration, 327
saliva levels; lack, effects, *H. influenzae* b meningitis, 67
Moxalactam disodium
comparison, clindamycin phosphate and gentamicin sulfate; prophylaxis, 316
saliva levels; lack, effects, *H. influenzae* b meningitis, 67
Mucolytic agents
acetylcysteine; atelectasis therapy, infants, 255
cystic fibrosis; therapy, review, 555
Myocardial diseases; levodopa; oral, therapy, 502

N

Naloxone hydrochloride; and clonidine hydrochloride; opiate withdrawal therapy, 100
National Institutes of Health
consensus development conference; anesthetics and sedatives use, dentistry, 357; obesity, risk factors, 367; osteogenic sarcoma, combined therapy, 485; postmenopausal breast neoplasms, 605
diarrhea; travelers', therapy recommendations, 141
Neuralgia; analgesics and antipyretics; postherpetic, therapy, 170
New Periodicals, 354, 706
News, 3, 123, 245, 357, 475, 595
Adjuvant chemotherapy useful in osteosarcoma, says NIH panel, 485
AIDS tests reach market as cases increase, 248
Allopurinol approved for management of recurrent calcium oxalate stones, 367
Applying pharmacodynamics in patient care, 3
Auranofin approved for second-line therapy of rheumatoid arthritis, 357
Captopril approved for all degrees of hypertension, 486
Cardioselective β blocker acebutolol approved by FDA, 142
Conference outlines challenges in the treatment of cocaine abuse, 595
Ceforanide approved for twice-daily dosing, 14
Ceftazidime reaches U.S. market, 486
Combination product approved for deep-vein thrombosis, 142
Data on dose-dumping of sustained-release theophylline published, 479
Dietary modifications recommended for reducing heart disease, 123
Drug-induced blood disorders very rare, 131
Haemophilus vaccine approved, 362
Health implications of obesity explored at consensus conference, 367
Injectable agent approved for urinary-tract infections, 142
Inosiplex available for AIDS patients, 367
Isotretinoin associated with new adverse effects, 142
I.V. indomethacin marketed for patent ductus arteriosus, 248
Leuprolide approved for palliative treatment of prostatic cancer, 611
Long-acting bronchodilator marketed, 142
Long-acting third-generation cephalosporin ceftriaxone reaches U.S. market, 134
Naltrexone approved by FDA, 134
News Briefs, 18, 144, 252, 367, 486
New β blocker for glaucoma approved by FDA, 614
New NIH recommendations for adjuvant therapy for breast cancer, 605
NIH panel recommends decreased use of frozen plasma, 14
Nomifensine, a second-generation antidepressant, approved by FDA, 134
Nonsedating antihistamine terfenadine approved by FDA, 357
Oral acyclovir approved for treatment of genital herpes, 141
Panel considers treatment of travelers' diarrhea, 141
Panel reviews sedation and anesthesia in the dental office, 357
Patients, professionals good guessers in double-blind trial, 252
Pentamidine now available commercially, 11
Phospholipids may hold key to allergic and immunologic reactions, 245
Researchers discuss promising drugs for AIDS at Atlanta conference, 475
Studies of bepridil in use against arrhythmias halted,

614
Study shows benefit in treating elderly hypertensive patients, 482
Study shows little change in microbial resistance patterns, 11
Synthetic THC approved by FDA, 479
Ticarcillin–clavulanic acid marketed by Beecham, 362
Tocainide marketed in U.S., 11
Wyeth's triphasic oral contraceptive marketed, 18
Nifedipine; effects; glucose intolerance, 649
Nitroglycerin
concomitant therapy; myocardial diseases, transdermal, 502
transdermal; efficacy, 453
Nomifensine maleate; depression; therapy, 673; therapy, review, 625
Norethindrone; combination, ethinyl estradiol; triphasic oral contraceptives, 24
Nutrition; diet; coronary disease prevention, 123; maldigestion therapy, review, 161
Nystatin; candidiasis; therapy, AIDS, review, 539

O

Obesity; patients; amikacin pharmacokinetics, surgery, 70; risk factors, 367
Opiate antagonists
clonidine hydrochloride and naloxone hydrochloride; withdrawal therapy, 100
naloxone hydrochloride and clonidine hydrochloride; withdrawal therapy, 100
Opiates
alone and with ibuprofen; cancer pain therapy, 53
diacetylmorphine; pain therapy, 80
pentazocine; Tourette's disease therapy, 494
withdrawal; therapy, 100
Osteomalacia; aluminum; toxicity, review, 434
Oxygen; bronchiolitis; viral, therapy, pediatrics, 297

P

Pain
ibuprofen; combined therapy, cancer patients, 53
morphine sulfate; postoperative, therapy, 48; therapy, patient-controlled i.v., 41
therapy; analgesics, 80
Pancreatic enzymes; cystic fibrosis; therapy, review, 555
Pancreatic insufficiency; therapy; review, 161
Pancreatin; formulations; Viokase, changes to pancrelipase, 388
Pancrelipase; formulations; powders, tablets, 388
Parkinson's disease; amantadine sulfate; i.v. therapy, 146
Parotitis; therapy; acute suppurative, 566
Patient care; pharmacodynamics; monitoring, 3
Patient education; drug administration; dobutamine injections, 195
Patient information; consultation; triphasic oral contraceptives, 24
Pediatrics
acetylcysteine; atelectasis therapy, 255
bronchiolitis; viral, therapy, 297
carbamazepine; allergies, 19
Haemophilus influenzae; type b, prevention, review, 637
indomethacin; patent ductus arteriosus therapy, 248
pentobarbital sodium; seizure therapy, neonate, 330
Penicillins
azlocillin sodium; pharmacokinetics, high dose, cystic fibrosis, 664
piperacillin; and gentamicin or moxalactam, therapy, 327
Pentamidine isethionate; pneumonia; *P. carinii,* therapy, review, 507
Pentazocine; Gilles de la Tourette's disease; and opiate withdrawal therapy, 494
Pentobarbital; blood levels; neonate, 330
Pentobarbital sodium; seizures; therapy, neonate, 330
Personnel; dentistry; anesthetics and sedatives use, 357
Pharmacodynamics
digoxin; relation, blood levels, 81
patient care; monitoring, 3
Pharmacogenetics; procainamide; toxicity, systemic lupus erythematosus, review, 657
Pharmacokinetics
acecainide; peritoneal dialysis clearance, 669
acyclovir; peritoneal dialysis, 320
amikacin; obesity, effects, surgery, 70
azlocillin sodium; high dose, cystic fibrosis, 664
aztreonam; review, 516
ceftriaxone; kidney failure, 177
drugs; arteriovenous hemofiltration, 620
enalapril maleate; review, 27
gentamicin; arteriovenous ultrafiltration, 327; effects, surgery, 182; prediction, 74; predictions, diabetes, 572
hydralazine; toxicity, systemic lupus erythematosus, review, 657
monitoring; drug therapy, limitations, 3; sampling time, blood levels, 84
nomifensine maleate; review, 625
procainamide; blood level prediction, 186; peritoneal dialysis clearance, 669
pseudoephedrine hydrochloride; availability, sustained-action suspensions, 199
ranitidine; lactation, 322
roentgenographic agents; intravascular, review, 527
theophylline; effects, excretion, 59; spinal cord injuries, 448
vancomycin; relation, creatinine clearance, 311
Pharmacy and therapeutics committee; phenytoin sodium, i.v. site recommendations, 618
Phenothiazines; and amitriptyline; postherpetic neuralgia therapy, 170
Phenytoin
and amitriptyline; postherpetic neuralgia therapy, 170
interactions; influenza vaccines, 191
Phenytoin sodium; intravenous; administration sites, toxicity, 618
Phytonadione; concomitant therapy, 316
Piperacillin; and gentamicin sulfate or moxalactam; therapy, ultrafiltration, 327
Plicamycin; alone and with etidronate disodium; hypercalcemia therapy, neoplasms, 204
Pneumonia; pentamidine isethionate; *P. carinii,* therapy, review, 507
Poisoning; overdose; trazodone, 97
Powders; pancrelipase; reformulation, 388
Prazosin; effects; glucose intolerance, 649
Procainamide
blood levels; prediction, 186
clearance; peritoneal dialysis, 669
lupus; erythematosus, systemic, toxicity, review, 657
Procainamide hydrochloride
metabolism; peritoneal dialysis clearance, 669
sustained-action; blood level prediction, 186
toxicity; hypotension, rapid i.v., 504; tachycardia, review, 675
Propranolol hydrochloride; toxicity; depression, psychosis, review, 214
Protozoan infections; therapy; AIDS, review, 539
Pruritus; theophylline anhydrous; adverse reactions, sustained-action, 334
Pseudoephedrine hydrochloride; availability; sustained-action suspensions, 199
Pseudomonas aeruginosa; resistance; gentamicin, parotitis, 566
Psychotherapeutic agents
carbamazepine; mental disorder therapy, review, 425
toxicity; tachycardia, review, 675
Psychotic disorders; propranolol hydrochloride; toxicity, review, 214
Publications; *Clinical Pharmacy;* ASHP journals, history, 82
Pulmonary embolism; therapy; review, 279
Purpura; globulin immune; thrombopenic, therapy, 206
Pyrimethamine; toxoplasmosis; therapy, AIDS, review, 539

Q

Quinacrine hydrochloride; protozoan infections; therapy, AIDS, review, 539
Quinidine; interactions; digoxin, review, 404
Quinidine sulfate; toxicity; tachycardia, review, 675

R

Radiation
and antineoplastic agents; osteogenic sarcoma therapy, 485
and cyclophosphamide; bone marrow transplantation, review, 149
Ranitidine; lactation; pharmacokinetics, 322
Ranitidine hydrochloride; lactation; pharmacokinetics, 322
Rate constants
excretion; gentamicin, 74; warfarin, short-bowel syndrome, 325
gentamicin; excretion, 182
procainamide; absorption, excretion, 186
trazodone; excretion, 97
Regulations
diacetylmorphine; pain therapy, 80
indomethacin; patent ductus arteriosus, FDA, 248
Release; pseudoephedrine hydrochloride; sustained-action suspensions, 199
Reserpine; effects; glucose intolerance, 649
Resistance; gentamicin sulfate; *P. aeruginosa,* parotitis, 566
Respiratory smooth muscle relaxants
aminophylline; theophylline excretion, 59; theophylline pharmacokinetics, paraplegics, 448
theophylline; overdose poisoning, 97
Resuscitation; ventricular fibrillation; procainamide toxicity, rapid i.v., 504
Ribavirin
acquired immunodeficiency syndrome; therapy, 475
bronchiolitis; viral, therapy, pediatrics, 297
Rifampin; *Haemophilus influenzae;* type b, prophylaxis, review, 637
Robins, A. H.; manufacturers; Viokase reformulation, 388
Roentgenographic agents
intravascular; review, 527
iothalamate sodium; pharmacokinetics, cystic fibrosis, 664
isosulfan blue; adverse reactions, anaphylaxis, 219

S

Saliva levels; moxalactam; lack, effects, *H. influenzae* b meningitis, 67
Sarcoma
antineoplastic agents and radiation; osteogenic, therapy, 485
radiation and antineoplastic agents; osteogenic, therapy, 485
Seizures; pentobarbital sodium; therapy, neonate, 330
Sex; patients; drug-induced systemic lupus erythematosus, review, 657
Short-bowel syndrome; warfarin; absorption, 325
Smoking; interactions; theophylline pharmacokinetics, paraplegics, 448
Sodium chloride; irrigating solutions; indwelling injection sites, 488
Solutions; dialysis; toxicity, aluminum-related osteomalacia, 434
Sorbitol; combination, charcoal activated; GI transit time, 446
Spinal cord injuries; effects; theophylline pharmacokinetics, 448
Spiramycin; protozoan infections; therapy, AIDS, review, 539
Steroids, cortico-; and albuterol; viral bronchiolitis therapy, 297
Streptokinase
thrombophlebitis; and pulmonary embolism therapy, review, 279
toxicity; vasculitis, 383
Structure-activity relationships
alprazolam; triazolo derivatives, 258
triazolam; triazolo derivatives, 258
Sulfadiazine; toxoplasmosis; therapy, AIDS, review, 539
Sulfamethoxazole; combination, trimethoprim; travelers' diarrhea therapy, 141; gonococcal urethritis therapy, 455; infection therapy, AIDS, review, 539
Sulfonamides
sulfadiazine; toxoplasmosis therapy, AIDS, review, 539
sulfamethoxazole, combination, trimethoprim; gonococcal urethritis therapy, 455; infection therapy, AIDS, review, 539
Suramin sodium; acquired immunodeficiency syndrome; therapy, 475
Surgery; effects; gentamicin pharmacokinetics, 182
Surgical supplies; administration sets; dobutamine injections, 195
Suspensions; pseudoephedrine hydrochloride; sustained-action, availability, 199
Sustained-action medications
procainamide hydrochloride; blood level prediction, 186
pseudoephedrine hydrochloride; suspensions, availability, 199
theophylline anhydrous; adverse reactions, 334
Sympatholytic agents
beta blockers; contraindications, glucose intolerance, 649
clonidine; Tourette's disease therapy, 494
Sympathomimetic agents
albuterol; and corticosteroids, bronchiolitis therapy, 297

bitolterol mesylate; aerosols, review, 393
dobutamine hydrochloride; congestive heart failure therapy, 195
effects; glucose intolerance, 649
fenoterol hydrobromide; aerosols, review, 393
isoproterenol hydrochloride; tachycardia therapy, review, 675
pseudoephedrine hydrochloride; sustained-action suspensions, 199

T

Tablets; pancrelipase; reformulation, 388
Tamoxifen; breast neoplasms; postmenopausal, combined therapy, 605
Testosterone; interactions; warfarin, 332
Testosterone propionate; interactions; warfarin, 332
Tests, laboratory; glucose; lack, effects, ceftazidime, 72
Tetracycline; blood levels; relation, metallic taste, 455
Tetracycline hydrochloride; toxicity; metallic taste, 455
Theophylline
excretion; factors affecting, 59
pharmacokinetics; spinal cord injuries, 448
poisoning; overdose, 97
Theophylline anhydrous; sustained-action; adverse reactions, 334
Thiazides; hypotensive agents; effects, glucose intolerance, 649
Thioridazine hydrochloride; toxicity; tachycardia, review, 675
Thrombocytopenia; carbamazepine; toxicity, 221
Thrombolytic agents
streptokinase; allergies, vasculitis, 383; therapy, review, 279
urokinase; therapy, review, 279
Thrombophlebitis; therapy; review, 279
Thyroid drugs; interactions; digoxin, review, 404
Time; sampling; blood levels, 84
Tobramycin sulfate; clindamycin phosphate and vancomycin hydrochloride; parotitis therapy, 566
Tolerance
morphine sulfate; patient-controlled analgesia, 41
nitroglycerin; transdermal, 453
Topical preparations; testosterone propionate; interactions, oral warfarin, 332
Toxicity
see also Drugs, adverse reactions
acetylcysteine; lack, 255
aluminum; osteomalacia, review, 434
amantadine sulfate; lack, i.v., 146
antibiotics; enterocolitis, 304
anticoagulants; review, 279
antineoplastic agents; enterocolitis, 304; vomiting, 102
aztreonam; review, 516
baclofen, lack, 93
bitolterol mesylate; aerosols, review, 393
carbamazepine; ataxia, 93; blood levels, review, 425; thrombocytopenia, 221
cardiac drugs; tachycardia, review, 675
cimetidine; alopecia, 145
clindamycin phosphate and gentamicin sulfate; lack, 316
clonazepam; sedation, 615
contraceptives, oral; triphasic, 24
cyclophosphamide; review, 149
digoxin; lack, relation, blood levels, 81
doxorubicin; myocardial diseases, 502
enalapril maleate; review, 27
fenoterol hydrobromide; aerosols, review, 393
gentamicin sulfate and clindamycin phosphate; lack, 316
hydralazine; systemic lupus erythematosus, review, 657
hypotensive agents; contraindications, glucose intolerance, 649
ibuprofen; lack, cancer pain therapy, 53
inhalation therapy; reservoir aerosols, 452
irrigating solutions; bowel cleansing, review, 414
isotretinoin; short terms, 142
metoclopramide hydrochloride; dystonic reactions, 102
morphine sulfate; i.m., i.v., 48
moxalactam disodium; lack, 316
nomifensine maleate, 673; review, 625
opiates; withdrawal symptoms, 100
pentamidine isethionate; review, 507
phenytoin sodium; i.v. injection sites, 618
procainamide; systemic lupus erythematosus, review, 657
procainamide hydrochloride; hypotension, rapid i.v., 504
propranolol hydrochloride; depression, psychosis, review, 214
psychotherapeutic agents; tachycardia, review, 675
ranitidine; lactation, 322
roentgenographic agents; intravascular, review, 527
streptokinase; vasculitis, 383
tetracycline hydrochloride; metallic taste, 455
thrombolytic agents; review, 279
trazodone hydrochloride; overdose poisoning, 97
triazolam; structure–activity relationships, 258
Toxicity, environmental; *Haemophilus influenzae;* type b, risks, pediatrics, 637
Toxoplasmosis; therapy; AIDS, review, 539
Transplantation; bone marrow; hematologic disease therapy, review, 149
Trazodone; poisoning; overdose, 97
Trazodone hydrochloride; poisoning; overdose, 97
Tremor; clonezepam; cerebellar, therapy, 615
Triazolam; structure–activity relationships; triazolo derivatives, 258
Triazolo derivatives; structure–activity relationships; alprazolam and triazolam, 258
Trifluoperazine hydrochloride; toxicity; tachycardia, review, 675
Trigeminal neuralgia
baclofen and carbamazepine; therapy, 93
carbamazepine; alone and with baclofen, therapy, 93
Trimethoprim
combination, sulfamethoxazole; gonococcal urethritis therapy, 455; infection therapy, AIDS, review, 539; travelers' diarrhea therapy, 141
diarrhea; travelers', therapy, 141

U

Urine levels
acecainide; peritoneal dialysis, 669
procainamide; peritoneal dialysis, 669
Urokinase; thrombophlebitis; and pulmonary embolism therapy, review, 279

V

Vaccines
Haemophilus b polysaccharide; type b, immunization, pediatrics, 637
influenza; interactions, phenytoin, 191
Valproate sodium; and amitriptyline; postherpetic neuralgia therapy, 170
Vancomycin
enterocolitis; therapy, review, 304
excretion; relation, creatinine clearance, 311
Vancomycin hydrochloride
clindamycin phosphate and gentamicin sulfate or tobramycin sulfate; parotitis therapy, 566
dosage; prediction methods, 311
Vasculitis; streptokinase; toxicity, 383
Vasodilating agents
amiodarone; interactions, digoxin, review, 404
effects; glucose intolerance, 649
interactions; digoxin, review, 404
nitroglycerin; transdermal, efficacy, 453
Vehicles; toxicity; phenytoin, i.v. sites, 618
Verapamil; effects; glucose intolerance, 649
Vitamins; cystic fibrosis; therapy, review, 555
Volume of distribution, see **Drugs, body distribution**
Vomiting; metoclopramide hydrochloride; therapy, 102

W

Warfarin
absorption; short-bowel syndrome, 325
concomitant therapy; pulmonary embolism, 383
interactions; testosterone ointment, 332
thrombophlebitis; and pulmonary embolism therapy, review, 279
Warfarin sodium
dosage; prediction methods, 440
therapy; anticoagulants, 325
Wounds; antibiotics; prophylaxis, costs, 316

Author Index

A

Akahoshi, Michael P. see Kloth, Dwight, D., 182
Alcalay, J. see Gadoth, N., 146
Amir, Jacob Acetylcysteine for severe atelectasis in premature infants (letter), 255
Amsel, Lewis P. see Graves, David A., 199
Applefeld, Mark M. see Roffman, David S., 195
Arnold, W. Stanley see Maddox, Ronald W., 502
Arrigo, Janice M. see Graves, David A., 41
Ashby, B. L. Origins of aztreonam resistance (letter), 23

B

Bailey, Robert T. Jr. see Dworzack, David L., 23
Baker, Karen A. Treatment of trigeminal neuralgia: use of baclofen in combination with carbamazepine, 93
Balfour, Henry H. Jr. see Fletcher, Courtney, 370
Barnhart, Glenn R. see Lehman, Mark E., 325
Barr, William H. see Lehman, Mark E., 325
Barriere, Steven L. Book review, 342
Bartelt, Margaret A. see Dworzack, David L., 23
Bartlett, Robert H. see Bollish, Stephen J., 48
Batenhorst, Randal L. see Graves, David A., 41
Baumann, Terry J. see Graves, David A., 41
Beam, Thomas R. Jr. Lack of effect of ceftazidime on serum glucose in patients with liver disease, 72
Beattie, B. Lynn see Levine, Marc, 191
Beatty, J. David see Kloth, Dwight D., 182
Bechar, M. see Gadoth, N., 146
Beck, Charles A. Jr. see Mendel, Stephen, 334
Beirne, Gregory J. see Raehl, Cynthia L., 669
Beirne, Gregory J. see also Schuna, Arthur A., 65
Berardi, Rosemary R. Book review, 113
Berardi, Rosemary R. Change in enzyme content and manufacturer of Viokase (letter), 388
Birkhimer, Lois J. Use of carbamazepine in psychiatric disorders, 425
Bivins, Brack A. see Crots, Larry D., 316
Blouin, Robert A. Amikacin pharmacokinetics in morbidly obese patients undergoing gastric-bypass surgery, 70
Blouin, Robert A. see also Michael, Katherine A., 572
Boike, Steve C. see Matzke, Gary R., 311
Bollish, Stephen J. Book review, 588
Bollish, Stephen J. Efficacy of patient-controlled analgesia versus conventional analgesia for postoperative pain, 48
Bones, Michelle see Thompson, Michael, 170
Bowden, Talmadge A. see Michael, Katherine A., 414
Bradley, Joan Marie Carbamazepine-induced thrombocytopenia in a young child, 221
Bressler, Linda R. see Shevrin, Daniel H., 204
Brink, Carla J. Conference outlines challenges in the treatment of cocaine abuse (News), 595
Brouwer, Kim L. Rowse see Blouin, Robert A., 70
Burnakis, Thomas G. Effect of warfarin on activated partial thromboplastin time (letter), 620

C

Camara, Daniel S. see Beam, Thomas R. Jr., 72
Canaday, Bruce R. see Sawyer, William T., 440
Carter, Barry L. Effect of warfarin on activated partial thromboplastin time (letter), 621
Carter, Barry L. Pathophysiology and treatment of deep-vein thrombosis and pulmonary embolism, 279
Carter, Barry L. see also True, Bev L., 372
Casto, Daniel T. Preventing *Haemophilus influenzae* type b disease, 637
Casto, Daniel T. Salivary penetration of moxalactam, 67
Check, William A. Researchers discuss promising drugs for AIDS at Atlanta conference (News), 475
Chinnock, Barbara see Fletcher, Courtney, 370
Chow, Moses S. S. see DiPersio, David M., 186
Collins, Carol L. see Bollish, Stephen J., 48
Colvin, Carol L. see Berardi, Rosemary R., 388
Conner, Dale P. see Vlasses, Peter H., 27
Corman, David see Levine, Marc, 191
Cosgrove, Ellen M. see Wordell, Cindy J., 206
Crots, Larry D. Twice-daily moxalactam versus gentamicin and clindamycin in patients with penetrating abdominal trauma, 316
Curry, Stephen H. Transdermal nitroglycerin patches (editorial), 453
Curtis, Judy L. see Birkhimer, Lois J., 425

D

Danziger, Larry H. Book review, 468
Dean, Terry Use of 0.9% sodium chloride injection without heparin for maintaining indwelling intermittent injection sites (letter), 488
DellaValle, Robert Metoclopramide-induced tetanus-like dystonic reaction, 102
Dick, Terry J. see Swanson, Dennis P., 527
DiPersio, David M. Predicting plasma procainamide concentrations resulting from a sustained-release preparation, 186
DiPiro, Joseph T. Book review, 114
DiPiro, Joseph T. see also Michael, Katherine A., 414
Drake, Susan Pentamidine isethionate in the treatment of *Pneumocystis carinii* pneumonia, 507
Driscoll, David F. Book review, 588
Dworzack, David L. Origins of aztreonam resistance (letter), 23

E

Earhart, Robert H. see Weingart, Wendy A., 53
Echols, Roger M. see Kowalsky, Steven F., 177
Edwards, Deborah L. see Casto, Daniel T., 637
Ellis, Michael D. Book review, 703
Ellison, Mark J. see Sawyer, William T., 440
Eltorai, Ibrahim M. see Segal, Jack L., 448
Epperson, Edward L. Use of 0.9% sodium chloride injection without heparin for maintaining indwelling intermittent injection sites (letter), 489
Ereshefsky, Larry Nomifensine: an antidepressant with a difference? (editorial), 673

F

Ferguson, Roger K. see Vlasses, Peter H., 27
Ferraro, Joseph M. Use of 0.9% sodium chloride injection without heparin for maintaining indwelling intermittent injection sites (letter), 488
Fitzgibbons, Robert J. Jr. see Dworzack, David L., 23
Fletcher, Courtney Oral acyclovir pharmacokinetics (letter), 370
Foster, Thomas S. see Graves, David A., 41
Furio, Melissa M. Treatment of infectious complications of acquired immunodeficiency syndrome, 539

G

Gadoth, N. I.V. amantadine sulfate for extrapyramidal crisis (letter), 146
Gal, Peter see Casto, Daniel T., 67
Gallagher, Jeff see Perry, Richard S., 161
Gaska, Janice A. see Wordell, Cindy J., 206
Goldhammer, G. see Gadoth, N., 146
Goldmann, Donald see Woolf, Roger A., 664
Gonzalez, Edgar R. Procainamide-induced hypotension during CPR (letter), 504
Goodfriend, Theodore L. see Schuna, Arthur A., 65
Goodman, Robert P. see McKenney, James M., 649
Gordon, Stanley K. see Segal, Jack L., 448
Graves, David A. Bioavailability assessment of a new liquid controlled-release pseudoephedrine product, 199
Graves, David A. Relationship between plasma morphine concentrations and pharmacologic effects in postoperative patients using patient-controlled analgesia, 41
Griffen, Ward O. Jr. see Blouin, Robert A., 70
Grochowski, Eugene C. see Melby, Michael J., 74
Gross, Mark H. Management of antibiotic-associated pseudomembranous colitis, 304
Grove, William R. see Roffman, David S., 195
Guanci, Robert F. see Ferraro, Joseph M., 488
Guay, David R. P. Aztreonam, a new monobactam antimicrobial, 516
Guzzardo, Michael M. see Longnecker, Stephen M., 219

H

Hassan, Erkan Book review, 342
Hassan, Erkan Toxicity and elimination of trazodone after overdose, 97
Haumschild, Mark J. Prediction of theophylline clearance using condition correction factors, 59
Hebert, Lee A. see Seth, Shiv K., 320
Heffron, Warren A. see Thompson, Robert F., 383
Heissler, Joseph F. see Melby, Michael J., 74
Hilman, Bettina C. see Woolf, Roger A., 664
Hinsvark, Orville N. see Graves, David A., 199
Holman, Philip W. Clonidine and naloxone in ultrashort opiate detoxification, 100
Hooymans, Piet M. Current status of cardiac glycoside drug interactions, 404
Horst, H. Mathilda see Crots, Larry D., 316
Hyneck, Martha L. How reliable are serum digoxin assays? (editorial), 81

J

Jann, Michael W. see Birkhimer, Lois J., 425
John, William see Blouin, Robert A., 70
Johnson, Curtis A. see Vick, Karen E., 434
Johnson, Julie A. see Nahata, Milap C., 297
Jones, Mark E. see Carter, Barry L., 279, 621

K

Kearns, Gregory L. Appearance of ranitidine in breast milk following multiple dosing, 322
Kelly, H. William New β-adrenergic agonist aerosols, 393
Kimbrough, Anthony C. see Bradley, Joan Marie, 221
Kinney, Janet L. Book review, 347
Kinney, Janet L. Nomifensine maleate: a new second-generation antidepressant, 625
Kirking, Duane M. see Bollish, Stephen J., 48
Klamerus, Karen J. Book review, 703
Kloth, Dwight D. Altered gentamicin pharmacokinetics during the perioperative period, 182
Kluza, Ronald B. see Kearns, Gregory L., 322
Kolb, Kenneth W. see Lehman, Mark E., 325, 327
Kong, Clifford see Kloth, Dwight D., 182
Koskoletos, Christopher see Guay, David R. P., 516
Koup, Jeffrey R. see Woolf, Roger A., 664
Kovarik, John M. see Matzke, Gary R., 311
Kowalsky, Steven F. Pharmacokinetics of ceftriaxone in subjects with renal insufficiency, 177
Krasny, Harvey C. see Seth, Shiv K., 320
Krenzelok, Edward P. Gastrointestinal transit times of cathartics used with activated charcoal, 446
Kriel, Robert L. see Welty, Timothy E., 330
Kuhn, Robert J. Therapeutic management of cystic fibrosis, 555
Kukla, Lawrence J. see Shevrin, Daniel H., 204
Kukreja, Subhash C. see Shevrin, Daniel H., 204

L

Lad, Thomas E. see Shevrin, Daniel H., 204
Lampasona, Victor see Drake, Susan, 507
Larijani, Ghassem E. see Vlasses, Peter H., 27
Leach, Stacie Hayase see Kloth, Dwight D., 182
Lehman, Mark E. Gentamicin elimination in a patient undergoing continuous ultrafiltration, 327
Lehman, Mark E. Warfarin absorption in a patient with short-bowel syndrome, 325
LeRoy, Marie see Raehl, Cynthia L., 675
Levine, Marc Phenytoin therapy and immune response to influenza vaccine, 191
Lilly, Gilbert E. see Baker, Karen A., 93
Lipman, Arthur G. Progress and problems with pain (editorial), 80
Longnecker, Stephen M. Life-threatening anaphylaxis following subcutaneous administration of isosulfan blue 1%, 219
Lorentz, Sarah McQuade Potentiation of warfarin anticoagulation by topical testosterone ointment, 332
Lucas, Bruce A. see Michael, Katherine A., 572

M

Maddox, Ronald W. Beneficial hemodynamic effects of oral levodopa in a patient with cardiomyopathy (letter), 502
Magnasco, Andrew J. see Magnasco, Louis D., 455
Magnasco, Louis D. Metallic taste associated with tetracycline therapy, 455
Matzke, Gary R. Evaluation of the vancomycin-clearance:creatinine-clearance relationship for predicting vancomycin dosage, 311
McConnell, Richard F. Jr. see Kearns, Gregory L., 322

McCue, Jack D. see Casto, Daniel T., 67
McGuire, Timothy R. see Yee, Gary C., 149
McGuire, William P. see Shevrin, Daniel H., 204
McKenney, James M. Use of antihypertensive agents in patients with glucose intolerance, 649
McLean, Donald M. see Levine, Marc, 191
McManus, Linda M. Phospholipids may hold key to allergic and immunologic reactions (News), 245
Melby, Michael J. Predicting serum gentamicin concentrations in patients undergoing hemodialysis, 74
Mendel, Stephen Dermatologic reaction to a sustained-release theophylline product, 334
Merkus, Frans W. H. M. see Hooymans, Piet M., 404
Michael, Katherine A. Failure of creatinine clearance to predict gentamicin half-life in a renal transplant patient with diabetes mellitus, 572
Michael, Katherine A. Whole-bowel irrigation for mechanical colon cleansing, 414
Miller, Delwyn D. see Hassan, Erkan, 97
Miller, Jane L. New NIH recommendations for adjuvant therapy for breast cancer (News), 605
Miller, Lucinda Glantz. Update on the new triphasic oral contraceptives (letter), 24
Mohler, James L. see Michael, Katherine A., 572
Moore, Fred H. see Patrias, John M., 77
Moorthy, A. Vishnu see Raehl, Cynthia L., 669
Moorthy, A. Vishnu see also Schuna, Arthur A., 65
Murphy, John E. see Haumschild, Mark J., 59

N

Nahata, Milap C. Management of bronchiolitis, 297
Nahata, Milap C. see also Kuhn, Robert J., 555
Newman, Kathryn A. see Roffman, David S., 195
Nicks, Harold L. see Drake, Susan, 507

O

Obeid, Farouck N. see Crots, Larry D., 316
Ornato, Joseph P. see Gonzalez, Edgar R., 504

P

Parker, Marie A. see Kowalsky, Steven F., 177
Parker, William A. Propranolol-induced depression and psychosis, 214
Pasko, Mary T. see Beam, Thomas R. Jr., 72
Patel, Ashvin K. see Raehl, Cynthia L., 675
Patrias, John M. Evaluation of two methods for predicting initial lithium dosages without measuring serum concentrations, 77
Perry, Richard S. Management of maldigestion associated with pancreatic insufficiency, 161
Perry, Richard S. Recognition and management of acute suppurative parotitis, 566
Picetti, George D. III see Dworzack, David L., 23
Pitterle, Michael E. see Raehl, Cynthia L., 669
Pitterle, Michael E. see also Schuna, Arthur A., 65
Plezia, Patricia M. see Blouin, Robert A., 70
Poe, Timothy E. see Sawyer, William T., 440
Posey, L. Michael Applying pharmacodynamics in patient care (News), 3
Posey, L. Michael Volume 4 (editorial), 82
Powell, Dwight A. see Nahata, Milap C., 297

R

Rackson, Joseph T. Venoconstriction by angiotensin II (letter), 266
Raehl, Cynthia L. Clearance of procainamide and *N*-acetylprocainamide in patients undergoing continuous ambulatory peritoneal dialysis, 669
Raehl, Cynthia L. Drug-induced torsade de pointes, 675
Rapp, Robert P. see Michael, Katherine, A., 572
Record, Kenneth E. see Blouin, Robert A., 70
Reed, William P. see Roffman, David S., 195
Reeme, Peter D. Phenytoin injection precautions (letter), 618
Reich, Jack W. see Dworzack, David L., 23
Reilly, Kathleen M. Book review, 589
Reisner, Salomon H. see Amir, Jacob, 255
Ridley, Pam see Dean, Terry, 488
Roberts, Mark A. see Tullio, Carl J., 145
Roffman, David S. Intermittent dobutamine hydrochloride infusions in outpatients with chronic congestive heart failure, 195
Rose, S. J. Severe hypersensitivity secondary to extended carbamazepine administration (letter), 19
Rotenberg, Keith S. see Graves, David A., 199
Rubino, Michael Drug clearance in patients undergoing continuous arteriovenous hemofiltration (letter), 620
Rumsfield, Jean A. see Mendel, Stephen, 334
Rybak, Michael J. see Matzke, Gary R., 311

S

Sagraves, Rosalie see Bradley, Joan Marie, 221
Sandyk, R. The opioid–nonadrenergic link in Gilles de la Tourette's syndrome (letter), 494
Sandyk, R. Potentiation of opiate analgesia with ibuprofen (letter), 505
Sandyk, R. Successful treatment of cerebellar tremor with clonazepam (letter), 615
Sawyer, William T. Multicenter evaluation of six methods for predicting warfarin maintenance-dose requirements from initial response, 440
Schmidt, Gary R. see Schuna, Arthur A., 65
Schumacher, Gerald E. Choosing optimal sampling times for therapeutic drug monitoring, 84
Schuna, Arthur A. Managing hypertension with captopril and hydrochlorothiazide using two versus three daily doses, 65
Schwarzmann, Stephen W. see Drake, Susan, 507
Segal, Jack L. Theophylline pharmacokinetics in paraplegic subjects, 448
Seth, Shiv K. Acyclovir pharmacokinetics in a patient on continuous ambulatory peritoneal dialysis, 320
Shevrin, Daniel H. Treatment of cancer-associated hypercalcemia with mithramycin and oral etidronate disodium, 204
Shor, Judi B. Book review, 583
Simms, Stuart M. see Swanson, Dennis P., 527
Sliger, Van Odell see Maddox, Ronald W., 502
Small, Ralph E. Book review, 704
Smith, Arnold L. see Woolf, Roger A., 664
Smith, Christopher M. see Segal, Jack L., 448
Sohn, Catherine Angell Book review, 235
Sorkness, Christine A. see Weingart, Wendy A., 53
Spooner, Jody A. see Beam, Thomas R. Jr., 72
Sroka, H. see Gadoth, N., 146
Stewart, Ronald B. Book review, 117
Stockmar, Richard A. see Melby, Michael J., 74
Stoneburner, Robert J. see Ferraro, Joseph M., 488
Stranz, Marc H. Book review, 113
Stratton, Mark A. Drug-induced systemic lupus erythematosus, 657
Stratton, Mark A. see also Thompson, Robert F., 383
Stubits, Elizabeth A. see Wordell, Cindy J., 206
Sutton, Frederick J. see Roffman, David S., 195
Swanson, Dennis P. Product selection criteria for intravascular ionic contrast media, 527

T

Talesnick, Barry S. see Roffman, David S., 195
Taniguchi, George Pharmacologic effects of the triazolo group (letter), 258
Tannenbaum, Renee P. Book review, 583
Tartaglione, Teresa A. Book review, 114
Taylor, Jerry E. see Baker, Karen A., 93
Taylor, Owen see DellaValle, Robert, 102
Tedesco, Francis J. see Michael, Katherine A., 414
Tegtmeier, Bernard R. see Kloth, Dwight, D., 182
Thompson, Michael Nontraditional analgesics for the management of postherpetic neuralgia, 170
Thompson Robert F. Hypersensitivity vasculitis associated with streptokinase (letter), 383
Thrall, James H. see Swanson, Dennis P., 527
Tietze, Karen J. Reservoir aerosol delivery systems (editorial), 452
Tietze, Karen J. see also Wordell, Cindy J., 206
Trang, John M. see Kearns, Gregory L., 322
True, Bev L. Oral acyclovir pharmacokinetics (letter), 372
Tullio, Carl J. Cimetidine-induced alopecia (letter), 145

V

Vaida, Allen J. Putting amoxicillin–potassium clavulanate in perspective (letter), 145
Van Voris, Lee P. see Longnecker, Stephen M., 219
Vick, Karen E. Aluminum-related osteomalacia in renal-failure patients, 434
Visconti, James A. see Seth, Shiv K., 320
Vlasses, Peter H. Enalapril, a nonsulfhydryl angiotensin-converting enzyme inhibitor, 27

W

Wagman, Lawrence D. see Lehman, Mark E., 325
Waickman, L. Anthony see Carter, Barry L., 279
Ward, Michael E. Book review, 228
Webb, C. Edwin see Sawyer, William T., 440
Weibert, Robert T. see Lorentz, Sarah McQuade, 332
Weiner, John S. see Sawyer, William T., 440
Weingart, Wendy A. Analgesia with oral narcotics and added ibuprofen in cancer patients, 53
Welsh, Olin H. Jr. Dietary modifications recommended for reducing heart disease (News), 123
Welty, Timothy E. Pentobarbital coma for treating intractable seizures in a neonate, 330
Wielenga, James L. see DellaValle, Robert, 102
Williams, Dennis M. see Sawyer, William T., 440
Williams-Warren, Judy see Woolf, Roger A., 664
Wilunsky, Eliahu see Amir, Jacob, 255
Woodworth, James R. see Graves, David A., 199
Woolf, Roger A. Pharmacokinetics of high-dose azlocillin sodium in patients with cystic fibrosis, 664
Wordell, Cindy J. Immune globulin in the treatment of autoimmune thrombocytopenic purpura, 206
Wordell, Cindy J. see also Furio, Melissa M., 539
Wright, Jackson T. Jr. see McKenney, James M., 649
Wulf, Bradley G. Book review, 238

Y

Yee, Gary C. Allogeneic bone marrow transplantation in the treatment of hematologic diseases, 149

Z

Zaia, John A. see Kloth, Dwight D., 182
Zelikovic, Israel see Amir, Jacob, 255
Zellmer, William A. see Posey, L. Michael, 82
Zumwalt, Alicia A. see Casto, Daniel T., 67

Advertising Index

A–B

Advanced Therapeutics Communications
Positions Available, 485
American Cancer Society
Institutional, 235
American College of Clinical Pharmacy
Call for Papers, 575
American Critical Care, Division of American Hospital Supply Corporation
Hespan, 492-494, 616-618
American Lung Association
Christmas Seals, 704
American Society of Hospital Pharmacists
American Hospital Formulary Service—Drug Information 85, Jan–Feb-IBC
Clinical Pharmacy, 26, 26A, 26B, 148, 148A, 148B, 354A, 354B, May–Jun-IBC, 468A, 468B, Jul–Aug-IBC, 590A, 590B, Sep–Oct-IBC, 624
Clinical Research Forum, 239, 267, 506
Guidelines for Administration of Intravenous Medications to Pediatric Patients, 339
Handbook on Injectable Drugs, 716
Positions Available, 92, 131, 621
Appalachian Regional Hospitals
Positions Available, 704
Beecham Laboratories
Ticar, 602–604
Timentin, 271–278, 375–382
Biotrack, Inc.
Warfcalc, 147, 341, 389
Bristol Laboratories, Division of Bristol-Myers Company
Cefadyl, 115–116, 143–144, 251–252
Precef, 16–18, 236–238, 348–350
Bristol-Myers Oncology Division
Mexate, 243–244, 373–374, 483–484, 593–594
Burroughs Wellcome Company
Zovirax, 472–474, 608–610

C–I

Cal Lab East
Analysis Programs, 383
Cambridge University Press
Publications, 25
Edlaw Preparations, Inc.
Colyte, 501–502
Emory University Hospital
Residency Training Programs, 705
Ingham Medical Center
Position Available, 347
International Pharmaceutical Federation
45th International Congress, 104, 227, 351

J–M

The Johns Hopkins Hospital
Position Available, 485
Lederle Laboratories, A Division of American Cyanamid Company
Maxzide, 9–10, 139–140, 249–250, 391–392, 477–478, 599–600
LyphoMed, Inc.
Institutional, 622–623
Midland Hospital Center
Position Available, 486
Mount Sinai Medical Center
Position Available, 578

N–T

Nash General Hospital
Position Available, 390
National Council on Patient Information and Education
Institutional, 223, 451, 565
Ochsner Foundation Hospital
Position Available, 390
Pfipharmecs, Division of Pfizer Corporation
Institutional, Mar–Apr-IBC, 619, Nov–Dec-IBC
Vibramycin, 387–388, 503–504
Roche Laboratories, Division of Hoffmann-La Roche, Inc.
Coactin, 121, 127–130, 253–254, 343–346, 363–366, 579–582
Institutional, 268–270, 360–361, 584–585
Rocephin, 229–234, 259–264, 457–462, 495–500, 697–702
Samford University
Positions Available, 390
Smith Kline & French Laboratories
Ancef, 15, Mar–Apr-IFC, 246–247, 358–359, 467, 487, 586–587, Nov–Dec-IFC, 606–607
Cefizox, Jan–Feb-IFC, 107–110, May–Jun-IFC, Jul–Aug-IFC, Sep–Oct-IFC
Monocid, 6–8, 135–138, 352–353, 368–369, 490–491, 596–598
Tagamet, 265–266, 371–372
E. R. Squibb & Sons, Inc.
Institutional, 4–5, 471
Stuart Pharmaceuticals, Division of ICI Americas, Inc.
Institutional, Jan–Feb-OBC, Mar–Apr-OBC, May–Jun-OBC, Jul–Aug-OBC, Sep–Oct-OBC, Nov–Dec-OBC

U–V

The University of Florida
Fellowship Program, 146
University of Massachusetts Medical Center
Position Available, 117
The University of Michigan
Positions Available, 347, 489
The Upjohn Company
Cleocin, 20–22, 124–126
Micronase, 12–14, 132–134, 256–258, 384–386, 480–482, 612–614
Veterans Administration
Positions Available, 390, 578, 705